Essential Cardiology

Essential Cardiology

PRINCIPLES AND PRACTICE

SECOND EDITION

Edited by

CLIVE ROSENDORFF, MD, PhD, FRCP

Professor of Medicine, Zena and Michael A. Wiener
Cardiovascular Institute, Mount Sinai School of Medicine,
New York, NY, and Veterans Affairs Medical Center, Bronx, NY

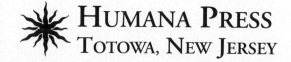

HUMANA PRESS
TOTOWA, NEW JERSEY

Cover design by Patricia F. Cleary
Cover illustration by Colin Richards. Used with permission of the artist.

For additional copies, pricing for bulk purchases, and/or information about other Humana titles, contact Humana at the above address or at any of the following numbers: Tel.: 973-256-1699; Fax: 973-256-8341; E-mail: orders@humanapr.com; or visit our Website: www.humanapress.com

This publication is printed on acid-free paper. ∞
ANSI Z39.48-1984 (American National Standards Institute) Permanence of Paper for Printed Library Materials.

Printed in the United States of America. 10 9 8 7 6 5 4 3 2 1

eISBN 1-59259-918-4

Library of Congress Cataloging-in-Publication Data
Essential cardiology : principles and practice / edited by Clive
Rosendorff.-- 2nd ed.
   p. ; cm.
  Includes bibliographical references and index.
  ISBN 1-58829-370-X (alk. paper)
  1. Heart--Diseases. 2. Cardiology.
  [DNLM: 1. Cardiovascular Diseases--Outlines. 2. Cardiovascular
Physiology--Outlines. WG 18.2 E78 2005] I. Rosendorff, Clive.
  RC681.E85 2005
  616.1'2--dc22
                                              2005006266

PREFACE

This second edition reflects the very rapid advances that have been made in our understanding and management of cardiovascular disease since the first edition was published in 2001. All of the chapters have been extensively reviewed and rewritten. There are now two chapters on acute coronary syndromes, reflecting the modern classification: one on unstable angina pectoris and non-ST-segment elevation myocardial infarction, and the other on ST-segment elevation myocardial infarction. Otherwise the format of the first edition has been retained, to include sections on epidemiology, cardiovascular function, examination and investigation of the patient, disorders of rhythm and conduction, heart failure, congenital heart disease, coronary artery disease, valvular heart disease, hypertension, and other conditions affecting the heart. I am also very happy to welcome Drs. Arnold M. Katz, Martin M. Goldman, David Benditt, Edward K. Kasper, and Roger J. Hajjar as new senior authors.

I wish also to thank Pedro Perez for his superb contributions to the artwork, my assistants, Maria Anthony and Anitra Collins, and Paul Dolgert, John Morgan, Patricia Cleary, and Donna Niethe, and the editorial, production, and composition departments of Humana Press for their encouragement and hard work.

Clive Rosendorff, MD, PhD, FRCP

PREFACE TO THE FIRST EDITION

"A big book," said Callimachus, the Alexandrian poet, "is a big evil!" Not always. There are some excellent, very big encyclopedias of cardiology, wonderful as works of reference. There are also many small books of cardiology, "handbooks" or "manuals," which serve a different purpose, to summarize, list, or simplify. This book is designed to fill a large gap between these extremes, to provide a textbook that is both substantial and readable, compact and reasonably comprehensive, and to provide an intelligent blend of molecular, cellular, and physiologic concepts with current clinical practice.

A word about the title. "Essential" is used here not in the sense of indispensable or absolutely required in all circumstances, for there is much more here than the generalist needs in order to practice good medicine, especially if there is easy access to a cardiology consultant. Rather, the word as used here denotes the essence or distillation or fundamentals of the mechanisms and practice of cardiology. The "Principles and Practice" subtitle affirms the idea that theory without a practical context may be academically satisfying but lacks usefulness, and practice without theory is plumbing. Good doctors understand the basic science foundation of what they do with patients, and great doctors are those who, as researchers or as teachers, see new connections between the basic sciences and clinical medicine.

I have been very fortunate to be able to assemble a team of great doctors who are outstanding physicians and scientists, most of them internationally recognized for their leadership position in their areas of specialization. They represent a careful blend of brilliance and experience, and, most of all, they all write with the authority of undoubted experts in their fields. They have all been asked to write up-to-date reviews of their respective areas of expertise, at a level that will be intelligible to noncardiologists as well as cardiologists, to medical students, internal medicine residents, general internists, and cardiology fellows. I believe that they have succeeded brilliantly, and I know that they are all very proud to have participated as authors in this project, the first textbook of cardiology of the new millennium. I am deeply grateful to all of them for the care and enthusiasm with which they carried out this task.

The organization of the book reflects pretty much the key issues that concern cardiologists and other internists at present; I have no doubt that the field will develop and change in time so that many of the modes of diagnosis and therapy described here will become much more prominent (such as gene therapy), while others may diminish or even disappear. This is what second or later editions of textbooks are for.

Clive Rosendorff, MD, PhD, FRCP

CONTENTS

CONTRIBUTORS

JONATHAN ABRAMS, MD • *Interim Section Chief of Cardiology, Professor of Medicine, University of New Mexico, School of Medicine, Albuquerque, NM*

SATYA REDDY ATMAKURI, MD • *Cardiology Fellow, The Methodist DeBakey Heart Center, Baylor College of Medicine, Houston, TX*

DAVID G. BENDITT, MD • *Professor of Medicine, Cardiovascular Division, University of Minnesota Medical School, Minneapolis, MN*

NIRAT BEOHAR, MD • *Assistant Professor of Medicine, Northwestern Cardiovascular Institute, Northwestern Memorial Hospital, Northwestern University, Chicago, IL*

ROBERT W. W. BIEDERMAN, MD, FACC • *Director Cardiac MRI, Allegheny General Hospital; Assistant Professor of Medicine, Drexel College of Medicine, Pittsburgh, PA*

DANIEL G. BLANCHARD, MD, FACC • *Professor of Medicine, University of California, San Diego, School of Medicine, and UCSD Medical Center; Director, Cardiology Fellowship Program and Chief of Clinical Cardiology, UCSD Thornton Hospital, San Diego, CA*

EDMUND A. W. BRICE, MB ChB, PhD, FCP (SA) • *Senior Lecturer, Department of Medicine, University of Stellenbosch; Cardiologist, Tygerberg Academic Hospital, Cape Town, South Africa*

JAMES F. BURKE, MD, FACC • *Clinical Assistant Professor of Medicine, Jefferson Medical College, Philadelphia; Director, Cardiovascular Disease Fellowship Program, The Lankenau Hospital, Wynnewood, PA*

CHRISTOPHER P. CANNON, MD • *Associate Professor of Medicine, Cardiovascular Division, Brigham and Women's Hospital, Harvard Medical School, Boston, MA*

SIMON CHAKKO, MD, FACP, FACC • *Chief, Cardiology Section, Miami Veterans Affairs Medical Center; Professor of Medicine, Department of Medicine, University of Miami School of Medicine, Miami, FL*

PATRICK M. COLLETTI, MD • *Professor of Radiology, University of Southern California, Keck School of Medicine; Chief of MRI, USC Imaging Science Center, Los Angeles, CA*

JACK M. COLMAN, MD, FRCPC, FACC • *Staff Cardiologist, University Health Network and Mount Sinai Hospitals; Staff Cardiologist, Toronto Congenital Cardiac Centre for Adults; Associate Professor (Medicine), University of Toronto, Toronto, Canada*

PATRICK J. COMMERFORD, MB ChB, FCP (SA) • *Professor and Head of the Division of Cardiology, University of Cape Town; New Groote Schuur Hospital, Cape Town, South Africa*

CHARLES J. DAVIDSON, MD • *Professor of Medicine, Northwestern Cardiovascular Institute, Northwestern Memorial Hospital, Northwestern University, Chicago, IL*

FEDERICA DEL MONTE, MD, PhD • *Cardiology Division, Harvard Medical School; Cardiology Laboratory of Integrative Physiology and Imaging, Massachusetts General Hospital; Cardiovascular Research Center, Charlestown, MA*

ANTHONY N. DEMARIA, MD • *Professor of Medicine, Judith and Jack White Chair in Cardiology, Division of Cardiovascular Medicine, University of California, San Diego, School of Medicine; Director, Cardiovascular Center, UCSD Medical Center, San Diego, CA*

RAJAT DEO, MD • *Cardiology Fellow, University of Texas Southwestern Medical Center, Dallas, TX*

TARA L. DIMINO, MD • *Cardiology Fellow, The Lankenau Hospital and Institute for Medical Research, Wynnewood, PA*

MARK DOYLE, PhD • *Cardiac MRI Physicist, Allegheny General Hospital, Pittsburgh, PA*

GREGORY ENGEL, MD • *Cardiology Fellow, Cardiac Electrophysiology, Division of Cardiovascular Medicine, Stanford University School of Medicine, Stanford, CA*

MURRAY EPSTEIN, MD • *Professor of Medicine, Department of Medicine, University of Miami School of Medicine, Miami, FL*

JOHN FARMER, MD • *Associate Professor of Medicine, Baylor College of Medicine; Chief, Section of Cardiology, Ben Taub Hospital, Houston, TX*

JONATHAN E. E. FISHER, MD • *Department of Medicine (Cardiology), Mount Sinai School of Medicine, New York, NY*

LEE A. FLEISHER, MD, FACC • *Robert D. Dripps Professor and Chair, Department of Anesthesia, University of Pennsylvania School of Medicine, Philadelphia, PA*

VICTOR FROELICHER, MD • *Professor of Medicine, Stanford University School of Medicine; Cardiology Division, VA Palo Alto Health Care Systems, Palo Alto, CA*

SEAN P. GAINE, MD, PhD, FRCPI • *Consultant Respiratory Physician, National Pulmonary Hypertension Unit, Mater Misericordiae Hospital, University College Dublin, Dublin, Ireland*

MICHAEL H. GOLLOB, MD, FRCPC • *Assistant Professor, Department of Medicine, University of Ottawa, Ottawa, Canada*

MARTIN E. GOLDMAN, MD • *Dr. Arthur and Hilda Master Professor of Medicine (Cardiology); Director, Echocardiography Laboratory, Zena and Michael A. Wiener Cardiovascular Institute, Marie-Josee and Henry R. Kravis Center for Cardiovascular Health, Mount Sinai School of Medicine, New York, NY*

STEPHEN S. GOTTLIEB, MD • *Professor of Medicine, University of Maryland School of Medicine; Director, Heart Failure and Transplantation, University of Maryland Hospital, Baltimore, MD*

ANTONIO M. GOTTO, JR., MD, DPhil • *The Stephen and Suzanne Weiss Dean, Professor of Medicine, Weill Medical College of Cornell University, New York, NY*

ROGER J. HAJJAR, MD, FACC • *Associate Professor of Medicine, Harvard Medical School; Director, Cardiology Laboratory of Integrative Physiology and Imaging, Massachusetts General Hospital, Cardiovascular Research Center, Charlestown, MA*

JONATHAN L. HALPERIN, MD • *Robert and Harriet Heilbrunn Professor of Medicine (Cardiology), Mount Sinai School of Medicine; Director, Clinical Cardiology Services, The Zena and Michael A. Weiner, Cardiovascular Institute, The Marie-Josée and Henry R. Kravis Center for Cardiovascular Health, New York, New York*

SIAN E. HARDING, PhD • *Professor, National Heart Lung Institute, Imperial College, London, United Kingdom*

ROBERT J. HENNING, MD, FACP, FCCP, FACC • *Professor of Medicine, Division of Cardiology, Department of Medicine, University of South Florida College of Medicine; James A. Haley Hospital, Moffitt Hospital, and Tampa General Hospital, Tampa, FL*

JULIEN I. E. HOFFMAN, MD • *Professor Emeritus, University of California, San Francisco, CA*

ERIC M. ISSELBACHER, MD • *Medical Director, Thoracic Aortic Center, Massachusetts General Hospital; Assistant Professor of Medicine, Harvard Medical School, Boston, MA*

ALEXANDER IVANOV, MD • *Attending, Somerset Medical Center, Somerville;
and Robert Wood Johnson University Hospital, New Brunswick, NJ*

SEI IWAI, MD • *Assistant Professor of Medicine, Weill Medical College of Cornell University,
New York, NY*

DIWAKAR JAIN, MD • *Professor of Medicine, Director, Nuclear Cardiology Laboratory, Section
of Cardiovascular Medicine, Drexel University College of Medicine, Philadelphia, PA*

JAMES J. JANG, MD • *Cardiology Fellow, Mount Sinai Medical Center, New York, NY*

WILLIAM B. KANNEL, MD, MPH, FACC • *Professor of Medicine and Public Health, Framingham
Study/Boston University School of Medicine, Framingham, MA*

NORMAN M. KAPLAN, MD • *Clinical Professor of Medicine, Department of Internal Medicine,
University of Texas Southwestern Medical Center, Dallas, TX*

ADOLF W. KARCHMER, MD • *Professor of Medicine, Harvard Medical School;Chief, Division
of Infectious Diseases, Beth Israel Deaconess Medical Center, Boston, MA*

EDWARD K. KASPER, MD, FACC • *Associate Professor of Medicine, Chief, Cardiology Division,
Johns Hopkins Bayview Medical Center, Baltimore, MD*

ARNOLD M. KATZ, MD, DMed (Hon), FACP, FACC • *Professor of Medicine Emeritus, University
of Connecticut School of Medicine, Farmington, CT; Visiting Professor of Medicine
and Physiology, Dartmouth Medical School, Hanover, NH*

EDDY KIZANA, MB BS, FRACP • *Department of Cardiology and Gene Therapy Research Unit,
Westmead Hospital, Westmead, New South Wales, Australia*

NEAL S. KLEIMAN, MD • *Associate Professor of Medicine, Director, Cardiac Catheterization
Laboratories, The Methodist DeBakey Heart Center, Baylor College of Medicine,
Houston, TX*

PETER R. KOWEY, MD, FACC • *Professor of Medicine, Jefferson Medical College, Philadelphia;
Chief, Division of Cardiovascular Disease, Main Line Health Heart Center, Lankenau,
Bryn Mawr; and Paoli Hospitals, Wynnewood, PA*

JAMES A. DE LEMOS, MD • *Coronary Care Unit Director, Parkland Memorial Hospital; Associate
Professor of Medicine, University of Texas Southwestern Medical Center, Dallas, TX*

BRUCE B. LERMAN, MD • *Hilda Altschul Master Professor of Medicine; Chief, the Maurice and
Corinne Greenberg Division of Cardiology; Director, Cardiac Electrophysiology Laboratory,
Weill Medical College of Cornell University, New York, NY*

FEI LÜ, MD, PhD • *Assistant Professor of Medicine, Cardiovascular Division, Department
of Medicine, University of Minnesota Medical School; Director, Cardiac Electrophysiology
Laboratory, Fairview-University Medical Center, Minneapolis, MN*

STEVEN M. MARKOWITZ, MD • *Associate Professor of Medicine, Assistant Director, Cardiac
Electrophysiology Laboratory, Weill Medical College of Cornell University, New York, NY*

DAVENDRA MEHTA, MD, PhD, FRCP, FACC • *Director, Cardiac Electrophysiology Section,
Cardiovascular Institute; Associate Professor of Medicine, Mount Sinai School
of Medicine, New York, NY*

MICHAEL MILLER, MD, FACC, FAHA • *Associate Professor of Medicine, Epidemiology, and
Preventive Medicine; Director, Center for Preventive Cardiology, University of Maryland
Medical Center, Baltimore, MD*

SUNEET MITTAL, MD • *Associate Professor of Medicine, Weill Medical College of Cornell
University, New York, NY*

YALE NEMERSON, MD • *Phillip J. and Harriet L. Goodhart Professor of Medicine, Professor
of Biochemistry, Mount Sinai School of Medicine, New York, NY*

DERMOT O'CALLAGHAN, MD • *Specialist Registrar in Respiratory Medicine, National Pulmonary Hypertension Unit, Mater Misericordiae University Hospital, University College Dublin, Dublin, Ireland*

RAY A. OLSSON, MD, FACP, FACC, Ch Chem, FRSC • *Professor of Medicine, Ed C. Wright Professor of Cardiovascular Research, Department of Internal Medicine, University of South Florida College of Medicine, Tampa, FL*

LIONEL H. OPIE, MD, DPhil, FRCP • *Professor of Medicine, Department of Medicine, University of Cape Town Medical School; Director, Hatter Institute, Cape Heart Center, Cape Town, South Africa*

JOSEPH P. ORNATO • MD, FACP, FACC, FACEP • *Professor and Chairman, Department of Emergency Medicine, Virginia Commonwealth University Medical Center, Richmond, VA*

FREDRIC J. PASHKOW, MD • *Clinical Professor of Medicine, Department of Medicine, John A. Burns School of Medicine, University of Hawaii; Senior Medical Director, Cardiovascular Thrombosis Medical Affairs, Sanofi-Aventis, Honolulu, HI*

GERALD M. POHOST, MD • *Chief of Cardiovascular Medicine, University of Southern California, Division of Cardiovascular Medicine, Los Angeles, CA*

PHILIP A. POOLE-WILSON, MD, FRCP, FESC, FACC • *Professor of Cardiology, Department of Cardiac Medicine, National Heart and Lung Institute, Imperial College, London, London, United Kingdom*

RICHARD A. PRESTON, MD, MBA • *Director, Division of Clinical Pharmacology, Department of Medicine, University of Miami School of Medicine, Miami, FL*

IAN F. PURCELL, MD, MRCP • *Consultant Cardiologist, Freeman Hospital, Newcastle upon Tyne, United Kingdom*

GAUTHAM P. REDDY, MD, MPH • *Assistant Professor of Radiology, University of California, San Francisco, San Francisco, CA*

MARK J. RICCIARDI, MD • *Assistant Professor of Medicine, Northwestern Cardiovascular Institute, Northwestern Memorial Hospital, Northwestern University, Chicago, IL,*

MICHAEL W. RICH, MD • *Associate Professor of Medicine, Cardiovascular Division, Department of Medicine, Washington University School of Medicine; Director, Cardiac Rapid Evaluation Unit, Barnes-Jewish Hospital, St. Louis, MO*

CLIVE ROSENDORFF, MD, PhD, FRCP, FACP, FACC • *Professor of Medicine, Zena and Michael A. Wiener Cardiovascular Institute, Mount Sinai School of Medicine, New York; VA Medical Center, Bronx, NY*

SCOTT SAKAGUCHI, MD • *Associate Professor of Medicine, Cardiovascular Division, Department of Medicine; Director, Cardiac Electrophysiology Fellowship Program, University of Minnesota Medical School, Minneapolis, MN*

RADHA J. SARMA, MD, FACC, FAHA, FACP • *Associate Professor of Clinical Medicine, University of Southern California, Keck School of Medicine; Director, Exercise Lab, and Associate Director of Echocardiography Lab, LAC and USC Medical Center, Los Angeles, CA*

JOSEPH SAVINO, MD • *Associate Professor, Department of Anesthesia, University of Pennsylvania School of Medicine, Philadelphia, PA*

MARK SCOOTE, MB BS, BSc, MRCP • *British Heart Foundation Clinical Research Fellow, Department of Cardiac Medicine, National Heart and Lung Institute, Imperial College London, London, United Kingdom*

PREDIMAN K. SHAH, MD • *Shapell and Webb Chair and Director, Division of Cardiology and Atherosclerosis Research Center, Cedars Sinai Medical Center; Professor of Medicine, David Geffen School of Medicine, UCLA, Los Angeles, CA*

SAMUEL C. B. SIU, MD, SM, FRCPC, FACC • *Staff Cardiologist, Toronto Congenital Cardiac Centre for Adults; Director of Echocardiography, University Health Network and Mount Sinai Hospitals; Associate Professor (Medicine), University of Toronto, Toronto, Ontario*

DAVID H. SPODICK, MD, DSc, FACC, FAHA, MACP • *Professor of Medicine, Cardiovascular Division, University of Massachusetts Medical School, Worcester, MA*

KENNETH M. STEIN, MD • *Associate Professor of Medicine, Associate Director, Cardiac Electrophysiology Laboratory, Weill Medical College of Cornell University, New York, NY*

ROBERT M. STEINER, MD • *Professor of Radiology, Temple University School of Medicine; Attending Radiologist Temple University Hospital, Philadelphia, PA*

H. J. C. SWAN, MD, PhD • *Professor of Medicine (Emeritus), UCLA School of Medicine; Director (Emeritus) Division of Cardiology, Cedars-Sinai Medical Center, Los Angeles, CA (Deceased)*

MARK B. TAUBMAN, MD • *Professor of Medicine and Chief of Cardiology; Director, Center for Cellular and Molecular Cardiology, University of Rochester School of Medicine and Dentistry, Rochester, NY*

BARRY L. ZARET, MD • *Robert W. Berliner Professor of Medicine, Professor of Diagnostic Radiology; Chief, Section of Cardiovascular Medicine; Associate Chairman for Clinical Affairs, Department of Internal Medicine, Yale University School of Medicine, New Haven, CT*

COLOR PLATES

Color Plates follow p. 268.

COLOR PLATE 1   Apical four-chamber images with color-flow Doppler during diastole and systole. Red flow indicates movement toward the transducer (diastolic filling); blue flow indicates movement away from the transducer (systolic ejection). RA, right atrium; RV, right ventricle; LV, left ventricle. (Chapter 9, Fig. 5; *see* full caption discussion on pp. 143–144. From ref. *1*, with permission.)

COLOR PLATE 2   Parasternal long-axis image showing a multicolored jet (indicating turbulent flow) of aortic regurgitation in the left ventricular outflow tract. The jet is narrow in width, suggesting mild regurgitation. AO, aorta; LA, left atrium; LV, left ventricle. (Chapter 9, Fig. 11A; *see* complete figure and caption on p. 151 and discussion on pp. 150–151. From ref. *1*, with permission.)

COLOR PLATE 3   Parasternal long-axis view in a case of severe mitral regurgitation. The color Doppler jet is directed posteriorly and is eccentric (black arrows). The jet "hugs" the wall of the left atrium (LA) and wraps around all the way to the aortic root (white arrows). LV, left ventricle. (Chapter 9, Fig. 13; *see* full caption on p. 154 and discussion on p. 152. From ref. *1*, with permission.)

COLOR PLATE 4   Apical four-chamber view of an ostium secundum atrial septal defect. On the left, a defect in the mid-atrial septum is present (arrows). On the right, there is color flow through the shunt. RA, right atrium; RV, right ventricle; LA, left atrium; LV, left ventricle. (Chapter 9, Fig. 22A; *see* complete figure and caption on p. 164 and discussion on pp. 162–163. From ref. *1*, with permission.)

COLOR PLATE 5   Exercise (Ex) and rest (R) ^{99m}Tc- sestamibi and exercise ^{18}FDG (Isch) images of a 67-yr-old man with angina and no prior myocardial infarction. There is a large area of partially reversible perfusion abnormality involving the septum, anterior wall, and apex (small arrows). Intense ^{18}FDG uptake is present in these areas (solid arrowheads). Coronary angiography showed 90% stenosis of the left anterior descending coronary artery and a 60% stenosis of the left circumflex artery. (Chapter 13, Fig. 10; *see* full caption on p. 239 and discussion on 238. Reproduced with permission from ref. *71*.)

COLOR PLATE 6   Right atrial electroanatomical mapping of automatic atrial tachycardia. Timing of atrial electrograms is color-coded. Red areas represent sites of early activation. Application of radiofrequency current (blue dots) at the earliest site lead to termination of tachycardia. (Chapter 17, Fig. 2; *see* full caption on p. 311 and discussion on p. 310.)

COLOR PLATE 7   Color-flow Doppler echocardiography demonstrates the high-velocity jet entering the left ventricle (arrow). (Chapter 30, Fig. 4; *see* full caption on p. 551 and discussion on p. 550.)

I

EPIDEMIOLOGY

Embryology

1

Multivariable Evaluation of Candidates for Cardiovascular Disease

William B. Kannel, MD, MPH

INTRODUCTION

A preventive approach to management of atherosclerotic cardiovascular disease (CVD) is needed because once CVD becomes manifest, it is often immediately lethal and those fortunate enough to survive seldom can be restored to full function. Prevention of the major atherosclerotic CVD events is now feasible because several modifiable predisposing risk factors have been ascertained that when corrected, can reduce the likelihood of such events occurring *(1,2)*. Multivariate risk formulations for estimating the probability of cardiovascular events conditional on the burden of a number of specified risk factors have been produced to facilitate evaluation of candidates for CVD in need of preventive management *(3–6)*.

The risk factor concept has become an integral feature of clinical assessment of candidates for initial or recurrent cardiovascular events. These risk factors represent associations that may or may not be causal. Most factors associated with an initial cardiovascular event are also predictive of recurrent episodes. The risk of a recurrent event is usually dominated by indicators of the severity of the first event, such as the number of arteries occluded or the amount of ventricular dysfunction, but other predisposing risk factors continue to play an important role. Risk factors enabling assessment of risk may be modifiable or nonmodifiable. The presence of nonmodifiable risk factors may nevertheless assist in risk assessment, and also may affect the degree of urgency for correction of modifiable risk factors (e.g., a strong family history of CVD).

Absent evidence from clinical trials, observational studies can provide evidence supporting a causal link between risk factors and CVD. Strong associations are less likely to be due to confounding and a causal relationship is more likely if exposure to the risk factor precedes the onset of the disease. Likewise, a causal relationship is likely if the association is dose-dependent and consistently demonstrated under diverse circumstances. Finally, the association should be biologically plausible.

Risk of CVD events is usually reported as a relative risk or as an odds ratio. Risk can also be expressed as an attributable risk by subtracting the rate in those without the risk factor from the rate in those who have it. For coronary disease risk factors, the absolute attributable risk increases with age, whereas the relative risk tends to decrease. The population-attributable fraction takes into account the prevalence of the risk factor as well as the risk ratio, assessing the impact of the risk factor on the incidence of disease in the population and the benefit of removing it from the population. An unimpressive risk-factor risk ratio can have a major public health impact because of its high prevalence in the general population.

Four decades of epidemiological research have identified a number of modifiable CVD risk factors that have a strong dose-dependent and independent relationship to the rate of development of atherosclerotic CVD *(2)*. Importantly, these risk factors can be readily ascertained from ordinary

From: *Essential Cardiology: Principles and Practice, 2nd Ed.*
Edited by: C. Rosendorff © Humana Press Inc., Totowa, NJ

Table 1
Risk of CVD Events According to Standard Risk Factors Framingham Study 36-Yr Follow-Up

	Age 35–64 yr				Age 65–94 yr			
	Rate/1000		Rel. risk		Rate/1000		Rel. risk	
CHD Risk Factors	Men	Women	Men	Women	Men	Women	Men	Women
High chol.	34	15	1.9^c	1.8^b	59	39	1.2^a	2.0^c
Hypertension	45	21	2.0^c	2.2^c	73	44	1.6^c	1.9^c
Diabetes	39	42	1.5^c	3.7^c	79	62	1.6^b	2.1^c
Smoking	33	13	1.5^b	1.1^d	53	38	1.0^d	1.2^d
ECG-LVH	79	55	3.0^c	4.6^c	134	94	2.7^c	3.0^c
ABI								
High chol.	3	2	1.0^d	1.1^d	10	12	1.0^d	1.0^d
Hypertension	7	4	5.7^c	4.0^c	20	17	2.0^c	2.6^c
Diabetes	7	4	3.0^c	2.4^a	20	28	1.6^d	2.9^c
Smoking	4	1	2.5^b	1.0^d	17	20	1.4^d	1.9^c
ECG-LVH	13	13	5.1^c	8.1^c	44	51	3.6^c	5.0^c
PAD								
High chol.	8	4	2.0^b	1.9^d	18	8	1.4^d	1.0^d
Hypertension	10	7	2.0^c	3.7^c	17	10	1.6^a	2.0^b
Diabetes	18	18	3.4^c	6.4^c	21	16	9.7^a	2.6^b
Smoking	9	5	2.5^c	2.0^b	18	11	8.5^b	1.8^a
ECG-LVH	16	17	2.7^b	5.3^c	36	14	23.7^b	2.2^a
CHF								
High chol.	7	4	1.2^d	1.1^d	21	18	1.0^d	1.0^d
Hypertension	14	6	4.0^c	3.0^c	33	24	1.9^c	1.9^c
Diabetes	23	21	4.4^c	8.0^c	40	51	2.0^c	3.6^c
Smoking	7	3	1.5^c	1.1^d	23	22	1.0^d	1.3^a
ECG-LVH	71	36	15.0^c	13.0^c	99	84	4.9^c	5.4^c

CHD, coronary heart disease; ABI, atherothrombotic brain infarction; PAD, peripheral artery disease; CHF, heart failure.

Rates are biennial per 1000 and age-adjusted. Risk ratios are age-adjusted.

Risk ratio, relative risk for persons with a risk factor versus those without it. For cholesterol >240 compared to <200 mg/dL. Hypertension >140/90 mmHg.

[a]$p < 0.05$.

[b]$p < 0.01$.

[c]$p < 0.001$.

[d]NS.

Source: ref. 41. Copyright 1996; with permission from Elsevier.

office procedures. Framingham Study epidemiological research has documented several classes of risk factors such as atherogenic personal traits, lifestyles that promote them, signs of organ damage, and innate susceptibility. Most of the relevant risk factors are easy to assess during an office visit and include systolic blood pressure, blood lipids, glucose tolerance, cigarette smoking, and left ventricular hypertrophy on the electrocardiogram (ECG) (2,7).

DISEASE-SPECIFIC EFFECTS

The impact of the standard established risk factors on atherosclerotic CVD events is displayed in Table 1. All the standard CVD risk factors contribute powerfully and independently to the rate of subsequent coronary disease in all its clinical manifestations. For atherothrombotic brain infarction, hypertension and ECG-left ventricular hypertrophy predominate and lipids appear to play a lesser role. For peripheral artery disease, glucose intolerance, left ventricular hypertrophy, and cigarette smoking are paramount, whereas cholesterol is less important. For heart failure, hyper-

Table 2
Development of Coronary Heart Disease
by Total/HDL Cholesterol Ratio Versus Total Cholesterol
According to Age 16 Yr Follow-up Framingham Study

AGE	Total/HDL-C ratio (Quintile 5/Quintile 1)			Total cholesterol (>240/<200 mg/dL)	
	49–59	60–69	70–81	35–64	65–94
Men	3.4[a]	2.9[a]	2.3[a]	1.9[c]	1.2[d]
Women	3.7[a]	6.7[a]	3.3[a]	1.8[b]	2.0[c]

[a]$p < 0.05$.
[b]$p < 0.01$.
[c]$p < 0.001$.
[d]NS.
Source: ref. *41*. Copyright 1996; with permission from Elsevier.

Table 3
Efficiency of Blood Lipids
and Ratios in Predicting Coronary Disease
Framingham Study Subjects Ages 50–80 Yr

	Age-adjusted Q_5/Q_1 risk ratios	
	Men	Women
Total cholesterol	1.9	2.5
LDL cholesterol	1.9	2.5
HDL cholesterol	0.4	0.5
Total/HDL cholesterol	2.5	3.1
LDL/HDL cholesterol	2.5	2.8

Q, quintiles of blood lipid distribution.
Source: ref. *42*. Copyright 1992; with permission from Elsevier.

tension, diabetes, and ECG-left ventricular hypertrophy (LVH) are all important, whereas total cholesterol appears to be unrelated (unless expressed as a total/HDL-cholesterol ratio). The standard risk factors also influence CVD rates with different strengths in men and women *(1,8,9)*. Some of the standard risk factors tend to have lower risk ratios in advanced age, but this reduced relative risk is offset by a high absolute incidence of disease in advanced age, making the standard risk factors highly relevant in the elderly.

REFINEMENTS IN STANDARD RISK FACTORS

The atherogenic potential of the serum total cholesterol derives from its LDL-cholesterol fraction, whereas its HDL component is protective and inversely related to the development of coronary disease *(10,11)*. The strength of the relation of total cholesterol to coronary disease declines after age 60 yr in men but the total/HDL-cholesterol ratio continues to predict events reliably in the elderly of both sexes (Table 2). It also predicts equally well at total cholesterol values above and below 240 mg/dL. This ratio has been found to be one of the most efficient lipid profiles for predicting cardiovascular events *(12,13)*. Comparing age-adjusted fifth to first quintile lipid CVD risk ratios for the individual lipids and their ratios it is evident that the total/HDL and LDL/HDL cholesterol ratios are much more powerful predictors of CHD than the individual lipids that comprise them (Table 3).

Table 4
Increment in Risk of CVD Events Per Standard Deviation Increase in Blood
Pressure Components Framingham Study 30-Yr Follow-Up

| Pressure component | Standardized increment in risk | | | |
| | Men | | Women | |
	35–64 Yr	65–94 Yr	35–64 Yr	65–94 Yr
Systolic	41%[a]	51%[a]	43%[a]	23%[a]
Diastolic	35%[a]	30%[a]	33%[a]	9%[b]
Pulse Pressure	29%[a]	42%[a]	36%[a]	22%[a]
Mean Arterial	41%[a]	44%[a]	42%[a]	18%[a]

[a] $p < 0.001$.
[b] p = NS.
Source: ref. 43. Copyright 2000; with permission from Elsevier.

Table 5
Risk of CVD Events According to Pulse Pressure
30-Yr Follow-Up Framingham StudyAge-Adjusted Rate Per 1000

| Pulse pressure (mmHg) | Age 35–64 | | Age 65–94 | |
	Men	Women	Men	Women
<40	9	4	2	17
40–49	13	6	16	19
50–59	16	7	32	22
60–69	22	10	39	25
>70	33	16	58	32
Increment per 10 mmHg	19.7%	20.9%	23.4%	10.5%

Source: ref. 43. Copyright 2000; with permission from Elsevier.

Evaluation of hypertension now places more emphasis on the systolic blood pressure component and recognizes isolated systolic hypertension as a hazard for development of CVD. At all ages in either sex, for all the atherosclerotic CVD outcomes, systolic blood pressure has been shown to have a greater impact than the diastolic pressure (Table 4) *(14)*. Isolated systolic hypertension by definition denotes increased pulse pressure and risk of CVD increases stepwise with the pulse pressure at all ages in each sex (Table 5). Framingham Study data suggest an important role of the pulse pressure at any level of systolic blood pressure *(15)*. Reliance on the diastolic blood pressure to evaluate the risk of CVD in the elderly with an elevated systolic blood pressure can be misleading because counter to expectations of those who do, risk *increases* the *lower* the accompanying diastolic pressure *(15)*.

Diabetes and obesity are now conceptualized as components of an "insulin resistance or metabolic syndrome" consisting of abdominal obesity, elevated blood pressure, dyslipidemia, hyperinsulinemia, glucose intolerance, and abnormal lipoprotein lipase levels *(16)*. The National Cholesterol Education Program (NCEP) Adult Treatment Panel (ATP III) guidelines identify the metabolic syndrome as a target for therapy in the management of dyslipidemia *(17)*. The diagnosis of metabolic syndrome is designated when three or more of the following risk factors are present: waist circumference exceeding 88 cm in women or 102 cm in men, triglycerides of 150 mg/dL or greater, HDL-C under 40 mg/dL (men) or under 50 mg/dL (women), blood pressure of 130/85 mmHg or greater, and fasting plasma glucose of 110 mg/dL or greater. Using this definition of the metabolic syndrome, analysis of National Health and Nutrition Examintion Survey (NHANES) II data suggest a 23.7% age-adjusted prevalence of this syndrome in the US *(18)*.

Table 6
Impact of Diabetes on CVD Events in Men and Women 36-Yr
Follow-Up Framingham Study Subjects Ages 35–64 Yr

CVD Events	Age-adjusted biennial rate per 1000		Age-adjusted risk ratio		Excess risk per 1000	
	Men	Women	Men	Women	Men	Women
CIID	39	21	1.5^a	2.2^b	12	12
PAD	18	18	3.4^b	6.4^b	13	15
CHF	23	21	4.4^b	7.8^b	18	18
STROKE	15	6	2.9^b	2.6^b	10	4
Total CVD	76	65	2.2^b	3.7^b	42	47

CHD, coronary heart disease; PAD, peripheral artery disease; CHF, heart failure.
[a]$p < 0.01$.
[b]$p < 0.001$.
Source: ref. *41*. Copyright 1996; with permission from Elsevier.

RISK FACTORS IN WOMEN

CVD risk factors are highly prevalent in middle-aged and elderly women. Two thirds of such women have at least one major risk factor. The national burden of atherosclerotic CVD is projected to increase substantially as elderly women constitute a progressively greater proportion of the US population. Women and men share the same CVD risk factors but some are more prevalent or exert a greater impact in women than in men. There are also some that are unique to women, such as early menopause and multiple pregnancies. With the exception of diabetes and ECG-LVH, the absolute risk for most risk factors is lower in women than men.

Because of the lower incidence of CVD in women than men, the most cost-effective preventive approach requires global risk assessment for targeting of high-risk women for preventive measures. Intensive risk factor screening is particularly needed for elderly women, African American women, and those of lower socioeconomic status. High total/HDL-cholesterol ratios, ECG-LVH, and diabetes markedly reduce the female coronary disease advantage *(9)*. Diabetes is clearly a greater CVD hazard for women than men virtually eliminating their advantage over men for coronary disease, heart failure, and peripheral artery disease (Table 6). Women with diabetes require comprehensive screening to detect the usually accompanying elevated triglyceride, reduced HDL cholesterol, hypertension, and abdominal obesity. Minority women and those with gestational diabetes, who are prone to develop an adverse coronary risk profile, deserve particular attention.

Reduced HDL cholesterol predicts coronary disease even better in women than in men. Women on average, have HDL-cholesterol levels that are 10 mg/dL higher than those in men throughout life so that it seems more appropriate to characterize "low" HDL cholesterol as under 50 mg/dL rather than 35 mg/dL, as was recommended in ATP II guidelines. Despite controversy about hypertriglyceridemia as an independent risk factor, it is an important marker for increased vulnerability to CVD for women as well as for men, and the combination of low HDL and high triglyceride, reflecting insulin resistance and presence of small-dense LDL, imparts an increased CVD risk. The majority of elderly women have hypertension, and isolated systolic hypertension is more prevalent in elderly women than in men. Its concordance with risk-enhancing high pulse pressure, obesity, dyslipidemia, and insulin resistance should be noted.

Risk factors unique to women include early menopause and bilateral oophorectomy. Estrogen replacement therapy has failed to eliminate the more than twofold increase in risk of coronary disease in this subgroup of women. Women who undergo early menopause require close surveillance for development of an adverse cardiovascular risk profile.

THE ELDERLY

The major modifiable risk factors remain relevant in the elderly. The strength of risk factors associated with CVD diminishes with advancing age, but this lower risk ratio is offset by a higher absolute risk. This makes risk factor control in the elderly at least as cost-effective as in the middle-aged. Epidemiologic research has quantified the impact of the standard CVD risk factors in the elderly *(19)*. Dyslipidemia, hypertension, glucose intolerance, and cigarette smoking all have smaller hazard ratios in advanced age, but this is offset by higher absolute and attributable risks. Diabetes operates more strongly in elderly women than men, further attenuating their waning advantage over men in advanced age (Table 1). Insulin resistance promoted by abdominal obesity in advanced age is an important feature of the CVD hazard of diabetes in the elderly. Hypertension, particularly the isolated systolic variety, is highly prevalent in the elderly, and is a safely modifiable hazard. Dyslipidemia, particularly the total/HDL cholesterol ratio, remains a major risk factor in the elderly that, in contrast to the total cholesterol, continues to be highly predictive in advanced age (Table 2). Left ventricular hypertrophy remains an ominous harbinger of CVD in the elderly, indicating an urgent need for attention to its promoters including hypertension, diabetes, obesity, and myocardial ischemia or valve disease. High-normal fibrinogen, C-reactive protein (CRP), and leukocyte counts in the elderly may indicate the presence of unstable atherosclerotic lesions. As in the middle-aged, all the major risk factors in the elderly tend to cluster so that the hazard of each one is powerfully influenced by the associated burden of the others. Multivariate risk assessment can quantify the joint effect of the burden of risk factors making it possible to more efficiently target elderly candidates for CVD for preventive measures *(3–6)*.

ATHEROSCLEROTIC COMORBIDITY

Atherosclerotic CVD is usually a diffuse process involving the heart, brain, and peripheral arteries. The presence of one clinical manifestation substantially increases the likelihood of having or developing others *(20)*. The major risk factors tend to affect all arterial territories and clinical atherosclerosis affecting the heart may also directly predispose to strokes and heart failure. Measures taken to prevent coronary disease should have an additional benefit in preventing atherosclerotic peripheral artery and stroke events as well as heart failure.

Coronary artery disease places a patient at considerable risk not only for a myocardial infarction, angina, sudden death, or heart failure, but also for transient ischemic attacks, strokes, and intermittent claudication because of concomitant atherosclerotic disease in the other vascular territories *(20)*. The incidence of other cardiovascular disease accompanying coronary disease is substantial *(21)*. The Framingham Study found that in men and women, respectively, an initial myocardial infarction is accompanied by intermittent claudication 9% and 10% of the time, by strokes or TIAs 5% and 8% of the time, and by heart failure 3% and 10% of the time *(21)*. Persons in the Framingham Study with intermittent claudication had a two- to threefold increased risk of developing coronary disease. Over 10 yr, 45% developed coronary heart disease. After an initial myocardial infarction, strokes and heart failure occurred at three to six times the rate of the general population. The 10-yr probability of a stroke or TIA was 16% in men and 24% in women, a rate three to four times that of the general population. Heart failure occurred in about 30% of patients who had experienced an MI, which represents a four- to sixfold increase in risk. After sustaining an atherothrombotic stroke, 25% to 45% developed coronary disease, a twofold increase in risk.

After an MI coexistence of intermittent claudication increased age-adjusted coronary mortality 1.7-fold in men and 1.5-fold in women, and of recurrent MI increased twofold in men and 1.6-fold in women *(21)*.

NOVEL RISK FACTORS

Because CVD often occurs in persons with what is considered acceptable or average standard risk factor values, novel risk factors are being sought. Among these are lipoprotein (a) (Lp[a]), homocysteine, fibrinogen, small-dense LDL, insulin resistance, fibrinolytic function assessed by tPA and PAI-1 antigens, platelet function, and inflammatory parameters such as CRP *(22–24)*. The novel risk factors under consideration are characterized as emerging because information about their relevance is incomplete. There is no consensus about sensitive and specific diagnostic tests for many of these risk factors so that it is difficult to make recommendations for screening to detect high-risk persons. For some there is lack of consistent prospective epidemiologic evidence indicating that the novel marker can be detected in healthy persons prior to the onset of an initial cardiovascular event. Fibrinogen, Lp (a), CRP, and homocysteine may increase after a myocardial infarction, making interpretation of retrospective data speculative. To date, consistent prospective data are available for fibrinogen, CRP, tPA, and PAI-1. Prospective studies for Lp (a) and homocysteine have been both positive and negative. It is also not clear whether these novel risk factors add to our ability to predict events over and above that already achievable using the established cardiovascular risk factors. To date, data demonstrating the additive value of Lp (a) and homocysteine are inconsistent, whereas the inflammatory parameters such as fibrinogen and CRP have been shown to improve prediction. An additional uncertainty relates to whether the novel risk factor is modifiable and whether such modification reduces the likelihood of a cardiovascular event. Randomized trials are needed to determine whether specific therapies to modify these novel markers actually reduce the risk of CVD events. Enthusiasm for screening for these emerging risk factors must be tempered and should not supersede the need to deal more effectively with the established risk factors where there is a widely available methodology of measurement, a high population prevalence of the risk factors, a consistent prospective connection with the rate of development of CVD, and demonstrated benefit of correction in terms of reduced morbidity and mortality.

MULTIVARIATE RISK STRATIFICATION

Atherosclerotic CVD events can be efficiently predicted from risk factors that are readily ascertained through routine office procedures and laboratory tests *(3–6)*. Optimal risk predictions require quantitative synthesis of the various independently contributing risk factors into a composite estimate. For this purpose, multivariable risk formulations are employed to quantify the combined effect of these interrelated risk factors. This concept takes into account the multifactorial elements of CVD risk and the continuous gradient of response. This allows identification of high-risk persons with multiple mild to moderate risk factor aberrations, from whom most of the coronary events emerge. Categorical assessment of risk by assignment of arbitrary values to designate the point at which a continuous risk variable is to be considered a "risk factor" has some pragmatic utility, but this approach is inefficient because it overlooks the substantial high-risk segment of the population with multiple marginal abnormalities. Global risk assessment is also essential because the major risk factors tend to cluster together at four to five times the rate expected by chance so that when confronted with any particular risk factor one is obliged to seek out the others. Isolated occurrence of the standard risk factors is uncommon, ranging from 11% to 38% (Table 7).

Multivariable risk formulations can quantify the global risk based on the actual risk factor values over a wide range. For office use, scoring systems have been devised based on Framingham Study multivariable risk formulations that provide estimates of global risk for any combination of risk factors. The standard risk factors to be ascertained are total and HDL cholesterol, systolic blood pressure, cigarette smoking, diabetic status, and age for each sex. From the estimated rate of disease, based on the risk-factor makeup of the patient, compared to the average rate for persons of the same age, the urgency for treatment can be estimated without needlessly alarming patients with only one "risk factor" in isolation or falsely reassuring patients at high risk because of multiple marginal abnormalities. These risk formulations have been shown to accurately predict disease in a variety of population samples *(25–27)*.

Other risk factor information, important in implementing therapy, includes triglycerides, weight, physical activity, and family history, but does not greatly enhance risk estimation. Weight gain and abdominal obesity are particularly important because they are major determinants of risk factor

Table 7
Risk Factor Clustering in the Framingham Study
Offspring Cohort Subjects Ages 18–74 Yr

Index quintile variable (sex-specific)		Percent with specified no. of additional risk factors	
	Sex	None	Two or more
High cholesterol	Men	29%	43%
	Women	26%	57%
Low HDL-cholesterol	Men	27%	45%
	Women	38%	36%
High BMI	Men	23%	48%
	Women	15%	54%
High systolic BP	Men	25%	46%
	Women	19%	53%
High triglyceride	Men	11%	61%
	Women	20%	50%
High glucose	Men	23%	45%
	Women	29%	44%

Risk factors: upper quintile of distribution of all variables except HDL-C (lowest quintile).
Source: ref. *44*.

Table 8
Risk Factor Clustering According to Body Mass Index in the Framingham Study
Offspring Cohort With Elevated Blood Pressure Subjects Ages 18–74 Yr

	Men		Women
$BMI\ (kg/m^{2})$	Avg. no. risk factors	$BMI\ (kg/m^{2})$	Avg. no. risk factors
<23.7	1.68	<20.8	1.80
23.7–25.5	1.85	20.8–22.3	2.00
25.6–27.2	2.06	22.4–23.9	2.22
27.3–29.5	2.28	24.0–26.8	2.20
>29.5	2.35	>26.8	2.66

Risk factors are top quintiles of systolic blood pressure, total cholesterol, triglycerides, and glucose; and bottom quintile of HDL-cholesterol.
Source: ref. *43*. Copyright 2000; with permission from Elsevier.

clustering by promoting insulin resistance. The average number of standard risk factors acquired increases with body mass index in both sexes (Table 8).

Coronary Risk Profile

Coronary heart disease is the most common outcome of the standard risk factors, equaling in incidence all the other atherosclerotic CVD outcomes combined (Fig. 1). Because it is the most common and most lethal of the atherosclerotic sequelae of the standard risk factors, prevention of coronary disease deserves the highest priority. Multivariable coronary risk formulations have been developed based on continuous variable relationships to coronary disease outcome, and more recently integrating categorical approaches that have become part of the framework of blood pressure (JNC-VII) and cholesterol (NCEP) programs in the US (28). This enables physicians to pull together all the relevant risk factor information into a composite estimate of the risk of having a coronary event and compare this to the average or optimal risk for persons of the same age and sex (Tables 9 and 10). The risk of developing coronary disease for any particular risk factor can be seen to vary widely depending on the burden of other associated risk factors in Fig. 2.

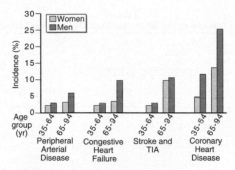

Fig. 1. Incidence of cardiovascular events by age and sex: Framingham Heart Study 36-yr follow-up. TIA, transient ischemic attack. (From ref. *41*. Copyright 1996; with permission from Elsevier.)

Stroke Risk Profile

A stroke, the most feared of the atherosclerotic diseases of the elderly, can also be risk-stratified in relation to the standard risk factors plus knowledge of the presence of coronary disease, heart failure, or atrial fibrillation (Table 11) *(4)*. The chief risk factor for a stroke is hypertension, but the risk associated with an elevated blood pressure varies over a 10-fold range depending on the degree of its coexistence with other risk factors that commonly accompany it (Fig. 3). Using the stroke risk profile table, it is possible to estimate the joint effect of any combination of the major predisposing factors in terms of the absolute and relative risk.

Heart Failure Profile

Heart failure is a lethal terminal stage of cardiac disease, with a survival experience resembling that of cancer *(29)*. A substantial reduction in the incidence and mortality from heart failure can be achieved only by the early detection and treatment of persons prone to left ventricular dysfunction so that it can be corrected before overt failure ensues. High-risk candidates for heart failure must be cost-effectively targeted for echocardiographic evaluation to detect the presence of left ventricular dysfunction. The Framingham Study has identified and quantified major contributing risk factors for the development of heart failure *(30)*. Using these, multivariable risk profiles have been developed that efficiently predict failure, providing risk estimates in those with the major predisposing conditions such as hypertension, coronary disease and valvular heart disease *(6)*. The ingredients of the profile consist of ECG-LVH, cardiomegaly on chest film, reduced vital capacity, heart rate, presence of heart murmurs, systolic blood pressure, and diabetes (Fig. 4). Using this risk assessment it is possible to identify high-risk candidates for heart failure who constitute good candidates for echocardiographic examination with a high likelihood of positive findings. Such persons stand to benefit from vigorous preventive measures such as therapy with angiotensin-converting enzyme (ACE)-inhibitors, cardiac revascularization, or valve surgery.

Profile for Peripheral Artery Disease

Using 38-yr follow-up data from the Framingham Study a risk profile for intermittent claudication was developed *(5)*. The variables needed are age, sex, serum cholesterol, blood pressure, cigarette smoking, diabetes, and coronary disease status (Table 12). Computation of multivariable risk using this risk profile allows physicians to identify high-risk candidates for development of peripheral artery disease and to educate such patients about modification of the cardiovascular risk factors. Identification of persons at risk of intermittent claudication is important not only because it limits mobility, and can lead to limb loss in those who develop it, but also because it is associated with a two- to fourfold excess of mortality, predominantly from CVD. The standard risk factors predict intermittent claudication even better than they predict coronary disease. Physicians can readily determine the probability of developing peripheral artery disease for each patient using a point score based on these risk factor data *(5)*.

Table 9
Coronary Heart Disease Score Sheet for Men Using TC or LDC-C Categories

Step 1 — Age

Years	LDL Pts	Chol Pts
30-34	−1	(−1)
35-39	0	(0)
40-44	1	(1)
45-49	2	(2)
50-54	3	(3)
55-59	4	(4)
60-64	5	(5)
65-69	6	(6)
70-74	7	(7)

Step 2 — LDL-C

(mg/dl)	(mmol/L)	LDL Pts
<100	<2.59	-3
100-129	2.60-3.36	0
130-159	3.37-4.14	0
160-190	4.15-4.92	1
≥190	≥4.92	2

Cholesterol

(mg/dl)	(mmol/L)	Chol Pts
<160	<4.14	(-3)
160-199	4.15-5.17	(0)
200-239	5.18-6.21	(1)
240-279	6.22-7.24	(2)
≥280	≥7.25	(3)

Step 3 — HDL-C

(mg/dl)	(mmol/L)	LDL Pts	Chol Pts
<35	<0.90	2	(2)
35-44	0.91-1.16	1	(1)
45-49	1.17-1.29	0	(0)
50-59	1.30-1.55	0	(0)
≥60	≥1.56	-1	(-2)

Key

Relative risk
- Very low
- Low
- Moderate
- High
- Very high

Step 4 — Blood Pressure

Systolic (mm Hg)	Diastolic (mm Hg) <80	80-84	85-89	90-99	≥100
<120	0 (0) pts				
120-129		0 (0) pts			
130-139			1 (1) pts		
140-159				2 (2) pts	
≥160					3 (3) pts

+ Note: When systolic and diastolic pressures provide different estimates for point scores, use the higher number

Step 5 — Diabetes

	LDL Pts	Chol Pts
No	0	(0)
Yes	2	(2)

Step 6 — Smoker

	LDL Pts	Chol Pts
No	0	(0)
Yes	2	(2)

Step 7 — Adding up the points

Age	___
LDL-C or Chol	___
HDL-C	___
Blood Pressure	___
Diabetes	___
Smoker	___
Point total	___

(sum from steps 1-6)

Step 8 — CHD Risk

LDL Pts Total	10 Yr CHD Risk	Chol Pts Total	10 Yr CHD Risk
<-3	1%		
-2	2%		
-1	2%	(<-1)	(2%)
0	3%	(0)	(3%)
1	4%	(1)	(3%)
2	4%	(2)	(4%)
3	6%	(3)	(5%)
4	7%	(4)	(7%)
5	9%	(5)	(8%)
6	11%	(6)	(10%)
7	14%	(7)	(13%)
8	18%	(8)	(16%)
9	22%	(9)	(20%)
10	27%	(10)	(25%)
11	33%	(11)	(31%)
12	40%	(12)	(37%)
13	47%	(13)	(45%)
≥14	≥56%	(≥14)	(≥53%)

(determine CHD risk from point total)

Step 9 — Comparative Risk

Age (years)	Average 10 Yr CHD Risk	Average 10 Yr Hard* CHD Risk	Low** 10 Yr CHD Risk
30-34	3%	1%	2%
35-39	5%	4%	3%
40-44	7%	4%	4%
45-49	11%	8%	4%
50-54	14%	10%	6%
55-59	16%	13%	7%
60-64	21%	20%	9%
65-69	25%	22%	11%
70-74	30%	25%	14%

(compare to average person your age)

Risk estimates were derived from the experience of the Framingham Heart Study, a predominantly Caucasian population in Massachusetts, USA

* Hard CHD events exclude angina pectoris   ** Low risk was calculated for a person the same age, optimal blood pressure, LDL-C 100-129 mg/dL or cholesterol 160-199 mg/dL, HDL-C 45 mg/dL for men or 55 mg/dL for women, non-smoker, no diabetes

The scoring uses age, TC (or LDL-C), HDL-C, blood pressure, diabetes, and smoking and estimates risk for CHD over a period of 10 yr based on Framingham experience in men 30 to 74 yr old at baseline. Average risk estimates are based on typical Framingham subjects, and estimates of idealized risk are based on optimal blood pressure, TC 160 to 199 mg/dL (or LDL 100 to 129 mg/dL), HDL-C of 45 mg/dL in men, no diabetes, and no smoking. Use of the LDL-C categories is appropriate when fasting LDL-C measurements are available. Pts indicates points. (TCA, total cholesterol; LDL-C, low-density lipoprotein cholesterol; HDL-C, high-density lipoprotein cholesterol; CHD, coronary heart disease.)

Source: ref. *45*. With permission from Lippincott Williams & Wilkins.

Risk Stratification of Existing Coronary Disease

Based on Framingham Study data, risk formulations have also been developed for predicting another coronary event, a stroke, or a death from cerebrovascular disease in persons who have already sustained a coronary event *(31)*. Risk of these adverse outcomes can be estimated from the

Table 10
Coronary Heart Disease Score Sheet for Women Using TC or LDL-C Categories

Step 1 — Age

Years	LDL Pts	Chol Pts
30-34	−9	(−9)
35-39	−4	(−4)
40-44	0	(0)
45-49	3	(3)
50-54	6	(6)
55-59	7	(7)
60-64	8	(8)
65-69	8	(8)
70-74	8	(8)

Step 2 — LDL-C

(mg/dl)	(mmol/L)	LDL Pts
<100	<2.59	-2
100-129	2.60-3.36	0
130-159	3.37-4.14	0
160-190	4.15-4.92	2
≥190	≥4.92	2

Cholesterol

(mg/dl)	(mmol/L)	Chol Pts
<160	<4.14	(-2)
160-199	4.15-5.17	(0)
200-239	5.18-6.21	(1)
240-279	6.22-7.24	(1)
≥280	≥7.25	(3)

Step 3 — HDL-C

(mg/dl)	(mmol/L)	LDL Pts	Chol Pts
<35	<0.90	5	(5)
35-44	0.91-1.16	2	(2)
45-49	1.17-1.29	1	(1)
50-59	1.30-1.55	0	(0)
≥60	≥1.56	-2	(-3)

Key

Relative risk

- Very low
- Low
- Moderate
- High
- Very high

Step 4 — Blood Pressure

Systolic (mm Hg)	Diastolic (mm Hg) <80	80-84	85-89	90-99	≥100
<120	-3 (-3) pts				
120-129		0 (0) pts			
130-139			0 (0) pts		
140-159				2 (2) pts	
≥ 160					3 (3) pts

+ Note: When systolic and diastolic pressures provide different estimates for point scores, use the higher number

Step 5 — Diabetes

	LDL Pts	Chol Pts
No	0	(0)
Yes	4	(4)

Step 6 — Smoker

	LDL Pts	Chol Pts
No	0	(0)
Yes	2	(2)

Step 7 — Adding up the points

Age	___
LDL-C or Chol	___
HDL-C	___
Blood Pressure	___
Diabetes	___
Smoker	___
Point total	___

(sum from steps 1-6)

Step 8 — CHD Risk

LDL Pts Total	10 Yr CHD Risk	Chol Pts Total	10 Yr CHD Risk
≤-2	1%	(≤-2)	(1%)
-1	2%	(-1)	(2%)
0	2%	(0)	(2%)
1	2%	(1)	(2%)
2	3%	(2)	(3%)
3	3%	(3)	(3%)
4	4%	(4)	(4%)
5	5%	(5)	(4%)
6	6%	(6)	(5%)
7	7%	(7)	(6%)
8	8%	(8)	(7%)
9	9%	(9)	(8%)
10	11%	(10)	(10%)
11	13%	(11)	(11%)
12	15%	(12)	(13%)
13	17%	(13)	(15%)
14	20%	(14)	(18%)
15	24%	(15)	(20%)
16	27%	(16)	(24%)
≥17	≥32%	(≥17)	(≥27%)

(determine CHD risk from point total)

Step 9 — Comparative Risk

Age (years)	Average 10 Yr CHD Risk	Average 10 Yr Hard* CHD Risk	Low** 10 Yr CHD Risk
30-34	<1%	<1%	<1%
35-39	<1%	<1%	1%
40-44	2%	1%	2%
45-49	5%	2%	3%
50-54	8%	3%	5%
55-59	12%	7%	7%
60-64	12%	8%	8%
65-69	13%	8%	8%
70-74	14%	11%	8%

(compare to average person your age)

Risk estimates were derived from the experience of the Framingham Heart Study, a predominantly Caucasian population in Massachusetts, USA

* Hard CHD events exclude angina pectoris

** Low risk was calculated for a person the same age, optimal blood pressure, LDL-C 100-129 mg/dL or cholesterol 160-199 mg/dL, HDL-C 45 mg/dL for men or 55 mg/dL for women, non-smoker, no diabetes

Scoring uses age, TC, HDL-C, blood pressure, diabetes, and smoking and estimates risk for CHD over a period of 10 yr based on Framingham experience in women 30 to 74 yr old at baseline. Average risk estimates are based on typical Framingham subjects, and estimates of idealized risk are based on optimal blood pressure, TC 160 to 199 mg/dL (or LDL 100 to 129 mg/dL), HDL-C of 55 mg/dL in women, no diabetes, and no smoking. Use of the LDL-C categories is appropriate when fasting LDL-C measurements are available. Pts indicates points. (TCA, total cholesterol; LDL-C, low-density lipoprotein cholesterol; HDL-C, high-density lipoprotein cholesterol; CHD, coronary heart disease.)

Source: ref. *45*. With permission from Lippincott Williams & Wilkins.

joint effect of age, diabetic status, total and HDL cholesterol, and systolic blood pressure. The 2-yr probability of these events conditional on the risk factor burden in survivors of coronary events can be estimated over a wide range and compared to the average risk.

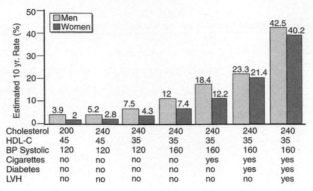

Fig. 2. Incidence of coronary heart disease: Framingham Heart Study 1972–1984, 42-yr-old adults. Reprinted from ref. *44*.

Table 11
Probability of a Stroke Within 10 Yr for Persons Age 55–85
Without a Previous Stroke Framingham Heart Study—Women

Points	0	+1	+2	+3	+4	+5	+6	+7	+8	+9	+10
Age	55	58	61	64	67	70	73	76	79	82	85
SBP	100	110	120	130	145	155	165	175	185	195	205
HypRx	No		M	F							
Diabetes	No		M	F							
Cigs	No			Yes							
CVD	No		F	M							
A.Fib.	No				M		F				
LVH	No				F		M				

Points	10-yr. prob	Age (yr)	Av. 10-yr prob
23	57%	60–64	5%
24	64%	65–69	7%
25	71%	70–74	11%
26	78%	75–79	16%
27	84%	80–84	24%

Source: ref. *4*; with permission from Lippincott Williams & Wilkins.

PREVENTIVE IMPLICATIONS

Comparison of the profiles for each of the various atherosclerotic CVD outcomes strongly suggests that correction of any particular set of risk factors imparts a bonus in reducing the risk of all outcomes. Reliance on single-risk-factor detection and treatment may be justified on a population basis, but is shortsighted on an individual basis. The goal in treating hypertension, diabetes, or dyslipidemia is not to simply correct these abnormalities but rather to prevent their CVD sequelae. They should be targeted for treatment from a multivariable risk profile and the goal of treatment should be to improve the global risk. Because of the tendency of all the established risk factors to cluster, it is imperative that physicians, when confronted with any particular risk factor, seek out the others likely to be present and take these into account in evaluating the risk and formulating the treatment regimen required.

A substantial proportion of the elderly warrant preventive measures because they are free of overt disease and active in their retirement years. Also, because of the aging of the general population it will be necessary to keep more of the elderly in the workforce, necessitating primary prevention of CVD. Because of the high average risk of CVD events in the elderly there is actually a great poten-

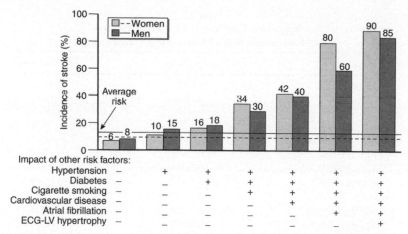

Fig. 3. The Framingham Heart Study: 10-yr probability of stroke, subjects aged 70 yr, systemic blood pressure 160 mmHg. ECG-LV, electrocardiographic left ventricular. (From ref. *4*; with permission from Lippincott Williams & Wilkins.)

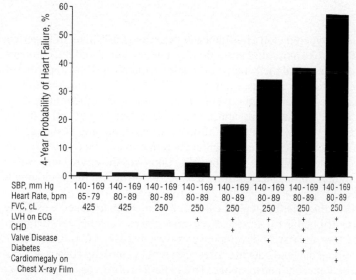

Fig. 4. Risk of heart failure in hypertensive men aged 60 to 64 yr by burden of associated risk factors after 38-yr follow-up in the Framingham Study. SBP indicates systolic blood pressure; FVC, forced vital capacity; LVH on ECG, left ventricular hypertrophy on electrocardiogram; and CHD, coronary heart disease. Plus sign indicates that patients in this category had this condition. (From ref. *6*. Copyright 1999 American Medical Association.)

tial benefit of preventive measures, but to avoid overtreatment it is important to assess multivariable risk and to take into account general heath status. There is little justification for pessimism about the efficacy of preventive measures in the elderly. The major risk factors can be safely modified without inducing intolerable side effects or adversely affecting the quality of the last years of life. The major risk factors remain highly relevant in the elderly not only for primary prevention but for secondary prevention as well.

Controlled trials have provided consistent evidence of the benefit of reducing elevated blood pressure and correcting dyslipidemia *(32,33)*. Lowering LDL and raising HDL cholesterol have been shown to slow progression of atherosclerosis. Primary prevention trials have shown consistent benefit for coronary disease by reducing LDL and raising HDL cholesterol even in persons with only average lipid values *(34,35)*.

Table 12
Regression Coefficients for Computation
of Multivariable Risk of Intermittent Claudication

Variable	β-coefficient	Standard error
Intercept	−8.9152	0.5241
Male sex	0.5033	0.1134
Age	0.0372	0.0063
Blood pressure		
Normal	Referent	
High normal	0.2621	0.1769
Stage 1 HBP	0.4067	0.1559
Stage 2+ HBP	0.7977	0.1519
Diabetes	0.9503	0.1360
Cigarettes per day	0.0314	0.0039
Cholesterol (mg/dL)	0.0048	0.0010
CHD	0.9939	0.1160

Source: ref. 5. With permission from Lippincott Williams & Wilkins.

Meta-analysis of hypertension trials indicates benefits of treatment of hypertension for overall vascular mortality, stroke morbidity and mortality, and fatal and nonfatal coronary events. Recent trials have also demonstrated the benefits of treating isolated systolic hypertension in the elderly for stroke, coronary disease, and heart failure (36,37). Antiatherogenic recommendations for diabetes now focus on correction of the metabolically linked dyslipidemia and hypertension that usually accompany it. Weight control appears to be an important preventive measure for avoiding atherosclerotic CVD (Table 8). Because of difficulty in achieving sustained weight reduction, there is as yet no direct evidence that weight reduction reduces the risk of clinical cardiovascular events despite convincing evidence that slimming improves the entire cardiovascular risk profile. Persons who maintain optimal weight have a 35–60% lower risk of developing CVD than those who become obese.

Meta-analysis of the benefits of physical activity for coronary disease estimates a 50% reduction in risk that is attributable to exercise. Even moderate exercise appears to improve both the predisposing risk factors and risk of developing coronary disease. Although controlled trial data are lacking, observational data indicate that after cessation of smoking coronary disease risk declines to half that of those who continue to smoke. This benefit is observed in a matter of months without regard to the amount smoked or the duration of smoking. Quitting smoking deserves a high priority in prevention of CVD because it is ranked as a leading preventable cause of the disease.

Meta-analysis of randomized trials conducted in persons with clinical vascular disease has shown that low-dose aspirin can reduce the incidence of subsequent myocardial infarction, stroke, or cardiovascular mortality by about 25%. In primary prevention trials initial myocardial infarctions were reduced 33%. As a result, aspirin has been recommended for primary prevention in men who are at high risk of coronary disease.

Two recent trials of the efficacy of hormone replacement therapy have challenged our understanding of the influence of the menopause and the alleged protective role of estrogen against atherosclerotic CVD (38,39). This confirmed the 1985 epidemiological prediction of the Framingham Study reported by Wilson et al. (40) who reported that despite control for the major CVD risk factors and a more favorable risk profile to begin with, women reporting estrogen use had a more than 50% excess of CVD morbidity and a two-fold increased risk of stroke. Increased myocardial infarction rates were also observed, particularly in those who smoked. Among nonsmokers, estrogen use was associated with a significant excess incidence of stroke. Importantly, the Framingham Study data did not show any CVD benefit of estrogen replacement therapy and concluded that "the potential drawbacks of postmenopausal estrogen therapy should be considered carefully before recommending its widespread use." This conclusion was ignored because most other observational studies suggested benefit.

Coronary heart disease and stroke mortality has declined over the past several decades but the incidence of new events has not, resulting in an increasing pool of persons with coronary disease, strokes, and heart failure. The specific challenges for the future are to implement comprehensive preventive programs using global risk stratification to target high-risk CVD candidates for preventive measures. The occurrence of an overt CVD event should come to be regarded as a medical failure rather than the first indication for treatment.

REFERENCES

1. Manson JE, Tosteson H, Ridker PM, et al. The primary prevention of myocardial infarction. N Engl J Med 1992;326: 1406–1416.
2. Kannel WB. Contribution of the Framingham Study to preventive cardiology. J Am Coll Cardiol 1990;15:206–211.
3. Anderson KM, Wilson PWF, Odell PM, et al. An updated coronary risk profile: a statement for health professionals. Circulation 1991;83:357–363.
4. Wolf PA, D'Agostino RB, Belanger AJ, et al. Probability of stroke: a risk profile from the Framingham Study. Stroke 1991;22:312–318.
5. Murabito JM, D'Agostino RB, Silbershatz H, Wilson PWF. Intermittent claudication: a risk profile from the Framingham Study. Circulation 1997;96:44–49.
6. Kannel WB, D'Agostino RB, Silbershatz H, et al. Profile for estimating risk of heart failure. Arch Intern Med 1999; 159:1197–1204.
7. Kannel WB, Sytkowski PA. Atherosclerosis risk factors. Pharmacol Ther 1987;32:207–235.
8. Kannel WB, McGee DL. Diabetes and glucose tolerance as risk factors for cardiovascular disease: The Framingham Study. Diabetes Care 1979;2:120–126.
9. Kannel WB, Wilson PWF. Risk factors that attenuate the female coronary disease advantage. Arch Intern Med 1995; 155:57–91.
10. NIH Consensus Development Panel. Triglyceride, high-density lipoprotein and coronary heart disease. JAMA 1993; 269:505–510.
11. Kannel WB. High-density lipoproteins: epidemiologic profile and risks of coronary artery disease. Am J Cardiol 1983;52:9B–12B.
12. Wilson PWF, Kannel WB. Hypercholesterolemia and coronary risk in the elderly: The Framingham Study. Am J Geriat Cardiol 1993;2:52–56.
13. Corti MC, Guralnic JM, Salive ME, et al. HDL cholesterol predicts coronary heart disease mortality in older persons. JAMA 1995;274:539–544.
14. Kannel WB, Dawber TR, McGee DL, et al. Perspectives on systolic blood hypertension: The Framingham Study. Circulation 1980;61:1179–1182.
15. Franklin SS, Kahn SA, Wong ND, et al. Is pulse pressure useful in predicting risk for coronary heart disease? The Framingham Heart Study. Circulation 1999;100:354–360.
16. Reaven GM. Banting Lecture 1988: role of insulin resistance in human disease. Diabetes 1988;37:1595–1607.
17. Expert Panel on Detection, Evaluation and Treatment of High Blood Cholesterol in Adults. Executive Summary of the Third Report of the National Cholesterol Education Program (NCEP) Expert Panel on Detection, Evaluation and Treatment of High Blood Cholesterol in Adults (ATP III). JAMA 2001;285:2486–2497.
18. Ford ES, Giles WH, Dietz WH. Prevalence of the metabolic syndrome among U.S. adults. JAMA 2002;287: 356–259.
19. Castelli WP, Wilson PWF, Levy D, Anderson K. Cardiovascular risk factors in the elderly. Am J Cardiol 1989; 63:12H–19H.
20. Kannel WB. Epidemiologic relationship of disease among the different vascular territories. In: Fuster V, Ross R, Topol EJ, eds. Atherosclerosis and Coronary Artery Disease, vol. II. Lippincott-Raven, Philadelphia, 1996, pp. 1591–1599.
21. Cupples LA, Gagnon DR, Wong ND, et al. Preexisting cardiovascular conditions and long-term prognosis after initial myocardial infarction. The Framingham Study. Am Heart J 1993;125:863–872.
22. Koenig W. Haemostatic risk factors for cardiovascular disease. Eur Heart J 1998;19(Suppl C):C39–C43.
23. Ridker PM, Cushman M, Stampfer MJ, et al. Inflammation, aspirin and the risk of cardiovascular disease. N Engl J Med 1997;336:973–979.
24. Welch GN, Loscalzo J. Homocysteine and atherothrombosis. N Engl J Med 1998;338:1042–1050.
25. Leaverton PE, Sorlie PD, Kleinman JC, et al. Representativeness of the Framingham risk model for coronary heart disease mortality: a comparison with a national cohort study. J Chronic Dis 1987;40:775–784.
26. Brand RJ, Rosenmann RH, Sholtz RI, et al. Multivariate prediction of coronary heart disease in the Western Collaborative Group Study compared to the findings of the Framingham Study. Circulation 1976;53:348–355.

27. Schulte H, Assmann G. CHD risk equations obtained from the Framingham Heart Study applied to PRO-CAM Study. Cardiovascular Risk Factors 1991;1:126–133.
28. Wilson PWF, D'Agostino RB, Levy D, et al. Prediction of coronary heart disease using risk factor categories. Circulation 1998;97:1837–1847.
29. Ho KL, Anderson KM, Grossman W, Levy D. Survival after onset of congestive heart failure in the Framingham Study. Circulation 1993;88:107–115.
30. Kannel WB, Belanger AJ. Epidemiology of heart failure. Am Heart J 1994;121:951–957.
31. Califf RM, Armstrong PW, Carver JR, et al. 27th Bethesda Conference: Matching the intensity of risk factor management with the hazard for coronary disease events. Task Force 5. Stratification of patients into high, medium and low risk subgroups for purposes of risk factor management. J Am Coll Cardiol 1996;5:1007–1019.
32. Manson JE, Tosteson H, Ridker PM, et al. The primary prevention of myocardial infarction. N Engl J Med 1992; 326:1406–1416.
33. Rich-Edwards JW, Manson JE, Hennekens CH, et al. The primary prevention of coronary heart disease in women. N Engl J Med 1995;332:1758–1766.
34. Sacks FM, Pfeffer MA, Moye LA, et al. The effect of pravastatin on coronary events after myocardial infarction in patients with average cholesterol levels. N Engl J Med 1996;335:1001–1009.
35. Downs JR, Clearfield M, Weis S, et al. For the AFCAPS/TexCAPS Research Group. Primary prevention of acute coronary events with lovastatin in men and women with average cholesterol levels: results of AFCAPS/TexCAPS. JAMA 1998;279:1615–1622.
36. Systolic Hypertension in the Elderly Program Cooperative Research Group. Prevention of stroke by antihypertensive drug treatment in older persons with isolated systolic hypertension: Final results of the Systolic Hypertension in the Elderly Program (SHEP). JAMA 1991;265:3255–3264.
37. Stassen JA, Fagard R, Thijs L, et al. Randomized double-blind comparison of placebo and active treatment for older patients with isolated systolic hypertension. The Systolic Hypertension in Europe (Syst-Eur) Trial investigators. Lancet 1997;350:757–764.
38. Risks and benefits of estrogen plus progestin in healthy postmenopausal women. Principal results from the Women's Health Initiative Randomized Controlled Trial. Writing group for the Women's Health Initiative investigators. JAMA 2002;288:321–333.
39. Hulley S, Grady D, Bush T, Furberg C, et al. Randomized trial of estrogen plus progestin for secondary prevention of coronary heart disease in postmenopausal women. For the Heart and Estrogen Progestin Replacement Study (HERS) Research Group. JAMA 1998;280:605–613.
40. Wilson PWF, Garrison RJ, Castelli WP. Postmenopausal estrogen, cigarette smoking and cardiovascular disease. The Framingham Study. N Engl J Med 1985;313:1038–1043.
41. Kannel WB, Wilson PWF. Comparison of risk profiles for cardiovascular events: implications for prevention. In: Abboud FM, ed. Advances in Internal Medicine. Mosby Yearbook, Chicago, 1997, pp. 39–66.
42. Kannel WB, Wilson PWF. Efficacy of lipid profiles in prediction of coronary disease. Am Heart J 1992;124:768–774.
43. Kannel WB. Elevated systolic blood pressure as a cardiovascular risk factor. Am J Cardiol 2000;85:251–255.
44. Kannel WB. Epidemiologic contributions to preventive cardiology and challenges for the 21st century. In: Wong, Black, Gardin, eds. Practical Strategies in Preventing Heart Disease. McGraw Hill, New York, 2000, pp. 3–20.
45. Wilson PW, D'Agostino RB, Levy D, et al. Prediction of coronary heart disease. Circulation 1998;97:1837.

II   CIRCULATORY FUNCTION

2

Molecular and Cellular Basis of Myocardial Contractility

Arnold M. Katz, MD, DMed (Hon)

INTRODUCTION

The heart's pumping action is made possible by interactions between myosin, the major protein of the thick filaments, and actin, which makes up the backbone of the thin filaments. These interactions, which are activated by calcium, are regulated by tropomyosin and troponins C, I, and T that are present along with actin in the thin filaments.

The signaling process that initiates cardiac systole, called excitation–contraction coupling, begins when an action potential depolarizes the plasma membrane. Opening of L-type calcium channels during the action potential plateau allows a small amount of calcium to enter the cytosol from the extracellular fluid. This calcium triggers the opening of calcium-release channels in the sarcoplasmic reticulum that admit a much larger amount of this activator to the cytosol from stores within this intracellular membrane system. Most of the calcium that binds to troponin C in the adult human heart is derived from the sarcoplasmic reticulum (intracellular calcium cycle); only a small fraction enters the cells from the extracellular fluid during the action potential (extracellular calcium cycle).

The heart relaxes when calcium is transported out of the cytosol. Most of this activator is transported back into the sarcoplasmic reticulum by an ATP-dependent calcium pump in the sarcoplasmic reticulum membrane. A smaller amount of calcium is transported from the cytosol into the extracellular space by a plasma membrane calcium pump and sodium/calcium exchanger.

Two mechanisms are traditionally viewed as regulating the heart's contractile performance. The first, length-dependent regulation (Starling's Law of the Heart), is brought about by variations in end-diastolic volume. The second, changes in myocardial contractility, occurs when the ability of the myocardium to do work is modified by factors other than altered fiber length. Most of the rapidly occurring changes in myocardial contractility are brought about by variations in the amount of calcium delivered to the contractile proteins during excitation–contraction coupling. Contractility is also regulated by posttranslational changes in the contractile proteins, ion channels, ion pumps and exchangers, and other structures that participate in excitation–contraction coupling and relaxation. Myocardial contractility is also modified by altered synthesis of the contractile proteins and membrane structures that participate in contraction, excitation–contraction coupling, and relaxation. These slowly evolving changes in contractility, which are important in hypertrophied and failing hearts, are mediated by altered transcriptional signaling.

MYOCYTE STRUCTURE

The working myocardial cells of the atria and ventricles are filled with cross-striated myofibrils that contain the heart's contractile proteins (Fig. 1). Excitation–contraction coupling and relaxation are regulated by the plasma membrane, which separates the cytosol from the extracellular

From: *Essential Cardiology: Principles and Practice, 2nd Ed.*
Edited by: C. Rosendorff © Humana Press Inc., Totowa, NJ

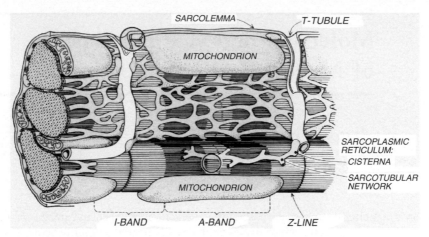

Fig. 1. Ultrastructure of the working myocardial cell. Contractile proteins are arranged in a regular array of thick and thin filaments (seen in cross-section at the left). The A-band represents the region of the sarcomere occupied by the thick filaments, while the I-band is occupied only by thin filaments that extend toward the center of the sarcomere from the Z-lines, which bisect each I-band. The sarcomere, the functional unit of the contractile apparatus, is defined as the region between two Z-lines, and contains two half I-bands and one A-band. The sarcoplasmic reticulum, a membrane network that surrounds the contractile proteins, consists of the sarcotubular network at the center of the sarcomere and the subsarcolemmal cisternae, which abut on the transverse tubular system (t-tubules) and the sarcolemma. The membrane surrounding the t-tubules is continuous with the sarcolemma, so that the lumen of the t-tubules carries the extracellular space toward the center of the myocardial cell. Mitochondria are shown in the central sarcomere and in cross-section at the left. (From Katz: N Engl J Med 1975;293:1184. Copyright 1975 Massachusetts Medical Society. All rights reserved.)

space, and by the internal membranes of the sarcoplasmic reticulum. Mitochondria, which are responsible for aerobic metabolism and oxidative phosphorylation, generate most of the adenosine triphosphate (ATP) that supplies the chemical energy for contraction and relaxation. Except under conditions of calcium overload, the mitochondria do not play an important role in controlling cytosolic calcium in the heart.

Myofibrils

The contractile proteins are organized into thick and thin filaments that are give rise to the characteristic cross-striations in cardiac myocytes (Fig. 1). The darker A-bands contain the thick filaments, while the more lightly staining I-bands are made up of the thin filaments (*see* next paragraph). Each I-band is bisected by a narrow, darkly staining Z-line, while a broad M-band occupies the center of the A-band. The morphological unit of striated muscle is the sarcomere, which lies between two Z-lines; each sarcomere therefore consists of a central A-band plus two adjacent half I-bands. A very large protein called titin runs through the thick filament from the Z-line and almost to the center of the A-band.

The thick filaments are composed largely of myosin, while the thin filaments are made up of two strands of polymerized actin along with tropomyosin and the troponin complex. In the resting heart at physiological sarcomere lengths the thin filaments extend from the Z-lines almost to the center of the A-band. Sarcomere shortening occurs when the thin filaments are pulled toward the center of the sarcomere by interactions between the thick and thin filaments. At short sarcomere lengths the thin filaments from the two I-bands at either side of the A-band cross in the center of the sarcomere.

Sarcomere shortening is effected by motion of cross-bridges that project from the thick filaments. These cross-bridges, which correspond to the heads of myosin molecules (*see* Myosin section below), interact with actin using energy provided by ATP hydrolysis. This process is controlled physiologically by calcium.

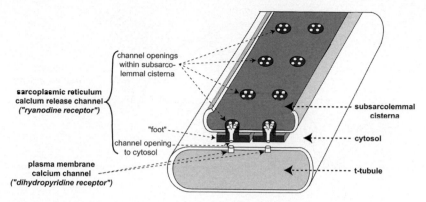

Fig. 2. Schematic diagram of a dyad showing the calcium release channels through which this activator leaves the subsarcolemmal cisternae of the sarcoplasmic reticulum. These intracellular calcium channels are closely approximated to plasma membrane L-type calcium channels. (Copyright © Arnold M. Katz, MD, modified from Katz, Physiology of the Heart, 3rd ed. Philadelphia, Lippincott Williams & Wilkins, 2001.)

Table 1
Contractile Proteins of the Heart

Protein	Location	Salient properties
Myosin	Thick filament	Hydrolyzes ATP, interacts with actin
Actin	Thin filament	Activates myosin ATPase, interacts with myosin
Tropomyosin	Thin filament	Modulates actin–myosin interaction
Troponin C	Thin filament	Binds calcium
Troponin I	Thin filament	Inhibits actin–myosin interactions
Troponin T	Thin filament	Binds troponin complex to the thin filament

Membranes

Two membrane systems regulate contraction and relaxation in the adult human heart: the plasma membrane and sarcoplasmic reticulum (Fig. 1). The plasma membrane (sarcolemma) surrounds the cell and so separates the cytosol from the extracellular space. Extensions of the plasma membrane, called the transverse tubular (t-tubular) system, penetrate the cell interior. The t-tubules open to the extracellular space so that their lumen contains extracellular fluid. The action potentials that activate contraction are propagated along the t-tubular membranes, which allows these structures to transmit the electrical signal into the cell interior. Special structures called dyads are formed by the plasma membrane and sarcoplasmic reticulum (Fig. 2). These structures regulate calcium release from intracellular stores during excitation–contraction coupling.

The cardiac sarcoplasmic reticulum includes subsarcolemmal cisternae, which contain the calcium release channels through which calcium enters the cytosol during excitation–contraction coupling, and a sarcotubular network that surrounds the contractile proteins. The subsarcolemmal cisternae also contain calcium-binding proteins that store this activator cation. The membranes of the sarcotubular network contain a densely packed array of calcium pump ATPase proteins that relax the heart by transporting calcium out of the cytosol into the lumen of the sarcoplasmic reticulum.

MYOCYTE FUNCTION
Contractile Proteins

Interactions between seven proteins are responsible for contraction and relaxation in the heart (Table 1). These proteins recognize the appearance of calcium in the cytosol as the signal for con-

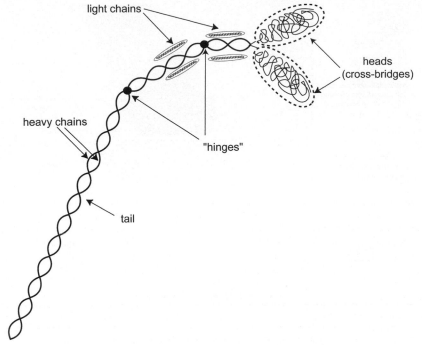

Fig. 3. Myosin is an elongated molecule consisting of two heavy chains and four light chains. The "tail" of the molecule, which is made up of α-helical regions of the heavy chains, extends into a paired globular "head" that makes up the cross-bridge. The hinges represent points of flexibility that allow for cross-bridge movement. (From Katz, Physiology of the Heart, 3rd ed. Philadelphia, Lippincott Williams & Wilkins, 2001.)

traction and use the chemical energy released by hydrolysis of the terminal phosphate bond of ATP to initiate the physicochemical changes that cause tension development and shortening.

MYOSIN

Myosin, the major protein of the thick filament, is a large, elongated molecule made up of a filamentous "tail" and a paired globular "head" (Fig. 3). Purified myosin is able to hydrolyze ATP so that this protein is an ATPase enzyme. When the myosin heads interact with actin, chemical energy is transduced into the mechanical energy that powers contraction.

Each myosin molecule contains two heavy chains and four light chains. The heavy chains extend the length of the molecule; in the head the heavy chains make up the cross-bridges that project from the thick filament. The myosin light chains are substrates for posttranslational phosphorylations that regulate the activity of the contractile proteins. Myosin heavy chains and light chains differ among different muscle types, between different regions of the heart, and between adjacent cells. Isoform shifts in these proteins play an important role in long-term changes in cardiac function, notably in hypertrophy and heart failure.

In the living muscle myosin is aggregated in the thick filaments where the tails are interwoven to form a rigid backbone and the heads project as the cross-bridges (Fig. 4). The cross-bridges in resting muscle are perpendicular to the long axis of the thick filament, whereas in active muscle their position shifts in a manner that allows the cross-bridges to "row" the thin filaments toward the center of the sarcomere (Fig. 5).

The heavy chains are the major determinants of myosin ATPase activity, muscle shortening velocity, and myocardial contractility. A high ATPase isoform, the α-myosin heavy chain, determines rapid shortening velocity, high contractility, and efficient contraction against light load, whereas a lower ATPase myosin isoform, called β heavy chain, is associated with lower shortening

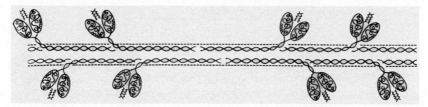

Fig. 4. Organization of myosin in the thick filament, in which the backbone—delineated by dashed lines— is made up of the tails of myosin molecules that have opposite polarities in the two halves of the sarcomere. The cross-bridges represent the heads of the individual myosin molecules, which project from the long axis of the thick filament. A bare area in the center of the thick filament, which is devoid of cross-bridges, occurs because of the tail-to-tail organization of myosin molecules unique to this region of the thick filament. (From Katz, Physiology of the Heart, 3rd ed. Philadelphia, Lippincott Williams & Wilkins, 2001.)

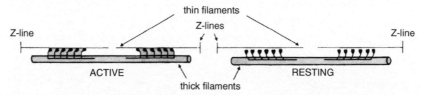

Fig. 5. In resting muscle (right) the cross-bridges project almost at right angles to the longitudinal axis of the thick filament. In active muscle (left), motion of the myosin cross-bridges pulls the thin filaments toward the center of the sarcomere. (From Katz, Physiology of the Heart, 3rd ed. Philadelphia, Lippincott Williams & Wilkins, 2001.)

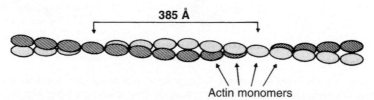

Fig. 6. Polymerized actin forms two strands of actin monomers (ovals) wound around each other. (The actin monomers in the two strands are identical; one strand is shaded here to illustrate the two-stranded structure of polymerized actin.) (From Katz, Physiology of the Heart, 3rd ed. Philadelphia, Lippincott Williams & Wilkins, 2001.)

velocity and contractility but a greater efficiency of tension development at high loads. The myosin heavy chains in the human atria are mostly a high-ATPase isoform, whereas the human ventricle contains only a small amount of the fast α-myosin heavy chain. Isoform shifts involving these proteins occur in diseased hearts; in heart failure, for example, increased expression of the β-myosin heavy chain isoform decreases myosin ATPase activity measured in vitro and reduces contractility in the intact heart.

Actin

Actin is a globular protein that, when polymerized, forms the double-stranded macromolecular helix that serves as the backbone of the thin filament (Fig. 6). The adult human heart contains mainly α-cardiac actin, along with a smaller amount of α-skeletal actin.

Tropomyosin

Tropomyosin is an elongated molecule made up of two helical peptide chains that can contain either or both of two isoforms, called α and β. In the thin filament one tropomyosin molecule lies in each of the two grooves between the two strands of actin (Figs. 7 and 8), where it regulates the interactions between the myosin cross-bridges and actin.

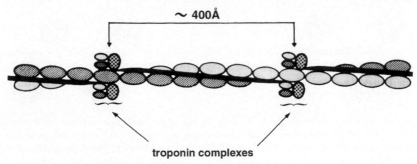

Fig. 7. Troponin complexes are distributed at intervals in the thin filament, along with actin and tropomyosin (dark lines in the grooves between the two actin strands). (From Katz, Physiology of the Heart, 3rd ed. Philadelphia, Lippincott Williams & Wilkins, 2001.)

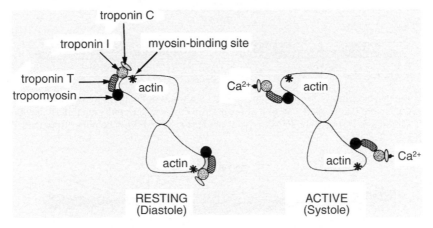

Fig. 8. Cross-section of a thin filament in resting (left) and active (right) muscle. At rest, the troponin complex holds the tropomyosin molecules toward the periphery of the groove between actin strands so as to prevent myosin-binding sites on actin (asterisks) from interacting with the myosin cross-bridges (not shown). In active muscle, calcium binding to troponin C weakens the bond linking troponin I to actin, which causes a structural rearrangement of the regulatory proteins that shifts the tropomyosin deeper into the groove between the strands of actin. This rearrangement exposes active sites on actin for interaction with the myosin cross-bridges. (From Katz, Physiology of the Heart, 3rd ed. Philadelphia, Lippincott Williams & Wilkins, 2001.)

THE TROPONIN COMPLEX

Troponin includes three discrete proteins (Figs. 7 and 8). In resting muscle troponin I, along with tropomyosin, reversibly inhibits the ability of the actin to interact with myosin. Troponin T binds the troponin complex to tropomyosin while troponin C, which is one of a family of high-affinity calcium-binding proteins that includes the myosin light chains and calmodulin, contains the high-affinity calcium-binding sites that allow this cation to initiate contraction. The latter occurs when calcium binding to troponin C reverses the inhibitory effect of troponin I, which allows actin to interact with the myosin cross-bridges (*see* "Calcium Binding to Troponin" section).

Troponin participates in several posttranslational changes that regulate cardiac performance. Phosphorylation of cardiac troponin I by cyclic AMP-dependent protein kinase (PK-A) reduces the calcium-sensitivity of troponin C, which facilitates calcium dissociation during relaxation. This effect, along with phosphorylation of phospholamban in the sarcoplasmic reticulum (*see* "Calcium Pump ATPases" below), contributes to the lusitropic effect of β-adrenergic stimulation. Isoform switches involving these regulatory proteins can modify contractility by altering the calcium-sensitivity of tension development.

REGULATION OF CONTRACTILE PROTEIN INTERACTIONS

The heart is a functional syncytium made up of myocytes whose contractions cannot be summated, so that cardiac performance is regulated largely by modifications of the interactions between the contractile proteins. Changes in calcium binding to troponin provide the major mechanisms for regulating myocardial contractility. Altered end-diastolic fiber length, by changing the lattice structure of the sarcomeres, represents a second mechanism that regulates cardiac performance.

Calcium Binding to Troponin

The most important of the mechanisms that regulate the interactions among the contractile proteins are changes in the amount of calcium made available for binding to troponin C. At the low cytosolic calcium concentrations in resting muscle, where the high-affinity calcium binding site on troponin C is unoccupied, interactions between actin and the myosin cross-bridges are inhibited by tropomyosin and the troponin complex. This inhibitory effect is reversed when calcium binding to troponin C initiates cooperative interactions in the thin filament that shift the position of the elongated tropomyosin molecules in the grooves between the two strands of polymerized actin (Fig. 8). In resting muscle, tropomyosin lies toward the outside of these grooves, where it blocks interactions between the thick and thin filaments. Calcium binding to troponin C, by shifting tropomyosin toward the center of the grooves, exposes active sites on actin that become able to interact with the myosin cross-bridges. The heart relaxes when calcium dissociation from troponin C returns tropomyosin to its inhibitory position.

The amount of calcium released into the cytosol during systole under basal conditions in the adult human ventricle is sufficient to occupy fewer than half of the high-affinity troponin C calcium-binding sites. Variations in the amount of calcium release during excitation–contraction coupling therefore represent a major determinant of myocardial contractility. The amount of calcium bound to troponin C can also be modified by changes in the calcium affinity of the troponin C binding site; these can occur as the result of posttranslational changes or isoform shifts involving the troponin complex.

Length-Dependent Changes: Starling's Law of the Heart

The second mechanism that regulates cardiac performance is initiated by changing end-diastolic volume (the Frank Starling relationship). This mechanism depends largely on length-dependent variations in the calcium sensitivity of the contractile proteins brought about by changes in the lattice structure of the sarcomeres. Length-dependent variations in calcium release from the sarcoplasmic reticulum play a minor role in the Frank-Starling relationship.

EXCITATION, EXCITATION–CONTRACTION COUPLING, AND RELAXATION

Excitation–contraction coupling, the process that initiates contraction, occurs when calcium becomes available for binding to troponin C. Unlike the more primitive myocytes found in smooth muscle and the embryonic heart, where calcium enters the cytosol from the extracellular space, most of this activator in the adult human heart is derived from intracellular stores within the sarcoplasmic reticulum. Contraction by the working cells of the adult myocardium is initiated when plasma membrane sodium channels are opened by an action potential propagated along the plasma membrane. The resulting movement of sodium into the cytosol generates an inward current that depolarizes the membrane, which opens plasma membrane L-type calcium channels. Calcium that enters the cell through these channels binds to and opens intracellular calcium release channels in the sarcoplasmic reticulum. The latter provide a much larger flux of calcium into the cytosol than calcium entry across the plasma membrane, so that most of the calcium that binds to troponin C in the adult heart is derived from intracellular stores.

The heart relaxes when energy-dependent calcium pumps and exchangers lower cytosolic calcium concentration, which causes calcium to dissociate from troponin C. Relaxation is not simply the reversal of the processes involved in excitation–contraction coupling, because different structures participate in calcium delivery to and calcium removal from the cytosol.

Energetics

The calcium concentration in the extracellular space and within the lumen of the sarcoplasmic reticulum is >1 mM, which is ~100 times greater than the calcium concentration needed to saturate troponin C (~10 µM) and ~5000 times higher than cytosolic calcium concentration in the resting heart (~0.2 µM). The calcium fluxes that activate contraction are therefore passive (downhill), whereas the calcium fluxes that relax the heart are active (uphill) and so require the expenditure of energy.

Relaxation, like contraction, also requires energy, but energy is used by different structures and in different ways during systole and diastole. The energy expended to perform mechanical work during systole is used by the contractile proteins for tension development and shortening, whereas the energy for the uphill calcium fluxes that relax the heart is utilized by energy-dependent ion pumps and exchangers to perform the osmotic work needed to transport this activator out of the cytosol.

Calcium Cycles in Excitation–Contraction Coupling and Relaxation

Calcium entry and removal from the cytosol, as noted at the beginning of this section, are not simply reversals of a single process; instead, they are effected by different structures. These processes can be viewed as two distinct calcium cycles (Fig. 9). In the "extracellular calcium cycle" calcium enters and leaves the cytosol by crossing the plasma membrane from what is, in effect, an unlimited calcium store in the extracellular fluid. In the "intracellular calcium cycle" the activator enters and leaves the cytosol from a much more limited store within the sarcoplasmic reticulum. Calcium that enters the cytosol from the extracellular space makes only a small contribution to the calcium that activates contraction; instead, the major role of the calcium flux through the L-type calcium channels is to trigger calcium release from the sarcoplasmic reticulum.

The functional link between plasma membrane depolarization (the action potential) and calcium release from intracellular stores is provided by the dyads (*see* "Membranes" section). Opening of L-type plasma membrane calcium channels by membrane depolarization admits a small amount of calcium into the cytosol. Much of the latter is "sprayed onto" the sarcoplasmic reticulum calcium release channels in the subsarcolemmal cisternae that in the dyads are adjacent to the plasma membrane L-type calcium channels (Fig. 2). Binding of this small amount of calcium opens the calcium release channels, which deliver a much larger amount of calcium into the cytosol from stores contained within the sarcoplasmic reticulum. This amplification, often referred to as "calcium-induced calcium release," provides most of the calcium that activates contraction.

Structures Involved in Excitation–Contraction Coupling and Relaxation

The L-type calcium channels found in the plasma membrane are structurally different from the calcium release channels in the sarcoplasmic reticulum (Table 2). Both membranes contain ATP-dependent calcium pumps that, although regulated differently, are members of a family of ion pump ATPases that also includes the sodium pump (Na/K ATPase). The major system that transports calcium out of the cytosol into the extracellular space is the sodium/calcium exchanger, which has no counterpart in the sarcoplasmic reticulum. Unlike the plasma membrane, where calcium fluxes generate an electrical current (i.e., are electrogenic), the sarcoplasmic reticulum membrane contains nonselective anion channels that neutralize the charge transfer associated with transmembrane calcium movements.

Plasma Membrane Ion Channels

Plasma membrane ion channels, which are generally named for the ions that they carry (Table 2), are oligomers that can contain as many as five subunits, called α_1, α_2, β, γ, and δ. Ions cross the hydro-

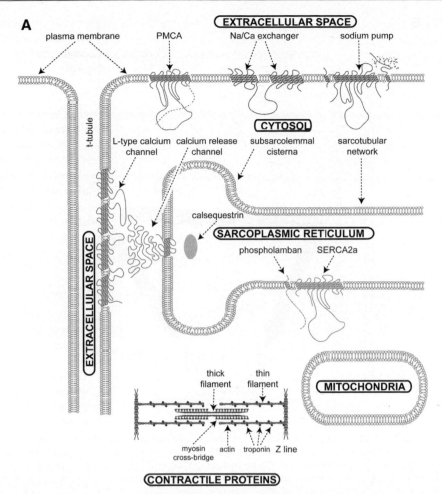

Fig. 9. Schematic diagram showing the key structures (**A**) and calcium fluxes (**B**) that control cardiac excitation–contraction coupling and relaxation. Calcium "pools" are in bold capital letters (**A**).

phobic core of the membrane bilayer through ion-selective pores contained within large proteins (called α or α_1 in different channels). Ion flux through these channels is controlled by changes in membrane potential. These voltage-dependent responses are controlled by structures generally referred to as activation and inactivation gates that open, close, and inactivate the channels (*see* below).

The α and α_1 subunits of sodium and calcium channels, and the delayed rectifier potassium channels (Fig. 10) are made up of four domains, each of which contains six α-helical transmembrane segments (Fig. 11). The channel "pores" are made up of the S_5 and S_6 α-helical transmembrane segments and intervening sequence of amino acids. The S_4 transmembrane segments, which are rich in positively charged amino acids, represent the "voltage sensors" that open the channel in response to membrane depolarization. Several classes of ion channel are inactivated by the intracellular peptide chain that links domains III and IV, which in the depolarized cell undergoes a conformational change to create an "inactivation particle" that blocks the inner mouth of the pore. The four domains of the α and α_1 subunits of most plasma membrane sodium and calcium channels are linked covalently in a single large protein (Fig. 10), whereas the domains of the delayed rectifier potassium channels, which also function as tetramers, are not covalently linked.

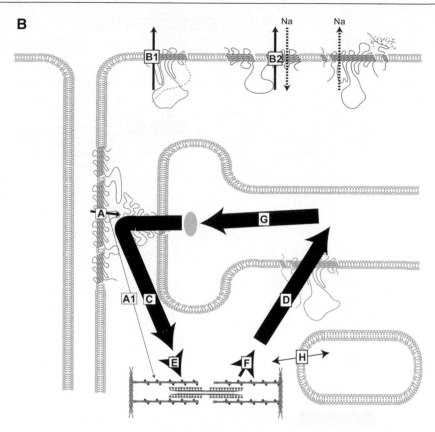

Fig. 9. *(Continued)* In **B**, the thickness of the arrows indicates the magnitude of the calcium fluxes, while their vertical orientations describe their "energetics": downward arrows represent passive calcium fluxes and upward arrows represent energy-dependent active calcium transport. Most of the calcium that enters the cell from the extracellular fluid via L-type calcium channels (arrow A) triggers calcium release from the sarcoplasmic reticulum; only a small portion directly activates the contractile proteins (arrow A1). Calcium is actively transported back into the extracellular fluid by the plasma membrane calcium pump ATPase (PMCA, arrow B1), and the sodium/calcium exchanger (arrow B2). The sodium that enters the cell in exchange for calcium (dashed line) is pumped out of the cytosol by the sodium pump. Two calcium fluxes are regulated by the sarcoplasmic reticulum: Calcium efflux from the subsarcolemmal cisternae via calcium release channels (arrow C) and calcium uptake into the sarcotubular network by the sarco(endo)plasmic reticulum calcium pump ATPase (arrow D). Calcium diffuses within the sarcoplasmic reticulum from the sarcotubular network to the subsarcolemmal cisternae (arrow G), where it is stored in a complex with calsequestrin and other calcium-binding proteins. Calcium binding to (arrow E) and dissociation from (arrow F) high-affinity calcium-binding sites of troponin C activate and inhibit the interactions of the contractile proteins. Calcium movements into and out of mitochondria (arrow H) buffer cytosolic calcium concentration. The extracellular calcium cycle consists of arrows A, B1, and B2, while the intracellular cycle involves arrows C, E, F, D, and G. (Modified from Katz, Physiology of the Heart, 3rd ed. Philadelphia, Lippincott Williams & Wilkins, 2001.)

There are several classes of plasma membrane calcium channels. In the heart, the most important are the L-type calcium channels, so named because of their relatively long-lasting openings. These channels bind the familiar classes of calcium channel blockers (dihydropyridines such as nifedipine, phenylalkylamines such as verapamil, and benzothiazepines such as diltiazem) and are sometimes called *dihydropyridine receptors* because of their high-affinity binding to this class of calcium channel blockers. A second class of calcium channel, called T-type channels, open only transiently; these channels play an important role in the SA node pacemaker but are virtually absent in working ventricular myocytes. The content of T-type channels increases in the hypertrophied heart, where they appear to participate in proliferative signaling.

Table 2
Structure–Function Relationships in Excitation–Contraction Coupling of Working Cardiac Myocytes

Structure	Role in systole	Role in diastole
Myofilaments		
Actin and myosin	Contraction	
Troponin C	Calcium receptor	
Other proteins	Regulation	
Plasma membrane		
Sarcolemma		
Sodium channels	Depolarization	
	Opens calcium channels	
Calcium channels	Action potential plateau	
	Calcium-triggered calcium release	
Calcium pump (PMCA)		Calcium removal
Sodium/calcium exchanger	Calcium entry	Calcium removal
Potassium channels		Repolarization
Sodium pump		Sodium gradient for the sodium/calcium exchanger
Transverse tubule		
Sodium channels	Action potential propagation	
Calcium channels	Calcium-triggered calcium release	
Sarcoplasmic reticulum		
Subsarcolemmal cisternae		
Calcium release channel	Calcium release	
Sarcotubular network		Calcium removal
Calcium pump (SERCA)		

The heart contains an even greater variety of potassium channels. These include the delayed rectifier potassium channels that exhibit outward rectification. The latter term refers to the ability of these channels to open in response to membrane depolarization, which generates a current that restores resting potential. Another class of potassium channels, called inwardly rectifying channels, are open in the resting cell but close in response to depolarization; closure of these channels prolongs the cardiac action potential and contributes to the characteristic plateau phase. The major subunits of inwardly rectifying potassium channels are smaller than those of the delayed rectifier potassium channels, and consist of regions homologous to the S_5 and S_6 α-helical transmembrane segments and intervening amino acid sequence that correspond to the pore region of the larger channel domains (Fig. 11).

INTRACELLULAR CALCIUM RELEASE CHANNELS

The intracellular calcium channels that control calcium flux out of the sarcoplasmic reticulum differ considerably from the calcium channels in the plasma membrane. The former, called calcium release channels, include at least two classes of related proteins. The *ryanodine receptors*, so named because they bind to this plant alkaloid, mediate excitation–contraction coupling by releasing calcium from the sarcoplasmic reticulum. A smaller class of intracellular calcium channels are activated by inositol trisphosphate ($InsP_3$), and so are called *$InsP_3$ receptors*. Both the ryanodine receptors and $InsP_3$ receptors are tetrameric structures in which the four subunits surround a central pore through which calcium moves when the channel is opened (Fig. 12).

The explosive contractile responses of cardiac and skeletal muscle are initiated by the opening of the ryanodine receptors, while the smaller $InsP_3$ receptors initiate the slower contractile responses in smooth muscle. In the heart, the slow calcium flux through the $InsP_3$ receptors may, like calcium entry through T-type calcium channels, regulate proliferative responses such as cell growth, differentiation, and programmed cell death (apoptosis).

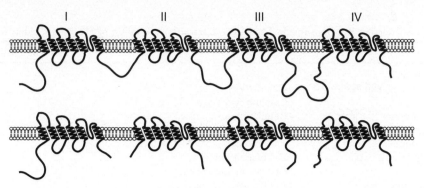

Fig. 10. Schematic representation of two types of voltage-gated ion channels. Top: Sodium and calcium channels are covalently linked tetramers made up of four homologous domains (numbered I–IV), each of which contains six α-helical transmembrane segments. Bottom: The major class of potassium channels is also made up of four homologous domains, except that unlike the channels shown in A, these domains are not linked covalently. (From Katz, Physiology of the Heart, 3rd ed. Philadelphia, Lippincott Williams & Wilkins, 2001.)

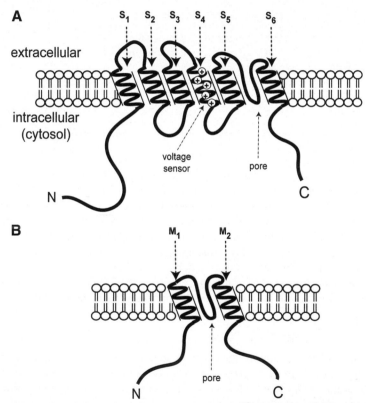

Fig. 11. Schematic representation of two types of ion channel domain. (**A**) The domains in sodium and calcium channels, and the delayed rectifier potassium channels, contain six transmembrane α-helices. The positively charged S_4 transmembrane segment in each of these domains provides the voltage sensor that responds to membrane depolarization by opening the channel. The "pore region" is made up of the S_5 and S_6 transmembrane segments and the intervening loop that "dips" into the membrane bilayer. (**B**) Inward rectifying potassium channels are made of smaller domains which are homologous to the S_5 and S_6 transmembrane segments of the larger domain shown in A. This domain is largely a pore, made up of the M_1 and M_2 transmembrane segments along with the intervening loop. The absence of a charged transmembrane segment homologous to S_4 explains why the response of inward-rectifying channels to membrane depolarization differs from that of channels made up of the larger domains depicted in A. (From Katz, Physiology of the Heart, 3rd ed. Philadelphia, Lippincott Williams & Wilkins, 2001.)

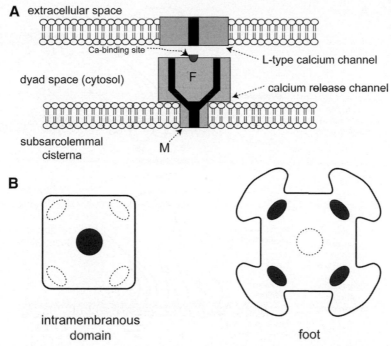

Fig. 12. Schematic representation of a calcium release channel (ryanodine receptor or foot protein) in a dyad. (**A**) View of a dyad in the plane of the bilayer showing the plasma membrane (above) and the subsarcolemmal cisterna (below). The former contains an L-type calcium channel that delivers calcium to a binding site on the sarcoplasmic reticulum calcium release channel. Each of the latter is a tetrameric structure that contains an intramembranous domain (M) and a large foot (F). Opening of the sarcoplasmic reticulum channel opens pores (dark areas). (**B**) Intracellular calcium release channel viewed from within the lumen of the subsarcolemmal cisterna, which faces the intramembranous domain (left), and from the cytosolic space within the dyad, which faces the foot. The intramembranous domain contains a central channel, while there are four radial channels within the foot. (From Katz, Physiology of the Heart, 3rd ed. Philadelphia, Lippincott Williams & Wilkins, 2001.)

CALCIUM PUMP ATPASES

The calcium pump ATPases found in cardiac myocytes are members of a family of P-type ion pumps made up of 10 membrane-spanning α-helices and a large peptide chain that projects into the cytosol (Fig. 13). The latter contains the ATPase site that provides chemical energy for active ion transport. P-type ion pumps utilize similar reaction mechanisms to couple the hydrolysis of the high-energy phosphate bond of ATP to ion transport. The cardiac plasma membrane calcium pump, called PMCA, is larger than the sarcoplasmic reticulum calcium pump, called SERCA (sarco[endo]plasmic reticulum calcium ATPase). The sarcoplasmic reticulum calcium pump is stimulated when cyclic AMP-dependent protein kinase (PK-A) catalyzes the phosphorylation of a small membrane protein called phospholamban that, when phosphorylated, accelerates calcium uptake by SERCA. Phospholamban phosphorylation mediates the inotropic and lusitropic effects of β-adrenergic stimulation by accelerating the pumping of calcium from the cytosol into the sarcoplasmic reticulum and increasing calcium stores in the sarcoplasmic reticulum, effects that contribute to the lusitropic and inotropic effects of sympathetic stimulation. Phospholamban can also be phosphorylated by calcium-calmodulin-dependent protein kinases (CAM kinases). The plasma membrane calcium pump ATPase is regulated by an inhibitory site located on the C-terminal domain of the molecule that, when bound to the calcium-calmodulin complex, stimulates calcium transport out of the cytosol. These calcium-activated responses promote the removal of calcium from the cytosol of calcium-overloaded cells.

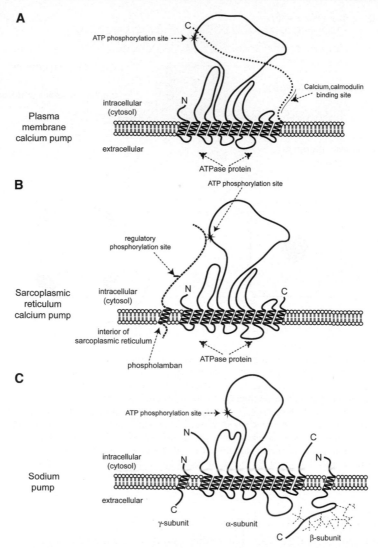

Fig. 13. Molecular structure of three P-type ATPase pump proteins. The plasma membrane calcium pump (**A**), sarcoplasmic reticulum calcium pump (**B**), and α-subunit of the sodium pump (**C**) contain 10 membrane-spanning α-helices within the plane of the membrane bilayer. In all three proteins a large cytosolic loop between the fourth and fifth membrane-spanning helices contains the active site that is phosphorylated by ATP to provide energy for active transport. In the plasma membrane calcium pump (**A**), a portion of the C-terminal peptide chain provides a regulatory site that binds the calcium/calmodulin complex. Phospholamban, which regulates the sarcoplasmic reticulum calcium pump (**B**), has a sequence similar to the C-terminal portion of the plasma membrane calcium pump. The sodium pump is made up of three subunits: the larger α-subunit contains the sodium-, potassium-, ATP-, and cardiac glycoside-binding sites. The glycosylated β-subunit and small γ-subunit regulate sodium pump activity. (From Katz, Physiology of the Heart, 3rd ed. Philadelphia, Lippincott Williams & Wilkins, 2001.)

SODIUM/CALCIUM EXCHANGER

Most of the calcium transport out of the cytosol into the extracellular space is effected by the sodium/calcium exchanger, which utilizes osmotic energy provided by the sodium gradient across the plasma membrane to provide the energy needed for uphill calcium transport. The ultimate energy source for calcium efflux via the exchanger is the sodium gradient established by the sodium pump (*see* below). The sodium/calcium exchanger, which differs structurally from the calcium pump ATPases, is a large-membrane protein containing 12 α-helical transmembrane segments.

Sodium/calcium exchange generates a small ionic current because the exchanger transports three sodium ions in exchange for one calcium ion. This electrogenicity has several important consequences. Because the negative intracellular potential in the resting heart tends to "pull" sodium into the cell, the exchanger favors calcium efflux during diastole; reversal of membrane potential during systole, when the cell interior becomes positively charged, has the opposite effect to favor calcium influx. The electrogenicity of the exchanger also plays an important role in causing arrhythmias in calcium-overloaded hearts, where increased calcium efflux generates an inward current that can cause afterdepolarizations. The latter, which occur during the "vulnerable period" at the end of the action potential, represent an important cause of sudden death in patients with heart failure.

Sodium Pump

The sodium pump (also called the sodium/potassium ATPase) is a P-type ion pump (Fig. 13) that transports sodium uphill out of the cell into the extracellular fluid in exchange for potassium that is brought into the cytosol. In addition to the osmotic work expended to pump sodium and potassium against their chemical gradients, energy is required to remove sodium ions out of the negatively charged interior of the resting cell. This electrical work is minimized because the pump exchanges sodium for potassium. Because the stoichiometry is three sodium ions pumped out of the cell for two potassium ions, the sodium pump generates a small outward (repolarizing) current.

The sodium pump removes the sodium that enters the cell during each action potential upstroke and brings potassium into the cell to replace the potassium that leaves during repolarization. The sodium gradient generated by the sodium pump is also coupled to the active transport of several molecules across the plasma membrane, notably calcium (*see* "Sodium/Calcium Exchanger" section). These additional functions of sodium influx explain why the pump exchanges more sodium than potassium.

Calcium Storage Proteins Within the Sarcoplasmic Reticulum

Some of the calcium stored in the sarcoplasmic reticulum is free (ionized), but much of this activator is associated with calcium-binding proteins that include calsequestrin, calreticulin, and a histidine-rich calcium-binding protein. These calcium-binding proteins are concentrated in the subsarcolemmal cisternae, where they provide a store of calcium that is available for release through the calcium release channels.

MITOCHONDRIA

Mitochondria, whose function in the heart is primarily to regenerate ATP, can also take up calcium. However the calcium affinity of mitochondrial calcium uptake is low, so that there is little mitochondrial calcium transport at physiological cytosolic calcium concentrations. Although these energy-producing structures do not normally play a role in excitation–contraction coupling, under conditions of calcium overload the mitochondria can take up some of the excess cytosolic calcium to protect the myocardium from the detrimental effects of excess calcium.

RECOMMENDED READING

Bers DM. Excitation-Contraction Coupling and Cardiac Contractile Force, 2nd ed. Kluwer, Dordrecht, The Netherlands, 2001.

Blanco G, Mercer RW. Isozymes of the Na-K-ATPase: heterogeneity in structure, diversity in function. Am J Physiol 1998;275:F633–F650.

Egger M, Niggli E. Regulatory function of Na-Ca exchange in the heart: milestones and outlook. J Memb Biol 1999;168: 107–130.

Hille B. Ionic Channels of Excitable Membranes, 3rd ed. Sinauer, Sunderland, MA, 2001.

Katz AM. Physiology of the Heart, 4th ed. Lippincott Williams & Wilkins, Philadelphia, 2006.

Langer GA, ed. The Myocardium. Academic Press, San Diego, 1997.

Opie LH. Heart Physiology: From Cell to Circulation, 4th ed. Lippincott Williams & Wilkins, Philadelphia, 2004.

Pogwizd SM, Bers DM. Na/Ca exchange in heart failure: contractile dysfunction and arrhythmogenesis. Ann NY Acad Sci 2002;976:454–465.

3 Ventricular Function

Lionel H. Opie, MD, DPhil

INTRODUCTION

Ventricular Contraction

The basic cardiac events of Wiggers' cycle (Fig. 1) are: (1) left ventricular (LV) contraction, (2) LV relaxation, and (3) LV filling. A natural starting point is with the arrival of calcium ions at the contractile protein that starts actin–myosin interaction and left ventricular contraction. During the initial phase of contraction, the LV pressure builds up until it exceeds that in the left atrium (normally 10 to 15 mmHg), whereupon the mitral valve closes. With the aortic and mitral valves both shut, the LV volume cannot change and contraction must be *isovolumic* (iso = the same) until the aortic valve is forced open as the LV pressure exceeds that in the aorta. Once the aortic valve is open, blood is vigorously ejected from the LV into the aorta, which is the phase of *maximal or rapid ejection.* The speed of ejection of blood is determined both by the pressure gradient across the aortic valve and by the elastic properties of the aorta, which undergoes systolic expansion.

Ventricular Relaxation

After the LV pressure rises to a peak, it starts to fall. As the cytosolic calcium is taken up into the sarcoplasmic reticulum under the influence of active phospholamban, more and more myofibers enter the state of relaxation. As a result, the rate of ejection of blood from the aorta falls (phase of *reduced ejection*). Although the LV pressure is falling, blood flow is maintained by aortic recoil. Next, the aortic valve closes as the pressure in the aorta exceeds the falling pressure in the LV. Now the ventricular volume is sealed, because both aortic and mitral valves are closed. The left ventricle therefore relaxes without changing its volume (*isovolumic relaxation*). Next, the filling phase of the cardiac cycle restarts as the LV pressure falls to below that in the left atrium, which causes the mitral valve to open and the filling phase to start.

Ventricular Filling Phases

The *first phase of rapid* or *early filling* accounts for most of ventricular filling. It starts very soon after mitral valve opening, as the LV pressure drops below that in the left atrium. In addition, some evidence shows that there is also active diastolic relaxation of the ventricle (*ventricular suction*) that also contributes to early filling. In the next phase, *diastasis* (i.e., separation), LV filling temporarily stops as pressures in the atrium and ventricle equalize. Thereafter atrial contraction (*atrial systole),* also called the *left atrial booster,* renews ventricular filling by increasing the pressure gradient across the open mitral valve.

Definitions of Systole and Diastole

In Greek, *systole* means "contraction" and *diastole* means "to send apart." For the physiologist, systole starts at the beginning of isovolumic contraction when LV pressure exceeds the atrial pressure. The start of cardiological systole, defined as mitral valve closure, corresponds reasonably well with the start of physiological systole, because mitral valve closure (M_1) actually occurs only

From: *Essential Cardiology: Principles and Practice, 2nd Ed.*
Edited by: C. Rosendorff © Humana Press Inc., Totowa, NJ

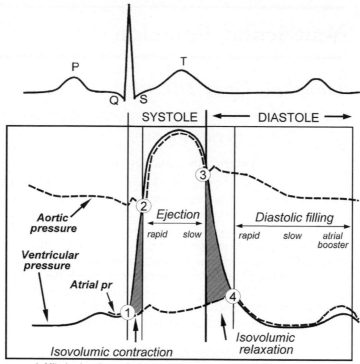

Fig. 1. The cardiac cycle, first assembled by Lewis in 1920, although conceived by Wiggers *(19)*. Systole and diastole relate to cardiological, not physiological, phases: (1) mitral valve closure that occurs shortly after the crossover point of atrial and ventricular pressures at the start of systole; (2) aortic valve opening; (3) aortic valve closure; and (4) mitral valve opening. Note the four phases of diastole: isovolumic relaxation and three filling phases.

about 20 ms after the onset of physiological systole at the crossover point of pressures. Thus in practice the term *isovolumic contraction* often also includes this brief period of early systolic contraction before the mitral valve shuts, when the heart volume does not change substantially.

Cardiological systole is demarcated by the interval between the first and second heart sounds (Fig. 1), lasting from the first heart sound (M_1) to A_2, the point of closure of the aortic valve *(1)*. The remainder of the cardiac cycle automatically becomes cardiological diastole. Thus cardiological systole starts fractionally later than physiological systole but ends significantly later. By contrast, from the physiological point of view, end-systole is just before the ventricle starts to relax, a concept that fits well with the standard pressure-volume curve. Thus, diastole commences as calcium ions are taken up into the sarcoplasmic reticulum, so that myocyte relaxation dominates over contraction, and the LV pressure starts to fall as shown on the pressure volume curve (Fig. 2).

In contrast stands another concept, argued by Brutsaert and colleagues *(2)*, namely that diastole starts much later than the moment at which relaxation starts or at which the aortic valve closes, and only when the whole of the contraction-relaxation cycle is over. According to this view, diastole would occupy only a small portion of the pressure volume cycle (Fig. 1). This definition of diastole, although not often used in cardiological practice, does help to remind us that abnormalities of left ventricular contraction often underlie defective relaxation.

Contractility versus Load

Contractility is the inherent capacity of the myocardium to contract independently of changes in the preload or afterload. Increased contractility means a greater rate of contraction, to reach a

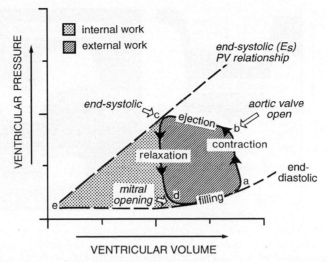

Fig. 2. Pressure-volume loop. Normal left ventricular pressure-volume relationship. The aortic valve opens at b and closes at c. The mitral valve opens at d and closes at a. External work is defined by a, b, c, d while potential energy (less accurately called internal work) is given by the triangle e, d, c. The pressure-volume area is the sum of external work and potential energy.

greater peak force. Often an increased contractility is associated with enhanced rates of relaxation, called the *lusitropic effect*. Alternate names for contractility are the *inotropic state* (*ino*, fiber; *tropos*, to move) or the *contractile state*. Contractility is an important regulator of the myocardial oxygen uptake. Factors that increase contractility include adrenergic stimulation, digitalis, and other inotropic agents. At a molecular level, an increased inotropic state is enhanced interaction between calcium ions and the contractile proteins. Such an interaction could result either from increased calcium transients or from sensitization of the contractile proteins to a given level of cytosolic calcium. Calcium-sensitizing drugs act by the latter mechanism, and conventional inotropes such as digitalis through an increase of internal calcium.

Preload and Afterload

Contractility is therefore a common part of the essential cardiological language. It is important to stress that any change in the contractile state must occur independently of the loading conditions. The two types of load are the *preload* and the *afterload*. The preload is the load present before contraction has started, at the end of diastole. The preload reflects the venous filling pressure that fills the atrium and hence the left ventricle during diastole. The afterload is the systolic load on the left ventricle after it has started to contract. When the preload increases, the left ventricle distends during diastole, and the stroke volume rises according to Starling's law (*see* next section). The heart rate also increases by stimulation of the atrial mechanoreceptors that enhance the rate of discharge of the sinoatrial node. Thus, the cardiac output (stroke volume times heart rate) rises.

Venous Return and Heart Volume: Starling's Law of the Heart

Starling (*3*) related the venous pressure in the right atrium to the heart volume in the dog heart-lung preparation (Fig. 3). He concluded that "[w]ithin physiological limits, the larger the volume of the heart, the greater the energy of its contraction and the amount of chemical change at each contraction."

Thus, assuming that an increased diastolic heart volume means that the end-diastolic fiber length increases, Starling's law is often paraphrased to mean that (1) an increased right atrial venous filling pressure translates into an increased left ventricular end diastolic fiber length, and (2) this

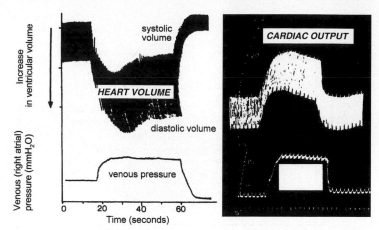

Fig. 3. Starling's law of the heart as applied to the preload (venous filling pressure). As the preload increases (bottom in both figures), the heart volume increases (left top), as does the cardiac output (right top). Starling's explanation was: "The output of the heart is a function of its filling; the energy of contraction depends on the state of dilatation of the heart's cavities" *(3)*.

increase in length increases the force of contraction and hence the stroke volume. Because the heart volume is difficult to determine even with modern echocardiographic techniques, the left ventricular diastolic *filling pressure* (the difference between the left atrial pressure and the left ventricular diastolic pressure) is often taken as a surrogate for heart volume. This is important because the venous filling pressure can be measured in humans, albeit indirectly, by the technique of Swan-Ganz catheterization (Fig. 4), as can the stroke volume. Nonetheless, there is a defect in this reasoning. The left ventricular pressure and volume are not linearly related because the myocardium cannot continue to stretch indefinitely. Rather, as the left ventricular end-diastolic pressure increases, so does the cardiac output reach a plateau. The LV volume can now be directly measured with two-dimensional echocardiography. Yet the value found depends on a number of simplifying assumptions such as a spherical LV shape and neglects the confounding influence of the complex anatomy of the left ventricle. In practice, the LV volume is not often measured. Therefore, although the Starling concept is valuable and underlies the hemodynamic management of those critically ill and receiving a Swan-Ganz catheter, several approximations are required to make these concepts clinically applicable.

Frank and Isovolumic Contraction

Starling emphasized that increasing the heart volume increased the initial length of the muscle fiber and thereby increased the stroke volume and cardiac output, which suggested but did not prove that diastolic stretch of the LV increased the force of contraction. In fact, his German predecessor, Frank, had already in 1895 *(4)* studied the relation between filling pressure and the force of contraction in an isolated heart (Fig. 5). He found that the greater the initial volume, the more rapid the rate of rise, the greater the peak pressure reached, the faster the rate of relaxation. Frank was therefore able to show that an increasing diastolic heart volume stimulated the ventricle to contract more rapidly and more forcefully, which is a positive inotropic effect. Thus the earlier observations of Frank could explain the contractile behavior of the heart during the operation of Starling's law. These findings of Frank and Starling are so complementary that they often referred to as the Frank-Starling Law. The beauty of the dual name is that between the two they described what accounts for the increased stroke volume of exercise, namely both the increased inotropic state *(4)* and the increased diastolic filling *(3)*.

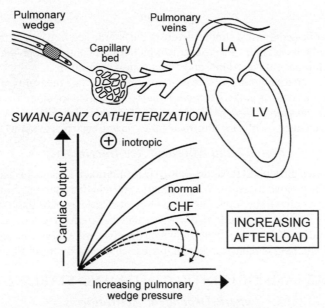

Fig. 4. A family of Starling curves with relevance to Swan-Ganz catheterization. Each curve relates the filling pressure (pulmonary capillary wedge pressure, PCWP) to the left ventricular (LV) stroke output and to the cardiac output. Note that the depressed inotropic state of the myocardium causes an abnormally low curve and that the downward limb can be related to an increased afterload. Clinically the measurements relating filling pressure to cardiac output are obtained by Swan-Ganz catheterization (a procedure presently undertaken less frequently than previously). Note the close association between LV diastolic dysfunction and pulmonary congestion. LA, left atrium; CHF, congestive heart failure (Copyright © L.H. Opie, 2004.)

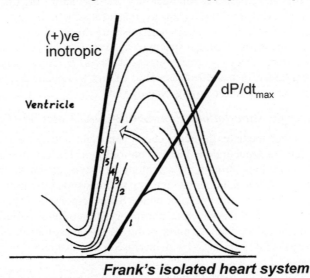

Frank's isolated heart system

Fig. 5. Frank's family of isometric (isovolumic) curves. Frank related heart volume to what would now be recognized as an index of contractility, a term not known then, as can be seen if two tangential lines are added to the curves of the original figure. In modern terms, these lines give the maximal rate of change of the intra-ventricular pressure (*dP/dt* max). Each curve was obtained at a greater initial filling of the left ventricle by an increased left atrial filling pressure. Then valves were shut to produce isovolumic conditions. Curve 6 has a greater velocity of shortening. Hence, the initial fiber length (volume of ventricle) can influence contractility. The line on curve 6 has the much steeper slope and, therefore, indicates a greater rate of contraction or a greater, in contrast to the line drawn on curve 1, which ascends more slowly and indicates a lower contractile state. (Figure based on author's interpretation of ref. *4*.)

Afterload

Starling and his colleagues gave a simple picture of the how an acute change in the afterload could influence an isolated muscle: *(3)*: "The extent to which it will contract depends on... the amount of the weight which it has to overcome" and "the tension aroused in it."

In clinical practice, arterial blood pressure is one of three important measures of the afterload, the others being any aortic stenosis and *aortic compliance*—the extent to which the aorta can "yield" during systole. *Aortic impedance* is an index of the afterload and is the aortic pressure divided by the aortic flow of that incidence, so that the afterload varies during each phase of the contraction cycle.

Preload and Afterload Are Interlinked

In practice, it is often difficult to separate preload from afterload. During the start of exercise, the venous return and the preload increase. When the left ventricle then starts to contract, the tension in the left ventricular wall will be higher because of greater distention of the left ventricle by the greater pressure. The load during systole also will rise, and the afterload will increase. Nonetheless, in general, the preload is related to the degree to which the myocardial fibers are stretched at the end of diastole, and the afterload is related to the wall stress generated by those fibers during systole.

CELLULAR BASIS OF CONTRACTILITY AND STARLING'S LAW

Length-Dependent Activation

How could an increased end-diastolic muscle length increase the force and rate of muscular contraction? Previously this effect of increased muscle length was ascribed to a more "optimal" overlap between actin and myosin. Intuitively, however, if actin and myosin are stretched further apart, there would be less rather than more overlap. Another earlier proposal—that troponin C, one of the contractile proteins, is the length sensor—is currently less favored. A more current view is that there is a complex interplay between anatomic and regulatory factors *(5)*, including the concept that an increased sarcomere length leads to greater sensitivity of the contractile apparatus to the prevailing cytosolic calcium. The major mechanism for this regulatory change, although not yet clarified, may reside in the interfilament spacing *(6)*. At short sarcomere lengths, as the lattice spacing increases, the number of strong cross bridges decreases *(7)*. Conversely, as the heart muscle is stretched, the interfilament distance decreases (Fig. 6), and, hypothetically, there is an increased rate of transition from the weak to the strong binding state.

β-Adrenergic Stimulation, Contractility, and Calcium (Fig. 7)

β-Adrenergic stimulation mediates the major component of its inotropic effect through increasing the cytosolic calcium transient and the factors controlling it. The following are all enhanced: the rate of entry of calcium ions through the sarcolemmal L-type channels, the rate of calcium uptake under the influence of phospholamban into the sarcoplasmic reticulum (SR), and the rate of calcium release from the ryanodine receptor on the SR in response to calcium entry, which in turn follows depolarization. Of all these factors, phosphorylation of phospholamban may be most important *(8)*, acting on the calcium uptake pump of the SR to increase the rate of uptake of calcium during diastole. Thereby the SR is preloaded with increased Ca so that more can be liberated during ensuing depolarizations.

Conversely, contractility is decreased whenever calcium transients are depressed, as when β-adrenergic blockade decreases calcium entry through the L-type calcium channel. Alternatively, there may be faulty control of the uptake and release of calcium ions by the SR, as when the SR is damaged in congestive heart failure. Anoxia or ischemia deplete the calcium uptake pump of the SR of the ATP required for calcium uptake, so that the contraction-relaxation cycle is inhibited.

Problems With the Contractility Concept

The concept of contractility has at least two serious defects, including first the absence of any potential index that can be measured *in situ* and is free of significant criticism, especially the absence

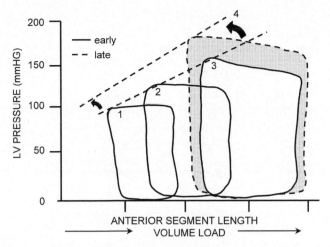

Fig. 6. Length-dependent activation. A volume load extends the anterior segment length, which corresponds to the diastolic volume in Starling's observations. The result is that the resting PV loop (loop 1) increases in area and in peak left ventricular systolic pressure (*see* loops 2 and 3). This is the Starling effect (*also see* legend to Fig. 9). After a few minutes (broken lines and shaded area) contractility increases modestly, pushing the length-pressure slope upwards and to the left, an example of length-dependent activation. (Figure based on data extracted from ref. *23* with permission of Lippincott Williams & Wilkins.)

of any acceptable noninvasive index; and second, the impossibility of separating the cellular mechanisms of contractility changes from those of load or heart rate. Thus, an increased heart rate acts by the sodium pump lag mechanism to give rise to an increased cytosolic calcium, giving the increased force of contraction of the Bowditch or treppe phenomenon. An increased preload involves increased fiber stretch, which in turn causes length activation, thought to be explicable in part by sensitization of the contractile proteins to the prevailing cytosolic calcium concentration. An increased afterload may indirectly, through stimulation of stretch-sensitive channels, increase cytosolic calcium. Thus, in relation to the underlying cellular mechanisms, there is a clear overlap between contractility (which should be independent of load or heart rate) and the effects of myocyte stretch and heart rate, which have some effects that could be called an increase in contractility.

In clinical terms, it nonetheless remains important to separate the effects of a primary increase of load or heart rate, on the one hand, from a primary increase in contractility, on the other. This distinction is especially relevant in congestive heart failure, where a decreased contractility could indirectly or directly result in increased afterload, preload, and heart rate, all of which could then predispose to a further decrease in myocardial performance. Because muscle length can influence contractility, the traditional separation of length and inotropic state into two independent regulators of cardiac muscle performance is no longer true if the end result is considered. However, it remains true that β-adrenergic stimulation has a calcium-dependent positive inotropic effect independent of loading conditions, which is therefore a true positive inotropic effect.

CARDIAC OUTPUT

The definition of *cardiac output* is the product of the stroke volume (SV) and the heart rate (HR):

Cardiac output = SV × HR (units = liters per minute)

The normal value is about 6–8 L/min, doubling or sometimes even trebling during peak aerobic exercise. The stroke volume is determined by the preload, the afterload, and the contractile state. Heart rate is also one of the major determinants of myocardial oxygen uptake. The heart rate responds to a large variety of stimuli, each of which thereby indirectly alters myocardial oxygen

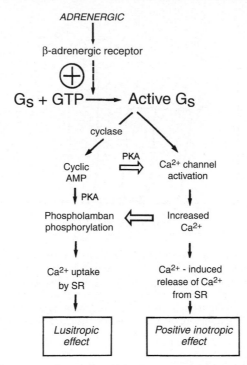

Fig. 7. β-Adrenergic signal systems, when activated, lead to changes in the cardiac calcium cycle that explain positive inotropic and lusitropic (enhanced relaxation) effects. When the β-adrenergic agonist interacts with the β-receptor, a series of G protein-mediated changes lead to activation of the stimulatory G protein, G_s, that interacts with GTP (guanosine triphosphate) that in turn activates adenylate cyclase (shown as cyclase) to form the adrenergic second messenger, cyclic adenosine monophosphate (cyclic AMP). The latter acts via protein kinase A (PKA) to phosphorylate phospholamban and to increase the activity of the calcium uptake pump on the sarcoplasmic reticulum (SR), hence decreasing cytosolic calcium and explaining the lusitropic (relaxant) effect of adrenergic stimulation. PKA also phosphorylates calcium channel protein. The result is an enhanced opening probability of the calcium channel, thereby increasing the inward movement of Ca^{2+} ions through the sarcolemma of the T tubule. Additionally, active Gs directly activates the calcium channel opening. More Ca^{2+} ions enter the cytosol, to release more calcium from the ryanodine release channel of the SR, rapidly to increase cytosolic calcium levels. The result is increased activation of troponin-C, explaining increased peak force development as result of adrenergic stimulation (positive inotropic effect). (Copyright © L.H. Opie, 2004.)

uptake. The three physiological factors most consistently increasing heart rate are exercise, waking up in the morning, and emotional stress.

Heart Rate

Each cycle of contraction and relaxation performs a certain amount of work and takes up a certain amount of oxygen. The faster the heart rate, the higher the cardiac output and the higher the oxygen uptake. Exceptions are: (1) when the heart rate is extremely fast, as may occur during a paroxysmal tachycardia, because an inadequate time for diastolic filling decreases the cardiac output; and (2) in coronary artery disease when lower degrees of tachycardia decrease the stroke volume because of ischemic failure of the left ventricle.

Force-frequency relation. An increased heart rate progressively increases the force of ventricular contraction even in an isolated papillary muscle preparation (*Bowditch staircase or treppe phenomenon*). In isolated human ventricular strips, increasing the stimulation rate from 60 to about 160 per minute stimulates force development. In strips from failing hearts, there is no such increase *(9)*. In the human heart *in situ*, pacing rates of up to 150 per minute can be tolerated, whereas higher rates cause AV block. Yet during exercise, a maximal heart rate of 170 beats per minute causes no block, presumably because of concurrent adrenergic stimulation of the AV node. Thus an excessive heart rate decreases rather than increases cardiac contraction and cardiac output. Relatively recently, tachycardia-induced cardiomyopathy has been recognized, being the result of excessive prolonged tachycardia (10).

To explain the staircase during rapid stimulation, the proposal is that each wave of depolarization brings more sodium ions into the myocardial cells than can be ejected by the sodium pump. Sodium overload leads to an increase of cytosolic calcium by the sodium-calcium exchanger, with an increased force of contraction. Too rapid a rate of stimulation causes the force of contraction to decrease by limiting the duration of ventricular filling and probably by calcium overload.

Loading Conditions and Cardiac Output

In general, when the afterload decreases, the cardiac output increases. Physiological examples of this principle exist during peripheral vasodilation induced by a hot bath or sauna or by a meal. In these conditions; however, there is also an accompanying tachycardia, as during drug-induced vasodilation. Conversely, when the afterload increases, there is initially a compensatory mechanism, possibly acting by increased end-diastolic fiber-stretch, to increase contractility (Fig. 5) and to maintain the stroke volume. If the afterload keeps rising, compensatory mechanisms cannot adapt, and eventually the stroke volume will fall. In exercise, although the peripheral vascular resistance decreases, systolic blood pressure rises, and the afterload increases. Thus, at really high rates of upright exercise, the stroke volume falls even though the cardiac output continues to rise, the latter as a result of heart rate increases (11). In congestive heart failure with a failing left ventricle, the stage at which the stroke volume and hence the cardiac output starts to fall in response to the excess "compensatory" peripheral arteriolar constriction is much sooner than with the normal left ventricle.

Contractility and Cardiac Output

During β-adrenergic stimulation or exercise, the contractile state is enhanced to contribute to the increased cardiac output. Conversely, during congestive heart failure or therapy with β-adrenergic blockade, decreased contractility means a decreased stroke volume.

EFFECTS OF EXERCISE

During dynamic exercise the cardiac output can increase severalfold (Fig. 8). There are three possible explanations: an increased heart rate, increased contractility, and an increased venous return. In humans, an increased heart rate provides most of the increased cardiac output, with the Starling mechanism and increased contractility playing lesser roles (11).

Tachycardia of Exercise

The mechanism of the increase in heart rate during exercise is a combination of withdrawal of inhibitory vagal tone and increased β-adrenergic stimulation. The signals for these changes come from the vasomotor center in the brainstem, which coordinates two types of input: one is from the cerebral cortex (e.g., the runner's "readiness to go" at the start of exercise), and the second is the Bainbridge reflex. The latter is stimulated by atrial distention, following the increased venous return during exercise. However, this is but a modest effect in humans. A tachycardia, from whatever cause, can further invoke a positive inotropic effect by the Bowditch (treppe) effect.

Venous Return During Exercise

Starling postulated (but did not measure) events at the start of exercise as follows: "If a man starts to run, his muscular movements pump more blood into the heart, so increasing the venous filling" (3). Because the cardiac output must equal the venous return, the increase in cardiac output during exercise must reflect an equal increase in the venous return. This increase does not, however,

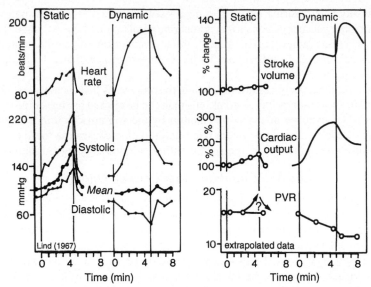

Fig. 8. Static vs dynamic exercise. Static exercise, at 30% of maximum voluntary contraction (MCV), caused a much larger rise in mean blood pressure than did dynamic exercise, first at oxygen consumption values of 28.5 mL/kg/min and then at 43.8 mL/kg/min. Conversely, dynamic exercise increased heart rate much more. For original data, *see* ref. *20*. Data on stroke volume are extrapolated from ref. *11*. Peripheral vascular resistance (PVR) for 0–2 min is based on ref. *21* and for 2–4 min on Lind and McNicol, shown above, in which the blood pressure rises markedly at 2–4 min of static exercise even when the rise in heart rate has leveled off; therefore the PVR must have increased. (Figure derived from author's analysis of conjoint data of above references.)

necessarily prove the operation of the Starling mechanism, which requires an increased venous filling pressure. If there were an increased contractility from β-adrenergic stimulation during exercise, then the venous filling pressure could actually fall, despite the increase in the venous return. To be sure of the events at the start of exercise in humans would need simultaneous measurements of venous return, of the venous filling pressure, and of the heart volume. Such data are missing. Nonetheless, the combination of increased venous return and sympathetic stimulation can give extrapolated explanations.

An increased venous return and filling pressure could explain the increased diastolic heart volume during exercise, as found in radionuclide studies *(12,13)*. Cardiac failure can be excluded, because the end-systolic volume decreases and the stroke volume increases. The Starling mechanism appears to operate in both supine and upright postures when low-level exercise is compared with rest *(12)*. This sequence is not inviolate, and may be altered by posture *(14)*, by exercise training *(15)*, and by increased contractility. Thus the three major changes during exercise are first, the increase in venous return, which increases the venous filling pressure when comparing the initiation of exercise with rest; second, this increase usually but not invariably evokes a Starling response; and third, sympathetic stimulation with an increased heart rate and contractility contribute variably but importantly. Once exercise has been initiated, the venous return must stay high and equal the cardiac output. The decrease in the systemic vascular resistance helps to keep the cardiac output and venous return high. The end result is that the increased venous return and increased cardiac output will have achieved a new enhanced equilibrium.

Regarding static exercise, the major hemodynamic differences from dynamic exercise are (1) the lesser rise in heart rate; (2) the greater rise in blood pressure; (3) the absence of increases in stroke volume and cardiac output (Fig. 8).

WALL STRESS

Myocardial wall stress or *wall tension* increases when the myofilaments slide over each other during cardiac contraction as they are squeezing blood out of the ventricles into the circulation. An analogy is the human effort required to squeeze a ball in the palm of the hand. A small rubber ball can be compressed easily. A larger rubber ball (tennis ball in size) is compressed less readily, and two large rubber balls—or one really large ball—could be compressed only with the greatest difficulty. As the size of the object in the hand increases, so does the force required to compress it. Intuitively, the stress on the hand increases as the ball increases in diameter. However, what is wall stress?

At this point it is appropriate to deviate briefly into a description of force, tension, and wall stress. *Force* is a term frequently used in studies of muscle mechanics. Strictly,

$$Force = mass \times acceleration$$

Thus when a load is suspended from one end of a muscle as the muscle contracts, it is exerting force against the mass of that load. In many cases, it is not possible to define force with such exactitude but, in general, force has the following properties. First, force is always applied by one object (such as muscle) on another object (such as a load). Second, force is characterized both by the direction in which it acts, and its magnitude. Hence, it is a vector, and the effect of a combination of forces can be established by the principle of vectors. Third, each object exerts a force on the other, so that force and counterforce are equal and opposite (Newton's third law of motion).

Tension exists when the two forces are applied to an object so that the forces tend to pull the object apart. When a spring is pulled by a force, tension is exerted; when more force is applied, the spring stretches, and the tension increases.

Stress develops when tension is applied to a cross-sectional area, and the units are force per unit area. According to the *Laplace law*:

$$Wall\ stress = \frac{pressure \times radius}{2 \times wall\ thickness}$$

The increased wall thickness due to hypertrophy balances the increased pressure, and the wall stress remains unchanged during the phase of compensatory hypertrophy. In congestive heart failure, the heart dilates to increase the radius factor, thereby elevating wall stress. Furthermore, because ejection of blood is inadequate, the radius stays too large throughout the contractile cycle, and both end-diastolic and end-systolic tensions are higher.

Wall Stress and Myocardial Oxygen Demand

At a fixed heart rate, the myocardial wall stress is the major determinant of the myocardial oxygen uptake. Because myocardial oxygen uptake ultimately reflects the rate of mitochondrial metabolism and ATP production, any increase of ATP requirement will be reflected in an increased oxygen uptake. It is not only external work that determines the requirement for ATP. Rather, tension development (increased wall stress) is oxygen-requiring even without external work being done. The difference between external work and tension developed can be epitomized by a man standing and holding a heavy suitcase, doing no external work yet becoming very tired, compared with the man lifting a much lighter suitcase, doing external work yet not tired. The greater the left ventricular chamber size, the greater the radius, the greater the wall stress. Hence, ejection of the same stroke volume from a large left ventricle against the same blood pressure will produce as much external work as ejection of the same stroke volume by a normal size left ventricle, yet with a much greater wall stress in the case of the larger ventricle. Therefore, more oxygen will be required. In clinical terms, heart size is an important determinant of myocardial oxygen uptake. In a patient with angina and a large left ventricle the appropriate therapy is to reduce left ventricular size, which will also lessen the myocardial oxygen demand.

The overall concept of wall stress includes afterload because an increased afterload generates an increased systolic wall stress. Wall stress also includes preload, which generates diastolic wall stress. Wall stress increases in proportion to the pressure generated and to the radius of the left ventricular cavity, factors that are responsive to increases in afterload and preload respectively. Wall stress allows for energy required for generation of muscular contraction that does not result in external work. Furthermore, in states of enhanced contractility, wall stress is increased. Thus, thinking in terms of wall stress provides a comprehensive approach to the problem of myocardial oxygen uptake. Apart from a metabolic component that is usually small but may be prominent in certain special circumstances, such as when circulating free fatty acids are abnormally high, changes in heart rate and wall stress account for most of the clinically relevant changes in myocardial oxygen uptake.

External versus Internal Work and Oxygen Demand

Bearing in mind that the major factor in cardiac work is the product of pressure and volume, it follows that external work can be quantified by the integrated pressure-volume area that represents the product of the systolic pressure and the stroke volume. To relate work to oxygen consumption, account must be taken of both the *external* work (a,b,c,d in Fig. 2) and *internal* work, which is the volume-pressure triangle joining the end-systolic volume-pressure point to the origin (c,d,e). The latter is more correctly called the *potential energy,* being the work generated in each contractile cycle that is not converted to external work.

Pressure versus Volume Work and Oxygen Demand

In analyzing the difference between oxygen cost of pressure work and volume work, the established clinical observation is that the myocardium can tolerate a chronic volume load better than a pressure load. Thus when cardiac work is chronically increased by augmenting the afterload, as during severe hypertension or narrowing of the aortic valve by aortic stenosis, the peak systolic pressure in the left ventricle must increase, and pressure power increases. However, because of the complex way in which the muscle fibers of the myocardium run, a greater proportion of the work is against the internal resistance. The result is that the efficiency falls. An extreme example of the loss of efficiency during pressure work would be if the aorta were completely occluded, so that none of the work would be external and all would be internal. Internal work is done against the noncontractile elements of the myocardium and is not useful work in terms of calculating efficiency.

When the heart is subject to a chronic volume load, as in mitral regurgitation, the increased work that the heart must perform is met by an increased end-diastolic volume. The myofibers stretch, and length-dependent activation occurs. The primary adaptation to increased heart volume is an increased fiber length and not increased pressure development, so that the amount of external work done is more, but that against the internal resistance is unchanged so that the efficiency of work rises. (The efficiency of work relates the amount of work performed to the myocardial oxygen uptake.)

LEFT VENTRICULAR FUNCTION

Maximal Rate of Left Ventricular Pressure Generation

In relation to the cardiac contraction-relaxation cycle, it is easiest to consider left ventricular function during the early period of isovolumic contraction. During this period of isovolumic contraction, the preload and afterload are constant, and the maximal rate of pressure generation should be an index of the inotropic state:

$$\text{inotropic index} = dP/dt \text{ max}$$

where P is left ventricular pressure, t is time, and d indicates rate of change. Unfortunately, this index, which has stood the test of years, is not fully load-independent—as Frank showed (Fig. 5), increasing the preload enhances the contractile state by length-activation.

In humans, the measurements required for dP/dt can be obtained only by left ventricular catheterization except in mitral regurgitation, when Doppler echocardiography can measure changes in the LV–atrial pressure gradient. Bearing in mind that left ventricular pressure is changing during the period of isovolumic contraction, some workers prefer to make a correction for the change in pressure by dividing dP/dt by a fixed developed pressure, e.g., $dP/dt(DP_{40})$ or by the pressure at the instant of the maximal rate of pressure development, $(dP/dt)/P$. Such corrections add little except complexity.

Ejection Phase Indices of Contractile State

During the ejection phase, the left ventricle contracts against the afterload. Hence, all indices of function in this period are afterload-dependent, a problem that is especially serious in the case of the failing myocardium, which is adversely affected by afterload increases *(16)*. The initial fiber length helps to determine contractility, which, in turn, influences the afterload, because a greater contractile state in the presence of a fixed peripheral (systemic) vascular resistance will increase the blood pressure and the afterload.

The *ejection fraction* of the left ventricle, measured by radionuclide or echocardiographic techniques, is one of the most frequently used indices and one of the least sensitive. The ejection fraction relates stroke volume to end-diastolic volume and is therefore an index of the extent of left ventricular fiber shortening. Nonetheless, this index is easy to obtain and particularly useful in evaluating the course of chronic heart disease. Because the ejection fraction measures the contractile behavior of the heart during systole, it is by definition afterload-sensitive. Another defect is that the ejection fraction relates the systolic emptying to the diastolic volume without measuring that volume, and the left ventricle could theoretically be markedly enlarged yet have reasonable systolic function by this measure. Thus, the correlation between the degree of clinical heart failure and the decrease in the ejection fraction is often only imperfect.

Echocardiographic Indices of Contractile State

The major advantages of echocardiographic indices is that the techniques are widely available and relatively rapid. *Fractional shortening* uses the percentage of change of the minor axis (defined in the next paragraph) of the left ventricular chamber during systole. An approximation often used by clinicians is to estimate the ejection fraction from fractional shortening. Despite obvious defects, this easily defined index is pragmatically useful in the management of heart failure. More accurately, ejection fraction can be determined from volume measurements.

The *end-systolic volume* reflects contractile state because the normal left ventricle ejects most of the blood present at the end of diastole (ejection fraction exceeds 55%). Impaired contractility, shown by an abnormally increased end-systolic volume, is a powerful predictor of adverse prognosis after myocardial infarction *(17)*. The *end-diastolic volume* is a less powerful predictor but essential for the accurate measurement of the ejection fraction.

Increasingly sophisticated and noninvasive measurements of the pumping function of the heart can be obtained with echocardiographic techniques. The velocity at which the circumference of the heart in its minor axis (the distance from the left side of the septum to the posterior endocardial wall) changes during systole is one useful index of myocardial contractility. The mean *velocity of circumferential fiber shortening* (mean V_{cf}) can be determined from echocardiographic measurements of the end-diastolic and end-systolic sizes and the rate of change. The difference between the calculated circumferences is divided by the duration of shortening, which is the ejection time. Even more sophisticated are the data now being generated by *tissue Doppler imaging*. This technique that records high-amplitude, low-frequency Doppler shifts, from which the endocardial and midmyocardial velocity of systolic change can be calculated, is currently one of the best indices of contractility of the human heart *in situ*.

Contractility Indices Based on Pressure-Volume Loops

There are two fundamental aspects of the Frank-Starling relationship that can be seen readily in a pressure-volume loop. First, as the preload increases, the volume increases. On the other hand,

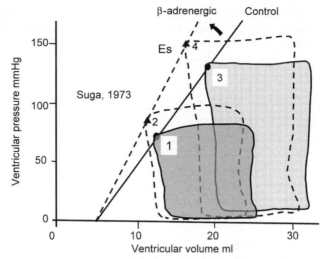

Fig. 9. β-Adrenergic versus volume effects on pressure-volume (PV) loops. Contrasting effects of β-adrenergic stimulation and effects of volume loading on the slope E_s (end-systolic point), which is a good index of contractility. Upon β-adrenergic stimulation, the control loop with its end-systolic point number 1 becomes the loop with point number 2. Likewise, the volume-loaded loop with point number 3 becomes the loop with point number 4 upon β-adrenergic stimulation. The mechanism of the volume response probably involves stretch of the molecular spring, titin *(22)*. Note that β-adrenergic stimulation induces a marked positive inotropic effect (increased contractility) as shown by the increased slope of the line E_s that joins the end-systolic points. By contrast, the effects of increased ventricular volume with increased PV loop area and increased external work occur with no early change in contractility as here, and with only a small delayed increase in contractility (Figs. 3–6). (Figure based on data extracted from ref. *24* with permission of Lippincott Williams & Wilkins.)

for any given preload (initial volume of contraction), a positive inotropic agent increases the amount of blood ejected, and for the same final end-systolic pressure, there is a smaller end-systolic volume. Thus, in response to beta-adrenergic stimulation the slope of the end-systolic pressure-volume relationship is increased at the same time that the venous return rises and the left ventricular end-systolic pressure increases (Fig. 9). It follows that relating pressure to volume is one way of assessing both the Starling effect and the contractility of the left ventricle.

Accordingly, measurements of pressure-volume loops remain among the best of the current approaches to the assessment of the contractile behavior of the intact heart, and hence the key to one of the major determinants of the myocardial oxygen demand. The end-systolic pressure-volume relation can be estimated noninvasively from the arterial systolic pressure and the end-systolic echocardiographic dimension. Invasive measurements of the left ventricular pressure are required for the full loop, which is an indirect measure of the Starling relationship between the force (as measured by the pressure) and the muscle length (measured indirectly by the volume). It is proposed that conditions associated with a higher contractile activity (increased inotropic state) will have higher end-systolic pressures at any for a given end-systolic volume, will have a steeper slope E_s and have correspondingly higher oxygen uptakes. Although useful, like all systolic phase indices, it is still not fully afterload-independent.

DIASTOLE AND DIASTOLIC FUNCTION

Among the many complex cellular factors influencing ventricular relaxation, four are of chief interest. First, the cytosolic calcium level must fall to cause the relaxation phase, a process requiring ATP and phosphorylation of phospholamban for uptake of calcium into the sarcoplasmic reticulum. Second, the inherent viscoelastic properties of the myocardium are of importance. In the hypertrophied heart, relaxation occurs more slowly. Third, increased phosphorylation of troponin

I enhances the rate of relaxation. Fourth, relaxation is influenced by the systolic load. The history of contraction affects crossbridge relaxation. Within limits, the greater the systolic load, the faster the rate of relaxation. This complex relationship has been explored in detail by Brutsaert *(2)*, but could perhaps be simplified as follows: When the workload is high, peak cytosolic calcium is also thought to be high. This high end-systolic cytosolic calcium means that the rate of fall of calcium will also be greater, provided that the uptake mechanisms are functioning effectively. In this way a systolic pressure load and the rate of diastolic relaxation can be related. Furthermore, a greater muscle length (when the workload is high) at the end of systole should produce a more rapid rate of relaxation by the opposite of length-dependent sensitization, so that there is a more marked response to the rate of decline of calcium in early diastole. Yet, when the systolic load exceeds a certain limit, then the rate of relaxation is delayed, perhaps because of too great a mechanical stress on the individual cross-bridges. Thus, in congestive heart failure caused by an excess systolic load, relaxation becomes increasingly afterload-dependent, so that therapeutic reduction of the systolic load should improve LV relaxation.

The *isovolumic relaxation* phase of the cardiac cycle is energy-dependent, requiring ATP for the uptake of calcium ions by the SR, which is an active, not a passive, process. Impaired relaxation is an early event in angina pectoris. A proposed metabolic explanation is that there is impaired generation of energy, which diminishes the supply of ATP required for the early diastolic uptake of calcium by the sarcoplasmic reticulum. The result is that the cytosolic calcium level, at a peak in systole, delays its return to normal in the early diastolic period. In other conditions, too, there is a relationship between the rate of diastolic decay of the calcium transient and diastolic relaxation, with a relation to impaired function of the sarcoplasmic reticulum. When the rate of relaxation is prolonged by hypothyroidism, the rate of return of the systolic calcium elevation is likewise delayed, whereas opposite changes occur in hyperthyroidism. In congestive heart failure, diastolic relaxation also is delayed and irregular, as is the rate of decay of the cytosolic calcium elevation. Most patients with coronary artery disease have a variety of abnormalities of diastolic filling, probably related to those also found in angina pectoris. Theoretically, such abnormalities of relaxation are potentially reversible because they depend on changes in patterns of calcium ion movement.

Phases of Diastole

Hemodynamically, diastole can be divided into four phases, using the clinical definitions of diastole according to which diastole extends from aortic valve closure to the start of the first heart sound. The first phase of diastole (*see* preceding section) is the isovolumic phase, which, by definition, does not contribute to ventricular filling (Fig. 10). The second phase of early (rapid) filling provides most of ventricular filling. The third phase of slow filling or diastasis accounts for only 5% of the total filling. The final atrial booster phase accounts for the remaining 15%.

Atrial Function

The left atrium, besides its well-known function as a blood-receiving chamber, also acts as follows: First, by presystolic contraction and its booster function, it helps to complete LV filling *(18)*. Second, it is the volume sensor of the heart, releasing atrial natriuretic peptide (ANP) in response to intermittent stretch. Third, the atrium contains receptors for the afferent arms of various reflexes, including mechanoreceptors that increase sinus discharge rate, thereby making in humans only a small contribution to the tachycardia of exercise as the venous return increases (*Bainbridge reflex*).

The atria have a number of differences in structure and function from the ventricles, having smaller myocytes with a shorter action potential duration as well as a more fetal type of myosin (both in heavy and light chains). Furthermore, the atria are more reliant on the phosphatidylinositol signal transduction pathway, which may explain the relatively greater positive inotropic effect in the atria than in the ventricles in response to angiotensin II. The more rapid atrial repolarization is thought to be due to increased outward potassium currents, such as I_{to} and I_{kACh}. In addition, some atrial cells have the capacity for spontaneous depolarization. In general, these histologic and

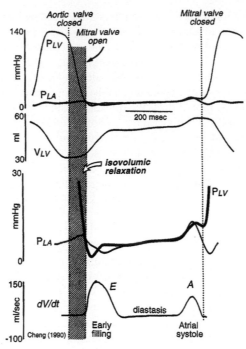

Fig. 10. Diastolic filling phases. *Top panel,* recording of left ventricular pressure (P_{LV}), left atrial pressure (P_{LA}), and left ventricular volume (V_{LV}). *Middle panel,* magnified scale of changes in P_{LV} and P_{LA}. *Lower panel,* rate of change of LV volume (*dV/dt*), an indication of the rate of left ventricular filling, which occurs early in diastole and then again during atrial systole in response to pressure gradient from the left atrium to the left ventricle. In between is the phase of slow filling or diastasis. The early diastolic pressure gradient shown in the middle panel is generated as LV pressure falls below left atrial pressure and the late diastolic gradient is generated as atrial contraction increases left atrial pressure above LV pressure. (Figure based on author's interpretation of data presented in ref. *25.*)

physiologic changes can be related to the decreased need for the atria to generate high intrachamber pressures, rather than being sensitive to volume changes, while retaining enough contractile action to help with LV filling and to respond to inotropic stimuli.

Diastolic Dysfunction in Hypertrophy and Failure

In *hypertrophic hearts,* as in chronic hypertension or severe aortic stenosis, abnormalities of diastole are common and may precede systolic failure, from which there are a number of important differences. The mechanism is not clear, although it is thought to be related to the extent of ventricular hypertrophy or indirectly to a stiff left atrium. Conceptually, impaired relaxation must be distinguished from prolonged systolic contraction with delayed onset of normal relaxation. Experimentally, there are several defects in early hypertensive hypertrophy, including decreased rates of contraction and relaxation and decreased peak force development. Loss of the load-sensitive component of relaxation may be due to impaired activity of the sarcoplasmic reticulum. Impaired relaxation is associated with an increase of the late (atrial) filling phase, so that the ratio E/A (early to atrial filling phases) on the mitral Doppler pattern declines. In time, with both increased hypertrophy and the development of fibrosis, LV chamber compliance decreases and the E wave again becomes more prominent. Thus is becomes difficult to separate truly normal from *pseudonormal* patterns of mitral inflow.

In *myocardial failure,* there are also multiple abnormalities that can be detected in the transmitral flow pattern, including an early change in the E/A ratio. It must be stressed that the E/A ratio changes considerably as LV failure progressively becomes more severe with late-phase pseudo-normalization.

COMPLIANCE

The diastolic volume of the heart is influenced both by the loading conditions and by the elastic properties of the myocardium that confer on it the stiffness that develops in response to stretch. In clinical practice, *stiffness* is taken as the ratio of dP/dV, that is, the rate of pressure change divided by the rate of volume change. This relation is curvilinear, and the initial slope of the change is gentle. As the pressure increases, the volume increases less and less so that there is a considerable increase of pressure for only a small increase of volume. Resting stiffness may in part be attributed to the unique myocardial collagen network, thought to counter the high systolic pressure normally developed in the ventricles. Pathological loss of compliance is usually due to abnormalities, of the myocardium. A true loss of muscular compliance occurs from a variety of causes: acute ischemia as in angina, fibrosis as after myocardial infarction, and infiltrations causing a restrictive cardiomyopathy. In angina, the increased temporary stiffness probably is caused by a combination of a rise of intracellular calcium and of altered myocardial properties. In myocardial infarction, the connective tissue undergoes changes after 40 min of occlusion. Eventually healing and fibrosis permanently increase stiffness. When muscle stiffness increases, so will *chamber stiffness* (the chamber referred to is the ventricle).

The opposite of stiffness is *compliance* (dV/dP)—as the heart stiffens, compliance falls. The term *diastolic distensibility* may be used instead of compliance. Distensibility refers not to the slope of the pressure-volume relation but to the diastolic pressure required to fill the ventricle to the same volume. Thus, when stiffness increases and compliance falls, the distensibility is less, as in the failing human heart. The compliance of the heart influences the Starling curve in that a stiffer heart will be on a lower Starling curve. The pressure-volume loop and the early diastolic filling rate of the heart will also change, while the baseline of the pressure-volume loop will rise upward more steeply, so that a higher left atrial pressure will be required for early diastolic filling. For these reasons, stiffness and compliance are fundamental mechanical properties of the heart.

CONTRACTILE PROPERTIES IN HUMAN HEART DISEASE

The failing human myocardium has many impaired mechanical properties. Thus even though the venous filling pressure is more than adequate, the Starling mechanism is upset and the stroke volume is reduced when compared with normal, so that the blood pressure tends to fall. An increased heart rate provides some compensation to help maintain the cardiac output and, thereby, the blood pressure. However, the normal treppe or Bowditch effect, whereby a faster stimulation rate increases the force of contraction, is severely diminished or even lost so that the tachycardia of exercise fails to increase the stroke volume in heart failure. Homeostatic mechanisms that come into play, such as renin-angiotensin-aldosterone system activation, sustain the blood pressure usually at a lower level than previously but with an increased afterload. The severely failing myocardium undertakes this challenge at the cost of decreased efficiency of work. Thus the pressure-volume loop changes so that internal work is increased relative to the lesser output of external work. Other defects include an impaired response to an increased preload, defective generation of cyclic AMP in response to β-adrenergic stimulation and numerous defects of the patterns of handling of intracellular calcium. These depend both on the abnormalities of the ryanodine receptor of the sarcoplasmic reticulum with hyperphosphorylation and on defects in the uptake of calcium from the cytosol by the calcium uptake pump. These changes result in a variety of different abnormalities of the patterns of contraction and relaxation of the failing myocardium, often with a delayed rise and fall in the calcium transients. Furthermore, when there is an increase in the afterload of isolated human trabecular myocardium from the severely failing human heart, the intracellular calcium transient becomes abnormally prolonged and exaggerated pattern of rise, despite poor generation of force *(16)*. This discrepancy between the patterns of the calcium transient and the contractile response of the severely failing heart could be explained by the abnormal mechanical properties of the myocytes, such as an increase in the stiffer isoform of titin.

REFERENCES

1. Katz AM. Physiology of the Heart, 2nd ed. Raven Press, New York, 1992, p. 453.
2. Brutsaert DL, Sys SU, Gilbert TC. Diastolic failure: pathophysiology and therapeutic implications. J Am Coll Cardiol 1993;22:318–325.
3. Starling EH. The Linacre Lecture on the Law of the Heart. Longmans, Green and Co., London, 1918.
4. Frank O. Zur dynamik des Herzmuskels. Z Biol 1895;32:370–447.
5. Fuchs F. Mechanical modulation of the Ca^{2+} regulatory protein complex in cardiac muscle. News Physiol Sci 1995; 10:6–12.
6. Solaro RJ, Rarick HM. Troponin and tropomysin: proteins that switch on and tune in the activity of cardiac myofilaments. Circ Res 1998;83:471–480.
7. Fitzsimons DP, Moss RL. Strong binding of myosin modulates length-dependent Ca^{2+} activation or rat ventricular myocytes. Circ Res 1998;83:602–607.
8. Luo W, Grupp IL, Harrer J, et al. Targeted ablation of the phospholamban gene is associated with markedly enhanced myocardial contractility and loss of beta-agonist stimulation. Circ Res 1994;75:401–409.
9. Mulieri LA, Leavitt BJ, Martin BJ. Myocardial force-frequency defect in mitral regurgitation heart failure is reversed by forskolin. Circulation 1993;88:2700–2704.
10. Fenelon G, Wijns W, Andries E, Brugada P. Tachycardiomyopathy: mechanisms and clinical implications. PACE 1996;19:95–105.
11. Flamm SD, Taki J, Moore R, et al. Redistribution of regional and organ blood volume and effect on cardiac function in relation to upright exercise intensity in healthy human subjects. Circulation 1990;81:1550–1559.
12. Poliner LR, Dehmer GJ, Lewis SE, et al. Left ventricular performance in normal subjects: a comparison of the responses to exercise in the upright and supine positions. Circulation 1980;62:528–534.
13. Iskandrian AS, Hakki AH, DePace NL, Manno B, Segal BL. Evaluation of left ventricular function by radionuclide angiography during exercise in normal subjects and in patients with chronic coronary heart disease. J Am Coll Cardiol 1983;1:1518–1529.
14. Upton M, Rerych SK, Roeback JR Jr, et al. Effect of brief and prolonged exercise on left ventricular function. Am J Cardiol 1980;45:1154–1160.
15. Bar-Shlomo B-Z, Druck MN, Morch JE, et al. Left ventricular function in trained and untrained healthy subjects. Circulation 1982;65:484–488.
16. Vahl CF, Bonz A, Timek T, Hagl S. Intracellular calcium transient of working human myocardium of seven patients transplanted for congestive heart failure. Circ Res 1994;74:952–958.
17. Schiller NB, Foster E. Analysis of left ventricular systolic function. Heart 1996;(Suppl 2)75:17–26.
18. Hoit BD, Shao Y, Gabel M, Walsh RA. In vivo assessment of left atrial contractile performance in normal and pathological conditions using a time-varying elastance model. Circulation 1994;89:1829–1838.
19. Wiggers CJ. Modern Aspects of Circulation in Health and Disease. Lea and Febiger, Philadelphia, 1915.
20. Lind AR, McNicol GW. Muscular factors which determine the cardiovascular responses to sustained and rhythmic exercise. Canad Med Ass J 1967;96:703–713.
21. Waldrop TG, Eldridge FL, Iwamoto GA, Mitchell JH. Central neural control of respiration and circulation during exercise. In: Rowell LB, Shepherd JT, eds. Handbook in Physiology, section 12. Oxford University Press, New York, 1996, pp. 333–380.
22. Granzier HL, Labeit S. The giant protein titin: a major player in myocardial mechanics, signaling, and disease. Circ Res 2004;94:284–295.
23. Lew WYW. Time-dependent increase in left ventricular contractility following acute volume loading in the dog. Circ Res 1988;63:635.
24. Suga H. Load independence of the instantaneous pressure-volume ratio of the canine left ventricle and effects of epinephrine and heart rate on the ratio. Circ Res 1973;32:314.
25. Cheng CP, et al. Effect of loading conditions, contractile state and heart rate on early diastolic left ventricular filling in conscious dogs. Circ Res 1990;66:814.

RECOMMENDED READING

Katz AM. Physiology of the Heart, 3rd ed. Chapters 8 and 11. Lippincott Williams & Wilkins, Philadelphia, 2001.
Opie LH. Heart Physiology: From Cell to Circulation. Chapter 12. Lippincott Williams & Wilkins, Philadelphia, 2004.
Opie LH. Mechanisms of cardiac contraction and relaxation. In: Zipes DP, Libby P, Bonow RD, Braunwald E, eds. Heart Disease, 7th ed. W. B. Saunders, Philadelphia, 2005, pp. 457–489.

4

Vascular Function

Clive Rosendorff, MD, PhD

INTRODUCTION

All blood vessels have an outer adventitia, a medial layer of smooth muscle cells, and an intima lined by endothelial cells. Contraction of the vascular smooth muscle causes changes in the diameter and wall tension of blood vessels. In the aorta and large arteries vascular smooth muscle contraction affects mainly the compliance (the reciprocal of stiffness) of the vessel. At the precapillary level, contraction of vascular smooth muscle will regulate blood flow to different organs, and contribute to the peripheral resistance. Compliance of large vessels and resistance of arterioles both contribute most of the impedance of the vascular circuit and therefore the afterload of the heart. The capacity of the circulation is determined by the degree of contraction of the veins ("capacitance vessels") especially in the splanchnic area; this will affect the venous filling pressure, or preload, of the heart.

TRANSMEMBRANE ION CONCENTRATIONS AND POTENTIALS

Potassium

Potassium ions *(1)* are transported into cells against their electrochemical gradient, by the ouabain-sensitive Na^+–K^+–adenosine triphosphatase (Na^+–K^+–ATPase), which expels three Na^+ ions in exchange for two entering K^+ ions. This ensures a 20-fold higher concentration of K^+ inside the cell than outside, and a 10-fold higher concentration of Na^+ outside the cell than inside.

The resting membrane potential (E_m) of excitable cells, including vascular smooth muscle cells, depends on the concentration gradients between the extracellular fluid (o) and the cytoplasm (i), and relative permeabilities (P), of Na^+, K^+ and Cl^- across the cell membrane, given by the Goldman constant field equation:

$$E_m = 61 \log \frac{P_{Na}[Na^+]_o + P_K[K^+]_o + P_{Cl}[Cl^-]_i}{P_{Na}[Na^+]_i + P_K[K^+]_i + P_{Cl}[Cl^-]_o}$$

In resting cells E_m is determined mainly by the K^+ permeability and gradient, because P_K is very much greater than P_{Na} and P_{Cl}. At rest, P_K is directly related to the whole-cell K^+ current $I_K = N i P_o$, where N is the total number of membrane K^+ channels, i is the single-channel current, and P_o is the open state probability of a K^+ channel. Thus when K^+ channels close, P_o, I_K, and P_K decrease, and the cell membranes depolarize toward their threshold for firing, (i.e., become more excitable). Conversely, anything that opens K^+ channels hyperpolarizes membranes and makes them less excitable.

In vascular smooth muscle cells (VSMC) this effect is amplified by the effect of the resting membrane potential on voltage-gated Ca^{2+} channels. When closure or inactivation of K^+ channels lowers E_m, voltage-gated Ca^{2+} channels open, producing vasoconstriction. Defective or attenuated K^+ chan-

From: *Essential Cardiology: Principles and Practice, 2nd Ed.*
Edited by: C. Rosendorff © Humana Press Inc., Totowa, NJ

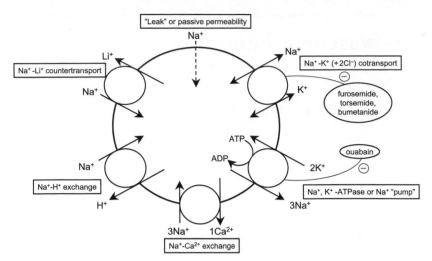

Fig. 1. Major cation transport pathways across cell membranes. For details, *see* text. ADP, adenosine diphosphate; ATP, adenosine triphosphate.

nels have been described in some types of essential hypertension, primary pulmonary hypertension, and hypoxia- or fenfluramine-induced pulmonary hypertension. The opposite is also true. Agents that open K^+ channels hyperpolarize cells and render them less excitable. In VSMC this translates to vasodilatation. Such agents include β-adrenergic agonists, muscarinic agonists, nitroglycerin, nitric oxide, prostacyclin, and "potassium-channel openers" such as cromokalim, now being developed as antihypertensive drugs.

Sodium (see *ref.* 2)

The major active transport pathway for Na^+ in mammalian cells is the Na^+ pump, or Na^+–K^+–ATPase-dependent Na^+–K^+ exchanger (Fig. 1). This results in large concentration gradients of Na^+ (outside greater than inside) and K^+ (inside greater than outside), which keeps the membrane polarized. There are also "passive" Na^+ transporters, which allows the movement of Na^+ from the outside the cell to the interior along a concentration gradient.

All these Na^+ fluxes have been studied intensively, mainly in red blood cells, in the context of human hypertension. In theory, any abnormality that reduces the electrochemical gradient for Na^+ across the vascular smooth muscle membrane (i.e., increases intracellular Na^+) lowers the threshold for those cells to contract. In the renal tubular cells, any increase in Na^+ influx (via passive Na^+ transport) on the luminal side of the cell, or of Na^+ efflux (via the Na^+–K^+–ATPase pump) on the abluminal side, causes Na^+ retention. Both vascular smooth muscle hypertonicity and renal Na^+ retention are important mechanisms of hypertension.

DISORDERS OF ACTIVE SODIUM TRANSPORT

Many studies have shown increased Na^+ content of red blood cells in patients with hypertension, a finding ascribed to a deficiency of the Na^+–K^+–ATPase pump. It has been suggested that this may be due to a circulating endogenous ouabain-like hormone. In vascular smooth muscle, the increased intracellular Na^+ concentration would reduce the resting membrane potential to lower the threshold of activation. Also, the increased cytosolic Na^+ slows Na^+–Ca^{2+} exchange, increasing intracellular free Ca^{2+} levels. The result is an increase in both cardiac and vascular smooth muscle contractility, and hypertension.

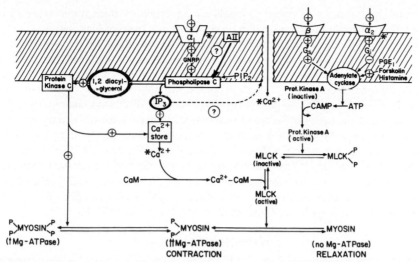

Fig. 2. Adrenergic receptors on vascular smooth muscle cells, with their downstream transduction mechanisms. α_1-Receptors, which mediate vasoconstriction, act via a guanine nucleotide regulatory protein (G protein) to activate phospholipase C, the enzyme that converts phosphatidylinositol bisphosphate (PIP_2) to 1,2-diacylglycerol and inositol 1,4,5-trisphospate (IP_3). IP_3 releases Ca^{2+} from the endoplasmic reticulum, and possibly also opens receptor-operated Ca^{2+} channels. Ca^{2+} forms complexes with calmodulin (CaM), and the complex activates myosin light chain kinase (MLCK), which in turn phosphorylates myosin to facilitate contraction. β-Receptors, mainly β_2, act via a stimulatory G protein (G_S) to activate adenylate cyclase, increase cyclic AMP (cAMP), and thus activate protein kinase A. Protein kinase A phosphorylates, and thus inactivates MLCK, causing relaxation of the smooth muscle cell. α_2-Receptors, via an inhibitory G protein (G_i), inhibit adenylate cyclase, and are therefore vasoconstrictors.

DISORDERS OF PASSIVE NA+ TRANPORT

Na+–H+ Exchange. The Na+–H+ antiporter (activated by several growth factors, including angiotensin II) raises intracellular pH. This is thought to be an important step in the sequence of events that leads to vascular smooth muscle hypertrophy/hyperplasia.

Na+–K+ (+ 2Cl−) Cotransport. This is inhibited by loop diuretics such as furosemide, torsemide, and bumetanide; some hypertensive patients have been shown to have abnormal cotransport activity.

Na+–Li+ Countertransport. Some studies have shown abnormalities of this quantitatively minor transport pathway in red blood cells—and by inference, in vascular smooth muscle cells. Since Na+–Li+ countertransport seems to be controlled by a single gene, this has given rise to much work on Na+–Li+ countertransport as a potential genetic marker for hypertension, marred by the finding that there is a considerable overlap between hypertensive and normotensive individuals.

Passive Na+ Transport. In some, but by no means all, patients with hypertension, there is increased passive (or "leak") inward Na+ flux.

VASCULAR SMOOTH MUSCLE CONTRACTION AND RELAXATION

The contractile activity of VSMC *(3)* depends largely on changes in the cytoplasmic calcium concentration, which, in turn, depends on calcium influx from the extracellular fluid or on release of calcium from intracellular stores, mainly the endoplasmic reticulum. At rest, the plasma membrane of VSMC is relatively impermeable to Ca^{2+}. On activation, calcium channels open, allowing influx of Ca^{2+} along a concentration gradient (Fig. 2). There are three types of calcium channels. The voltage-operated (or potential-operated) calcium channels are regulated by changes in membrane potential, and receptor-operated channels are governed by transmitter–receptor or drug–receptor reactions. The third, much smaller, component is a passive leak pathway.

Release of Ca^{2+} from the sarcoplasmic reticulum (SR) is activated by two mechanisms. First, influx Ca^{2+} through transmembrane Ca^{2+} channels causes an increase in cytosolic calcium, called Ca^{2+}-*induced* Ca^{2+} *release*, which amplifies the increase in cytosolic Ca^{2+} produced by Ca^{2+} flux across the membrane. Second, Ca^{2+} release from the sarcoplasmic reticulum is controlled by a receptor on the SR, the inositol trisphosphate (IP_3) receptor, discussed later.

The Ca^{2+} released into the cytoplasm forms a complex with calmodulin, and this complex binds to and activates the catalytic subunit of myosin light chain kinase, which, in turn, phosphorylates the myosin light chain, permitting ATPase activation of myosin cross-bridges by actin.

Relaxation of vascular smooth muscle may occur by any combination of the following mechanisms: (1) hyperpolarization of the vascular smooth muscle membrane; (2) inhibition of Ca^{2+} entry; (3) increase in the cytoplasmic concentration of cyclic 3',5'-adenosine monophosphate (cAMP); and (4) increased formation of cyclic 3',5'-guanosine monophosphate (cGMP).

Hyperpolarization

The resting membrane potential in VSMC, as in all cells, depends on the transmembrane gradient of diffisible ions, particularly Na^+ and K^+. Changes in the resting membrane potential may effect the gating of calcium channels in the plasma membrane, or may modify Na^+–Ca^{2+} exchange. Hyperpolarization can be produced by activating the Na^+–K^+–ATPase system, whereby three Na^+ are extruded from the cell in exchange for two K^+ pumped in. This will reduce calcium influx via voltage operated calcium channels, and also stimulate Na^+–Ca^{2+} countertransport, to promote Ca^{2+} efflux. This may be the mechanism of the relaxation induced by the endothelium-derived hyperpolarizing factor (EDHF). Another mechanism for hyperpolarization involves increased membrane permeability to K^+, which allows greater efflux of K^+ along its concentration gradient, producing a greater (more negative) resting membrane potential. This action is the basis of the development of a new class of antihypertensive and vasodilator drugs, such as cromokalim, pinacidil and nicorandil, known as K^+ *channel openers*.

Inhibition of Ca^{2+} Entry

Calcium channel blockers, or calcium antagonists, block receptor-activated or voltage-activated Ca^{2+} influx. They do not inhibit intracellular release of Ca^{2+}, reduce passive Ca^{2+} entry (Ca^{2+} leak) or stimulate Ca^{2+} extrusion (Ca^{2+}–ATPase and Na^+–Ca^{2+} countertransport).

Increase in Cyclic Adenosine Monophosphate

β-Adrenergic receptors on the plasma membrane promote the conversion of intracellular adenosine triphosphate (ATP) to cyclic adenosine monophosphate (cAMP) via the enzyme adenylate cyclase. Adenylate cyclase is coupled to the receptor by a guanine nucleotide-binding protein (G protein). In the cell, cAMP binds to and activates cAMP-dependent protein kinase, which, in turn, phosphorylates myosin light chain kinase, thus blocking contraction, and therefore reducing vasomotor tone (Fig. 2).

ADRENERGIC NEUROTRANSMITTERS

Figure 3 shows the biosynthetic pathway of the synthesis of the catecholamines, dopamine, norepinephrine (NE) and epinephrine (E), all of which play very important roles in cardiovascular functions *(4,5)*. This biosynthesis occurs in adrenergic nerves (up to the NE stage) and in the adrenal medulla.

Catecholamines are stored in adrenergic nerve terminals and in adrenal chromaffin cells in storage vesicles together with ATP and storage proteins called *chromogranins*. Catecholamine concentrations in vesicles are continually being replenished by *de novo* synthesis from precursors (dopamine β-hydroxylase is localized within the vesicle), and by neuronal reuptake of released NE (called

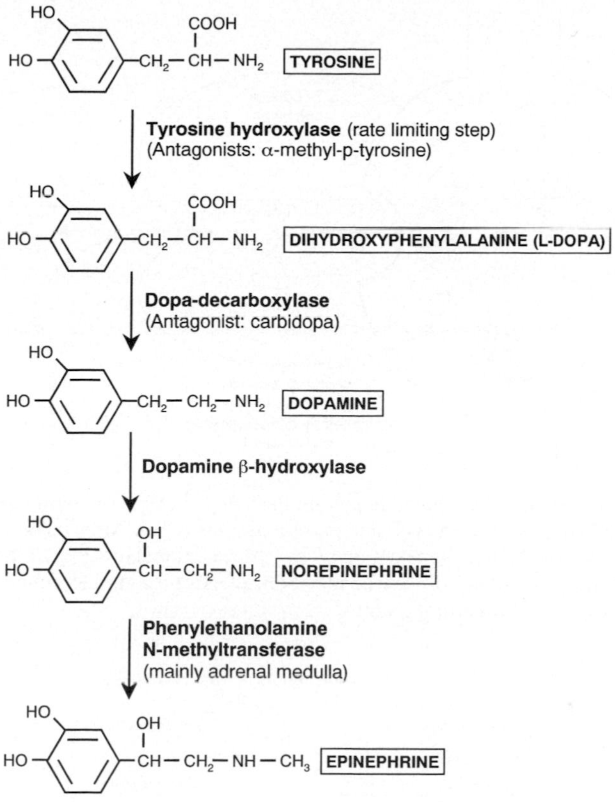

Fig. 3. Biosynthesis of catecholamines.

uptake 1). NE release and reuptake are described in Fig. 4, and the metabolism of NE in Fig. 5. Of the three enzymes principally responsible for the metabolism of NE, two have inhibitors that are used clinically. Monoamine oxidase (MAO) inhibitors work to treat depression by blocking NE metabolism in the central nervous system, and the MAO inhibitor seligiline is used as an adjunct to L-dopa to treat Parkinson's disease. For patients taking an MAO inhibitor, ingestion of tyramine (as in cheese) can cause a life-threatening hypertensive crisis. Catechol-*O*-methyl transferase inhibitors are used with L-dopa for Parkinson's disease. Measurements of catecholamines, such as epinephrine, norepinephrine and dopamine, and their metabolites, such as metanephrine, nonmetanephrine, and vanillylmandelic acid, in blood or urine, are used in the diagnosis of pheochromocytoma (*see* Chapter 32).

Adrenergic Receptors

The main adrenergic receptors, α and β, are generally subdivided into α_1, α_2, β_1, and β_2. In fact, nine subtypes are known, designated $\alpha_{1A,B,C}$, $\alpha_{2A,B,C}$, and $\beta_{1,2,3}$ (*6*). In VSMC there are α_1, α_2, and β_2 receptors. In all three types, the actions on the VSMC are mediated by guanine nucleotide-binding regulating proteins (G proteins).

Receptors designated α_1 are more sensitive to NE than E and are vasoconstrictors. Their action is mediated by a G_{qa} protein, with activation of phospholipase C, but also to direct activation of Ca^{2+} channels, activation of Na^+–H^+ and Na^+–Ca^{2+} exchange, and inhibition of K^+ channels. Phospholipase C catalyzes the conversion of phospatidyl inositol bisphosphate (PIP$_2$) to inositol trisphosphate (IP$_3$) and 1,2-diacylglycerol (DAG). IP$_3$ acts on an IP$_3$ receptor on the sarcoplasmic membrane to release Ca^{2+} into the cytoplasm, which binds with calmodulin (CaM) to form a Ca^{2+}–CaM complex. This complex activates myosin light chain kinase (MLCK), to phosphorylate myosin and thus

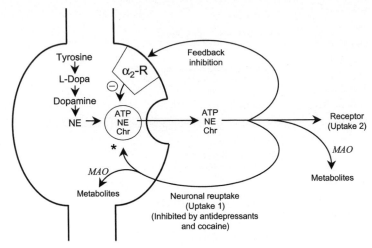

Fig. 4. Biosynthesis and release of catecholamines from the sympathetic nerve terminal. Norepinphrine (NE) is stored in vesicles and coreleased with ATP and chromogranins (Chr). After release the NE may activate an adrenergic receptor (uptake 2), may be taken up by the neurone (uptake 1), may inhibit, via prejunctional α_2-receptors, the further release of NE, or may be metabolized extra- or intraneuronally. *, vesicular uptake of NE. Blocked by reserpine. Chr, chromogranins.

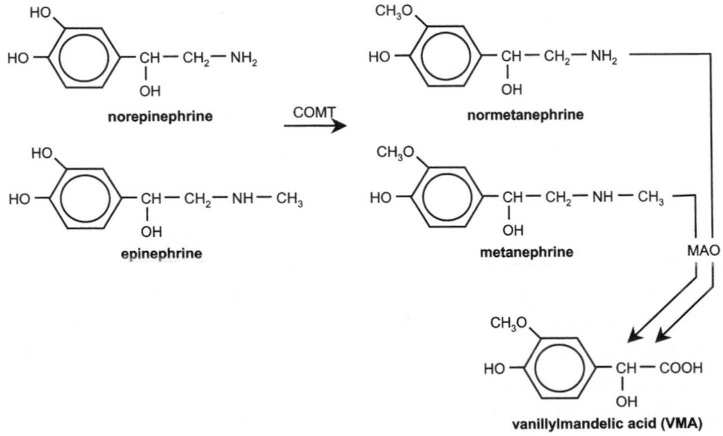

Fig. 5. Metabolism of norepinephrine and epinephrine.

cause contraction. DAC activates protein kinase C (PKC). In addition to initiating VSMC contraction, sustained stimulation of α_1 receptors also switches on cell processes that lead to hypertrophy or hyperplasia, via the released Ca^{2+} and the PKC, both of which stimulate growth and proliferation through a variety of mechanisms, including the MAP-kinase system (*see* The Renin–Angiotensin System below).

Vascular β-receptors, mainly β_2, are linked to a $G_{s\alpha}$ (stimulatory) protein; the $G_{s\alpha}$ protein activates adenylate cyclase, which converts ATP to cAMP. cAMP activates protein kinase A (PKA), which phosphorylates, and therefore inactivates, MLCK. Stimulation of β-receptors thus causes vasodilatation. β-Adrenergic-blocking drugs are therefore directly vasoconstrictor (and so are relatively contraindicated in patients with severe peripheral vascular disease); their antihypertensive action is due to their actions on the heart, to reduce cardiac output, and on the kidney, to block renin release.

α_2-Receptors have a potency order E > NE, and, like α_1 receptors, are also vasoconstrictors, but via a different mechanism. α_2-Receptors couple with inhibitory G proteins ($G_{i\alpha}$) to inhibit membrane–related adenylate cyclase, and therefore have inhibitory actions on the formation of cAMP, activated PKA and phosphorylated MLCK, causing vasoconstriction. There are also α_2-ARs as autoreceptors on postganglionic sympathetic nerve terminals, which synthesize and release NE. These pre-junctional α_2-ARs respond to released (or circulating) catecholamines by inhibiting the further release of NE. Also, activation of brain α_2-ARs reduces sympathetic outflow, and stimulation of these receptors with clonidine and similar α_2-agonists lowers blood pressure.

Dopamine

Dopamine *(7)* is not only a precursor of NE and E; it is also a neurotransmitter in its own right. VSMC contain both D_1- and D_2-receptors. D_1-receptors are located in the heart (myocardial cells and coronary vessels), VSMC, adrenal cortex (zona glomerulosa cells), and kidney tubule cells. Stimulation of D_1-receptors, as by dopamine, dobutamine or fenoldopam, causes vasodilation by increasing adenylase cyclase and cAMP-dependent PKA, resembling in this respect the β_2 receptor. It also causes natriuresis and diuresis by inhibiting Na^+–K^+ antiport activity, to decrease Na^+ reabsorption.

D_2-receptors are found in the endothelial and adventitial layers of blood vessels, where their function is unknown; on pituitary cells where they inhibit prolactin secretion, and where bromocriptine, a D_2-receptor agonist acts to reduce hyperprolactinemia; and in the zona glomerulosa of the adrenal gland, where they inhibit aldosterone secretion. There are also D_2-receptors on the sympathetic nerve terminal, where they inhibit NE release.

THE RENIN–ANGIOTENSIN SYSTEM

The major components of the renin–angiotensin system *(7–9)* are angiotensinogen, renin, angiotensin I (Ang I), angiotensin-converting enzyme (ACE), and angiotensin II (Ang II).

Angiotensinogen, a large globular protein, is synthesized in the liver. The enzyme renin cleaves a leucine-valine bond in the N-terminal region of human angiotensinogen to produce the decapeptide Ang I. The major source of renin is the juxtaglomerular cells of the afferent arterioles of the kidneys. Translation of renin mRNA in these cells produces pre-prorenin, which in turn is converted to prorenin. Juxtaglomerular cells convert prorenin to renin, and both are secreted. Prorenin is the more abundant circulating form of renin; however, the major site of conversion of prorenin to renin is unknown. Prorenin mRNA is expressed at very low levels or is absent in blood vessels, but vascular tissue avidly takes up prorenin, which suggests that blood vessels may be the principal site of the formation of renin from circulating prorenin. Some controversy exists as to whether renin is synthesized to any significant extent in cardiovascular tissue or is derived entirely from plasma uptake.

ACE converts Ang I to the octopeptide Ang II, and also inactivates bradykinin. Bradykinin stimulates the release of vasodilating protaglandins and nitric oxide and may be responsible for ACE inhibitor-induced cough.

Some enzymatic pathways independent of ACE (tissue-type plasminogen activator [t-PA], cathepsin, tonin, and elastase) allow for the formation of Ang II directly from angiotensinogen. Enzymes other than ACE (t-PA, tonin, cathepsin G, chymase, and a chymostatin-sensitive angiotensin II-generating enzyme [CAGE]) catalyze the formation of Ang II from Ang I. The importance of these pathways is obscure; in particular, it is not known whether these non-ACE pathways are present in vivo, or whether they are activated only when the conventional ACE pathway is blocked. Also, there is little or no experimental evidence that ACE-independent pathways contribute substantially to Ang II biosynthesis or to vascular hypertrophy.

Another pathway of interest is the conversion of Ang I to a seven-peptide angiotensin (Ang 1–7) by several endopeptidases. Ang 1–7 is an endogenous competitive inhibitor of Ang II. Ang 1–7 is degraded to the inactive Ang 1–5 by ACE, therefore Ang 1–7 is increased during ACE-inhibitor therapy, and may have vasodepressor and antigrowth functions.

Angiotensin II Receptors

Two major Ang II receptor types exist: AT_1 and AT_2. The AT_1 receptors are found in vascular and many other tissues, and are almost certainly the receptors that transduce Ang II-mediated cardiovascular actions, as discussed in the next section.

Less is known about AT_2 receptors. The fact that AT_2 binding sites are much more abundant in fetal and neonatal tissue than in adult tissue suggests that AT_2 receptors have a role in development. Localization is mainly in the brain, adrenal medulla, and the kidney. It is probable, therefore, that AT_2 receptors have little to do with the acute cardiovascular actions of Ang II. Also, as described later, most of the growth-promoting effects of Ang II on arteries seem to be mediated by AT_1 receptors. Some recent evidence, however, indicates that AT_2 receptor expression is related to the suppression of VSMC growth, in contrast to the growth-promoting effect of stimulating AT_1 receptors (10).

Angiotensin II Signal Transduction Pathways for Mitogenesis and Growth

The AT_1 receptors are present in vascular and many other tissues and seem to mediate the vaso-constricting and growth stimulating effects of Ang II in vascular smooth muscle. Like the α_1-receptor, the AT_1 receptor is coupled to a G protein that activates phosphatidyl inositol bisphosphate (PIP_2) to inositol 1,4,5-trisphosphate (IP_3) and 1,2-diacylglycerol (DAG) (Fig. 6). IP_3, acting through the IP_3 receptor (IP_3R) on the endoplasmic reticulum, stimulates the mobilization of Ca^{2+} from intracellular stores, a process accelerated also by the influx of Ca^{2+} through voltage-dependent Ca^{2+} channels during activation. The increase the cytosolic Ca^{2+} concentration is an essential component of both the activation of the contractile proteins of vascular smooth muscle and of the mediation of the growth-promoting actions of Ang II and other growth factors, at least partially through protein kinase C (PKC) activation.

An alternative pathway for the formation of DAG is the hydrolysis of phosphatidylcholine (PC) by phospholipase C (PLC) or by phospholipase D (PLD). Both DAG and Ca^{2+} activate a PKC that has many actions. PKC affects transmembrane Na^+–K^+ exchange to alkalinize the cytoplasm, which is important in mitogenesis. PKC activates a serum response element (SRE) found on the promoter region of c-*fos*, an early-response protooncogene activated by Ang II, which is thought to be a major factor in initiating the nuclear events that result in cell proliferation and growth.

There are alternative signal transduction pathways for Ang II. One of these is the mitogen-activated protein (MAP) kinase cascade. Although many components of this pathway have been identified, it is not known how Ang II (which binds to a G protein-coupled receptor that lacks intrinsic tyrosine kinase activity) feeds into the MAP kinase phosphorlyation cascade. One possibility is through PKC regulation of Raf-1 kinase. Convincing evidence, nevertheless, shows that the MAP-kinase pathway mediates some of the vascular growth-promoting actions of Ang II. This and related pathways are shown in Fig. 6.

We still do not know to what extent these signal transduction pathways are shared by receptors, such as AT_1, α_1-adrenergic, and endothelin receptors, all of which mediate vasoconstriction and vascular hypertrophy. We also do not know much about the physiologic specificity of these pathways, such as which ones are essential for cell hypertrophy versus hyperplasia, which activate c-*fos*, c-*jun*, or c-*myc* selectively, and which of the myriad intracellular events activated by Ang II depend on which pathway. It is obvious, however, that this is an area of research in which there is enormous potential for the development of new and very precise gene and drug therapies for many clinical problems.

Atherogenic Effects of Angiotensin II

Depending on which model is studied, Ang II can produce VSMC hypertrophy alone, hypertrophy and DNA synthesis without cell division (polyploidy), or DNA synthesis with cell division (hyperplasia). These different effects of Ang II on different cell and animal models of hypertension are difficult to explain. Several lines of evidence suggest, however, that angiotensin II stimulates

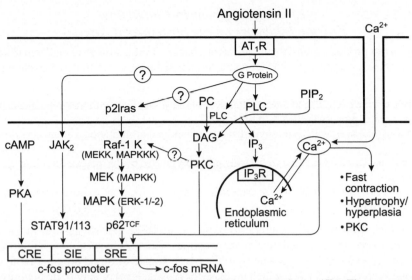

Fig. 6. Signal transduction pathways for the angiotensin II receptor (subtype AT_1). The receptor is coupled to a guanine nucleotide-binding regulatory protein (G protein), which activates phospholipase C (PLC). PLC catalyzes the hydrolysis of phosphatidyl-inositol bisphosphate (PIP_2) to inositol 1,4,5-trisphosphate (IP_3) and 1,2-diacylglycerol (DAG). Inositol 1,4,5-trisphosphate, acting through the IP_3 receptor (IP_3R) on the endoplasmic reticulum, stimulates the mobilization of Ca^{2+} from intracellular stores, a process also accelerated by the influx of Ca^{2+} through voltage-dependent Ca^{2+} channels during activation (Ca^{2+}-dependent Ca^{2+} release). Free cytosolic Ca^{2+} has many actions relating to contractility and cell hypertrophy or hyperplasia including the activation of protein kinase C (PKC). An alternative pathway for the formation of DAG is through the hydrolysis of phosphatidylcholine (PC) by PLC. DAG activates PKC, which in turn may induce hypertrophy or hyperplasia through several mechanisms, one of which is the activation of a serum response element (SRE) on the c-*fos* promoter. The SRE also interacts with products of the mitogen-activated protein (MAP) kinase phosphorylation cascade. Both PKC and a small-molecular-weight guanine-nucleotide-binding protein, p21ras, regulate the serine/threonine kinase Raf kinase (Raf-1K) which acts as a MEK kinase (or MAP kinase kinase kinase). MEK (**M**AP/**E**RK **k**inase) is a MAP kinase kinase, and MAP kinase has two active isoforms, extracellular-signal-regulated kinases-1 and -2 (ERK-1 and -2). Activated MAP kinase substrates include the transcription factor p62^{TCF}, which forms a complex on the c-*fos* promoter (SRE). Angiotensin II also stimulates the phosphorylation and activity of STAT 91 and STAT 113 through the action of **J**anus **k**inase 2 (JAK_2); this interacts with a sis-inducing element (SIE) on the c-*fos* promoter. Another c-*fos* promoter element is a **c**AMP **r**esponse **e**lement (CRE), which is sensitive to protein kinase A (PKA). The significance of this pathway in angiotensin II cell signaling is not known. (From ref. *8.*)

both proliferative and antiproliferative cell processes. The proliferative actions include stimulation via AT_1 receptors of the growth factors platelet-derived growth factor-A chain (PDGF-A) and basic fibroblast growth factor (bFGF), possibly via AT_1 receptor. The antiproliferative processes include transforming growth factor-β1 (TGF-β1). Another antiproliferative mechanism is the ability of the AT_2 receptor to mediate programmed cell death (apoptosis) by dephosphorylation of MAP kinase, or to inhibit guanylate cyclase.

Ang II also has a profound effect on the composition of the extracellular matrix of VSMC, including the synthesis and secretion of thrombospondin, fibronectin, and tenascin. Other processes of atherogenesis are stimulated by angiotensin II, such as migration of VSMC, the activation, release of tumor necrosis factor-α (TNF-α), the adhesion to endothelial cells by human peripheral blood monocytes, and thrombosis. Ang II increases plasminogen activator inhibitor type 1 (PAI-1). All these actions increase the probability that Ang II is atherogenic and prothrombotic, and that ACE inhibitors or angiotensin II antagonists may exert some protective effect through these mechanisms.

Effect of Angiotensin-Converting
Enzyme Inhibitors on the Structure of Arteries

Hypertension produces consistent and major changes in the structural and functional properties of arteries and arterioles, which increase arterial resistance and stiffness. The changes include these:

- Reductions in the external and internal diameter of the vessel wall without any increase in its cross-sectional area, a process known as *remodeling*.
- Altered wall thickness, with medial hypertrophy, myointimal proliferation, and an increase in collagen content.
- Increased passive stiffness of the vessel wall, probably caused by the increase in collagen and smooth muscle mass.
- Increased active vascular muscle tone, caused by a variety of local and extrinsic metabolic and neurohormonal factors.

Many studies show that ACE inhibitors counteract all these mechanisms. Is the prevention of vascular hypertrophy by ACE inhibitors in these animal models of hypertension unique to this class of antihypertensive agents, or is it a nonspecific consequence of blood pressure reduction? Pure vasodilators, such as hydralazine, which increase the plasma level of Ang II, do not prevent vessel wall thickening, despite the normalization of blood pressure, and ACE inhibitors have been shown to be more effective that other antihypertensive agents (α-blockers, vasodilators) in decreasing vascular hypertrophy, despite similar decreases in blood pressure.

Angiotensin II Receptor Antagonists

A major advance in antihypertensive drug therapy has been the development of nonpeptide Ang II receptor antagonists, sometimes called angiotensin receptor blockers, or ARBs (losartan, irbesartan, candesartan, valsartan, olmasartan, telmasartan), selective for the AT_1 receptor subtype, which mediates the vasoconstrictor actions of Ang II. A critical question is whether the hypertrophic action of Ang II can also be inhibited by selective AT_1 receptor antagonists. These drugs block Ang II-induced DNA and protein synthesis and intracellular Ca^{2+} mobilization in VSMC, whereas AT_2 receptor antagonists have no effect. In intact animals, results have been consistent with those from cell culture: there is a reduction of medial thickness in the aorta and arteries of hypertensive rats treated with these agents.

ENDOTHELIN

Endothelin *(11,12)* is a 21-amino-acid peptide (Fig. 7) with three isoforms: endothelin-1 (ET-1), endothelin-2 (ET-2), and endothelin-3 (ET-3). First discovered as products of endothelial cells, these peptides have since been shown to be also produced by other cells, including cardiac, renal tubule, and vascular smooth muscle cells. "Big ET" (39 amino acids) is formed from proendothelin (39 amino acids) by the action of the endothelin-converting enzyme (ECE); ECE then cleaves big ET to form the active 21-amino-acid ET. Many factors stimulate endothelin release, including hormones (Ang II, vasopressin, catecholamines, insulin), growth factors (transforming growth factor-β, insulin-like growth factors), metabolic factors (glucose, low-density lipoprotein cholesterol), hypoxia, and changes in shear stress on the vascular wall (Fig. 8).

There are two endothelin receptors, ET_A and ET_B. These are G-protein-coupled receptors that activate phospholipase C, which, in turn, mobilizes intracellular calcium, activates protein-kinase C, stimulates Na^+–H^+ exchange to raise intracellular pH, and activates MAP kinase and the proto-oncogenes, c-*fos*, c-*jun*, and c-*myc*. ET_A receptors respond mainly to ET-1, are found mainly on vascular smooth muscle cells, and mediate vasoconstriction, proliferation, and cell hypertrophy. ET_B receptors have two subtypes, an endothelial receptor activating the release of nitric oxide (NO) and a vascular smooth muscle receptor mediating vasoconstriction. The ET_A receptor is the predominant type in adult cardiomyocytes. ETs have both chronotropic and inotropic effects on cardiac

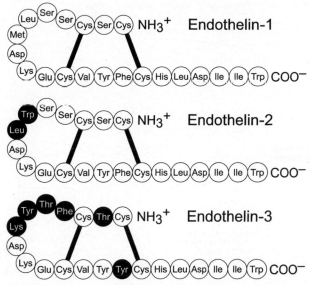

Fig. 7. Molecular structure of endothelin-1, -2, and 3. (From ref. *12*.)

muscle. There are no ET_B receptors in the coronary circulation, so that endothelins are coronary vasoconstrictors.

The downstream events initiated by the binding of endothelin to the ET_A receptor (Fig. 8) involve (G-protein-dependent) activation of phospholipase C to hydrolyze phosphatidylinositol bisphosphate to form IP_3 and DAG. IP_3 promotes the release of Ca^{2+} from endoplasmic reticulum stores, and IP_3 and G-proteins may also open voltage-dependent calcium channels in the cell membrane, resulting in an increase in the cytosolic Ca^{2+} concentration, which is essential both for the activation of the contractile proteins in the cell and for cell growth and proliferation. These signal transduction mechanisms of endothelin receptors are shared with α_1-receptors and Ang II receptors in the vasculature.

In addition to the pivotal role of cytosolic Ca^{2+} in cell proliferation, the activation of PKC by DAG may also result in upregulation of the genes concerned with cell growth in both VSMC and cardiac myocytes. This effect may be mediated through a rise in intracellular pH and/or the activation of MAP kinases. MAP kinases are known to induce the phosphorylation of nuclear proteins; thus, the PKC-MAP kinase pathway could be a plausible signaling system that links angiotensin II and endothelin activation of cell surface receptors with changes in nuclear activity. ET_A receptors may also mediate atherosclerosis by stimulating inflammatory mediators (such as NFκB), adhesion molecules (intercellular adhesion molecule-1 [ICAM-1] and vascular cell adhesion molecule-1 [VCAM-1], and chemokines (such as monocyte chemoattractant protein-1).

Endothelin in Hypertension

Convincing evidence for the role of endothelin in hypertension should include demonstration of increased levels of the peptide in plasma or in vascular tissue; potentiation of vasoconstrictor responses, because of increased responsiveness of vascular smooth muscle or of a vascular proliferative effect; sustained increase in blood pressure during chronic intravenous infusion; or a normalization of elevated blood pressure by endothelin receptor antagonists.

Plasma immunoreactive ET-1 concentration is very slightly increased or normal in most models of hypertension in the rat. In hypertensive humans, plasma endothelin levels have been reported as normal or slightly raised or definitely elevated. This does not preclude an important role for

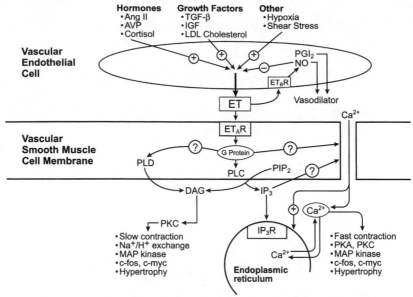

Fig. 8. Stimuli to endothelin (ET) release and ET signal transduction pathways. Hormones, such as angiotensin II (Ang II), arginine vasopressin (AVP), and cortisol; the growth factors, transforming growth factor-β (TGF-β), insulin-like growth factor (ILGF), and LDL cholesterol; and other factors, such as hypoxia and shear stress, all stimulate ET production and release by the vascular endothelial cell. The endothelial cell has ET_B receptors (ET_BR), which may mediate vasodilation by the release of nitric oxide (NO) and prostacyclin (PGI_2). NO also inhibits endothelial ET release. The predominant endothelin receptor in the vascular smooth muscle cell membrane is the ET_A type, which is coupled to a guanine nucleotide-binding regulatory protein (G-protein), which activates phospholipase C (PLC). PLC catalyzes the hydrolysis of phosphatidyl-inositol bisphosphate (PIP_2) to inositol 1,4,5-trisphospate (IP_3) and 1,2-diacylglycerol (DAG). IP_3, acting via the IP_3 receptor (IP_3R) on the endoplasmic reticulum membrane, stimulates the release of Ca^{2+} into the cytosol, a process also accelerated by the influx of Ca^{2+} through L-type voltage-dependent Ca^{2+} channels during activation (Ca^{2+}-dependent Ca^{2+} release). Free cytosolic Ca^{2+} has several actions that relate to contractility and cell hypertrophy, possibly involving PKA, PKC, MAP kinase, and protooncogenes, such as c-*fos* and c-*myc*. DAG may be formed by the action of PLC or PLD, and alkalinizes the cytoplasm (Na^+/H^+ exchange), activates MAP kinase and protooncogenes, and thus contributes to hypertrophy. (From ref. *12*.)

endothelin in the pathogenesis of hypertension, because it has been suggested that endothelin release is mainly abluminal, that is, the paracrine release is from the endothelial cell toward the vascular media, and little if any spills over into the circulation.

Increased plasma endothelin levels (and sympathetic activity and plasma norepinephrine levels) in the offspring of hypertensive parents, but not in the offspring of normotensive parents, suggest a genetically determined dysregulation of endothelin release and of the sympathetic nervous system in response to to certain stressful stimuli in the former group. The data on vascular responsiveness to endothelin in hypertension are not straightforward. In some animal models of hypertension responsiveness to endothelin is enhanced, but in sodium and fluid overload models of hypertension in rats, and in human hypertension, the ET-1 responses are attenuated. This may be due to downregulation of endothelin receptors in response to the increased production of endothelin.

Chronic intravenous infusion of ET-1 causes sustained hypertension in conscious rats, and endothelin receptor antagonists block the rise of blood pressure in some, but not all, rat models of hypertension. Nonpeptide receptor-selective antagonists are now available; these will help to establish the importance of endothelin in human hypertension and may lead to the development of an important new class of antihypertensive drugs. Early clinical studies are already under way.

Cardiac Hypertrophy and Heart Failure

In addition to causing coronary vasoconstriction and myocardial ischemia in hypertension, ET-1, like Ang II, is a growth factor for cardiac myocytes, and may be involved in myocardial hypertrophy. In heart failure, the neurohormonal activation includes the ET system. ET receptor antagonists improve cardiac function and hemodynamics in experimental animals and humans, but this may be simply due to blockade of ET-dependent systemic vasoconstriction, with reduction of left ventricular afterload.

Atherosclerosis

All the main cell components of atherosclerotic lesions—endothelial cells, smooth muscle cells, and macrophages—can express ET-1. In atherosclerosis, ET-1 mRNA expression is increased, and ET-1 accumulates and acts as a chemoattractant for monocytes. In animals selective ET_A receptor blockade decreases the number and size of macrophage-foam cells and reduces neointima formation.

Coronary Artery Disease

Coronary atherosclerotic tissue has increased tissue endothelin–like immunoreactivity in smooth muscle cells, macrophages, and endothelial cells. Local ET-1 is also increased after coronary angioplasty, particularly in the neointima. ET_A receptors predominate, although there is also an increased population of ET_B receptors, and there is some evidence to suggest that both are involved in neointima formation.

Pulmonary Hypertension

Both ET-1 mRNA expression and ET-1 immunoreactivity have been documented in the lungs of patients with both primary and secondary pulmonary hypertension, and ET_A receptor antagonists prevent and reverse chronic hypoxia-induced pulmonary hypertension in rats. Bosentan, a nonselective ET_A- and ET_B-receptor inhibitor, is used in the treatment of WHO Class III and IV pulmonary arterial hypertension, although its use is limited by significant hepatotoxicity and teratogenicity.

Conclusion

ET-1 is generated by the endothelin-converting enzyme (ECE) in endothelial and VSMC, and cardiac myocytes. In the vasculature ET-1 is a vasoconstrictor, activating the PLC–DAG–Ca^{2+} axis, with significant "crosstalk" with the tyrosine-kinase-dependent pathways. ET promotes proliferation of VSMC in hypertension and atherosclerosis, and promotes smooth muscle cell migration, intimal hyperplasia, and monocyte recruitment. These atherogenic effects could, theoretically, be blocked by endothelin receptor antagonists or ECE inhibitors, but we do not yet know whether these drugs are effective.

NITRIC OXIDE (13–15)

In 1980, Furchgott and Zawadzki showed that simple mechanical disruption of the vascular endothelium (as by rubbing the endothelial surface with a cotton swab) abolished the vasodilator effect of acetylcholine, and they proposed that the normal response to acetylcholine involved release of an endothelium–derived relaxing factor (EDRF). Moncada and colleagues showed later that the EDRF is NO. In 1998 both Furchgott and Moncada received the Nobel Prize.

The enzyme nitric oxide synthase (NOS) catalyses the conversion of l-arginine to l-citrulline and NO in endothelial and vascular smooth muscle cells and in neurons (Fig. 9). Three NOS isoforms have been identified. Endothelial cells produce a constitutive NOS (eNOS), and nNOS is found in neurons; both require calcium and calmodulin for activity. Inducible NOS (iNOS) isoforms, mainly in VSMC and macrophages, are calcium-independent and can produce high, sustained levels of NO. Shear stress exerted by blood flow in arteries induces NO production; other stimuli include the activation of α_2, 5-HT$_{1D}$, ET_B, B_2, and adenosine receptors.

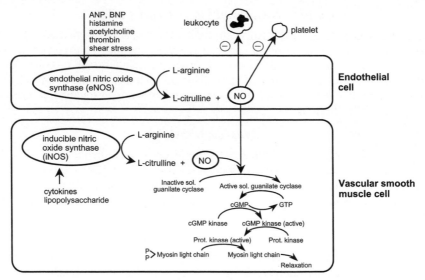

Fig. 9. The nitric oxide and cyclic guanosine monophosphate (cGMP) signal transduction mechanism. Constitutive endothelial nitric oxide synthase (eNOS) synthesizes nitric oxide (NO) from L-arginine. eNOS activity is stimulated by many factors, shown on the figure. NO inhibits leukocyte and platelet activation and adhesion. NO diffuses to the subjacent vascular smooth muscle cell, where it activates a cascade of events, including cGMP and an activated cGMP-dependent protein kinase, to cause vasodilation. NO may also be synthesized by inducible nitric oxide synthase (iNOS) in vascular smooth muscle cells exposed to cytokines and/or lipolysaccharides. ANP, atrial natriuretic peptide; BNP, brain natriuretic peptide. (Modified from ref. *14*.)

Both endothelial cell and VSMC NO activate VSMC-soluble guanylate cyclase, stimulating the conversion of guanosine triphosphate to cyclic guanosine monophosphate (cGMP). cGMP activates c-GMP-dependent protein kinases, which do several things, including extruding intracellular calcium via a membrane-associated $Ca^{2+}-Mg^{2+}-ATPase$ pump, opening K^+ channels to hyperpolarize the cell membrane, and inhibiting PLC and Rho-kinase. All of these effects cause smooth muscle relaxation, and thus vasodilation.

There is some evidence that a underproduction of NO can cause hypertension in animals and in humans. Overproduction of NO by iNOS in macrophages and VSMC exposed to cytokines and/ or lipopolysaccharide contributes to the vasodilation and hypotension of septic shock.

There is also some evidence that NO is antiatherogenic. In animals, inhibitors of NOS, such as N-nitro-L-arginine methyl ester (L-NAME), accelerate the development of atherosclerotic lesions, and L-arginine slows it. The progress of the endothlial dysfunction associated with developing arteriosclerosis can be followed in patients by measuring the vasodilator response to infused acetylcholine. Acetylcholine releases NO from the endothelium to relax VSMC, but acts directly on VSMC to constrict them. The net effect in persons with a normal functioning endothelium is that the vasodilator effect predominates. In patients with damaged endothelial cells, as in atherosclerosis, endothelial NO production is deficient, so there is a blunting of the normal endothelium-dependent vasodilation, and, in severe cases, there is an unopposed vasoconstrictor effect of acetylcholine on VSMC directly. Vasodilator responses to nitroglycerin are normal, since nitroglycerine acts directly on vascular smooth muscle.

What are the mechanisms of atherogenesis? First, NO inhibits LDL oxidation in vitro. This is true of the continuous generation of NO by the constitutive eNOS; however, when NO is present with superoxide or at a low pH, as occurs in the atherosclerotic lesions, both NO and its oxidized metabolite peroxynitrite ($ONOO^-$) oxidize LDL, which is proatherogenic. The second proposed mechanism is the inhibition by NO of platelet activation and adhesion. NO also negatively regu-

Table 1
Factors Released by the Endothelium

Vasodilators	Vasoconstrictors
Nitric oxide	Angiotensin II
Bradykinin	Endothelin
Prostacyclin	Thromboxane A_2, serotonin[a], arachidonic
Endothelium-derived hyperpolarizing factor	acid, prostaglandin H_2, thrombin
Serotonin[a], histamine, substance P	
C-type natriuretic peptide	
Inhibitors of smooth muscle cell growth	Promoters of smooth muscle cell growth
Nitric oxide, prostacyclin, bradykinin	Platelet-derived growth factor
Heparan sulfate	Basic fibroblast growth factor
Transforming growth factor-β	Insulin-like growth factor-I
C-type natriuretic peptide	Endothelin, angiotensin II
Inhibitors of inflammation or adhesion	Promoters of inflammation or adhesion
Nitric oxide	Superoxide radicals
	Tumor necrosing factor-α
	Endothelial leukocyte adhesion molecule
	Intercellular adhesion molecule
	Vascular cell adhesion molecule
Thrombolytic factors	Thrombotic factors
Tissue-type plasminogen activator	Plasminogen activator inhibitor-1

[a]Serotonin functions mostly as a vasodilator in normal blood vessels, but it produces paradoxical vasoconstriction when the endothelium is impaired by hypertension, hypercholesterolemia, or other risk factors for cardiovascular disease.

lates leukocyte chemotaxis and adhesion, limiting monocyte migration to the intima and macrophage and foam cell formation. NO also inhibits vascular smooth muscle proliferation.

The mechanism of restenosis after percutaneous angioplasty may be due to denudation of the endothelium with poor NO production; leukocytes and platelets adhere to the damaged surface and release growth factors that lead to VSMC proliferation and migration into the intima. Several studies have shown slowing of neointimal formation by NO donors (such as L-arginine) or by the transfer in vivo of the eNOS gene. Vascular injury also stimulates the expression of iNOS, which is a damage-limiting response.

All these data suggest a promising therapeutic approach to a number of cardiovascular problems—particularly hypertension, atherosclerotic disease, coronary spasm, and postangioplasty restenosis—that involve strategies for increasing vascular NO production. This could be achieved (1) by supplementing the NOS substrate, L-arginine, or cofactors, such as tetrahydrobiopterin, (2) by using NO donor compounds (of which the most commonly used are nitrates) or inhibiting the conversion of NO to superoxide by superoxide dismutase, or (3) by overexpression of the NOS gene using intravascular gene therapy techniques. However, none of these approaches has yet been shown to be successful in slowing or reversing atherosclerosis in humans. More successful has been treatment of endothelial dysfunction with cholesterol-lowering agents, particularly statins, and with antioxidant therapy, or a combination of both.

ENDOTHELIUM AND ARTERIOSCLEROSIS

It is clear, then, that the endothelium plays a critical role in maintaining vascular health, by secreting vasodilators, inhibitors of smooth muscle growth, and thrombolytic factors, as listed in Table 1.

It is also well known that conditions such as hypertension, diabetes, dyslipidemia, and smoking cause the physiologic and structural changes in the vessel that lead to vascular disease. It has been suggested that one of the earliest changes to occur in each of these conditions is an alteration of the oxidative metabolism of the endothelium, with increased oxidative stress. This causes endothelial dysfunction, manifested by a decrease in vasodilators, inhibitors of growth, and thrombolytic factors, and an increase in the synthesis and release of vasoconstrictor substances (which promote smooth muscle growth), adhesion molecules, and prothrombotic factors.

In particular, there is a decrease in NO formation, and activation of vascular ACE and endothelin. The result is vasoconstriction, vascular hypertrophy and/or hyperplasia (vascular remodeling) due to Ang II, endothelin, and other growth factors, and also inflammatory changes including monocyte adhesion and infiltration, due to adhesion molecules (VCAM, ICAM) and cytokines. Eventually, if the patient is unlucky, the plaque ruptures due to proteolysis, and thrombosis is caused by tissue factor and excess plasminogen activator inhibitor-1 (PAI-1) release from the atherosclerotic plaque.

ACETYLCHOLINE

Acetylcholine (ACh) *(16)* is the neurotransmitter for postganglionic parasympathetic neurons (acting on muscarinic receptors), both sympathetic and parasympathetic preganglionic neurons (acting on nicotinic receptors), preganglionic autonomic neurons innervating the adrenal medulla, motor end plates in skeletal muscle, and some neurons in the central nervous system. ACh is synthesized by acetylation of choline, stored in vesicles, and then released from cholinergic nerves when these are depolarized. After acting on the ACh receptor, ACh is rapidly degraded by acetylcholinesterase.

Muscarinic Receptors

At least five subtypes of muscarinic receptors are known, M_1 to M_5. Although several vascular effects of ACh have been described—notably the release of nitric oxide from endothelial cells to produce vasodilation—the administration of atropine, a muscarinic antagonist, has no significant effect on vascular resistance. It is therefore unlikely that ACh has a major role in vascular homeostasis. However, the intense negative cardiac inotropic and chronotropic effects of parasympathetic (vagal) stimulation, opposed by atropine, are well known.

Nicotinic Receptors

All autonomic ganglionic neurotransmission is mediated by nicotinic cholnergic receptors. Ganglion-blocking drugs, such as trimethophan and mecamylamine, were once among the few agents available for the treatment of hypertension. They caused blood pressure to fall, but what is effectively a blockade of the efferent pathway of the baroreceptor reflex frequently caused profound postural hypotension, dizziness, and syncope. These drugs are no longer used.

SEROTONIN

Serotonin, or 5-hydroxytryptamine (5-HT) *(17)*, is found in the central and peripheral nervous system, in the enterochromaffin cells of the gastrointestinal tract, and in platelets. It is synthesized by the hydroxylation of tryptophan to 5-hydroxytryptophan, then by decarboxylation to 5-HT. The cardiovascular actions of 5-HT are complex. At least 14 different 5-HT receptors exist. Activation of the central nervous system 5-HT_{1A} receptors lowers blood pressure. 5-HT_{1B} receptors cause decreased ACh and NE release from nerve terminals and 5-HT_{1A} receptors mediate endothelium–dependent vasodilation. Receptors for 5-HT_2 are involved with direct arterial and venous constriction, and 5-HT_3 receptor activation causes bradycardia and hypotension. Intravenous serotonin causes a brief depressor phase mediated by 5-HT_3 receptors, followed by a brief pressor effect due to 5-HT_2 receptors in the renal, splanchnic, and cerebral circulation. Next, there is a more prolonged fall in blood pressure, due to vasodilation in skeletal muscle, probably mediated by 5-HT_{1A} receptors. Ketanserin is a 5-HT_2 (and α_1-adrenergic) receptor antagonist, which is used as an antihypertensive agent.

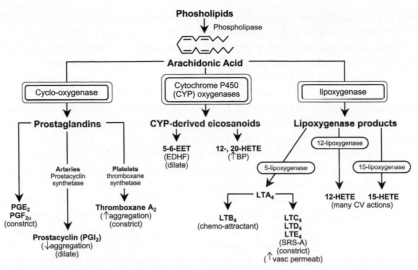

Fig. 10. The biosynthesis of protaglandins, cytochrome P450-derived eicosanoids and lipoxygenase products from arachidonic acid. PG, prostaglandin. For other abbreviations, *see* text.

ADENOSINE

Adenosine *(18)*, made up from adenine and D-ribose, is distributed throughout all body tissues, and aside from its importance in AMP, ADP and ATP, is a potent vasodilator with a short half-life of not more than 6 s. It also has negative inotropic and chronotropic effects on the heart, and is used to treat supraventricular tachycardias. There are four adenosine receptors: A_1, A_{2a}, A_{2b}, and A_3. A_1 and A_3 receptors in the heart inhibit adenylate cyclase and activate K^+ channels to decrease inotropy and to suppress sinus mode automaticity and atrioventricular nodal conduction. Vasodilation is mediated via A_{2a} and A_{2b} receptors, which activate adenylate cyclase via a G_S protein. Adenosine is also used as a test agent for coronary artery disease; by causing vasodilatation of normal coronary arteries, it produces a "steal" effect, revealing any area of myocardial ischemia.

γ-AMINOBUTYRIC ACID

γ-Aminobutyric acid (GABA) *(19)* is an inhibitory amino acid found throughout the central nervous system. GABAergic neurons in the posterior hypothalamus and ventral medulla exert a tonic inhibitory effect on blood pressure, and GABA antagonists raise blood pressure.

ENDOGENOUS OUABAIN

The plant glycoside, ouabain *(20)*, has digitalis-like actions, particularly inotropic effects. Recently an endogenous ouabain-like (EO) steroid hormone was discovered, which is a high-affinity, selective inhibitor of Na^+–K^+–ATPase, is positively inotropic, and is a vasopressor. All these actions would be expected cause hypertension, and this has been shown with sustained infusions of EO in rats. Elevated EO levels have been described in 30 to 45% of humans with hypertension. The primary site of EO production seems to be the adrenal zona glomerulosa, and EO release can be stimulated by adrenocorticotrophin (ACTH) and by Ang II via AT_2 receptors.

EICOSANOIDS *(21,22)*

Prostacyclin (PGI_2) is an eicosanoid prostaglandin (Fig. 10) that is rapidly released from endothelial cells in response to a variety of humoral and mechanical stimuli. PGI_2 is the major product of arachidonic acid metabolism through the cyclooxygenase pathway in blood vessels. It is a vaso-dilator, but also retards platelet aggregation and adhesion. This action is the opposite to that of the major metabolite of arachidonic acid in platelets, thromboxane A_2, which is a vasoconstrictor and stimulates platelet aggregation. Although the PGI_2 receptor is present in the arterial vascular wall, PGI_2 is not constitutively expressed and therefore is not involved in the regulation of systemic vascular tone. Rather, it is released in response to short-term perturbations of tone. Recently, however, an enzyme, prostaglandin H synthase II (PHS-II), has been identified. This is an inducible form of a key enzyme in PGI_2 synthesis, which provides a mechanism for the sustained production of PGI_2 in chronic inflammation and vascular injury.

Other physiologically important eicosanoids are synthesized from arachidonic acid by cytochrome P450 oxygeneses. These are (1) 5,6-epoxy-eicosatrienoic acid (5,6-EET), which is the endothelium-derived hyperpolarizing factor, which, like PGI_2, is a vasodilator; (2) 12(R)-hydroxyeicosatetraenoic acid (12R-HETE) which inhibits Na^+–K^+–ATPase; and (3) 20-HETE, which elevates blood pressure via several different mechanisms, both directly and via the kidney.

The third enzyme pathway for the production of vasoactive arachidonic acid products is via lipoxygenases, of which there are three, designated 5-, 12-, and 15-lipoxygenase. The 5-lipoxygenase pathway produces leukotriene A_4 (LTA_4), which is then converted to LTB_4, a potent chemoattractant substance that causes polymorphonuclear cells to bind to vessel walls, and may therefore be important in atherogenesis. LTA_4 can also be converted to LTC_4, LTD_4, or LTE_4, formerly collectively known as "slow-reacting substance of anaphylaxis" (SRS-A), made by mast cells, neutrophils, eosinophils, and macrophages, and which are potent vasoconstrictors and cause increased microvascular permeability. The 12- and 15-lipoxygenase pathways produce 12-HETE and 15-HETE, respectively, in VSMC and endothelial cells. Also, platelets, adrenal glomerulosa cells, and renal mesangial and glomerular cells can make 12-HETE, and monocytes can make 15-HETE. These two lipoxygenase products have several potential roles in vascular disease. The eicosenoid 12-HETE may activate MAP kinase, suggesting a role in cell proliferation and atherogenesis. Both 12- and 15-HETE inhibit prostacyclin synthesis and vasoconstrict certain vascular beds. They are growth-promoting on vascular smooth muscle cells, may increase monocyte adhesion to endothelial cells, and may be involved in the oxidation of LDL-cholesterol.

KININS

Kinins *(23)* are vasodilator peptides that are released from substrates known as *kininogens* by serine protease enzymes known as *kininogenases*. There are two main kininogenases, plasma and tissue kallikrein, and these produce bradykinin and lysyl-bradykinin from the high- or low-molecular-weight kininogens, made in the liver and circulating in the plasma (Fig. 11). Kinins are broken down by enzymes known as *kininases*, one of which is kininase II, also known as the angiotensin-converting enzyme (ACE). Others include neutral endopeptidases (NEP) 24.11 and 24.15. Most kininases are found in the endothelial cells of capillaries.

Kinins activate B_1 and B_2 receptors. B_1 receptors are involved with inflammatory responses to bacterial endotoxins. B_2 receptors mediate vasodilator responses. In the kidney, kinins are vasodilatory, natriuretic, and diuretic, actions that are possibly mediated by the kinin-induced release of prostaglandin E_2 and nitric oxide. In children a low urinary kallikrein excretion is an important genetic marker for primary hypertension, so kinins may play some role in hypertension. At least some of the antihypertensive actions of both ACE inhibitors and NEP inhibitors may be due to potentiation of the effect of kinins.

Tissue kallikrein is present in heart, arteries, and veins. Kinin production is increased in myocardial ischemia, may be an important mediator of myocardial preconditioning (protection from damage during subsequent ischemic episodes), and may contribute to the beneficial effect of ACE inhibitors in reversing ventricular remodeling and in improving cardiac function. Kinins also have several important functions in hemostasis. Plasma kallikrein and high-molecular-weight kininogen are involved with the intrinsic pathway of blood coagulation. Kinins also promote NO and

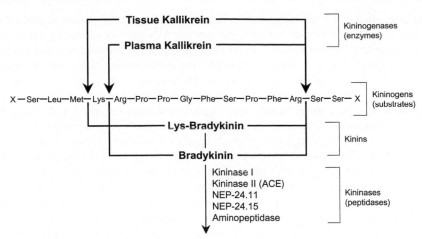

Fig. 11. Biosynthesis and metabolism of kinins. For description, *see* text.

prostacyclin (PGI$_2$) formation, both of which inhibit platelet aggregation and adhesion, and kinins stimulate the release of tissue plasminogen activator to promote fibrinolysis. All these effects are enhanced by inhibitors of kininases, such as ACE inhibitors and NEP inhibitors.

ENDOGENOUS NATRIURETIC PEPTIDES

There are three structurally and functionally similar natriuretic peptides *(24)*: atrial natriuretic peptide (ANP), brain natriuretic peptide (BNP), and C-type natriuretic peptide (CNP), which all induce natriuresis and are vasodilators. ANP is released from atrial and ventricular myocytes in response to stretch (making the heart a true endocrine organ). The ANP prohormone contains 126 amino acids, and is cleaved in cardiac myocytes to two fragments. The C-terminal 28-amino-acid peptide is the active hormone. BNP, structurally similar to ANP, is synthesized and stored in the brain and in cardiac myoctyes, and is also released in response to atrial and ventricular stretch, although at lower concentrations than is ANP. The third member of the group, CNP, is made not in the heart but in the endothelium of blood vessels, and probably acts not as a circulating hormone but in a paracrine manner, acting on adjacent VSMC as a vasodilator and antimitogenic agent.

ANP and BNP bind to the natriuretic peptide receptor-A (NPR-A) receptor, which is found on vascular endothelial cells and renal epithelial cells. CNP binds to the NPR-B receptor, on VSMC. Both ANPR-A and ANPR-B receptors activate guanilyl cyclase and cyclic GMP to cause natriuresis, diuresis, and vasodilation. They inhibit the renin–angiotensin system, endothelin, and sympathetic function, and are antimitogenic in VSMC.

ANP and BNP levels are elevated in congestive heart failure, and can be used for the diagnosis and as a guide to the management of that condition. New agents are in development that will enhance ANP and BNP activity, particularly drugs that inhibit the enzyme that degrades the peptides, neutral endopeptidase. One such drug is omapatrilat, which inhibits both angiotensin-converting enzyme and neutral endopeptidase, and which has been shown to be effective in both high-renin and low-renin forms of hypertension. Unfortunately omapatrilat may cause angioedema, because of the potentiation of bradykinin by the NEP inhibition and because its development has been stopped. Infusions of BNP (nesiritide) have been used, successfully, for the treatment of heart failure.

VASOPRESSIN

Arginine vasopressin (AVP) *(25)*, also known as the antidiuretic hormone (ADH), is released from the posterior pituitary in response to (1) increased plasma osmolality, via osmoreceptors in the hypothalamus; (2) reduced blood volume, sensed by atrial stretch receptors; and (3) decreased blood pressure, via aortic and carotid baroreceptors. In addition to its action in promoting water reabsorbtion in renal collecting ducts (via V_2 receptors), AVP activates blood vessel V_{1a} receptors to cause vasoconstriction, but it also stimulates hepatic glycogenolysis and renal tubular prostaglandin E_2 generation. The V_{1a} receptors are coupled to membrane G proteins, phosphatidylinositol phosphate (PIP), phospholipase C (PLC), and increased free cytosolic Ca^{2+} released from the endoplasmic reticulum. The V_2 receptors, mediating water permeability of the collecting ducts and also vasodilation in skeletal muscle, are coupled to adenylate cyclase and cyclic-AMP.

The normal concentration of AVP is 1–3 pg/mL (10–12 mol/L), and concentrations within the physiologic range (10–20 pg/mL), can produce significant vasoconstriction in skin, splanchinic, renal, and coronary beds, and some V_2-receptor mediated skeletal muscle vasodilation, with variable effects on arterial blood pressure. AVP also enhances sympathoinhibitory responses to baroreceptor stimulation, so that quite high plasma AVP concentrations are not accompanied by hypertension, which allows the antidiuretic action of AVP to occur unopposed by any pressure-induced diuresis. The role of AVP in human hypertension is not clear. In a small percentage of patients with primary hypertension (30% of males, 7% of females) there is a significant elevation (5–20 pg/mL) of plasma AVP, but it is not known whether these changes in AVP concentrations are primary or secondary. These concentrations are lower than those required to increase blood pressure in normal humans, but may contribute to the fluid retention and volume expansion seen in many hypertensive patients. There is, however, the phenomenon of "vasopressin escape"—the AVP-induced pressure diuresis overcomes the fluid-retaining effects of AVP, so that, after a few weeks, extracellular fluid volumes return to normal.

NEUROPEPTIDE Y

Neuropeptide Y (NPY) *(26)* is a 36-amino-acid vasoconstrictor peptide, which is coreleased with norepinephrine and ATP from sympathetic nerve terminals innervating small arteries, heart, and kidney. It is also abundant in the brain (hypothalamus, ventrolateral medulla, and locus coeruleus) and in sympathetic ganglia. Y_1 receptors in blood vessels inhibit adenylate cyclase and increase intracellular free Ca^{2+} to cause vasoconstriction. The Y_2 receptors are on the sympathetic nerve terminal, and mediate feedback inhibition of neurotransmitter release.

In the central nervous system NPY probably acts to lower blood pressure and heart rate. Unlike most other vasoconstrictor agents, NPY is diuretic and natriuretic. Plasma concentrations of NPY are elevated in some patients with hypertension, but the significance of this is unknown.

ADIPOCYTE HORMONES *(27)*

Leptin is a 167-amino-acid protein produced by adipocytes. Leptin binds to leptin receptors in the hypothalamus, where it decreases appetite and increases thermogenesis. In obese people circulating leptin levels are elevated, suggesting some leptin resistance. Leptin also activates the sympathetic nervous system, so hyperleptinemia may explain the frequent association between obesity and hypertension. Other actions of leptin include endothelial NO formation, angiogenesis, natriuresis, diuresis, and platelet aggregation.

Other adipocyte-derived hormones are (1) resistin, which inhibits insulin-stimulated glucose uptake; and (2) adiponectin, which normalizes insulin resistance, and is antiinflammatory in vessel walls.

PLASMINOGEN ACTIVATOR INHIBITOR-1

Plasminogen activator inhibitor-1 (PAI-1) *(29)* is found in the vascular endothelium, platelets, adipose tissue, and the liver. It binds to vitronectin in the extracellular matrix of blood vessels. PAI-1 is an acute-phase reactant, induced by inflammatory cytokines such as interleukin-1 (IL-1) and tumor necrosis factor-α (TNF-α), by growth factors such as transforming growth factor-β (TGF-β) and epidermal growth factor, and by hormones like Ang II and aldosterone. Plasma levels of PAI-1 are increased in hypertension, and PAI-1 is present in atherosclerotic plaques, contributing to the development of atherosclerotic cardiovascular disease.

PEROXISOME PROLIFERATOR-ACTIVATED RECEPTORS (30)

Peroxisomes are organelles that oxidize various molecules, including long-chain fatty acids. Peroxisome proliferators (which activate peroxisome proliferator-activated receptors [PPAR]) are agents that increase the size and number of peroxisomes. There are three PPARs, named PPAR α,γ, and δ. PPAR-α is widely expressed, is activated by fibrates such as gemfibrozil and fenofibrate, and regulate fatty acid and apolipoprotein A-1 and lipoprotein lipase activation. PPAR-α also inhibits vascular inflammatory cytokines and tissue factor. PPAR-γ, expressed mainly in adipose tissue and the vasculature, is activated by the thiazolidinediones (proglitazone and rosiglitazone) to increase insulin sensitivity, also to repress several stages in the atherosclerotic process, including cytokine-induced chemokines, monocyte cytokines, matrix metalloproteinases and VSMC proliferation. The ubiquitous PPAR-δ is activated by fatty acids and prostacyclin, and increases HDL-cholesterol.

REFERENCES

1. Nelson MT, Quayle JM. Physiological roles and properties of potassium channels in arterial smooth muscle. Am J Physiol 1995;268:C799–C822.
2. Lijnen P. Alterations in sodium metabolism as an etiological model for hypertension. Cardiovasc Drugs Ther 1995;9:377–399.
3. Stamler JS, Dzau VJ, Loscalzo J. The vascular smooth muscle cell. In: Loscalzo J, Creager MA, Dzau VJ, eds. Vascular Medicine: A Textbook of Vascular Biology and Diseases, 1st ed. Little Brown, Boston, 1992, pp. 79–132.
4. Insel PA. Adrenergic receptors: evolving concepts and clinical applications. N Engl J Med 1996;334:580–585.
5. Day MD. Autonomic Pharmacology, Experimental and Clinical Aspects. Churchill Livingstone, Edinburgh, 1979.
6. Alexander SPH, Peters JA. Receptor and Ion Channel Nomenclature Supplement. 12th ed. TIPS 2001, pp. 9–13.
7. Rosendorff C. The renin-angiotensin system and vascular hypertrophy. JACC 1996;28:803–812.
8. Rosendorff C. Vascular hypertrophy in hypertension. Role of the renin-angiotensin system. Mt Sinai J Med 1998; 65:108–117.
9. Atlas SA, Rosendorff C. The renin-angiotensin system-from Tigerstedt to Goldblatt to ACE inhibition and beyond. Mt Sinai J Med 1998;65:81–86.
10. Touyz RM, Schiffrin EL. Signal transduction mechanisms mediating the physiological and pathophysiological actions of angiotensin II in vascular smooth muscle cells. Pharmacol Rev 2000;52:639–672.
11. Horiuchi M, Akashita M, Dzau VJ. Recent progress in angiotensin II type 2 receptor research in the cardiovascular system. Hypertension 1999;33:613–621.
12. Rosendorff C. Endothelin, vascular hypertrophy and hypertension. Cardiovasc Drugs Ther 1996;10:795–802.
13. Schiffrin EL. Role of endothelin-1 in hypertension. Hypertension 1999;34(Part 2):876–881.
14. Lloyd-Jones DM, Bloch KD. The vascular biology of nitric oxide and its role in atherogenesis. Annu Rev Med 1996; 47:365–375.
15. Radomski MW, Moncada S. The biological and pharmacological role of nitric oxide in platelet function. In: Authi KS, ed. Mechanisms of Platelet Activation and Control. Plenum, New York, 1993, pp. 251–264.
16. Vanhoutte PM. Endothlial function and vascular disease. In: Panza JA, Cannon RO III, eds. Endothelium, Nitric Oxide and Atherosclerosis. From Basic Mechanisms to Clinical Implications. Futura Publishing, New York, 1999, pp.79–95.
17. Lefkowitz RJ, Hoffman BB, Taylor P. Neurohumoral transmission: the autonomic and somatic motor nervous systems. In: Gilman AG, Rall TW, Nies AS, Taylor P, eds. The Pharmacologic Basis of Therapeutics, 8th ed. Pergamon Press, New York, 1992, pp. 84–121.
18. Hollenberg N. Serotonin and vascular responses. Ann Rev Pharmacol Toxicol 1988;28:41–59.
19. Olah ME, Stiles GL. Adenosine receptor subtypes: characterization and receptor regulation. Annu Rev Pharmacol Toxicol 1995;35:581–606.
20. Peng YJ, Gong QL, Li P. GABA (A) receptors in the rostral ventrolateral medulla mediate the depressor response induced by stimulation of the greater splanchnic nerve afferent fibres in rats. Neurosci Lett 1998;249:95–98.
21. Schoner W. Endogenous cardiotonic steroids. Cell Mol Biol 2001;47(2):273–280.
22. Nasjletti A. The role of eicosanoids in angiotensin-dependent hypertension. Hypertension 1997;31:194–200.
23. Nasjletti A, McGiff JC. Prostaglandins and P450 metabolites. In: Izzo JL, Black HR, eds. Hypertension Primer, 3rd ed. American Heart Association and Lippincott Williams & Wilkins, Philadelphia, 2003, pp. 55–58.
24. Margolius HS. Kallikreins and kinins. Some unanswered questions about system characteristics and roles in human disease. Hypertension 1995;26(2):221–229.
25. Levin ER, Gardner DG, Samson WK. Natriuretic peptides. N Engl J Med 1998;339:321–328.

26. Cowley AW Jr, Michalkiewicz M. Vasopressin and neuropeptide Y. In: Izzo JL, Black HR, eds. Hypertension Primer, 3rd ed. American Heart Association and Lippincott Williams & Wilkins, Philadelphia, 2003, pp. 37–39.
27. Michel MC, Rascher W. Neuropeptide Y: a possible role in hypertension. J Hypertens 1995;13:385–395.
28. Ahima RS, Flier JS. Adipose tissue as an endocrine organ. Trends Endocrinol Metab 2000;11:327–333.
29. Vaughn DE. Plasminogen activator inhibitor-1: a common denominator in cardiovascular disease. J Invest Med 1998;46:370–376.
30. Bishop-Bailey D. Peroxisome proliferator-actived receptors in the cardiovascular system. Br J Pharmacol 2000;129: 823–834.

RECOMMENDED READING

Cines DB, Pollak ES, Buck CA, Loscalzo J, et al. Endothelial cells in physiology and in the pathophysiology of vascular disorders. Blood 1998;91:3527–3561.
O'Rourke ST, Vanhoutte PM. Vascular pharmacology. In: Loscalzo J, Creager MA, Dzau VJ, eds. Vascular Medicine: A Textbook of Vascular Biology and Diseases, 1st ed. Little Brown, Boston, 1992, pp. 133–156.
Stamler JS, Dzau VJ, Loscalzo J. The vascular smooth muscle cell. In: Loscalzo J, Creager MA, Dzau VJ, eds. Vascular Medicine: A Textbook of Vascular Biology and Diseases, 1st ed. Little Brown, Boston, 1992, pp. 79–132.
Pepine CJ, ed. A Symposium: Endothelial Function and Cardiovascular Disease: Potential Mechanisms and Interventions. Amer J Cardiol 1998;82(10A):1S–64S.

5 Thrombosis

Yale Nemerson, MD and Mark B. Taubman, MD

INTRODUCTION

Thrombosis and hemostasis are similar processes, the former being pathologic and involving intravascular formation of aggregates of platelets and fibrin, and the latter resulting in the cessation of bleeding after external injury to the vasculature. While it is not clear that these processes involve precisely the same biochemical and biophysical events, they appear to be sufficiently similar to be considered as a single process that results in quite different structures owing to the local environment, either within a vessel or at the site of bleeding.

The initial event in both instances likely is the exposure of tissue factor (TF) at the site of injury (1,2). In arterial thrombosis, the most frequent initiating event appears to be rupture or fissuring of an atheromatous plaque, which exposes TF; an event that enables the circulating blood to contact TF, thus activating the coagulation cascade (3).

BRIEF VIEW OF THE MECHANISM OF BLOOD COAGULATION

Although for many years it was thought that coagulation was initiated via the so-called intrinsic system (so named because it was believed that all the components required for coagulation were "intrinsic" to the blood), it is generally recognized that this system was an artifact of glass activation (1). The prevailing view is that coagulation via the TF pathway is the principal means of thrombin production. Some patients who are deficient in factor XI, however, have some hemorrhagic symptoms. Until recently, it was thought that factor XI was activated mainly when the blood contacted glass or a similar surface by a mechanism independent of TF. Two findings, however, offer alternative schemes, each consistent with TF being the only physiologic activator of the coagulation system. First, it was shown that factor XI could be activated on platelets via a mechanism independent of factor XII or glass. Interestingly, platelet factor XI is an alternatively spliced form of plasma factor XI (4), and its synthesis is independent (5). Alternatively, the major catalyst of factor XI activation may be thrombin, which activates this zymogen via limited proteolysis (6). Formation of a thrombus involves many circulating proteins, blood platelets, and damage to the arterial wall with consequent exposure of TF. Because of this complexity, it is difficult to describe the entire process precisely. The clinical efficacy of anticoagulant and antiplatelet agents indicates that perhaps all these components are necessary but that none alone is sufficient for thrombus formation.

TF forms a complex with activated factor VII (VIIa), thereby forming a holoenzyme that initiates the coagulation cascade by activating factors IX and X (Fig. 1). The TF:VIIa complex has a regulatory subunit, TF, and a catalytic subunit, VIIa. The latter is a serine protease that has essentially no procoagulant activity unless it is in complex with TF. This theme—the assembly of holoenzymes from regulatory and enzymatic species—is central to the understanding of coagulation, because is occurs three times in this process.

The vast majority of circulating factor VII is in the zymogen, or unactivated form, but small amounts of VIIa also circulate (7,8), and it is probably responsible for the initial activity of the

From: *Essential Cardiology: Principles and Practice, 2nd Ed.*
Edited by: C. Rosendorff © Humana Press Inc., Totowa, NJ

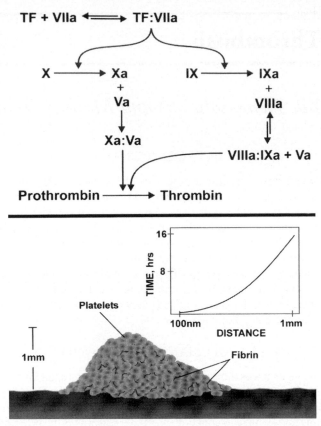

Fig. 1. (Upper panel) Schematic view of blood coagulation with tissue factor (TF) as the initiating species. TF is shown as a complex with activated factor VII (VIIa) and that small amounts of this enzyme are present in normal blood. (Lower panel) Schematic view of a thrombus. The inset indicates the relationship between the time it takes a diffusing molecule to traverse a given distance. This relationship is such that as the distance doubles, the time to capture is squared.

TF complex. When factor VII is bound to TF, it has little or no enzymatic activity; however, in the bound state (whose crystal structure has been described [9]), zymogen factor VII is in a conformation that renders it liable to limited proteolysis that results in its conversion to its active enzymatic form, VIIa (10,11). The complex of TF:VIIa has two substrates, factors IX and X. Their activated forms, IXa and Xa, respectively, form complexes with two circulating regulatory proteins; IXa with the antihemophilic factor, factor VIII, and Xa with factor V, forming the so-called prothrombinase complex. These complexes are similar to the TF:VIIa complex inasmuch as each contains a serine protease (factors IXa and Xa, respectively) and a regulatory protein (factors VIIIa and Va, respectively). Both factors VIII and V circulate as "pro-cofactors" and must be activated via limited proteolysis to function in these complexes. Thrombin is likely the enzyme that is mainly responsible for activating these cofactors; thus, strong positive feedback results in explosive formation of thrombin. The last event in this cascade is the cross-linking of fibrin via the action of factor XIII, which, after being activated by thrombin, crosslinks the fibrin monomers. Once cross-linked, fibrin becomes resistant to lysis by plasmin, which is one explanation for lytic therapy losing efficacy over time.

This concert of events, during which the platelets become activated, enables them to support coagulation and to form a nidus for thrombus formation via the action of the IIb/IIIa receptor that facilitates the formation of platelet masses by interacting with fibrin. The IIb/IIIa receptor is the target of the clinically effective antithrombotic monoclonal antibody Rheopro®. Leukocytes are also involved in thrombus formation. It is noteworthy that a blocking antibody to P selectin inhibited fibrin formation in an arteriovenous shunt model in vitro *(12)*. P selectin is a protein stored in platelet granules that translocates to the plasma membrane upon platelet activation. When on the platelet surface, P selectin interacts with its cognate ligand, CD-15, on the surface of leukocytes. This observation raises the issue of the role of leukocytes in thrombus formation, which is addressed later.

NATURAL ANTICOAGULANT SYSTEMS

Natural anticoagulant systems can conveniently be divided into two classes: those that circulate as inhibitory species and those that are activated during coagulation. Of those that require activation, that best studied is protein C, which, like factors VII, and X, is a vitamin K-dependent zymogen that must be activated by limited proteolysis (for a review, *see* ref. *13)*. The activation of protein C is accomplished by thrombin that is complexed with an endothelial surface protein, thrombomodulin. When thrombin is in this complex, the substrate specificity of thrombin is altered so that it activates protein C and thrombin-activatable fibrinolysis inhibitor (TAFI) *(14)* but does not clot fibrinogen. Activated protein C is a serine protease that attacks activated factors V and VIII, thus shutting down the coagulation cascade. Factor V Leiden is a genetic variant of factor V that is resistant to proteolysis by activated protein C. Those with this mutation exhibit increased thrombosis, mostly venous, although serious arterial thrombosis is also increased *(15–17)*. This is a reasonably common mutation: some 5 to 6% of Caucasians possess it *(18)*. Deficiencies of protein C are associated mainly with venous thromboembolic disease, although instances of arterial thrombosis have been reported *(19)*.

TAFI is a recently described fibrinolysis inhibitor that is a form of procarboxidase B. When activated by thrombin or (>1000-fold faster) by thrombomodulin-thrombin complex, the resultant enzyme attacks the carboxy-terminal residues of proteins, resulting, in this case, in reduced plasmin/plasminogen and tissue plasminogen activator (tPA) binding to fibrin *(20)*. Thus, the formation of the thrombin-thrombomodulin complex results in the generation of an anticoagulant, activated protein C, and the antifibrinolytic (prothrombotic) species TAFI. Clearly, sorting out these phenomena with respect to thrombogenesis will be most difficult.

The blood also contains an inhibitory protein, tissue factor pathway inhibitor (TFPI), whose functioning is complex: TFPI has modest affinity for TF and thus it is not directly inhibitory. TFPI is in its most effective form when it is bound to factor Xa; this binary complex then attacks TF:VIIa, with which it forms an inactive quaternary complex, thus damping TF-initiated coagulation *(21, 22)*. No clinical deficiency states of TFPI have yet been reported, so it is difficult to assess its role in preventing thrombosis. It is noteworthy, however, that mice whose gene for TFPI has been knocked out die *in utero (23)*.

The other major circulating anticoagulant is antithrombin III, which forms a stable complex with several of the coagulation enzymes, most prominently thrombin, and activated factor X. This reaction is markedly accelerated by heparin and similar compounds and is the mechanism by which heparin exerts its anticoagulant activity *(24)*. Like deficiencies of protein C, antithrombin III deficiencies are associated mainly with venous thrombosis, although recent data indicate that low levels of this protein are predictive of future cardiac events *(25)*.

FIBRINOLYSIS

Just as coagulation involves multiple enzymatic and regulatory proteins, fibrinolysis, the process by which fibrin is lysed to reestablish blood flow, involves multiple proteins and reactions, the details of which are beyond the scope of this chapter. Plasminogen is the circulating zymogen of plasmin, a serine protease that has high specificity for fibrin. It is activated in vivo by plasminogen activators that are released from tissue stores by ischemia. The activators generate plasmin, the active fibrinolytic enzyme, from the zymogen plasminogen. Plasminogen activation inhibitors 1 and 2 oppose the activation of plasmin and thus are prothrombotic *(26–28)*. These inhibitors appear to be the major components of the fibrinolytic system that are associated with thrombotic risk.

Interestingly, while hemophilia A patients are protected against myocardial infarction *(29)*, hereditary absence of factor XI affords no such protection *(30)*.

TISSUE FACTOR AND ATHEROSCLEROTIC PLAQUE

As noted above, occlusive thrombi of the coronary arteries are thought to be a consequence of plaque rupture and are the leading cause of death in the Western world; because of this and because TF in plaques is felt to be necessary for thrombosis, many studies have focused on the presence of this protein in plaques. As early as 1972, TF was detected in plaque by immunostaining, although the antibody was undoubtedly polyspecific *(31)*. Subsequent experiments with antibodies raised against pure TF confirmed these findings *(32)*, as did results obtained with monoclonal antibodies and the use of haptene-labeled factor VIIa, a specific probe for TF *(33)*. Because immunostaining reflects only localization of antigen, and binding of VIIa to TF the localization of TF-binding sites, it follows that neither of these techniques demonstrates TF activity in plaque. Direct enzymatic assay of TF harvested from plaque has been reported, and the majority of samples demonstrated activity *(34,35)*. The activity, however, was low, and it is not certain that the specimens contained only plaque; thus, the meaning of these findings is somewhat questionable. What clearly is required to demonstrate unambiguously active TF in plaque is an enzyme histochemical assay for TF, which, however, has not been reported.

Circulating Tissue Factor: A Thrombogenic Species

Recent experiments have demonstrated that native, normal human blood forms TF-dependent thrombi on collagen-coated glass slides in a laminar flow chamber. The fact that these thrombi contain fibrin indicates that the deposited TF is biochemically active; furthermore, inclusion of active site-inhibited VIIa (a potent TF inhibitor) essentially abolished both fibrin and thrombus formation on the collagen surface *(36)*. This finding contradicts many statements in the literature, including our own, that circulating TF is of no consequence. Further, these experiments suggest that exposure of collagen on blood vessels may be sufficient to initiate thrombus formation, although it seems likely that vessel wall TF initiates thrombus formation, whereas circulating TF may be responsible for its propagation. The apparent mechanism by which blood-borne TF can initiate thrombosis ex vivo works as follows: The first event appears to be binding of platelets to collagen; thereafter, neutrophils and monocytes bind to the platelets (probably via P selectin and other molecules as yet to be identified). The leukocytes, which contain TF, apparently deposit TF-containing membranous structures on the platelets, thus rendering them highly thrombogenic. These experiments were designed to mimic thrombosis in vivo in the sense that they involved laminar flow at arteriolar shear rates (1000 to 2000/s). We imagine that the shear field, which is also encountered in mildly stenosed coronary arteries, favors (1) delivery of leukocytes to the nascent thrombus and (2) their fragmentation *in situ*. Thus, as the thrombus grows the platelets become surrounded with TF-containing vesicles and membranous structures that are competent to initiate coagulation and support thrombus propagation.

Encryption of Cell Surface Tissue Factor: What Is the Biologically Active Species?

The fact that blood-borne TF is active in experimental thrombogenesis suggests that there is a mechanism for controlling its activity in blood cells, One possibility is that cell surface TF in vivo is entirely encrypted, by which we mean that while it is capable of binding VIIa and specific antibodies, cell surface TF is catalytically inactive. The phenomenon of encryption or dormancy on the cell surface was suggested many years ago *(37)* and was subsequently explored and documented using contemporary techniques *(38–40)*. It has been suggested that on the cell surface TF exists as inactive dimers and that it must be monomerized to exhibit procoagulant activity *(41)*. Quantitative studies using cultured cells have shown that the majority of surface TF is encrypted

(40). One possibility that is difficult to explore is that, in vivo, cell-surface TF is inactive; if so, that fact raises the question of the state of the active species. Extracellular TF has been noted in arterial adventitia and in the plaque, which raises the possibility that it is the active pool *(42)*. It is well documented that, for optimal activity, TF requires acidic phosphatides to be exposed. It is presumed that normally these molecules are on the inner leaflets of plasma membranes and render these membranes more or less inactive. Extracellular TF, however, is present on membrane fragments and vesicles, which lack the energy necessary to maintain phospholipid asymmetry; therefore, one expects acidic phosphatides to be randomly distributed, the net result being that extracellular TF quite likely is procoagulant.

Tissue Factor in Arterial Injury

In addition to its association with acute coronary syndromes such as myocardial infarction and unstable angina, thrombosis is also a concomitant of acute arterial injury, such as that produced by coronary angioplasty, directional atherectomy, and coronary artery stenting *(43,44)*. TF antigen is induced in the smooth muscle cells near the intimal border in rat *(45)*, rabbit *(46–48)*, and porcine *(49)* models of arterial injury; the significance of this induction is subject to the same concerns raised earlier in the discussion of the atherosclerotic plaque. It has been demonstrated that TF activity in the injured rat aortic media increased coordinately with TF mRNA and antigen *(45)*; however, activity was measured in homogenized aortic sections and therefore could have come from encrypted or intracellular stores not capable of initiating coagulation in vivo.

The relevance of TF induction after balloon injury can be questioned on the grounds that injury to normal rat and rabbit arteries does not result in deposition of macroscopic fibrin, the end product of TF activation, even when medial smooth muscle is injured. However, fibrin deposition occurs rapidly when previously injured rabbit arteries are subjected to a second injury 1 to 2 wk later. Fibrin deposition and microthrombi were not seen at any time after single injuries to normal rat aortas but were present on the luminal surface within 30 min of a second injury. TF antigen was not detectable in the endothelium or media during the first 4 h after injury; TF antigen was abundant in the media by 24 h and then declined to baseline levels over the next 2 d. TF antigen subsequently accumulated in the developing intima and was abundant throughout the intima after 2 wk, at the time of the second injury. Whole-mount preparations showed minimal TF antigen on the surface of uninjured or once-injured vessels, but the second injury rapidly exposed surface TF antigen. Rapid exposure of intimal TF to the circulation may be necessary to generate fibrin and produce thrombosis.

Other studies have suggested that the induction of TF by arterial injury is functionally important. Antibodies to TF inhibited the variations in cyclic flow in rabbits subjected to arterial injury and mechanical stenosis and inhibited thrombus formation in a rabbit femoral artery eversion graft preparations. TFPI has also been shown to inhibit angiographic restenosis and intimal hyperplasia in balloon-injured atherosclerotic rabbits and to attenuate stenosis in balloon-injured hyperlipidemic pigs. Once again, the precise location of the functionally important TF remains to be determined and awaits the development of an *in situ* activity assay.

REFERENCES

1. Nemerson Y. Tissue factor and hemostasis [published erratum appears in Blood 1988 Apr;71:1178]. Blood 1988;71: 1–8.
2. Edgington TS, Ruf W, Rehemtulla A, Mackman N. The molecular biology of initiation of coagulation by tissue factor. Curr Stud Hematol Blood Transfus 1991;58:15–21.
3. Fuster V. Present concepts of coronary atherosclerosis-thrombosis, therapeutic implications and perspectives. Arch Mal Coeur Vaiss 1997;90 Spec No 6:41–47.
4. Hsu TC, Shore SK, Seshsmma T, et al. Molecular cloning of platelet factor XI, an alternative splicing product of the plasma factor XI gene. J Biol Chem 1998;273:13,787–13,793.
5. Hu CJ, Baglia FA, Mills DC, et al. Tissue-specific expression of functional platelet factor XI is independent of plasma factor XI expression. Blood 1998;91:3800–3807.
6. Gailani D, Broze GJ Jr. Factor XI activation in a revised model of blood coagulation. Science 1991;253:909–912.

7. Wildgoose P, Nemerson Y, Hansen LL, et al. Measurement of basal levels of factor VIIa in hemophilia A and B patients. Blood 1992;80:25–28.
8. Morrissey JH. Plasma factor VIIa: measurement and potential clinical significance. Haemostasis 1996;26(Suppl 1): 66–71.
9. Banner DW, D'Arcy A, Chene C, et al. The crystal structure of the complex of blood coagulation factor VIIa with soluble tissue factor [see comments]. Nature 1996;380:41–46.
10. Nemerson Y, Repke D. Tissue factor accelerates the activation of coagulation factor VII: the role of a bifunctional coagulation cofactor. Thromb Res 1985;40:351–358.
11. Rao LV, Rapaport SI. Activation of factor VII bound to tissue factor: a key early step in the tissue factor pathway of blood coagulation. Proc Natl Acad Sci USA 1988;85:6687–6691.
12. Palabrica T, Lobb R, Furie BC, et al. Leukocyte accumulation promoting fibrin deposition is mediated in vivo by P-selectin on adherent platelets. Nature 1992;359:848–851.
13. Esmon CT, Gu JM, Xu J, et al. Regulation and functions of the protein C anticoagulant pathway. Haematologica 1999; 84:363–368.
14. Bajzar L, Morser J, Nesheim M. TAFI, or plasma procarboxypeptidase B, couples the coagulation and fibrinolytic cascades through the thrombin-thrombomodulin complex. J Biol Chem 1996;271:16,603–16,608.
15. Heresbach D, Pagenault M, Gueret P, et al. Leiden factor V mutation in four patients with small bowel infarctions. Gastroenterology 1997;113:322–325.
16. Rosendaal FR. Thrombosis in the young: epidemiology and risk factors. A focus on venous thrombosis. Thromb Haemost 1997;78:1–6.
17. Eskandari MK, Bontempo FA, Hassett AC, et al. Arterial thromboembolic events in patients with the factor V Leiden mutation. Am J Surg 1998;176:122–125.
18. Heijmans BT, Westendorp RG, Knook DL, et al. The risk of mortality and the factor V Leiden mutation in a population-based cohort. Thromb Haemost 1998;80:607–609.
19. Coller BS, Owen J, Jesty J, et al. Deficiency of plasma protein S, protein C, or antithrombin III and arterial thrombosis. Arteriosclerosis 1987;7:456–462.
20. Bajzar L, Nesheim M, Morser J, Tracy PB. Both cellular and soluble forms of thrombomodulin inhibit fibrinolysis by potentiating the activation of thrombin-activable fibrinolysis inhibitor. J Biol Chem 1998;273:2792–2798.
21. Broze GJ Jr, Miletich JP. Characterization of the inhibition of tissue factor in serum. Blood 1987;69:150–155.
22. Rapaport SI. The extrinsic pathway inhibitor: a regulator of tissue factor-dependent blood coagulation. Thromb Haemost 1991;66:6–15.
23. Huang ZF, Higuchi D, Lasky N, Broze GJ Jr. Tissue factor pathway inhibitor gene disruption produces intrauterine lethality in mice. Blood 1997;90:944–951.
24. Rosenberg RD. Biochemistry of heparin antithrombin interactions, and the physiologic role of this natural anticoagulant mechanism. Am J Med 1989;87:2S–9S.
25. Thompson SG, Fechtrup C, Squire E, et al. Antithrombin III and fibrinogen as predictors of cardiac events in patients with angina pectoris. Arterioscler Thromb Vasc Biol 1996;16:357–362.
26. Geppert A, Graf S, Beckmann R, et al. Concentration of endogenous tPA antigen in coronary artery disease: relation to thrombotic events, aspirin treatment, hyperlipidemia, and multivessel disease. Arterioscler Thromb Vasc Biol 1998; 18:1634–1642.
27. Zhu Y, Carmeliet P, Fay WP. Plasminogen activator inhibitor-1 is a major determinant of arterial thrombolysis resistance. Circulation 1999;99:3050–3055.
28. Cushman M, Lemaitre RN, Kuller LH, et al. Fibrinolytic activation markers predict myocardial infarction in the elderly. The Cardiovascular Health Study. Arterioscler Thromb Vasc Biol 1999;19:493–498.
29. Rosendaal FR, Varekamp I, Smit C, et al. Mortality and causes of death in Dutch haemophiliacs, 1973–1986. Br J Haematol 1989;71:71–76.
30. Salomon O, Steinberg DM, Dardik R, et al. Inherited factor XI deficiency confers no protection against acute myocardial infarction. J Thromb Haemost 2003;1:658–661.
31. Zeldis SM, Nemerson Y, Pitlick FA, Lentz TL. Tissue factor (thromboplastin): localization to plasma membranes by peroxidase-conjugated antibodies. Science 1972;175:766–768.
32. Wilcox JN, Smith KM, Schwartz SM, Gordon D. Localization of tissue factor in the normal vessel wall and in the atherosclerotic plaque. Proc Natl Acad Sci USA 1989;86:2839–2843.
33. Thiruvikraman SV, Guha A, Roboz J, et al. In situ localization of tissue factor in human atherosclerotic plaques by binding of digoxigenin-labeled factors VIIa and X. Lab Invest 1996;75:451–461.
34. Annex BH, Denning SM, Channon KM, et al. Differential expression of tissue factor protein in directional atherectomy specimens from patients with stable and unstable coronary syndromes. Circulation 1995;91:619–622.
35. Marmur JD, Thiruvikraman SV, Fyfe BS, et al. Identification of active tissue factor in human coronary atheroma. Circulation 1996;94:1226–1232.
36. Giesen PL, Rauch U, Bohrmann B, et al. Blood-borne tissue factor: another view of thrombosis. Proc Natl Acad Sci USA 1999;96:2311–2315.
37. Maynard JR, Heckman CA, Pitlick FA, Nemerson Y. Association of tissue factor activity with the surface of cultured cells. J Clin Invest 1975;55:814–824.
38. Bach R, Rifkin DB. Expression of tissue factor procoagulant activity: regulation by cytosolic calcium. Proc Natl Acad Sci USA 1990;87:6995–6999.

39. Le DT, Rapaport SI, Rao LV. Relations between factor VIIa binding and expression of factor VIIa/tissue factor catalytic activity on cell surfaces. J Biol Chem 1992;267:15,447–15,454.
40. Schecter AD, Giesen PL, Taby O, et al. Tissue factor expression in human arterial smooth muscle cells. TF is present in three cellular pools after growth factor stimulation. J Clin Invest 1997;100:2276–2285.
41. Bach RR, Moldow CF. Mechanism of tissue factor activation on HL-60 cells. Blood 1997;89:3270–3276.
42. Carrozza JP Jr, Baim DS. Complications of directional coronary atherectomy: incidence, causes, and management. Am J Cardiol 1993;72:47E–54E.
43. Losordo DW, Rosenfield K, Pieczek A, et al. How does angioplasty work? Serial analysis of human iliac arteries using intravascular ultrasound. Circulation 1992;86:1845–1858.
44. Nath FC, Muller DW, Ellis SG, et al. Thrombosis of a flexible coil coronary stent: frequency, predictors and clinical outcome. J Am Coll Cardiol 1993;21:622–627.
45. Marmur JD, Rossikhina M, Guha A, et al. Tissue factor is rapidly induced in arterial smooth muscle after balloon injury. J Clin Invest 1993;91:2253–2259.
46. Pawashe AB, Golino P, Ambrosio G, et al. A monoclonal antibody against rabbit tissue factor inhibits thrombus formation in stenotic injured rabbit carotid arteries. Circ Res 1994;74:56–63.
47. Speidel CM, Eisenberg PR, Ruf W, et al. Tissue factor mediates prolonged procoagulant activity on the luminal surface of balloon-injured aortas in rabbits. Circulation 1995;92:3323–3330.
48. Speidel CM, Thornton JD, Meng YY, et al. Procoagulant activity on injured arteries and associated thrombi is mediated primarily by the complex of tissue factor and factor VIIa. Coron Artery Dis 1996;7:57–62.
49. Gertz SD, Fallon JT, Gallo R, et al. Hirudin reduces tissue factor expression in neointima after balloon injury in rabbit femoral and porcine coronary arteries. Circulation 1998;98:580–587.

RECOMMENDED READING

Belting M, Dorrell MI, Sandgren S, et al. Regulation of angiogenesis by tissue factor cytoplasmic domain signaling. Nat Med 2004;10:502–509.
Bogdanov VY, Balasubramanian V, Hathcock J, et al. Alternatively spliced human tissue factor: a circulating, soluble, thrombogenic protein. Nat Med 2003;9:458–462.
Degen JL. Genetic interactions between the coagulation and fibrinolytic systems. Thromb Haemost 2001;86:130–137.
Mackman N. The role of the tissue factor-thrombin pathway in cardiac ischemia-reperfusion injury. Semin Vasc Med 2003; 3:193–198.
Mackman N. Role of tissue factor in hemostasis, thrombosis, and vascular development. Arterioscler Thromb Vasc Biol 2004;24:1015–1022.
Ruf W, Dorfleutner A, Riewald M. Specificity of coagulation factor signaling. J Thromb Haemost 2003;1:1495–1503.

III EXAMINATION AND INVESTIGATION OF THE PATIENT

6

The Medical History
and Symptoms of Heart Disease

H. J. C. Swan, MD, PhD*

INTRODUCTION

The medical history and physical examination provide the most fundamental information regarding personal health and the need for specific medical care. It is the purpose of this chapter, first, to restate and underscore the objective of the taking of a medical history in general, and then to consider the nature of complaints that may be associated with cardiovascular disease in the adult patient. Specific symptom profiles and presentations are best discussed in association with specific clinical entities, including the chapters on ischemic heart disease, acute myocardial infarction, and congestive heart failure. Symptoms related to congenital malformations with associated cardiac lesions, including "failure to thrive," cyanosis, and heart failure in the neonate will not be considered in this chapter. The principal symptoms are summarized in tables, followed by a short comment on general issues. The onset and severity of a principal complaint may dominate the initial history taking, and relief of distressing symptoms becomes a first priority. However, it is then essential to return to obtain a complete and comprehensive medical and cardiac history. Because of the overall primacy of atherosclerosis *(1,2)* as a cause of vascular and heart disease, specific inquiries must be made to include a risk evaluation for atherosclerosis, not only for the coronary arteries but also for the aorta and its principal branches. (The factors currently deemed most important are listed in Table 1.) Gender offers no specific protection, as heart disease is the most frequent cause of death in women although later in life than men. Women are equally prone to congenital and rheumatic heart disease, arrythmias, and the less common diseases such as cardiac tumor.

The medical history gives the physician the ability to define the more likely diagnoses, and to achieve a level of confidence sufficient to allow logical action—additional testing, treatment, optimal management decisions, including reassurance, and lifestyle modification. Each conceptual step must be a "what if" and "if–then" form of clinical reasoning. However, more advanced testing strategies must follow, and not precede, a careful consideration of the initial history, the physical examination, electrocardiogram, chest X-ray, and basic blood and urine testing. A physician who claims to be "objective" with an intellectual, or strictly academic, approach may not meet a fundamental emotional need of the individual patient. In his epic "The Ballad of Reading Gaol" *(3)*, Oscar Wilde wrote: "Something was dead in each of us, and what was dead was hope," that never-to-be-forgotten or ever-to-be-ignored yearning of each and every person. Many years ago, the famed surgeon, William James Mayo of Rochester, Minnesota, characterized his fellow doctors: "One meets with many men who have been fine students, and have stood high in their classes, who have had great knowledge of medicine but very little wisdom in its application. They have mastered the science and have failed in their understanding of the human being" *(4)*.

---

*Jeremy Swan died before the publication of this edition. He was a giant of cardiology, and a gracious and generous friend.

From: *Essential Cardiology: Principles and Practice, 2nd Ed.*
Edited by: C. Rosendorff © Humana Press Inc., Totowa, NJ

Table 1
Atherosclerosis Risk

Age and gender
Past cardiovascular events
  Stable angina pectoris, unstable angina, acute myocardial infarction, revascularization procedures,
  prior testing for ischemia, previous emergency room visit for chest pain, positive family history of
  premature cardiovascular events (history of a major cardiovascular event in a first-degree relative,
  by age 50 yr for males and 55 yr for females)
Present symptoms and medications
  Chest discomfort/pain requiring antianginal medications
  Blood pressure requiring antihypertensive medications
  Familial hyperlipidemia
Conventional metabolic and endocrinological factors
  Blood lipids, elevated LDL-C, low HDL-C, elevated triglycerides
  Elevated blood glucose, and glucose intolerance
  Thyroid status, menopausal status
  Body weight, obesity
Personal habits
  Cigarette smoking—never, former, current, how many?
  Dietary composition
  Activity level—sedentary, ordinarily active, exercise program
  Alcohol usage—for how long, how much
Personality profile
  Socioeconomic status
  Psychosocial, familial, and occupational stress and coping

THE HISTORY *(5)*

The fundamental objective of this encounter is to initiate a process of interaction and confidence-building between patient and physician. The purpose is to include the most likely possible causes of complaint, along with other aspects relevant to the patient's well-being. History-taking is far more an art than a science *(6)*. It is an exercise in unstructured probabilistics, and should be so regarded. In all this, the opportunity to establish a sense of trust and confidence between physician and patient is paramount. After all, it is the patient who has "hired" you, not the contrary. As Claude Bennett put it, "the good doctor becomes a friend and resource for his patient in regard to family, suffering, aging and dying" *(7)*. In a commentary, "Humility and the Practice of Medicine," James Li suggests that the overconfident physician who believes that medical science and technology are sufficient subordinates the patient-physician relationship. Competency, concern, compassion, and caring are the hallmark of best medical practice, but there is a place for the honest "I don't know," tactfully put *(8)*.

Initial Presentation

The history-taking in a "first visit" patient is a vital part of the practice of medicine and of its subspecialties, including cardiology. Clearly, medical history-taking differs for an initial elective, a follow-up, a "consultation," or the emergent presentation of a patient. In a "first visit" the physician will assess the general health of the patient and develop impressions as to educational and intellectual background and thus the accuracy and credibility of the patient's "story." The attitudinal, social, and emotional makeup of the patient is clarified by nonverbal as well as verbal communication. At the same time, the prudent patient will assess not only the physician's professional competence but also his or her communicative ability to address the patient's needs and concerns appropriately. While personalities and attitudes differ widely among patients and physicians, every patient must feel that the physician is "on my side."

The Complaint

A complaint is defined as "an expression of discontent, regret, pain, censure, resentment, or grief" *(9)*. Each of these elements enters into the complaint and thus into the analysis of symptoms. However, the fundamental objective remains: to effect reductions or enhancements of the probability or possibility of a specific organic or functional cause for the complaint. "The nature of man is best understood by the company he keeps." So it is with the medical history. The commitment of appropriate time for an initial history is essential. The patient expects to be listened to, and his or her concerns respected and understood. A careful and complete history is the shortcut to appropriate additional testing and the defense against waste of resources. Specific complaints must be considered against the background and demography of the patient, if their significance is to be analyzed effectively. The initial history for any patient must include and record with accuracy the elements of age, gender, racial origin, education, occupation, socioeconomic status, family status, and physical activities.

The noncardiovascular history must be incorporated since many complaints commonly associated with cardiovascular disease may be due to other disorders—for example, dyspnea in emphysema and bronchitis, or ankle edema in patients with renal insufficiency, obesity, or venous varicosities. A detailed inquiry into past and current medication must be made. All medications taken by the patient must be listed. From time to time patients referred for a "cardiology" consultation feel that medications for other noncardiovascular complaints may not be relevant and therefore these may go unreported. Likewise, the family history requires careful exploration, since, in the US, many patients are far removed from their place of origin. A spouse or other family member may provide unexpected information—for example, a history of prior premature heart disease or death in genetically related individuals. In regard to specifics of complaints in cardiovascular disease, consideration centered only on the chief complaint of the patient is likely to result in significant error. Observation of nonverbal communication between spouses may be a useful guide to future compliance with recommended treatment. In all these matters, a physician's behavior influences a patient's response. Patients who suspect or are suspected of heart disease come with a sense of uncertainty or even fear. The simple open-ended questions, "Tell me how you feel" and "How can I help you?" are important, as they imply physician concern, invite the patient to express himself or herself in a personal way, and then allow the physician to inquire further concerning the complaint. While every effort must be made not to "lead the patient," it is essential to understand the intrinsic limitations of the patient's understanding of medical questions, necessitating specific direct inquiry. A good example is the heart failure patient who no longer complains of shortness of breath because his activity level has now been reduced to a degree appropriate to his residual ventricular function. It is a useful exercise to "live through a day" with the patient by a brief verbal "diary" of his or her activities and attitudes. A knowledge of the issues that disturb or please the patient assists in the overall assessment. It also provides information concerning physical activity. In patients with existing disabilities, the impact of emotional, social, and functional limitations in matters large and small have become the continued living experience of the patient. In many, prior testing for heart disease may have been done, including exercise stress testing, angiography, cardiovascular intervention procedures, and vascular scanning, including estimation of the state of the carotid and systemic arteries. Tests for the presence of coronary calcification are now available and increasingly common, and may be the precipitating reason for a patient visit. Each test should be documented with care and entered in the medical record. Whenever possible, original copies of such reports must be obtained.

Follow-Up, Emergent, and Consulting Visits

While the initial visit provides the bedrock of understanding, the circumstances of presentation determine the nature and purpose of the later medical history. Follow-up visits are usually structured to document responses to treatment, since in an effective practice, an accurate prior profile should exist and should be available for comparison. The physician time commitment of an initial visit may not be required. A careful record of current medications and laboratory and other test results may be made by a specialty nurse and, when appropriate, reported to the patient. But such a visit is always worth a "How are you doing?" from the physician, with a specific inquiry as to changes in a principal complaint, a new event, new test results, or response to medication. Emergent visits assume the availability of at least a minimum of prior information; usually the issues at hand are specific. When patient survival is in question, the obtaining of full historical details will, of necessity, be deferred. In contrast, a formal consultation requires a clearly defined purpose—diagnosis, management, procedure, and reassurance. Here the interview establishes, in great detail and with precision, the nature and significance of complaints, and the relation of physical examination and other data relevant to an optimal strategy.

Questionnaires, Nurse Practitioners, and Physician Extenders

The history taking may be facilitated by a questionnaire, which is best sent to a patient several days before a first visit. A questionnaire raises important general issues in a patient's mind and provides opportunity for unhurried thought and discussion with family members. Also, it promotes the careful completion of essential demographics, the inclusion of secondary complaints, and a considered review by the patient and spouse of family and past histories and medications. A trained physician assistant may review the responses and obtain clarification when necessary. The interview must be unhurried, with the patient receiving sufficient time for self-expression and for clarifications of uncertainties in his or her own mind. Because accurate and specific information is required and patients may be unfamiliar with symptoms and their significance, direct inquiry is usually necessary. Patients feel (properly) unsatisfied if the duration of the initial consultation is such that many of their concerns go unassessed and unanswered. There may be important advantages if a spouse or family member is involved in an initial interview, or at least be present for the physician's summation and recommendations. When physicians interview a patient, absent a spouse, symptoms and other important information may go unreported. On the other hand, the presence of a spouse may inhibit an open interview with some patients. Elements of family history may be denied or forgotten and the interspousal and personal dynamics, possibly relevant to future management and compliance, will become evident. Also, in elderly patients, a younger party may provide a more accurate reporting of specific complaints. This is even more essential for patients whose primary language is not that of the physician. While an interpreter may translate, the actual meaning of the words can be confused. An experienced physician assistant or nurse practitioner can inform a patient of the findings, but the conclusion of an initial interview is best addressed directly by the physician —and always when conducted by consulting subspecialists. The needs of the poor and underserved pose a major challenge to providers, and require innovative approaches. The important and expanding role of nurse practitioners in primary care, follow-up, and extended caregiving is predicated on the confidence of the patient regarding a "team support" approach embedded in prompt physician participation.

The Medical Record

Clinical information and its meaning are subject to scrutiny regarding their accuracy, precision, variability, sensitivity, and specificity (11). In this respect the veracity of the medical record is paramount. To record is "to set down in writing of the like, as to the purpose of presenting evidence" (12). This definition implies that the facts be described accurately and be complete, inclusive, and, when proper, available to and understandable by persons of similar backgrounds to the originator of the record. Also, the record should be readily available when required for a specific purpose. Current medical records seldom fulfill these criteria, are usually incomplete, not easily available, frequently handwritten, and many times only partially legible. This is a particular problem with emergency room reports, which may be a critical part of the admission or call for an immediate cardiac consultation. In legal disputes, a physician may be required to read his or her notes into the court record to allow for reasonable interpretation by counsel or by other physicians. It

Table 2
Symptoms Associated With Cardiovascular Disease

Pain (in the chest and elsewhere)
Dyspnea on effort, orthopnea, paroxysmal nocturnal dyspnea
Fatigue on exertion, at rest
Embolic manifestations
Complaints related to systemic disorders with a possible cardiovascular cause or relationship

is essential that this serious deficiency of record completeness and legibility be corrected, as an accurate record is vital to the provision of both immediate and long-term medical care. Desktop and handheld automated devices now exist for the effective collection of diagnostic information of all sorts, including a detailed medical history. Thus reliable, computerized patient records have been successfully introduced into hospital-based and office-based services, and a variety of software packages are available. These provide a computerized and totally integrated record system, which includes notes, order entry, laboratory, and other data, and lists of medications. Some also include drug interactions, risk analyses, and clinical guidelines. There are also some excellent physician dictation systems. While these all offer great advantages with respect to legibility, accessibility, and integration, it should be recognized that some physicians believe that the computer is a greater obstruction to easy physician-patient interaction than are pen and paper. This is changing rapidly as the enormous benefits of computerized patient record systems become better known.

After the History

An effective history is followed by the inclusion of other factual observations, including the findings on physical examination, the standard 12-lead electrocardiogram, the chest X-ray, and basic laboratory data, including a blood lipid panel and blood glucose. Each of these contributes to the ongoing process of qualitative, unstructured probabilistics relative to a specific anatomic or functional diagnosis. Physicians must recognize the intrinsic reality of such a process, and apply scientific reasoning whenever possible. This will allow conclusions as to appropriate areas for further investigation, in order to improve or cast doubt on the direction of diagnostic inquiry. In particular, such an analytic approach usually allows a physician to exclude the least probable causes and to proceed logically to a correct diagnosis.

CARDIAC SYMPTOMS

The principal symptoms associated with cardiovascular disorders are listed in Table 2. Each will be considered briefly regarding relevant causation. Also, it is essential to distinguish between the far more frequent noncardiac and the far more serious cardiac causations. Symptoms associated with heart disease are frequently activity-related, as in angina pectoris and heart failure and certain dysrhythmias. But a particular symptom, or its absence, may serve to favor certain possibilities over others.

Chest Pain or "Discomfort in the Chest"

The principal causes of chest pain are listed in Table 3. Table 4 lists the characteristics of chest pain that should be recorded. Chest pain is one of the most frequent symptoms leading to a visit to a physician or cardiologist. It is the most common, and possibly the most important, symptom associated with heart disease, yet it is neither highly sensitive nor specific for a specific diagnosis. Chest pain may range from brief, transient, mild discomfort to continuous, excruciating pain. In general, the more severe the pain, the greater is the likelihood of important underlying pathology.

Table 3
Causes of "Discomfort in the Chest"

Chest Wall
    Cervical/thoracic spine osteoarthritis
    Intervertebral disk disease
    Intercostal neuritis
    Rib fracture
    Costochrondritis
    Herpes zoster
Intrathoracic—Cardiovascular
    Vascular
        Aortic dissection
        Pulmonary hypertension
    Myocardial
        Stable angina pectoris
        Unstable angina
        Prolonged myocardial ischemia
        Acute myocardial infarction
    Pericardial
        Acute, subacute pericarditis
        Malignancy
    Other
        Mitral valve prolapse
        Hypertrophic cardiomyopathy
Intrathoracic—Pulmonary
    Acute pneumothorax
    Pleurisy and pleural effusion
    Pneumonia
    Pulmonary embolism
Referred from other organs
    Gastroesophageal reflux
    Esophagitis and esophageal spasm
    Peptic ulcer disease
    Pancreatitis
    Gall bladder disease

Table 4
Characteristics of "Discomfort in the Chest"

Intensity: severity, continuous/discontinuous, easing/worsening
Quality: visceral, superficial, pressure, crushing, stabbing, burning, tearing
Location: retrosternal, suprasternal, epigastric
Referral to: chest wall, back, right shoulder, right arm, both arms, jaw, occiput, head, epigastric, right, left subcostal, abdominal
Onset: sudden, gradual, precipitating cause (if any)
Worsened by: activity, breathing, position
Associated with: anxiety, coughing, dyspnea, nausea, vomiting, diarrhea, sweating, pallor, cold extremities, abnormal heart rate

CARDIAC ISCHEMIA

Although many forms of heart disease are associated with discomfort in the chest, by far the most important is that due to coronary atherosclerosis. Ischemic pain is the sensation caused by an imbalance between available oxygen supply and the metabolic demand of working myocardium. The afferent pathway is complex and the resulting symptoms also are complex and variable in regard to intensity, location, and radiation. Is the pain continuous or intermittent?

The "onset" characteristics may be defining. Transient substernal chest discomfort or discomfort on activity or climbing stairs, excitement, anxiety, postprandial, or cold, favor angina pectoris. Fever, tachycardia, or anemia may precipitate "new" angina or worsen existing angina. In general, the pain of angina pectoris recurs at a repeatable level of activity or emotional stress, rapidly regresses when the activity ceases, and is reproducible under comparable circumstances. The duration of effort-related angina is usually short and self-limited, and described as "pressure," "constrictions," "squeezing," and "unlike anything I have ever experienced." Severe unrelenting pain is suggestive of ongoing severe myocardial ischemia and acute myocardial infarction. Intermittent recurrent pain may be associated with stable or unstable angina pectoris. Other qualitative descriptors of angina pectoris include "new," "accelerated," "progressive," "preinfarction," and "nocturnal."

An "angina equivalent" refers to dyspnea as an alternative symptom that occurs under similar circumstances to common angina pectoris. Stable angina occurs predictably following a certain and constant level of exercise. "Unstable angina" includes angina of new onset (less than 1 mo), symptoms increasing in severity, frequency, and intensity, precipitated by less exercise load than before, or changing pattern of radiation, without enzymatic evidence of infarction. This entity is due to partial and transient thrombotic occlusion of a diseased vessel and may progress to a completed infarction.

LOCATION AND RADIATION

Ischemic chest pain is usually substernal with varying radiation patterns, the most common of which is into the left shoulder and the ulnar aspect of the left arm. Pain is usually perceived as pressing, constricting, and heavy, frequently associated with activity but not necessarily so. Although classically centrally located pain characterizes ischemia, pain may be solely in the neck and jaw, left shoulder or left arm, and may not radiate. Atypical distribution patterns are not unusual and include the right chest alone and the epigastrium without radiation to the neck or arms. However, in a high-risk individual, e.g., a male 60 yr of age or older, the presence of any chest pain raises a possibility of underlying coronary disease. Other causes of chest pain—the acute tearing of aortic dissection or aneurysm and pain associated with respiration as in acute pneumothorax, pleurisy, pneumonia, pericarditis, or pulmonary embolus—may be identified on the basis of their specific characteristics. The initial pain of aortic dissection may be described as "the worst possible," and may be located in or radiate to the back. Pleuritic chest pain is worsened on inspiration or coughing. The severity and duration of pain are useful indicators, with rapid relief in angina pectoris; more prolonged, yet with relief in unstable angina; and persistent and perhaps increasing with acute infarction. The association of nausea, vomiting, sweating, and anxiety with chest pain is suggestive of evolving myocardial infarction. Angina at rest is usually caused by severe prolonged myocardial ischemia, may be spontaneous, and often occurs at night, waking the patient from sleep. Chest pain associated with nausea, vomiting, palpitations, a feeling of weakness, and fear is common in acute infarction.

NONCARDIAC CHEST PAIN

Pain secondary to peptic ulcer, gall bladder disease, gastric reflux, and esophagitis, as well as spinal disease and costochondritis, is much more frequent than cardiac chest pain. In these conditions pain may be spontaneous, may be related to meals associated with recumbency (reflux), and may be relieved by antacids or by food itself. The pain and discomfort of esophageal spasm may be relieved by nitroglycerin. Chest pain associated with ingestion of food, swallowing, coughing, and position changes is less likely to be of cardiac origin. Musculoskeletal pain, if variable, differs in location and severity, and is worsened by respiration, other movements and localized pressure. Attention to simple demographics (age, gender, prior history) will usually, but not always, serve to clarify the complaint. Even though, for example, acute infarction is uncommon in younger women, the assumption "it could not be" has resulted in tragic outcomes. Ischemia should always be considered in older patients reporting new-onset chest pain. The key in differential diagnosis is an awareness of such possibilities, but in many cases a diagnosis as to causation can be established with confidence based on history alone. Anxiety (which frequently is justified) can color the symptom presentation. Pain due to pneumothorax, pleurisy, pneumonia, or pulmonary embolism is worsened on inspiration, and patients will minimize the effort of breathing with unilateral chest splinting. Pain of pulmonary origin, in general, does not radiate and is localized to one side or the other and is seldom substernal. The discomfort associated with other forms of heart diseases—mitral valve prolapse, pulmonary hypertension, and hypertrophic cardiomyopathy—is usually not sufficient to cause severe distress. Functional chest pain associated with fear of heart disease or due to an anxiety state is usually described as acute, sharp, and stabbing, and frequently located to the cardiac apex. At times, it is associated with hyperventilation, but is not usually exercise-related. However, it may subside relatively rapidly.

Factors associated with relief of pain are all important. Relief with cessation of activity and nitroglycerin suggest angina pectoris. Worsening or an unchanged level of pain under those circumstances is consistent with unstable angina or myocardial infarction, or with aortic dissection. Acute pericarditis may be relieved by leaning forward. In brief, any complaint that includes chest pain is deserving of careful interrogation and analysis.

Dyspnea

Dyspnea is defined as an uncomfortable awareness of the necessity of breathing. It is a common symptom in both cardiac and pulmonary disorders, as well as a reaction to anxiety. It is frequently associated with an increase in pulmonary venous pressure. The principal causes are listed in Table 5.

Dyspnea, in and of itself, is not abnormal, as this symptom is universal at several levels of exercise, including treadmill testing, and even trained athletes may experience it. However, an awareness of an abnormal need for breathing under conditions of mild or moderate exertion or at rest is significant. Acute-onset dyspnea is usually of pulmonary cause—for example, acute pneumothorax, pleurisy, pneumonia, or pulmonary embolus—but may also be a major, early feature of an extensive myocardial infarction, acute valve regurgitation, and pericarditis. The dyspnea of congestive heart failure is experienced at decreasing levels of external work, and finally, under resting conditions. Dyspnea may be associated with cardiac causes for chest pain. A prior history of smoking or other disorders, including recurrent chest infections, bronchitis and emphysema, congestive heart failure, and the associated presence of acute myocardial infarction serve to define the cause of this symptom. Again, relief of dyspnea should occur when the precipitating cause is removed or alleviated. Several factors contributing to dyspnea include deconditioning and obesity, as well as fever, tachycardia, or anemia. Of interest, anxiety-induced hyperventilation is commonly misinterpreted as dyspnea.

Orthopnea indicates a severe level of dyspnea in which the patient is unable to lie flat and must sit in an upright position. Paroxysmal nocturnal dyspnea is usually associated with chronic heart failure. Beginning shortly after sleeping flat, it is relieved by attaining the upright position. The common mechanism is an increase in pulmonary venous pressure due to mitral valve disease or left ventricular dysfunction. Acute pulmonary edema is an expression of pulmonary venous hypertension with transudation of large quantities of fluid into the alveoli, precipitating severe coughing with expectoration of frothy fluid that may be blood-stained. "Functional" dyspnea often occurs at rest and is associated with apical stabbing or prolonged chest-wall pains.

Fatigue

This is a transient weariness during exertion, due to an imbalance between the metabolic demands of working skeletal muscle and the availability of blood flow to deliver oxygen and remove products of muscle metabolism. The symptom may be due to deconditioning, as in prolonged bed rest, or the presenting symptom in anemia of any causation. When cardiac output is reduced from any cause and cannot increase, the response to skeletal muscle metabolic demand during activity cannot be

Table 5
Causes of Dyspnea

Pulmonary Disease
  Acute
    Spontaneous pneumothorax
    Pulmonary embolus
    Pneumonia
    Airway obstruction
  Subacute
    Chronic obstructive lung disease
    Emphysema
    Pulmonary fibrosis
    Chronic bronchitis
    Bronchiectasis
Cardiac Disease
  Acute
    Pulmonary edema
    Aortic/mitral valve insufficiency
    Prosthetic valve dysfunction
    Left atrial thrombus
    Left atrial myxoma
  Subacute
    Heart failure
    Myocardial infarction
    Pericardial effusion
    Constrictive pericarditis
Other Causes
    Intrathoracic malignancies
    Rib fracture, chest trauma
    Anxiety state
    Hyperventilation

met. The presence of obstructive vascular disease also limits the availability of blood flow and is a common cause of limb fatigue and of intermittent claudication.

Palpitations

This is an awareness of an unusual beating of the heart. Palpitations are common and may be benign or indicative of important heart disease. In general, the term refers to an awareness of an irregularity of the heartbeat. A patient also may be aware of either severe tachycardia or bradycardia, and the associated symptoms of lightheadedness or even syncope. As with the other symptoms of heart disease, the nature of the occurrence, precipitating and continuing factors, and the prior medical history are vital. The underlying causes of palpitations include ectopic beats, transient atrial fibrillation, and heart block. A sudden onset or offset favors paroxysmal atrial tachycardia or atrial flutter/fibrillation. "Flip-flops" favor premature ventricular contractions. A moderate unexplained increased in heart rate may favor an anxiety state. Again, the influence of other factors including fever, anemia, or hyperthyroidism must be considered.

Syncope

Syncope is defined as a loss of consciousness due to underperfusion of the brain. It may be due heart block, or in response to ventricular flutter or fibrillation. Syncope following effort occurs

Table 6
Other Conditions and Symptoms Associated With Heart Disease

General Symptoms of Infection—fever, sweating, malaise
   Rheumatic fever
   Infective endocarditis
   Atrial myxoma
General Manifestations of Connective Tissue Diseases
   Systemic lupus erythematosus
   Scleroderma
   Polymyositis
   Polyarteritis nodosa
   Muscular dystrophies
   Progressive, myotonic, Freidrich's ataxia
Embolic disorders
   Cerebral
      Hemiparesis
      Transient/persistent visual disorder
Manifestations of septic emboli occurring in:
   Skin, digits, nail beds, spleen, kidney, limbs

in association with aortic stenosis, but also in patients with hypertrophic cardiomyopathy and pulmonary hypertension. The differential diagnosis includes the common faint (vasovagal attack) and seizure disorders. This is discussed fully in Chapter 18.

Other Symptoms

Other symptoms of heart and vascular disease are listed in Table 6. Although these associations may not be frequent in regard to the specific symptom, such a possibility is important to consider. Embolic stroke always requires a search for an intracardiac source, particularly atrial fibrillation and infective endocarditis, but also in patients post-myocardial infarction or with carotid artery disease. Embolic sources include left atrium, left ventricle, mitral and aortic valves, and the aorta and carotid arteries. Paradoxical embolism occurs by way of a patent foramen ovale.

Systemic findings of fever, rigors, and tachycardia associated with a new or changing murmur suggest infective endocarditis, but also may be due to rheumatic fever or atrial myxoma. Cardiac involvement may occur in a number of systemic disorders, including rheumatoid arthritis, lupus erythematosus, and scleroderma. Hematologic disorders affecting the heart include polycythemia vera, sickle cell anemia, and thalassemia. Cardiac involvement is common in cancer patients as a group. Acute leukemia, malignant melanoma, and Hodgkin's disease are frequent causes of cardiac symptoms, as are interthoracic malignancies, in particular bronchogenic carcinoma and metastatic breast disease. Infiltrative disorders of the myocardium include amyloidosis and hemochromatosis.

CONCLUSION

The evaluation of the complaints of any patient reduces to a form of detection, a "who done it." The astute clinician considers the medical history "the primary evidence" and then seek new clues—"forensic tests" and the like. Perhaps he or she revisits "the scene of the crime" with a second interview: "I did not understand how your father died. Please tell me." We all rely on probabilistic or likelihood considerations, structured or unstructured, intuitive, instinctive, or scientifically derived. Nevertheless, the taking of a medical history is somewhat of an art—a learned experience. It is application of a true "uncertainty principle"—inexactitudes in action. Yet from the patient's perspective, "the verdict"—a solution to a specific issue, "the complaint"—is the purpose. This also is basic to our purpose as physicians and as to whether or not our derived conclusions are correct and our recommended treatments effective. But that is not the only outcome to be fostered. It also should be the basis for a continuing interaction between doctor and patient so as to result in a net gain in individual personal health, which is the fundamental purpose of medical practice.

REFERENCES

1. Wilson PWF, D'Agostino RB, Levy D, et al. Prediction of coronary heart disease using risk factor categories. Circulation 1998;97:1837–1847.
2. American College of Cardiology 27th Bethesda Conference. Matching the intensity of risk factor management with the hazard for coronary disease. J Amer Coll Cardiol 1996;27:958–1047.
3. Wilde O. The balade of Reading Gaol. The Works of Oscar Wilde. The Wordsworth Poetry Library, Hants, Ware, UK, 1994, pp. 136–152.
4. Mayo WJ. Aphorism # 78. In: Willius FW, ed. Aphorisms, 2nd ed. Rochester MN, Mayo Foundation, 1990, p. 67.
5. Swartz MH. The art of interviewing. In: Textbook of Physical Diagnosis, History and Examination, 3rd ed. W. B. Saunders, Philadelphia, 1998, pp. 1–81.
6. Smith LH Jr. Medicine as an art. In: Cecil's Textbook of Medicine. W. B. Saunders, Philadelphia, 1992, pp. 6–9.
7. Bennett JC. The social responsibilities and humanistic qualities of "the good doctor." In: Cecil's Textbook of Medicine. W. B. Saunders, Philadelphia, 1992, pp. 2–6.
8. Li JTC. Humility and the practice of medicine. Mayo Clin Proc 1999;74:529–530.
9. Webster's College Dictionary. Random House, New York, 1992.

RECOMMENDED READING

Bickley LS, Szilagyi PG. Bates' Guide to Physical Examination, 8th ed. Lippincott, Philadelphia, 2003.
Meador CK. A Little Book of Doctors' Rules. Hanley and Belfus, Philadelphia, 1992.
Swartz MH. Textbook of Physical Diagnosis, History and Examination, 3rd ed. W. B. Saunders, Philadelphia, 1998.
Seidel HM, ed. Mosby's Guide to Physical Examination, 5th ed. Mosby, St. Louis, 2003.
RA Gross. Making Medical Decisions. An Approach to Clinical Decision Making American College of Physicians-American Society of Internal Medicine, Philadelphia, 1999.

7

Physical Examination of the Heart and Circulation

Jonathan Abrams, MD

CARDIAC EXAMINATION

The examination of the heart and circulation has a long and rich tradition in clinical medicine. Most of the cardinal signs of cardiovascular disease detectable on the physical examination were described and documented by master physicians during the 19th and early 20th centuries. Subsequently, echocardiography and cardiac catheterization have demonstrated that the presumed pathogenesis of many to most cardiovascular abnormalities on the physical examination were accurately and presciently described before these modern techniques became available. In the past, generations of internists and cardiologists were well trained in the skills of cardiac examination; the absence of our current ultrasound technology providing "immediate" answers contributed to the emphasis of expertise in cardiac physical diagnosis. Unfortunately, clinical skills in this area are no longer emphasized in medical education, in part due to the burgeoning of other aspects of medical science that must be taught in the medical student curriculum. The advent of readily available two-dimensional echocardiography has clearly contributed to the demise of cardiac physical diagnosis capability among physicians, a phenomenon well documented in recent published studies.

This chapter will highlight the core components of the cardiac physical examination, and will focus on a practical assessment of the heart and circulation in health and disease. The author's assumption is that the reader will already possess a basic knowledge of one cardiac exam and structural heart disease. It is hoped that physicians will redouble their efforts in applying the well-known components of the cardiac examination to their patients. The rewards are many—in particular, a feeling of real satisfaction in making a diagnosis of organic heart disease with one's hands and ears.

Limitation of the Cardiac Examination

Echocardiography has clearly demonstrated that much cardiovascular disease is not detectable or accurately quantifiable, even to the expert, on the physical examination. For instance, mitral and aortic regurgitation are often missed; left ventricular function may be significantly depressed without a detectable abnormality on examination. Thus, it is best to consider the physical examination and the echo as complementary. For the experienced clinician, the findings on the cardiac exam often predict what will be noted on the echo. Nevertheless, if significant heart disease is suspected, a complete 2-D echo-Doppler examination is often indicated. Conversely, with a negative cardiac physical examination in the setting of a normal electrocardiogram, an echo can be avoided in many instances.

The Cardiac Exam

The components of the cardiac physical examination are standard (Table 1). As with the more general physical examination, physicians are urged to conduct the cardiac exam in a systematic

From: *Essential Cardiology: Principles and Practice, 2nd Ed.*
Edited by: C. Rosendorff © Humana Press Inc., Totowa, NJ

Table 1
Cardiac Pysical Examination

Overall assessment of the patient
    General features, e.g., dyspnea, cyanosis, edema
    Special features, e.g., unusual facies, lipid deposits
Blood pressure
    Supine, upright
    Leg pressure (if coarctation suspected)
Arterial pulses
    Contour, volume
Precordial motion
    LV apex impulse (PMI)
    RV activity
    Ectopic impulses
    Thrills (loud murmur)
Heart Sounds
    Characteristics of S_1, S_2
    Is an S_3 or S_4 present?
    Ejection or nonejection clicks
    Opening snap
Heart Murmurs
    Systolic
    Diastolic
    Continuous
    Timing in cardiac cycle
    Quality
    Length
    Radiation

Table 2
Blood Pressure and Peripheral Arterial Examination Clues to Cardiovascular Disease

Coarctation of aorta	Hypertension in upper extremities; brachial–femoral delay
Aortic regurgitation	Wide pulse pressure with increased systolic and decreased diastolic pressure
	Increased volume, rate of rise of arterial pulses with exaggerated collapse
Pulsus or mechanical alternans	Beat-to-to beat alternation in peak pressure and pulse volume (detect by palpation, not cuff)
Pulsus paradoxus	Exaggerated inspiratory decline (>10 mmHg) in peak systolic pressure measured carefully by cuff; palpation may pick up if severe
Hypertension	Elevated systolic and diastolic pressure; increased systolic pressure with normal diastolic (isolated systolic hypertension of the elderly)

and sequential fashion. After a general assessment of the patient, the arterial pulses and pressure and venous pulsations are evaluated, followed by careful inspection and palpation of the precordium. Auscultation is the last but most important component of the cardiac exam.

EVALUATION OF ARTERIAL PULSE

An accurate determination of arterial pressure is part of the cardiac physical examination. Careful attention to the details of the technique of taking blood pressure are important. Abnormalities of blood pressure are not usually a component of structural heart disease except in selected instances (Table 2). Assessment of the severity of aortic regurgitation or detection of pulsus paradoxus are two situations in which the blood pressure can provide important information.

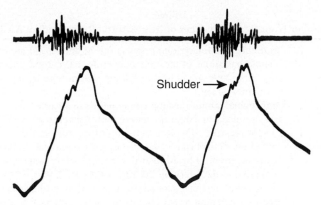

Fig. 1. The arterial pulse in aortic stenosis. Note the delayed upstroke and the jagged contour representing a palpable shudder or transmitted thrill. The pulse volume is usually decreased as well.

The Examination

The physician must become familiar with the normal volume and rate of rise of the arterial pulse. In general, the carotid artery is the only artery that should be utilized for detection of cardiovascular abnormalities. Because of delay of transmission of the pulse wave in the periphery, as well as the distal decrease in arterial diameter, assessment of the radial or brachial arterial pulses usually is of little value (except in the assessment of pulsus alternans, pulsus paradoxus, and cardiogenic shock). In hypertensive patients, simultaneous assessment of the brachial and femoral arterial pulses is useful to rule out a significant coarctation of the aorta. In such cases, the femoral peak of the pulse wave peak will *clearly follow* the palpable brachial artery impulse; a delay indicates a probable obstruction in the aorta.

The contour of the aortic pulse is important in the assessment of aortic valve disease. *Aortic stenosis* characteristically produces a small volume, late peaking, or delayed carotid upstroke, often with a palpable shudder or thrill (anacrotic notch, transmitted murmur) (*see* Fig. 1). Remember that in the healthy older subject, decreased compliance and increased arterial stiffness typically result in an increase in the arterial pulse amplitude as well as the pulse pressure. This can readily mask the typical abnormalities of aortic stenosis. Aortic regurgitation, when significant (e.g., 2+/4), typically results in an arterial pulse with an increased amplitude and rate of rise and a collapsing quality. In severe aortic regurgitation, the aortic pulsations are abnormal throughout the arterial system (*see* Table 3). A prominent (often visible), high-amplitude, full-volume carotid arterial pulse, coupled with a wide pulse pressure (diastolic blood pressure 60 mmHg) is highly suggestive of severe aortic regurgitation. A double peaking or bisferiens pulse is common in advanced aortic regurgitation (Fig. 2).

PULSUS PARADOXUS

A greater-than-normal difference in systolic blood pressure between inspiration and expiration is known as pulsus paradoxus. This is common whenever there are major fluctuations of intrathoracic pressure or in pericardial tamponade. *Careful palpation and auscultation is mandatory to detect significant pulsus paradoxus (>10 mmHg).* Normally, there is a slight physiologic respiratory difference between inspiration and expiration, typically 6 to 8 mmHg or less during quiet respiration. Pulsus paradoxus may be detected in severe congestive heart failure, decompensated chronic obstructive lung disease, asthma, and in an occasional very obese individual.

PULSUS ALTERNANS

In setting of severe left ventricular systolic dysfunction, beat-to-beat alteration in the peak amplitude of the arterial pulse may be noted (Fig. 3). This can be palpated in the brachial or radial

Table 3
Peripheral or Nonauscultatory Signs of Severe Aortic Regurgitation: A Glossary

Bisferiens pulse	A double or bifid systolic impulse felt in the carotid arterial pulse.
Corrigan's sign	Visible pulsations of the supraclavicular and carotid arteries.
Pistol shot of Traube	A loud systolic sound heard with the stethoscope lightly placed over a femoral artery.
Palmar click	A palpable, abrupt flushing of the palms in systole.
Quincke's pulse	Exaggerated sequential reddening and blanching of the fingernail beds when light pressure is applied to the tip of the fingernail. A similar effect can be induced by pressing a glass slide to the lips.
Duroziez's sign	A to-and-fro bruit heard over the femoral artery when light pressure is applied to the artery by the edge of the stethoscope head. This bruit is caused by the exaggerated reversal of flow in diastole.
DeMusset's sign	Visible oscillation or bobbing of the head with each heartbeat.
Hill's sign	Abnormal accentuation of leg systolic blood pressure, with popliteal pressure 40 mmHg or higher than brachial artery pressure.
Water-hammer pulse	The high-amplitude, abruptly collapsing pulse of aortic regurgitation. (This term refers to a popular Victorian toy producing a slapping impact on being turned over.)
Miller's sign	Visible pulsations of the uvula.

arteries. This phenomenon, usually undetected, is most likely to be associated with a left ventricular heave and third heart sound. Careful palpation of the radial artery is recommended.

Determination of pulsus paradoxus and/or mechanical pulsus alternans are two exceptions to the rule of always using the carotid arteries for arterial pulse analysis. Table 2 lists the conditions where arterial pulse wave analysis is particularly valuable.

EVALUATION OF VENOUS PULSE

Most physicians do a poor job of the venous examination and many are intimidated by the presumed difficulty in assessment of the jugular venous pulse (JVP). The following key points should help make the JVP examination straightforward:

1. The A wave (produced by right atrial contraction) is normally larger or taller than the V wave in normal subjects. Expect to visualize a dominant A wave in most instances (Fig. 4).
2. Conditions of decreased right ventricular compliance, such as right ventricular hypertrophy or pulmonary disease, may augment the A wave amplitude and prominence, particularly the setting of pulmonary hypertension.
3. Detection of the A wave is easy if one remembers that it immediately precedes the palpable carotid arterial pulse (one must use simultaneous inspection and palpation of the carotid upstroke). Conversely, the V wave of the jugular venous pulse occurs simultaneous with the carotid upstroke (systolic in timing).
4. When the V wave is the predominant wave form and is greater than the A wave (in the absence of atrial fibrillation), it is likely that significant tricuspid regurgitation is present even in the absence of a typical murmur of tricuspid regurgitation.
5. Mean jugular pressure is relatively easy to measure (Fig. 5). It is most important to determine if the mean venous pressure is normal or elevated; quantification of the precise degree of venous pressure elevation is less important, although this can be often accomplished.

Dr. Gordon Ewy has emphasized the use of abdominal or hepatic compression to bring out latent or borderline elevation of the jugular venous pressure, which may be important to assess if a volume overload state or heart failure is suspected. The technique is simple and employs steady

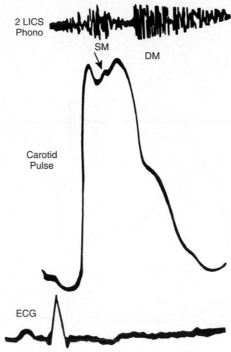

Fig. 2. Bisferiens pulse of aortic regurgitation. Note the bifid systolic pulse wave, which is best detected using light finger pressure over the carotid arteries. This contour is usually associated with an increased pulse volume. The bisferiens pulse must be differentiated from a transmitted systolic murmur or palpable thrill. Note the soft S_1 and S_2. SM, systolic murmur; DM, diastolic murmur; 2 LIC, 2nd left intercostal space.

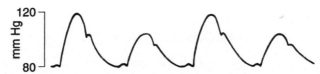

Fig. 3. Pulsus alternans. Note that every other beat has a lower systolic pressure. The rate of rise of the second pulse wave is slower, relating to decreased contractile force in alternate beats. Pulsus alternans is an important sign of severe left ventricular dysfunction. It is best detected in a peripheral vessel, such as the radial artery. Heart sounds and murmurs may also alternate in intensity.

pressure with the hand over the upper abdomen for 60 s while carefully observing the jugular venous pulsations. The normal response is a brief rise and a decline in the mean jugular venous pressure. An abnormal test consists of progressive and sustained rise in the mean venous pressure for up to 1 min.

Remember that abnormalities of the venous contour or pressure reflect right heart events. While it is true that left heart disease, particular left ventricular failure, is the most common cause of right ventricular failure, *an increased level of venous pressure does not necessarily imply left ventricular systolic failure*. Fluid or volume overload in the setting of normal cardiac function, left ventricular diastolic dysfunction, pulmonary hypertension, severe tricuspid regurgitation, or isolated right heart failure (cor pulmonale) can all produce an increase in jugular venous pressure in the absence of left ventricular pathology. Nevertheless, an increased jugular venous pressure is one of the hallmarks of congestive heart failure, usually a left heart problem in adults.

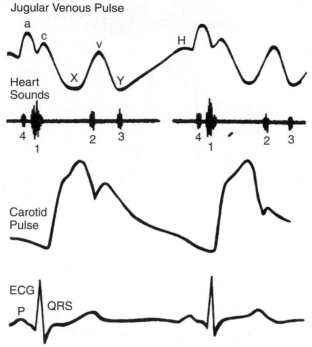

Jugular Venous Pulse

Fig. 4. Normal jugular venous pulse. Note the biphasic venous waveform with a large A wave immediately preceding the carotid arterial upstroke and roughly coinciding with S_1, and a smaller V wave that peaks almost coincident with S_2. The jugular X descent occurs during systole and in some individuals may be quite prominent. The Y descent occurs during early diastole; the nadir of the Y descent times with S_3. The C wave and H wave are not visible to the eye but are often recordable in venous pulse tracings.

PRECORDIAL MOTION

Left Ventricle

By far the most important aspect of inspection and palpation of the heart is a determination as to whether the left ventricle is grossly normal or abnormal. Left ventricular hypertrophy and dilation are the commonest causes of an abnormal PMI (point of maximal impulse—an old-fashioned term that is still useful), also known as the left ventricular apical impulse. The normal left ventricle is felt over a small area (<3 cm), not displaced beyond the midclavicular line, not sustained into late systole, and not hyperdynamic (Table 4, Fig. 6). Often, the left ventricle is not palpable in the supine position; the examiner must then ask the patient to turn onto the left side with the left arm elevated for optimal assessment of the precordium (Fig. 7). Commonly, the left ventricular impulse will then become apparent in this position, although not always. Older subjects (>50 years of age), those with large chests, prominent musculature or obesity, or large breasts, all have a decreased likelihood of a detectable the PMI.

Abnormalities of the apical impulse are listed in Table 5. Palpable third and fourth heart sounds are more commonly present than physicians realize (particularly in the left lateral position), and represent important findings suggesting abnormal left ventricular size, function, or compliance. In coronary artery disease, an ectopic or bifid (double) left ventricular impulse is related to dyskinesis/akinesis caused by a prior myocardial infarction. A palpable S_4 is an important observation in aortic valve disease (suggesting severe aortic stenosis or regurgitation), as well as coronary artery disease (suggesting decreased LV compliance).

A meticulous search for the impulse can be quite rewarding, and may suggest increased LV size or LV hypertrophy with high specificity. Absence of an abnormal left ventricular impulse in a thin

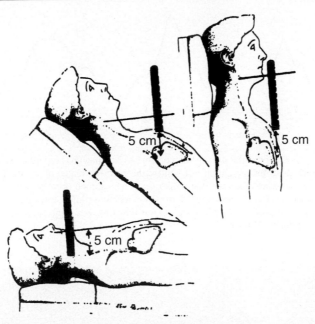

Fig. 5. Estimation of mean venous pressure. The right atrium is approximately 5 cm below the sternal angle of Louis with the subject in any body position. Thus with a patient supine or erect, the height of the venous pulsations from the sternal angle can be measured; by adding 5 cm to this value, one can estimate the actual venous pressure. The thorax and neck should be positioned until the peak of the venous column is readily identified. In subjects with a normal venous pressure, only the peaks of the A and V waves may be seen when the patient is sitting up at 45 degrees or greater; the neck veins are often in this position. When the venous pressure is abnormally high, the thorax and head must be elevated in order to accurately identify the true peak of the venous column.

Table 4
Normal Supine Apical Impulse

A gentle, nonsustained tap
Early systolic anterior motion that ends before the last third of systole
Located within 10 cm of the midsternal line in the fourth or fifth left intercostal space
A palpable area <2 to 2.5 cm^2 and detectable in only one intercostal space
Right ventricular motion normally not palpable
Diastolic events normally not palpable
May be completely absent in older persons

individual is useful in *excluding* significant aortic stenosis, hypertrophic cardiomyopathy, or severe mitral regurgitation in an individual with a prominent systolic murmur.

Right Ventricle

Right ventricular activity is not usually detectable in normal subjects, except in young or thin individuals where a gentle parasternal impulse may be found. Technique is important in the detection of a right ventricular impulse; firm pressure over the lower parasternal region is the key, with the hand held in end-expiration (Fig. 8). The examining hand should be observed for an upward or anterior motion, which can be quite subtle. Subxiphoid palpation with two or three fingers may be employed in patients with a large chest or chronic obstructive pulmonary disease (COPD).

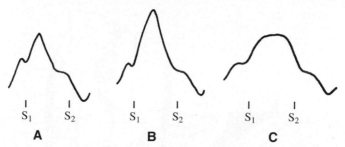

Fig. 6. Major variants of left ventricular precordial motion. (**A**) Normal. (**B**) Hyperdynamic. (**C**) Sustained. With the patient in the supine position, sustained left ventricular activity detectable in the latter half of systole is distinctly abnormal. Some experts believe that palpation of a sustained impulse when patients are in the left lateral decubitus position may have less specificity for underlying left ventricular enlargement. (Adapted from Abrams J. Precordial palpation. In: Horwitz LD, Groves BM, eds. Signs and Symptoms of Cardiology. J. B. Lippincott, Philadelphia, 1985.)

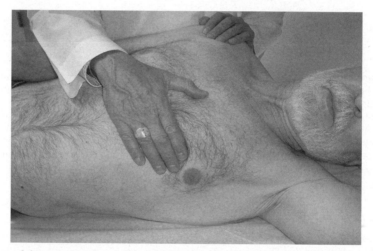

Fig. 7. Palpation of the apex impulse, left lateral decubitus position. This maneuver should be used in any patient with suspected left ventricular disease. The patient should be turned 45 to 60 degrees onto the left side with the left arm extended above the head.

Table 5
Causes of Palpable Precordial Abnormalities

Left ventricular hypertrophy and/or dilation
Left ventricular wall motion abnormalities (fixed or transient)
Increased force of left atrial contraction (palpable S_4)
Accentuated diastolic rapid filling (palpable S_3)
Anterior thrust of the heart from severe mitral regurgitation
Right ventricular hypertrophy and/or dilation
Loud murmurs (thrills)
Loud heart sounds (normal and abnormal)
Dilated or hyperkinetic pulmonary artery
Dilated aorta

Detection of right ventricular hypertrophy generally implies pulmonary hypertension in an adult. Severe mitral regurgitation can occasionally result in a recoil phenomenon related to left atrial expansion, with the regurgitant jet of blood "pushing" the heart forward.

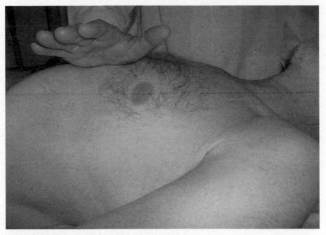

Fig. 8. Precordial palpation for detection of parasternal or right ventricular activity. Use firm downward pressure with the heel of the had while the patient's breath is held in end-expiration.

Palpable Heart Sounds

The experienced examiner is familiar with palpable heart sounds that can be felt with the hand or fingers as discrete deflections. Thus, a loud S_1, S_2, or opening snap are often palpable. An S_3 or S_4 may be detectable in the left lateral position. For instance, mitral stenosis can be strongly suspected solely by detection of a palpable S_1, opening snap, diastolic apical thrill, and a right ventricular lift.

HEART SOUNDS

Normal and Abnormal

Abrupt intracardiac pressure changes and the subsequent valve motion related to alterations hemodynamic are responsible for most normal and abnormal heart sounds. Thus, closure of the A-V and semilunar valves (S_1, S_2) and the opening motion of thickened and noncompliant aortic and mitral valve leaflets (aortic ejection click, mitral opening snap) produce commonly heard sounds. The S_3 and S_4 are due to left ventricular filling transients produced by left atrial contraction (S_4) and passive left ventricular inflow after mitral valve opening (S_3). These sounds are low-frequency and dull, and are best heard with the bell of the stethoscope (light pressure) with the patient in the left lateral position. Conversely, the first and second heart sounds, aortic and pulmonary ejection clicks and opening snap, are high-frequency, and best heard with the diaphragm of the stethoscope (firm pressure).

First Heart Sound (S_1)

The S_1 is directly related to vibrations of the A-V valves and myocardium produced by A-V closure and in general has little diagnostic usefulness. A loud S_1 is common in mitral stenosis and in individuals with a short PR interval. A soft S_1 is common in individuals with decreased left ventricular systolic function or first-degree AV block.

Second Heart Sound (S_2)

Although assessment of respiratory movement and intensity of the two components of S_2 is a well-emphasized aspect of auscultation, for practical purposes, analysis of S_2 is helpful in relatively few conditions (Table 6). The physician should focus on the relative intensity of aortic and pulmonary components (A_2, P_2) and the possible presence of reversed or paradoxic splitting, characterized by inspiratory narrowing and expiratory widening of the two components of S_2. Paradoxic

Table 6
Assessment of Second Heart Sound (S$_2$): A Practical Approach

Character[a]	Significance
Abnormalities of respiratory variation	
Wide splitting, inspiratory increase	Right ventricular conduction delay (e.g., incomplete or
in A$_2$–P$_2$ interval	total right bundle branch block—important clue)
	Idiopathic dilation of pulmonary artery
	Small atrial septal defect (unusual)
	Pulmonic stenosis
Wide splitting, fixed A$_2$–P$_2$ interval	Atrial septal defect (important clue)
Single S$_2$	Often normal in older patients
	Aortic stenosis
	Mild left ventricular conduction delay
	Severe pulmonary hypertension
	(A$_2$ "masked")
Reversed or paradoxical splitting	Left bundle branch block (important clue)
	Left ventricular systolic dysfunction (important in acute
	ischemia)
Abnormalities of intensity	
Loud A$_2$	Dilated aorta
	Hypertension
	Tetralogy of Fallot
Loud P$_2$	Pulmonary hypertension (important clue)
	Atrial septal defect
	Dilated pulmonary artery
Soft A$_2$	Aortic sclerosis or stenosis
	Hypotension
Soft P$_2$	Pulmonic stenosis

[a]The physician must differentiate between decreased intensity of *all* cardiac sounds vs a *selective* decrease in the loudness of A$_2$ or P$_2$.

splitting is an important clue to an underlying left bundle branch block or significant aortic stenosis in a patient with a systolic ejection murmur. A loud P$_2$, particularly when P$_2$ is louder than A$_2$ at the base and apex, is predictive of significant pulmonary hypertension.

Third Heart Sound (S$_3$)

The low-pitched early diastolic third heart sound can be a normal finding or a significant cardiovascular abnormality. The S$_3$ is most easily heard by turning the patient into the left lateral position, identifying the apex impulse with a finger, and carefully applying the bell of the stethoscope with light pressure (Fig. 7).

Fourth Heart Sound (S$_4$)

The atrial sound or S$_4$ is caused by augmentation of late LV diastolic filling resulting from left atrial contraction. Audibility is correlated with increased left ventricular stiffness or decreased compliance; thus, S$_4$ is a useful finding in hypertension, or coronary artery disease, where its presence suggests increased LV end-diastolic pressure and/or LV hypertrophy. The S$_4$ (and S$_3$) may be palpable. The S$_4$ is felt as a *presystolic* outward thrust just before the palpable LV impulse, and is noted as a double early systolic left ventricular impulse. It is important to use the left lateral position for optimal detection by palpation or auscultation of both the S$_3$ and S$_4$ (Fig. 7).

Ejection Sounds

These are high-frequency, discrete audible sounds that occur immediately after S$_1$ (Fig. 9). They are usually caused by stiff or malformed semilunar leaflets, such as a bicuspid aortic valve,

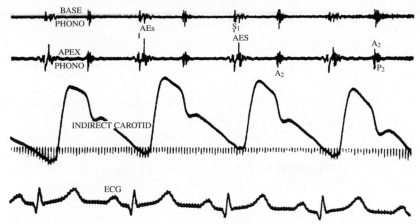

Fig. 9. Aortic ejection sound. This phonocardiogram and carotid arterial pulse tracing demonstrates a prominent, discrete aortic ejection sound that is better heard and recorded at the apex than at the base. This is characteristic of aortic ejection sounds or clicks. Note the prominent separation of the ejection sound from S_1 by approx 40 to 50 ms. (Adapted from Shaver JA, Griff FW, Leonard JJ. Ejection sounds of left-sided origin. In: Leon DF, Shaver JA, eds. Physiologic Principles of Heart Sounds and Murmurs. American Heart Association Monograph No. 46, 1975.)

or a valvar pulmonic stenosis. Importantly, ejection sounds may be detected in the setting of a dilated great vessel (aorta or pulmonary artery), particularly if systolic pressure is elevated. An isolated ejection sound or click in a patient with or without a systolic ejection murmur suggests a congenitally deformed aortic valve, typically biscuspid.

HEART MURMURS

Physicians are more knowledgeable about heart murmurs than about any other aspect of the cardiac physical examination. Nevertheless, recent studies confirm that physician skills in cardiac auscultation are poor, probably worse than in earlier decades. The widespread availability and utilization of two-dimensional echocardiography certainly is a significant factor relating to this decline in expertise. In addition, the teaching of the cardiac physical examination in medical schools takes up an increasingly limited amount of the curriculum.

Murmurs are a result of turbulence of blood flow; thus, systolic murmurs are by far the most common and are related to ejection of blood across the aortic and pulmonic valves in the normal or structurally abnormal heart. Abnormal similar valves frequently produce systolic ejection murmurs that must be differentiated from functional or flow murmurs. Mitral valve incompetence with regurgitation of blood into the left or right atrium commonly produces audible cardiac sound. Thus, a systolic murmur may be normal or abnormal. On the other hand, all diastolic murmurs are abnormal, as there is no physiologic explanation for normal flow of sufficient turbulence during diastole to produce a heart murmur.

Classification of Murmurs (Fig. 10)

SYSTOLIC MURMUR

The classic heart murmur is a systolic ejection murmur, characterized by a crescendo contour and a gap between the end of audible sound and S_2. This sound-free period represents the critical distinction from a regurgitant systolic murmur, in which sound continues up to S_2 (holosystolic, pansystolic) (Fig. 11). Distinguishing between the two is not always possible, even by an expert in cardiac physical diagnosis. Nevertheless, the large majority of systolic murmurs can be identified correctly by a careful cardiac examination.

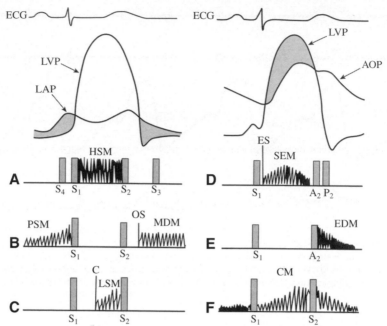

Fig. 10. Intracardiac pressures and heart murmurs of the major cardiac valve abnormalities. *See* text for discussion of specific murmurs. LVP, left ventricular pressure; LAP, left atrial pressure; AOP, aortic pressure; HSM, holosystolic murmur; PSM, presystolic murmur; OS, opening snap; MDM, mid-diastolic murmur; C, mid-systolic click; LSM + late systolic murmur; ES, ejection sound; SEM, systolic ejection murmur; EDM, early diastolic murmur; CM, continuous murmur. (Adapted from Crawford MH, O'Rourke RA. A systematic approach to the bedside differentiation of cardiac murmurs and abnormal sound. Curr Prob Cardiol 1979;1:1.)

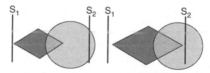

Fig. 11. Importance of late systole in evaluation of systolic murmurs. It is essential to assess the last part of systole to determine whether a murmur is ejection in nature or is holosystolic. On the left, an early peaking murmur ends before the last third of systole. This is the rule in functional murmurs or with mild semilunar valve stenosis. On the right, a long ejection murmur is shown, which peaks later in systole. Sound vibrations extend to S_2, suggesting severe obstruction to ventricular outflow. In severe semilunar valve stenosis, the vibrations may extend beyond S_2.

The *functional heart murmur*, also known as an *innocent* or *physiologic murmur*, is usually not very loud (grade 1–2 intensity), is best heard at or near the base of the heart, and is unassociated with other cardiac abnormalities. It is thought that functional murmurs are related to normal turbulent blood flow across semilunar valves. Thus, anxiety, fever, anemia, excitement, pregnancy, or exercise can all accentuate murmur intensity. Younger individuals (children, teens, young adults) commonly have innocent or functional systolic murmurs.

DIASTOLIC MURMUR

The most common audible diastolic murmur is the blowing or high-pitched decrescendo murmur of aortic regurgitation (Fig. 2). This can be difficult to hear and should be sought out by the clinician. Examination in a quiet room with the subject sitting up and leaning forward with the

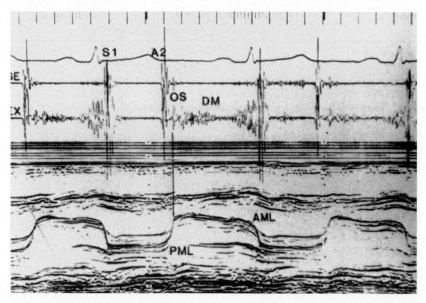

Fig. 12. Echocardiographic correlates of the loud first sound and opening snap in mitral stenosis. S_1 is produced by mitral valve closure and is accentuated and delayed due to elevation of left atrial pressure and the loss of valve compliance. A prominent presystolic diastolic murmur merges with S_1; this represents augmented transmitral flow with left atrial contraction. The opening snap (OS) times precisely with the maximum opening excursion of the anterior leaflet of the mitral valve and is produced by tensing of the valve cusps during early diastole. Left ventricular filling and the resultant early to mid-diastolic murmur (DM) follows the OS. (From Reddy PS, Salerni R, Shaver JA. Normal and abnormal heart sounds in cardiac diagnosis. Part II. Diastolic sound. Curr Prog Cardiol 1985;10:1.)

breath held in end-expiration will enhance detection of these murmurs, which can be quite soft and are typically high-frequency. Thus, the inexperienced or distracted physician will often miss a grade 1–2 aortic regurgitation murmur. Furthermore, echocardiography confirms that mild to moderate aortic regurgitation is often silent to examination.

Mitral stenosis produces with a diastolic murmur, which is different from the murmur of aortic regurgitation. The classic "mitral rumble" is low-frequency, begins after the early diastolic opening snap, and is often heard *only* at the cardiac apex in the left lateral position (Fig. 12).

CONTINUOUS MURMUR

These unusual murmurs are caused by late systolic flow and persistent blood flow from one cardiac chamber or great vessel to another after ventricular ejection has been completed. Thus, a continuous murmur typically is heard in late systole extending into diastole. These murmurs are often phasic in intensity and may be audible at sites away from the classic valve areas. Table 7 lists some of the more common continuous murmurs. The murmur of a patent ductus arteriosus is usually very loud and harsh, maximal at the upper left infraclavicular area and left scapular area. Aortic valve disease with both stenosis and regurgitation may simulate a continuous murmur, especially at fast heart rates.

CARDIAC PHYSICAL EXAMINATION
IN SPECIFIC CARDIOVASCULAR CONDITIONS

The cardinal physical findings in a variety of common cardiac syndromes and conditions are summarized below. It is important to recognize that typical or classic features of structural heart disease on examination are not always present. In many instances, atypical characteristics or no

Table 7
Common Causes of a Continuous Murmur[a]

Patient ductus arteriosus
Arteriovenous fistula, congenital or acquired, systemic or pulmonary
Ruptured aneurysm of the sinus of Valsalva (communication usually into right atrium or right ventricle)
Venous hum (innocent finding in children)
Anomalous origin of the coronary artery from the pulmonary artery
Coronary arteriovenous fistula
"Mammary soufflé" of pregnancy
Systemic arterial-pulmonary arterial collaterals or bronchial arterial collaterals in congenital defects
Coarctation of the aorta: coarctation site and/or collateral vessel flow

[a]Pseudocontinuous murmur suggests aortic stenosis and regurgitation.

specific features may be present (e.g., "silent" valve disease), resulting in considerable diagnostic confusion or error.

Congestive Heart Failure

Overt or decompensated heart failure is a very common clinical condition; the cardiac physical examination can confirm this diagnosis suggested by the patient's history. Importantly, the absence of features of heart failure on examination may suggest another etiology for the patient's complaints, such as chronic obstructive lung disease or pneumonia.

GENERAL APPEARANCE

The patient is often tachypneic and orthopneic, with lower extremity peripheral edema. Rales may be heard at the lung bases; percussion dullness and decreased breath sounds suggest pleural effusions.

JUGULAR VENOUS PULSE

Elevation of the mean venous pulse is the *sine qua non* of right heart failure. The A-wave may be prominent, suggesting right arterial (and right ventricular) pressure elevation (Fig. 4). Tricuspid regurgitation in subjects with heart failure is common and may produce a dominant systolic jugular V wave, typically seen simultaneous with the palpable carotid arterial upstroke (Fig. 13). A large systolic V wave is often present in heart failure, but is frequently missed by the examiner.

PRECORDIAL IMPULSE

The examiner should actively seek out an abnormally prominent LV impulse and/or a parasternal heave. Look for findings on the examination that confirm structural heart disease and/or cardiac enlargement. On occasion, an S_3 can be palpated in the left lateral position. In the presence of hypertensive heart disease or coronary artery disease, a hypertrophic or dilated LV may result in a prominent LV thrust. Displacement of the PMI leftward indicates LV enlargement. Remember, heart failure may be due to diastolic dysfunction (a stiff left ventricle with normal systolic function).

HEART SOUNDS

An S_4 or S_3 are common. The latter has adverse prognostic implications. Conversely, an S_4 (audible or palpable) indicates decreased LV compliance and LV hypertrophy. S_1 may be diminished in heart failure.

MURMURS

Mitral and tricuspid regurgitation are common in heart failure, but often these regurgitant murmurs are nondescript or inaudible. If congestive heart failure is due to an underlying valve lesion, specific features of that structural abnormality may be prominent. Remember that in the setting of heart failure due to decreased left ventricular systolic function, the murmur of severe

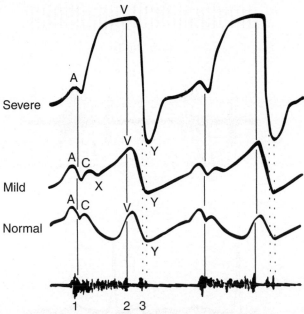

Fig. 13. The large V wave of tricuspid regurgitation. As reflux across the tricuspid wave increases in severity, the systolic V wave becomes higher as well as broader. The X descent disappears and the Y descent is progressively accentuated with increasing severity of tricuspid regurgitation. With severe tricuspid regurgitation, the systolic wave may be so dominant as to mimic the carotid arterial pulsations; the entire lower neck will swell with each right ventricular systole.

aortic regurgitation, aortic stenosis, or mitral regurgitation may be unimpressive or even inaudible, in spite of a major hemodynamic burden due to the valve lesion.

Coronary Artery Disease

Unless there is left ventricular damage from prior infarction or episodes of prior myocardial stunning and/or hibernation, the cardiac exam in patients with coronary disease is usually unremarkable. Signs of hypercholesterolemia should be sought, such as arcus senilus, xanthelasma, or tendon xanthomata. In patients with left ventricular dysfunction, an ectopic cardiac impulse or enlarged apical impulse may be noted. An S_4 is common, but this finding is not specific enough to be diagnostically helptful. A third heart sound may be heard, but only if severe LV dysfunction is present. Mitral regurgitation is common in patients with depressed systolic function; the late systolic murmur of papillary muscle dysfunction should be sought. It is important to examine all subjects with coronary heart disease in the left lateral position to "bring out" the left ventricular impulse as well as the third and fourth heart sounds (Fig. 7).

Mitral Stenosis

Mitral stenosis is easily identified by the experienced examiner but is usually missed by the inexperienced practitioner. The classic features include a very loud S_1, often palpable, as well as an increased P_2, and an early diastolic sound, the opening snap. The typical murmur of mitral stenosis is a mid-late diastolic, low-frequency "rumble," that is best (or only) heard at the left ventricular apex in the left lateral position (Fig. 10). A right ventricular lift is common; in pure mitral stenosis, the LV impulse is not abnormal and may be undetectable. Coexisting mitral regurgitation may confuse the auscultatory findings, usually producing an apical murmur that is typically holosystolic. Many physicians have difficulty assessing the timing of the acoustic events in mitral stenosis, confusing systole for diastole.

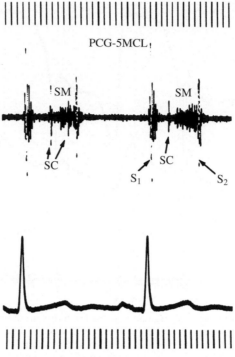

Fig. 14. The classic late systolic murmur of mitral valve prolapse. Note the crescendo configuration of the murmur, which begins in midsystole following the first systolic click. The frequency of this murmur is usually relatively pure. SM, systolic murmur; SC, systolic click. (Adapted from Delman AJ, Stein E. Dynamic cardiac auscultation and phonocardiography. W. B. Saunders, Philadelphia, 1979.)

Mitral Regurgitation

This lesion is ubiquitous and occurs in many forms. In longstanding severe mitral regurgitation, the left ventricle dilates. Thus, careful evaluation of the apical impulse is important, with the examiner seeking a left ventricular heave, palpable S_3, or apical systolic thrill. A right ventricular lift is common in chronic severe mitral regurgitation. The murmur of mitral regurgitation is typically holosystolic at the apex, but variants of the classic murmur can confuse the picture. Myxomatous mitral valve prolapse may produce a mid-late systolic murmur that can radiate to the aortic area in the setting of selective posterior leaflet prolapse. Mitral regurgitation murmur may be variable in intensity, particularly in the setting of left ventricular dysfunction; when mitral regurgitation is secondary to left ventricular disease, the murmur is loudest during the decompensated heart failure state. Conversely, organic mitral regurgitation murmurs are usually loudest after heart failure has been effectively treated and left ventricular function has improved.

MITRAL VALVE PROLAPSE

The cardinal features of mitral valve prolapse include a mid-late systolic murmur and one or more mid-late systolic clicks (Fig. 14). The latter may or may not be present, or can be variably heard from day to day. The clicks are often confusing to the uninitiated; they may be "close to the ear," quite high-frequency, sounding like extracardiac events. Typically the systolic murmur begins well after S_1 and may be variable in length and intensity, especially with specific maneuvers that alter left ventricular volume or systemic resistance (e.g., going from supine to upright position, squatting, Valsalva maneuver, sustained hand grip).

Aortic Stenosis

Classic features of valvar aortic stenosis include a small and slow-rising carotid arterial upstroke (Fig. 1); a left ventricular lift; a palpable S_4; a palpable basal systolic thrill; and a loud, often harsh systolic murmur at the aortic area radiating into the neck. The murmur of aortic stenosis is often more high-frequency and pure pitched at the apex (where it is often confused with mitral regurgitation). The length of the murmur is key; functional or aortic sclerosis murmurs are not very long and late-peaking; moderate to severe aortic stenosis murmurs typically take up much of systole and their peak intensity is later than normal. These murmurs can be quite harsh and grunting above the right clavicle, and usually radiate into the carotids.

HYPERTROPHIC CARDIOMYOPATHY

These patients have an extremely prominent left ventricular heave, a very loud and usually palpable fourth heart sound, and a loud, long systolic murmur that is best heard at the left sternal region and apex. The murmur classically changes with body position, Valsalva, or following post-ventricular contraction (PVC). The murmur often has characteristics of mitral regurgitation and aortic stenosis. The carotid upstrokes are brisk and not delayed. Experienced examiners should be able to differentiate valvular aortic stenosis from hypertrophic cardiomyopathy.

Aortic Regurgitation

The first clue to the recognition of significant aortic regurgitation is an abnormal carotid arterial pulse, characterized by a full-volume, high-amplitude impulse, often with a double or bisferiens contour (Fig. 2). Signs of left ventricular enlargement signify a major degree of regurgitation. A third heart sound is a poor prognostic finding. Fourth heart sounds are commonly heard. A high-frequency blowing decrescendo diastolic murmur beginning with S_2 is the typical finding in aortic regurgitation. This valve or aortic root lesion uncommonly produces a loud murmur.

Careful technique is necessary to hear the often-soft murmur of aortic regurgitation; the optimal patient position for examination is sitting up, leaning forward, with the breath held in end-expiration. An accompanying aortic systolic murmur is common.

RECOMMENDED READING

Roldan C, Abrams J. Evaluation of the Patient with Heart Disease: Integrating the Physical Exam and Echocardiography. Lippincott Williams & Wilkins, Philadelphia, 2002.

Abrams J. Synopsis of Cardiac Physical Diagnosis. Butterworth Heinemann, Boston, 2001.

Otto C. Valvular Heart Disease, W. B. Saunders, Philadelphia, 1999.

Don, Michael A. Auscultation of the Heart: A Cardiophonetic Approach. McGraw Hill, New York, 1998.

Criley J. Beyond Heart Sounds, vol. 1 (CD-ROM). Armus (www.armus.com), 2000.

8

Electrocardiography

Tara L. DiMino, MD, Alexander Ivanov, MD, James F. Burke, MD, and Peter R. Kowey, MD

INTRODUCTION

The electrocardiogram (ECG) records electric potential changes in the electrical field produced by the heart. Although it records only the *electrical* behavior of the heart, it can be used to identify numerous metabolic, hemodynamic, and anatomic changes. Electrocardiography is considered a gold standard for the diagnosis of arrhythmias (*see* Chapter 17). In this chapter, mostly nonarrhythmic ECG changes will be reviewed. Abbreviations and acronyms used in this chapter can be found in Table 1.

ECG LEADS

The standard 12-lead ECG traditionally consists of tracings obtained from the bipolar limb leads (I, II, and III), unipolar limb leads (aVR, aVL, and aVF), and usually six unipolar chest or precordial leads (V_1 through V_6). The *bipolar limb leads* I, II, and III register the potential differences between the right arm and left arm, the right arm and left leg, and the left arm and left leg, respectively. The axis of a bipolar lead is an imaginary vector directed from the electrode assumed to be negative to the electrode assumed to be positive (Fig. 1). To record *unipolar limb leads*, the above three extremities are connected to a central terminal used as the indifferent electrode. The exploring electrode (called positive) can then be placed on one of the three extremities to register the potentials transmitted to that particular limb. The letter V denotes a unipolar lead. The letters *R, L*, and *F* identify the right arm, left arm, and left leg (foot), respectively. The letter "*a*" means that the potential difference was electrically augmented (*1*). The axis of a unipolar lead is an imaginary vector directed from the indifferent electrode to the exploring (positive) electrode.

By combining the bipolar and unipolar limb leads, one may view the entire electrical picture of the heart in the frontal plane. With the heart at the center, this essentially creates a circle that is bisected by six imaginary vectors. These vectors, by the nature of their position, allow determination of the precise electrical axis of the heart. This information aids in the diagnosis of many conditions such as bundle branch block, improper lead placement, and axis shifts (Fig. 2).

Table 2 describes the placement of the precordial ECG leads, and Fig. 3 demonstrates their axes. When an exploring electrode is situated on the chest, it records potentials from that particular site on the chest wall. Typically, limb leads record electrical forces from the anatomic frontal plane, and precordial leads reflect potentials from the horizontal plane. Therefore, when approached as a whole, the ECG may provide an electrical map that corresponds to specific territories of the heart. For example, the inferior limb leads (II, III, and aVF) preferentially record the electrical activity from the inferior wall of the heart because of their proximity to that wall.

From: *Essential Cardiology: Principles and Practice, 2nd Ed.*
Edited by: C. Rosendorff © Humana Press Inc., Totowa, NJ

Table 1
Abbreviations and Acronyms

ARVD	Arrhythmogenic right ventricular dysplasia	LPFB	Left posterior fascicular block
		LV	Left ventricle
AV	Atrioventricular	LVH	Left ventricular hypertrophy
bpm	Beats per minute	MI	Myocardial infarction
CAD	Coronary artery disease	mm	Millimeter
cm	Centimeter	mV	Millivolt
CNS	Central nervous system	RAA	Right atrial abnormality
COPD	Chronic obstructive pulmonary disease	RBBB	Right bundle branch block
		RV	Right ventricle
ECG	Electrocardiogram	RVH	Right ventricular hypertrophy
ICS	Intercostal space	QTc	QT interval corrected for heart rate
LAA	Left atrial abnormality	SA	Sinoatrial
LAD	Left axis deviation	s	Second
LAFB	Left anterior fascicular block	VT	Ventricular tachycardia
LBBB	Left bundle branch block	WPW	Wolff-Parkinson-White syndrome

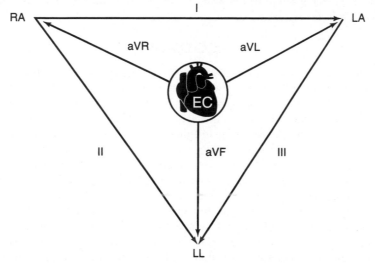

Fig. 1. Frontal lead axes. Leads I, II, and III are formed by connecting the right arm (RA) to the left arm (LA), the right arm to the left leg (LL), and LA to LL, respectively. Arrows indicate the axes of these leads in relation to the theoretical electrical center (EC) of the heart. The indifferent electrode of the unipolar system is obtained by connecting RA, LA, and LL into a central terminal.

GENERATION OF ECG TRACING

Before attempting to understand the electrical activity of the heart as an organ, one should appreciate its function on a cellular level (Fig. 4). A resting or polarized muscle strip is positively charged on the outside and negatively charged inside. Therefore, there is no potential difference along the uniformly charged surface of the resting muscle strip. Electrical activation at any given site of the strip produces depolarization. Depolarization causes a charge shift that results in a negative charge outside the depolarized portion of the membrane. During spread of the depolarization wave, a potential difference develops between already depolarized (negative) and still polarized (positive or resting) portions of the membrane. An electric current flows from the negatively charged (depolarized) portions of the membrane to the positively charged ones. This current may be represented by a dipole or vector.

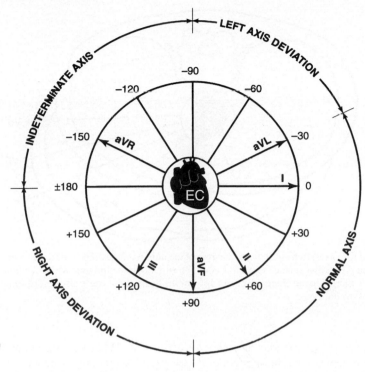

Fig. 2. The frontal plane hexaxial reference system. This represents the limb leads where axes are drawn with intersection at the electrical center (EC) of the heart. (Modified from refs. *1* and *11*.)

Table 2
Precordial Lead Placement

Name	Leads	Location
Septal	V_1–V_2	V_1 is in the fourth intercostal space (ICS) to the right of the sternum. V_2 is in the fourth ICS to the left of the sternum.
Anterior (transitional or mid-precordial)	V_3–V_4	V_3 is midway between V_2 and V_4. V_4 is in the fifth ICS at the midclavicular line.
Lateral	V_5–V_6	V_5 is at the anterior axillary line at the same horizontal level as V_4 (but not necessarily in the same ICS). V_6 is at the midaxillary line at the level of V_4.
Right-sided	V_1, V_2, V_3R, V_4R, V_5R, V_6R	The same as standard precordial but on the right side of the chest.

Depending on the anatomical position of the heart in the thorax, these leads may vary in which area they represent. For example, leads V_3 and V_4 may also represent potentials from the septum in a vertically oriented heart.

A vector moves along the muscle strip from the point of excitation, and it reflects the constantly changing electrical activity of the strip *(1)*. Vector size is directly proportional to the number of depolarized muscle strips. The magnitude and direction of these changes can be recorded as positive or negative deflections from the baseline of an ECG tracing. By convention, a positive deflection is recorded if the vector that is directed from the negative to the positive portion of the muscle strip points in the *same* direction as the axis of the recording lead. A negative deflection is recorded if the vector points in the direction *opposite* to the axis of the recording lead. No deflection is

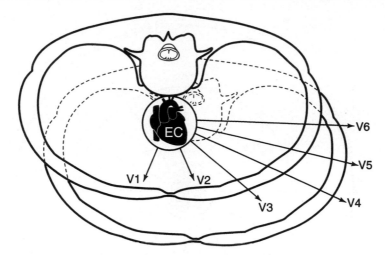

Fig. 3. Horizontal lead axes. Arrows indicate the axes of the unipolar leads. The indifferent electrode is obtained by connecting the precordial surface leads to a central terminal. Since the precordial electrodes are placed at different levels in relation to the electrical center (EC) of the heart, these leads also record some frontal vectors in addition to horizontal ones.

produced if the vector is perpendicular to the axis of the lead. At any given moment, the magnitude of the deflection depends on the strength of the electrical source; the distance from that source; and the cosine of the angle between the vector and the axis of the recording lead *(1)*.

Repolarization restores muscle cells to their resting state: negative intracellularly, positive extracellularly. During this process, a wave of positivity proceeds in the same direction as the original wave of depolarization. However, it has the opposite potential vector in reference to the recording lead. This occurs because positive potentials produced outside the membrane during repolarization spread from the site of *initial* depolarization toward the still depolarized portion of the membrane (Fig. 4). Thus, the net area of the deflection caused by repolarization equals the area of depolarization *(1)*.

In the intact ventricles, the subendocardial action potential normally lasts longer than the subepicardial. Therefore, repolarization proceeds from the subepicardium to the subendocardium in a direction approximately opposite to that of depolarization. In other words, since the subepicardium has a shorter action potential, it is ready to repolarize *before* the subendocardium. Consequently, the vector of repolarization has a direction more or less similar to that of the depolarization vector. The ECG deflections of depolarization and repolarization (represented by the QRS complex and T wave, respectively) therefore have the same polarity despite unequal shapes and areas under the curve. Furthermore, since the intact heart contains more than one muscle strip, the net ECG tracing reflects contributions of all such portions of the myocardium *(1)*.

In the thin-walled atria, action potential duration of the subendocardium and subepicardium are equal. The ECG deflections of depolarization and repolarization therefore have opposite polarities. The deflection of atrial *de*polarization is called the P wave. The wave of atrial *re*polarization is usually hidden within the large QRS complex of ventricular depolarization.

AXIS DETERMINATION

The amplitude of an ECG deflection, measured conventionally in millivolts, depends on the magnitude of the electrical source as well as the angle between the axis of the electrical vector and the axis of the recording lead. This means that the heart chamber with the most significant electrical contribution will produce the largest deflection, especially if the recording lead is very close

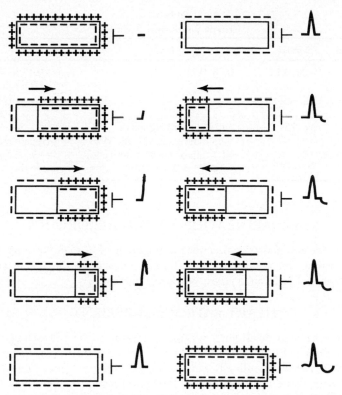

Fig. 4. Potential generated during depolarization (left vertical sequence) and repolarization (right vertical sequence) recorded with an exploring electrode located at one end of the muscle strip. (Modified from ref. *1.*)

to that chamber. A lead whose axis is most parallel to the electrical vector of the heart will record the largest ECG deflection. As illustrated in Fig. 2, the approximate spatial orientation of the lead axes is known. Therefore, by comparing the amplitude of deflections in different leads, one can infer the direction and amplitude of the electrical vector at any given moment.

Summation of *instantaneous* vectors of atrial or ventricular depolarization or repolarization over time is reflected by ECG deflections such as the P waves, QRS complexes, and T waves (*see* "Generation of ECG Tracing"). The direction of the *mean* vector of these deflections is called the *axis* of that deflection. The axis of a wave is easy to calculate; it can therefore be used in everyday practice to assess relative electrical contribution of the atria or ventricles throughout depolarization or repolarization. Relative contribution of the chambers to electrical events in the heart commonly changes in the presence of abnormalities of those chambers or of the metabolic, anatomic, or hemodynamic milieu of the body.

By convention, the axes of the P, QRS, and T waves are calculated using the *hexaxial system* of the frontal plane leads (Fig. 2). The following two rules are frequently utilized to calculate an electrical axis. First, the axis of an ECG deflection is perpendicular to the axis of the lead with the algebraic sum of deflections equaling zero (*isoelectric* complexes). Second, the axis is parallel to and has the same direction as the axis of the lead with the largest positive deflection. Combining these rules improves the accuracy of axis determination.

For axis determination, the *area* of the deflection is more important than the *amplitude*. The normal QRS axis is the frontal plane is −30 to +90 degrees. When the R wave equals the S wave in all three bipolar limb leads, the QRS axis is considered indeterminate. This relationship allows the ECG to provide useful information in many different clinical situations.

Table 3
Criteria for Normal P Wave

	Normal	RAA	LAA
Duration (s)	0.08–0.11	0.08–0.11	≥0.12 in leads II, III, aVF (morphology is notched) negative deflection $V_1 > 1$ mm and ≥0.04 s
Axis (degree)	0 to 75°	>+75° (rightward axis)	—
Amplitude (mm)	—	>2.5 mm in leads II, III, aVF >1.5 mm of positive deflection on V_1 or V_2	Negative deflection in $V_1 ≥ 1$ mm and ≥ 0.04 s

STANDARDIZATION OF ECG RECORDING

Most often, millimeters are used to describe the amplitude of ECG deflections. When potentials registered by the leads are recorded on paper, a 10-mm vertical deflection on the paper usually represents a 1-mV potential difference unless otherwise indicated.

HEART RATE MEASUREMENT

The heart rate can be easily determined by using several rules. The first assumes that the distance between two thick lines on ECG paper equals 0.5 cm, and the standard paper speed is 2.5 cm/s. If the distance between two consecutive R waves equals 0.5 cm (two thick lines), the heart rate is 300 bpm. If the distance is 1 cm, the heart rate is 150 bpm; 1.5 cm, 100 bpm; 2 cm, 75 bpm; 2.5 cm, 60 bpm; 3 cm, 50 bpm; 3.5 cm, 43 bpm; 5 cm, 30 bpm.

The above method is not accurate when the heart rhythm is irregular. To estimate the heart rate when the rhythm is irregular, the number of QRS complexes between the 3-s marks (7.5 cm apart) on the paper can be measured and multiplied by 20. This method is not accurate for slow heart rates.

P WAVE

Normal P Wave

Atrial depolarization begins within the SA node in the subendocardium and spreads through the right atrium, then to the interatrial septum, and then to the left atrium. Therefore, the mean vector of normal atrial depolarization is directed leftward and downward, producing a positive ECG deflection in the leads with the same axis (such as I and II). The vector of atrial repolarization, which is opposite to the vector of depolarization, produces an ECG deflection in the opposite direction (see "Generation of the ECG Tracing"). This small wave may be seen occasionally after the P wave in long PR interval when the QRS complex does not obscure it. Table 3 lists the criteria for the normal P wave.

Right Atrial Abnormality/Enlargement

Right atrial abnormality (RAA) implies RA hypertrophy, dilation, or primary intraatrial conduction abnormality (Table 3). In this situation, electrical forces of the RA, which is located anteriorly, rightward, and inferiorly to the LA, dominate forces of the LA.

Left Atrial Abnormality/Enlargement

Left atrial abnormality (LAA) implies LA hypertrophy, dilation, or primary intraatrial conduction abnormality (Table 3). In this situation, electrical forces of the LA, which is located posteriorly, leftward, and slightly superiorly, dominate forces of the RA. If evidence of LAA and RAA appears simultaneously, biatrial enlargement can be suspected.

Table 4
Criteria for Normal QRS Complex[a]

1. Duration 0.06 to 0.10 s
2. Axis −30 to approx +100°
3. Transitional zone between V_2 and V_4

[a]Transitional zone is the precordial lead having equal positive and negative deflections.

NORMAL PR INTERVAL

The normal PR interval represents the time from the beginning of atrial activation to the beginning of ventricular activation. During this time, the impulse travels from the sinoatrial node through the atria, the atrioventricular (AV) node, and the His-Purkinje network toward the ventricular myocytes. Normal PR duration is 0.12 to 0.20 s. It increases with slower heart rates and advanced age. It shortens with preexcitation and certain disease states.

QRS COMPLEX

Normal QRS

Ventricular excitation begins predominantly in the middle third of the left side of the interventricular septum. From there, the initial wave of depolarization spreads toward the right side of the septum. A small resultant vector that is rightward, anterior, and either superior or inferior produces the initial QRS deflection of the ECG. Next, the impulse spreads throughout the apex and free walls of both ventricles from the endocardium to the epicardium. Because of the larger mass of the left ventricle, the resultant mean vector is leftward and inferior. This vector produces the major deflection of the QRS complex. Finally, the wave of depolarization arrives at the posterobasal LV wall and the posterobasal septum. A small resultant vector is directed posteriorly and superiorly, producing the latest QRS deflection (2). Criteria for a normal QRS complex may be found in Table 4.

Low Voltage

An amplitude of an entire QRS complex (R plus S) less than 5 mm in all limb leads and less than 10 mm in all precordial leads describes a low-voltage ECG. This abnormality is associated with chronic lung disease, pleural effusion, myocardial loss due to multiple myocardial infarctions, cardiomyopathy, pericardial effusion, myxedema, and obesity.

Axis Deviation

In patients with left axis deviation (LAD), the QRS axis is −30 to −90 degrees. Common causes of LAD include left ventricular hypertrophy, left anterior fascicular block, and an inferior wall MI (when superior and leftward forces dominate). In patients with right axis deviation, the QRS axis is +90 to +180 degrees. Common causes include right ventricular hypertrophy, a vertically oriented heart, COPD, and a lateral wall MI.

R Wave Progression

R wave progression and transition refers to the pattern of QRS complexes across the precordial leads (V_1–V_6). With properly placed leads, the R waves *in a normal heart* should become progressively larger in amplitude as the S waves become smaller when looking from V_1 to V_6. The transition zone, defined as the lead where the positive R wave deflection equals that of the negative S wave, should usually be between V_2 and V_4.

In *early R wave progression*, there is a shift of the transitional zone to the right of V_2 (counterclockwise rotation of the heart when looking up from the apex). R is bigger than S in V_2 and possibly in V_1. The differential diagnosis of early R wave progression includes lead malposition, normal

Table 5A
Romhilt-Estes Scoring System for LVH

1. R or S in any limb lead $\geq$ 2 mV (20 mm)	3 points[a]
or S in lead V_1 or V_2	
or R in lead V_5 or V_6 $\geq$ 3 mV (30 mm)	
2. Left ventricular strain	
ST segment and T wave in opposite direction to QRS complex	
without digitalis	3 points
with digitalis	1 point
3. Left atrial enlargement	
Terminal negativity of the P wave in lead V_1 is $\geq$ 1 mm in depth	3 points
and $\geq$ 0.04 s in duration	
4. Left axis deviation of $\geq$ −30?	2 points
5. QRS duration $\geq$ 0.09 s	1 point
6. Intrinsicoid deflection in lead V_5 or V_6 $\geq$ 0.05 s	1 point
TOTAL	13 points

[a]LVH, 5 points; probable LVH, 4 points.
Reproduced with permission from ref. *11*.

Table 5B
Sokolow-Lyon Criteria for LVH

S wave in lead V_1 + R wave in lead V_5 or V_6 > 35 mm
or
R wave in lead V_5 or V_6 > 26 mm

Reproduced with permission from ref. *11*.

Table 5C
Cornell Voltage Criteria for LVH

Females	R wave in lead aVL + S wave in lead V_3 > 20 mm
Males	R wave in lead aVL + S wave in lead V_3 > 28 mm

Reproduced with permission from ref. *11*.

variant, right ventricular hypertrophy (RVH), and posterior wall MI. Some congenital malformations and deformations such as dextrocardia may also exhibit this. In *late* or *poor R wave progression*, the transitional zone shifts to the left of V_4 (clockwise rotation). Here, the differential includes lead malposition, mild RVH (as in COPD), left bundle branch block (LBBB), left anterior fascicular block (LAFB), left ventricular hypertrophy (LVH), and anteroseptal MI.

Left Ventricular Hypertrophy

Leftward and posterior electrical forces increase when LV mass increases. Delay in completion of subendocardial-to-subepicardial *de*polarization may result in *re*polarization that begins in the subendocardium instead of the subepicardium. Reversal of repolarization forces ensues; this causes inversion of the T waves and sometimes of the QRS complexes (*see* Table 5 for common LVH criteria) *(3,4)*.

In subjects younger than 30 yr or when LVH is accompanied by LBBB or right bundle branch block (RBBB), the usual voltage criteria for LVH no longer apply. However, research into these and other special circumstances has yielded some acceptable criteria for accurate diagnosis. For example, the sum of an S in V_2 plus an R in V_6 greater than 45 mm has been shown to have 86% sensitivity and 100% specificity for LVH in LBBB *(3)*.

In Table 5D, ranges of sensitivity are listed for four separate LVH criteria. These data were collected from patients with LVH who had either coronary artery disease (CAD), hypertension, car-

Table 5D
Other Criteria for Left Ventricular Hypertrophy

1. Amplitude of R wave in lead aVL >11 mm
2. Amplitude of R wave in lead I >13 mm (0–25% sensitivity)
3. Amplitude of Q or QS wave in lead aVR >14 mm
4. Amplitude of R wave in lead aVF >20 mm
5. Sum of R wave in lead I and the S wave in lead III >25 mm
6. Sum of R wave in V_5 or V_6 and S wave in V_1 >35 mm (6–67% sensitivity)
7. Amplitude of R wave in V_5 or V_6 >26 mm (2–44% sensitivity)
8. Sum of maximum R wave and deepest S wave in the precordial leads >40 mm (14–78% sensitivity)

Modified with permission from ref. 6.

Table 6
Criteria for Right Ventricular Hypertrophy

1. RAD ≥ +110°
2. R > S in V_1
3. R < S in V_6
4. QR in V_1 without prior anteroseptal myocardial infarction
5. Right atrial abnormality
6. Secondary ST–T changes, namely, downsloping ST depression with upward convexity and asymmetric T wave inversion in the right precordial and inferior leads
7. S_I, S_{II}, S_{III} pattern (R ≥ S in I, II, and III)

diomyopathy, or valvular disease. Overall, the criteria seemed to be more sensitive in each case for those patients with hypertension or valvular disease *(5)*.

Right Ventricular Hypertrophy

In RVH, anterior and rightward forces increase when RV masses increases. Usually these forces are masked by LV forces unless RVH is significant. Occasionally, posterior and rightward forces also increase secondary to a posterior tilt of the cardiac apex. Delay in completion of subendocardial-to-subepicardial depolarization may cause repolarization to begin in the subendocardium instead of the subepicardium. Consequently, the ECG manifests this delay of depolarization and reversal of repolarization as QRS complexes and T waves opposite their normative vectors.

The diagnosis of RVH requires two or more criteria to be present *(3)*, and the sensitivity and specificity of these criteria span a wide range. Most likely this is secondary to the population observed in the study. *See* Table 6 for RVH criteria.

Biventricular Hypertrophy

In a patient with combined RVH and LVH, LV and RV forces may cancel each other. Because of its relatively larger size, LV forces usually predominate. EKG criteria for biventricular hypertrophy, however, are only 24.6% sensitive and 86.4% specific *(5)*.

Right Bundle Branch Block

The right bundle branch does not contribute significantly to septal activation. Therefore, the *early* part of the QRS complex is unchanged in RBBB. LV activation proceeds normally. The RV, which is located anteriorly and to the right of the LV, is activated late and from left to right. Therefore, terminal forces are directed anteriorly and rightward. In addition, this late (terminal) depolarization of the RV propagates by slow, cell-to-cell conduction without using the right-sided His-Purkinje system. This phenomenon gives wide and slurred terminal deflections of the QRS. Repolarization proceeds from the subendocardium to the subepicardium secondary to alteration of the recovery process (*see* "Generation of ECG Tracing" for comparison to *normal* repolarization). Thus, the ST

Table 7
Criteria for Right Bundle Branch Block

1. Prolonged QRS (≥0.12 s)
2. R' (secondary R wave) taller than the initial R wave in the right precordial leads
3. Wide S wave in I, V_5, V_6
4. Axis of initial 0.06–0.08 s of QRS should be normal
5. Secondary ST–T changes (downsloping ST depression with upward convexity and asymmetric T inversion) in inferior and posterior leads

In incomplete RBBB, QRS complex has typical RBBB morphology but QRS duration is only 0.09–0.11 s.

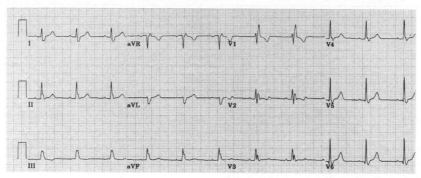

Fig. 5. ECG demonstrating typical complete right bundle branch block.

and T vectors are opposite to the terminal part of the QRS. Table 7 lists the RBBB criteria. The diagnosis requires all the criteria to be present (*see* Fig. 5, for example) *(3,4).*

Any discussion of RBBB would be incomplete without mention of two entities that most likely represent a continuum of disease: the Brugada syndrome and arrhythmogenic RV dysplasia (ARVD). The Brugada syndrome describes a persistent combination of ST-T elevation in the precordial leads, RBBB, and sudden cardiac death. Occasionally, ST-T segment elevation is not apparent at baseline; it may require provocation with procainamide in the electrophysiology laboratory. This syndrome has been described predominantly in young men. Families of probands should be evaluated.

Arrhythmogenic RV dysplasia, a rare cardiomyopathy caused by progressive fibro-fatty infiltration of the RV, may also present with RBBB and/or T-wave inversion in leads V_1 through V_3. This disease also seems to afflict young men most commonly, and it is associated with sudden cardiac death as well. Once again, family members of the proband should be evaluated.

RSR' Pattern in V_1

RSR' pattern in V_1 is a common ECG pattern. It may be seen as a normal variant, or it may be present in association with abnormalities of the RV or the posterior wall of the LV.

Left Anterior Fascicular Block

The left anterior fascicle travels toward the anterolateral papillary muscle (i.e., superiorly, anteriorly, and leftward). Thus, in LAFB, the *initial* depolarization is directed inferiorly, posteriorly, and rightward through the posterior fascicle. *Delayed* depolarization of both anterior and lateral walls is directed leftward and superiorly. Therefore, leftward and superior terminal forces of the LV free wall are unopposed and prominent. The LAFB criteria may be found in Table 8 *(3,4).*

Left Posterior Fascicular Block

True left posterior fascicular block is rare. Differential diagnosis includes asthenia, COPD, RVH, and extensive lateral wall MI. The transitional zone is often displaced leftward which may cause

Table 8
Criteria for Left Anterior Fascicular Block

1. Mean QRS axis of −45° to −90° (S_{II} amplitude is less than S_{III} amplitude)
2. QR complex (or a pure R wave) in I and aVL; RS complex in leads II, III, and aVF
3. Normal to slightly prolonged QRS duration (0.08–0.12 s)
4. Deep S waves may be seen in the left precordial leads secondary to occasional extreme superior deviation of the mean QRS vector in the frontal plane.

Table 9
Criteria for Left Posterior Fascicular Block

1. Frontal plane QRS axis of +100° to +180°
2. $S_I Q_{III}$ pattern (as opposed to left anterior fascicular block)
3. Normal or slightly prolonged QRS duration (0.08–0.12 s)

Table 10
Criteria for Left Bundle Branch Block[a]

1. Prolonged QRS duration (≥0.12 s)
2. Broad, monophasic R in leads I, V_5, or V_6 that is usually notched or slurred
3. Absence of any Q waves in I and V_5–V_6
4. Direction of the ST segment shift and the T wave is opposite to that of the QRS complex. T waves in "lateral" leads (i.e., I, aVL, V_4–V_6) may become tall (Fig. 7E)

[a]See Fig. 6.

the Q waves in the left precordial leads to disappear. This happens because the mean QRS vector is directed posteriorly in the horizontal plane (see Fig. 3). Table 9 lists the LPFB criteria (4).

Left Bundle Branch Block

Normally, the left bundle *does* contribute to septal activation. Thus, in LBBB, septal activation develops late. Therefore, early forces manifested on ECG originate from the RV apex, which is located to the left, in front of, and below the electrical center of the heart. Depolarization spreads from the subendocardium of the RV apex to the subepicardium. Consequently, the resultant vector is directed leftward, forward, and down. Leftward orientation of the forces remains as depolarization progresses. Terminal depolarization proceeds by slow, cell-to-cell conduction. This causes slurring and widening of the terminal deflection. *Repolarization* proceeds from the subendocardium to the subepicardium secondary to changes in the course of the recovery process (see "Generation of ECG Tracing"). Thus, the ST and T vectors are opposite to the terminal part of the QRS (Fig. 6). Table 10 lists LBBB criteria. All criteria should be present to diagnose LBBB (3,4).

Other Types of Block

Nonspecific intraventricular conduction disturbance is characterized by QRS duration greater than 0.11 s when the QRS morphology does not satisfy all criteria for either LBBB or RBBB. Common causes of other various blocks below the AV node include coronary artery disease, hypertensive heart disease, aortic valve disease, cardiomyopathy, sclerosis of the conduction tissue or cardiac skeleton (usually seen in elderly people), and surgical trauma (3). Heart rate-related RBBB (and less commonly LBBB) or other conduction abnormalities are not rare in clinical practice.

Abnormal/Pathological Q Wave

Electrically inert myocardium, like that affected by previous MI, fails to contribute to normal electrical forces. Thus, the vector of the opposite wall takes over. The Q wave is larger, and the R wave may become smaller. Larger S waves are often obscured by ST changes. Table 11 lists the criteria for abnormal Q waves.

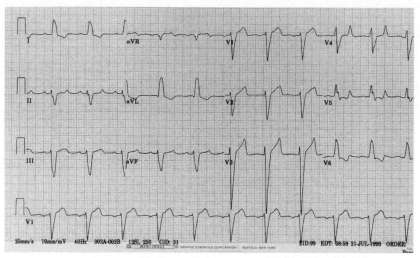

Fig. 6. ECG demonstrating typical complete left bundle branch block.

Table 11
Criteria for Q Wave Abnormality*

1. Duration of the Q wave ≥0.04 s
2. Amplitude of the Q wave in the limb leads ≥4 mm or ≥25% of the R wave in that lead (even deeper required for leads III, aVF and aVL)
3. Normally, QRS in V_2–V_4 begins with the R wave. Thus, even small Q waves are abnormal if seen in V_2–V_4 (unless the transitional zone is markedly shifted secondary to another cause)

*Note that a new myocardial infarction may mask ECG changes from a previous one.

Table 12
Electrocardiographic Localization of Q Wave Myocardial Infarction[a]

Site of infarct	Signs of electrically inert myocardium
Anteroseptal	Pathological Q or QS in V_1–V_3 and sometimes V_4
Anterior	Absence of Q in V_1; QS or QR in V_2–V_4; and
	Late R progression or reversal of R progression in precordial leads may also be present
Anterolateral	Abnormal Q in V_4–V_6
Lateral	Abnormal Q in V_5–V_6
Extensive anterior	Abnormal Q in V_1–V_6
High lateral	Abnormal Q in I and aVL
Inferior	Pathological Q in II, III, aVF (Q in III and aVF >25% of the amplitude of the R wave)
Inferolateral	Abnormal Q in II, III, aVF, V_5–V_6
Posterior	Initial R wave in V_1 and V_2 longer than 0.04 s with R larger than S

[a]This is based on a normal anatomic position of the heart.

In a normally positioned heart, the right-sided precordial leads V_3R and V_4R are located over the mid-RV. The usual lead V_1 is located over the high RV or septum and opposite to the posterior LV wall. V_2 is placed over the septum and opposite to the posterior LV wall. Leads V_3 and V_4 cover the middle anterior LV. V_5 and V_6 are situated over the low lateral LV, and I and aVL are across the high lateral LV. Leads II, III, and aVF are closest to the inferior LV. Therefore, the location of an infarction may be deduced from the location of abnormal Q waves (Table 12).

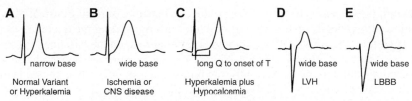

Fig. 7. Some examples of tall T waves.

In a posterior MI, reciprocal changes of the ST segment (i.e., depression in the anteroseptal leads) are often seen in acute ischemia/injury. When diagnosing posterior MI, one should rule out juvenile ECG changes, early R wave progression, and RVH. RV infarction is characterized by ST elevation more than 10 mm in the right precordial lead(s). V_4R is considered more sensitive and specific than V_1 for this diagnosis.

ST SEGMENT/T WAVE CHANGES

The normal ST segment reflects steady membrane polarization from the end of depolarization to the beginning of repolarization. Its vertical baseline is that of the T-to-Q interval. Usually, the ST segment is almost absent because the ascending limb of the T wave begins right at the J point (the junction of the end of the QRS complex and the beginning of the ST segment).

Normal T waves represent ventricular repolarization. As previously described, longer action potential duration in the ventricular subendocardium as compared to the subepicardium causes repolarization to proceed in the direction opposite that of depolarization (i.e., it begins in the subepicardium and spreads toward the subendocardium; *see* "Generation of ECG Tracing"). Therefore, the vector of repolarization (T wave) has the same direction as the vector of depolarization (QRS). Usually, the T wave is asymmetric: the ascending limb is longer than the descending one. It is at least 5 mm tall in I, II, and the left precordial leads *(3)*, but it may be slightly inverted or biphasic in other leads.

Juvenile T waves are a normal variant characterized by persistence of negative T waves in V_1 to V_3 after approx 20 years of age. They are usually neither symmetric nor deep. The degree of T wave inversion decreases progressively from V_1 to V_4. In normal tracings from subjects with this ECG pattern, however, the T waves are always upright in I, II, and the left precordial leads.

Peaked T waves may also be seen as a normal variant. In this case, the T wave is more than 6 mm high in the limb leads or more than 10 mm in the precordial leads (Fig. 7A) *(1)*. Early repolarization is due to a dominant parasympathetic effect on the heart *(7)*. This normal variant (Fig. 7A) is characterized by (1) an elevated J point and ST segment; (2) a distinct notch or slur on the downstroke of the R wave; and (3) upward *concavity* of the ST segment. There are no reciprocal changes of the ST segment in the leads with opposite axes. *Increased vagal tone* is accompanied by tall, peaked T waves. It is usually associated with a characteristic ST elevation; this is called early repolarization.

Nonspecific ST segment and/or T wave abnormalities may show either (1) slight ST depression or elevation (less than 1 mm) or (2) flattening, decreased amplitude, or slight inversion of the T wave. On a normal ECG, the T wave should be at least 5 mm tall in I, II, and the left precordial leads. These ST-T changes may be local or diffuse. Numerous physiologic and pathologic conditions can cause this.

ST Segment and T Wave Changes in Ischemia/Injury

Any ischemic area exhibits prolonged repolarization which causes a difference of potentials between ischemic and nonischemic areas during phase III of action potential repolarization. This results in QT prolongation and T wave changes *(6)*. Consequently, a difference in potential between injured and uninjured areas is formed which produces a diastolic or resting current of injury. The ECG machine automatically adjusts for this baseline shift by shifting the tracing in the opposite direction. Therefore, the whole QRS-T complex is shifted to keep the baseline (TQ segment) at the same level. This causes the ST segment to look elevated or depressed depending on what layer of the myocardial wall it involves. Secondly, the injured area shows early completion of repolarization or diminished depolarization. Thus, phase II, the plateau phase of the action potential, is shortened. Systolic difference in potentials between the injured and uninjured area ensues. The second mechanism, systolic current of injury, plays a lesser role *(1)*.

T-wave abnormalities suggesting *myocardial ischemia* may include (1) abnormally tall, upright T waves (*see* Fig. 7 for common types of tall T waves); (2) symmetrically and/or deeply inverted T waves; (3) "pseudonormalization" of inverted T waves (when previously inverted T waves become positive secondary to ischemia-induced changes in repolarization); and (4) nonspecific T-wave abnormalities. Hyperacute T waves may be seen occasionally in the earliest stage of coronary occlusion. They are tall, symmetric or asymmetric, and peaked or blunted *(1,3)*. More often, however, T waves on the initial ECG are isoelectric, biphasic, or inverted. The T-wave changes of angina may be transitory or persistent.

ST segment abnormalities suggesting *myocardial injury* may be pronounced or subtle. These abnormalities include acute ST segment elevation with upward convexity in the leads facing the area of transmural or subepicardial injury (Fig. 8B). There may be reciprocal ST depression. Posterior wall transmural or subepicardial injury may cause ST segment depression in V_1–V_3. In clinical as opposed to experimental coronary occlusion, any ST or T changes may reflect CAD. The ECG may also be completely normal. Subendocardial injury, ischemia, and necrosis commonly cause horizontal or downsloping ST segment depression and/or flattening with or without the T wave changes described above (*see* Figs. 8B–D for some examples). Usually, the depressed ST segment is flat or sagging in contrast to the upward convexity of the "strain pattern." To diagnose CAD, ECG changes should be present in at least two contiguous leads.

QT INTERVAL

The QT interval represents the duration of electrical systole. The normal QT corrected for the heart rate is less than 0.44 s. It is usually less than half of the preceding RR interval. A prolonged QT interval may be caused by dyssynchrony or prolongation of ventricular repolarization. The prolonged corrected QT interval is associated with numerous pathological conditions. These include ischemia and infarction, the most common causes, and central nervous system (CNS) disorders. In hypokalemia, prominent U waves merge with T waves and result in *pseudo*-QT prolongation. In this case, "bifid T waves" may be present. A shortened QT interval is most often caused by digitalis or hypercalcemia.

U WAVE

The normal U wave represents afterpotentials of the ventricular myocardium or delayed repolarization of the Purkinje fibers. Normally, it should be upright in all leads except aVR. Prominent, clinically significant U waves often have an amplitude larger than 25% of the T wave in the same lead, or they are larger than 1.5 mm. Common causes include bradycardia, hypokalemia, and LVH. *U wave inversion* is highly specific for organic heart disease.

NORMAL ECG

Normal variants of the ECG include early repolarization; juvenile T waves; occasionally, the $S_I S_{II} S_{III}$ pattern; rSR' in V_1; Parkinson's tremor; and the "athlete's heart." The mechanism of ECG changes in the "athlete's heart" reflects increased vagal tone, RVH or LVH, and asymmetry of ventricular repolarization. In this condition, one may see sinus bradycardia with a junctional escape rhythm; first-degree or second-degree type I AV block; and increased P wave and QRS amplitude. Early repolarization is also more common in athletes. T waves in the precordial leads may be tall,

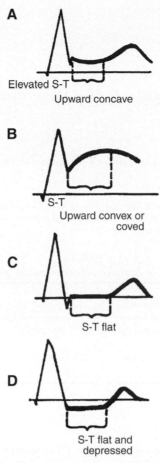

A Elevated S-T
Upward concave

B S-T
Upward convex or
coved

C S-T flat

D S-T flat and
depressed

Fig. 8. Early repolarization and the ST segment changes in injury/ischemia. (Modified from ref. *14*.)

inverted, or biphasic. Parkinson's tremor can simulate atrial flutter or ventricular tachycardia with a rate of 330 bpm.

Incorrect electrode placement in a normal healthy person may produce characteristic ECG changes. The most common error is reversal of the right and left arm leads, which causes P, QRS, and T inversion in leads I and aVL.

MYOCARDIAL INFARCTION

Distinction between *Q wave* and *non-Q wave MI* may be less relevant clinically than once thought. Subendocardial or nontransmural MI often shows abnormal Q waves whereas transmural MI may not.

The typical evolution of the ECG in acute Q wave MI includes these stages:

1. *Tall T waves* (Fig. 7B) may appear within the first minutes or hours, but more often isoelectric, negative, or biphasic T waves are seen on presentation.
2. *ST segment elevation* (Fig. 8B) appears within hours after coronary occlusion and may last approx 2 wk. If it lasts longer than 2 wk, ventricular aneurysm, pericarditis, or concomitant early repolarization should be considered.
3. *Abnormal Q waves* appear within hours or days after MI and persist indefinitely.

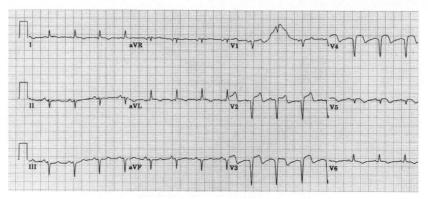

Fig. 9. Acute extensive anterior MI. Note upward convexity of the ST segment elevation in leads V_4 and V_5, which is typical for myocardial injury. Also note that upward convexity is obscured by acute T waves in lead V_2. Motion artifact is apparent in lead V_1.

Table 13
Results of the Univariate Analysis of Electrocardiographic Criteria in LBBB

Criterion	Sensitivity (95% CI)	Specificity (95% CI)
ST segment elevation ≥1 mm and concordant with QRS complex	73 (64–80)	92 (86–96)
ST segment depression ≥1 mm in lead V_1, V_2, or V_3	25 (18–34)	96 (91–99)
ST segment elevation ≥5 mm and discordant with QRS complex	31 (23–39)	92 (85–96)
Positive T wave in lead V_5 or V_6	26 (19–34)	92 (86–96)

Modified with permission from ref. 9.

4. *Decline in ST elevation* occurs simultaneously with or after the onset of the T wave inversion. In acute pericarditis, in contrast, the ST segment becomes isoelectric before the T wave becomes inverted.
5. *Isoelectric ST segment with symmetric T wave inversion* may last months to years or persist indefinitely.

The ECG interpretation of myocardial infarction may be complicated by the fact that the QRS wave, ST segment, and T wave may normalize transiently in the course of its evolution. If the ST segment is elevated, the infarction is probably recent or acute (within approx 2 wk) (Fig. 9). If there is no ST segment elevation, the infarction is probably old or of indeterminate age. Traditional teaching also holds that T wave changes reflect ischemia; ST segment changes reflect injury; and abnormal Q waves reflect necrosis. This is an overly simplistic and artificial approach. Both T wave and ST segment changes may be due to ischemia, injury, or necrosis. The Q wave may reflect temporary electrical silence and not necessarily necrosis.

The presence of LBBB on the baseline ECG has presented a challenge in the face of an acute MI. This was recognized more than fifty years ago when Cabrera studied the tracings of such patients in 1953 *(15)*. Other investigators followed suit, but none of their proposed signs have gained widespread acceptance *(9)*.

In order to aid in this diagnosis, criteria have been proposed based on a review of ECGs from patients enrolled in the Global Utilization of Streptokinase and Tissue Plasminogen Activator for Occluded Coronary Arteries (GUSTO) trial (*see* Table 13). This provides some guidelines, but continued research is needed in this area.

Recent publications suggest predictive and prognostic value in ST-segment elevation in lead aVR during a first acute, non-ST segment elevation MI. One study published in 2003 suggests that

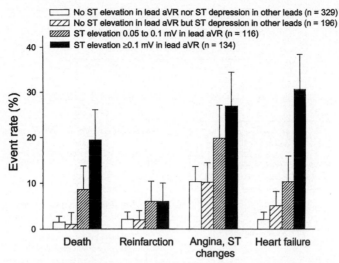

Fig. 10. Rates of major in-hospital adverse events in patients with and without ST segment depression ≥0.1 mV on admission after stratifying for ST segment elevation in lead aVR. This latter variable identified a high-risk subgroup, whereas the remaining patients had low complication rates irrespective of ST segment depression in other leads. Error bars represent the upper limits of the 95% CIs. (Reproduced with permission from ref. *12*.)

≥1 mm ST segment elevation in lead aVR correlates positively with adverse events, including death (Fig. 10). Another significantly smaller study stated that acute left main coronary artery obstruction may be predicted using a similar criterion *(10)*. Based on these new findings, lead aVR should be carefully scrutinized on any ECG suspicious for infarction.

Prompt identification of the culprit artery during a myocardial infarction can help the clinician to choose the appropriate acute therapies for patients. Historically, the electrocardiogram has played a major role in locating the vessel. Variations in coronary artery anatomy, both subtle and obvious, can occasionally make this diagnosis quite difficult. For example, the His bundle may receive dual blood supply from septal perforators from the LAD as well as the AV nodal artery from the posterior descending artery. An inferior MI could therefore cause a LAFB pattern on the ECG *(5)*. Figure 11 is an algorithm for ECG identification of the infarct-related artery in inferior MI.

DIFFERENTIAL DIAGNOSIS OF MYOCARDIAL INFARCTION

A QS pattern in the right precordial leads or late R wave progression may indicate *LVH*. In LVH, however, this pseudoinfarction pattern is not present in the chest leads if they are recorded one intercostal space lower than usual. The "strain" pattern of LVH may also mimic or mask ischemia or injury. Ischemia or subendocardial injury is favored over hypertrophy with the strain pattern when (1) the ST segment changes are disproportional to the R wave amplitude in the same lead; (2) ST segment depression is present without T wave inversion; and (3) T wave inversion is symmetric.

In *RVH*, T wave inversion in the inferior or right precordial leads may imitate CAD. However, other ECG changes often suggest this diagnosis. In patients with *pulmonary disease*, late R wave progression in the precordial leads may be mistaken for an anterior MI. However, in COPD and cor pulmonale this "abnormality" disappears when the leads are placed one intercostal space lower than usual. With pulmonary diseases there may also be other signs of RV involvement. Sometimes patients with diseases exhibit abnormal Q waves in the inferior leads that may mimic inferior infarction. Abnormal Q waves are rarely seen in lead II, but they may appear along with ST segment and T wave changes in myocardial diseases secondary to localized fibrosis and in repolarization abnormalities.

In *Wolff-Parkinson-White (WPW) syndrome*, preexcitation of a ventricle significantly changes the initial QRS forces. The resultant *delta wave* can mimic an abnormal Q wave if it is negative.

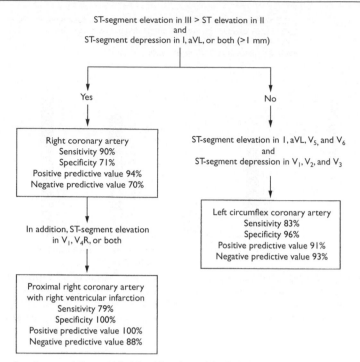

Fig. 11. Algorithm for electrocardiographic identification of the infarct-related artery in inferior myocardial infarction. (Reproduced with permission from ref. *13*. Copyright 2003 Massachusetts Medical Society.)

An upward or positive delta wave may mask abnormal Q waves. The degree of preexcitation and ST/T change may vary in any given person, a finding that mimics evolutionary changes of an acute ischemic event. In WPW syndrome, however, the PR interval is usually short, and the QRS complex is wide with initial slurring. Marked ST segment elevation in the leads with an upright QRS complex or ST depression in the leads with a downward QRS complex is also very unlikely in WPW syndrome.

Among *CNS disorders*, ECG changes are most often present in subarachnoid or intracranial hemorrhage. One can observe ST elevation or depression; large, wide, inverted, or upright T waves; a long QT segment; and occasionally, abnormal Q waves. Often only the clinical picture helps to make a definitive diagnosis.

In *hyperkalemia*, the T wave is tall, and the ST segment may be elevated or depressed. In contrast to ischemia, the QT is normal or shortened (only if there is no QRS complex prolongation or other reasons for QT lengthening). In addition, the T wave is narrow-based (Fig. 7A). ST segment depression slopes upward, not horizontal or downward as it does in ischemia. Presence of a U wave tends to rule out hyperkalemia.

Patients with *acute pericarditis* very often have ST segment elevation that mimics acute injury. In pericarditis, however, ST segment elevation is usually present in almost all leads on the ECG, and there is no reciprocal ST segment depression. In contrast to MI, the ST segment elevation in pericarditis has an upward concavity, and it is rarely greater than 5 mm from the baseline *(5)*. T wave inversion tends to be less pronounced but more diffuse in pericarditis than in ischemia.

Digitalis effect or *toxicity* may cause horizontal or downsloping ST segment depression that looks similar to MI. Digitalis-induced ST depression often has a sagging, upwardly concave shape. In addition, the QT interval is often shortened.

In *RBBB*, the initial forces of depolarization are not altered. In MI, they are abnormal. Therefore, RBBB usually does not interfere with signs of MI. In *LAFB* and *LPFB*, the initial forces may occasionally be altered. Thus, both LAFB and LPFB can imitate or mask MI. Abnormal Q waves may also be prominent if the precordial leads are recorded one intercostal space higher than usual.

Both *LBBB* and *pacing* cause significant alteration of initial and late QRS forces. Therefore, both LBBB and pacing may imitate or mask MI. In the presence of these conditions, correct diagnosis of MI from the ECG alone may be impossible. Occasionally, MI can be diagnosed in the presence of LBBB or pacing by the presence of (1) pathologic Q waves; (2) ST-T deflections that have the same direction as the QRS complex; (3) ST segment elevation disproportionate to the amplitude of the QRS complex (greater elevation is required for leads V_1–V_2); or (4) notched upstroke of the S wave in two precordial leads.

DRUG EFFECTS: DIGITALIS

Many classes of drugs have the potential to affect the appearance of the ECG. Antiarrhythmics directly interfere with molecular myocardial conduction channels; diuretics may alter serum electrolyte concentrations. These changes may cause subtle variations in myocardial depolarization and repolarization, and the resultant ECG will reflect these variations. The altered ECG may mimic certain disease states, and recognition is therefore essential. Because of its well-described findings, only digitalis will be discussed here.

Digitalis increases vagal tone as well as the amount of calcium in myocytes. The drug may also improve bypass tract conduction should one exist. The *digitalis effect* may be accompanied by QT interval shortening, PR interval lengthening, and increased U wave amplitude. Another characteristic finding is a sagging ST segment depression with upward concavity. This may also be seen in CAD.

In *digitalis toxicity*, there is increased automaticity of the myocytes and/or impaired conduction in the His-Purkinje system. Ventricular premature depolarizations are common. Tachyarrhythmias with different degrees of AV block are considered diagnostic.

METABOLIC ABNORMALITIES

In *hyperkalemia*, the main electrophysiological abnormality is shortening of phase III of the action potential. This phase generates the T wave on the ECG. Therefore, the earliest and most prominent ECG findings involve the T waves. In *hypokalemia*, phase III of the action potential is prolonged. Therefore, many of the ECG changes are opposite to those of hyperkalemia. Prominent U waves with decreased T wave amplitude are typical.

In *hypercalcemia*, the main electrophysiologic finding is shortening of phase II of the action potential. This "plateau" phase is not usually accompanied by significant deflections on the ECG tracing. The ST segment is shortened or nearly absent, and the entire QT interval consequently shortens. There is usually little effect on the QRS complex or the P or T waves. *Hypocalcemia* is usually accompanied by the opposite ECG changes (i.e., a prolonged QT interval due to a long ST segment). The combination of hyperkalemia and hypercalcemia (often seen in renal disease) causes QT prolongation combined with peaked T waves, which may occasionally be exceptionally tall.

PULMONARY DISEASES

Chronic Lung Disease

In patients with lung disease, ECG changes may possibly be caused by a vertical heart position (due to hyperinflation of the lungs), RVH, or RAA. The ECG criteria for pulmonary disease are listed in Table 14.

Acute Cor Pulmonale Including Pulmonary Embolism

One mechanism of ECG change in acute cor pulmonale involves sudden RV dilatation. Dilatation causes RV myocardial conduction abnormalities. On ECG, this may manifest as a vertically positioned heart with counterclockwise rotation in the precordial leads. ECG abnormalities in these patients are frequently transitory. *See* Table 15 for the diagnostic criteria *(4)*.

Table 14
Criteria for Chronic Obstructive Pulmonary Disease

1. The P wave axis is farther right than +75°
2. Any of the right ventricular hypertrophy criteria (increased R/S ratio in V_1 is the least common right ventricular pattern in COPD)
3. Late R wave progression in precordial leads
4. Low voltage
5. Abnormal Q waves in the inferior or anterior leads
6. Supraventricular arrhythmias, especially atrial tachycardia, multifocal atrial tachycardia, and atrial fibrillation

Table 15
Criteria for Acute Cor Pulmonale

1. Sinus tachycardia (most common ECG sign)
2. Transient right bundle branch block (incomplete or complete)
3. Inverted T waves in V_1–V_3
4. $S_I Q_{III}$ or $S_I Q_{III} T_{III}$ pattern with pseudoinfarction in the inferior leads
5. Right axis deviation
6. Right atrial abnormality with various supraventricular tachyarrhythmias

ACUTE PERICARDITIS

ECG changes in pericarditis reflect subepicardial myocarditis with subepicardial injury. Typically, the ECG in acute pericarditis has the following evolution:

Stage 1: The ST segment elevates (upward concave) in almost all leads except aVR. Reciprocal changes are absent.
Stage 2: The ST segment returns to the baseline, and the T wave amplitude begins to decrease. At this point, the ECG may look completely normal.
Stage 3: The T wave inverts.
Stage 4: Electrocardiographic resolution may occur.

Other clues may also help in diagnosis. In the early stages, PR segment depression reflects atrial injury (as ST elevation reflects ventricular injury). Low-voltage QRS complexes and electrical alternans of ECG waves may occur in the presence of a pericardial effusion, which may or may not be associated with pericarditis. Sinus tachycardia and atrial arrhythmias are very common *(4)*.

The differential diagnosis of acute pericarditis should include early repolarization. Absence of serial ST/T changes, the presence of tall T waves, and a characterisitic notching of the terminal QRS favor early repolarization. PR segment depression in *both* limb and precordial leads (as opposed to *either* limb or precordial leads) favor pericarditis. In addition, ST segment depression in lead V_1, occasionally present in pericarditis, is not present in early repolarization.

PERICARDIAL EFFUSION

As mentioned above, *pericardial effusion* may cause electrical alternans on ECG. It may also cause low-voltage QRS complexes that are defined as complexes less than 5 mm in amplitude in all limb leads and less than 10 mm in all precordial leads.

CENTRAL NERVOUS SYSTEM DISORDERS

The most common CNS disorders associated with ECG abnormalities are subarachnoid and intracranial hemorrhage. The mechanism of ECG changes in these patients includes altered auton-

Table 16
Criteria for Wolff-Parkinson-White Syndrome

1. Normal P wave with a PR interval generally <0.12 s
2. Initial slurring of the QRS (delta wave)
3. Wide QRS interval >0.10 s (except with septal insertion of a bypass tract)
4. Secondary ST/T changes (similar to the "strain pattern")
5. Atrioventricular reentrant tachycardias (most common arrhythmias)
6. Atrial fibrillation or flutter with a wide QRS complex and a rate >200 bpm is suggestive

omic tone with resultant changes in repolarization. The most common ECG findings are deeply inverted T waves and a markedly prolonged QT_C interval. Occasionally, the T waves may be upright and tall.

PREEXCITATION (WOLF-PARKINSON-WHITE) SYNDROME

In WPW syndrome, one or more accessory AV pathways allow the atrial impulse to bypass the AV node and activate the ventricles prematurely. AV delay is shortened. Ventricular activation may follow the usual course through the normal conduction system, or it may begin from the site of attachment of the bypass tract within one of the ventricles. Commonly, both pathways contribute to the QRS complex. Refer to Table 16 for WPW criteria.

CONGENITAL AND ACQUIRED HEART DISEASE

Although beyond the scope of this chapter, no reference in electrocardiography could be complete without at least a brief word on congenital and acquired heart disease. Many defects and malformations have very specific findings on ECG: incomplete RBBB, a rightward axis, and precordial changes of a secundum atrial septal defect; the reversal of normal septal activation in L-transposition of the great vessels; the possible RVH with persistent truncus arteriosus. Similarly, acquired disease, including valvular disease such as mitral stenosis, has specific characteristics. Recognition of these abnormalities will undoubtedly aid in following the clinical course.

SUMMARY

Electrocardiography offers a glimpse into many aspects of cardiac function. When combined with a clinical scenario, physical examination, and other methods of diagnosis, it permits a fuller understanding of both acute and chronic disease states in the heart. Its use has proven invaluable in the practice of modern medicine.

REFERENCES

1. Fisch C. Electrocardiography. In: Braunwald E, ed. Heart Disease: A Textbook of Cardiovascular Medicine, 5th ed. W. B. Saunders, Philadelphia, 1997, pp. 108–152.
2. Durrer D, et al. Total excitation of the isolated human heart. Circulation 1970;41:899.
3. Chou TC, Knilans TK. Electrocardiography in Clinical Practice: Adult and Pediatric, 4th ed. W. B. Saunders, Philadelphia, 1996.
4. O'Keefe JH Jr, et al. ECG Board Review and Study Guide: Scoring Criteria and Definitions. Futura Publishing, Armonk, NY, 1994.
5. In Surawicz B, Knilans TK, eds. Chou's Electrocardiography in Clinical Practice: Adult and Pediatric, 5th ed. W. B. Saunders, Philadelphia, 2001, p. 56.
6. Murphy ML, et al. Sensitivity of electrocardiography criteria for left ventricular hypertrophy according to type of cardiac disease. Am J Cardiol 1985;55:545–549.
7. Mason JW, et al. ECG-SAP. American College of Cardiology, 1995.
8. Antzelevitch C, Sicouri S, Lukas A, et al. Clinical implications of electrical heterogeneity in the heart: the electrophysiology and pharmacology of epicardial, M, and endocardial cells. In: Podrid PJ, Kowey PR, eds. Cardiac Arrhythmia: Mechanisms, Diagnosis and Management. Williams & Wilkins, Baltimore, 1995, pp. 88–107.

9. Sgarbossa EB, et al. Electrocardiographic diagnosis of evolving acute myocardial infarction in the presence of left bundle branch block. N Engl J Med 1996;334:481–487.
10. Yamaji H, et al. Prediction of acute left main coronary artery obstruction by 12-lead electrocardiography: ST segment elevation in lead aVR with less ST segment elevation in lead V_1. J Am Coll Cardiol 2001;38:1348–1354.
11. Wagner GS. Marriott's Practical Electrocardiography, 9th ed. Williams & Wilkins, Philadelphia, 1994.
12. Barrabes JA, et al. Prognostic value of lead aVR in patients with a first non-ST segment elevation acute myocardial infarction. Circulation 2003;108:814–819.
13. Zimetbaum PJ, Josephson ME. Use of the electrocardiogram in acute myocardial infarction. N Engl J Med 2003;348: 933–940.
14. Constant J. Learning Electrocardiography: A Complete Course, 2nd ed. Little, Brown, Boston, 1981.
15. Wackers FJT. The diagnosis of myocardial infarction in the presence of left bundle branch block. Cardiol Clin 1987;5:393.

RECOMMENDED READING

Antzelevitch C, Sicouri S, Lukas A, et al. Clinical implications of electrical heterogeneity in the heart: the electrophysiology and pharmacology of epicardial, M, and endocardial cells. In: Podrid PJ, Kowey PR, eds. Cardiac Arrhythmia: Mechanisms, Diagnosis and Management. William & Wilkins, Baltimore, 1995.
O'Keefe JH Jr, et al. ECG Board Review and Study Guide: Scoring Criteria and Definitions. Futura Publishing, Armonk, NY, 1994.
Surawicz B, Knilans TK, eds. Chou's Electrocardiography in Clinical Practice: Adult and Pediatric, 5th ed. W. B. Saunders, Philadelphia, 2001.
Wagner GS. Marriott's Practical Electrocardiography, 9th ed. Williams & Wilkins, Philadelphia, 1994.
Zimetbaum PJ, Josephson ME. Use of the electrocardiogram in acute myocardial infarction. N Engl J Med 2003;348: 933–940.

9   Echocardiography

Daniel G. Blanchard, MD
and Anthony N. DeMaria, MD

INTRODUCTION

Echocardiography is the evaluation of cardiac structures and function utilizing images produced by ultrasound (US) energy. Echocardiography started as a crude one-dimensional technique but has evolved into one that images in two and three dimensions (2-D, 3-D) and that can be performed from the chest wall, from the esophagus, and from within vascular structures. Clinically useful M-mode recordings became available in the late 1960s and early 1970s. In the mid-1970s, linear-array scanners that could produce 2-D images of the beating heart were developed. Eventually, these evolved into the phased-array instruments currently in use. In addition to 2-D imaging, the Doppler examination has become an essential component of the complete echocardiographic evaluation. Doppler US technology blossomed in the early 1980s with the development of pulsed-wave (PW), continuous-wave (CW), and 2-D color-flow imaging. The field of cardiac US continues to grow rapidly: recent clinical additions include 3-D imaging, harmonic imaging, and contrast echocardiography.

PHYSICS AND PRINCIPLES

US is sonic energy with a frequency higher than the audible range (greater than 20,000 Hz). US is created by a transducer that consists of electrodes and a piezoelectric crystal that deforms when exposed to an electric current. This crystal creates US energy and then generates an electrical signal when struck by reflected US waves. US is useful for diagnostic imaging because, like light, it can be focused into a beam that obeys the laws of reflection and refraction. A US beam travels in a straight line through a medium of homogeneous density but if the beam meets an interface of different acoustic impedance, part of the energy is reflected. This reflected energy can then be evaluated and used to construct an image of the heart *(1)*.

Because the velocity of sound in soft tissue is relatively constant (approx 1540 m/s), the distance from the transducer to an object that reflects US can be calculated using the time a sound wave takes to make the round trip from the transducer to the reflector and back again. Sophisticated computers can examine reflections from multiple structures simultaneously and display them on a screen as 1-D images. If the US beam is then electronically swept very rapidly across a sector, a 2-D image can be generated.

Several characteristics of US are important in obtaining high-quality images. High-frequency US energy yields excellent resolution, and such beams tend to diverge less over distance than low-frequency signals. High-frequency beams, however, tend to reflect and scatter more as they pass through tissue and are thus subject to greater attenuation than low-frequency signals. Therefore, echocardiographic examinations should utilize the highest frequency that is capable of obtaining signals from the targets in the US field of interest *(1)*.

From: *Essential Cardiology: Principles and Practice, 2nd Ed.*
Edited by: C. Rosendorff © Humana Press Inc., Totowa, NJ

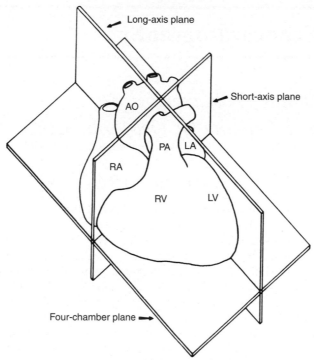

Fig. 1. The three basic tomographic imaging planes used in echocardiography: long-axis, short-axis, and four-chamber. LV, left ventricle; LA, left atrium; RV, right ventricle; RA, right atrium; PA, pulmonary artery; AO, aorta. (From ref. *1*, with permission.)

TWO-DIMENSIONAL ECHOCARDIOGRAPHY: STANDARD EXAMINATION

A US beam can image the heart from multiple areas on the chest wall. Several years ago, M-mode imaging (which detects motion along a single beam of US) was the primary tool of clinical echocardiography. M-mode has been largely supplanted by 2-D imaging. To help standardize the 2-D examination, the American Society of Echocardiography recognizes three orthogonal imaging planes: the long-axis, the short-axis, and the four-chamber planes (Fig. 1) *(2)*. *It is important to remember that the long and short axes are those of the heart, not of the entire body.* These three planes can be imaged in four basic transducer positions: parasternal, apical, subcostal, and suprasternal (Fig. 2). From these parasternal positions, the transducer angle can be modified to obtain views of the mitral valve, the base of the heart, the tricuspid valve, and the right ventricular outflow tract (Fig. 3A,B). From the apical and subcostal transducer positions, both ventricles and all cardiac valves can be examined (Fig. 3C–E). The transducer can also be placed in the suprasternal position to image the thoracic aorta and great vessels.

A complete examination utilizing these imaging planes and transducer positions visualizes the cardiac valves, chamber sizes, and ventricular function in the great majority of cases. Echocardiography is an accepted method for evaluating cardiac systolic function, and assessments of ejection fraction and regional ventricular dysfunction correlate well with those made with angiographic and radionuclide methods. In occasional patients, however, examination is limited owing to US artifacts, marked obesity, severe lung disease (with lung tissue interposed between chest wall and heart), or chest wall deformities.

An additional advance that has improved imaging quality is *harmonic imaging*. Until recently, all US transducers transmitted and received signals at the same frequency. With harmonic imag-

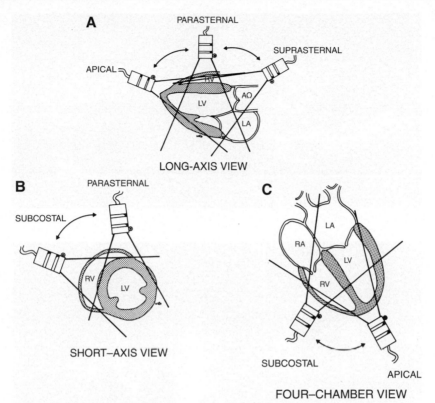

Fig. 2. Visualization of the heart's basic tomographic imaging planes by various transducer positions. The long-axis plane (**A**) can be imaged in the parasternal, suprasternal, and apical positions; the short-axis plane (**B**) in the parasternal and subcostal positions; and the four-chamber plane (**C**) in the apical and subcostal positions.

ing, the transducer transmits at a given (fundamental) frequency but receives at the higher harmonic frequency (for example, transmission at a frequency of 2.5 MHz and reception at 5 MHz). This technology helps to limit artifacts and often improves visualization of regional ventricular function and cardiac anatomy *(3)*.

DOPPLER ECHOCARDIOGRAPHY

Two-dimensional imaging provides abundant information about cardiac structure but no direct data on blood flow. This important area of cardiac imaging is addressed by Doppler echocardiography. When a sound signal strikes a moving object, the frequency of the reflected signal is altered in a way that is proportional to the velocity at which the object is moving and to its direction. The velocity of the moving object can be calculated by the Doppler equation:

$$v = f_d \cdot c/2f_o \ (\cos \theta),$$

where v is the velocity of red blood cells under examination, f_d is the Doppler frequency shift recorded, f_0 the transmitted frequency, and c the velocity of sound *(4)*. The angle θ is the angle between the US beam and the direction of red blood cell flow (i.e., if the US beam is directed parallel to blood flow, the angle is 0 degrees). The importance of this angle cannot be overstated, as echocardiography computer systems assume it to be zero degrees. If the angle θ is greater than 20 degrees, significant errors in velocity calculation occur *(5)*.

Thus, the echocardiography system evaluates the change in frequency (the Doppler shift) of US reflected by red blood cells and translates this into velocity of blood flow. By convention,

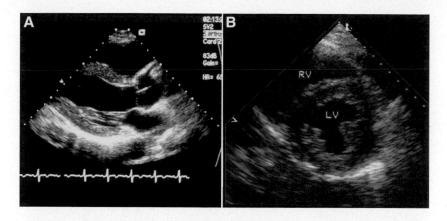

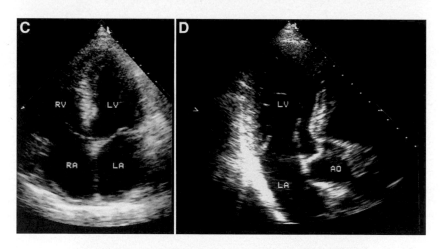

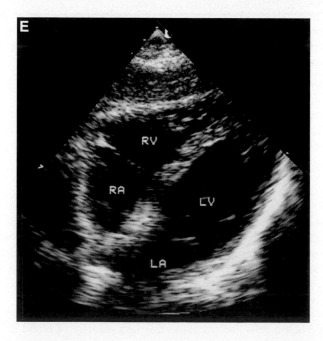

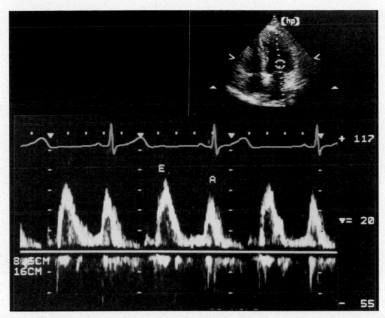

Fig. 4. Normal pulsed-wave Doppler tracing from the left ventricular inflow tract displays the early rapid filling (E) and atrial contraction (A) phases of diastolic flow. The transducer is in the apical position, and the sample volume is at the mitral leaflet tips. (From ref. *1*, with permission.)

spectral Doppler tracings (1) plot velocity with respect to time and (2) display blood flow toward the transducer above an arbitrary "zero" line and flow away from the transducer below this line. As an example, Fig. 4 shows a normal Doppler tracing of blood flow through the mitral valve and the typical early filling (E) and late filling from atrial contraction (A). In this example, the transducer is in the apical position.

There are three main forms of Doppler imaging: PW, CW, and color-flow Doppler. Through a technique called *range gating,* PW Doppler can examine flow in discrete, specific areas in the heart and vasculature. This capability is extremely useful in assessing local flow disturbances, but because of the phenomenon of "aliasing," high velocities cannot be accurately recorded (for a more complete discussion of this phenomenon, the reader is referred to refs. *5* and *6*). The normal velocity of flow through the tricuspid valve is 0.3 to 0.7 m/s and through the pulmonary artery 0.6 to 0.9 m/s. Normal flow velocity through the mitral valve is 0.6 to 1.3 m/s and 1.0 to 1.7 m/s through the LV outflow tract.

Unlike PW Doppler, CW Doppler records all blood flow velocities encountered along the Doppler US beam. Therefore, there is ambiguity of flow location, but CW Doppler is free from "aliasing" and can successfully record very high flow velocities. Color-flow imaging, a major advance in echocardiography, is an extension of PW Doppler. This technique assesses the velocity of flow in multiple sample volumes along multiple beam paths and then assigns a color to each velocity. This color "map" is then superimposed on the 2-D image to obtain a real-time, moving description of blood flow. By convention, flow moving toward the transducer is color coded in

Fig. 3. (*Opposite page*) (**A**) Two-dimensional image of the heart in the parasternal long-axis view. The cardiac chambers correlate with the diagram in Fig. 2A. (**B**) Short-axis plane through the heart at the level of the papillary muscle. (**C**) Two-dimensional image of the apical four-chamber plane. (**D**) Two-dimensional image of the apical three-chamber plane. (**E**) Two-dimensional image of the subcostal four-chamber plane. RA, right atrium; RV, right ventrical; LV, left ventrical; LA, left atrium; AO, aorta. (From ref. *1*, with permission.)

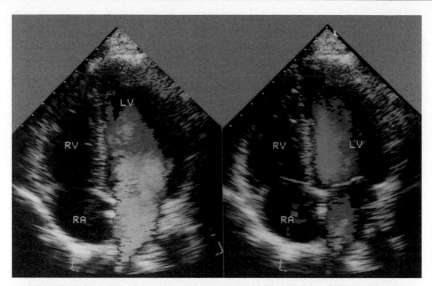

Fig. 5. Apical four-chamber images with color-flow Doppler during diastole and systole. Red flow indicates movement toward the transducer (diastolic filling); blue flow indicates movement away from the transducer (systolic ejection). RA, right atrium; RV, right ventricle; LV, left ventricle. (*See* Color Plate 1, following p. 268. From ref. *1*, with permission.)

shades of red, flow moving away from the transducer in blue (Fig. 5). Very high-velocity flow is assigned a speckled or green color. Color-flow Doppler is an essential part of the complete echocardiographic examination and is an excellent tool for both screening and semiquantitation of valvular regurgitation and stenosis.

Recently, there has been much interest in using mitral inflow velocity patterns to evaluate left ventricular (LV) diastolic function *(7)*. Normally, the E wave is larger than the A wave (*see* Fig. 4). In cases of LV relaxation impairment, the early diastolic transmitral pressure gradient is blunted, causing a decrease in the peak E wave velocity and the rate of flow deceleration. Accompanying this, the peak A wave velocity increases (Fig. 6A). In patients with advanced diastolic dysfunction and markedly increased left atrial pressure and LV stiffness, the E/A ratio becomes abnormally high and the E wave develops a very rapid deceleration of flow velocity (i.e., a short deceleration time). This is the so-called "restrictive" filling pattern (Fig. 6B). In general, the former "relaxation" abnormality (small E, large A) represents mild diastolic dysfunction, whereas the "restrictive" pattern indicates severe diastolic dysfunction and significantly elevated left atrial pressure. This restrictive pattern can occur in restrictive cardiomyopathy, advanced LV systolic dysfunction, pericardial disease, and severe valvular disease (e.g., severe mitral or aortic regurgitation). The restrictive pattern also has been associated with increased risk of death in patients with advanced heart failure.

Despite the utility of transmitral flow patterns in assessing diastolic properties, these should not be interpreted as pathognomonic findings of diastolic dysfunction but rather as a component of a complete clinical and echocardiographic evaluation. In this regard, pulmonary vein flow patterns and tissue Doppler imaging of the mitral annulus are also quite useful and may help detect elevated left atrial pressure when mitral inflow patterns are equivocal or (falsely) appear normal (Fig. 6C) *(7)*. The reader is referred to ref. *7* for a complete discussion of the use of US in diastolic function.

Bernoulli and Continuity Equations

The *modified Bernoulli equation* states that the gradient across a discrete stenosis in the heart or vasculature can be estimated thus:

Pressure gradient = 4 ([Stenotic orifice velocity]^2 − [Proximal velocity]^2).

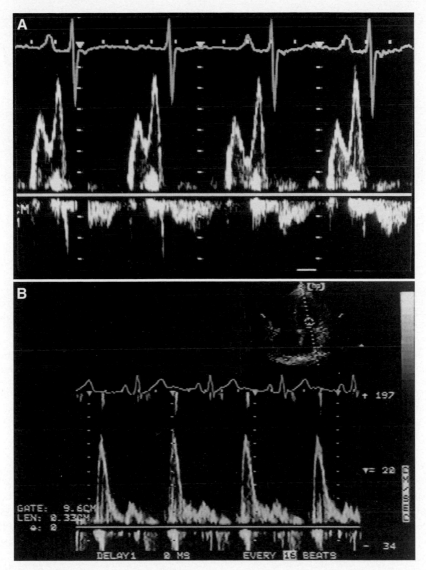

Fig. 6. (A) Pulsed-wave Doppler tracing of diastolic relaxation abnormality. The transducer is in the apical position with the sample volume at the mitral leaflet tips. **(B)** Pulsed-wave Doppler tracing of diastolic restrictive abnormality. (From ref. *1*, with permission.)

If the blood velocity proximal to the stenosis is less than 1.5 m/s, this proximal velocity term can be ignored. The resulting equation states that the pressure gradient across a discrete stenosis is four times the square of the peak velocity through the orifice. This equation can be used to calculate pressure gradients across any flow-limiting orifice (8). In addition, if valvular regurgitation is present, the Bernoulli equation can be used to calculate pressure gradients across the tricuspid and mitral valves. This is quite helpful in measuring pulmonary artery pressure, as the peak right ventricular (RV) and pulmonary artery pressures equal 4 (peak TR velocity)^2 plus the right atrial pressure (which can be estimated on physical examination).

The *continuity equation* states that the product of cross-sectional area and velocity is constant in a closed system of flow:

$$A_1V_1 = A_1V_2$$

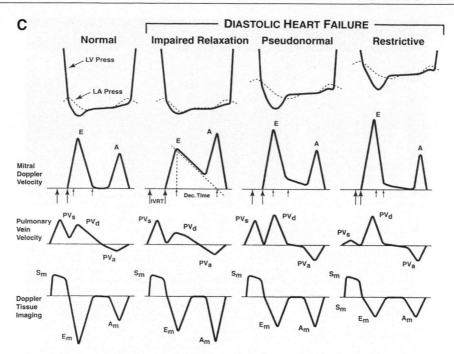

Fig. 6. *(Continued)* **(C)** Doppler assessment of progressive diastolic dysfunction utilizing transmitral pulsed-wave Doppler, pulmonary venous Doppler, and mitral annular tissue Doppler imaging. IVRT, isovolumic relaxation time; Dec. Time, E wave deceleration time; E, early LV filling velocity; A, atrial component of LV filling; PVs, systolic pulmonary vein velocity; PVd, diastolic pulmonary vein velocity; Pva, pulmonary vein velocity resulting from atrial contraction; $\dot{S}_m$, systolic myocardial velocity; E_m, early diastolic myocardial velocity; A_m, myocardial velocity during LV filling produced by atrial contraction. (From ref. 7, with permission.)

The most common use of the continuity equation is calculating aortic valve area, where the product of the cross-sectional area and flow velocity of the LV outflow tract (LVOT) equals the product of the cross-sectional area and velocity of the aortic valve orifice *(9)*. LVOT area is defined as $\pi(d/2)^2$. This area is multiplied by the LVOT peak systolic velocity (measured by PW Doppler) and then divided by the peak velocity through the stenotic orifice (measured by CW Doppler) to obtain the aortic valve area.

TRANSESOPHAGEAL AND HANDHELD ECHOCARDIOGRAPHY

Occasionally transthoracic echocardiography (TTE) does not provide adequately detailed information regarding cardiac anatomy. This is most often true in the evaluation of posterior cardiac structures (e.g., the left atrium and mitral valve), prosthetic cardiac valves, small vegetations or thrombi, and the thoracic aorta. Transesophageal echocardiography (TEE) is well-suited for these situations, as the esophagus is, for much of its course, immediately adjacent to the left atrium and the thoracic aorta *(10)*.

TEE images can be recorded from a variety of positions, but most authorities recommend three basic positions: (1) posterior to the base of the heart, (2) posterior to the left atrium, and (3) inferior to the heart (Fig. 7A,B). There are several specific instances in which TEE is recommended. These include assessment and evaluation of (1) cardiac anatomy when TTE is inadequate, (2) valvular vegetations and infective intracardiac abscesses (Fig. 8A), (3) prosthetic valve function, (4) cardiac embolic sources, including atrial appendage thrombi (Fig. 8B), patent foramen ovale, and interatrial septal aneurysm, and (5) aortic dissection and atherosclerosis *(11)*.

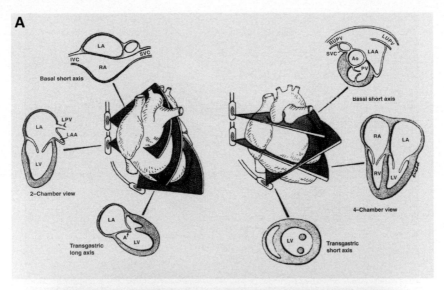

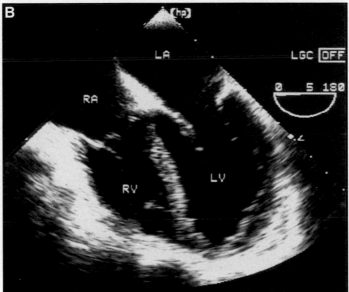

Fig. 7. (A) Standard TEE imaging planes in transverse and longitudinal axes. **(B)** Transverse four-chamber TEE plane; SVC, IVC, superior and inferior vena cava; LAA, left atrial appendage; RUPV, LUPV, right and left upper pulmonary vein; LA, left atrium; LV, left ventricle; RA, right atrium; RV, right ventricle. (From ref. *1*, with permission.)

Recent technologic advances have led to production of small, lightweight (5–6 lb) echocardiographic units. These handheld devices are very portable, and facilitate point-of-care echo evaluation by the physician. The quality of images from these scanners, however, still does not equal that of state-of-the-art standard ultrasound instruments. In addition, current handheld scanners have marginal spectral and color Doppler capabilities. The appropriate use of these scanners is currently controversial, and recommendations will evolve over time. Several studies have shown benefits from handheld scanning in detection of cardiac and aortic pathology, while other reports have shown a relative lack of utility, especially in critically ill patients.

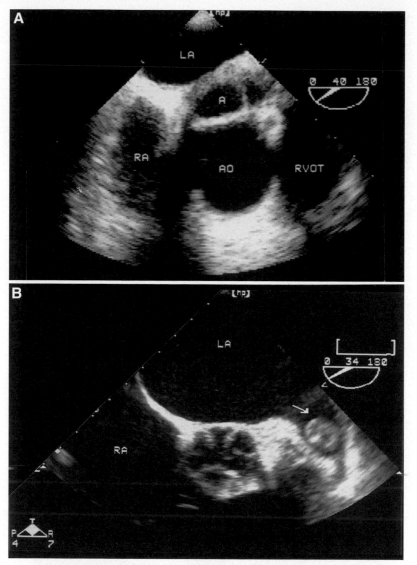

Fig. 8. (A) Short-axis TEE image through the cardiac base. A large septated abscess cavity (A) is present between the aortic root (AO) and the left atrium (LA). **(B)** TEE image of a thrombus in the left atrial appendage (arrow). RVOT, right ventricular outflow tract. (From ref. *1*, with permission.)

This area is definitely in flux, but at this time it may be best to view handheld and limited echo examinations as extensions of the stethoscope. Performed by a competent individual, the diagnostic capability of handheld scanning is at least the equal of auscultation, and probably significantly superior *(12)*.

CONTRAST ECHOCARDIOGRAPHY

Contrast echocardiography has grown explosively in the last few years. For many years, the main agent used for echocardiographic "contrast" injection was agitated saline, which contains numerous air microbubbles that are strong reflectors of US energy. When injected intravenously, agitated saline produces dense opacification of the right heart structures and is an excellent method

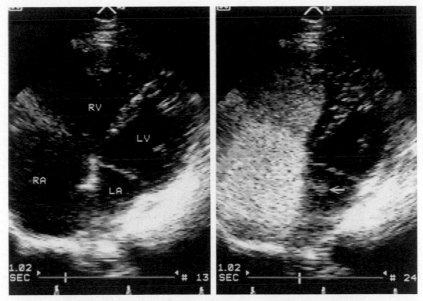

Fig. 9. Contrast microbubble injection demonstrating a shunt (arrow) from the right atrium (RA) to the left atrium (LA). RV, right ventricle; LV, left ventricle. (From ref. *1*, with permission.)

for detecting intracardiac shunts. As the air microbubbles dissolve rapidly into the bloodstream, they do not pass through the pulmonary circulation. Therefore, any air microbubbles entering the left side of the heart must arrive there through a shunt (Fig. 9).

Direct injection of agitated saline into the aorta or left ventricle produces US opacification of the myocardium and LV cavity, respectively *(13)*. LV opacification markedly enhances US images and endocardial border definition, but intraarterial contrast injection is clearly impractical for routine use. Extensive research in the past few years has resulted in the creation of several echocardiographic contrast agents (including Optison™, Definity®, and Imagent™) that survive transit through the pulmonary circulation and reach the left side of the heart after intravenous injection. The current generation of these agents have microbubbles filled with various perfluorocarbon gases instead of air. Because these gases are dense and much less soluble in blood than air, they can persist in the circulation, producing consistent and dense opacification of the LV cavity. These microbubbles also flow along with blood through the coronary vessels, and new technology now permits quantitation of myocardial bloodflow by measuring contrast transit characteristics through the myocardium. In addition, harmonic imaging enhances the US backscatter from contrast microbubbles (which resonate in an US field) while it decreases the signal returning from the myocardium (which does not resonate) *(14)*. Echocontrast agents are especially useful in stress echocardiography, as the enhanced LV endocardial border definition improves detection of regional dysfunction. Recent studies have also shown that regional abnormalities in myocardial perfusion can be assessed during stress testing.

VALVULAR HEART DISEASE

Aortic Valve

Aortic Stenosis

The thin leaflets of the aortic valve are usually well-visualized by echocardiography. Aortic valve disease is often best imaged from the parasternal views. In cases of acquired (calcific) aortic stenosis (AS), the valve leaflets are markedly thickened and calcified, and their motion severely

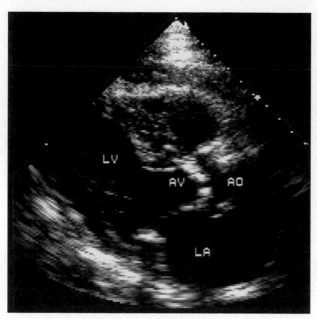

Fig. 10. Parasternal long-axis view demonstrates a thickened, stenotic aortic valve (AV). AO, aorta; LV, left ventricle; LA, left atrium. (From ref. *1*, with permission.)

restricted (Fig. 10). In congenital AS, systolic "doming" of the leaflets is seen, often along with congenital anomalies of the valve leaflets (e.g., bicuspid, unicuspid). Attempts at valve area planimetry by transthoracic echocardiography have generally been unsuccessful, although planimetry with TEE has yielded better results. Thus, standard 2-D imaging accurately detects AS, but not its severity.

The cornerstone of quantification is the Doppler examination. CW Doppler can record the peak velocity of blood flow through the aortic valve, which then can be used to calculate the peak instantaneous systolic gradient with the modified Bernoulli equation. As mentioned above, the aortic valve orifice area is then calculated via the continuity equation in the following manner:

First, the area of the LVOT just proximal to the aortic valve is calculated using this equation: π r^2, where r is half of the diameter of the LVOT measured in the parasternal long axis view; next, the velocity of flow in the LVOT is measured using PW Doppler; finally, the area of the valve orifice is calculated by multiplying the LVOT area by the LVOT velocity and dividing the result by the peak flow velocity through the stenotic orifice *(9,10)*. These calculations correlate quite well with catheterization-derived values and are valid as long as the LVOT flow velocity is less than 1.5 in/s.

AORTIC INSUFFICIENCY

Two-dimensional imaging may show a normal aortic valve in cases of aortic insufficiency (Al), but it can also demonstrate leaflet abnormalities, aortic root enlargement, LV dilation, and diastolic "flutter" of the anterior mitral valve leaflet. In acute severe Al, M-mode imaging can reveal early diastolic closure of the mitral valve (an uncommon but extremely important finding). Although 2-D imaging provides clues to the presence of Al, the Doppler examination is much more useful and easily detects the abnormal flow. Indeed, color-flow Doppler is a very rapid screening tool that detects Al with nearly 100% sensitivity. Quantitation of Al, however, is considerably more difficult.

There are several approaches for semiquantitation of Al by echocardiography. The first utilizes color-flow imaging. In the parasternal views, severity can be estimated by the diameter (or cross-sectional area) of the color jet in the LVOT. Mild Al generally has a jet diameter smaller than 25%

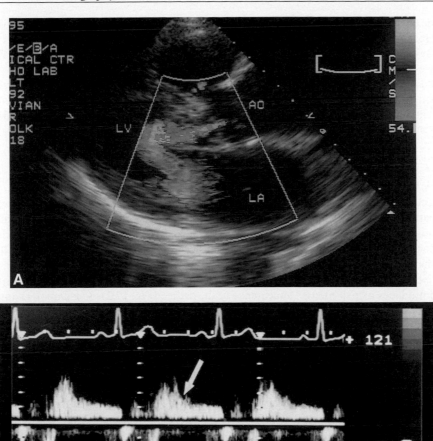

Fig. 11. (A) Parasternal long-axis image showing a multicolored jet (indicating turbulent flow) of aortic regurgitation in the left ventricular outflow tract. The jet is narrow in width, suggesting mild regurgitation. (*See* Color Plate 2, following p. 268.) **(B)** Pulsed-wave Doppler tracing (from the suprasternal transducer position) in a case of severe aortic regurgitation. The sample volume is in the descending thoracic aorta, and holodiastolic flow reversal (arrow) is present. AO, aorta; LA, left atrium; LV, left ventricle. (From ref. *1*, with permission.)

of the outflow tract diameter (Fig. 11A), whereas a severe AI color jet often occupies more than 75% of the outflow tract during diastole. Findings with moderate AT fall between these.

A second method uses CW Doppler to calculate the AI "pressure half-time" (*see* "Mitral Stenosis" section). This parameter is a function of the gradient between the aorta and left ventricle during diastole. In severe AI, this gradient decreases very quickly (producing a short pressure half-time) but with mild AI it decreases much more slowly (producing a long pressure half-time). In general, a pressure half-time of 200 to 250 ms or less strongly suggests severe aortic insufficiency.

In the third method, PW Doppler is utilized to detect diastolic reversal of flow in the descending aorta. Holodiastolic flow reversal suggests severe AI (Fig. 11B). Several other techniques for evaluating severity of AI (e.g., calculation of regurgitant flow volume and orifice area using flow convergence measurements) are beyond the scope of this chapter *(1)*.

Although echocardiographic assessment of aortic stenosis is quantitative and generally accurate, assessment of AI is semiquantitative at best. Therefore, clinical examination and correlation are essential. Despite this, echocardiography is quite useful with aortic valve disease and can help to determine proper timing of valve surgery.

Mitral Valve

MITRAL STENOSIS

Detection of mitral stenosis (MS) was one of the earliest clinical applications of cardiac US. Rheumatic MS is characterized by tethering and fibrosis of the mitral leaflets, principally at the distal tips. The leaflets are sometimes calcified and usually are thickened and display characteristic "doming" during diastole (Fig. 12A). The posterior leaflet of the valve may be pulled anteriorly during diastole secondary to commissural fusion with the longer anterior leaflet. The left atrium is almost always enlarged. In the parasternal short-axis view, the commissural fusion is apparent and produces a "fish-mouth" appearance of the orifice (Fig. 12B) *(15)*. Doppler examination reveals abnormally high diastolic flow velocity through the mitral valve and often detects coexistent mitral regurgitation.

Echocardiographic quantitation of MS severity is done in two ways. First, the mitral orifice area can be measured directly via planimetry in the parasternal short-axis view. Gain artifacts must be avoided, and care must be taken to find the smallest orifice area at the distal end of the leaflets. Properly done, this technique is accurate and correlates well with catheterization data. The second commonly used technique is the "pressure half-time" method. The pressure half-time is the interval required for transmitral flow velocity to decrease from its maximum to the velocity that represents half of the pressure equivalent. As the severity of MS increases, the rate of flow deceleration decreases (i.e., the pressure gradient between left atrium and LV remains high during diastole), prolonging the pressure half-time. The pressure half-time method also correlates well with planimetry measurements, but is not accurate immediately after mitral valvuloplasty.

In addition to valve area quantitation, echocardiography is useful in predicting success of percutaneous mitral valvuloplasty. A score based on four variables (mitral valvular thickening, calcification, mobility, and subvalvular involvement) has been devised and tested. Each variable is rated on a scale of 1 to 4 (where 4 is most severe) and the individual components are summed. A score of 8 to 12 or greater predicts a poor response to valvuloplasty and an increased risk of complications.

MITRAL REGURGITATION

As it is for AI, echocardiography is extremely accurate for detecting mitral regurgitation (MR), but quantitation is more difficult. Two-dimensional imaging in MR may reveal thickened, abnormal mitral valve leaflets (for example, in cases of rheumatic disease, myxomatous degeneration, mitral valve prolapse, or ruptured mitral chordae tendineae). With severe MR, the left atrium and ventricle are often enlarged. Doppler echocardiography is the primary method of semiquantitation of MR. Color-flow imaging shows a jet of aliased flow in the left atrium during systole, and the size of this color jet correlates roughly with angiographic MR severity (Fig. 13; *see* Color Plate 3, following p. 268) *(17)*. Eccentrically directed MR, however, may produce a color jet of misleadingly small cross-sectional area on US imaging, even when left ventriculography demonstrates severe MR.

Volumetric analysis with PW Doppler can be used to calculate regurgitant volumes, but its accuracy is limited. PW Doppler interrogation of the pulmonary veins (by TTE or TEE) is helpful in quantifying MR, as systolic flow reversal within the vein is quite specific for severe regurgitation. Recent work has shown that flow convergence is a useful marker in cases of valvular regurgitation *(18)*. With significant MR, there is often a large zone of high-velocity (aliased) color flow proxi-

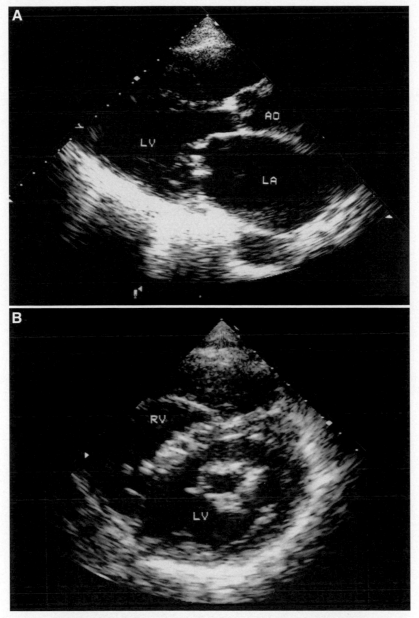

Fig. 12. (A) Parasternal long-axis view of mitral stenosis. The left atrium (LA) is enlarged, mitral opening is limited, and "doming" of the anterior mitral leaflet is present. **(B)** Parasternal short-axis plane in mitral stenosis. RV, right ventricle; LV, left ventricle; AO, aorta. (From ref. *1*, with permission.)

mal to the mitral valve leaflets. This finding (even with a relatively small color jet in the left atrium) often indicates MR of at least moderate severity.

MITRAL VALVE PROLAPSE

Echocardiography is the diagnostic procedure of choice for mitral valve prolapse. This condition is defined by the bulging back of the mitral valve leaflets into the left atrium, with a portion of the leaflets passing the level of the mitral valve annulus on the parasternal long-axis view (Fig. 14). M-mode imaging also can detect mitral valve prolapse, but it is less sensitive than 2-D imaging.

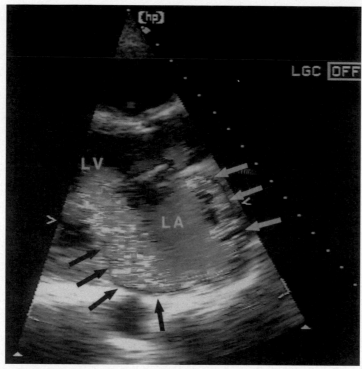

Fig. 13. Parasternal long-axis view in a case of severe mitral regurgitation. The color Doppler jet is directed posteriorly and is eccentric (black arrows). The jet "hugs" the wall of the left atrium (LA) and wraps around all the way to the aortic root (white arrows). LV, left ventricle. (*See* Color Plate 3, following p. 268. From ref. *1*, with permission.)

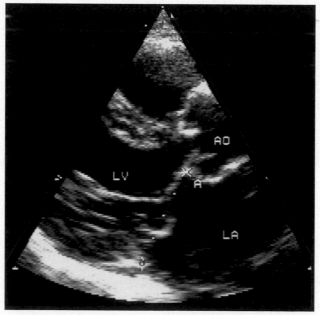

Fig. 14. Parasternal long-axis image through the mitral valve in late systole. The plane of the annulus (A) is drawn in a dotted line. The posterior leaflet prolapses past the level of the annulus. LA, left atrium; AO, aorta; LV, left ventricle. (From ref. *1*, with permission.)

Rupture of a chordae tendineae is well-visualized by US. Imaging usually reveals the involved chord and leaflet as well as the severity of MR. TEE is especially beneficial for assessing the feasibility of mitral valve repair.

PROSTHETIC CARDIAC VALVES

Echocardiography can assess the anatomy and function of bioprosthetic and mechanical heart valves. In general, however, evaluation is considerably more limited than that of native valves. Because of acoustic shadowing, the areas distal to prosthetic (especially mechanical) valves are obscured, limiting detection of valvular regurgitation, thrombi, and vegetations. Because of this, TEE has become indispensable in the evaluation of prosthetic valve dysfunction and associated abnormalities.

Right-Sided Valvular Disease and Pulmonary Hypertension

Two-dimensional echocardiography can detect rheumatic involvement of the tricuspid and pulmonic valves and congenital pulmonic stenosis. Color-flow imaging detects and helps to semiquantify tricuspid and pulmonic regurgitation, similar to insufficiency of the mitral and aortic valves. Measurement of the peak tricuspid regurgitation velocity by CW Doppler is helpful for estimating peak systolic pulmonary artery and right ventricular pressures (via the modified Bernoulli equation) *(9)*.

The 2-D findings associated with right ventricular overload and pulmonary hypertension include enlargement of the right ventricle and right atrium, dilation of the pulmonary artery and inferior vena cava, flattening of the interventricular septum (with loss of the normal curvature toward the right), and hypertrophy of the right ventricular free wall. Doppler examination often shows moderate to severe tricuspid regurgitation in these cases.

DISEASES OF THE AORTA

Aortic Dissection

In the last several years, echocardiography has fundamentally changed the diagnostic approach to suspected aortic dissection. TTE is a reasonably accurate screening tool for ascending aortic dissection (type A) but is not sensitive for detecting descending aortic dissection (type B). Diagnostic findings include a dilated aorta with a thin, linear mobile signal in the lumen representing the dissected intimal flap. Color Doppler imaging may reveal normal or high-velocity flow in the true lumen and slow (stagnant) flow in the false channel. Occasionally, the entrance into the false channel is defined. Although TTE is sometimes helpful, TEE has become a diagnostic procedure of choice for aortic dissection *(12)*. Its sensitivity and specificity rival those of magnetic resonance imaging, and TEE has the advantage of being portable and rapid. In addition, LV and valvular function can be defined during the examination. TEE can also help detect thrombosis of the false lumen, traumatic transection of the aorta, and intramural aortic hematoma (an increasingly recognized disorder with a prognosis similar to that of dissection) *(19)*.

Aortic Aneurysm and Atherosclerosis

Aneurysms of the aorta may appear saccular or fusiform, and on echocardiography are seen as focal or diffuse areas of aortic enlargement. TTE is useful for detecting ascending aortic dilation and can sometimes visualize descending thoracic and abdominal aortic aneurysms (Fig. 15). Sinus of Valsalva aneurysms (asymmetric dilations of the aortic root) are also well-visualized, and the aortic insufficiency or shunts often associated with these aneurysms are well-defined. Echocardiography has been used extensively to aid decision making on the timing of aortic valve and root replacement in patients with Marfan's syndrome *(12)*.

TEE has played a major role in the detection of aortic atherosclerosis. This disease has been underappreciated in the past but appears to be a powerful risk factor for stroke and peripheral

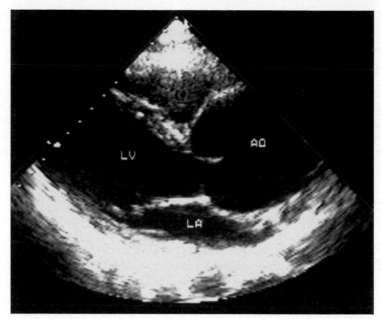

Fig. 15. Parasternal long-axis image demonstrates severe aortic root (AO) enlargement. LA, left atrium; LV, left ventricle. (From ref. *1*, with permission.)

emboli. TEE is currently the procedure of choice for detecting aortic atheromas, which characteristically appear as asymmetric, calcified plaques that protrude into the aortic lumen *(12)*.

INFECTIVE ENDOCARDITIS

Echocardiography is an integral part of the diagnosis and management of infective endocarditis. Clearly, the diagnosis remains a clinical one, but echocardiographic detection of vegetations is now included in most modern diagnostic algorithms and strategies. The hallmark of endocarditis is an infective valvular vegetation (Fig. 16), and TTE detects these with reasonable sensitivity (although as many as 20% of patients with proven native valve endocarditis may have unremarkable TTE findings).

TEE is considerably more accurate than TTE for visualizing vegetations and is significantly better in detecting valvular abscesses and prosthetic valve endocarditis (*see* Fig. 8A) *(20)*. Echocardiography also helps visualize associated abnormalities such as valvular regurgitation, purulent pericarditis, and intracardiac fistulae. Accurate visualization of these abnormalities helps guide management and is useful in assessing the need for cardiac surgery. A common clinical dilemma concerns the appropriate use of TEE in persons with endocarditis. It seems reasonable to use TTE as the first screening test for most patients with suspected endocarditis. If the study is technically limited or findings are equivocal or diagnostic of vegetations in patients at high risk for perivalvular complications, TEE should be performed. If TTE findings are unremarkable or vegetations are detected in patients at low risk for complications, TEE is probably unnecessary. Patients at high risk (e.g., those with prosthetic cardiac valves, congenital heart disease, or infection with virulent organisms) should undergo TEE if endocarditis is strongly suspected, even if TTE results are unremarkable *(20)*.

Despite all technologic advances, infective endocarditis remains a clinical diagnosis, and the utility of echocardiography should not be overestimated. Myxomatous valvular degeneration can masquerade as vegetations, and an old, healed vegetation can be mistaken for an active lesion. Therefore, echocardiographic results should be integrated with all available clinical data.

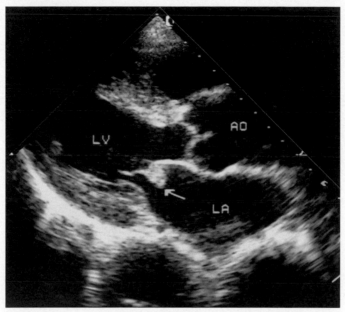

Fig. 16. Parasternal long-axis view demonstrates a vegetation (arrow) on the anterior mitral valve leaflet. AO, aorta; LV, left ventricle; LA, left atrium. (From ref. *1*, with permission.)

ISCHEMIC HEART DISEASE

Echocardiography is an important technique for detecting and analyzing myocardial ischemia and infarction (MI). LV ischemia quickly produces dysfunction and hypokinesis of the involved ventricular segment. If coronary flow is not restored, permanent damage occurs with resulting akinesis and thinning of the affected myocardial segment. If the region of dysfunctional myocardium is identified, the infarct-related coronary artery often can be inferred *(21)*. Echocardiography detects these abnormalities, along with the LV dilation and depression of ejection fraction that accompany severe ischemic heart disease. The LV myocardium can be divided into 16 wall segments according to a format adopted by the American Society of Echocardiography (Fig. 17) *(21)*. By grading the contraction of each of these segments, a semiquantitative wall motion score can be calculated. This parameter has been used to assess prognosis for both acute MI and chronic ischemic heart disease.

Although echocardiography can help estimate the extent of damage in acute MI, the technique is also valuable for detecting post-MI complications. Easily visualized findings include pericardial effusion (from pericarditis or LV free wall rupture), ventricular septal rupture, mitral regurgitation (from LV enlargement or papillary ischemia), LV pseudoaneurysm, and RV dysfunction associated with inferior wall MI. Long-term LV remodeling and aneurysm formation can also be assessed (Fig. 18) *(22)*.

Stress Echocardiography

Echocardiography can been combined with stress testing to increase the accuracy of ischemia detection *(23)*. In this technique, side-by-side cine loops of 2-D images made before and after (or during) stress are displayed on a computer monitor. Normally, the LV myocardium becomes hypercontractile with exercise, and end-diastolic LV cavity size decreases. Stress-induced segmental hypo-kinesis is abnormal, and the affected coronary artery can be predicted from which particular area(s) exhibit inducible ventricular dysfunction. Multiple wall segment abnormalities and LV dilation with stress are ominous findings that suggest severe stenoses in multiple coronary arteries and widespread ischemia *(23)*.

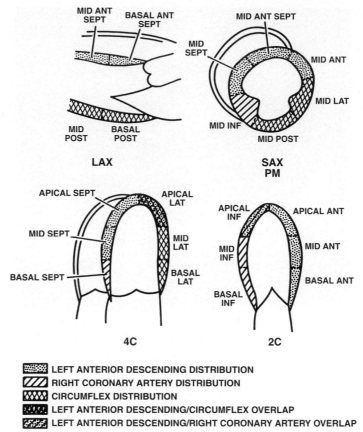

Fig. 17. Sixteen-segment format for identification of left ventricular wall segments. Coronary arterial territories are also included. LAX, parasternal long-axis; SAX PM, short-axis at papillary muscle level; 4C, apical four-chamber; 2C, apical two-chamber; ANT, anterior; SEPT, septal; POST, posterior; LAT, lateral; INF, inferior. (From ref. *21*.)

Stress echocardiography can be performed with either exercise or a graded infusion of dobutamine. In general, both types of stress are safe and are tolerated well, and accuracy rates are comparable with those of nuclear stress imaging. Stress echocardiography tends to be slightly less sensitive than nuclear stress imaging but slightly more specific. Dobutamine echocardiography has assumed an important role in the detection of myocardial viability and the phenomenon of "hibernation" *(24)*. Technical innovations such as harmonic imaging and contrast echocardiography have increased the accuracy and applicability of stress echocardiography. In addition, US contrast agents help facilitate the direct quantitation of myocardial perfusion during stress.

CARDIOMYOPATHIES

Cardiomyopathies are generally separated into three categories: dilated (DCM), hypertrophic (HCM), and restrictive (RCM). Echocardiography plays an important role in the clinical evaluation, providing information on cavity size, ventricular wall thickness, valvular lesions, and systolic function. In cases of classic HCM, echocardiography alone may be diagnostic. In cases of dilated, restrictive, and nonclassic HCM, however, additional clinical information may be needed to arrive at a firm diagnosis. These diseases are discussed in further detail in Chapter 33. In this section, we focus primarily on their US features.

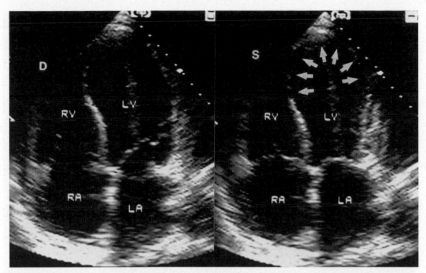

Fig. 18. Apical four-chamber images of a large apical infarction with aneurysm. Diastole (D) is displayed on the left, systole (S) on the right. During systole, the base on the ventricle contracts but the apex is dyskinetic (arrows). RA, right atrium; RV, right ventricle; LV, left ventricle; LA, left atrium. (From ref. *1*, with permission.)

Hypertrophic Cardiomyopathy

HCM is a primary abnormality of the myocardium that exhibits unprovoked hypertrophy and often affects the septum disproportionately. The first and fundamental echocardiographic abnormality is LV hypertrophy, which is often severe. Classically, the septum is involved more extensively than other areas (Fig. 19A), but the hypertrophy may also be concentric or apical. Asymmetric septal hypertrophy leads to the second classic US feature of HCM: dynamic LVOT obstruction. This is associated with systolic anterior motion (SAM) of the mitral valve (*see* arrow, Fig. 19A). Systolic encroachment of the abnormally thickened septum into the LVOT creates a pressure drop via the Venturi effect, which then draws the mitral leaflets toward the septum, causing dynamic obstruction. Like severe LVH, SAM is not pathognomonic for HCM and can occur in other conditions such as hypovolemia and hyperdynamic states *(1)*.

The third manifestation of classic HCM is mid-systolic partial closure of the aortic valve. This occurs only in obstructive HCM cases and is probably a manifestation of the sudden late systole pressure drop caused by SAM. Therefore, when this sign is present, significant LVOT obstruction is likely *(25)*. The fourth sign of HCM is seen on CW Doppler imaging through the LVOT. Normally, flow velocity in this area peaks early during systole and has a maximum of 1.7 m/s. In HCM with outflow tract obstruction, the peak systolic flow velocity is abnormally high. As opposed to valvular aortic stenosis, however, the CW spectral tracing of obstructive HCM peaks late in systole, creating a characteristic "sabertooth" pattern (Fig. 21B). Catheterization data would predict this type of tracing, as the outflow tract gradient is not severely elevated in early systole but rises in mid- and late systole because of dynamic obstruction. The peak CW velocity can be used to calculate the systolic gradient via the modified Bernoulli equation, although recent studies have suggested that this calculation may not be consistently accurate in HCM.

Dilated Cardiomyopathy

Echocardiographic findings in DCM include four-chamber cardiac dilation and marked LV enlargement. Systolic function is depressed, often severely. In addition, the LV walls are often thin, with concomitant left atrial enlargement, limited mitral and aortic valve opening (due to low stroke

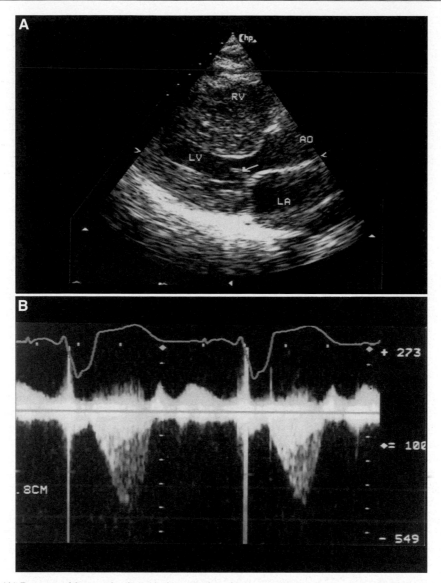

Fig. 19. (A) Parasternal long-axis view (during systole) of hypertrophic cardiomyopathy (HCM). Asymmetric septal hypertrophy is present, as well as systolic anterior motion of the anterior mitral leaflet (arrow). **(B)** Continuous-wave Doppler tracing through the left ventricular outflow tract (from the apical transducer position) in hypertrophic obstructive cardiomyopathy. In comparison to valvular aortic stenosis, the rise in velocity is delayed (reflecting dynamic rather than fixed outflow obstruction). LV, left ventricle; LA, left atrium; RV, right ventricle; AO, aorta. (From ref. *1*, with permission.)

volume), and mitral annular dilation (with secondary mitral regurgitation) *(26)*. Unfortunately, these findings are not specific for DCM and can be caused by severe ischemic heart disease, viral myocarditis, cardiac toxins, and nutritional deficiencies. Ischemic heart disease can often be predicted by the presence of regional LV dysfunction, but, again, this finding is not always reliable. Diastolic dysfunction is common in DCM, and Doppler interrogation of mitral inflow may show an abnormal relaxation, restrictive, or "pseudonormal" pattern, depending on left atrial pressure and loading conditions. A restrictive pattern of inflow is associated with poor prognosis for DCM.

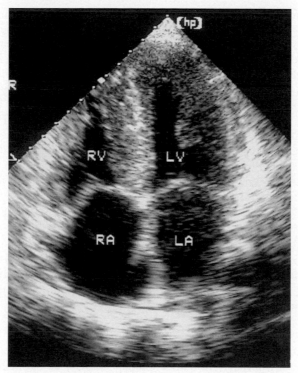

Fig. 20. Apical four-chamber view of cardiac amyloid. RV, right ventricle; RA, right atrium; LA, left atrium; LV, left ventricle. (From ref. *1*, with permission.)

Restrictive Cardiomyopathy

RCM is a fairly rare condition that is characterized on US by (1) a diffuse increase in LV wall thickness in the absence of severe cavity dilation and (2) marked biatrial enlargement *(27)*. Systolic function may be normal or modestly decreased. Doppler examination may show a mitral inflow relaxation abnormality early in the course of RCM, but this tends to evolve into a restrictive pattern as the disease progresses. RCM may be idiopathic or secondary to infiltrative diseases such as hemochromatosis and hypereosinophilic endocardial disease. The most common canse of RCM, however, is amyloidosis, which causes biventricular hypertrophy and diffuse thickening of the interatrial septum and cardiac valves (Fig. 20). A "ground-glass" or speckled appearance of the myocardium has been described with amyloid, but this sign has minimal clinical usefulness. As with the other cardiomyopathies, the echocardiographic findings in RCM are often helpful but ultimately nonspecific.

CARDIAC MASSES

Echocardiography has become the procedure of choice for the detection of intracardiac thrombi, vegetations, and tumors. It also visualizes a number of "pseudo-masses" or benign anatomic variants (e.g., prominent eustachian valve, Chiari network, prominent right ventricular moderator band, and LV false chordae tendineae). US can also detect intracardiac foreign bodies, including pacemaker leads, intracardiac catheters, and endomyocardial bioptomes.

Intracardiac Thrombi

Thrombi can develop in any chamber of the heart and may cause embolic events *(28)*. The major predisposing factors for intracardiac thrombus formation include low cardiac output, localized stasis of flow, and myocardial injury. The echocardiographic appearance of thrombi is quite variable: thrombi can be freely mobile or attached to the endocardium, and they may be laminar and homogeneous in density or heterogeneous with areas of central liquefaction or calcification. Thrombi typically have identifiable borders on US and should be visible in multiple imaging planes *(28)*.

Thrombi within the right heart are often laminar but can be quite mobile (especially venous thromboemboli that have migrated to the right side of the heart), and they increase the risk of pulmonary embolism. Left atrial thrombi occur most often in the setting of LV systolic dysfunction, mitral stenosis, atrial fibrillation, and severe left atrial enlargement. TEE is clearly superior to TTE for detecting these thrombi, especially those within the left atrial appendage (*see* Fig. 8B). Because approx 50% of left atrial thrombi are limited to the appendage, TEE is the procedure of choice for detecting them. Left atrial thrombi are often accompanied by spontaneous US contrast (or "smoke") in the left atrium, which indicates stagnant flow and increased likelihood of embolic events.

LV thrombi usually occur in settings of systolic dysfunction *(28)*, including DCM, acute MI, and chronic LV aneurysm. Most LV thrombi are located in the apex and thus are best visualized in the apical views. LV thrombi may be laminar and fixed, protruding or mobile, and homogeneous or heterogeneous in US density. Artifacts can sometime mimic apical thrombi. A true LV thrombus has a density that is distinct from that of the myocardium, moves concordantly with the underlying tissue, and is visible in multiple imaging planes. Finally, an LV thrombus rarely occurs in areas of normally functioning myocardium.

Cardiac Tumors

Cardiac tumors can be benign or malignant; malignancies may be primary, metastatic, or the result of direct extension from adjacent tumors. Although primary cardiac malignancies are exceedingly rare, metastatic spread to the heart from lung cancer, breast cancer, lymphoma, or melanoma is fairly common, especially in the later stages of disease. Such tumors may be seen within the cardiac chambers, but pericardial or epicardial involvement is more common.

Myxomas are by far the most common primary cardiac tumors, and about 75% are found in the left atrium *(29)*. On 2-D imaging, these tumors generally appear gelatinous, speckled, and sometimes globular. Tissue heterogeneity is frequently seen, but calcifications are rare. Although they can originate from any portion of the atrial wall, myxomas are usually attached by a pedicle to the interatrial septum. Large myxomas are almost always mobile and may move back and forth into the mitral annulus. Doppler examination may demonstrate valvular regurgitation, obstruction, or both. TTE accurately detects most large myxomas (*see* Fig. 21), but TEE is superior for delineating small tumors *(29)*. Less common benign primary cardiac tumors include rhabdomyomas (associated with tuberous sclerosis), fibromas (which tend to grow within the LV myocardial wall), and papillary fibroelastomas (which grow on valves and tend to embolize systemically).

CONGENITAL HEART DISEASE

In this section we focus primarily on the echocardiographic recognition of the more common congenital lesions seen in adults.

Atrial Septal Defect

Most ostium secundum and ostium primum atrial septal defects (ASD) are easily seen with TTE *(30)*. Sinus venosus defects, however, can be difficult to detect without TEE. As the normal interatrial septum is thin and parallel to the US beam from the apical position, artifactual "dropout" in the area of the fossa ovalis can be mistaken for ASD. Therefore, subcostal imaging is usually superior. Ostium secundum defects (the most common form of ASD) are distinguished by localized absence of tissue in the middle portion of the interatrial septum (Fig. 22A; *see* Color Plate 3, following p. 268). The absence of any septal tissue interposed between the defect and the base of the interventricular septum together with the loss of normal apical displacement of the

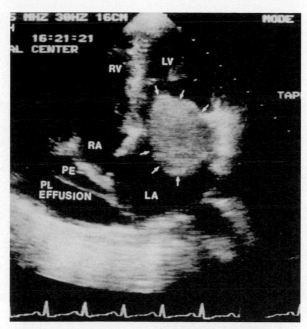

Fig. 21. Apical four-chamber view of a large left atrial myxoma (arrows) that is attached to the lateral wall of the left atrium (LA). RA, right atrium; RV, right ventricle; LV, left ventricle; PE, pericardial effusion; PL, pleural. (From ref. *1*, with permission.)

tricuspid annulus suggests an ostium primum defect. Cleft anterior mitral valve leaflet, mitral regurgitation, and inlet ventricular septal defect often occur with ostium primum ASDs. Sinus venosus ASDs are seen in the superior and posterior portions of the interatrial septum and are usually associated with anomalous drainage of one or more pulmonary veins into the right atrium *(1)*.

Additional 2-D findings seen in ASD include right atrial and RV enlargement, flattening of the interventricular septum, and paradoxical septal motion. Doppler interrogation often demonstrates blood flow though the defect, but atrial inflow from the vena cava and pulmonary veins sometimes mimics ASD. To prevent misdiagnosis of ASD, intravenous injection of agitated saline is recommended (*see* "Contrast Echocardiography"). Finally, Doppler and 2-D imaging can be used to estimate roughly the pulmonary-to-systemic blood flow ratio in patients with ASD or other intracardiac shunts.

Ventricular Septal Defect

The majority of VSDs in adults are perimembranous. Inlet (AV canal), trabecular, and outlet (supracristal) defects are much rarer. Although large VSDs are often visible on 2-D imaging alone (Fig. 22B), color-flow imaging is essential for detection of small defects *(31)*. CW Doppler measurement of peak systolic flow velocity through a VSD can be used to estimate the pressure gradient between the two ventricles via the modified Bernoulli equation (the estimated RV systolic pressure is the systolic arterial pressure minus the calculated Bernoulli gradient) *(9)*. Associated 2-D and Doppler findings include cardiac enlargement (possibly with RV pressure overload), mitral and tricuspid valvular abnormalities and regurgitation, coexistent ASD (most often with inlet VSD), ventricular septal aneurysms, and aortic insufficiency (especially with supracristal VSD). During intravenous injection of agitated saline, "negative" contrast jets are sometimes seen at the right ventricular aspect of the VSD.

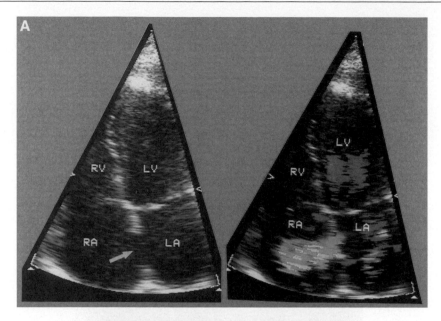

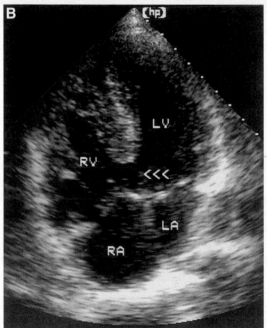

Fig. 22. (A) Apical four-chamber view of an ostium secundum atrial septal defect. On the left, a defect in the mid-atrial septum is present (arrows). On the right, there is color flow through the shunt. RA, right atrium; RV, right ventricle; LA, left atrium; LV, left ventricle. (*See* Color Plate 4, following p. 268.) **(B)** Apical four-chamber image of an inlet ventricular septal defect. RV, right ventricle; RA, right atrium; LA, left atrium; LV, left ventricle. (From ref. *1*, with permission.)

Patent Ductus Arteriosus

Patent ductus arteriosus (PDA) is a connection between the distal portion of the aortic arch and the pulmonary artery (usually just to the left of its bifurcation). Two-dimensional imaging occasionally detects a PDA, but color Doppler interrogation is considerably more likely to demonstrate the

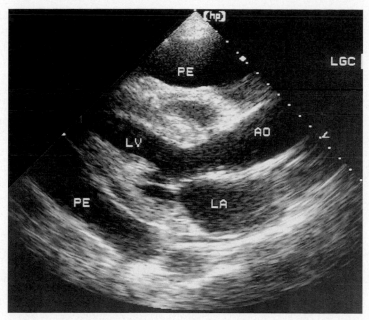

Fig. 23. Parasternal long-axis image of a large pericardial effusion (PE). LV, left ventricle; LA, left atrium; AO, aorta. (From ref. *1*, with permission.)

characteristic high-velocity diastolic flow in the proximal pulmonary artery *(32)*. Additional 2-D findings include LV enlargement and volume overload. If "Eisenmenger" physiology supervenes, the right side of the heart enlarges and LV dilation may reverse to some degree. Therefore, absence of LV or RV enlargement suggests a small shunt.

Conotruncal and Aortic Abnormalities

The most common congenital cardiac anomaly in adults is a bicuspid aortic valve (prevalence of 1 to 2% in men and somewhat less in women). This anomaly is often associated with aortic insufficiency or stenosis, as well as coarctation of the aorta. Tetralogy of Fallot is one of the more frequent conotruncal abnormalities. The classic echo features include a large perimembranous VSD, pulmonic stenosis, RV enlargement and hypertrophy, and anterior displacement of the aortic valve. Coarctation of the aorta, which is often associated with a bicuspid aortic valve, is best visualized from the suprasternal position. Two-dimensional imaging sometimes detects the coarctation, but acoustic shadowing and dropout may limit evaluation of the descending aorta. Doppler examination is more reliable and shows abnormally high flow velocity in the descending aorta. A classic finding in coarctation is holodiastolic antegrade flow in the descending aorta, indicating a pressure gradient throughout diastole and, therefore, severe coarctation. Another congenital abnormality seen occasionally in adult patients is Ebstein's anomaly. Two-dimensional imaging in classic cases reveals a deformed tricuspid valve, including an elongated anterior leaflet and an apically displaced septal leaflet. Associated findings include enlargement of the right side of the heart and tricuspid regurgitation. ASDs are present in a significant minority of cases.

PERICARDIAL DISEASE

Echocardiography is an accurate, reliable tool for the detection of pericardial effusion, intra-pericardial masses, and cardiac tamponade. Pericardial fluid is identified as a "dark" or echo-free space immediately adjacent to the epicardium (Fig. 23). Pericardial effusions may be concentric or loculated and vary much in size. Large, nonloculated effusions generally contain at least 400 mL of fluid and often allow free motion of the heart within the pericardial space. Multiple fibrinous strands in the pericardial effusion raise the possibility of infection, hemorrhage, or malignancy.

There are several echocardiographic clues to the presence of tamponade. Collapse of the right atrial wall (especially with associated tachycardia) is a sensitive, although not specific, sign of increased pericardial pressure. A more specific sign of tamponade is RV free wall diastolic collapse or compression, which indicates marked elevation of intrapericardial pressure. Finally, PW Doppler interrogation of mitral inflow in cardiac tamponade demonstrates an abnormal respiratory variation of peak velocity *(33)*. A respiratory variation in peak E velocity greater than 20% suggests cardiac tamponade when an effusion is present (and pericardial constriction when an effusion is absent or minimal). This Doppler finding is useful for differentiating constrictive pericarditis from restrictive cardiomyopathy, as exaggerated respiratory variation of mitral inflow velocity is not seen in the latter *(34)*.

REFERENCES

1. DeMaria AN, Blanchard DG. The echocardiogram. In: Fuster V, Alexander RW, O'Rourke R, et al., eds. Hurst's The Heart, 11th ed. McGraw-Hill, New York, 2004, pp. 351–465.
2. Henry WL, DeMaria A, Gramiak R, et al. Report of the American Society of Echocardiography: nomenclature and standards in two-dimensional echocardiography. Circulation 1980;62:212.
3. Thomas JD, Rubin DN. Tissue harmonic imaging: why does it work? J Am Soc Echocardiogr 1998;11:803–805.
4. Burns PM. The physical principles of Doppler and spectral analysis. J Clin Ultrasound 1987;15:567–590.
5. Nishimura RA, Miller FA Jr, Callahan MJ, et al. Doppler echocardiography: theory, instrumentation, technique, and application. Mayo Clin Proc 1985;60:321–343.
6. Bom K, deBoo J, Rijsterborgh H. On the aliasing problem in pulsed Doppler cardiac studies. J Clin Ultrasound 1984; 12:559–567.
7. Zile MR, Brutsaert DL. New concepts in diastolic dysfunction and diastolic heart failure: Part I. Circulation 2002; 105:1387–1393.
8. Hegrenaes L, Hatle L. Aortic stenosis in adults. Noninvasive estimation of pressure differences by continuous wave Doppler echocardiography. Br Heart J 1985;54:396–404.
9. Richards KL, Cannon SR, Miller JF, Crawford MH. Calculation of aortic valve area by Doppler echocardiography: a direct application of the continuity equation. Circulation 1986;73:964–969.
10. Daniel WG, Mugge A. Transesophageal echocardiography. N Engl J Med 1995;332;1268–1279.
11. Blanchard DG, Kimura BJ, Dittrich HC, DeMaria AN. Transesophageal echocardiography of the aorta. JAMA 1994;272:546–551.
12. Seward JB, Douglas PS, Erbel R, et al. Hand-carried cardiac ultrasound (HCU) device: recommendations regarding new technology. A report from the echocardiography task force on new technology of the nomenclature and standards committee of the American Society of Echocardiography. J Am Soc Echocardiogr 2002;15:369–373.
13. Gramiak R, Shah PM. Echocardiography of the aortic root. Invest Radiol 1968;3:356–366.
14. Galiuto L, DeMaria AN, May-Newman K, et al. Evaluation of dynamic changes in microvascular flow during ischemia-reperfusion by myocardial contrast echocardiography. J Am Coll Cardiol 1998;32:1096–1101.
15. Glover MU, Warren SE, Vieweg WVR, et al. M-mode and two-dimensional echocardiographic correlation with findings at catheterization and surgery in patients with mitral stenosis. Am Heart J 1983;105:98–102.
16. Hatle L, Angelsen B, Tromsdal A. Noninvasive assessment of atrioventricular pressure half-time by Doppler ultrasound. Circulation 1979;60:1096–1104.
17. Spain MG, et al. Quantitative assessment of mitral regurgitation by Doppler color flow imaging: angiographic and hemodynamic correlations. J Am Coll Cardiol 1989;13:585.
18. Bargiggia CS, Tronconi L, Sahn DJ, et al. A new method for quantitation of mitral regurgitation based on color flow Doppler imaging of flow convergence proximal to regurgitant orifice. Circulation 1991;84:1481–1489.
19. Sawhney NS, DeMaria AN, Blanchard DG. Aortic intramural hematoma: an increasingly recognized and potentially fatal entity. Chest 2001;120:1340–1346.
20. Yvorchuk KJ, Chan K-L. Application of transthoracic and transesophageal echocardiography in the diagnosis and management of infective endocarditis. J Am Soc Echocardiogr 1994;14:294–308.
21. Segar DS, Brown SC, Sawada SC, et al. Dobutamine stress echocardiography: correlation with coronary lesion severity as determined by quantitative angiography. J Am Coll Cardiol 1992;19:1197–1202.
22. Matsumoto M, Watanabe E, Gotto A, et al. Left ventricular aneurysm and the prediction of left ventricular enlargement studied by two-dimensional echocardiography: quantitative assessment of aneurysm size in relation to clinical course. Circulation 1985;72:280–286.
23. Quinones MA, Verani MS, Haichin RM, et al. Exercise echocardiography versus T1-201 single photon emission computerized tomography in evaluation of coronary artery disease. Analysis of 292 patients. Circulation 1992;85: 1026–1031.

24. Bax JJ, Comel JH, Visser FC, et al. Prediction of recovery of myocardial dysfunction after revascularization: comparison of fluorine-18 fluorodeoxyglucose/thallium-201 SPECT, thallium-201 stress-reinjection SPECT and dobutamine echocardiography. J Am Coll Cardiol 1996;28:558–564.
25. Wigle ED, Rakowski H, Kimball BP, Williams WG. Hypertrophic cardiomyopathy: clinical spectrum and treatment. Circulation 1995;92:1680–1692.
26. Shah PM. Echocardiography in congestive or dilated cardiomyopathy. J Am Soc Echocardiogr 1985;1:20–27.
27. Picano E, Pinamonti B, Ferdeghini EM, et al. Two-dimensional echocardiography in myocardial amyloidosis. Echocardiography 1991;8:253–262.
28. Haugland JM, Asinger RW, Mikeil FL, et al. Embolic potential of left ventricular thrombi: detection by two-dimensional echocardiography. Circulation 1984;70:588–598.
29. Reynen K. Cardiac myxomas. N Engl J Med 1995;1610–1617.
30. Shub C, Dimopoulos IN, Seward JB, et al. Sensitivity of two-dimensional echocardiography in the direct visualization of atrial septal defect utilizing the subcostal approach: experience with 154 patients. J Am Coll Cardiol 1983;2: 127–135.
31. Linker DT, Rossvoll O, Chapman JV, Angelsen B. Sensitivity and speed of color Doppler flow mapping compared with continuous wave Doppler for the detection of ventricular septal defects. Br Heart J 1991;65:201–203.
32. Liao P-K, Su W-J, Hung J-S. Doppler echocardiographic flow characteristics of isolated patent ductus arteriosus: better delineation by Doppler color flow mapping. J Am Coll Cardiol 1988;12:1285–1291.
33. Appleton CP, Hatle LK, Popp RL. Cardiac tamponade and pericardial effusion: respiratory variation in transvalvular flow velocities studied by Doppler echocardiography. J Am Coll Cardiol 1988;11:1020–1030.
34. Oh JK, Hatle LK, Seward JB, et al. Diagnostic role of Doppler echocardiography in constrictive pericarditis. J Am Coll Cardiol 1994;23:154–162.
35. Fisher EA, Stahl JA, Budd JH, Goldman ME. Transesophageal echocardiography: procedures and clinical applications. J Am Coll Cardiol 1991;18:1333–1348.

RECOMMENDED READING

DeMaria AN, Blanchard DG. The echocardiogram. In: Fuster V, Alexander RW, O'Rourke R, et al., eds. Hurst's The Heart, 11th ed. McGraw-Hill, New York, 2004, pp. 351–465.
Blanchard DG, DeMaria AN. Cardiac and extracardiac masses: echocardiographic evaluation. In: Skorton DJ, Schelbert HR, Wolf CL, Brundage BH, eds. Marcus' Cardiac Imaging, 2nd ed. W. B. Saunders, Philadelphia, 1996, pp. 452–480.
Nishimura RA, Miller FA Jr, Callahan MI, et al. Doppler echocardiography: theory, instrumentation, technique, and application. Mayo Chin Proc 1985;60:321–343.

10 Exercise Testing

Gregory Engel, MD and Victor Froelicher, MD

INTRODUCTION

Exercise can be considered the true test of the heart because it is the most common everyday stress that humans undertake. The exercise test is the most practical and useful procedure in the clinical evaluation of cardiovascular status.

Despite the many recent advances in technology related to the diagnosis and treatment of cardiovascular disease, the exercise test remains an important diagnostic modality. Its many applications, widespread availability, and high yield of clinically useful information continue to make it an important gatekeeper for more expensive and invasive procedures. The numerous approaches to the exercise test however, have been a drawback to its proper application. Excellent guidelines have been developed based on a multitude of research studies over the last 20 yr, and have led to greater uniformity in methods.

ADVANTAGES AND DISADVANTAGES OF EXERCISE TESTING

The standard exercise test surprisingly has characteristics not dissimilar from newer, more expensive tests. Table 1 lists its disadvantages and advantages.

INDICATIONS

The common clinical applications of exercise testing to be discussed in this chapter are diagnosis and prognosis. The other applications listed in Table 2 are discussed elsewhere (1). The ACC/AHA Guidelines will be followed in regard to diagnosis and prognosis (2).

METHODS

Safety Precautions and Risks

The safety precautions outlined by the American Heart Association are very explicit in regard to the requirements for exercise testing. Everything necessary for cardiopulmonary resuscitation must be available, and regular drills should be performed to ascertain that both personnel and equipment are ready for a cardiac emergency. The classic survey of clinical exercise facilities by Rochmis and Blackburn (3) showed exercise testing to be a safe procedure, with approximately one death and five nonfatal complications per 10,000 tests. Perhaps due to an expanded knowledge concerning indications, contraindications, and endpoints, maximal exercise testing appears safer today than 20 yr ago. Gibbons et al. (4) reviewed 71,914 tests conducted over 16 yr and reported a complication rate of only 0.8 per 10,000 tests. The risk of exercise testing in coronary artery disease patients cannot be disregarded, however, even with its excellent safety record. Cobb and Weaver (5) estimated that the risk of arrhythmic events may be 100 times higher in the recovery period.

From: *Essential Cardiology: Principles and Practice, 2nd Ed.*
Edited by: C. Rosendorff © Humana Press Inc., Totowa, NJ

Table 1
Advantages and Disadvantages of the Standard Exercise Test

Advantages
  Low cost
  Convenience
  Availability of equipment
  Ready availability of trained personnel
  Exercise capacity determined
  Patient acceptability
  Takes less than an hour to accomplish
Disadvantages
  Relatively limited sensitivity and specificity
  No localization of ischemia or coronary lesions
  No estimate of LV function
  Not suitable for certain groups
  Requires cooperation and the ability to walk strenuously

Table 2
Additional Applications of the Exercise Test

Treatment evaluation
Exercise capacity determination
After myocardial infarction
Screening
Cardiac rehabilitation
Exercise prescription
Arrhythmia evaluation
Intermittent claudication
Preoperative evaluation

Most problems can be prevented by having an experienced physician, nurse, or exercise physiologist standing next to the patient, measuring blood pressure, and assessing patient appearance during the test. The exercise technician should operate the recorder and treadmill, take the appropriate tracings, enter data on a form, and alert the physician to any abnormalities that may appear on the monitor. If the patient's appearance is worrisome, if systolic blood pressure drops or plateaus, if there are alarming electrocardiographic abnormalities, if chest pain occurs and becomes worse than the patient's usual pain, or if a patient wants to stop the test for any reason, the test should be stopped, even at a submaximal level. In most instances, a symptom-limited maximal test is preferred, but is usually advisable to stop if 2 mm of additional ST segment elevation occurs, or if 2 mm of flat or downsloping ST depression occurs. In some patients estimated to be at high risk because of their clinical history, it may be appropriate to stop at a submaximal level since it is not unusual for severe ST segment depression, dysrhythmias, or both to occur only after exercise. If the measurement of maximal exercise capacity or other information is needed, it is better to repeat the test later, once the patient has demonstrated a safe performance of a submaximal workload.

Exercise testing should be an extension of the history and physical examination. A physician obtains the most information by being present to talk with, observe, and examine the patient in conjunction with the test. A physical examination should always be performed to rule out significant obstructive aortic valvular disease. In this way, patient safety and an optimal yield of information are assured. In some instances, such as when asymptomatic, apparently healthy subjects are being screened, or a repeat treadmill test is being done on a patient whose condition is stable, a physician need not be present, but should be in close proximity and prepared to respond promptly. The physician's reaction to signs or symptoms should be moderated by the information the patient gives regarding his or her usual activity. If abnormal findings occur at levels of exercise that the patient

Table 3
Contraindications to Exercise Testing

Absolute
    Acute myocardial infarction (within 2 d)
    Unstable angina not stabilized by medical therapy
    Uncontrolled cardiac arrhythmias causing symptoms or hemodynamic compromise
    Symptomatic severe aortic stenosis
    Uncontrolled symptomatic heart failure
    Acute pulmonary embolus or pulmonary infarction
    Acute myocarditis or pericarditis
Relative[a]
    Left main coronary stenosis or its equivalent
    Moderate stenotic valvular heart disease
    Electrolyte abnormalities
    Severe arterial hypertension[b]
    Tachyarrhythmias or bradyarrhythmias
    Hypertrophic cardiomyopathy and other forms of outflow tract obstruction
    Mental or physical impairment leading to inability to exercise adequately
    High-degree atrioventricular block

---

[a]Relative contraindications can be superseded if benefits outweigh risks of exercise
[b]In the absence of definitive evidence, a systolic blood pressure of 200 mmHg and a diastolic blood pressure of 110 mmHg seem reasonable criteria.

usually performs, then it may not be necessary to stop the test for them. Also, the patient's activity history should help determine appropriate work rates for testing.

Contraindications

Table 3 lists the absolute and relative contraindications to performing an exercise test. Good clinical judgment should be foremost in deciding the indications and contraindications for exercise testing. In selected cases with relative contraindications, testing can provide valuable information even if performed submaximally.

Patient Preparation

Preparations for exercise testing include the following:

1. The patient should be instructed not to eat or smoke at least 2 to 3 h prior to the test, and to come dressed for exercise.
2. A history and physical examination (particularly for systolic murmurs) should be accomplished to rule out any contraindications to testing.
3. Specific questioning should determine which drugs are being taken, and potential electrolyte abnormalities should be considered.
4. If the reason for the exercise test is not apparent, the referring physician should be contacted.
5. A 12-lead electrocardiogram should be obtained in both the supine and standing positions. A baseline abnormality may prohibit testing.
6. There should be careful explanations of why the test is being performed, of the testing procedure including its risks and possible complications, and of how to perform the test. The patient should be told that he or she can hold on initially, but later on should use the rails only for balance.

β-Blockers

With patients subgrouped according to β-blocker administration as initiated by their referring physician, no differences in exercise score test performance were found in a consecutive group of males being evaluated for possible coronary artery disease; however, if only ST segment elevation/depression criteria are to be used then 0.5 mm is needed to maintain sensitivity (6). Though perhaps optimal, for routine exercise testing it is unnecessary for physicians to accept the risk of stopping

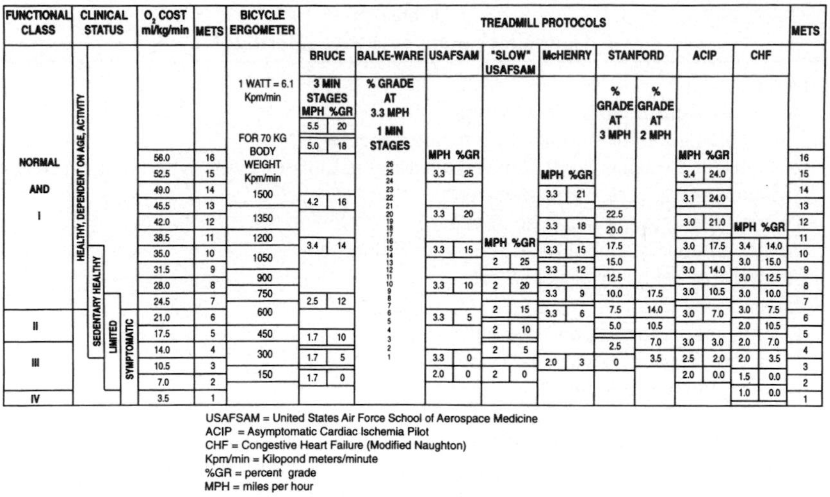
FUNCTIONAL CLASS
CLINICAL STATUS
O2 COST ml/kg/min
METS
BICYCLE ERGOMETER
TREADMILL PROTOCOLS
BRUCE
BALKE-WARE
USAFSAM
"SLOW" USAFSAM
McHENRY
STANFORD
ACIP
CHF
USAFSAM = United States Air Force School of Aerospace Medicine
ACIP = Asymptomatic Cardiac Ischemia Pilot
CHF = Congestive Heart Failure (Modified Naughton)
Kpm/min = Kilopond meters/minute
%GR = percent grade
MPH = miles per hour

Fig. 1. The most common protocols, their stages, and the predicted oxygen cost of each stage are illustrated.

β-blockers before testing. Because of the life-threatening rebound phenomena associated with discontinuing β-blockers, if they are going to be stopped, it should be done gradually with careful supervision of the tapering process by a physician or nurse.

Protocols

The many different exercise protocols in use have led to some confusion regarding how physicians compare tests between patients and serial tests in the same patient. The most common protocols, their stages, and the predicted oxygen cost of each stage are illustrated in Fig. 1. When treadmill and cycle ergometer testing were first introduced into clinical practice, practitioners adopted protocols used by major researchers, i.e., Balke *(7)*, Astrand *(8)*, Bruce *(9)*, and Ellestad *(10)* and their co-workers. In 1980, Stuart and Ellestad surveyed 1375 exercise laboratories in North America and reported that of those performing treadmill testing, 65.5% use the Bruce protocol for routine clinical testing *(11)*. This protocol uses relatively large and unequal 2 to 3 metabolic equivalent (MET) increments in work every 3 min. Large and uneven work increments such as these have been shown to result in a tendency to overestimate exercise capacity *(12)*. Investigators have since recommended protocols with smaller and more equal increments *(13,14)*.

Ramp Testing

An approach to exercise testing that has gained interest is the ramp protocol, in which work increases constantly and continuously (Fig. 2). The recent call for "optimizing" exercise testing would appear to be facilitated by the ramp approach, as work increments are small, and, because it allows for increases in work to be individualized, a given test duration can be targeted.

To investigate this, our laboratory compared ramp treadmill and bicycle tests to protocols more commonly used clinically *(15)*. Ten patients with chronic heart failure, 10 with coronary artery disease who were limited by angina during exercise, 10 with coronary artery disease who were asymptomatic during exercise, and 10 age-matched normal subjects performed three bicycle tests (25 W/2 min stage, 50 W/2 min stage, and ramp) and three treadmill tests (Bruce, Balke, and ramp) in randomized order on different days. For the ramp tests on the bicycle and treadmill, ramp rates were individualized to yield a test duration of approx 10 min for each subject. Maximal oxygen uptake was significantly higher (18%) on the treadmill protocols versus the bicycle protocols collectively, confirming previous observations. Only minor differences in maximal oxygen uptake, however, were observed between the treadmill protocols themselves or between the cycle ergometer protocols themselves.

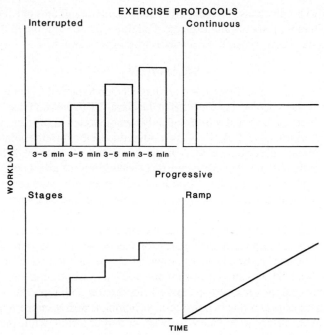

Fig. 2. An approach to exercise testing that has gained interest is the ramp protocol, in which work increases constantly and continuously.

Because this approach appears to offer several advantages, we currently perform all our clinical and research testing using the ramp. This approach is empirical and more data from other laboratories are needed to confirm its utility. A number of equipment manufacturers have developed treadmills that can perform ramping but simple individual manual stepping up of the grade and speed is possible with any device.

HEMODYNAMIC RESPONSES

Age-predicted maximal heart rate targets are relatively useless for clinical purposes. A consistent finding in population studies has been a relatively poor relationship of maximal heart rate to age. Correlation coefficients of −0.4 are usually found with a standard error of the estimate of 10 to 25 beats/min. Since prediction of maximal heart rate is an inaccurate science, exercise should be symptom-limited and not targeted on achieving a certain heart rate.

Exertional hypotension, best defined as a drop in systolic blood pressure below standing rest or a drop of 20 mmHg after a rise, is very predictive of severe angiographic coronary artery disease (CAD) and a poor prognosis. A failure of systolic blood pressure to rise is particularly worrisome after an MI. Until automated devices are adequately validated, we strongly recommend that blood pressure be taken manually with a cuff and stethoscope.

Exercise Capacity

The MET is a unit of basal oxygen consumption equal to approx 3.5 mL O_2 per kilogram of body weight per minute and is the approximate amount of oxygen required to sustain life in the resting state. An individual's maximal oxygen uptake is normally estimated from the workload reached using a formula based on speed and grade. Maximal oxygen uptake is most precisely determined by direct measurement using ventilatory gas-exchange techniques. In certain circumstances where precision is important, such as in athletics, research studies, and patients considered for cardiac transplantation, a direct measurement is essential.

Exercise capacity should always be reported in METs and not minutes of exercise. In this way, the results from different protocols and exercise modalities can be compared directly. Achieved workload in METs has been shown to be a major prognostic variable.

ST Analysis

ST segment depression is a representation of global subendocardial ischemia, with a direction determined largely by the placement of the heart in the chest. ST depression does not localize coronary artery lesions. V_5 is the lead that most frequently demonstrates significant ST depression. ST depression in the inferior leads (II, AVF) is most often due to the atrial repolarization wave that begins in the PR segment and can extend to the beginning of the ST segment. When ST depression is isolated to these leads and there are no diagnostic Q waves, it is usually a false-positive. ST segment depression limited to the recovery period does not generally represent a "false-positive" response. Inclusion of analysis during this time period increases the diagnostic yield of the exercise test.

When the resting ECG shows Q waves of an old MI, ST elevation can be due to wall motion abnormalities, whereas accompanying ST depression can be due to a second area of ischemia or reciprocal changes. When the resting ECG is normal, ST elevation is due to severe ischemia (spasm or a critical lesion). Such ST elevation is uncommon and very arrhythmogenic. Exercise-induced ST elevation (not over diagnostic Q waves) and ST depression both represent ischemia, but they are quite distinctive: *elevation* is due to transmural ischemia, is arrhythmogenic, has a 0.1% prevalence, and localizes the artery where there is spasm or a tight lesion, while *depression* is due to subendocardial ischemia, is not arrhythmogenic, has a 5 to 50% prevalence, is rarely due to spasm, and does not localize. Figure 3 illustrates the various patterns. The standard criterion for abnormality is 1 mm of horizontal or downsloping ST depression below the PR isoelectric line or 1 mm further depression if there is baseline depression.

The most important times to look for ST depression are during maximal exercise in lead V_5 and 3 min into recovery *(16)*. Patients should be placed supine as soon as possible after exercise, avoiding a cool-down walk, to maximize sensitivity for ST abnormalities. ECG recordings should continue for 5 min in recovery or until any new changes from baseline normalize.

Nonsustained ventricular tachycardia is uncommon during routine clinical treadmill testing (prevalence less than 2%), is well tolerated, and its prognosis is determined by any accompanying ischemia or LV damage *(17)*.

DIAGNOSTIC USE OF EXERCISE TEST
The ACC/AHA Guidelines

The task force to establish guidelines for the use of exercise testing met and produced guidelines in 1986, 1997, and 2002 *(2)*. Over the years some dramatic changes have occurred, including the recommendation that the standard exercise test be the first diagnostic procedure in women and in most patients with resting ECG abnormalities rather than performing imaging studies. The following is a synopsis of the recommendations from these evidence-based guidelines for the use of exercise testing to diagnose obstructive coronary artery disease.

Class I.   Conditions for which there is evidence and/or general agreement that the standard exercise test is useful and effective.

• Adult male or female patients (including those with complete right bundle branch block or with less than 1 mm of resting ST depression) with an intermediate pretest probability* of coronary artery disease (specific exceptions are discussed in Class II and III sections).

---

*Pretest probability was determined from the Diamond-Forrester estimates by age, symptoms, and gender (*see* Table 4).

When the ST level begins at or above the isoelectric line (A and B):

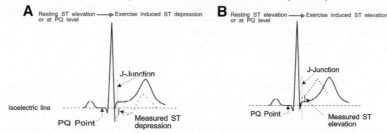

When the ST level begins below the isoelectric line (C and D):

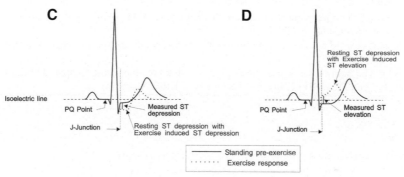

Fig. 3. The various patterns of exercise ST shifts possible with ischemia. ST amplitude measurement depends on the ST level at baseline.

Table 4
Pretest Probability of Coronary Disease by Symptoms, Gender, and Age[a]

Age[b]	Gender	Typical/definite angina pectoris	Atypical/probable angina pectoris	Nonanginal chest pain	Asymptomatic
30–39	Males	Intermediate	Intermediate	Low	Very low
	Females	Intermediate	Very low	Very low	Very low
40–49	Males	High	Intermediate	Intermediate	Low
	Females	Intermediate	Low	Very low	Very low
50–59	Males	High	Intermediate	Intermediate	Low
	Females	Intermediate	Intermediate	Low	Very low
60–69	Males	High	Intermediate	Intermediate	Low
	Females	High	Intermediate	Intermediate	Low

[a]High = >90%, intermediate = 10–90%, low = <10%, and very low = <5%.
[b]There are no data for patients younger than 30 or older than 69 but it can be assumed that coronary artery disease prevalence increases with age.

Class IIa. Conditions for which there is conflicting evidence and/or a divergence of opinion that the standard exercise test is useful and efficacious. Weight of evidence/opinion is in favor of usefulness/efficacy.

• Patients with vasospastic angina

Class IIb. Conditions for which there is conflicting evidence and/or a divergence of opinion that the standard exercise test is useful and efficacious. Usefulness/efficacy is less well established by evidence/opinion.

Table 5
Definitions and Calculation of the Terms Used to Quantify Test Diagnostic Accuracy

True-positive (TP) = number of patients with the disease and a positive result
False-negative (FN) = number of patients with the disease but with a negative result
True-negative (TN) = number of patients without the disease and a negative result
False-positive (FP) = number of patients without the disease but with a positive result
Total population = TP + TN + FP + FN
Sensitivity = percentage of those with the disease who test positive: $TP / (TP + FN) \times 100$
Specificity = percentage of those without the disease who test negative: $TN / (TN + FP) \times 100$
Positive predictive value (PV+) = percentage of those with a positive test result who have the disease:
  $TP / (TP + FP) \times 100$
Negative predictive value (PV–) = percentage of those with a negative test who do not have the disease:
  $TN / (TN + FN) \times 100$
Predictive accuracy (PA) = percentage of correct classifications, both positive and negative:
  $(TP + TN) /$ Total population $\times 100$
Range of characteristics (ROC) curve = plot of sensitivity vs specificity for the range of measurement
  cutpoints
Risk ratio (RR) = The ratio of the disease rate in those with a positive result compared to those with a
  negative result : $TP/(TP + FP) / FN/(FN + TN) = PV+ / FN/(FN + TN)$

- Patients with a high pretest probability of coronary artery disease.*
- Patients with a low pretest probability of coronary artery disease.*
- Patients taking digoxin with less than 1 mm of baseline ST depression.
- Patients with ECG criteria for left ventricular hypertrophy with less than 1 mm of baseline ST depression.

Class III.   Conditions for which there is evidence and/or general agreement that the standard exercise test is not useful or efficacious and in some cases may be harmful.

- Patients who demonstrate the following baseline ECG abnormalities:
  - Preexcitation (Wolff-Parkinson-White) syndrome
  - Electronically paced ventricular rhythm
  - More than 1 mm of ST depression
  - Complete left bundle branch block
- Patients who have had a well-documented myocardial infarction or significant disease demonstrated on coronary angiography.

Test Performance Definitions

Sensitivity and specificity are the terms used to define how reliably a test distinguishes diseased from nondiseased individuals. They are parameters of the accuracy of a diagnostic test. Sensitivity is the percentage of times that a test gives an abnormal ("positive") result when those with the disease are tested. Specificity is the percentage of times that a test gives a normal ("negative") result when those without the disease are tested. This is quite different from the colloquial use of the word "specific." The methods of calculating sensitivity, specificity, and other test characteristics are shown in Table 5. Table 6 presents an example in which test performance characteristics are calculated and the effects of differences in the prevalence of disease are demonstrated.

Standards for Studies of Diagnostic Test Performance

Reid, Lachs, and colleagues updated the seven "methodological standards" for diagnostic tests in 1995 *(18)*. The standards are: (1) specify spectrum of evaluated patients, (2) report test indexes for clinical subgroups, (3) avoid workup bias, (4) avoid review bias, (5) provide numerical pre-

Table 6
Example of Calculating Test Performance and the Effect of Differences in the Population Tested

CAD prevalenve	Subjects	Test characteristics	Number with abnormal test result	Number with normal text result	Predictive value of a positive result
5%	500 with CAD	50% sensitive	250 (TP)	250 (FN)	250/250 + 950
	9500 w/o CAD	90% specific	950 (FP)	8550 (TN)	= 21%
50%	5000 with CAD	50% sensitive	2500 (TP)	2500 (FN)	2500/3000
	5000 w/o CAD	90% specific	500 (FP)	4500 (TN)	= 83%

Disease prevalence sensitivity/specificity	Predictive value of an abnormal test		Risk Ratio	
	5%	50%	5%	50%
70/90%	27%	88%	27×	3×
90/70%	14%	75%	14×	5×
90/90%	32%	90%	64×	9×
66/84%	18%	80%	9×	3×

Calculation of the predictive value of an abnormal test (positive predictive value) using a test with a sensitivity of 50% and a specificity of 90% in two populations of 10,000 patients: one with a coronary artery disease prevalence of 5% and the other with 50% prevalence. This demonstrates the important influence that prevalence has on the positive predictive value.

cision for test indexes, (6) report frequency and management of indeterminate results when calculating test indexes, and (7) specify test reproducibility. In their evaluation of 112 studies, there was limited application of the standards with only one standard being fulfilled by more than half the studies, demonstrating inadequate evaluation of most diagnostic tests. The purpose of refining these standards was to improve patient care, reduce health care costs, improve the quality of diagnostic test information, and to eliminate useless tests or testing methodologies.

Some of the logical and easily appreciated ways to conform to diagnostic test standards in evaluating exercise testing are by blinding to test interpretation, exclusion of patients with prior MIs, and classifying chest pain. Two subtle standards that are least understood but affect test performance drastically and are most commonly not fulfilled are *limited challenge* and *workup bias*. Limited challenge could be justified as the first step of looking at a new measurement or test. An investigator may choose both healthy and sick persons, test them using a new measurement, and see if they are different. If no difference were noted then further investigation would not be indicated. This approach favors the measurement and a better test would be performed in consecutive patients presenting for evaluation. A measurement or test may function well to separate the extremes but fail in a clinical situation. Workup bias means that the decision of who goes to catheterization is made by the physician using the test results and his/her clinical acumen. So the patients in the study are different from patients presenting for evaluation before this selection process occurs. This can only be avoided by having patients agree to both procedures (an exercise test and a cardiac catheterization) prior to performing any testing.

Populations chosen for test evaluation that fail to avoid limited challenge will result in predictive accuracy and range of characteristics (ROC) curves greater than truly associated with the test measurement. Workup bias can affect the calibration of the measurement cutpoints. That is, a score or ST measurement can have a different sensitivity and specificity for a particular cutpoint when workup bias is present.

The two studies that have removed workup bias by protocol have included 2000 patients and have considerably different test characteristics *(19)*.

Meta-Analysis of Exercise Testing Studies

Gianrossi et al. investigated the variability of the reported diagnostic accuracy of the exercise electrocardiogram by performing a meta-analysis *(20)*. One hundred forty-seven consecutively published reports, involving 24,074 patients who underwent both coronary angiography and exercise testing, were summarized. Details regarding population characteristics and methods were evaluated including number of ECG leads, exercise protocol, pre-exercise hyperventilation, definition of an abnormal ST response, exclusion of certain subgroups, and blinding of test interpretation. Wide variability in sensitivity and specificity was found (the mean sensitivity was 68% with a range of 23 to 100% and a standard deviation of 16%; the mean specificity was 77% with a range of 17 to 100% and a standard deviation of 17%). The median predictive accuracy (percentage of total true calls) is approx 73%.

To more accurately portray the performance of the exercise test, only the results in 41 studies out of the original 147 were considered *(21)*. These 41 studies removed patients with a prior MI from this meta-analysis, fulfilling one of the criteria for evaluating a diagnostic test, and provided all the numbers for calculating test performance. These 41 studies, including nearly 10,000 patients, demonstrated a lower mean sensitivity of 68% and a lower mean specificity of 74%; this means that there also is a lower predictive accuracy of 71%. In several studies in which workup bias has been lessened, fulfilling another major criterion, the sensitivity is approximately 50% and the specificity 90%; the predictive accuracy is 70% *(22)*. *This demonstrates that the key feature of the standard exercise test is high specificity and that low sensitivity is a problem.*

Effects of Digoxin, LVH, and Resting ST Depression

LVH, resting ST depression, and digoxin were evaluated in the meta-analysis done as part of the guidelines *(2)*. Only those studies that provided sensitivity, specificity, and total patient numbers and included more than 100 patients were considered. The conclusion from this analysis was that only digoxin had a major effect on test performance.

Gender

There has been controversy regarding the use of the standard exercise ECG test in women. In fact, some experts have recommended that only imaging techniques be used for testing women because of the impression that the standard exercise ECG did not perform as well as it did in men. The recent ACC/AHA guidelines reviewed this subject in detail and came to another conclusion. This position was based on evidence from meta-analysis as well as 15 studies that considered only women. Exercise testing for the diagnosis of significant obstruction coronary disease in adult patients including women, with symptoms or other clinical findings suggestive of intermediate probability of coronary artery disease is a Class I indication (i.e., definitely indicated). Women with intermediate pretest probability are those age 30 to 59 with typical or definite angina pectoris, 50 to 69 with atypical or probable pectoris, and 60 to 69 with nonanginal chest pain (*see* Table 4).

Exercise Test Scores

Improved exercise test characteristics can be obtained by considering additional information in addition to the ST response. Studies have confirmed that this approach is effective *(23)*. The Duke score, originally developed for prognostic use, has been extended to diagnosis *(24)*. Simplified scores derived from multivariable equations have been developed to determine the probability of disease and prognosis. All variables are coded with the same number of intervals so that the coefficients will be proportional. For instance, if 5 is the chosen interval, dichotomous variables are 0 if not present and 5 if present. Continuous variables such as age and maximum heart rate are coded into groups associated with increasing prevalence of disease. The relative importance of the selected variables is obvious and the health care provider merely compiles the variables in the score, multiples by the appropriate number and then adds up the products. Calculation of the "simple" exercise test score can be done using Fig. 4 *(25)* for men and Fig. 5 *(26)* for women.

Variable	Circle response	Sum	Men
Maximal Heart Rate	Less than 100 bpm = 30		
	100 to 129 bpm = 24		
	130 to 159 bpm = 18		
	160 to 189 bpm = 12		
	190 to 220 bpm = 6		
Exercise ST Depression	1-2mm = 15		<40 =
	> 2mm = 25		Low
Age	>55 yrs = 20		Probability
	40 to 55 yrs = 12		
Angina History	Definite/Typical = 5		40-60 =
	Probable/atypical = 3		Intermediate
	Non-cardiac pain = 1		Probability
Hypercholesterolemia?	Yes = 5		
Diabetes?	Yes = 5		>60 =
Exercise Test Induced Angina?	Occurred = 3		High
	Reason for stopping = 5		Probability
	Total Score:		

Fig. 4. Calculation of the simple exercise test score for men.

Variable	Circle response	Sum	Women
Maximal Heart Rate	Less than 100 bpm = 20		
	100 to 129 bpm = 16		
	130 to 159 bpm = 12		
	160 to 189 bpm = 8		
	190 to 220 bpm = 4		
Exercise ST Depression	1-2mm = 6		<37 =
	> 2mm =10		Low
Age	>65 yrs = 25		Probability
	50 to 65 yrs = 15		
Angina History	Definite/Typical - 10		37-57 =
	Probable/atypical = 6		Intermediate
	Non-cardiac pain = 2		Probability
Hypercholesterolemia?	Yes = 10		
Diabetes?	Yes = 10		>57 =
Exercise Test Induced Angina?	Occurred = 9		High
	Reason for stopping =15		Probability
Estrogen Status	Positive=-5, Negative=5		
	Total Score:		

Fig. 5. Calculation of the simple exercise test score for women.

COMPARISON WITH OTHER DIAGNOSTIC TESTS

Nuclear Perfusion and Echocardiography

The performances of exercise echocardiography and exercise nuclear perfusion scanning in the diagnosis of coronary artery disease were compared in a meta-analysis of 44 studies published between 1990 and 1997 (27). Articles were included if they discussed exercise echocardiography and/or exercise nuclear imaging with thallium or sestamibi for detection and/or evaluation of coronary artery disease, if data on coronary angiography were presented as the reference test, and if the absolute numbers of true-positive, false-negative, true-negative, and false-positive observations were available or derivable from the data presented. Studies performed exclusively in patients

Table 7
Comparison of Exercise Testing Subgroups and Different Test Modalities

Grouping	Studies	Patients (n)	Sensitivity (%)	Specificity (%)	Predictive accuracy
Meta-analysis of standard ETT	147	24,047	68%	77%	73%
Meta-analysis w/o MI	58	11,691	67%	72%	69%
Meta-analysis of treadmill scores	24	11,788			80%
Consensus treadmill score	1	2000	85%	92%	88%
Electron beam computed tomography	4	1631	90%	45%	68%
Thallium scintigraphy	59	6038	85%	85%	85%
SPECT w/o MI	27	2136	86%	62%	74%
Persantine thallium	11		85%	91%	87%
Exercise ECHO	58	5000	84%	75%	80%
Exercise ECHO w/o MI	24	2109	87%	84%	85%
Dobutamine ECHO	5		88%	84%	86%

after myocardial infarction, after percutaneous transluminal coronary angioplasty, after coronary artery bypass grafting, or with recent unstable coronary syndromes were excluded. When the discriminatory abilities of exercise echo and exercise nuclear were compared to exercise testing without imaging, both echo and nuclear performed significantly better than the exercise ECG.

Predictive Accuracy

Some test results are dichotomous (normal vs abnormal, positive vs negative) rather than continuous like a score. Predictive accuracy (true positive plus true negatives divided by the total population studied) can be used to compare dichotomous test results. Any score can also be dealt with as a dichotomous variable by choosing a cutpoint. An advantage of predictive accuracy is that it provides an estimate of the number of patients correctly classified by the test out of 100 tested. However, when predictive accuracy is used to compare tests, populations with roughly the same prevalence of disease should be considered. Table 7, based on published meta-analyses, summarizes the sensitivity, specificity, and predictive accuracy of the major diagnostic tests for coronary artery disease currently available (28). While the nonexercise stress tests are very useful, the results shown are probably better than their actual performance because of patient selection. For studies of diagnostic characteristics, patients with a prior MI should be excluded, as diagnosis of coronary disease is not an issue in them.

PROGNOSTIC USE OF EXERCISE TEST

ACC/AHA Guidelines (2)

Indications for exercise testing to assess risk and prognosis in patients with symptoms or a prior history of coronary artery disease:

Class I.   Conditions for which there is evidence and/or general agreement that the standard exercise test is useful and effective.

• Patients undergoing initial evaluation with suspected or known CAD. Exceptions are noted below in Class IIb.
• Patients with suspected or known CAD previously evaluated with significant change in clinical status.
• Low-risk unstable angina patients 8–12 h after presentation who have been free of active ischemic or heart failure symptoms.
• Intermediate-risk unstable angina patients 2–3 d after presentation who have been free of active ischemic or heart failure symptoms.

Class IIa. Conditions for which there is conflicting evidence and/or a divergence of opinion that the standard exercise test is useful and efficacious. Weight of evidence/opinion is in favor of usefulness/efficacy.

- Intermediate-risk unstable angina patients who have initial and 6–12 h cardiac markers that are normal, a repeat ECG without significant change, and no other evidence of ischemia.

Class IIb. Conditions for which there is conflicting evidence and/or a divergence of opinion that the standard exercise test is useful and efficacious. Usefulness/efficacy is less well established by evidence/opinion.

- Patients who demonstrate the following ECG abnormalities:
  - Pre-excitation (Wolff-Parkinson-White) syndrome
  - Electronically paced ventricular rhythm
  - More than 1 mm of resting ST depression
  - QRS duration greater than 120 ms
- Periodic monitoring to guide management of patients with a stable clinical course.

Class III. Conditions for which there is evidence and/or general agreement that the standard exercise test is not useful or efficacious and in some cases may be harmful.

- Patients with severe comorbidity likely to limit life expectancy and/or candidacy for revascularization.
- High-risk unstable angina patients.

Prognostic Scores

The DUKE and VA predictive equations represent the "state of the art" in prognostication.

DUKE TREADMILL SCORE AND NOMOGRAM

Mark et al. studied 2842 consecutive patients who underwent cardiac catheterization and exercise testing and whose data were entered into the Duke computerized medical information system *(29)*. The median follow-up for the study population was 5 yr and 98% complete. All patients underwent a Bruce protocol exercise test and had standard ECG measurements recorded. A treadmill angina index was assigned a value of 0 if angina was absent, 1 if typical angina occurred during exercise, and 2 if angina was the reason the patient stopped exercising. Before the test, 54% of the patients had taken propranolol and 11% had taken digoxin. ST measurements considered were sum of the largest net ST depression and elevation, sum of the ST displacements in all 12 leads, the number of leads showing ST displacement of 0.1 mV or more, and the product of the number of leads showing ST displacement and the largest single ST displacement in any lead. This nomogram and an example are shown in Fig. 6.

VA PREDICTIVE EQUATION

On the basis of clinical and exercise test data, patients with signs and symptoms of coronary heart disease can be classified into low- and high-risk categories. The latter clearly should be considered for cardiac catheterization, while the former should not, unless their symptoms dictate otherwise. The problem lies in justifying intervention to improve survival for patients whose symptoms are satisfactorily managed medically. Cardiac catheterization is not needed to do so in the majority of such patients.

The VA predictive rules demonstrate that simple noninvasive clinical indicators can stratify these patients with stable coronary artery disease into high- or low-risk groups. In our VA population, a simple score based on one item of clinical information (history of congestive heart failure or digoxin use) and three exercise test responses (ST depression, exercise capacity, and change in systolic blood pressure) can identify a group of patients at high risk for cardiovascular death *(30)*. Clinical judgment must be applied to decide whether intervention is likely to improve survival in our high-risk patients.

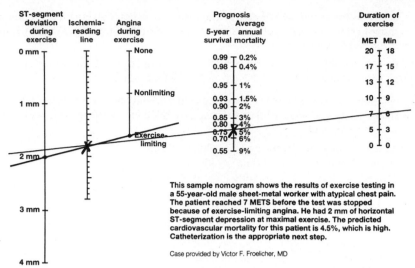

Fig. 6. The Duke Treadmill prognostic nomogram and an example.

Recovery Heart Rate

Heart rate usually falls rapidly at the end of a bout of progressive exercise. While the rate of the drop in heart rate is related to fitness, more recently it has been shown to be inversely related to survival *(31)*. In general, a decline in heart rate of less than 20 bpm by the first or second minute of recovery is associated with an increased risk of death *(32)*.

SUMMARY

The exercise test is relatively inexpensive and readily available. It can be performed in the doctor's office and does not require injections or exposure to radiation. It can provide diagnostic and prognostic information and can also help determine functional capacity and degree of disability. Many physicians have learned from experience that the exercise test complements the medical history and the physical exam as no other test can, so it remains the second most commonly performed cardiology procedure next to the routine ECG. The renewed efforts to control costs will undoubtedly win more over to this group of enlightened physicians. Convincing evidence that treadmill scores enhance the diagnostic and prognostic power of the exercise test will add this movement.

The ACC/AHA guidelines for exercise testing clearly indicate the correct uses of exercise testing. Since the last guidelines, exercise testing has been extended as the first diagnostic test in women and in individuals with right bundle branch block and resting ST segment depression. When diagnostic scores and prognostic scores are used with exercise testing, test characteristics approach that of the nuclear and echocardiographic add-ons to the exercise test.

The following rules are important to follow for getting the most information from the standard exercise test:

- The exercise protocol should be progressive, with even increments in speed and grade whenever possible; consider using a manual or automated ramp protocol.
- The treadmill protocol should be adjusted to the patient; one protocol is not appropriate for all patients.
- Report exercise capacity in METs, not minutes of exercise.
- ST-segment measurements should be made at ST_0 (J-junction) and ST segment depression should be considered abnormal only if horizontal or downsloping.
- Raw ECG waveforms should be considered first and then supplemented by computer-enhanced (filtered and averaged) waveforms when the raw data are acceptable.

- The recovery period is critical to include in analysis of the ST segment response.
- Patients should be placed supine as soon as possible after exercise.
- Measurement of systolic blood pressure during exercise is extremely important and exertional hypotension is ominous; manual blood pressure measurement techniques are preferred.
- Age-predicted heart rate targets are largely useless because of the wide scatter for any age; exercise tests should be symptom-limited.
- A treadmill score should be calculated for every patient; use of multiple scores or a computerized consensus score should be considered as part of the treadmill report.

To ensure the safety of exercise testing, the following list of the most dangerous circumstances in the exercise testing lab should be considered:

- Testing patients with aortic valvular disease should be done with great care because these patients can have a cardiovascular collapse.
- ST segment elevation without diagnostic Q waves is due to transmural ischemia and can be associated with dangerous arrhythmias and infarction.
- Exertional hypotension accompanied by ischemia (angina or ST depression) can be an ominous sign.
- A cool-down walk is advisable in any high-risk patient where ST segment changes are not critical to diagnosis or the evaluation purpose.

REFERENCES

1. Froelicher VF, Myers J. Exercise and the Heart, 4th ed. Saunders/Mosby Year Book Medical Publishers, 1999.
2. Gibbons RJ, Balady GJ, Bricker JT, et al. ACC/AHA 2002 guideline update for exercise testing: a report of the American College of Cardiology/American Heart Association Task Force on Practice Guidelines (Committee on Exercise Testing). Circulation 2002;106:1883–1892.
3. Rochmis P, Blackburn H. Exercise tests: a survey of procedures, safety, and litigation experience in approximately 170,000 tests. JAMA 1971;217:1061–1066.
4. Gibbons L, Blair SN, Kohl HW, Cooper K. The safety of maximal exercise testing. Circulation 1989;80:846–852.
5. Cobb LA, Weaver WD. Exercise: a risk for sudden death in patients with coronary heart disease. J Am Coll Cardiol 1986;7:215–219.
6. Gauri AJ, Raxwal VK, Roux L, et al. Effects of chronotropic incompetence and beta-blocker use on the exercise treadmill test in men. Am Heart J 2001;142:136–141.
7. Balke B, Ware R. An experimental study of physical fitness of air force personnel. US Armed Forces Med J 1959; 10:675–688.
8. Astrand PO, Rodahl K. Textbook of Work Physiology. McGraw-Hill, New York, 1986, pp. 331–365.
9. Bruce RA. Exercise testing of patients with coronary heart disease. Ann Clin Res 1971;3:323–330.
10. Ellestad MH, Allen W, Wan MCK, Kemp G. Maximal treadmill stress testing for cardiovascular evaluation. Circulation 1969;39:517–522.
11. Stuart RJ, Ellestad MH. National survey of exercise stress testing facilities. Chest 1980;77:94–97.
12. Sullivan M, McKirnan MD. Errors in predicting functional capacity for postmyocardial infarction patients using a modified Bruce protocol. Am Heart J 1984;107:486–491.
13. Webster MWI, Sharpe DN. Exercise testing in angina pectoris: the importance of protocol design in clinical trials. Am Heart J 1989;117:505–508.
14. Panza JA, Quyyumi AA, Diodati JG, et al. Prediction of the frequency and duration of ambulatory myocardial ischemia in patients with stable coronary artery disease by determination of the ischemic threshold from exercise testing: importance of the exercise protocol. J Am Coll Cardiol 1991;17:657–663.
15. Myers J, Buchanan N, Walsh D, et al. A comparison of the ramp versus standard exercise protocols. J Am Coll Cardiol 1991;17:1334–1342.
16. Lachterman B, Lehmann KG, Abrahamson D, Froelicher VF. "Recovery only" ST-segment depression and the predictive accuracy of the exercise test. Ann Intern Med 1990;112:11–16.
17. Yang JC, Wesley RC, Froelicher VF. Ventricular tachycardia during routine treadmill testing. Risk and prognosis. Arch Internal Med 1991;151:349–353.
18. Reid M, Lachs M, Feinstein A. Use of methodological standards in diagnostic test research. JAMA 1995;274:645–651.
19. Froelicher VF, Lehmann KG, Thomas R, et al. The electrocardiographic exercise test in a population with reduced workup bias: diagnostic performance, computerized interpretation, and multivariable prediction. Veterans Affairs Cooperative Study in Health Services β016 (QUEXTA) Study Group. Quantitative Exercise Testing and Angiography. Ann Intern Med 1998;128:965–974.
20. Gianrossi R, Detrano R, Mulvihill D, et al. Exercise-induced ST depression in the diagnosis of coronary artery disease: A meta-analysis. Circulation 1989;80:87–98.

21. Marcus R, Lowe R, Froelicher VF, Do D. The exercise test as gatekeeper. Limiting access or appropriately directing resources? Chest 1995;107:1442–1446.
22. Morise A, Diamond GA. Comparison of the sensitivity and specificity of exercise electrocardiography in biased and unbiased populations of men and women. Am Heart J 1995;130:741–747.
23. Yamada H, Do D, Morise A, Froelicher V. Review of studies utilizing multivariable analysis of clinical and exercise test data to predict angiographic coronary artery disease. Progress in CV Disease 1997;39:457–481.
24. Shaw LJ, Peterson ED, Shaw LK, et al. Use of a prognostic treadmill score in identifying diagnostic coronary disease subgroups. Circulation 1998;98:1622–1630.
25. Raxwal V, Shetler K, Do D, Froelicher V. A simple treadmill score. Chest 2000;113:1933–1940.
26. Morise AP, Lauer MS, Froelicher VF. Development and validation of a simple exercise test score for use in women with symptoms of suspected coronary artery disease. Am Heart J 2002;144:818–825.
27. Fleischmann KE, Hunink MG, Kuntz KM, Douglas PS. Exercise echocardiography or exercise SPECT imaging? A meta-analysis of diagnostic test performance. JAMA 1998;280:913–920.
28. O'Rourke RA, Brundage BH, Froelicher VF, et al. American College of Cardiology/American Heart Association Expert Consensus Document on electron-beam computed tomography for the diagnosis and prognosis of coronary artery disease. J Am Coll Cardiol 2000;36:326–340.
29. Mark DB, Hlatky MA, Harrell FE, et al. Exercise treadmill score for predicting prognosis in coronary artery disease. Ann Int Med 1987;106:793–800.
30. Morrow K, Morris CK, Froelicher VF, Hideg A. Prediction of cardiovascular death in men undergoing noninvasive evaluation for CAD. Ann Int Med 1993;118:689–695.
31. Cole CR, Blackstone EH, Pashkow FJ, et al. Heart-rate recovery immediately after exercise as a predictor of mortality. N Engl J Med 1999;341:1351–1357.
32. Shetler K, Marcus R, Froelicher VF, et al. Heart rate recovery: validation and methodologic issues. J Am Coll Cardiol 2001;38:1980–1987.

RECOMMENDED READING

Ashley EA, Froelicher V. The post myocardial infarction exercise test: still worthy after all of these years. Eur Heart J 2001;22:273–276.
Ashley EA, Myers J, Froelicher V. Exercise testing in clinical medicine. Lancet 2000;356:1592–1597.
Atwood JE, Do D, Froelicher VF, et al. Can computerization of the exercise test replace the cardiologist? Am Heart J 1998;136:543–552.
Do D, Marcus R, Froelicher VF, et al. Predicting severe angiographic coronary artery disease using computerization of clinical and exercise test data. Chest 1998;114:1437–1445.
Do D, West JA, Morise A, Froelicher VF. A consensus approach to diagnosing coronary artery disease based on clinical and exercise test data. Chest 1997;111:1742–1749.
Fletcher GF, Froelicher VF, Hartley LH, et al. Exercise standards. A statement for health professionals from the American Heart Association. Circulation 1990;82:2286–2321. Revised, Circulation 1995;91:580–632.
Froelicher VF. Manual of Exercise Testing, 2nd ed. Mosby Year Book Medical Publishers, 1995.
Froelicher VF, Myers J. Research as part of clinical practice: use of Windows-based relational data bases. Veterans Health System Journal March 1998:53–57.
Froelicher VF, Quaglietti S. Handbook of Exercise Testing, Little, Brown, Boston, 1995.
Morrow K, Morris CK, Froelicher VF, Hideg A. Prediction of cardiovascular death in men undergoing noninvasive evaluation for CAD. Ann Int Med 1993;118:689–695.
www.cardiology.org

11 Radiology of the Heart

Gautham P. Reddy, MD, MPH,
and Robert M. Steiner, MD

INTRODUCTION

Imaging plays a critical role in the diagnosis of heart disease. In the past 25 to 30 yr, advanced imaging modalities such as digital angiography, echocardiography, magnetic resonance imaging (MRI), computed tomography (CT), and nuclear cardiology have become important in the evaluation of the heart. However, the conventional radiographic examination remains the mainstay of cardiac imaging. This chapter will discuss the role of the chest radiograph in the diagnosis of cardiac disease in adults, with an emphasis on both normal cardiovascular anatomy and pathoanatomy in a variety of diseases. Correlation will be made with cross-sectional imaging in order to illustrate important anatomic points.

NORMAL ANATOMY

The standard radiographic examination of the chest consists of upright frontal (posteroanterior) and lateral projections (Fig. 1). If a patient is acutely ill or is unable to stand upright, an anteroposterior frontal radiograph may be obtained with the patient in the supine position, and the lateral radiograph is usually omitted. It is important to ensure that the patient is properly positioned in the both the frontal and lateral views so that cardiac structures can be evaluated accurately. In the past left and right anterior oblique projections were obtained routinely, often with contrast medium in the esophagus. With the advent of echocardiography, however, the current role of oblique radiographs is limited.

In the normal chest radiograph, there is excellent inherent contrast between the air-filled lungs, pulmonary vessels, and mediastinum. The chest film therefore is the primary imaging study for evaluation of the lung parenchyma and vessels. However, the components of the mediastinum, including the heart, the blood, and the fat, have similar radiographic densities and cannot be easily distinguished on chest radiographs. Nevertheless, the margins of the heart and mediastinal vessels are clearly demarcated, and variation from the normal appearance suggests the presence of disease.

Left Subclavian Artery

On the frontal chest radiograph, the left subclavian artery forms the superior portion of the left mediastinal border above the aortic arch (Fig. 1A). This artery usually forms a concave border with the lung, although a convex border may be seen if there is increased blood flow, such as in coarctation of the aorta, or if the vessel is tortuous because of atherosclerosis or hypertension. A persistent left superior vena cava is suggested by a straight or convex left supraaortic border.

Aorta

On the frontal view, the ascending aorta forms a convex margin above the right heart border (Fig. 1A). When the ascending aorta enlarges, it projects farther to the right. On the lateral view,

From: *Essential Cardiology: Principles and Practice, 2nd Ed.*
Edited by: C. Rosendorff © Humana Press Inc., Totowa, NJ

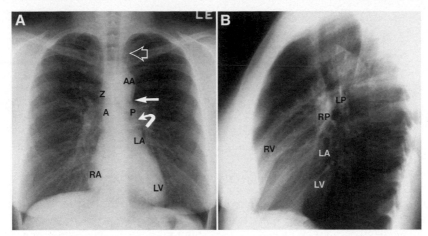

Fig. 1. Normal chest radiograph in a 36-year-old woman. (**A**) Posteroanterior frontal projection. (**B**) Lateral projection. A, ascending aorta; AA, aortic arch; LA, left atrium; LP, left pulmonary artery; LV, left ventricle; P, main pulmonary artery; RA, right atrium; RP, right pulmonary artery; RV, right ventricle; Z, azygos vein. Open arrow = left subclavian artery; straight arrow = aorticopulmonary window; curved arrow = left mainstem bronchus.

the anterior margin of the ascending aorta lies above the right ventricle but is not seen in the normal individual due to an abundance of mediastinal fat.

The aortic arch or "knob" forms a convex border just below the left subclavian artery on the frontal radiograph (Fig. 1A). The aortic arch displaces the trachea slightly to the right. In a patient with a right aortic arch, the trachea is deviated slightly to the left *(1)*. The arch is usually small in the young, healthy individual. An enlarged aortic arch is higher and wider than the normal aorta.

The ascending aorta or arch may be enlarged on the frontal view in individuals with aortic aneurysm, aortic regurgitation, systemic hypertension, or atherosclerosis.

Immediately below the aortic arch along the left mediastinal border, there is an indentation known as the aorticopulmonary window, bordered by the lower margin of the aortic arch and by the superior margin of the left pulmonary artery (Fig. 1A). Convex bulging of the aorticopulmonary window may reflect a ductus diverticulum, lymphadenopathy, or other mass *(2)*.

Pulmonary Vasculature

The main pulmonary artery forms a slightly convex border along the left side of the mediastinum between the aortic knob and the left atrial appendage (Fig. 1A). A prominent convex bulge in this location indicates enlargement of the main pulmonary artery. A large main pulmonary artery may be related to pulmonary arterial hypertension; increased blood flow, as in anemia or a left-to-right shunt; or turbulent flow, as in patients with pulmonary valvular stenosis. On the other hand, the main pulmonary artery border may be flat or convex in patients with transposition of the great vessels, truncus arteriosus, tetralogy of Fallot, or pulmonary atresia. On the lateral projection the anterior border of the main pulmonary artery, located above the right ventricle, is not clearly seen due to the presence of mediastinal fat.

The left pulmonary artery is visualized as a smooth arc just inferior to the aorticopulmonary window. The left pulmonary artery arches over the left mainstem bronchus, as seen on the lateral projection (Fig. 1B). On the other hand, the right pulmonary artery is a round or oval opacity anterior to the right mainstem bronchus on the lateral view (Fig. 1B).

The intrapulmonary branch arteries parallel the airways, and gradually decrease in size toward the lung periphery. The arteries and bronchi are of approximately the same size at any given level; comparison of arterial and bronchial diameters is therefore useful when assessing increase or redistribution of blood flow. When a patient is upright, lower-lobe vessels are larger than upper-lobe vessels due to differences in blood flow, partly due to the effects of gravity *(3)*.

Heart

On the posteroanterior frontal radiograph, the normal heart usually occupies no more than 50% of the transverse diameter of the thorax *(4)*. The respective widths of the heart and the chest can be measured to determine the "cardiothoracic ratio," calculated as the maximum transverse diameter of the heart divided by the maximum width of the thorax *(4)*. In practice, the size of the heart is usually assessed subjectively. Low lung volumes, lordotic projection of the radiograph, or pectus excavatum deformity can cause the heart to appear larger than it really is. A large heart may appear to be of normal size if the lungs are hyperinflated, as in patients with emphysema, or if the cardiac apex is displaced inferiorly. When evaluating the size of the heart, it should be kept in mind that anteroposterior frontal projections result in magnification of the cardiac silhouette by 10 to 13% *(5)*.

LEFT ATRIUM

The left atrial appendage is identified as a smooth, slightly concave segment of the left heart border immediately inferior to the left mainstem bronchus in the frontal view (Fig. 1A). When the left atrial border is straightened or convex, atrial enlargement is suggested. It is important to recognize that noncardiac pathology, such as a pericardial cyst or lymphadenopathy, may mimic enlargement of the left atrial appendage on the frontal radiograph. The right-side margin of the normal left atrium is visualized deep to the right atrial border as an convex "double" density. If the left atrium is severely dilated, the left atrial border may project lateral to the margin of the right atrium *(6)*. Elevation of the left mainstem bronchus is another sign of left atrial enlargement *(7)*. On the lateral projection, the normal left atrium forms a slight bulge at the upper posterior cardiac border (Fig. 1B). Enlargement of the left atrium results in posterior displacement of the esophagus, most easily seen when the esophagus is filled with contrast medium.

LEFT VENTRICLE

The borders of the left ventricle blend with the left atrial margins on both the frontal and lateral radiographs (Fig. 1). On both projections, the slightly convex left ventricular border extends to the diaphragm. The cardiac apex can be displaced inferiorly and laterally when the left ventricle is dilated due to aortic or mitral regurgitation. When the ventricle is hypertrophied because of aortic stenosis or hypertrophic cardiomyopathy, it may be rounded and the apex may be elevated.

RIGHT ATRIUM

The right atrium forms a gentle convex border with the right lung (Fig. 1A). The margins of the right atrium blend with the inferior and superior vena cavae. The border of the inferior vena cava below the right atrium is usually straight *(8)*. On the lateral view, the right atrium is not seen directly because this chamber does not form the cardiac border.

RIGHT VENTRICLE

The right ventricle cannot be visualized directly on the frontal projection because it is not border-forming in the frontal projection. A large right ventricle can displace the left ventricle posteriorly and to the left, causing widening of the cardiac silhouette on the frontal view. On the lateral view, the right ventricle comprises the anterior margin of the heart in the subxyphoid area, occupying the inferior one-third of the thorax (Fig. 1B). A dilated right ventricle will extend further superiorly into the retrosternal space *(9)*.

Azygos Vein

The azygos vein is an oval structure seen in the frontal radiograph at the right tracheobronchial angle (Fig. 1A). The size of the azygos vein is a good marker of cardiovascular dynamics. It enlarges in left and right heart failure, obstruction of the superior vena cava, and absence of the intrahepatic

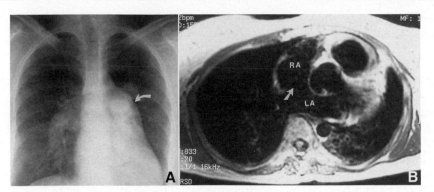

Fig. 2. Pulmonary arterial hypertension secondary to Eisenmenger syndrome in a 32-yr-old woman with atrial septal defect. (**A**) Frontal chest radiograph. The main (arrow), left, and right pulmonary arteries are enlarged. (**B**) Transverse electrocardiographically gated spin echo MRI image shows a large defect (arrow) of the atrial septum. LA, left atrium; RA, right atrium.

segment of the inferior vena cava *(10)*. A change in size of the azygos vein will parallel changes in pulmonary venous pressure, making it a useful radiographic indicator of congestive heart failure.

SPECIFIC ABNORMALITIES

Abnormal Pulmonary Blood Flow and Pulmonary Edema

Pulmonary blood flow reflects the hemodynamics of the heart itself. Increased, decreased, or asymmetrical pulmonary blood flow can be recognized on chest radiographs and correlated with other signs of disease.

The size of the pulmonary arteries is related both to blood flow and blood pressure or to pressure alone *(4)*. Enlarged pulmonary arteries are present in a variety of conditions, including left-to-right shunt, increased cardiac output due to chronic anemia or pregnancy, and pulmonary arterial hypertension, which may be primary or may be secondary to conditions such as chronic interstitial lung disease, emphysema, Eisenmenger's syndrome, or chronic thromboembolism (Fig. 2). Central pulmonary artery calcification indicates chronic, severe pulmonary arterial hypertension *(11)*.

Elevation of pulmonary venous pressure can be due to left ventricular failure, mitral stenosis, and other causes of vascular obstruction distal to the pulmonary arterial bed. When pressure rises to between 12 and 18 mmHg, there is a redistribution of pulmonary blood flow to the upper lobes, which manifests radiographically as enlargement of the upper lobe vessels ("cephalization") *(12)*. As pulmonary venous pressure increases above 18 mmHg, pulmonary interstitial edema occurs. Radiographically, thin horizontal interlobular septal lines, called "Kerley B lines," are visible at the lung bases (Fig. 3) *(13)*. With elevation of pulmonary venous pressure above 25 mmHg, alveolar edema ensues. In the setting of alveolar edema, chest radiographs demonstrate opacities that typically involve the central portions of the lungs, sometimes producing a "batwing" appearance. If the pulmonary edema is related to heart failure, the cardiac silhouette is enlarged (Fig. 3).

Valvular Heart Disease

Stenosis of the aortic valve is most frequently related to a congenital bicuspid valve. Less commonly a tricuspid aortic valve can undergo degeneration, which can be due to rheumatic valvulitis. Aortic stenosis of a mild to moderate degree causes left ventricular hypertrophy. Radiographically, the valve may be calcified, and typically the right side of the ascending aorta bulges due to poststenotic dilation. The left ventricular border may be rounded or the cardiac apex may be elevated due to concentric hypertrophy of the left ventricle *(14)*. More severe narrowing of the valve can lead to enlargement of the left ventricle and atrium *(15)*, in proportion to the degree of stenosis

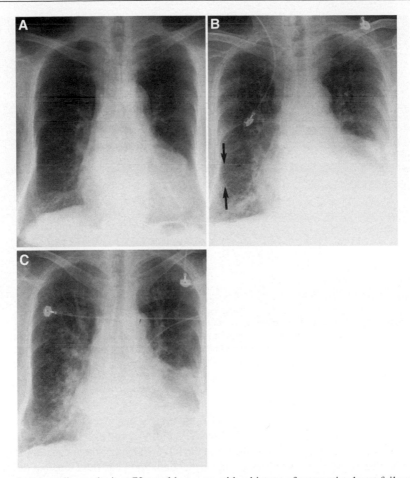

Fig. 3. Frontal chest radiographs in a 72-yr-old woman with a history of congestive heart failure. (**A**) Baseline film demonstrates moderate enlargement of the heart. (**B**) Radiograph performed when the patient was in acute cardiac decompensation. The cardiac silhouette has increased in size, and there is cephalization of the pulmonary vasculature. Kerley B lines (between arrows) are identified in the right lower lobe, indicating pulmonary interstitial edema. (**C**) Film obtained the next day shows progression of pulmonary edema with alveolar opacities.

and the severity of associated mitral regurgitation. Pulmonary venous hypertension and pulmonary edema also can develop in patients with severe aortic stenosis.

Aortic regurgitation can develop in a stenotic bicuspid valve, or it can be due to rheumatic valvulitis, infective endocarditis, or annular dilation resulting from enlargement of the ascending aorta in conditions such as annuloaortic ectasia. Aortic dissection also can cause aortic insufficiency. With mild aortic regurgitation, the heart size usually remains normal, and the ascending aorta is normal or mildly dilated. Enlargement of the left atrium suggests coexisting mitral regurgitation. In patients with moderate or severe aortic regurgitation, the left ventricle and the aorta are enlarged. In contrast to aortic stenosis, diffuse dilation of the aorta can occur in patients with aortic regurgitation. When aortic regurgitation is secondary to annuloaortic ectasia, the aortic root is disproportionately enlarged. Valve calcification often occurs in patients with aortic insufficiency due to a congenital bicuspid valve or rheumatic valve disease. In chronic aortic regurgitation, the left ventricle becomes enlarged, but the lungs appear essentially normal *(16)*. When aortic regurgitation is acute, such as in trauma or dissection, chest radiographs demonstrate pulmonary venous hypertension and pulmonary edema without left ventricular enlargement.

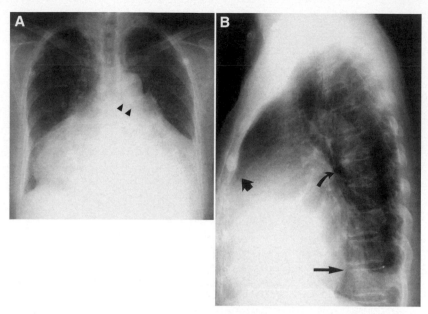

Fig. 4. Severe tricuspid and mitral regurgitation. (**A**) Frontal projection reveals a markedly enlarged cardiac silhouette with global cardiomegaly. The prominent right heart border indicates severe right atrial dilation. The elevation of the left mainstem bronchus (arrowheads) suggests left atrial enlargement. (**B**) Lateral view demonstrates enlargement of the right ventricle (short, wide arrow), left ventricle (long, straight arrow), and left atrium (curved arrow).

Mitral stenosis is most commonly secondary to rheumatic heart disease. Mild enlargement of the left atrium is one of the initial radiographic manifestations of mitral stenosis. When the stenosis is more severe, the left atrium dilates further, and the left atrial appendage can enlarge disproportionately (17). Pulmonary venous hypertension and cephalization can develop, and the central pulmonary arteries can enlarge. The mitral valve is frequently calcified. The left ventricle appears normal in most patients with mitral stenosis.

Chronic mitral regurgitation can be due to a variety of causes, including ischemic cardiomyopathy, rheumatic heart disease, valve prolapse due to myxomatous degeneration, and calcification of the mitral annulus. Chest radiographs exhibit enlargement of both the left atrium and left ventricle (Fig. 4). Because of volume overload and elevated pressure, chamber enlargement can be severe. Acute mitral regurgitation can be caused by rupture of the chordae tendineae or papillary muscles, ischemic dysfunction, and bacterial endocarditis. Although the heart may be normal in size, these patients have left heart failure, which causes severe pulmonary alveolar edema. Occasionally asymmetric pulmonary edema, more severe in the right upper lobe, can result from selective retrograde flow from the mitral valve into the right upper lobe pulmonary veins (18). The valve can be evaluated and the regurgitant flow can be quantified with either echocardiography or MRI.

Tricuspid valve regurgitation (Fig. 4) can be due to ischemic cardiomyopathy, rheumatic heart disease, Ebstein's anomaly, and other causes. Typically the right-sided chambers enlarge, and the right atrium can be disproportionately dilated (19). Patients with tricuspid regurgitation can have massive cardiac enlargement, known as a "wall-to-wall heart."

Ischemic Heart Disease

Several imaging techniques can be used for evaluation of ischemic heart disease, including coronary angiography, radionuclide scintigraphy, echocardiography, electron-beam CT, and MRI. In patients with ischemic cardiomyopathy, the chest films can be completely normal, even in patients who have severe disease. However, many of these patients have cardiomegaly, especially left ventricular enlargement. These patients may also have a left ventricular aneurysm. Pulmonary edema may be present, especially in patients who are acutely short of breath.

Dressler syndrome, or postmyocardial infarction syndrome, manifests radiographically as enlargement of the cardiac silhouette due to pericardial effusion. Pleural effusion (usually unilateral on the left side) is common, and consolidation is present in a minority of patients (20).

Occasionally left ventricular aneurysm can develop after myocardial infarction. A true aneurysm is most frequently located at the cardiac apex or on the anterior ventricular wall. On chest radiographs, the aneurysm appears as a focal bulge along the left heart border (21). A thin rim of calcification is sometimes seen within the aneurysm. A false aneurysm can arise after left ventricular rupture secondary to acute transmural infarction (22). Although most patients with cardiac rupture die immediately, in a small percentage the rupture is contained by the surrounding soft tissues, resulting in a false aneurysm. Chest films can be normal or can demonstrate a contour abnormality, most commonly along the posterior or diaphragmatic aspect of the heart (22). Definitive diagnosis is made by MRI, CT, or echocardiography. Cross-sectional imaging can differentiate a false aneurysm, with its narrow neck, from a true aneurysm, which has a wide neck communicating with the ventricular chamber.

Papillary muscle rupture is an unusual complication of myocardial infarction. Chest radiographs demonstrate a wide spectrum of findings, from no abnormality to marked cardiomegaly and pulmonary edema. Echocardiography or MRI can be performed to diagnose the abnormal mitral valve leaflets and to quantify the severity of mitral regurgitation (23).

In patients with dilated cardiomyopathy and ischemic cardiomyopathy, the left ventricular ejection fraction is decreased. Left ventricular and later biventricular failure develop in most of these patients. Radiographic presentation can vary from a normal heart to diffuse globular enlargement, which may simulate a large pericardial effusion. Ventricular hypokinesis and dilation of the left atrium and left ventricle are the findings at echocardiography.

Coronary artery calcification is an indicator of atherosclerosis, and the quantity of calcification correlates with the total atherosclerotic burden (24). Coronary artery calcification can be identified by various imaging modalities including radiography, fluoroscopy, and CT. CT has the highest diagnostic accuracy for detection of coronary artery calcification (24). In the past several years, electron-beam CT and multidetector helical CT have been investigated for identification of coronary atherosclerosis. Evidence from several recent studies seems to support the use of electron-beam CT and multidetector helical CT for risk stratification in asymptomatic individuals and for diagnosis of coronary artery disease in patients with atypical chest pain (25,26).

Pericardial Disease

On the lateral chest radiograph, the normal pericardium can be seen in some patients as a curved linear opacity between the pericardial fat and the subpericardial fat. Because of their excellent contrast resolution, CT and MRI depict the pericardium more readily than plain radiographs do (27,28).

A small pericardial effusion often is not seen on chest radiographs. As the quantity of pericardial fluid increases, the cardiac silhouette may acquire a "water bottle" or globular configuration (Fig. 5). The normal bulges and indentations of the cardiac borders may become obscured, and the contours of the heart may become blunted and featureless. Because a pericardial effusion can cause enlargement of the cardiac silhouette (28), it may be difficult to distinguish pericardial effusion from cardiomegaly. Since the pericardium extends to the main pulmonary artery, a large pericardial effusion can obscure the hilar vessels, which should not occur with cardiomegaly alone. Occasionally, pericardial effusion may been seen on a lateral chest radiograph as an opaque band between the pericardial fat and the subpericardial fat, known as the "fat pad sign" (Fig. 5C). Although this sign is specific for a pericardial effusion, its sensitivity is limited.

Echocardiography is more sensitive than plain radiographs for the diagnosis of pericardial effusion (29). When a pericardial effusion is suggested by clinical or radiographic findings, echocardiography

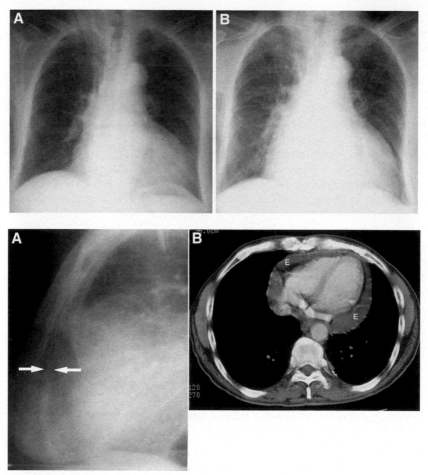

Fig. 5. Pericardial effusion in a 52-yr-old woman on hemodialysis. (**A**) Baseline frontal chest film. (**B**) and (**C**) Films performed two days later just before dialysis. (**B**) The cardiac silhouette has increased in size. (**C**) The lateral view shows the "fat pad sign." There is a dense layer of fluid (between arrows) between the lucent epicardial and pericardial layers of fat. (**D**) Contrast-enhanced CT scan demonstrates a large pericardial effusion (E).

can be used for more definitive evaluation. CT and MRI also can identify pericardial effusion and are useful for the identification of a hemorrhagic effusion (Fig. 5D) *(30)*.

Constrictive pericarditis may occur as a result of open heart surgery, radiation therapy, viral or tuberculous infection, or hemopericardium *(31)*. The cardiac silhouette usually is normal or small, and the right heart border may be flattened *(32)*. A pericardial effusion is present in the majority of these patients, and enlargement of the left atrium and azygous vein in a minority. In a small proportion of patients with pericardial constriction, calcification of the pericardium may be seen. Most often due to tuberculous pericarditis, such calcification may be seen most readily along the anterior and inferior borders of the heart and in the atrioventricular and interventricular grooves (Fig. 6).

Because constrictive pericarditis and restrictive cardiomyopathy may have overlapping clinical presentations and findings, MRI and CT can play an important role in distinguishing the two diagnoses. Pericardial thickening of at least 4 mm is highly sensitive and specific for constrictive pericarditis *(30)*. Ancillary findings of constrictive pericarditis include enlargement of the right atrium, inferior vena cava, and hepatic veins, in addition to a narrowed, "tubular" configuration of the

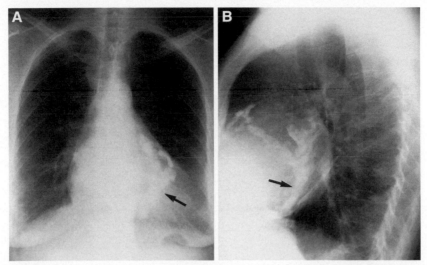

Fig. 6. Calcific pericarditis in a patient with a history of tuberculosis. (**A**) Frontal and (**B**) lateral radiographs demonstrate dense calcium (arrows) in the interventricular groove.

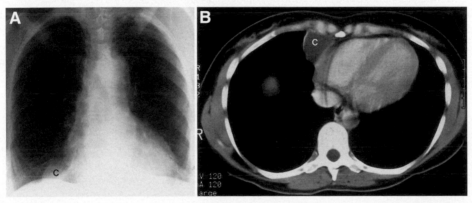

Fig. 7. Pericardial cyst. (**A**) Frontal chest film reveals a smoothly marginated round mass in the right cardiophrenic angle. (c) (**B**) Contrast-enhanced CT scan demonstrates a well-circumscribed, thin-walled mass of fluid density.

right ventricle. Although pericardial calcification and thickening indicate chronic pericardial inflammation and can be used to support the diagnosis of pericardial constriction, the diagnosis must be based on clinical criteria in addition to imaging findings.

When a mediastinal mass is identified on chest radiography, CT or MRI may be performed for more precise evaluation (Fig. 7). A pericardial cyst appears as a smooth, well-margined fluid-filled paracardiac structure. Because they are benign and generally asymptomatic, these cysts may be clinically important only because cross-sectional imaging must be performed to differentiate a cyst from a solid mass. Echocardiography also can be used to make the diagnosis of a pericardial cyst.

Congenital Heart Disease in the Adult

There are three groups of adults with congenital heart disease: those who were treated surgically in childhood, those who were diagnosed as children but did not receive surgical intervention, and those whose disorder was not recognized until adulthood.

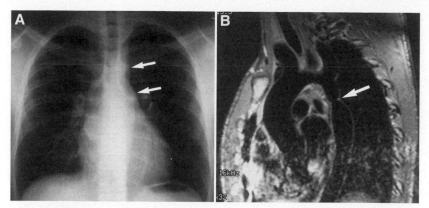

Fig. 8. Young man with hypertension. (**A**) Frontal chest radiograph shows a "figure 3" sign (arrows), consistent with coarctation of the aorta. Rib notching is not seen in this film. (**B**) Oblique sagittal electrocardiographically gated spin echo MRI image demonstrates a severe discrete postductal narrowing of the aorta.

COARCTATION OF AORTA

In adults, a focal juxtaductal stenosis is most common. Chest radiographs may demonstrate a characteristic abnormal contour of the aortic arch, known as the "figure 3" sign, which is a double bulge immediately above and below the region of the aortic knob (Fig. 8A) *(33)*. Bilateral symmetrical rib notching in an older child or adult is diagnostic of coarctation. In recent years, MRI has been used for the evaluation of coarctation of the aorta before and after surgical repair or angiography (Fig. 8B) *(34)*. Because it a noninvasive technique that provides complete anatomic and functional evaluation of the coarctation, MRI can usually be performed in place of diagnostic angiography.

LEFT-TO-RIGHT SHUNTS

Ostium secundum atrial septal defect (ASD) is the most common left-to-right shunt diagnosed in adult life, accounting for more than 40% of adult congenital heart defects *(35)*. Although the chest radiograph may be normal in a patient with a small shunt, typically the main pulmonary artery, the peripheral pulmonary branches, the right atrium, and right ventricular borders are enlarged (Fig. 2A). Echocardiography can delineate the size and location of the ASD, as well as associated abnormalities such as mitral valve prolapse. MRI can be performed if echocardiography does not reveal the ASD (Fig. 2B).

If a ventricular septal defect (VSD) is small, the chest film is normal. However, the pulmonary arteries, both ventricles, and the left atrium are enlarged if the left-to-right shunt is large or if there is secondary pulmonary hypertension,. Echocardiography usually will demonstrate the site of the defect. MRI is performed in certain cases to evaluate associated abnormalities or to define certain lesions such as a supracristal VSD, which may be difficult to image by echocardiography *(36)*.

REFERENCES

1. Steiner RM, Gross G, Flicker S, et al. Congenital heart disease in the adult patient. J Thorac Imaging 1995;10:1–25.
2. Danza FM, Fusco A, Breda M. Ductus arteriosus aneurysm in an adult. AJR 1984;143:131–133.
3. West JB. Regional differences in gas exchange in the lung in erect man. J Appl Physiol 1962;17:893–898.
4. Kabala JE, Wilde P. Measurement of heart size in the anteroposterior chest radiograph. Br J Radiol 1987;60: 981–986.
5. Milne ENC, Burnett K, Aufrichtig D, et al. Assessment of cardiac size on portable chest films. J Thorac Imaging 1988; 3:64–72.
6. Higgins CB, Reinke RT, Jones WE, et al. Left atrial dimension on the frontal thoracic radiograph: a method for assessing left atrial enlargement. AJR 1978;130:251–255.
7. Carlsson E, Gross R, Hold RG. The radiological diagnosis of cardiac valvar insufficiencies. Circulation 1977;55: 921–933.
8. Jefferson K, Rees S. Clinical Cardiac Radiology, 2nd ed. Butterworths, London, 1980, pp. 3–24.

9. Murphy ML, Blue LR, Ferris EJ, et al. Sensitivity and specificity of chest roentgenogram criteria for right ventricular hypertrophy. Invest Radiol 1988;23:853–856.
10. Berdon WE, Baker DH. Plain film findings in azygos continuation of the inferior vena cava. AJR 1968;104:452–457.
11. Gutierrez FR, Moran CJ, Ludbrook PA, et al. Pulmonary arterial calcification with reversible pulmonary hypertension. AJR 1980;135:177–178.
12. Harrison MO, Conte, PJ, Heitzman ER. Radiological detection of clinically occult cardiac failure following myocardial infarction. Br J Radiol 1971;44:265–272.
13. Grainger RG. Interstitial pulmonary oedema and its radiological diagnosis. A sign of pulmonary venous and capillary hypertension. Br J Radiol 1958;31:201–217.
14. Higgins CB. Radiography of acquired heart disease. In: Higgins CB, ed. Essentials of Cardiac Radiology and Imaging. J. B. Lippincott, Philadelphia, 1992, pp. 1–48.
15. Lasser A. Calcification of the myocardium. Hum Pathol 1983;14:824–826.
16. Follman DF. Aortic regurgitation. Identifying and treating acute and chronic disease. Postgrad Med 1993;93:83–90.
17. Green CE, Kelley MJ, Higgins CB. Etiologic significance of enlargement of the left atrial appendage in adults. Radiology 1982;142:21–27.
18. Gurney JW, Goodman LR. Pulmonary edema localized in the right upper lobe accompanying mitral regurgitation. Radiology 1989;172:397–399.
19. Stanford W, Galvin JR. The radiology of right heart dysfunction: chest roentgenogram and computed tomography. J Thorac Imaging 1989;4:7–19.
20. Watanabe AM. Ischemic heart disease. In: Kelly NW, ed. Essentials of Internal Medicine. J. B. Lippincott, Philadelphia, 1994, pp. 1511–1512.
21. Higgins CB, Lipton MJ. Radiography of acute myocardial infarction. Radiol Clin North Am 1980;18:359–368.
22. Higgins CB, Lipton MJ, Johnson AD, et al. False aneurysms of the left ventricle. Identification of distinctive clinical, radiographic, and angiographic features. Radiology 1978;127:21–27.
23. Kotler MN, Mintz GS, Panidis I, et al. Noninvasive evaluation of normal and abnormal prosthetic valve function. J Am Coll Cardiol 1983;2:151–173.
24. Wexler L, Brundage B, Crouse J, et al. Coronary artery calcification: pathophysiology, epidemiology, imaging methods, and clinical implications. A statement for health professionals from the American Heart Association. Circulation 1996;94:1175–1192.
25. Rumberger JA, Sheedy PF, Breen JF, et al. Electron beam computed tomography and coronary artery disease: scanning for coronary artery calcification. Mayo Clin Proc 1996;71:369–377.
26. Thompson BH, Stanford W. Imaging of coronary calcification by computed tomography. J Magn Reson Imaging 2004;19:720–733.
27. Olson MC, Posniak HV, McDonald V, et al. Computed tomography and magnetic resonance imaging of the pericardium. Radiographics 1989;9:633–649.
28. Steiner RM, Rao VM. Radiology of the pericardium. In: Grainger RG, Allison J, eds. Diagnostic Radiology. Churchill Livingstone, London, 1986, pp. 675–689.
29. Engel PJ. Echocardiography in pericardial disease. Cardiovasc Clin 1983;13:181–200.
30. Sechtem U, Tscholakoff D, Higgins CB. MRI of the abnormal pericardium. AJR 1986;147:245–252.
31. Vaitkus PT, Kussmaul WG. Constrictive pericarditis versus restrictive cardiomyopathy: a reappraisal and update of diagnostic criteria. Am Heart J 1991;122:1431–1441.
32. Carsky EW, Mauceri RA, Azimi R. The epicardial fat pad sign: analysis of frontal and lateral chest radiographs in patients with pericardial effusion. Radiology 1980;137:303–308.
33. Chen JTT, Khoury M, Kirks DR. Obscured aortic arch on the lateral view as a sign of coarctation. Radiology 1984;153:595–596.
34. Von Schulthess GK, Higashino SM, Higgins SS, et al. Coarctation of the aorta: MR imaging. Radiology 1986;158:469–474.
35. Whittemore R, Wells JA, Castellsague X. A second generation study of 427 probands with congenital heart disease and their 837 children. J Am Coll Cardiol 1994;23:1459–1467.
36. Bremerich J, Reddy GP, Higgins CB. MRI of supracristal ventricular septal defects. J Comput Assist Tomogr 1999;23:13–15.

RECOMMENDED READING

Lipton MJ, Boxt LM. How to approach cardiac diagnosis from the chest radiograph. Radiol Clin North Am 2004;42:487–495.
Miller SW, ed. Cardiac Radiology. The Requisites (2nd ed.). Elsevier, Philadelphia, 2004.
Steiner RM. Radiology of the heart and great vessels. In: Braunwald E, Zipes DP, Libby P, eds. Heart Disease. A Textbook of Cardiovascular Medicine (6th ed.). W. B. Saunders, Philadelphia, 2001, pp. 237–272.

12

Cardiac Catheterization and Coronary Angiography

Mark J. Ricciardi, MD, Nirat Beohar, MD, and Charles J. Davidson, MD

INTRODUCTION

In 1929, Werner Forssman performed the first human cardiac catheterization when he passed a urethral catheter from his left antecubital vein into the right side of his heart *(1)*. The introduction of left heart catheterization by Zimmerman *(2)* and Limon Lason *(3)* and selective coronary arteriography by Sones in the 1950s *(4,5)* began the modern era of coronary artery disease management and revascularization. In each of the decades subsequent to the introduction of coronary arteriography, major advances in revascularization therapy were introduced: coronary artery bypass graft surgery by Favolaro in the late 1960s *(6)*, percutaneous balloon coronary angioplasty by Gruentzig in the late 1970s *(7,8)*, and coronary stent implantation by Sigwart in the late 1980s *(9)*.

INDICATIONS

Cardiac catheterization remains an indispensable diagnostic tool to determine the presence and severity of diseases of the heart. Identification and quantification of coronary artery disease are the most common indications for cardiac catheterization in adults. Indications for coronary angiography are given in Table 1 *(10)*.

In addition to coronary imaging, cardiac catheterization allows for the assessment of ventricular function, valve stenosis and regurgitation, aortic root imaging, right and left heart hemodynamics, intracardiac shunts, and pharmacologic interventions.

RELATIVE CONTRAINDICATIONS

The relative contraindications to cardiac catheterization are listed in Table 2. Efforts should be made to ameliorate factors that increase procedural risk before procedure initiation. Persons at increased risk, for whom special precautions are recommended, are listed in Table 3.

PRECATHETERIZATION PROTOCOL

Prior to the procedure, a standardized preoperative protocol should be followed. A sample protocol follows:

- Highlights of the technical aspects of the procedure and its purpose, risks, benefits, and alternatives are fully explained to the patient and family.
- Preprocedure history with special attention to:
  - Prior cardiac catheterization (catheters used, difficulty with arterial access or coronary cannulation);
  - Prior revascularization procedures (coronary artery bypass grafting, number of grafts, graft type, and vessels bypassed, percutaneous coronary interventions, vessels treated, equipment used, adjunctive medications);

From: *Essential Cardiology: Principles and Practice, 2nd Ed.*
Edited by: C. Rosendorff © Humana Press Inc., Totowa, NJ

Table 1
Class I and II Indications for Coronary Angiography

Known or Suspected* Coronary Disease Who Are Currently Asymptomatic or Have Stable Angina
Asymptomatic or Stable Angina
   Class I
     Evidence of high risk on noninvasive testing.
     Canadian Cardiovascular Society (CSS) class III or IV angina on medical treatment.
     Patients resuscitated from sudden cardiac death or with sustained monomorphic VT or nonsustained
       polymorphic VT.
   Class IIa
     CCS class III or IV angina that improves to class I or II on medical therapy.
     Serial noninvasive testing showing progressive abnormalities.
     Patient with disability or illness that cannot be stratified by other means.
     CCS Class I or II with intolerance or failure to respond to medical therapy.
     Individuals whose occupation involves safety of others (e.g., pilots, bus drivers) with abnormal
       stress test results or high-risk clinical profile.
Nonspecific Chest Pain
   Class I
     High-risk findings on noninvasive testing
   Class IIa
     None.

Unstable Coronary Syndromes
   Class I
     High or intermediate risk for adverse outcome in patients with unstable angina refractory to initial
       adequate medical therapy, or recurrent symptoms after initial stabilization.
     Emergent catheterization is recommended.
     High risk for adverse outcome in patients with unstable angina. Urgent catheterization is
       recommended.
     High- or intermediate-risk unstable angina that stabilizes after initial treatment.
     Initially low short-term-risk unstable angina that is subsequently high-risk on noninvasive testing.
     Suspected Prinzmetal's variant angina.
   Class IIa
     None.

Patients with Postrevascularization Ischemia
   Class I
     Suspected abrupt closure or subacute stent thrombosis after percutaneous revascularization.
     Recurrent angina or high-risk criteria on noninvasive evaluation within 9 mo of percutaneous
       revascularization.
   Class IIa
     Recurrent symptomatic ischemia within 12 mo of CABG.
     Noninvasive evidence of high-risk criteria occurring at any time postoperatively.
     Recurrent angina inadequately controlled by medical means after revascularization.

During the Initial Management of Acute MI
(MI Suspected and ST Segment Elevation or Bundle Branch Block Present)
Coronary Angiography Coupled with Intent to Perform Primary PTCA
   Class I
     As an alternative to thrombolytic therapy in patients who can undergo angioplasty of the infarct-
       related artery within 12 h of the onset of symptoms or beyond 12 h if ischemic symptoms
       persist, *if performed in a timely fashion by individuals skilled in the procedure and supported by*
       experienced personnel in an appropriate laboratory environment.

Table 1 (Continued)

In patients who are within 36 h of an acute ST elevation Q wave or new LBBB MI who develop
  cardiogenic shock, who are younger than 75 yr, and in whom revascularization can be performed
  within 18 h of the onset of the shock.
Class IIa
  As a reperfusion strategy in patients who are candidates for reperfusion but who have a contra-
    indication to fibrinolytic therapy, if angioplasty can be performed as outlined earlier in class I.
Early Coronary Angiography in Patient with Suspected MI
  (ST Segment Elevation or Bundle Branch Block Present) Who Has Not Undergone Primary PTCA
  Class I
    None.
  Class IIa
    Cardiogenic shock or persistent hemodynamic instability.
Early Coronary Angiography in Acute MI (MI Suspected but No ST Segment Elevation)
  Class I
    Persistent or recurrent (stuttering) episodes of symptomatic ischemia, spontaneous or induced, with or
      without associated ECG changes.
    Presence of shock, severe pulmonary congestion, or continuing hypotension.
  Class IIa
    None.
Coronary Angioplasty During Hospital Management Phase
  (Patients with Q Wave and Non-Q-Wave Infarction)
  Class I
    Spontaneous myocardial ischemia or myocardial ischemia provoked by minimal exertion, during
      recovery from infarction.
    Before definitive therapy of a mechanical complication of infarction such as acute mitral regurgitation,
      ventricular septal defect, pseudoaneurysm, or left ventricular aneurysm.
    Persistent hemodynamic instability.
  Class IIa
    When MI is suspected to have occurred by a mechanism other than thrombotic occlusion at an
      atheroslcerotic plaque (e.g., coronary embolism, arteritis, trauma, certain metabolic or hematologic
      diseases or coronary spasm).
    Survivors of acute MI with left ventricular EF < 0.40, CHF, prior revascularization, or malignant
      ventricular arrhythmias.
    Clinical heart failure during the acute episode, but subsequent demonstration of preserved left
      ventricular function (left ventricular EF > 0.40).
During the Risk-Stratification Phase (Patients with All Types of MI)
  Class I
    Ischemia at low levels of exercise with ECG changes (1-mm ST segment depression or other
      predictors of adverse outcome) and/or imaging abnormalities.
  Class IIa
    Clinically significant CHF during the hospital course.
    Inability to perform an exercise test with left ventricular EF ≤ 0.45.
Perioperative Evaluation Before (or After) Noncardiac Surgery
  Class I: Patients with suspected or known CAD
    Evidence for high risk of adverse outcome based on noninvasive test results.
    Angina unresponsive to adequate medical therapy.
    Unstable angina, particularly when facing intermediate- or high-risk noncardiac surgery.
    Equivocal noninvasive test result in high-clinical-risk patient undergoing high-risk surgery.
  Class IIa
    Multiple-intermediate-clinical risk markers and planned vascular surgery.
    Ischemia on noninvasive testing but without high-risk criteria.   *(continued)*

Table 1 (Continued)

Equivocal noninvasive test result in intermediate-clinical-risk patient undergoing high-risk noncardiac surgery.

Urgent noncardiac surgery while convalescing from acute MI.

Patients with Valvular Heart Disease
Class I

Before valve surgery or balloon valvotomy in an adult with chest discomfort, ischemia by noninvasive imaging, or both.

Before valve surgery in an adult free of chest pain but with many risk factors for CAD.

Infective endocarditis with evidence of coronary embolization.

Class IIa

None.

Patients with Congenital Heart Disease
Class I

Before surgical correction of congenital heart disease when chest discomfort or noninvasive evidence is suggestive of associated CAD.

Before surgical correction of suspected congenital coronary anomalies such as congenital coronary artery stenosis, coronary arteriovenous fistula, and anomalous origin of the left coronary artery.

Forms of congenital heart disease frequently associated with coronary artery anomalies that may complicate surgical management.

Unexplained cardiac arrest in a young patient.

Class IIa

Before corrective open heart surgery for congenital heart disease in an adult whose risk profile increases the likelihood of coexisting CAD.

Patients with CHF
Class I

CHF due to systolic dysfunction with angina or with regional wall motion abnormalities and/or scintigraphic evidence or reversible myocardial ischemia when revascularization is being considered.

Before cardiac transplantation.

CHF secondary to postinfarction ventricular aneurysm or other mechanical complications of MI.

Class IIa

Systolic dysfunction with unexplained cause despite noninvasive testing.

Normal systolic function, but episodic heart failure raises suspicion if ischemically mediated left ventricular dysfunction.

Other Conditions
Class I

Diseases affecting the aorta when knowledge of the presence or extent of coronary artery involvement is necessary for management (e.g., aortic dissection or aneurysm with known CAD).

Hypertrophic cardiomyopathy with angina despite medical therapy when knowledge of coronary anatomy might affect therapy.

Hypertrophic cardiomyopathy with angina when heart surgery is planned.

Class IIa

High risk for CAD when other cardiac surgical procedures are planned (e.g., pericardiectomy or removal of chronic pulmonary emboli).

Prospective immediate cardiac transplant donors whose risk profile increases the likelihood of CAD.

Asymptomatic patients with Kawasaki's disease who have coronary artery aneurysms on echocardiography.

Before surgery for aortic aneurysm/dissection in patients without known CAD.

Recent blunt chest trauma and suspicion of acute MI, without evidence of preexisting CAD.

CABG, coronary artery bypass graft; CAD, coronary artery disease; CHF, congestive heart failure; ECG, electrocardiographic; EF, ejection fraction; LBBB, left bundle branch block; MI, myocardial infarction; PTCA, percutaneous transluminal coronary angioplasty.

*Known, previous myocardial infarction, coronary bypass surgery or PTCA; suspected; Rest- or exercise-induced ECG abnormalities suggesting silent ischemia.

Table 2
Relative Contraindications to Coronary Angiography

Unexplained fever, untreated infection	Digitalis toxicity
Severe anemia (Hb < 8 g/dL)	Prior contrast allergy without pretreatment
Severe electrolyte imbalance	Active or recent stroke (<1 mo)
Active bleeding	Progressive renal insufficiency
Uncontrolled systemic hypertension	Pregnancy

Table 3
Factors That Increase Risk of Complications

Increased general medical risk
    Age >70 yr
    Complex congenital heart disease
    Morbid obesity
    General debility or cachexia
    Uncontrolled glucose intolerance
    Arterial oxygen desaturation
    Severe chronic obstructive lung disease
    Chronic renal insufficiency with creatinine >1.5 mg/dL
Increased cardiac risk
    Known three-vessel coronary artery disease
    Known left main coronary artery disease
    NYHA functional class IV
    Significant mitral or aortic valve disease or mechanical prosthesis
    Low ejection fraction (<35%)
    High-risk exercise treadmill test results (hypotension or severe ischemia)
    Pulmonary hypertension
    Pulmonary artery wedge pressure >25 mmHg
Increased vascular risk
    Anticoagulation or bleeding diathesis
    Uncontrolled systemic hypertension
    Severe peripheral vascular disease
    Recent stroke
    Severe aortic insufficiency
    Extremely large or small body size

- - Peripheral vascular disease and surgeries;
  - Presence of diabetes mellitus;
  - Contrast medium intolerance/allergy;
  - Chronic anticoagulation;
  - Renal insufficiency;
  - Stroke;
  - Bleeding diathesis.
- Physical examination with special attention to volume status, cardiorespiratory examination, and peripheral circulation.
- Laboratory evaluation:
  - Complete blood count with platelets;
  - Basic chemistries including blood urea nitrogen, creatinine, and glucose;
  - Prothrombin time, partial thromboplastin time (if necessary);
  - EGG.
  Chest films are not mandated unless indicated by the preoperative evaluation.
- Patient fasts for at least 6 h.
- All cardiac medicines, including aspirin but not anticoagulants, should be continued.

Table 4
Metformin Management Prior to Angiography

Day of angio:	Hold metformin
48 h post-angio:	Check renal function
	Resume medication, if normal

Table 5
Recommended Premedication for Known Contrast Allergy

Elective oral regimen	Acute intravenous regimen
13, 7, and 1 h prior	Hydrocortisone 100 mg
Prednisone 50 mg	Diphenhydramine 25–50 mg
1 hr prior	Cimetidine 300 mg
Diphenhydramine 25–50 mg	
? Cimetidine, 300 mg	
? Albuterol 4 mg	

Special patient subgroups include the chronically anticoagulated, those on metformin, and those with contrast allergy:

• Patients should discontinue warfarin for at least 48 h before the procedure to ensure an international normalized ratio (INR) less than 1.8. Patients at high risk for thromboembolism should be admitted for heparinization as the effects of oral anticoagulation wane.
• Because metformin (glucophage)-associated lactic acidosis can be precipitated by contrast nephropathy, patients on metformin require special care (Table 4).
• Patients known to have contrast allergy need either oral or intravenous prophylaxis for 24 h before the procedure (Table 5).

CORONARY ANGIOGRAPHY

Coronary angiography is the reference standard for coronary artery imaging and provides the most reliable information for making treatment decisions about medical therapy, angioplasty, or bypass surgery. When properly performed, there is little or no patient discomfort and procedure time is usually less than 15 min.

TECHNIQUE

Because of its relative ease, speed, reliability, and low complication rate, the Judkins technique has become the most widely used method of left-heart catheterization and coronary arteriography. After local anesthesia with 1% lidocaine, percutaneous entry of the femoral artery is achieved by puncturing the vessel 2–3 cm (2 fingerbreadths) below the inguinal ligament (which is easily palpated in thin persons and is located on a plane between the anterior superior iliac crest and the cephalad aspect of the pubic bone). Patients with truncal obesity require careful palpation of the bony landmarks and fluoroscopic visualization of the femoral head, which marks the level of the inguinal ligament. This ligament, not the inguinal crease, should be used as the landmark. A transverse skin incision is made over the femoral artery with a scapel. Using a modified Seldinger's technique, an 18-gage thin-walled needle is inserted at a 30- to 45-degree angle into the femoral artery, and a 0.035 or 0.038-in. J-tip Teflon-coated guidewire is advanced through the needle into the artery. An arterial sheath with proximal one-way valve and side arm is placed over the wire and allows multiple catheter exchanges. Sheath diameter is at least equal to coronary catheter diameter (typically 4–6 French sheaths are used). The outer diameter of the catheter is specified using French units, where one French unit (F) = 0.33 mm.

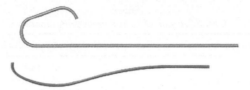

Fig. 1. Judkins left (top) and right (bottom) coronary catheters used for selective left and right coronary angiography.

Left ventricular systolic and end-diastolic pressures are obtained by advancing a pig-tail catheter retrograde into the left ventricle. To perform left ventriculography, 30-degree right anterior oblique and 45- to 60-degree left anterior oblique views are obtained during automated power injection of 30 to 40 mL of contrast medium over a period of 3 to 4 s into the ventricle via the pigtail catheter.

Intubation of the left and right coronary arteries for coronary angiography entails advancing the Judkins left and right catheters (Fig. 1) retrograde to the level for coronary sinuses. The Judkins left 4 (JL4) is shaped to allow easy access to the left main artery with minimal manipulation once in the left coronary sinus. Smaller or larger curves on the end of the catheter may be needed depending on aortic root size. The Judkins right 4 (JR4) catheter is used in the majority of cases to access the right coronary artery. Unlike the JL, the JR catheter requires clockwise rotation to swing the end of the catheter into the right coronary sinus and artery. Again, different shaped JR catheters can be used depending on aortic and coronary anatomy. Less frequently used are the Amplatz, multi-purpose, and no-torque right coronary catheters.

At procedure completion, manual compression is most commonly used for hemostasis after removal of the indwelling femoral artery sheath. Adequate compression of the femoral artery against the femoral head (just cephalad to the puncture site) is adjusted according to the presence or absence of bleeding and the presence or absence of pulses distally. Typically, compression over the femoral area for 15 to 20 min achieves hemostasis. With 4F or 5F catheters, 2 h of flat bed rest is usually sufficient to maintain hemostasis and allow for safe ambulation. 6F catheters may require 3 to 4 h. Recently, "hemostasis patches," cloth pads impregnated with substances to enhance hemostasis, have been used to shorten femoral compression and bed-rest times. Studies to determine efficacy are on-going. Because arterial compression can precipitate vasovagal reactions, atropine should be available for immediate administration.

Alternatively, mechanical vascular closure devices (the two most commonly used devices utilize collagen and suture for arteriotomy closure), may be applied in lieu of manual compression. In select patients, these devices allow earlier ambulation and permit immediate sheath removal. *See* "Complications" section below.

The percutaneous brachial approach is less commonly used and is typically reserved for persons with severe lower-extremity vascular disease. The brachial cutdown is similarly used and has the benefit of direct arterial visualization and arteriotomy closure. The radial approach has become the access site of choice in some centers. Before using the radial artery, a positive Allen's test of ulnar artery patency should be demonstrated (whereby, after manual compression of both the radial and ulnar arteries during fist clenching, normal color returns to the relaxed hand after pressure over the ulnar artery is released). The higher risk of thromboembolism with upper extremity arterial access warrants bolus administration of low-dose intravenous or intraarterial heparin.

COMPLICATIONS

The risk of major adverse outcomes after coronary angiography is small. A proper history, physical examination, and review of all laboratory, ECG, and imaging studies select out many persons at risk for untoward events. The published incidence of complications associated with cardiac catheterization is shown in Table 6 *(10–12)*. The incidence of death or myocardial infarction for the

Table 6
Complications of Coronary Angiography

Complication	Approximate incidence
Death	1:1000
Myocardial infarction	5:10,000
Cerebrovascular accident	5:10,000
Arrhythmia	5:1000
Vascular complications	5:1000
Contrast reactions	3:1000
Total of major complications	1–2:100

patient having elective cardiac catheterization in an experienced lab is exceedingly rare. Cerebro-vascular accident, especially transient loss of neurological function, is somewhat more common. Vascular complications and contrast-induced nephropathy deserve special mention.

Vascular Complications

Arterial access site bleeding accounts for the majority of complications encountered after cardiac catheterization and is often avoidable. The most common vascular complications are sub-cutaneous hematoma, pseudoaneurysm formation, arteriovenous fistula, retroperitoneal bleeding, and rectus sheath hematoma. Persons of advanced age, extreme body habitus (large and small), bleeding diathesis, and those receiving anticoagulant or antiplatelet drugs are at greatest risk. Care and attention to detail are critical at the time of arterial puncture and sheath removal to avoid vascular misadventures.

Proper management of the arterial sheath once in place is important in avoiding complications. Since sheath dwell times correlate with vascular access complication rates, all sheaths are removed as soon as possible. Hemodynamic and anticoagulation issues are addressed before the sheath is removed (the blood pressure must not be excessively low or high and persons recently exposed to heparin should have an activated clotting time [ACT] of less than 170 s). The newer mechanical arterial closure devices mentioned above may allow for earlier sheath removal and ambulation times but their ability to lessen vascular complication rates has not been established compared to careful and judicious manual compression. In fact, they may introduce new catheterization-related complications such as intravascular device infection and vessel occlusion.

Contrast Media-Related Renal Toxicity

Contrast media-related renal toxicity occurs in 1.4% to 2.3% of patients who receive contrast media *(13)*. Predictors of contrast-mediated renal insufficiency are (1) baseline renal dysfunction, (2) dehydration, (3) contrast volume used, (4) diabetes mellitus, and (5) congestive heart failure. Diabetics with renal insufficiency appear to present the greatest risk of toxicity.

Periprocedural hydration with saline, minimizing total contrast volume to less than 30 cc, and substituting for nonionic, low-osmolar or isoosmolar contrast agents have all been shown to reduce the risk of renal toxicity in patients with baseline renal insufficiency. Forced diuresis with manni-tol and furosemide appears to be less effective than simple intravenous saline hydration *(14)*. Several studies have suggested that the orally administered antioxidant *n*-acetylcysteine reduces the inci-dence of contrast-induced nephropathy, while others have not shown a beneficial effect. Partly because of ease of use and low risk of side effects, its use has found its way into clinical practice pend-ing the results of larger randomized trials.

A reasonable approach to the patient with renal insufficiency undergoing coronary angiography includes:

- Ensure adequate hydration prior to procedure. Consider IV hydration (1 L 0.9 NS over 12–24 h before and after the procedure).
- Use biplane angiography if available.
- Limit contrast dose to <30 cc for diagnostic studies and <100 cc for percutaneous coronary intervention (PCI).
- Perform "staged" procedure, whereby intervention is performed at later date (usually at least 48 h).
- Administer low or iso-osmolar contrast media.
- Discontinue potentially nephrotoxic medications (e.g., nonsteroidal antiinflammatory medications), if possible.
- Hold metformin prior to the procedure and do no restart until serum creatinine has returned to normal 48 h post procedure.
- Avoid repeated contrast exposure during recovery phase of acute tubular necrosis.
- Consider administering *n*-acetylcysteine 600 mg po BID for 2 d.

CORONARY ARTERY ANATOMY

The heart is supplied by the left and right coronary arteries, which usually originate from the left and right sinuses of Valsalva, respectively.

Coronary Dominance

The term *dominance* is applied to the artery that supplies the posterior diaphragmatic portion of the interventricular septum (the posterior descending artery [PDA]) and the diaphragmatic surface of the left ventricle (the posterior LV [PLV]). When these branches originate from the right coronary artery (RCA), the system is said to be *right-dominant;* if they arise from the left circumflex artery (LCx), it is *left-dominant* (the AV nodal artery also arises from the LCx in this case). Mixed or codominance occurs when these circulations are shared by the RCA and LCx. The coronary circulation is right-dominant in approx 85% of humans, left-dominant in 8%, and codominant in 7%. Dominance, in the absence of coronary disease, has no particular clinical significance.

Normal Coronary Anatomy (Fig. 2)

The *left main coronary artery* (LMCA) arises from the upper portion of the left sinus of Valsalva, is 3 to 6 mm in diameter and up to 10 mm long, and courses behind the right ventricular outflow tract before bifurcating into the left anterior descending (LAD) and LCx branches.

The *LAD artery* courses along the anterior interventricular groove toward the cardiac apex and gives off septal perforator and diagonal branches. The first septal perforator demarcates the junction between proximal and mid-LAD segments. In a minority of patients, the LMCA trifurcates, with a *ramus intermedius* artery arising between the LCx and LAD. This vessel supplies the free wall along the lateral aspect of the left ventricle.

The *LCx* originates at the bifurcation (or trifurcation) of the LMCA (or occasionally from a separate ostium of the left coronary sinus) and travels in the left atrioventricular (AV) groove. Obtuse marginal arteries arise from the LCx and supply the LV lateral wall. The origin of the first marginal artery demarcates the junction between the proximal and mid LCx artery segments. When dominant, the LCx gives rise to PDA, PLV, and frequently AV nodal arteries. A large left atrial branch arises proximally from the LCx in a third of people and gives rise to the sinus node artery. In disease states, it can be an important conduit for collateral flow to the RCA.

The *RCA* arises from the right coronary sinus at a point somewhat lower than the origin of the LCA from the left sinus. It travels along the right AV groove toward the crux (a point on the diaphragmatic surface of the heart where the right AV groove, the left AV groove, and the posterior AV groove come together). The first branch of the RCA, the conus artery, can serve as a source of collateral circulation in patients with LAD occlusion. The sinus node artery originates from the proximal RCA in two thirds of patients and arises just distal to the conus artery. It supplies the sinus

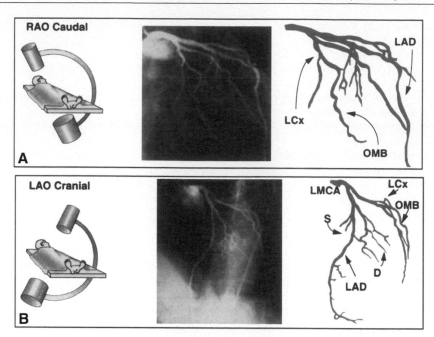

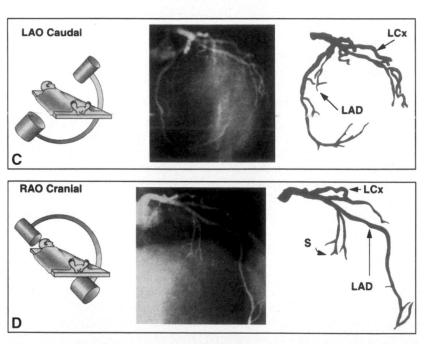

Fig. 2. Representative angiographic views of the left and right coronary systems are shown. The image intensifier position, as it relates to the patient, is used to describe the different views. *Left coronary artery views*: The RAO (right anterior oblique) caudal view shows the mid- and distal left main (LM), the proximal left anterior descending (LAD), and most of the left circumflex (LCx) and obtuse marginal branches (OMB). The LAO (left anterior oblique) cranial view demonstrates the mid- and distal LAD and its septal (S) and diagonal (D) branches, as well as the proximal LCx and its obtuse marginal branches. The LAO caudal or "spider" view shows the proximal LM and proximal LAD and LCx. The RAO cranial view demonstrates the mid- and distal LAD and its S and D branches.

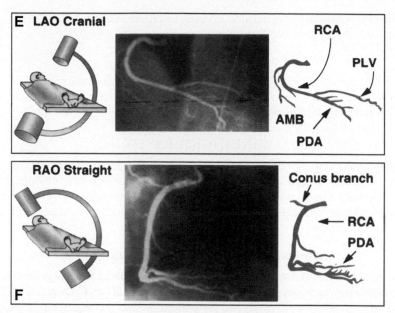

Fig. 2. *(Continued) Right coronary artery views*: The LAO cranial view shows the body of the right coronary artery (RCA) and especially the "crux" or distal RCA bifurcation into the posterior left ventricular (PLV) and posterior descending artery (PDA) branches. The acute marginal branch (AMB) is also well seen. The RAO straight view also demonstrates the body of the RCA, the conus branch, and the mid- and distal PDA. (From ref. *35*; with permission from Elsevier.)

node, usually the right atrium, or both atria. Like the LCx, which also travels in the AV groove, the RCA gives rise to marginal arteries, the first of which marks the junction between the proximal and mid-RCA segments. Occlusion of the RCA proximal to the RV marginal can result in RV infarction and its hemodynamic sequelae. At the distal crux, the RCA birfurcates into PDA and PLV arteries. Several small septal perforator arteries arise from the PDA and supply the lower third of the septum. As with the LAD, the right angle origin of the septal perforators helps to identify the PDA. The apex of the bend in the PLV is often the origin of the AV nodal arteries.

Coronary Artery Anomalies

Knowledge of the commonly encountered coronary anomalies is essential to performing cardiac catheterization. Coronary anomalies are found on 1 to 1.5% of coronary angiograms *(15)* and are usually benign. The most common anomaly of coronary anatomy is separate origins for the LAD and LCx arteries (i.e., absence of the LMCA). This benign anomaly occurs in 0.4 to 1% of patients and may be associated with a bicuspid aortic valve. The second most common anomaly is the LCx arising from the RCA or from the right coronary sinus.

Of the clinically significant anomalies, the most common is the LMCA or LAD arising from the right sinus of Valsalva or the RCA from the left sinus. A subset of these may course between the aorta and the pulmonary artery, predisposing to kinking and coronary insufficiency. In tetralogy of Fallot, the LAD arises from the RCA in 4% of patients. Less commonly, the LMCA, LAD, or RCA may originate from the pulmonary artery. Nearly 90% of these patients die in infancy unless there is left-to-right shunting with retrograde filling through coronary collaterals.

Coronary Fistula

The majority of coronary artery fistulas involve the RCA and empty into the right ventricle, right atrium, or coronary sinus. Generally, the shunt is small and the patients asymptomatic. If the shunt is large, however, pulmonary hypertension, congestive failure, bacterial endocarditis, myocardial ischemia, and (rarely) rupture can occur *(16)*.

Myocardial Bridging

In 5 to 12% of humans, the LAD descends from the epicardium to the submyocardium, where it is prone to systolic contraction and narrowing *(17)*. Although most of the coronary flow is diastolic, myocardial ischemia or infarction may result.

CINEANGIOGRAPHY

The primary aim of coronary angiography is lumen opacification of all segments of the epicardial coronary arteries and their branches (and any bypass grafts) in at least two orthogonal planes. Stenoses of the coronary arteries must be seen without foreshortening and without overlap of vessels. Coronary arteriography visualizes the major epicardial vessels and their second-, third-, and perhaps fourth-order branches.

Terminology of Angiographic Views (Fig. 2)

In most cardiac catheterization laboratories the X-ray tube is under the patient table and the image intensifier, with its coupled video and cinecamera, over the patient on a C-shaped arm. The relationship between the image intensifier (II) and the patient defines the angiographic projection. For example, if the image intensifier is oblique and on the patient's left, it is called *left anterior oblique* (LAO). In the caudal projection, the II is tilted toward the patient's feet. The degree of angulation of the image intensifier is noted in degrees (e.g., 45 degrees LAO, 20 degrees caudal).

Angiographic Projections

The coronary arteries lie in one of two orthogonal planes. The LAD and PDA lie in the plane of the interventricular septum, and the RCA and LCx in the plane of the AV valves. The best angiographic projections to visualize these arteries in profile are the oblique views. The 60-degree LAO view looks down the plane of the interventricular septum. The 30-degree RAO looks down the plane of the AV valves and the plane of the interventricular septum is seen *en face*. Shortcomings caused by foreshortening and overlapping in the straight RAO and LAO views necessitate the addition of cranial or caudal angulation. Often, a combination of cranial or caudal and right and left oblique projections is used.

Coronary Artery Bypass Graft Angiography

Coronary artery graft attrition and native vessel disease progression often warrant coronary and graft opacification in patients with coronary artery bypass grafts. Most aorto-coronary grafts are cannulated with a right Judkins catheter or specially designed left and right bypass catheters. Internal mammary catheters are also available for selective cannulation of the left and right internal mammary arteries. Views used to demonstrate the native vessels typically are also used for graft visualization. It is important to profile the proximal anastomosis to avoid misinterpreting poor catheter engagement as graft occlusion or disease. The body of the graft should be seen from at least two projections. The distal anastomosis should be projected free of overlapping vessels, as it is frequently a site of stenosis.

Pitfalls of Coronary Angiography

Most of the pitfalls in coronary angiography involve errors of omission whereby stenoses or anomalies are not appreciated. The most common angiographic pitfalls are:

*   *Unrecognized LMCA stenosis.* The LMCA should be viewed in several projections with the vessel unobscured by the spine. Catheter pressure damping (a result of "wedging" into a stenosed vessel

causing a damped waveform) and the absence of contrast reflux into the aorta suggest the presence of ostial LMCA disease. Several factors make adequate assessment of ostial LM stenosis challenging; they include the inherent difficulty of assessing aorto-ostial disease, vulnerability to catheter-induced vasospasm (*see* below), the high degree of interobserver variability of LMCA stenosis severity, and the prognostic significance of over- or underestimating LMCA lesion severity.

- *Too few projections.* Eccentric lesions and those obscured by overlap will go unnoticed unless additional projections are made. Detection of eccentric stenoses requires that the short axis of the stenotic lumen is projected.
- *Inadequate opacification.* Inadequate opacification can result in streaming and give the impression of ostial stenosis, missing side branches, thrombus, and stenosis over- or under-estimation. Properly sized catheters and injection rates avoid this problem.
- *Aorto-ostial lesions.* If an aorto-ostial lesion is suspected by partial ventricularization or pressure damping, injecting during withdrawal of the catheter from the ostium may be useful.
- *Failure to recognize occlusions.* Occlusions at branch origins tend to escape detection and may be recognized only by late filling of the distal segment by collateral circulation.
- *Catheter tip-induced spasm.* Catheter tip-induced spasm can occur at or within 1 cm of the catheter tip. It is caused by mechanical irritation and reflex contraction of the artery. Intracoronary or sublingual nitroglycerin should be given before the injection is repeated.
- *Congenital variants.* Variations in the origin or distribution of the coronary branches may confuse the operator. It is useful to remember that acquired atherosclerotic coronary artery disease is far more common than unusual anatomic variants. Before an unusual vessel is accepted as a variant, an occlusion or large collateral channel should be ruled out.

Angiographic Lesion Quantification

Under stress conditions, normal coronary artery flow can increase three- to fourfold (coronary flow reserve of 3 to 4). With luminal diameter reductions of greater than 50% (75% cross-sectional area reduction), the ability to normally increase coronary flow reserve may be impaired (i.e., less than 50% diameter narrowing is usually hemodynamically insignificant). Greater than 70% diameter stenosis (90% cross-sectional area) severely limits the ability to increase flow above resting level. A 90% diameter stenosis may reduce antegrade blood flow at rest *(18–20)*. Also important is lesion length, whereby a 50% narrowed 10-mm lesion will be less hemodynamically significant than a 50% narrowed 30-mm lesion.

The capability of coronary angiography to quantify the degree of stenosis is limited by the fact that the image is a "lumenogram." Stenoses can be evaluated only by comparison to adjacent reference segments, which are presumed to be disease-free. The majority of arteries will have disease in the reference segment, leading to underestimation of stenosis severity. In addition, vessel segments adjacent to areas of denser contrast (e.g., an overlying branch artery) are prone to perceptual artifact due to the Mach effect *(21)*, a consequence of the physiologic process of lateral inhibition. These neuroinhibitory interactions in the retina and central nervous system of the observer cause artery segments adjacent to the denser overlying artery to appear less dense and simulate stenosis.

To enhance quantification of vessel size, the absolute diameter of the coronary artery can be compared to the size of the diagnostic catheter. This approach to lesion quantification is limited by its dependence on visual estimation and suffers from significant operator variability *(22)*. To overcome these limitations, digital calipers and quantitative coronary angiography (QCA) have been developed, as have several computer-assisted approaches to quantitative angiography *(23)*.

Angiographic Assessment of Myocardial Blood Flow

The severity of the stenosis and the status of the microvasculature determine flow in the distal artery. The Thrombolysis in Myocardial Infarction (TIMI) study group first proposed a scheme for quantifying coronary perfusion, which has proved useful in predicting outcome after myocardial infarction *(24,25)*. The TIMI classification for coronary flow follows:

Grade 0: No perfusion.

No antegrade flow of contrast is detected beyond the point of occlusion.

Grade 1: Penetration without perfusion.

Contrast passes through the point of obstruction but antegrade flow fails to opacify the distal portion of the vessel at any time.

Grade 2: Partial perfusion.

Contrast penetrates the point of obstruction but enters the distal vessel at a rate slower than that for nonobstructed arteries in the same patient.

Grade 3: Complete perfusion.

Antegrade flow into the distal coronary bed is rapid and complete.

The TIMI frame count can be used to quantify angiographic coronary artery perfusion. An automated frame counter counts the number of cinefilm frames that elapse before the involved artery is opacified. Although TIMI frame count is more labor-intensive, it is more objective and more reproducible, and correlates more closely with clinical outcomes than conventional methods *(26)*.

Coronary Collateral Circulation

Collaterals usually cannot be demonstrated at coronary angiography unless the recipient vessel has developed at least 90% diameter stenosis. A common method of quantifying collateral filling is the Cohen and Rentrop grading system *(27)*:

Grade 0: No collaterals present.

Grade 1: Barely detectable collateral flow.

Contrast medium passes through the collaterals but fails to opacify the recipient epicardial vessel.

Grade 2: Partial collateral flow.

Contrast medium enters but fails to completely opacify the target epicardial vessel.

Grade 3: Complete collateral flow.

Contrast enters and completely opacifies the target epicardial vessel.

The development and genetic manipulation of collateral formation in patients with obstructed coronary arteries is an area of intensive investigation. In some persons, collateral circulation is the only conduit for perfusion of certain myocardial territories. This very important "safety valve" for coronary obstruction has significant interpatient variability and can account for very different patient outcomes in both acute and chronic disease. In patients with total occlusions, regional LV contraction has been shown to be significantly better in segments supplied by adequate collaterals than in those with inadequate collateral circulation.

Coronary Artery Spasm

Coronary spasm can play an important role in exercise-induced angina, unstable angina, acute myocardial infarction, and sudden death and often requires coronary angiography to establish the diagnosis and rule out atherosclerotic disease. Provocative testing in the cardiac catheterization lab was once fairly common but is now rarely performed. When contemplated, all vasodilators are withdrawn for at least 24 h. Intravenous ergonovine maleate or intacoronary acetylcholine, potent arterial vasoconstrictors with proven utility in diagnosing variant angina, may be used *(28)*. The test is considered positive if focal spasm occurs and is associated with clinical symptoms and/or ECG ST segment changes. Induced coronary spasm is reversed by administering intracoronary nitroglycerin. The diagnostic yield of provocative testing depends on the population studied. Catheter tip-induced spasm should not be confused with vasospastic coronary disease.

Intravascular Ultrasonography

Although coronary angiography is considered the reference standard for coronary artery imaging, it detects only arterial disease that impinges on the luminal column of contrast medium. It has

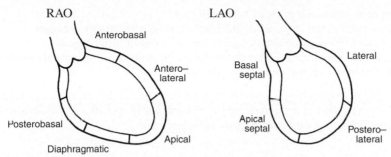

Fig. 3. The left ventricle, as viewed from the right anterior oblique (RAO) and left anterior oblique (LAO) views. This "biplanar" assessment allows for segmental analysis of ventricular function.

limited ability to detect plaque content or the disease process itself. In contrast, intravascular ultrasonography (IVUS) provides tomographic assessment analogous to histologic cross-sections and provides information about plaque morphology, vessel wall structure, and luminal and vessel area. IVUS offers the following advantages over angiography:

- Clarification of angiographically equivocal or intermediate lesions. This is especially helpful with left main lesions, which can be difficult to quantitate with angiography.
- Assessment of coronary stenoses before and after catheter-based coronary interventions. IVUS has proven useful in determining true vessel size prior to stent implantation and appropriate stent strut apposition after stent implantation.
- In cardiac transplant recipients, coronary artery disease is best studied by IVUS because of the diffuse nature of atherosclerosis that develops after transplantation.

LEFT VENTRICULOGRAPHY

Left ventriculography entails the opacification of the ventricle with contrast medium and is an important part of left heart catheterization. Indications for left ventriculography include assessment of wall motion abnormalities, ejection fraction, and the presence and severity of mitral regurgitation. The osmolarity and vasodilatory effects of bolus injection of contrast medium during ventriculography can make it poorly tolerated is certain persons. Those at high risk for complications during left ventriculography include patients with (1) severe symptomatic aortic stenosis, (2) severe congestive heart failure or angina at rest, (3) LV thrombus, especially if mobile or protruding into the LV cavity, and (4) left-sided endocarditis.

Segmental Wall Motion Analysis and Ejection Fraction

Biplane assessment of LV wall motion provides an excellent means of assessing LV function. The LV is divided into anterobasal, anterolateral, apical, diaphragmatic, and inferobasal segments in the RAO projection and into lateral, posterolateral, apical septal, and basal septal segments in the LAO projection (Fig. 3). Wall motion is classified qualitatively as hyperdynamic; normal; mildly, moderately, or severely hypokinetic; akinetic (no systolic contraction); or dyskinetic (paradoxic motion during systole). Overall ejection fraction (EF) is visually estimated or determined by computerized quantitative analysis. The most commonly used is the center line method, which uses end-diastolic and end-systolic contours to assess shortening fraction of the cardiac segments.

Visual Assessment of Regurgitation

Valvular regurgitation can be assessed visually by determining the relative amount of contrast medium that opacifies the chamber proximal to the chamber injected. The original classification devised by Sellers et al. (29) remains the standard in most catheterization laboratories and can be used to assess mitral regurgitation during left ventriculography:

1+ Minimal regurgitant jet that clears with each beat.
2+ Moderate opacification of proximal chamber, clearing with subsequent beats.
3+ Intense opacification of proximal chamber, equal to that of distal chamber.
4+ Intense opacification of proximal chamber, becoming more dense than distal chamber. Opacification often persists over the entire series of images.

The main pitfall of this classification is the lack of control for different-sized proximal chambers (e.g., mitral regurgitation of a given degree more completely opacifies a normal-sized left atrium than one that has undergone compensatory enlargement).

Regurgitant Fraction

Although not commonly used in clinical practice, angiographically derived volumes can be used to calculate regurgitant fraction (RF). Unlike visual assessment of regurgitation severity, this method provides a quantitative assessment of valvular regurgitation. The RF is that portion of the angiographic stroke volume that does not contribute to the net cardiac output (CO):

$$RF = \frac{RSV}{SV}$$

where RSV is regurgitant stroke volume (angiographic stroke volume – forward stroke volume), and SV is forward stroke volume. The forward stroke volume is CO (determined Fick or thermodilution method) divided by heart rate.

A comparison of RF and regurgitation assessed visually follows a 20/40/60 rule:

RF less than 20% is equivalent to 1+ regurgitation.
RF between 21% and 40% is equivalent to 2+ regurgitation.
RF between 41% and 60% is equivalent to 3+ regurgitation.
RF greater than 60% is equivalent to 4+ regurgitation.

SUPRAVALVULAR AORTOGRAPHY

In 1929, Dos Santos and coworkers first described aortography (30) by direct needle puncture of the abdominal aorta. We now use peripheral arterial access, which, like ventriculography, requires high-pressure injection of a large volume of contrast over a short time. Indications for supravalvular (or root) aortography include:

- *Aortic regurgitation.* The appearance of contrast in the left ventricle during supravalvular aortography confirms the diagnosis of AR. The Sellers classification described above for mitral regurgitation assessment is also used to quantitate aortic regurgitation severity.
- *Coronary artery bypass grafts.* When bypass graft location or number is not known or a "flush" proximal occlusion is suspected, supravalvular aortography can be used for nonselective graft opacification.
- *Aortic aneurysms.* Although a number of noninvasive techniques are now available, including transesophageal echocardiography, contrast CT, and magnetic resonance imaging (MRI), thoracic aortography remains a widely used diagnostic tool for aortic ascending aortic aneurysm evaluation.
- *Aortic dissection.* Aortography can accurately identify aortic dissection by showing an intimal flap, opacification of the false lumen, and deformity of the true lumen. The choice of test for dissection (transesophageal echocardiography, CT, MRI, or aortography) depends on local expertise and the hemodynamic stability of the patient.
- *Aortic coarctation.* Aortography assumes an important role, as it can distinguish complete aortic interruption and hypoplastic aortic segment from the most common type of coarctation involving a stenosis at the site of the isthmus distal to the left subclavian artery. Again, centers with expertise in CT and MRI can achieve similar diagnostic yield noninvasively.

HEMODYNAMIC EVALUATION

The hemodynamic component of the cardiac catheterization procedure largely focuses on pressure and flow measurements, and stenotic valve orifice and intracardiac shunt calculations.

Pressure Measurement

Intravascular pressures are typically measured using a fluid-filled catheter attached to a pressure transducer, which detects the pressure wave within the catheter. The majority of pressure transducers used are electrical strain gauges. The pressure wave distorts the diaphragm or wire within the transducer; this energy is converted to an electrical signal proportional to the pressure being applied using the principle of the Wheatstone bridge. This signal is then amplified and recorded as an analog signal. The pressure transducer must be calibrated against a known pressure, and the establishment of a zero reference is established at the start of the catheterization procedure. To "zero" the transducer, the tranducer is placed at the level of the atria, which is approximately mid-chest.

Potential sources of error include catheter whip artifact (motion of the tip of the catheter within the measured chamber), end pressure artifact (an end-hole catheter measures an artificially elevated pressure due to streaming or high velocity of the pressure wave), catheter impact artifact (when the catheter is impacted by the walls or valves of the cardiac chambers), and catheter tip obstruction within small vessels or valvular orifices occurring because of the size of the catheter itself. The use of micromanometer catheters, which have the pressure transducer mounted at their tip, greatly reduces measurement errors. Because of expense, device fragility, and time needed for calibration, they are now rarely used.

Cardiac Output

Volumetric flow or cardiac output (CO, expressed in liters per minute) can be measured by several methods. The Fick and thermodilution methods will be briefly discussed here. Other measures of CO include the indicator-dilution technique, angiographic CO and the Doppler flow velocity method.

The Fick principle dictates that the amount of an indicator substance in the blood leaving the circulation must equal the amount of that substance entering plus any amount added to the circulation during transit. The total amount of a substance passing any point in the circulation per unit of time is the product of its concentration and flow rate. CO by Fick *(31)* is calculated thus:

$$\text{Fick CO (L/mm)} = \frac{O_2 \text{ consumption (mL/min)}}{\text{A-V } O_2 \text{ difference (mL/100 mL)} \times O_2\text{-carrying capacity (mL/100 mL)} \times 10}$$

$$= \frac{O_2 \text{ consumption (mL/min)}}{(\text{Art sat} - \text{MV sat}) \times \text{Hb (g/100 mL)} \times 1.36 \times 10}$$

where (A-V) O_2 is the difference in O_2 content between arterial and mixed venous blood, expressed as milliters of O_2 per 100 mL of blood. O_2-carrying capacity (mL/100 mL) is calculated by multiplying the hemoglobin (in g/100 mL) by 1.36.

The Fick method is limited by the relatively cumbersome measurement of O_2 consumption and tends to underestimate cardiac output in the presence of significant tricuspid regurgitation. Estimated O_2 consumption based on patient height and weight is often used to calculate an estimated Fick cardiac output.

The thermodilution method requires injection of a bolus of liquid (saline or dextrose), the temperature of which differs from the body temperature, into the proximal port of the catheter. The resultant change in temperature in the liquid is measured by a thermistor mounted on the distal end of the catheter. CO is inversely related to the area under the thermodilution curve, plotted as a function of temperature versus time, with a smaller area indicating a higher CO. This method has

Table 7
Normal Intracardiac Pressures

Chamber	Pressure (mmHg)
Right atrium	3–5
Right ventricle	20–25/3–5
Pulmonary artery	20–25/10–15
Pulmonary capillary wedge	10–15
Left ventricle	100–140/10–15
Aorta	100–140/60–80

become standard practice because it is easy to use. It is less accurate than the Fick method in the setting of irregular rhythm and low CO states.

Right Heart Catheterization

Right heart catheterization provides important hemodynamic information not often available with noninvasive methods. It is performed using balloon flotation (Swan-Ganz) catheters that afford easy entry into the right atrium, right ventricle, and pulmonary artery via the internal jugular, subclavian, brachial, or femoral veins.

Atrial Pressure Waveforms

The right and left atrial pressures are venous waveforms representing diastolic filling. There are three positive deflections (*a, c,* and *v waves*) and two negative deflections (*x* and *y descents*).

- The *a wave* reflects atrial contraction and follows the ECG p wave.
- The *x descent* follows the *a* wave and represents relaxation of the atrium and downward pulling of the tricuspid annulus by right ventricular contraction.
- The *c wave* interrupts the *x* descent and is caused by protrusion of the closed tricuspid valve into the right atrium.
- The second pressure peak is the *v wave*, which is caused by blood returning to the atrium from the periphery and reflects atrial compliance.
- The *y descent* follows the *v* wave and reflects tricuspid valve opening and right atrial emptying into the ventricle. (For normal intracardiac pressures and waveforms, *see* Table 7 and Fig. 4, respectively.)

Ventricular Pressure Waveforms

Right and left ventricular waveforms are similar in morphology. Ventricular systole occurs at the time of the T wave on the simultaneous ECG. Ventricular diastolic pressure is characterized by an early rapid filling wave during which most of the ventricle fills, a slow filling phase, and the *a* wave denoting atrial systole. End-diastolic pressure is generally measured at the onset of iso-volumic contraction and occurs at the time of the R wave on the simultaneous ECG.

Vascular Resistance

Resistance to flow across both the pulmonary and systemic circuits is easily calculated and provides important information in many disease states, including pulmonary hypertension, congestive heart failure, and valvular heart disease. It is calculated using Ohm's Law ($V = IR$) (Table 8). Resistance is calculated in Wood units and is often converted to dynes $\times$ s/cm^3 by multiplying by 80.

Intracardiac Shunts

Intracardiac shunts can be left to right (oxygenated blood from the left heart mixes with systemic venous blood), right to left (unoxygenated venous blood mixes with arterial blood), or mixed. The following terms are helpful in describing complex shunts and for shunt calculations (*see* Table 8):

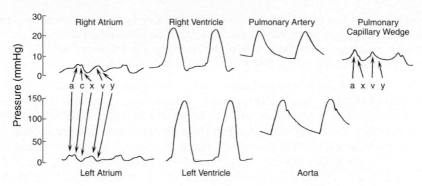

Fig. 4. Representative right and left heart waveforms. *See* text for details.

Table 8
Commonly Used Hemodynamic Formulae

Fick CO (L/min)	$\dfrac{VO_2 \text{ (mL/min)}}{(\text{Art-MV } O_2 \text{ sat}) \times Hb \text{ (mg/dL)} \times 13.6}$
SVR (Wood units)	$\dfrac{\text{mAO (mmHg)} - \text{RA (mmHg)}}{\text{CO (L/min)}}$
PVR (Wood units)	$\dfrac{\text{mPA (mmHg)} - \text{mPCWP (mmHg)}}{\text{CO (L/min)}}$
Qef (L/min)	$\dfrac{VO_2 \text{ (mL/min)}}{(PVO_2 \text{ sat} - MVO_2 \text{ sat})}$
Q recirculated systemic (Qrsf, L/min)	Qs (L/min) – Qef (L/min)
Q recirculated pulmonary (Qrpf, L/min)	Qp (L/min) – Qef (L/min)
Qp (L/min)	$\dfrac{VO_2 \text{ (mL/min)}}{(PVO_2 \text{ sat} - PAO_2 \text{ sat})}$
Qs (L/min)	$\dfrac{VO_2 \text{ (mL/min)}}{(ArtO_2 \text{ sat} - MVO_2 \text{ sat})}$
MVO_2 sat (%)	$\dfrac{3 \text{ SVC sat} + \text{IVC sat}}{4}$
% Left-to-right shunt	$\dfrac{\text{Q recirc pulm (L/min)}}{\text{Q tot pulm (L/min)}}$
% Right-to-left Shunt	$\dfrac{\text{Q recirc syst (L/min)}}{\text{Q tot sys (L/min)}}$

CO, cardiac output; VO_2, oxygen consumption; Art, arterial; MV, mixed venous; Sat, saturation, expressed as a fraction; Hb, hemoglobin (mg/dL); SVR, systemic vascular resistance; mAO, mean aortic pressure; RA, right atrial pressure; PVR, pulmonary vascular resistance; MPA, mean pulmonary artery pressure; mPCWP, mean pulmonary capillary wedge pressure; Q, flow; Qs, systemic flow; Qef, effective flow; Qp, pulmonary flow; PV, pulmonary venous; SVC, superior vena cava; IVC, inferior vena cava.

Effective flow (Qef) is the quantity of systemically mixed venous blood that circulates through the lungs, is oxygenated, and then circulates through systemic capillaries.

Recirculated systemic flow (Qrsf) is the amount of relatively desaturated, systemically mixed venous blood that recirculates directly into the aorta without being oxygenated by the lungs.

Recirculated pulmonary flow (Qrpf) is the quantity of fully saturated pulmonary venous blood that recirculates to the pulmonary artery without passing through the systemic capillaries.
Total pulmonary flow (Qp) is the effective flow plus recirculated pulmonary flow.
Total systemic flow (Qs) is the effective flow plus recirculated systemic flow.

To quickly assess for the presence of left-to-right intracardiac shunting, serial O_2 saturation samplings are performed. A "step-up" in O_2 saturation indicates an abnormal increase in O_2 content between the chambers proximal and distal to the level of shunting. A significant left-to-right shunt is present when the step-up is greater than 7% at the atrial level and greater than 5% at the ventricular or pulmonary level. The degree of shunting is typically reported as a ratio of pulmonary to systemic flow (Qp/Qs). Qp/Qs > 1 suggests left-to-right shunting; Qp/Qs < 1, right-to-left shunting. The degree of shunting can also be reported as a percentage of right-to-left or left-to-right shunt and is used when bidirectional shunting is present (*see* Table 8).

Evaluation of Stenotic Valvular Lesions

Calculation of valve area based on hemodynamic measurements is derived from the Bernoulli principle and was conceived by Gorlin and Gorlin.

MITRAL STENOSIS

Mitral stenosis (MS) causes a diastolic gradient between the left atrium and the left ventricle. The mean mitral valve gradient (MVG) depends on the degree of MS, cardiac output, and the diastolic filling period (DFP). MVG can be measured directly from catheters placed in the left atrium and left ventricle. More commonly, pulmonary capillary wedge pressure (PCWP) is used instead of the left atrial (LA) pressure. This requires a properly estimated wedge pressure using an end-hole catheter, fluoroscopic guidance, and/or confirmation by oxygen saturation (PCWP and LA saturations are normally 97% or greater).

Mitral valve area (MVA) can be calculated thus using the Gorlin formula: *(32)*

$$\text{MVA (cm}^2) = \frac{1000 \times \text{CO (L/mm)}}{37.7 \times \sqrt{\text{MVG (mmHg)}} \times \text{HR (beats/min)} \times \text{DFP (s/beat)}}$$

where MVA is mitral valve area, and DFP is diastolic filling period. The MVA calculation can be erroneous in the setting of both low and high heart rates and concomitant mitral regurgitation. MS is severe when the MVA is less than approx 1.3 cm^2.

AORTIC STENOSIS

Like the MVG, the aortic valve gradient (AVG) depends on the CO and severity of valvular stenosis. While the peak-to-peak gradient between aorta and left ventricle is commonly used to describe aortic stenosis (AS), it is a nonphysiologic measurement that is obtained from nonsimultaneous pressure tracings. The mean AVG, on the other hand, is physiologic and is the preferred measurement for providing information about severity of obstruction. In practice, the peak-to-peak gradient often closely matches the true mean gradient in the absence of low-output states or irregular rhythms. The optimal method for obtaining AVG is to simultaneously measure aortic and ventricular pressures using catheters in each chamber.

Aortic valve area (AVA) can be calculated using the Gorlin formula: *(32)*

$$\text{AVA} = \frac{1000 \times \text{CO (L/mm)}}{44.3 \times \sqrt{\text{AVG (mmHg)}} \times \text{HR (beats/min)} \times \text{SEP (s/beat)}}$$

where AVG is the mean aortic gradient, and SEP the systolic ejection period. AVA calculations can be inaccurate in the presence of low or high heart rates, low CO, and significant aortic regurgitation. An AVA less than 1.0 cm^2 is consistent with severe AS; less than 0.75 cm^2 suggests critical AS.

Both mitral and aortic valve areas can be estimated using the simplified formula of Hakki *(33)*:

$$\text{Valve area (cm}^2) = \frac{\text{CO (L/min)}}{\sqrt{\text{mean gradient}}}$$

Restrictive and Constrictive Heart Disease

Both myocardial restriction and pericardial constriction are conditions of abnormal diastolic filling. Diastolic dysfunction in restriction results from a noncompliant ventricular myocardium, whereas scarring and consequent loss of pericardial sac elasticity is the culprit in constrictive heart disease. Abnormal filling in both conditions produces equalization of diastolic RV and LV pressures with a characteristic "dip and plateau" or "square root sign" ($\sqrt{}$) on the ventricular diastolic filling tracing. This diastolic filling pattern results from early emptying of the atrium into the ventricle followed by a rapid rise and plateau due to abnormal late ventricular filling. On the right atrial pressure tracing, both the normally dominant y descent and the x descent become more pronounced, producing a "W" or "M" configuration.

A significant difference between the two conditions concerns ventricular interaction or interdependence. In constriction, the septum is not involved and can therefore bulge toward the LV, allowing changes in RV hemodynamics (e.g., inspiratory increase in volume) to be transmitted to the LV. In restrictive cardiomyopathy, the stiff septum does not allow for this interaction. Despite this, hemodynamic analysis often fails to reliably differentiate the two conditions. In the majority of cases, clues from the clinical history, ECG, and chest imaging distinguish the two. For example, the presence of concomitant disease known to cause cardiac infiltration (e.g., amyloid), or low voltage or conduction disease on ECG, is strongly favors the diagnosis of restriction in the appropriate hemodynamic setting. A history of pericardial disease or pathologic conditions known to affect the pericardium (tuberculosis, pericarditis, cancer, etc.) in conjunction with pericardial calcium on chest films (or thickened pericardium on computed tomography [CT]) favors constrictive disease.

When the history and simple diagnostic measures fail to clearly separate constriction from restriction, the following hemodynamic findings are helpful:

Constriction	Restriction
RVEDP = LVEDP within 5 mmHg	LVEDP > RVEDP by 5 mmHg
RVEDP > 1/3 RVSP	RVEDP < 1/3 RVSP
RVSP < 60 mmHg, often < 40	RVSP > 40 mmHg, occasionally > 60
RVSP, LVSP discordance with respiration	RVSP, LVSP concordance with respiration

Cardiac Tamponade

Cardiac catheterization is invaluable in establishing the hemodynamic importance of pericardial effusion. Cardiac tamponade is a condition in which pericardial fluid causes constraint and severely impaired filling, leading to hypotension, tachycardia, and diminished stroke volume *(34)*. Cardiac catheterization demonstrates several findings:

1. Elevated RA pressure with a characteristic preserved systolic x descent and absence of or a diminutive diastolic y descent (suggesting that RA emptying is impaired by compression of the right ventricle early in diastole).
2. Elevation and equalization of intrapericardial and RA pressures. The right ventricular (RV) diastolic pressure equals the intrapericardial and RA pressures and lacks the dip and plateau configuration of constrictive disease. Tamponade physiology occurs when RV and LV filling is limited by the inability of the heart to distend adequately during diastole. If intrapericardial pressure is not elevated and RA and intrapericardial pressures are not virtually identical, the diagnosis of cardiac tamponade is questionable.
3. Exaggerated inspiratory elevation of RA pressure and depression of systemic pressure (pulsus paradoxus). Normally, inspiration increases venous return to the right heart, resulting in increased RV

end-diastolic volume. The enlarged RV causes the interventricular septum to bulge into the LV, resulting in a slightly lower LV end-diastolic volume, stroke volume, and systolic blood pressure. In tamponade, the compression of the RV exaggerates leftward septal bulging and amplifies the reduction in systolic blood pressure during inspiration (>10 mmHg during quiet breathing).

Hypertrophic Obstructive Cardiomyopathy (HOCM)

A dynamic LV outflow tract gradient in the presence of LV hypertrophy suggests the presence of HOCM. Various physiological maneuvers that take advantage of the dynamic outflow obstruction in HOCM can be easily performed in the cardiac catheterization lab and provide useful information. While simultaneously measuring aortic and LV pressure, an increase of the subaortic pressure gradient in the HOCM patient can be demonstrated using the following maneuvers: *Valsalva maneuver* (forced expiration against closed glottis), *Brockenbrough's maneuver* (introduction of a premature ventricular contraction though LV catheter manipulation), or *pharmacologic maneuvers* (amyl nitrate, nitroglycerin).

Maneuver	Mechanism
Valsalva maneuver	Decreased venous return accentuates gradient by decreasing LV volume and size
Amyl nitrate/nitroglycerin	Decreased preload accentuates gradient by decreasing LV volume and size
Brockenbrough's maneuver	Vigorous contraction of post-premature beat accentuates gradient and decreases aortic pulse pressure*

*In the non-HOCM patient, premature ventricular contractions increase the pulse pressure of the subsequent ventricular beat. Brockenbrough's maneuver also may accentuate the spike-and-dome configuration of the aortic pressure waveform.

SUMMARY

Invasive hemodynamic and radiographic contrast interrogation of the heart and related structures remain central to the evaluation of patients with cardiovascular disease. Many of the methods described in this chapter are the gold standard for cardiovascular assessment against which newer and less invasive tools are measured.

REFERENCES

1. Forssman W. Die Sondierung des rechien Herzens. KIm Wochenschr 1929;8:2085.
2. Zimmerman HA, Scott RW, Becker ND. Catheterization of the left side of the heart in man. Circulation 1950;1:357.
3. Limon Lason R, Bouchard A. El cateterismo intracardico; Cateterizacion de las caridades izquierdas en el hombre intracaretanos. Arch Inst Cardiol Mexico 1950;21:271.
4. Sones FM Jr, Shirey EK, Prondfit WL, Westcott RN. Cinecoronary arteriography (abstract). Circulation 1959;20: 773.
5. Sones FM Jr. Cine coronary arteriography. In: Hurst JW, Logue RB, eds. The Heart, 2nd ed. McGraw-Hill, New York, 1970, pp. 377.
6. Favaloro RG. Saphenous vein autograft replacement of severe segmental coronary artery occlusion: operative technique. Ann Thorac Surg 1968;5:334.
7. Gruentzig A, et al. Coronary transluminal angioplasty. Circulation 1977;56:II, 319.
8. Gruentzig A, Senning A, Siegenthaler WE. Nonoperative dilation of coronary artery stenosis. Percutaneous transluminal coronary angioplasty. N Engl J Med 1979;301:61.
9. Sigwart U, Urgan P, Golf S, et al. Emergency stenting for acute occlusion after coronary balloon angioplasty. Circulation 1988;78:1121–1127.
10. Scanlon PJ, Faxon DP, Audet A, et al. ACC/AHA guidelines for coronary angiography: a report of the American College of Cardiology/American Heart Association Task Force on Practice Guidelines (Committee on Coronary Angiography). J Am Coll Cardiol 1999;33:1756–1824.
11. Davis K, Kennedy JW, Kemp HG, et al. Complications of coronary arteriography from the Collaborative Study of Coronary Artery Surgery (CASS). Circulation 1979;59:1105.

12. Johnson LW, Lozner EC, Johnson S, et al. Coronary arteriography 1984–1987: a report of the Registry of the Society for Cardiac Angiography and Interventions. I. Results and complications. Cathet Cardiovasc Diagn 1989; 17:5.
13. Shehadi WH. Contrast media adverse reactions: occurrence, recurrence and distribution patterns. Radiology 1982; 143:11.
14. Solomon R, Werner C, Mann D, et al. Effects of saline, mannitol, and furosemide on acute decrease in renal function induced by radiocontrast agents. N Engl J Med 1994;331:1416.
15. Yamanaka O, Hoobs RE. Coronary artery anomalies in 126,595 patients undergoing coronary arteriography. Cathet Cardiovasc Diagn 1990;21:28.
16. Levin DC, Fellows KE, Abrams HL. Hemodynamically significant primary anomalies of the coronary arteries: angiographic aspects. Circulation 1978;58:25.
17. Kramer JR, Kitazurne H, Proudflt WL, Sones FM Jr. Clinical significance of isolated coronary bridges: benign and frequent condition involving the left anterior descending artery. Am Heart J 1982;103:282.
18. Gould KL, et al. Physiologic basis for assessing critical coronary stenosis—instantaneous flow response and regional distribution during coronary hyperemia as measures of flow reserve. Am J Cardiol 1974;33:87.
19. Wilson RE, Marcus ML, White CW. Prediction of physiologic significance of coronary arterial lesions by quantitative lesion geometry in patients with limited coronary artery disease. Circulation 1987;75:723.
20. Uren NG, et al. Relation between myocardial blood flow and the severity of coronary artery stenosis. N Engl J Med 1994;330:1782.
21. Randall PA. Mach bands in cine coronary arteriography. Radiology 1978;129:65.
22. Gibson CM, Safian RD. Limitations of cineangiography—impact of new technologies for image processing and quantitation. Trends Cardiovasc Med 1992;2:156.
23. Gronenschild E, Jannsen J, Thjdent F. CAAS II: a second generation system for off-line and on-line quantitative coronary angiography. Cathet Cardiovasc Diagn 1994;33:61.
24. TIMI Study Group. The Thrombolysis in Myocardial Infarction (TIMI) trial: phase I findings. N Engl J Med 1985; 312:932.
25. The GUSTO Angiographic Investigators. The effects of tissue plasminogen activator, streptokinase, or both on coronary artery patency, ventricular function, and survival after acute myocardial infarction. N Engl J Med 1993;32: 1615.
26. Gibson CM. TIMI frame count: a new standardization of infarct-related artery flow grade, and its relationship to clinical outcomes in TIMI-4 trial. Circulation 1994;90:I-220.
27. Cohen M, Rentrop P. Limitations of myocardial ischemia by collateral circulation during sudden controlled coronary artery occlusion in human subjects. Circulation 1986;74:469.
28. Heupler FA, et al. Ergonovine maleate provocative test for coronary arterial spasm. Am J Cardiol 1978;41:631.
29. Sellers RD, Levy MJ, Amplatz K, Lillehei CW. Left retrograde cardioangiography in acquired cardiac disease: technique, indications and interpretation in 700 cases. Am J Cardiol 1964;14:437.
30. Dos Santos R, Lamas AC, Pereira-Caldas J. Arteriografla da aorta e dos vasos abdonmialis. Med Contemp 1929;47:93.
31. Fagard R, Conway J. Measurement of cardiac output: Fick principle using catheterization. Eur Heart J 1990;11:1.
32. Gorlin R, Gorlin SG. Hydraulic formula for calculation of the area of stenotic mitral valve, other cardiac valves, and central circulatory shunts. Am Heart J 1951;41:1.
33. Hakki AH. A simplified valve formula for the calculation of stenotic cardiac valve areas. Circulation 1981;63:1050.
34. Reddy PS, Curtis EI, O'Toole JD, Shaver JA. Cardiac tamponade: hemodynamic observations in man. Circulation 1978;58:265.
35. Bittle JA, Popma J. Coronary arteriography. In: Braunwald F, ed. Heart Disease: A Textbook of Cardiovascular Medicine, 6th ed. W. B. Saunders, Philadelphia, 2001.

RECOMMENDED READING

Grossman's Cardiac Catheterization, Angiography and Intervention, 6th ed. Baim DS, ed. Lippincott Williams & Wilkins, Philadelphia, PA, 2000.
Braunwald E, Zipes DP, Libby P, eds. Heart Disease: A Textbook of Cardiovascular Medicine, 7th ed. W. B. Saunders, Philadelphia, PA, 2004.

13 Nuclear Imaging in Cardiovascular Medicine

Diwakar Jain, MD and Barry L. Zaret, MD

INTRODUCTION

Nuclear imaging harnesses the unique properties of radiopharmaceuticals in allowing us to non-invasively image physiological phenomena, anatomical structures, and metabolic reactions, as well as various physiological spaces and compartments in patients *(1)*. Nuclear imaging plays an important role in the noninvasive evaluation of patients with established or suspected coronary artery disease. A number of different radiopharmaceuticals and scintigraphic imaging techniques are available for obtaining important diagnostic and prognostic information about myocardial perfusion, metabolism, cardiac function, and myocardial necrosis in patients with cardiovascular disorders. This chapter briefly describes various cardiac nuclear imaging techniques, their applications in clinical practice, and the recent developments in this field.

MYOCARDIAL PERFUSION IMAGING

Of various techniques in nuclear cardiology, myocardial perfusion imaging is the most widely used technique.

Physiological Considerations

Coronary artery disease is characterized by luminal narrowing of the coronary arteries due to the deposition of atheromatous material in its walls. This complex process evolves slowly over several decades. Symptoms occur relatively late in the course of disease and appear only after significant narrowing of coronary arteries has already occurred. Coronary arterial narrowing interferes with myocardial perfusion downstream. With partial narrowing of the lumen, myocardial perfusion may be normal at rest, but fails to increase appropriately during conditions of increased demand such as physical exertion or pharmacological vasodilation. This results in regional flow heterogeneity, which can be imaged by injecting radiotracers that are extracted by the myocardium, proportional to the regional blood flow.

Radiotracers

THALLIUM-201

Thallium-201 (^{201}Tl) is the conventional perfusion tracer *(2)*. ^{201}Tl behaves like a potassium analog and enters the myocytes through Na^+/K^+ ATPase channels. Two to three mCi of ^{201}Tl is injected intravenously at peak exercise or during pharmacological stress. ^{201}Tl is rapidly extracted from the blood pool by the myocardium, skeletal muscle, and several organs within the next few minutes. Approximately 2 to 4% of the injected dose of ^{201}Tl goes to the myocardium. Myocardial uptake is proportional to the regional blood flow. Cardiac imaging is started soon after completion

From: *Essential Cardiology: Principles and Practice, 2nd Ed.*
Edited by: C. Rosendorff © Humana Press Inc., Totowa, NJ

of exercise. Myocardial segments perfused by narrowed coronary arteries or with scarring due to prior myocardial infarction show diminished tracer uptake on these images. [201]Tl shows a continuous redistribution after initial tissue extraction. Stress images are followed by redistribution images 3 to 4 h later to detect reversibility in segments with stress related perfusion abnormalities. Perfusion abnormality due to ischemia reverses on redistribution images whereas that due to scarring remains unchanged. Segments characterized by scar and ischemia show partial reversibility of the perfusion abnormality.

Stress ^{201}Tl imaging has a sensitivity of nearly 85 to 92% and a specificity of 90% or above for the detection of coronary artery disease (3). However, redistribution of ^{201}Tl in somewhat unreliable and unpredictable. In a significant proportion of defects due to ischemia, ^{201}Tl redistribution may be incomplete (4). Thus the standard stress-redistribution ^{201}Tl imaging may underestimate the true extent of myocardial ischemia. A number of different strategies have been proposed for overcoming this limitation (5). A second injection of ^{201}Tl at rest, either on the same day or on a separate day, appears to be the most satisfactory way of overcoming this limitation in selected cases (4–7). However, a routine second injection of ^{201}Tl to all patients irrespective of the presence or absence of perfusion abnormalities on the stress images is unnecessary and inadvisable.

Other limitations of ^{201}Tl include its long physical half-life (3 d), which limits the dose that can be used safely without causing undue radiation exposure to the patients. [201]Tl emits low-energy photons (69–83 KeV), which are prone to attenuation by the thoracic wall and the soft tissue lying anterior to the heart. The attenuation can be particularly troublesome in obese patients and in women.

TECHNETIUM-99M-LABELED TRACERS

[201]Tl was used extensively for nearly two decades after its introduction in the 1970s. [201]Tl has now been largely replaced by technetium-99m (^{99m}Tc)-labeled myocardial perfusion tracers. However, ^{201}Tl is still used for the detection of myocardial viability, as will be discussed later, and also for dual-isotope perfusion imaging, where ^{201}Tl is used for rest perfusion imaging and a ^{99m}Tc-labeled perfusion tracer is used for stress perfusion imaging.

[99m]Tc has a shorter half-life (approx 6 h) and emits slightly higher energy photons (140 KeV), and its chemical structure allows its incorporation into a number of different chemicals or ligands, which can be used for studying the anatomy, perfusion, and metabolism of various organs. ^{99m}Tc-labeled agents can be used in much higher doses and provide better-quality images. Three agents: sestamibi (Cardiolite, Bristol Myers Squibb, Princeton, NJ), teboroxime (Cardiotech, Bracco Inc., Princeton) and tetrofosmin (Myoview, GE Healthcare, Princeton) are approved by the FDA (8–11). Sestamibi and tetrofosmin are lipophilic cationic agents. They are taken up by the myocardium because of their lipophilicity and positive charge. Their myocardial uptake is not mediated by the Na^+/K^+ ATPase pump. In the myocytes, they are localized mainly in the mitochondria. These agents are tightly bound to the myocardium and show little or no clearance or redistribution from the myocardium after initial cardiac uptake.

The mechanism of tissue clearance of ^{99m}Tc-sestamibi has recently been elucidated (11). ^{99m}Tc-sestamibi is a substrate for p-glycoproteins, which belong to a large group of cell membrane transporters. Whereas these transporters are abundantly expressed in the liver, intestinal mucosa, and several other organs, they are not expressed in the myocardium (11). A lack of these transporters in the myocardium explains a relative lack of clearance of ^{99m}Tc-sestamibi from the myocardium. With the use of cationic ^{99m}Tc perfusion tracers, two separate injections are required for stress and rest imaging. Teboroxime is a neutral compound and shows very rapid washout after initial myocardial uptake. This is an important drawback and therefore this agent is not currently in clinical use. Another new ^{99m}Tc-labeled agent, Noet (Berlex, Montville, NJ) is undergoing clinical evaluation but is not yet available for routine clinical use (12). Table 1 gives a summary of different myocardial perfusion imaging agents.

The perfusion images are gated to the electrocardiogram. This provides information about left and right ventricular function and wall motion. Another advantage of ^{99m}Tc-labeled agents is that first-pass imaging can also be carried out during injection of the radiotracer during stress or rest (13).

Table 1
Different Agents for Myocardial Perfusion Imaging and Their Salient Features

Agent	Physical half life	Chemical structure	Site of myocellular localization	Myocardial retention	Redistribution	Main route of excretion
Tl-201	72 h	Element	Cytosol	Good	Yes	Renal
99mTc-sestamibi	6 h	Isonitrile	Mitochondria	Good	Minimal	Hepatobiliary
99mTc-teboroxime	6 h	Boronic acid derivative	Sarcolemma	Poor	Yes	Hepatobiliary
99mTc-tetrofosmin	6 h	Diphosphine	Mitochondria	Good	None	Hepatobiliary/Renal
99mTc-N-Noet[a]	6 h	Dithiocarbamate	Sarcolemma	Good	Yes	Hepatobiliary

[a]Not approved by the FDA for routine clinical use.

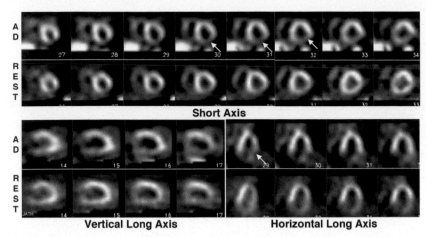

Fig. 1. Adenosine stress (AD) and rest ^{99m}Tc-sestamibi SPECT images of a 62-yr-old woman with end-stage renal disease, diabetes, hypertension, and hyperlipidemia who underwent angioplasty and stenting of her RCA 6 mo earlier because of angina. She had recurrence of her chest pain. There was no chest pain or ST-segment depression during adenosine infusion. There is a large area of ischemia involving the inferior and lateral walls (arrows). In addition, transient post-stress LV dilation is noticed. The left ventricular ejection fraction was 37% on the post stress images with hypokinesia of the inferior and lateral wall, and 52% on the rest images with normal wall motion. Coronary angiography showed 100% occlusion of the first obtuse marginal branch of the left circumflex coronary artery and long 80% in-stent restenosis of the RCA. Successful revascularization of the RCA and OM1 were carried out.

However, both ^{99m}Tc-sestamibi and ^{99m}Tc-tetrofosmin suffer from several limitations: liver and gastrointestinal uptake, which can degrade the image quality and produce artifacts; and relatively low first-pass myocardial extraction, which can potentially result in an underestimation of myocardial ischemia, particularly in myocardial segments perfused by coronary arteries with lower grade of narrowing. An ideal ^{99m}Tc myocardial perfusion tracer should have minimal or no hepatic and gastrointestinal uptake and should have a high first-pass myocardial extraction that linearly tracks the myocardial blood flow over a wide range.

Instrumentation

Planar imaging was used extensively in the past, but this has now largely been replaced with single photon emission computed tomography (SPECT) imaging. Planar imaging was limited to the acquisition of images in anterior, left anterior oblique, and left lateral views, whereas SPECT imaging provides a series of cross-sectional images of the heart in multiple axes. SPECT imaging allows a better anatomic delineation of the perfusion abnormalities and a better angiographic correlation than planar imaging. For SPECT imaging, 32 to 64 images are acquired in a 180–360° orbit around the heart. These images are processed in a manner similar to that for CT images so that the left ventricular myocardium is displayed in a series of slices of varying thickness (Figs. 1–3). SPECT cameras are available with a single, double, or triple heads. Double and triple heads reduce the imaging time.

The SPECT images are gated with ECG (gated SPECT) to assess left ventricular wall motion, thickening, and ejection fraction from the same study. Thus simultaneous assessment of myocardial perfusion and function can be carried out from a single study. Since myocardial ischemia and left ventricular function are the two most important determinants of optimal therapy and short-term as well as long-term prognosis, gated SPECT perfusion imaging is currently the single most powerful diagnostic and prognostic modality in cardiovascular medicine.

Soft-tissue attenuation continues to be another major source of artifacts in myocardial perfusion imaging. As soft tissue attenuation is nonuniform and varies from patient to patient, a relatively

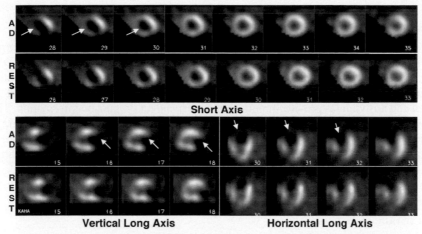

Fig. 2. Adenosine stress and rest ^{99m}Tc-sestamibi SPECT images of a 66-yr-old woman who sustained an anterior wall myocardial infarction 8 yr earlier. The left ventricle is dilated with a large, dense fixed defect involving the anterior wall, apex and distal septum consistent with a large scar (arrows). There is no reversible perfusion abnormality on this study. On gated SPECT the anterior wall is akinetic and the apex is dyskinetic indicative of an apical aneurysm.

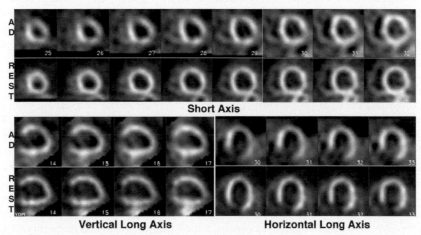

Fig. 3. Adenosine stress and rest ^{99m}Tc-sestamibi SPECT images of a 44-yr-old woman with exertional chest pain and progressively worsening shortness of breath. She has a history of breast cancer treated with surgery, chemotherapy (epirubicin and cytoxan), and radiotherapy. There is no regional perfusion abnormality but the LV and RV are markedly enlarged with global severe hypokinesia and LVEF of 19%. She has cardiomyopathy related to chemotherapy with epirubicin.

sophisticated approach is required for its correction. Attenuation correction is carried out with the use of a simultaneously acquired transmission map using an external source of radiation such as gadolinium. A three-dimensional attenuation map is created from these transmission images for pixel-by-pixel correction of the attenuation. Recently, SPECT imaging has been combined with CT imaging for attenuation correction. However, because of several inadequately resolved technical issues, attenuation correction is not yet a widely accepted and routinely used technique. With technological improvements, wider use of attenuation correction is anticipated in the future.

Choice of Stress

EXERCISE

Exercise is the preferred method of stress testing. In the US, treadmill exercise is the preferred exercise modality, whereas in Europe, bicycle exercise is preferred. Information about exercise capacity, changes in heart rate and blood pressure, adverse symptoms such as chest pain and undue fatigue, and electrocardiographic changes such as the magnitude and duration of ST segment depression and arrhythmias provide important and independent prognostic information. The radiotracer is injected close to the peak exercise and exercise is continued for another 2 min to allow radiotracer extraction by the myocardium at peak exercise. It is important for the patients to reach an adequate workload, which can be judged from the peak heart rate, product of the heart rate and blood pressure at peak exercise (peak double product), or oxygen consumption at peak exercise. A peak heart rate above 85% of the age-predicted maximum heart rate or a double product >25 K is used to determine the adequacy of the exercise level.

PHARMACOLOGICAL STRESS

In patients who are unable to exercise or unable to reach an adequate workload due to noncardiac limitations (peripheral vascular disease, musculoskeletal disorders, or pulmonary disease) pharmacological stress should be used. Dipyridamole and adenosine (Adenoscan®, Fujisawa Inc.) are the most widely used agents for this purpose *(14–18)*. Following intravenous administration, these agents cause marked coronary vasodilation and can increase myocardial blood flow three to four times the resting flow. However, blood flow increase is blunted in myocardial segments perfused by narrowed coronary arteries. This produces flow heterogeneity and results in apparent perfusion abnormalities on the perfusion images. True ischemia is rare and occurs in patients with severe coronary artery disease where collateral circulation contributes significantly toward myocardial perfusion. Dipyridamole and adenosine may induce a coronary steal in such cases. At a cellular level, dipyridamole acts by inhibiting the intracellular uptake of adenosine. Thus adenosine is more directly acting than dipyridamole and has more predictable effect on the coronary blood flow *(15)*.

Adenosine has an extremely short half-life and its side effects are transient. Side effects are common with dipyridamole or adenosine infusion, but generally are minor and self-limiting in nature. The most common side effects are nausea, headache, flushing of face, and hypotension. Transient high-grade AV block can also occur with adenosine infusion. Chest pain occurs in approx 25% of cases but is not specific for myocardial ischemia. The exact mechanism of dipyridamole- or adenosine-induced chest pain is not clear; perhaps they act directly on the pain receptors. ST segment depression occurs rarely but if it occurs, it is indicative of severe coronary artery disease. If possible, dipyridamole or adenosine infusion should be combined with low-level exercise *(15,18)*. This reduces adverse effects such as hypotension, nausea, and flushing and also reduces radiotracer uptake in the liver and other splanchnic organs, which improves the image quality. Addition of low-level exercise to adenosine infusion also improves the sensitivity and specificity for the detection of coronary artery disease *(15)*.

Theophylline derivatives, including caffeine, act as antagonists of dipyridamole and adenosine at the cellular level and should be stopped prior to performing dipyridamole or adenosine stress perfusion imaging. Aminophylline can be given intravenously if the side effects of dipyridamole are persistent and bothersome to the patient. Because of the extremely short half-life, side effects of adenosine generally disappear with the discontinuation of its infusion and aminophylline is only very rarely required. Figures 1 and 2 are examples of markedly abnormal adenosine stress and rest ^{99m}Tc-sestamibi studies.

Apart from coronary vasodilation, adenosine also results in systemic vasodilation and slowing of conduction in the AV node, which are undesirable side effects for pharmacological stress testing. A number of adenosine analogs, which are highly selective for adenosine receptors in coronary vessels (adenosine A2a receptors), are being developed for pharmacological stress perfusion imaging *(19,20)*. It is anticipated that these agents will have fewer adverse effects and a better safety profile than adenosine, particularly in sicker patient populations.

Intravenous dobutamine can also be used for stress imaging *(21)*. This acts by increasing the heart rate and myocardial oxygen demand. This can be used in patients where dipyridamole or adenosine are contraindicated, such as in patients with severe bronchopulmonary disease or congestive heart failure or in those where theophylline can not be stopped. Arbutamine is a dobutamine analog, which results in a greater chronotropic response compared to dobutamine, but its sensitivity and specificity for the detection of perfusion abnormalities are similar to that of dobutamine *(22)*. Table 2 lists various pharmacological agents for myocardial perfusion imaging and their important characteristics.

For myocardial perfusion imaging, adenosine or dipyridamole are preferable over dobutamine or arbutamine because of a greater increase in myocardial blood flow and flow heterogeneity with these agents.

Interpretation of Perfusion Images

Interpretation of myocardial perfusion images requires experience and skill and an adequate understanding of the cardiac physiology, pathology, and applied physics, as well as awareness of the possible sources of artifacts. Perfusion images are prone to artifacts due to attenuation from structures overlying the heart or in proximity to the heart. The diaphragm and liver can attenuate the inferior wall. In women, the breast can cause attenuation. Proximity of the liver to the inferior wall of the heart is also an important source of artifacts. Tracer activity in the liver can result in artifactually higher counts in the inferior wall due to scattered counts. Conversely, during image reconstruction, oversubtraction of counts from the structures in close proximity of the hot liver can result in artifactually lower counts in the inferior wall. SPECT imaging is also prone to a variety of other artifacts, such as patient motion during imaging and tracer activity in the gut and other subdiaphragmatic structures. ^{99m}Tc-sestamibi and ^{99m}Tc-tetrofosmin produce high activity in the liver, gall bladder, and gut, particularly in the rest and pharmacological stress images. Sometimes bowel loops with significant radiotracer activity may overlap the heart, which can substantially degrade the image quality and in the worst scenario can render the images uninterpretable. If bowel loops with radioactivity are noticed to overlap the heart during image acquisition, the image acquisition should be aborted and recommenced after repositioning the patient few minutes later. Administration of fatty food prior to imaging does not enhance clearance of radiotracer from the liver. On the other hand, this can increase the amount of radioactivity in the gut because of dumping of gall bladder activity in the gut. Artifacts can also appear during various stages of processing of the raw data to the processed images. A meticulous effort is required to prevent false interpretation of the images due to these artifacts *(23)*.

A number of techniques are currently under development for the correction of attenuation artifacts during SPECT imaging. Attenuation is nonuniform, being dependent on the density and thickness of the tissue around the heart. A three-dimensional spatial map of attenuation coefficients using an external transmission source is obtained. These attenuation maps are unique for each patient and are used for correcting the emission images *(24,25)*.

Imaging patients in the prone position can also help in the differentiation of attenuation artifacts from true perfusion abnormalities in the inferior wall. However, prone imaging does not replace standard supine imaging. Prone images are acquired in addition to the standard supine images. This increases the time required to image the patients.

The perfusion images can be interpreted visually. However, quantitative analysis of the images is more reliable. Subtle abnormalities can be better appreciated with quantitative analysis. Quantitative analysis can be performed using a simple circumferential analysis program or with the use of a polar map. To obtain a circumferential profile, a region of interest is drawn around the cardiac contour, the myocardium is divided into 36 radial sectors, and the counts in these sectors are plotted and compared with the normal database. In a polar plot, the short-axis myocardial slices from SPECT images are displayed as a series of concentric rings in a single display. These rings are displayed on a color scale, so that the myocardial segments with abnormally low radiotracer uptake are shown in a different color from the normal myocardium. Quantitative analysis can also provide an estimate

Table 2
Different Agents for Pharmacological Stress Perfusion Imaging

Agent	Mode of action	Effect on HR	Effect on SBP	Effect on double product
Dipyridamole	Coronary vasodilation	Slight increase	Decrease	Minimal change
Adenosine	Coronary vasodilation	Slight increase	Decrease	Minimal change
Binodenoson[a] (MRE 0473)	Selective coronary vasodilation	Minimal increase	Minimal decrease or no change	Minimal or no change
Regadenoscan (CVT 5131)[a]	Selective coronary vasodilation	Minimal increase or no change	Minimal decrease	Minimal or no change
Dobutamine	Increased myocardial oxygen demand	Significant increase	Increase or no change	Increase

[a]Not approved for routine clinical use (undergoing clinical evaluation).

of the extent or severity of myocardial ischemia, which is important if serial studies are used to follow the disease progress. Quantitative analysis also minimizes the intra- and interobserver variability of the image interpretation (23).

A systematic approach is required for the comprehensive interpretation of myocardial perfusion studies. The raw images should be examined to look for any potential sources of artifacts and overall image quality. Sometimes important extracardiac abnormalities, such as tumors in lungs, mediastinum or breasts or pleural effusion, can be detected on raw images. Gastrointestinal abnormalities such as hiatal hernias or ascites can also be observed on raw images. Many times, these abnormalities are detected for the first time as incidental findings during perfusion imaging but nevertheless are important for the management of the patients (26). The patient's gender, body weight, and body habitus, the radiopharmaceutical used and its dose, the interval between tracer injection and imaging, and the type of stress used should be taken into consideration while viewing the raw images. With ^{201}Tl, the lung fields should be examined for any evidence of increased lung tracer uptake on stress images, which is an indicator of high-risk study. The processed images should be interpreted qualitatively as well as quantitatively. Clinical history, pretest likelihood of coronary artery disease, details of stress testing, and electrocardiographic changes should be taken into consideration while performing the final interpretation.

Clinical Applications of Myocardial Perfusion Imaging

Detection of Coronary Artery Disease

Myocardial perfusion imaging is useful for establishing the diagnosis of coronary artery disease in patients presenting with chest pain or in those with a high clinical suspicion of coronary artery disease because of the presence of one or more risk factors for coronary artery disease. This is an important noninvasive test for identifying patients who should be considered for further invasive studies. Addition of myocardial perfusion imaging to exercise ECG increases the sensitivity as well as specificity of the test for the detection of coronary artery disease (27). The sensitivity and specificity of exercise ECG alone are 50 to 60% and 60% respectively for the detection of coronary artery disease, whereas myocardial perfusion imaging has a sensitivity of 85 to 90% and specificity of 90% or above for the detection of coronary artery disease. Myocardial perfusion imaging has a particular advantage over exercise ECG in patients with left ventricular hypertrophy, left bundle branch block (LBBB), therapy with digoxin, and other abnormalities interfering with proper interpretation of ST-segment changes on exercise.

Myocardial perfusion imaging is an important and cost-effective gatekeeper for the identification of patients who should undergo further invasive cardiac workup (27). In a study involving more than 4000 patients who underwent stress myocardial perfusion imaging for the evaluation of coronary artery disease, the subsequent cardiac catheterization rates over a mean follow-up period of 9 mo were 32% in those with reversible perfusion abnormality and only 3.5% in those without reversible perfusion abnormality (28). Furthermore, in the reversible perfusion abnormality group, cardiac catheterization rate was 60% in those with high-risk studies (reversible perfusion abnormality of the left anterior descending coronary artery territory, multiple areas of ischemia or increased lung tracer uptake), compared with 9% in the remaining patients with reversible perfusion abnormalities. The findings on myocardial perfusion imaging were far more predictive of subsequent cardiac catheterization than clinical and treadmill exercise ECG variables alone or in combination, indicating the important role of stress myocardial perfusion imaging for initial evaluation of patients with suspected coronary artery disease.

Risk Stratification of Patients With CAD

Information about the severity, location, and extent of myocardial ischemia is useful for risk stratification of patients with known coronary artery disease. Large areas or multiple areas of perfusion abnormality identify patients at high risk for cardiovascular events on follow-up. Increased lung tracer uptake and transient left ventricular dilation on stress images are indicative of severe coronary

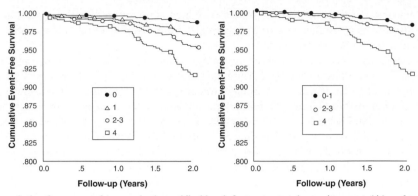

Fig. 4. Cumulative 2-yr event-free survival stratified by defect extent and severity score (**A**) and reversibility score (**B**), $p < 0.001$ for each. (Reproduced with permission from ref. *33*.)

artery disease and are predictive of poor prognosis *(29,30)*. Both of these findings are due to a transient left ventricular dysfunction during stress. The magnitude of ST depression on symptom-limited exercise testing does not correlate with the extent of ischemia on perfusion imaging *(31)*. The quantitative extent and severity of myocardial ischemia determined from stress-rest perfusion imaging correlates with the subsequent occurrence of unstable angina, acute myocardial infarction, and cardiac death. Of various clinical and laboratory variables including electrocardiographic and coronary angiographic variables, myocardial perfusion imaging provides the most powerful prognostic information in all groups of patients with coronary artery disease. Based on the quantitative extent and severity of perfusion abnormalities on stress perfusion images and the extent of reversibility on stress-rest perfusion imaging, patients with coronary artery disease can be categorized into low- to high-risk categories for the occurrence of adverse cardiac events on follow-up (Fig. 4) *(32,33)*. Patients with a negative myocardial perfusion study have an excellent prognosis; several large clinical studies have shown these patients to have a less than 0.6% annual cardiac event rate *(32,33)*. A normal myocardial perfusion study, even in the presence of angiographically documented coronary artery disease, is associated with an excellent long-term prognosis and a very low incidence of cardiac events on follow-up.

POST-MYOCARDIAL INFARCTION EVALUATION

Submaximum stress perfusion imaging is an established technique for risk stratification of patients with uncomplicated myocardial infarction prior to hospital discharge *(35)*. Patients with fixed defects have a low incidence of adverse cardiac events, whereas those with reversible defects have a higher incidence of adverse cardiac events. This test can be used to identify patients with recent myocardial infarction who can benefit from cardiac catheterization and revascularization. With the current practice of the routine use of revascularization with percutaneous interventions in patients with acute myocardial infarction and unstable angina, predischarge stress perfusion imaging is less commonly needed these days. However, stress perfusion imaging plays an important role in determining the need of subsequent revascularization in the presence of additional noncritical coronary lesions of unclear significance and in patients with recurrence of symptoms of chest pain following revascularization for acute myocardial infarction *(36)*. Myocardial perfusion imaging is very helpful for long-term follow-up of patients undergoing revascularization for acute myocardial infarction.

TRIAGING OF PATIENTS WITH CHEST PAIN OF UNCERTAIN ORIGIN

With greater public education and awareness for presenting immediately to the nearest emergency department in case of chest pain or any other symptoms suspicious of a myocardial infarc-

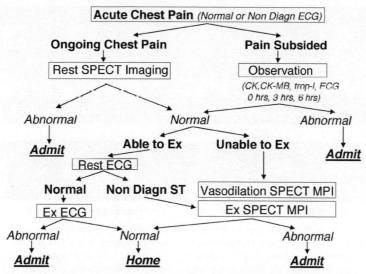

Fig. 5. A schematic representation of the proposed algorithm for early triaging of patients presenting with acute chest pain using myocardial perfusion imaging. (Reproduced with permission from ref. *38*.)

tion, a large number of patients with chest pain are seen in the emergency departments these days. Acute chest pain is the second most common condition seen in emergency departments in the US *(37)*. In the US, nearly 6 million patient visits for chest pain occur annually to the emergency department. Fewer than 15% of these patients turn out to have acute coronary syndrome. On the other hand, a small but significant proportion of patients with acute coronary syndrome may have only atypical symptoms with no overt electrocardiographic or biochemical abnormalities at presentation, which may prompt an early but inappropriate discharge from the emergency department with a mistaken conclusion of noncardiac chest pain. Most large emergency departments now have a dedicated chest pain center for an effective, reliable, and prompt triage of patients with chest pain. A combination of serial electrocardiograms, cardiac enzymes, and noninvasive cardiac imaging is used for triaging these patients *(37–40)*. Resting and stress myocardial perfusion imaging can be used quite effectively in chest pain centers. Despite an upfront cost associated with instrumentation and training of personnel and recurring cost associated with each study, an appropriate use of myocardial perfusion imaging in emergency departments is associated with significant reductions in the time required to arrive at a definitive diagnosis, hospital admission rate, average hospital stay, and overall per-patient cost *(37,40)*. The presence of perfusion abnormalities in patients with chest pain in the absence of prior myocardial infarction is indicative of an acute coronary syndrome and warrants admission to the coronary care unit and appropriate treatment. Absence of perfusion abnormalities points more toward a noncardiac cause of chest pain. Patients with negative resting perfusion images can further undergo stress perfusion imaging within a short period of time to detect the presence of exercise-induced myocardial ischemia. Figure 5 shows a proposed scheme for the utilization of myocardial perfusion imaging in chest pain centers *(38)* and Fig. 6 shows rest perfusion images of a patient who presented with atypical chest pain and turned out to have severe CAD.

RISK STRATIFICATION PRIOR TO NONCARDIAC SURGERY

Adverse cardiac events are an important cause of morbidity and mortality following noncardiac surgery, particularly in elderly patients and in those with known coronary artery disease or with risk factors for coronary artery disease *(41–43)*. Appropriate use of nuclear imaging techniques can significantly lower the incidence this complication. The frequency of occurrence of adverse cardiac events in the perioperative period depends on a number of factors: the prevalence and severity

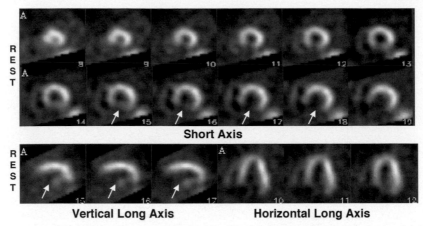

Fig. 6. Rest myocardial perfusion images of 43-yr-old male patient with multiple risk factors for CAD, who presented with atypical chest pain and no electrocardiographic changes or increase in cardiac enzymes. The patient had no history of prior myocardial infarction. There is a large area of perfusion abnormality involving the inferior and inferoseptal walls. Coronary angiography showed completely occluded RCA with a large thrombus and 90% narrowing of the LCx. There was a significant reduction of the perfusion abnormality following immediate revascularization the RCA and LCx.

of coronary artery disease and left ventricular dysfunction in this patient population and the nature and severity of hemodynamic stress during the perioperative period. Patients with a high prevalence of coronary artery disease, either symptomatic or occult, and with impaired left ventricular function, are particularly vulnerable to cardiac events. Prolonged vascular surgery involving cross-clamping of the aorta, major shifts between intravascular and extravascular fluid compartments, and hypotension impose significant stress on the cardiovascular system and can result in arrhythmias, pulmonary edema, or myocardial infarction in the perioperative period in patients with coronary artery disease. Patients with peripheral vascular disease have a high prevalence of coronary artery disease and are at a high risk of perioperative cardiac events. Even after peripheral vascular surgery, these patients continue to have very high morbidity and mortality due to cardiac events. A number of studies have established the role of pharmacological stress perfusion imaging for identifying patients at high risk for perioperative cardiac events *(42)*. Dipyridamole and adenosine are particularly suitable because of the inability of these patients to exercise. Abnormalities of dipyridamole perfusion imaging are predictive not only of perioperative morbidity and mortality but also of long-term mortality and morbidity *(43)*.

DETECTION OF MYOCARDIAL VIABILITY

The impairment in left ventricular function and regional wall motion abnormalities in many patients with coronary artery disease may be reversible to varying extents with proper utilization of revascularization procedures. This can result in improvement in left ventricular function and symptoms of heart failure, as well as well prognosis, and can potentially avoid or delay the need for cardiac transplantation in some patients with advanced heart failure. However, identification and differentiation of this viable but dysfunctional myocardium with a potential for recovery in contractility and left ventricular dynamics from the irreversibly scarred myocardium with no potential for recovery in function poses a major challenge in current practice of cardiology. Symptoms, clinical examination, electrocardiogram, and conventional techniques for functional assessment are often not helpful. A number of techniques such as dobutamine echocardiography and magnetic resonance imaging have been employed with varying success, but nuclear imaging techniques, conventional perfusion imaging as well as positron emission tomography, have played a crucial role in this field

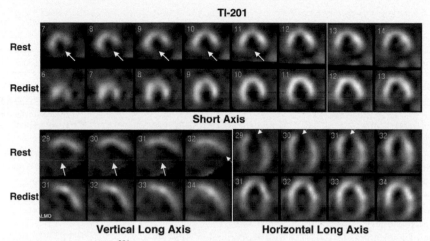

Fig. 7. Rest and 4-h redistribution ^{201}Tl images of a patient with old myocardial infarction and congestive heart failure. The left ventricle is enlarged with a large dense scar involving the inferior and lateral walls with no viability (solid arrows). There is apical reversible perfusion abnormality indicating viability (dotted arrows). The anterior wall and septum are normally perfused at rest indicating preserved viability. The inferior and lateral walls are akinetic and the remaining ventricle is hypokinetic on gated SPECT with an LVEF of 21%. LAD had 70% proximal lesion and RCA had 100% occlusion. Based on the presence of viability in the anterior wall, septum and apex, the LAD was revascularized.

(4). Myocardial uptake and retention or washout of perfusion tracers is dependent on the structural and metabolic integrity of the myocytes. Rest-redistribution ^{201}Tl imaging can be used for the detection of myocardial viability. Presence of significant myocardial uptake on quantitative analysis ($\geq$50% uptake compared to the normal myocardial segments) or redistribution on delayed imaging are indicative of myocardial viability and predictive of functional improvement after revascularization in abnormal myocardial segments (Fig. 7) *(44).* Resting ^{99m}Tc-sestamibi or ^{99m}Tc-tetrofosmin can also provide information about myocardial viability using a quantitative approach. Similar to ^{201}Tl, $\geq$50% uptake of ^{99m}Tc-sestamibi or ^{99m}Tc-tetrofosmin in abnormal myocardial segments is predictive of myocardial viability *(45).*

Recent studies indicate a promising role of nitrate administration prior to the injection of myocardial perfusion imaging tracers for the detection of myocardial viability. Viable myocardial segments with resting hypoperfusion show an improvement in perfusion following nitrate administration; this change is predictive of functional improvement after revascularization *(46).* PET imaging techniques for myocardial viability are based on the demonstration of metabolic activity in the dysfunctional myocardial segments. This will be described in a later section of this chapter.

EVALUATION OF PATIENTS WITH CONGESTIVE HEART FAILURE

Currently, there are more than 4.5 million patients with congestive heart failure in the United States, and more than 500,000 new patients are diagnosed with congestive heart failure every year. A detailed and often expensive workup is required to determine its etiology, assess its severity and optimize its treatment. Myocardial perfusion imaging can be used to differentiate between ischemic and nonischemic cardiomyopathy and for the assessment of left and right ventricular function (Fig. 3). This is highly cost-effective and can potentially avoid invasive tests in a substantial proportion of patients with heart failure. In patients with ischemic cardiomyopathy, perfusion imaging can be used quite effectively for the detection of myocardial viability, which may warrant a consideration for revascularization. Furthermore, as described below, nuclear imaging techniques can be used for an accurate, reliable, and highly reproducible serial assessment of left ventricular and right ventricular function in these patients. This is critical because an appropriate use of angiotensin-

Table 3
Indications of Myocardial Perfusion Imaging
and the Most Appropriate Imaging Technique(s) and Radiotracer(s)

Indication	Imaging technique(s)	Radiotracer(s)
Detection of coronary artery disease	Gated stress[a]-rest SPECT	^{201}Tl/^{99m}Tc tracers (prefer ^{99m}Tc tracers for women and overweight males)
Risk stratification of patients with known CAD	Gated stress[a]-rest SPECT	^{99m}Tc tracers
Post myocardial infarction evaluation	Gated stress[a]-rest SPECT	^{99m}Tc tracers
Patients with acute chest pain of uncertain origin	Gated rest SPECT	^{99m}Tc tracers
Evaluation prior to noncardiac surgery	Gated pharmacological stress-rest SPECT	^{99m}Tc tracers
Detection of myocardial viability	Rest-redistribution SPECT/ gated rest SPECT (preferably with nitrates)	^{201}Tl/^{99m}Tc tracers
Congestive heart failure	Rest/redistribution-stress SPECT	^{201}Tl-^{99m}Tc-tracers

^{99m}Tc-tracers, ^{99m}Tc-sestamibi or ^{99m}Tc-tetrofosmin.
[a]Exercise is the preferred stress modality. Choose pharmacological stress for those unable to exercise to an adequate workload.

converting enzyme inhibitors and β-blockers can result in an improvement in left ventricular function in a significant proportion of patients with congestive heart failure.

Table 3 provides a summary of the indications of myocardial perfusion imaging and the optimal imaging techniques and radiotracers for each indication.

ASSESSMENT OF LEFT VENTRICULAR FUNCTION

Although a number of techniques such as echocardiography, contrast ventriculography, and magnetic resonance imaging can be used for the assessment of ventricular function, nuclear imaging techniques offer a distinct advantage in several clinical situations. With nuclear imaging techniques, left ventricular function can be assessed by first-pass imaging, equilibrium radionuclide angiocardiography, or gated SPECT imaging.

First-Pass Imaging

First-pass imaging is done by dynamic imaging of the passage of radioactivity from the superior vena cava to the right heart, lungs, and then to the left heart after injecting a bolus of radiotracer into the peripheral vein. Right and left ventricular ejection fraction can be calculated from these data. An important advantage of the newer ^{99m}Tc-labeled myocardial perfusion imaging agents is that dynamic first-pass imaging can be carried out during the injection of these agents either at rest or during exercise. Thus information about perfusion and function can be obtained from the same injection of radiopharmaceutical *(13)*. The wide spread use of ^{99m}Tc-labeled myocardial perfusion imaging agents in current clinical practice has revived interest in first-pass imaging *(47)*.

Equilibrium Radionuclide Angiocardiography

Equilibrium radionuclide angiocardiography (ERNA), also commonly known as multigated acquisition (MUGA), is performed by labeling the blood pool with ^{99m}Tc-pertechnetate. ^{99m}Tc-pertechnetate, when injected after the administration of pyrophosphate, binds to red blood cells. The ECG gated images of the heart are acquired in three standard views (anterior, left anterior oblique, and left lateral) to assess left ventricular wall motion and to calculate left ventricular ejection fraction. A time activity curve reflecting the temporal changes in left ventricular volumes during the cardiac cycle can also be obtained from these images. From this curve, left ventricular ejection fraction can be calculated. The slopes of this curve during rapid ejection phase in systole and during the rapid filling phase in diastole provide the peak ejection and peak filling rates. Left ventricular ejection fraction (LVEF) is the most widely used index of left ventricular function. SPECT imaging can also be used with equilibrium radionuclide angiocardiography. This may provide a more detailed assessment of the regional left ventricular function.

With the wider acceptance of gated SPECT myocardial perfusion imaging, gated SPECT perfusion imaging is the most widely used technique for determining the left ventricular ejection fraction in patients with coronary artery disease.

In patients with coronary artery disease, left ventricular ejection fraction is an important determinant of long-term prognosis (48). Measurement of left ventricular ejection fraction also has important therapeutic implications in patients with coronary artery disease. Progressive spontaneous deterioration of LVEF occurs in patients with moderately impaired LVEF (EF < 40%) due to ventricular remodeling. This process can be arrested by appropriate use of angiotensin-converting enzyme inhibitors (49).

Serial LVEF monitoring is also useful for the prevention of overt heart failure in cancer patients undergoing chemotherapy with anthracyclines. Congestive heart failure is the most significant complication of doxorubicin and other anthracycline derivatives. However, anthracycline-induced congestive heart failure is preceded by a progressive deterioration in left ventricular function, which in the initial stages is asymptomatic, but nevertheless provides an opportunity for the prevention of overt heart failure by discontinuation of anthracyclines at an early stage with only a subclinical left ventricular dysfunction. This requires a highly reliable, reproducible, and accurate technique for the serial monitoring of left ventricular function. Because of its high reproducibility and accuracy, ERNA is ideal for detecting changes in left ventricular ejection fraction at an early stage during the course of doxorubicin chemotherapy. In contrast, echocardiography provides an approximation of left ventricular ejection fraction, which is suboptimal for detecting early changes in left ventricular ejection fraction on serial studies. With the appropriate use of guidelines for performing serial ERNA in various subsets of patients, it is possible to reduce the incidence of doxorubicin-induced congestive heart failure from 20% to 2–3% (50–53).

Exercise ERNA

ERNA can also be carried out during exercise. This has been used for the detection of coronary artery disease. A drop in left ventricular ejection fraction of 5% or more compared to the pre-exercise ejection fraction and/or appearance of new wall motion abnormalities during exercise is indicative of the presence of CAD (54). However, the sensitivity and specificity both are relatively modest. With the widespread use of myocardial perfusion imaging, exercise radionuclide angiocardiography is rarely used these days for detecting coronary artery disease. Exercise perfusion imaging has better sensitivity and specificity and provides more quantitative information about the presence, location, and severity of CAD. Perfusion-based imaging techniques are preferable and more reliable than wall motion-based imaging techniques for the detection and quantification of CAD.

Ambulatory Left Ventricular Function Monitoring

This technique is unique for nuclear imaging of the heart. A combination of equilibrium radionuclide angiocardiography with Holter monitoring has resulted in a device for the continuous ambulatory monitoring of left ventricular function over several hours (55). This device uses a miniature radiation detector that is positioned on the chest after blood pool labeling with ^{99m}Tc-pertechnetate, which monitors and records the left ventricular blood pool activity on a modified Holter monitor. This technique has been used for studying the effects of interventions such as mental stress on left ventricular function and for detecting spontaneous changes in left ventricular function in patients with coronary artery disease *(56)*. Figure 8 shows left ventricular ejection fraction, heart rate, and relative end-diastolic and end-systolic volume trends at baseline, with mental stress and with exercise in a patient with chronic stable angina. This patient shows a significant fall in left ventricular ejection fraction with two different forms of mental stress, which was not accompanied by any symptoms or ST-segment depression. Mental-stress-induced left ventricular dysfunction is predictive of adverse cardiac events in patients with chronic stable angina *(57)*. Figure 9 shows the incidence of adverse cardiac events over 1 yr in coronary artery disease patients with and without mental-stress-induced left ventricular dysfunction. Mental-stress-positive patients had a threefold higher incidence of adverse cardiac events over 1 yr compared with mental-stress-negative patients *(57)*. Several subsequent studies have confirmed the adverse prognostic implications of mental-stress-induced changes in left ventricular wall motion or ejection fraction *(58,59)*.

MYOCARDIAL NECROSIS IMAGING

^{99m}Tc-pyrophosphate was used for imaging acute myocardial necrosis in the 1970s and 1980s. However, due to several technical drawbacks, this is only very rarely used these days. Indium-111 (^{111}In)-labeled Fab fraction of antibody against cardiac myosin (^{111}In-antimyosin) (Centocor Inc.) is highly selective for imaging the necrotic myocardium. This has high sensitivity and specificity for diagnosing acute myocardial infarction. ^{111}In-antimyosin imaging can be used for confirming the diagnosis of acute myocardial infarction in patients with atypical clinical presentation or in those where electrocardiographic changes are absent or unreliable for diagnosing of acute myocardial infarction *(60)*. However, because of its slow clearance from the blood pool and slow localization in the necrotic myocardium, an interval of 24 to 48 h is needed between ^{111}In-antimyosin injection and imaging. This significantly limits the clinical utility of this technique for the detection of acute myocardial infarction. ^{111}In-antimyosin is more useful for diagnosing acute myocarditis and cardiac transplant rejection *(61–63)*. These conditions are characterized by a diffuse myocardial uptake of ^{111}In-antimyosin. ^{111}In-antimyosin has also been used for evaluating doxorubicin cardiotoxicity *(51,52)*. Most of the patients show an abnormal myocardial uptake of ^{111}In-antimyosin after receiving intermediate doses of doxorubicin even in the absence of any fall in left ventricular ejection fraction. However, an intense ^{111}In-antimyosin uptake pattern after intermediate doses of doxorubicin even with normal left ventricular ejection fraction is predictive of an impending fall in left ventricular ejection fraction and congestive heart failure, if doxorubicin therapy is continued. Currently, ^{111}In-antimyosin is no longer commercially available in the US because of limited demand.

The ^{99m}Tc-labeled agents ^{99m}Tc-glucarate and ^{99m}Tc-annexin V are also infarct avid agents *(64–67)*. Glucaric acid is a simple 6-carbon dicarboxylic acid sugar that can be labeled with ^{99m}Tc. This localizes in the infarcted myocardium as early as 2 to 4 h after its injection and also clears rapidly from the blood pool. Abnormal ^{99m}Tc-glucarate uptake can be seen as early as 3 to 4 h after the onset of myocardial infarction. This would allow acute infarct imaging within a relatively short period of time and is potentially promising for use in chest pain centers *(65)*. ^{99m}Tc-Annexin is a normally circulating protein, which binds to the outer membrane of the cells undergoing apoptosis or necrosis. This agent has been used extensively for imaging apoptosis in tumors and in myocardium under various pathological conditions. Apart from imaging apoptotic myocardium, this also binds to acutely necrotic myocardium and has been used quite successfully for imaging acute myocardial infarction *(66)*. However, with the wider availability of reliable and simpler biochemical markers of acute myocardial injury and because of the need to intervene early, acute myocardial infarction imaging is unlikely to gain a wide acceptance in clinical practice.

POSITRON EMISSION TOMOGRAPHY

Positron emission tomography (PET) involves the use of positron-emitting isotopes (^{11}C, ^{18}F, ^{13}N, ^{15}O). Positrons disintegrate into two γ rays released at 180°, which can be detected as coincident photons by an array of detectors placed around the patient. PET images are of very high technical

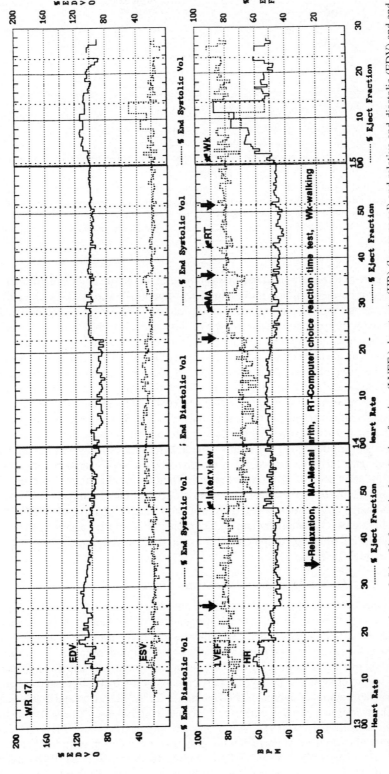

Fig. 8. Continuous data trend over 2.5 h of left ventricular e;ection fraction (LVEF), heart rate (HR) (lower panel) and relative end-diastolic (EDV) and end-systolic volumes (ESV) (upper panel) of a patient with chronic stable angina. The EF and HR are normal at baseline. After a period of stabilization patient underwent psychological interview. This was accompanied by a minimal increase in HR, a significant fall in EF and increase in ESV. Mental arithmetic (MA), another form of mental stress, produced similar changes. In contrast, computer choice reaction time (RT), a nonstressful task, produced no change in EF or HR. Walking (Wk) resulted in an increase in HR but no change in EF.

237

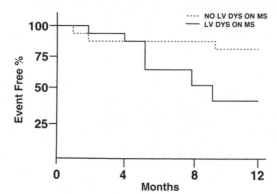

Fig. 9. Cardiac event-free survival rate in two groups of patients with chronic stable angina. One group of patients had left ventricular dysfunction in response to mental stress and the other group had no left ventricular dysfunction in response to mental stress. A significantly greater proportion of patients with mental stress induced left ventricular dysfunction developed cardiac events over 1 year. (Reproduced with permission from ref. *72*.)

quality. These tracers are of relatively short half-life and require an on-site cyclotron for their production. PET traces can be incorporated into a number of metabolic substrates such as deoxyglucose, fatty acids, acetate, and sympathomimetic amines and are useful for studying the metabolic and adrenergic neuronal activity of the myocardium *(68)*. ^{15}O-water and ^{13}N-ammonia can be used for myocardial perfusion imaging. A major advantage of PET perfusion imaging is that, apart from a qualitative assessment, an accurate quantitative assessment of the regional myocardial blood flow per gram of myocardial tissue at rest and under various physiological conditions can be carried out. ^{18}F-fluorodeoxyglucose (^{18}FDG) imaging is useful for studying myocardial viability. Chronically ischemic but viable myocardial segments are characterized by a preferential uptake of ^{18}FDG that is disproportionately higher compared to the regional perfusion. This is the classical paradigm for viability with PET imaging. However, ^{18}FDG imaging for viability requires a strict control of metabolic milieu and is of limited value in patients with diabetes or recent myocardial infarction.

Recently ^{18}FDG imaging has been carried out using conventional SPECT cameras after making alterations in the scintillation crystals and collimators *(69)*. Dual-head cameras with thicker scintillation crystals can also be used in coincidence imaging mode, similar to standard PET imaging. Alternatively, a high-energy collimator can be used for standard SPECT imaging of ^{18}FDG. ^{18}FDG is currently being used extensively for tumor imaging. The rapid growth of PET oncology has resulted in wider availability of PET imaging equipment. This would result in greater availability of PET imaging in cardiovascular medicine.

Direct Myocardial Ischemia Imaging

Recently, ^{18}FDG has been used for imaging exercise-induced myocardial ischemia. Myocardial ischemia results in a metabolic shift: There is a suppression of fatty acid uptake and metabolism and a substantial increase in glucose uptake with the onset of myocardial ischemia. Enhanced glucose uptake persists for several hours after an episode of myocardial ischemia. This prompted an exploration of the use of ^{18}FDG for imaging exercise-induced myocardial ischemia to detect the presence and assess the severity of CAD *(70–72)*. A preliminary study by He, Jain, and colleagues has shown a remarkable potential of exercise ^{18}FDG imaging for the detection and quantification of CAD. Whereas the overall sensitivity of exercise ^{18}FDG and exercise-rest ^{99m}Tc-sestamibi imaging was similar for the detection of CAD (91% vs 82%, p = ns), the sensitivity of ^{18}FDG was significantly higher than that of exercise-rest perfusion imaging for the detection of individual vessels with ≥50% luminal narrowing (67% vs 49%, p < 0.01). Figure 10 shows exercise ^{18}FDG and exercise-rest perfusion images of a patient with coronary artery disease. Clearly further large-scale studies are warranted to explore this concept further. (*See* Color Plate 5, following p. 268.)

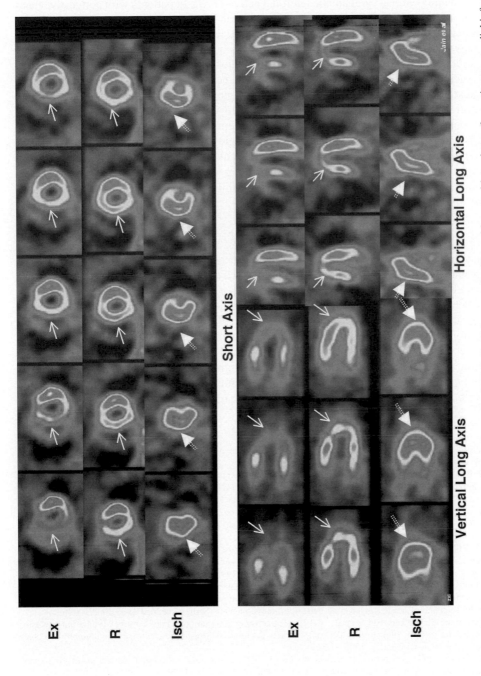

Short Axis

Vertical Long Axis

Horizontal Long Axis

Ex

R

Isch

Ex

R

Isch

Fig. 10. Exercise (Ex) and rest (R) ^{99m}Tc-sestamibi and exercise ^{18}FDG (Isch) images of a 67-yr-old man with angina and no prior myocardial infarction. There is a large area of partially reversible perfusion abnormality involving the septum, anterior wall, and apex (small arrows). Intense ^{18}FDG uptake is present in these areas (solid arrowheads). Coronary angiography showed 90% stenosis of the left anterior descending coronary artery and a 60% stenosis of the left circumflex artery (*See* Color Plate 5, following p. 268. Reproduced with permission from *71*.)

239

NEW RADIOTRACERS

A number of new radiotracers are in various stages of clinical development. Metaiodobenzyl-guanidine (MIBG) labeled with iodine-123 and parafluorobenzylguanidine labeled with ^{18}F can be used for imaging cardiac sympathetic neuronal activity *(73)*. In patients with congestive heart failure, there is activation of the sympathetic activity, and the extent of sympathetic activation cor-relates negatively with the prognosis of these patients. Therefore, cardiac uptake of ^{123}I-MIBG correlates inversely with the prognosis of patients with heart failure and this technique has the potential for understanding the mechanism of various interventions in these patients. ^{123}I-labeled fatty acids such as iodophenylpentadecanoic acid (IPPA) and 15-(*p*-iodophenyl)3R, S-methylpenta-decanoic acid (BMIPP) have been used for studying regional myocardial fatty acid metabolism. This is useful in studying the extent of myocardial viability and is also undergoing evaluation as a possible ischemia memory marker *(74)*. Radiopharmaceuticals targeted against various compo-nents of atheroma are being developed for atheroma imaging *(75–77)*. In the future, it may become possible to radiolabel various adhesion molecules, interleukins, and other mediators of endothelial dysfunction, intimal injury, and atherogenesis in experimental models. This is likely to emerge as an interesting approach for understanding the pathophysiology of endothelial dysfunction, intimal injury, and atherosclerosis.

CONCLUSION

Radionuclide imaging techniques have greatly enhanced our understanding of cardiovascular physiology and pathology. These techniques have played a crucial role in the evaluation of patients with definite or suspected coronary artery disease and for optimal and cost-effective utilization of various therapeutic options. Myocardial perfusion imaging is the most important and most widely used nuclear imaging technique. This provides important diagnostic and a very powerful prognos-tic information in males as well as in females and in all subsets of the patient population: suspected coronary artery disease, known coronary artery disease, and following acute myocardial infarction. New imaging techniques, radiopharmaceuticals, and imaging paradigms are emerging to meet the challenge of changing practice of cardiovascular medicine. Direct myocardial ischemia imaging with exercise ^{18}FDG is very exciting and is likely to be used more extensively in the future.

REFERENCES

1. Jain D, Strauss HW. Introduction to nuclear cardiology. In: Dilsizian V, Narula J, eds. Atlas of Nuclear Cardiology. London, Current Science 2003, pp. 1–18.
2. Kaul S, Boucher CA, Newell JB, et al. Determination of the quantitative thallium imaging variables that optimize detection of coronary artery disease. J Am Coll Cardiol 1986;7:527–537.
3. Wackers FJTh, Fetterman RC, Mattera JA, Clements JP. Quantitative planar thallium-201 stress scintigraphy: a critical evaluation of the method. Sem Nucl Med 1985;15:46–66.
4. Jain D, Zaret BL. Nuclear imaging techniques for the assessment of myocardial viability. Cardiol Clin 1995;13; 43–57.
5. Wackers FJTh. The maze of myocardial perfusion imaging protocols in 1994. J Nucl Cardiol 1994;1:180–188.
6. Dilsizian V, Rocco T, Freedman N, et al. Enhanced detection of ischemic but viable myocardium by the reinjection of thallium after stress-redistribution imaging. N Engl J Med 1990;323:141–146.
7. Kayden DS, Sigal S, Soufer R, et al. Thallium-201 for assessment of myocardial viability: quantitative comparison of 24-hour redistribution imaging with imaging after reinjection at rest. J Am Coll Cardiol 1991;18:1480–1486.
8. Jain D. ^{99m}Technetium labeled myocardial perfusion imaging agents. Semi Nucl Med 1999;29;221–236.
9. Zaret BL, Rigo P, Wackers FJTh, et al., and the Tetrofosmin International Trial Group. Myocardial perfusion imaging with technetium-99m tetrofosmin: comparison to thallium-201 imaging and coronary angiography in a phase III multicenter trial. Circulation 1995;91:313–319.
10. Jain D, Wackers FJTh, Mattera J, et al. Biokinetics of ^{99m}Tc-tetrofosmin: myocardial perfusion imaging agent: implications for a one day imaging protocol. J Nucl Med 1993;34:1254–1259.
11. Joseph B, Bhargava KK, Kandimala J, et al. The nuclear imaging agent sestamibi is a substrate for both MDR1 and MDR2 p-glycoprotein genes. Eur J Nucl Med 2003;30:1024–1031.
12. Vanzetto G, Fagret D, Pasqualini R, et al. Biodistribution, dosimetry, and safety of myocardial perfusion imaging agent 99mTcN-NOET in healthy volunteers. J Nucl Med 2000;41:141–148.

13. Iskandrian AS, Heo J, Kong B, et al. Use of technetium-99m isonitrile in assessing left ventricular perfusion and function at rest and during exercise in coronary artery disease and comparison with coronary angiography and exercise thallium-201 SPECT imaging. Am J Cardiol 1989;64:270–275.

14. Eagle KA, Singer DE, Brewster DC, et al. Dipyridamole-thallium scanning in patients undergoing vascular surgery: optimizing preoperative evaluation of cardiac risk. JAMA 1987;257:2185–2189.

15. Samady H, Wackers FJ, Zaret BL, et al. Pharmacological stress perfusion imaging with adenosine: role of simultaneous low level treadmill exercise. J Nucl Cardiol 2002;9:188–196.

16. Taillefer R, Amyot R, Turpin S, et al. Comparison between dipyridamole and adenosine as pharmacologic coronary vasodilators in detection of coronary artery disease with thallium 201 imaging. J Nucl Cardiol 1996;3:204–211.

17. Lette J, Tatum JL, Fraser S, et al. Safety of dipyridamole testing in 73,806 patients: the Multicenter Dipyridamole Safety Study. J Nucl Cardiol 1995;2:3–17.

18. Holly TA, Satran A, Bromet DS, et al. The impact of adjunctive adenosine infusion during exercise myocardial perfusion imaging: results of the Both Exercise and Adenosine Stress Test (BEAST) trial. J Nucl Cardiol 2003;10: 291–296.

19. Glover DK, Ruiz M, Takehana K, et al. Pharmacological stress myocardial perfusion imaging with the potent and selective A(2A) adenosine receptor agonists ATL193 and ATL146e administered by either intravenous infusion or bolus injection. Circulation 2001;104:1181–1187.

20. Udelson JE, Heller GV, Wackers FJ, et al. Randomized, controlled dose-ranging study of the selective adenosine A2A receptor agonist binodenoson for pharmacological stress as an adjunct to myocardial perfusion imaging. Circulation 2004;109:457–464.

21. Calnon DA, Glover DK, Beller GA, et al. Effects of dobutamine stress on myocardial blood flow, ^{99m}Tc sestamibi uptake, and systolic wall thickening in the presence of coronary artery stenoses: implications for dobutamine stress testing. Circulation 1997;96:2353–2360.

22. Shehata AR, Ahlberg AW, Gillam LD, et al. Direct comparison of arbutamine and dobutamine stress testing with myocardial perfusion imaging and echocardiography in patients with coronary artery disease. Am J Cardiol 1997;80: 716–720.

23. Wackers FJ. Science, art, and artifacts; how important is quantification for the practicing physician interpreting myocardial perfusion studies? J Nucl Cardiol 1994;1:S109–S117.

24. Ficaro EP, Corbett JR. Advances in quantitative perfusion SPECT imaging. J Nucl Cardiol 2004;11:62–70.

25. Heller GV, Links J, Bateman TM, et al. American Society of Nuclear Cardiology and Society of Nuclear Medicine joint position statement: attenuation correction of myocardial perfusion SPECT scintigraphy. J Nucl Cardiol 2004; 11:229–230.

26. Panjrath G, Jain D. Myocardial perfusion imaging in a patient with chest pain. J Nucl Cardiol 2004;11:515–517.

27. Wackers FJ, Zaret BL. Radionuclide stress myocardial perfusion imaging: the future gatekeeper for coronary angiography [editorial]. J Nucl Cardiol 1995;2:358–359.

28. Bateman TM, O'Keefe JH, Dong VM, et al. Coronary angiographic rates after stress single photon emission computed tomographic scintigraphy. J Nucl Cardiol 1995;2:217–223.

29. Jain D, Lahiri A, Raftery EB. Lung thallium uptake on rest, stress and redistribution cardiac imaging: state-of-the-art-review. Am J Card Imag 1990;4:303–309.

30. Gill JB, Ruddy TD, Newell JB, et al. Prognostic importance of thallium uptake by the lungs during exercise in coronary artery disease. N Engl J Med 1987;317:1485–1489.

31. Taylor AJ, Sackett MC, Beller GA. The degree of ST-segment depression on symptom-limited exercise testing: relation to the myocardial ischemic burden as determined by thallium-201 scintigraphy. Am J Cardiol 1995;75: 228–231.

32. Iskander S, Iskandrian AE. Risk assessment using single-photon emission computed tomographic technetium-99m sestamibi imaging. J Am Coll Cardiol 1998;32:57–62.

33. Thomas GS, Miyamoto MI, Morello P, et al. Technetium-99m sestamibi myocardial perfusion imaging predicts clinical outcome in the community outpatient setting: The Nuclear Utility in the Community (NUC) Study. J Am Coll Cardiol 2004;43:213–223.

34. Raiker K, Sinusas AJ, Wackers FJ, Zaret BL. One-year prognosis of patients with normal planar or single-photon emission computed tomographic technetium 99m labeled sestamibi exercise imaging. J Nucl Cardiol 1994;1:449–456.

35. Gibson RS, Watson DD, Craddock GB, et al. Prediction of cardiac events after uncomplicated myocardial infarction: a prospective study comparing predischarge exercise thallium-201 scintigraphy and coronary angiography. Circulation 1983;68:321–336.

36. Jain D, Wackers FJTh, Zaret BL. Radionuclide imaging techniques in the thrombolytic era. In: Becker R, ed. Modern Era of Coronary Thrombolysis, 1st ed. Kluwer Academic Publishers, Norwell, MA, 1994, pp. 195–218.

37. Udelson JE, Beshansky JR, Ballin DS, et al. Myocardial perfusion imaging for evaluation and triage of patients with suspected acute cardiac ischemia: a randomized controlled trial. JAMA 2002;288:2693–2700.

38. Abbott BG, Abdel-Aziz I, Nagula S, et al. Selective use of single-photon emission computed tomography myocardial perfusion imaging in a chest pain center. Am J Cardiol 2001;87:1351–1355.

39. Abbott BG, Jain D. Nuclear cardiology in the evaluation of acute chest pain in the emergency department. Echocardiography 2000;17:597–604.

40. Abbott BG, Jain D. Impact of myocardial perfusion imaging on clinical management and the utilization of hospital resources in suspected acute coronary syndromes. Nucl Med Comm 2003;24:1061–1069.

41. Jain D, Fleisher LA, Zaret BL. Diagnosing perioperative myocardial infarction in noncardiac surgery. Int Anesthesiology Clin 1992;30:199–216.
42. Leppo JA. Preoperative cardiac risk assessment for noncardiac surgery. Am J Cardiol 1995;75:42D–51D.
43. Fleisher LA, Rosenbaum SH, Nelson AH, et al. Preoperative dipyridamole thallium imaging and Holter monitoring as a predictor of perioperative cardiac events and long term outcome. Anesthesiology 1995;83:906–917.
44. Ragosta M, Beller GA, Watson DD, et al. Quantitative planar rest-redistribution ^{201}Tl imaging in detection of myocardial viability and prediction of improvement in left ventricular function after coronary bypass surgery in patients with severely depressed left ventricular function. Circulation 1993;87:1630–1641.
45. Caner B, Beller GA. Are technetium-99m-labeled myocardial perfusion agents adequate for detection of myocardial viability? Clin Cardiol 1998;4:235–242.
46. He ZX, Verani MS, Liu XJ, Nitrate-augmented myocardial imaging for assessment of myocardial viability [editorial]. J Nucl Cardiol 1995;2:352–357.
47. Borges-Neto S, Shaw LJ, Kesler KL, et al. Prediction of severe coronary artery disease by combined rest and exercise radionuclide angiocardiography and tomographic perfusion imaging with technetium 99m-labeled sestamibi: a comparison with clinical and electrocardiographic data. J Nucl Cardiol 1997;4:189–194.
48. Lee KL, Proyer DB, Pieper KS, et al. Prognostic value of radionuclide angiography in medically treated patients with coronary artery disease: a comparison with clinical and catheterization variables. Circulation 1990;82:1705–1717.
49. The SOLVD Investigators. Effect of enalapril on mortality and the development of heart failure in asymptomatic patients with reduced left ventricular ejection fractions. N Engl J Med 1992;327:685–691.
50. Schwartz RG, McKenzie B, Alexander J, et al. Congestive heart failure and left ventricular dysfunction complicating doxorubicin therapy: seven-year experience using serial radionuclide angiocardiography. Am J Med 1987;82:1109–1118.
51. Jain D, Zaret BL. Antimyosin cardiac imaging: will it play a role in the detection of doxorubicin cardiotoxicity? (editorial) J Nucl Med 1990;31:1970–1975.
52. Jain D. Cardiotoxicity of doxorubicin and other anthracyclines derivatives. J Nucl Cardiol 2000;7:53–62.
53. Mitani I, Jain D, Joska TM, et al. Doxorubicin cardiotoxicity: prevention of congestive heart failure with serial cardiac function monitoring with equilibrium radionuclide angiocardiography in the current era. J Nucl Cardiol 2003;10:132–139.
54. Bonow RP, Kent KM, Rosing DR, et al. Exercise-induced ischemia in mildly symptomatic patients with coronary artery disease and preserved left ventricular function: identification of subgroups at risk of death during medical therapy. N Engl J Med 1984;311:1339–1345.
55. Zaret BL, Jain D. Monitoring of left ventricular function with miniaturized non-imaging detectors. In: Zaret BL, Beller GA, eds. Nuclear Cardiology: State of the Art and Future Directions, 2nd ed. Mosby Year Book, St. Louis, 1999, pp. 191–200.
56. Burg MM, Jain D, Soufer R, et al. Role of behavioral and psychological factors in mental stress induced silent left ventricular dysfunction in coronary artery disease. J Am Coll Cardiol 1993;22:440–448.
57. Jain D, Burg MM, Soufer RS, Zaret BL. Prognostic significance of mental stress induced left ventricular dysfunction in patients with coronary artery disease. Am J Cardiol 1995;76:31–35.
58. Jiang W, Babyak M, Krantz DS, et al. Mental stress-induced myocardial ischemia and cardiac events. JAMA 1996;275:1651–1656.
59. Krantz DS, Santiago HT, Kop WJ, et al. Prognostic value of mental stress testing in coronary artery disease. Am J Cardiol 1999;84:1292–1297.
60. Jain D, Lahiri A, Raftery EB. Immunoscintigraphy for detecting acute myocardial infarction without electrocardiographic changes. Br Med J 1990;300:151–153.
61. Dec GW, Palacios I, Yasuda T, et al. Antimyosin antibody cardiac imaging: its role in the diagnosis of myocarditis. J Am Coll Cardiol 1990;16:97–104.
62. Ballester M, Bordes R, Tazelaar HD, et al. Evaluation of biopsy classification for rejection: relation to detection of myocardial damage by monoclonal antimyosin antibody imaging. J Am Coll Cardiol 1998;31:1357–1361.
63. Carrio I, Estorch M, Berna L, et al. Indium-111-antimyosin and iodine-123-MIBG studies in early assessment of doxorubicin cardiotoxicity. J Nucl Med 1995;36(11):2044–2049.
64. Narula J, Petrov A, Pak C, et al. Hyperacute visualization of myocardial ischemic injury: comparison of Tc-99m glucarate, thallium-201 and indium-111-antimyosin. J Am Coll Cardiol 1994;23:317.
65. Mariani G, Villa G, Rossettin PF, et al. Detection of acute myocardial infarction by 99mTc-labeled D-glucaric acid imaging in patients with chest pain. J Nucl Med 1999;40:1832–1839.
66. Hofstra L, Liem IH, Dumont EA, et al. Visualisation of cell death in vivo in patients with acute myocardial infarction. Lancet 2000;356:209–212.
67. Blankenberg F, Mari C, Strauss HW. Imaging cell death in vivo. Q J Nucl Med 2003;47:337–348.
68. Schelbert HR. Positron emission tomography as a biochemical probe for human myocardial ischemia. In: Zaret BL, Kaufman L, Dunn R, Berson A, eds. Frontiers of Cardiac Imaging. Raven Press, New York, 1993, pp. 53–70.
69. Bax JJ, Patton JA, Poldermans D, et al. 18-Fluorodeoxyglucose imaging with positron emission tomography and single photon emission computed tomography: cardiac applications. Semin Nucl Med 2000;30:281–298.
70. Jain D, McNulty PH. Exercise-induced myocardial ischemia: can this be imaged with F-18-fluorodeoxyglucose? (editorial) J Nucl Cardiol 2000;7:286–288.

71. He ZX, Shi RF, Wu YJ, et al. Direct imaging of exercise induced myocardial ischemia in coronary artery disease. Circulation 2003;108:1208–1213.

72. Gould KL, Taegtmeyer H. Myocardial ischemia, fluorodeoxyglucose, and severity of coronary artery stenosis: the complexities of metabolic remodeling in hibernating myocardium (letter to the editor and response). Circulation 2004;109:e167–e170.

73. Berry CR, Garg PK, DeGrado TR, et al. Para-[18F]fluorobenzylguanidine kinetics in a canine coronary artery occlusion model. J Nucl Cardiol 1996;3:119–129.

74. Morita K, Tsukamoto E, Tamaki N. Perfusion-BMIPP mismatch: specific finding or artifact? Int J Cardiovasc Imaging 2002;18:279–282.

75. Narula J, Petrov A, Bianchi C, et al. Noninvasive localization of experimental atherosclerotic lesions with mouse/human chimeric Z2D3 F(ab')2 specific for the proliferating smooth muscle cells of human atheroma. Imaging with conventional and charge-modified antibody fragments. Circulation 1995;92:474–484.

76. Jain D, Kulkarni P, Kolodgie FD, et al. Noninvasive imaging of atherosclerotic plaques with In-111 labeled lipid-seeking coproporphyrin. J Am Coll Cardiol 2000;35(Suppl A):493–A.

77. Kietselaer BL, Reutelingsperger CP, Heidendal GA, et al. Noninvasive detection of plaque instability with use of radiolabeled annexin-5 in patients with carotid-artery atherosclerosis. N Engl J Med 2004;350:1472–1473.

RECOMMENDED READING

Dilsizian V, Narula J, eds. Atlas of Nuclear Cardiology, 1st ed. Current Medicine, 2003.

Gerson MC. Cardiac Nuclear Medicine, 3rd ed. McGraw-Hill, New York, 1997.

Heller GV, Hendel RC. Nuclear Cardiology: Practical Applications, 1st ed. McGraw-Hill, New York, 2004.

Iskandrian AS, Verani MS. New Developments in Cardiac Nuclear Imaging, 1st ed. Futura Publishing, 1998.

Zaret BL, Beller GA, eds. Nuclear Cardiology: State of the Art and Future Directions, 3rd ed. Mosby Year Book, St. Louis, 2005.

14

Cardiovascular Magnetic Resonance and X-Ray Computed Tomography

Gerald M. Pohost, MD, Radha J. Sarma, MD, Patrick M. Colletti, MD, Mark Doyle, PhD, and Robert W. W. Biederman, MD

INTRODUCTION

There have been considerable advances in cardiovascular cross-sectional imaging techniques. These include cardiac magnetic resonance imaging (CMR) and computed tomography (CT)—electron beam CT (EBCT) and multidetector CT (MDCT). EBCT generates a cross-sectional scan through the chest within a fraction of a second. It is widely used as a means of detecting calcium in the coronary arteries and providing evidence of atherosclerotic disease. This application is presently controversial, as to date, the available data do not yet support the utility of EBCT-detected coronary artery calcium as a diagnostic or prognostic indicator of ischemic heart disease. EBCT has several other potential uses, however, which will be discussed in this chapter.

Magnetic resonance (MR) methods are among the newest of the imaging technologies. While magnetic resonance generates images with high resolution and high contrast without the need for contrast agent administration, most magnetic resonance systems available today must be gated to acquire high-quality images that demonstrate cardiac contraction. Newer systems, only recently available, allow acquisition of images at high speed, obviating the need for electrocardiographic synchronization. However, at present, gated studies offer superior resolution and image contrast, but either gated or "real-time" magnetic resonance images are optimally suited to visualize the heart and its contractile function. Magnetic resonance angiography (MRA) is excellent for rapidly evaluating the aorta and the peripheral arteries and can be acquired and displayed in 2-D and 3-D. Magnetic resonance spectroscopy (MRS) allows assessment of the biochemical character of the myocardium by generating spectra from the hydrogen and the phosphorus nuclei. Phosphorus spectroscopy can generate spectra showing the relative concentrations of the two high-energy phosphates adenosine triphosphate (ATP) and phosphocreatine (PCr). A relative decrease in PCr to ATP indicates a myocardial insult such as ischemia.

MAGNETIC RESONANCE METHODS

Principle of Nuclear Magnetic Resonance

When an atomic nucleus contains an odd number of subatomic particles (i.e., protons plus neutrons) it possesses a property known as "spin." The nucleus can be imagined to spin around its axis in a manner similar to the rotation of the earth. When electrical charges (in this case, the atomic nucleus) move, a magnetic field is generated. Intrinsic magnetic fields of atomic nuclei can interact

From: *Essential Cardiology: Principles and Practice, 2nd Ed.*
Edited by: C. Rosendorff © Humana Press Inc., Totowa, NJ

with externally applied magnetic fields. Sensitive atomic nuclei placed within an extrinsic magnetic field will align either *with* or *against* that field. Quantum mechanical considerations dictate that for any macroscopic amount of material, slightly more nuclei will align with the field than will be antialigned. Thus material placed in an external magnetic field will attain a bulk magnetic field strength. Stronger fields generate higher numbers of nuclei that preferentially align. If the nucleus is disturbed—for example, by applying a radiofrequency (RF) field—it will displace from alignment with the extrinsic magnetic field. When the RF energy is terminated, the disturbed nuclei continue to precess. *Precession* is the relatively slow "wobbling" phenomenon that is observed with a child's spinning top or a gyroscope. In a similar manner, nuclei with intrinsic "spin" and a magnetic moment will precess in an external magnetic field. The frequency of precession depends on the strength of the magnetic field (B_0) and the nuclear characteristics (gyromagnetic ratio, γ) of a given element. The RF field has to be applied at the precession frequency (i.e., at the resonance frequency for the system, which is also known as the Larmor frequency). The phenomenon of nuclear MR (NMR) is manifested when a substance with magnetically sensitive nuclei (e.g., the nucleus of hydrogen-1 [proton], phosphorus-31, fluorine-19, or sodium-23) that is placed in a strong magnetic field is momentarily pulsed with RF energy at the resonance frequency. The nuclei of all these atoms are naturally abundant and stable (i.e., not radioactive). While virtually all MR images are derived from the hydrogen nucleus (ubiquitous in water), researchers have created cardiac images of less-abundant signal sources, such as the natural sodium-23 distribution. During the process of free precession (i.e., after termination of the RF field), nuclei give off a detectable signal. This RF signal is detected by an RF coil placed close to the sample *(1)*.

The units of magnetic field strength are the gauss (G) and the tesla (T). The strength of the earth's magnetic field is on the order of 0.5 G. A typical commercial MR system useful for cardiovascular studies has a field strength of 15,000 to 30,000 G. It is customary to express field strength with NMR in tesla units (1 T = 10,000 G). Thus, 15,000 G is equivalent to 1.5 T.

Importance of Radio Waves or Radiofrequency

RF pulses are delivered at the resonant or Larmor frequency:

$$\omega = \gamma B_0$$

For protons, $\gamma = 42.58$ MHz/T. Typical spin-echo pulses reorient the net magnetism of the nuclear spins by 90 or 180 degrees. Faster and newer imaging techniques used for cardiovascular MR apply pulses of short duration, with net spin reorientation of less than 90 degrees. Following the RF pulse, the net magnetization precesses at the Larmor frequency. As individual spins precess, they emit an RF signal, which is detected by an RF coil. The frequency of these radio waves is characteristic for a given atomic nucleus and is affected by the chemical milieu. The detected radio waves are digitized and converted into signal peaks, or spectra, by application of the mathematical process known as *Fourier transformation*. The chemical milieu can cause the location of a resonance peak in the spectra to appear at a slightly different position than indicated by the field strength, B_0, a phenomenon known as chemical shift. Thus, the three peaks of adenosine triphosphate (ATP) are located in different spectral positions on phosphorus spectroscopy, and the hydrogen nuclei of water and of fat are in different spectral locations with proton spectroscopy.

The intrinsic magnetic field produced by the tissue will gradually reorient and realign with the extrinsic field after perturbation by the RF pulse and is said to "*relax*." There are two relaxation times: T1 (or spin-lattice relaxation), which is related to the time required for the net magnetization of the sample to realign with the main magnetic field by 63% (i.e., $1 - 1/e$); and T2 (or spin-spin relaxation time), which is related to the time required for spins that were originally in phase with the applied RF pulse to lose phase coherence by 63% (i.e., $1 - 1/e$). The concentration of the nuclei (spin density) and the relaxation times T1 and T2 determine the magnitude of a peak in the spectrum, or the intensity of a pixel in an image. Other variables that affect signal intensity are motion, flow, chemical shift, and magnetic susceptibility.

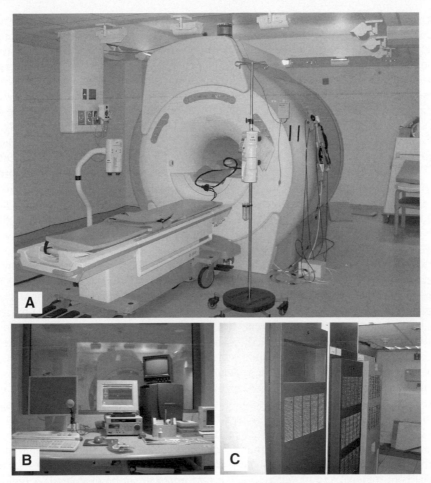

Fig. 1. Composite photograph of major components of a typical MRI system. (**A**) Scanner magnet and patient table; the table accommodates patient entry, exit, and positioning within the magnet bore. (**B**) Operator's console, which is remote from the scanner, allows control of scanner functions and incorporates an image and physiologic data viewing station. (**C**) Bulky hardware to power the scanner is typically located in a separate room; components include gradient and RF power units and the controlling computer.

Whereas spectroscopy utilizes sample-dependent differences in the magnetic field, imaging utilizes externally applied magnetic field gradients. The key to imaging is to vary the magnetic field strength as a function of spatial location. This is accomplished by applying a linear magnetic gradient along each axis in which spatial differentiation is required. Each gradient either adds to or subtracts from the main magnetic field, producing a continuous variation in resonance frequency along the sample. Application of the Fourier transform to signals acquired in the presence of linear gradients directly translates this range of frequency information into spatial intensity data and forms the basis of imaging and angiography. Control of the gradients allows slice selection to be achieved in any orientation.

Instrumentation for Magnetic Resonance Studies

A CMR system consists of a large (typically cylindrical) superconducting magnet, an RF coil that fits within the bore of the magnet; RF receiver coils, gradient coils that generate the magnetic fields needed to create images; and an image-processing computer (Fig. 1). The large magnet contains multiple coils of niobium titanium, which has essentially no resistance to electrical current when it is supercooled. Such supercooling takes place when the coils in the magnet are bathed in liquid helium at 4 K or −269°C. While permanent, "open" magnets are also available for CMR, high-field superconducting magnets are preferable for cardiac applications. The imaging gradient coils are located within the magnet bore and are used to vary the magnetic field in a precisely controlled manner. They introduce controlled variations in magnetic field related to the position of an organ or a portion of an organ within the magnet. Having the ability to rapidly switch the gradient coils on and off allows rapid acquisition of cardiovascular images. The cylindrical body RF coil also fits concentrically within the bore of a cylindrical magnet and transmits the radio waves needed to create a spectrum or an image. A smaller multielement coil placed over the heart or vascular bed of interest is used to receive the RF signal with high sensitivity. Naturally, coordination of this complex system requires extensive computer control of the gradient and RF amplifiers and the vast array of associated electronic components. Typically, an operator's console is placed in a room adjacent to the scan room, allowing visual contact with the patient environment via a window. The console provides a convenient means to alter the acquisition methods, RF pulse sequence, and view selection.

A spin echo image of the heart typically is acquired with high spatial resolution in which moving blood appears as a signal void or as a "dark blood" region. A gradient echo pulse sequence typically generates images at higher speed and with "bright blood." The dark-blood approach is ideal for assessing cardiac morphology, whereas the bright-blood approach is appropriate for assessing ventricular function. When turbulence occurs in the bloodstream, bright-blood images demonstrate a localized reduction in brightness directly associated with the turbulence. For example, the jet associated with mitral or aortic regurgitation is visualized as a dark region against otherwise bright blood, owing to signal dephasing. Newer systems have higher-speed imaging capabilities such as "echoplanar" and spiral imaging, which are capable of generating an image in under 30 ms, but presently, these images are of generally low resolution. Both dark-blood and bright-blood imaging can be performed with cardiac gating to freeze heart motion at certain phases in the cardiac cycle, thus allowing higher-resolution images to be acquired, but at the expense of increased scan time. Typically, in cardiac gated sequences, 20–30 frames representing the cardiac cycle are acquired. In general, cardiac cine sequences are based on bright blood gradient recalled echo (GRE) approaches. In this way both regional and global ventricular performance can be evaluated. A typical GRE sequence requires 10 to 15 s acquisition time, and can be acquired within a breath-hold. Using GRE methods, a series of images can be acquired throughout the cardiac cycle and then assembled in sequence in the computer as a cine loop that can be replayed repeatedly to allow evaluation of wall motion (Fig. 2).

Recently, steady-state-free precession (SSFP) imaging approaches have been introduced that effectively combine the gradient and spin echo components to increase blood signal contrast. These approaches, variously termed FIESTA, True FISP and balanced FFE, result in excellent blood-myocardial contrast, almost independently of blood flow characteristics. Both dark-blood and bright-blood imaging sequences are performed in conjunction with cardiac gating to effectively freeze the heart motion at distinct phases within the cardiac cycle.

Older CMR systems have rather long cylindrical magnets. Some patients (as many as 5%) are unable to tolerate such an enclosure due to claustrophobia. Anxious patients can be given a mild sedative such as benzodiazepine. Most modem systems have shorter-bore magnets and are more "patient-friendly." Again, on older systems, the gradients can be quite noisy. This is especially true for the fast imaging sequences used in cardiovascular MR. Earplugs are always required to protect the patient from noise-related hearing damage. Newer systems incorporate substantial sound dampening to isolate the gradient vibrations from the system, thus reducing noise. An intercom system is used to maintain verbal contact between system operator and patient. This is important, to inform the patient of important events during the examination such as table movements, injections of contrast agents, or stress agents. Verbal communication is especially important to direct the patient with the appropriate timing for breath-holding during image acquisition. Special MR-

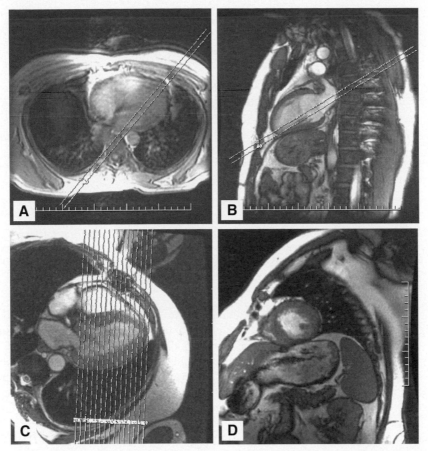

Fig. 2. Sequence of scans required to obtain standard cardiac views. (**A**) A noncardiac triggered spin echo transverse scout is obtained, and is used to plan the two-chamber view. (**B**) The two-chamber view of the left ventricle is in turn used to plan the four-chamber view. (**C**) The four-chamber view is in turn used to plan the multiple-slice short-axis views. (**D**) A short-axis view of the left and right ventricles. Views B–D were obtained in cine mode using steady-state free precession imaging.

compatible systems are required for physiological monitoring of the cardiac MR patient during an examination. This is especially important if the patient receives pharmacological stress while within the magnet.

While a uniform body coil is required to optimally transmit RF energy into the body, the most important characteristic for signal reception is maximization of the signal-to-noise ratio. This can be accomplished by positioning a receiver coil system on the body's surface. A typical reception system consists of a number of separate coils that are essentially positioned or wrapped around the thorax (for cardiac imaging). This composite coil is made up of a number of smaller subcoils, each requiring its own signal reception electronics, and is referred to as a phased array system. Importantly, recent advances have allowed reduction in scan time by separately processing the signal from each coil to essentially construct a separate part of each full image. These approaches cause a slight reduction in signal-to-noise ratio, but typically can reduce the scan time by factors of 2 or 4. These approaches are generically termed parallel imaging, and are known under the trade names of ASSET, SMASH, and SENSE.

In addition to the inherent contrast produced by each imaging sequence, it is possible to augment contrast by means of "spin preparation pulses." Preparation pulses are typically applied to

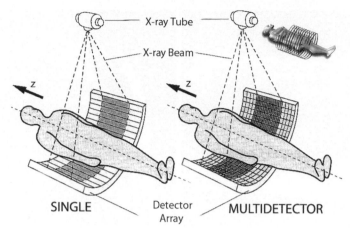

Fig. 3. Multidetector CT. Comparison of single-slice and multidetector CT. Multidetector CT uses an array of detectors to improve resolution (smaller pixels) and temporal (more slices) coverage of the heart and great vessels. Cardiac CT has shown continued improvement as detector arrays have increased from 1 to 2, 4, 8, 16, 40, and 64.

produce contrast dependent on the T1 relaxation process. At 1.5 T the T1 value of myocardium (water signal) is approximately 850 ms, while that of fat tissue is about 300 ms. Application of an RF pulse to invert the spin system will initially invert both the water and fat signals. However, as the spin system relaxes to its equilibrium condition, the fat signal relaxes faster than the water signal. By carefully selecting the time following the inversion pulse at which to perform the imaging sequence, it is possible to "null" either the fat or the water signal. The process of inverting the signal and waiting for it to partially recover before performing imaging is referred to as "inversion recovery" (IR).

Further, it is possible to alter the T1 of tissue by administration of a contrast agent. These nonionic agents typically contain a gadolinium chelate, which, when it comes in close contact with tissue, effectively reduces the tissue's T1 by introducing a highly localized, randomly varying, magnetic field gradient. Contrast agents have application areas varying from allowing visualization of myocardial perfusion, imaging the vasculature, differentiating between masses, and identifying viable and nonviable myocardium with high accuracy.

COMPUTED TOMOGRAPHY

There are two types of CT systems used for cardiovascular diagnosis: multidetector CT (MDCT) and electron beam CT (EBCT). MDCT devices use a slip-ring, continuously rotating X-ray source and circular arrays of stationary detectors (Fig. 3). MDCT is performed with the table continuously in motion during scanning, generating multiple (4, 8, 16, 32, 64, up to 256) spiral slices per 400 ms revolution, with excellent ($0.5 \times 0.5 \times 0.5$ mm^3) spatial resolution. MDCT cardiac acquisitions must be ECG-triggered and coupled with a breath hold of 5 to 20 s. Partial rotational data may be subsegmentally reconstructed to produce cardiac images with an effective temporal resolution for MDCT images of from 50 to 200 ms.

EBCT employs an electron gun and a fixed tungsten target, as opposed to a standard X-ray tube. The produced X-ray beam is collimated through the patient to an array of high-grade crystal silicon photodiode detectors (Fig. 4). This permits the rapid acquisition of tomographic images of the heart, allowing for multislice imaging in a temporal sequence coordinated with cardiac motion. Again, scans are usually acquired during breath-holding, and acquisitions are triggered using the ECG signal to reduce the potentially blurring effect of heart motion. Typically, a series of transaxial EBCT images can be obtained with a temporal resolution of 30 to 50 ms with a scan slice thickness of 3 mm.

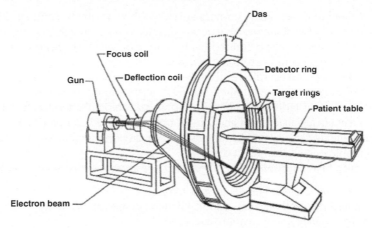

Fig. 4. Diagrammatic display of an electron beam computed tomographic imaging system. (Courtesy of Imatron.)

Cardiovascular CT spatial resolution is considerably better than MR. While the spatial resolution of EBCT is inferior to that of MDCT, the temporal resolution is superior. MDCT is difficult to perform effectively in patients with a heart rate over 90 beats/min. Heart rate reduction using a β-blocker such as propranolol (20–40 mg) prior to EBCT for coronary artery examinations is desirable *(2)*. EBCT has somewhat less patient radiation exposure as compared with MDCT. Currently available MDCT techniques allow for better control of the X-ray tube output, so that there is now little difference in exposure compared with EBCT, but depending on the technology used, MDCT could be four to five times the dose of EBCT. MDCT does not spare the radiation exposure compared to angiography. When angiographic intervention procedures are performed, they generate considerably more radiation exposure for patients and personnel *(3,4)*.

Because the relative radiographic densities of the myocardium and the blood pool are nearly identical, other than for the evaluation of coronary artery calcification, there is an absolute need to administer iodinated radiopaque contrast medium with CT *(5)*. Some patients may be allergic to radiopaque contrast media and administration of contrast medium could precipitate renal failure in patients with borderline renal function or idiosyncratically in those with normal function. Finally, the osmotic load required to generate important diagnostic information could precipitate an episode of pulmonary edema in patients with congestive heart failure. The use of low osmolality nonionic contrast agents is required in such patients but does not reduce the incidence of renal impairment.

CURRENT APPLICATIONS

CMR and MRA are excellent for assessing both morphology and function. CMR has the unique ability to acquire images of the heart in any tomographic plane that is preselected by the operator at the console. However, it is customary to acquire imaging planes through the vertical long axis (two-chamber view), the horizontal long axis (four-chamber view), and the short axis (Fig. 2). At the present time, magnetic resonance imaging and angiography are excellent for assessing global and regional left and right ventricular size and performance; for evaluating the abnormal morphology and physiology found in congenital heart disease, including intracardiac shunt quantification; for characterizing myocardial tissue, such as in arrhythmogenic myocardial dysplasia; for assessing myocardial wall thickness and ventricular volumes and geometries in the cardiomyopathies and in valvular heart disease, particularly to interrogate velocities; for the assessment of the pericardium, particularly differentiation of constrictive pericarditis from restrictive myocardial disease; for cardiac/paracardiac masses; for comprehensive evaluation of aortic dissection and aortic aneurysms; and for assessment of the larger arterial branches from the aorta such as the carotids, renals, and ileofemorals, and more recently, coronary arteries with and without contrast. CMR has been demonstrated to be effective in myocardial perfusion and is considered to be the gold standard for myocardial viability. MRI has the unique ability to acquire images of the heart in any tomographic plane, as selected by the operator from the console.

Cardiac chamber size, myocardial wall thickness, and mass are readily assessed from CMR images. Chamber morphology, orientation, and relationships to the great vessels and viscera are easily assessed. In addition, atrioventricular, venoatrial, and ventriculoarterial connections can readily be defined and evaluated in terms of anatomy and hemodynamics. Three-dimensional contrast-enhanced cardiac views can be rotated and viewed from any orientation. Such capability is ideal for assessing complex congenital heart disease.

Many of the current applications of EBCT and MDCT are similar to those described for CMR.

- Global and regional left and right ventricular function
- Assessing myocardial wall thickness and ventricular volumes and cardiomyopathies
- Assessment of coronary artery anatomy and stenosis
- Assessment of coronary calcium to detect atherosclerosis
- Assessment of myocardial ischemia and infarction
- Assessment of aorta and the larger arterial branches
- Comprehensive evaluation of aortic dissection and aortic aneurysms
- Evaluating congenital heart disease, anatomy, and conduit patency
- Assessing cardiac and paracardiac masses
- Assessing the pericardium and pericardial effusion or constriction

Table 1 contrasts/compares these technologies in their respective applications.

Ventricular Function Chamber Size and Wall Thickness

CMR TECHNIQUES

Global and regional right and left ventricular function can be assessed using cine GRE, SSFP, or other rapid acquisition sequences such as echoplanar imaging (6). Ventricular volumes can be measured at end-diastole and end-systole using traditional area-length approaches from the long-axis images or using Simpson's rule with serial short-axis images (7). Simpson's rule is the common method of computing volumes of continuous objects by summing the areas of cross-sections obtained at a discrete number of points. While most current techniques acquire contiguous slices, gaps between sampled cross-sections are treated as if they were represented by the average of the nearest cross-sectional views. In essence, the area is found by summing each cross-sectional area and multiplying it by the sum of the slice thickness and the interslice gap. Stroke volume and ejection fraction can be readily determined from the end-systolic and end-diastolic volumes. In addition to the geometrically simple left ventricle, the more irregularly shaped right ventricle can also be studied using a Simpson's rule approach with serial short-axis views from base to apex. The three-dimensional coverage of CMR images makes possible calculation of highly accurate right ventricular volumes and ejection fractions (8). By evaluating size, shape, and the regional contractile ability of the left ventricle, lesions such as ventricular aneurysm and pseudoaneurysm, dilated and hypertrophic cardiomyopathy, myocardial thinning, and remodeling can readily and comprehensively be evaluated. Since the myocardium is clearly visualized, it is easy to measure wall thickness and to evaluate wall thickening (9). Furthermore, global and regional myocardial mass can be measured (10).

In addition to functional evaluation with conventional contrast imaging, two other methods are available for cardiovascular MR studies: phase-velocity mapping and RF tagging. Phase-velocity mapping is analogous to Doppler echocardiography. In phase-velocity mapping, the phase of each pixel in the MR image is related to the voxel's velocity. Unlike Doppler echocardiography, it is not dependent on exact angulation and it measures accurately in all three dimensions (typically within 7%). Phase-velocity mapping has a plethora of applications, including blood flow visualization and determination of stroke volume and cardiac output at the aortic valve and in evaluating ventral-

Table 1
CMR EBCT and MDCT: Respective Clinical Applications

	MRI	*EBCT and MDCT*
Cardiac morphology	Excellent intrinsic soft tissue and blood contrast allows delineation of anatomic features with good resolution. No external contrast required.	Requires administration of contrast agent to delineate blood pool features, but provides good anatomic depiction.
Cardiac function	Excellent temporal and spatial resolution with any orientation allows optimal evaluation of contractile function. RF tags provide further delineation of regional wall function.	Requires contrast agent to distinguish blood pool, limited angulation available, but 3-D images can be generated with good resolution.
Coronary anatomy	Breath-hold techniques allow coronary artery location to be traced to origin.	Contrast techniques allow coronary artery trajectory to be traced to origin.
Coronary stenosis detection	Limited ability at present to reliably detect stenosis due to decreased signal within the artery related to turbulence. New techniques promise improved results not requiring contrast agent.	Limited ability at present to detect stenosis, but new techniques promise improved results requiring contrast agent.
Myocardial perfusion	Techniques being developed to detect myocardial perfusion, in later stages of development	Techniques being developed to assess myocardial perfusion by tracking a bolus of radiopaque contrast.
Pericardial disease	Allows differentiation between restrictive and constrictive disease (i.e., generally, myocardial vs pericardial). MR is a "gold standard" for assessing pericardial thickness. Able to determine physiologic significance, even in absence of thickened pericardium.	MDCT is able to distinguish between myocardium and pericardium similar to CMR.
Valvular assessment	Can assess valve function and visualize turbulent flow to approximate the severity of regurgitation and stenosis.	Unable to visualize turbulence; must rely on ancillary data (quantifying differences in stroke volumes between LV and RV.
Metallic artifacts	Signal void.	Streak artifacts.
Cardiac masses	Can be easily detected, may be an important role for T1 and T2 tissue characterization.	Can be identified after a contrast bolus.
Contrast agent	Chelates of Gadolinium and Dysprosium with no known adverse effects.	Iodinated contrast-many adverse side effects: renal failure, anaphylaxis or pulmonary edema
Angiography of the arterial system:	No need for contrast agent although early data suggests contrast markedly shortens acquisition time and further increases resolution.	Radiopaque iodinated contrast agent required.
Aorta	++++	+++
Arch	++++	+++
Carotids	++++	++
Peripheral	++++	+++
Coronary calcification	Not well visualized; calcium is not visualized due to its solid state.	Easily visualized without contrast administration.
Ionizing radiation	No	Yes

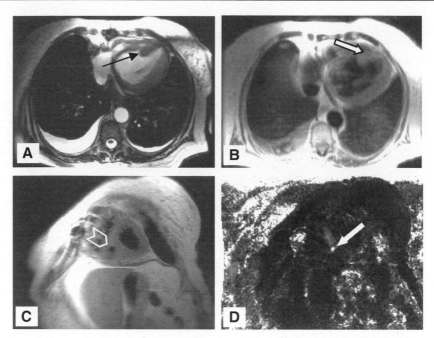

Fig. 5. A 54-yr-old female with progressive dyspnea 6 mo following an anterior septal MI. A murmur was heard prompting an MRI evaluation. (**A**) A septal defect in the interventricular myocardium is seen. (**B**) The high-velocity flow between the LV and RV was diagnostic of a post-infarct VSD. (**C**) Selective breath-hold imaging reveals the distinct septal hole, allowing for measurement. (**D**) Phase velocity imaging allowed quantitation of the Qp:Qs of 2.2, primarily left to right. As the patient was turned down for surgical repair, she underwent compassionate use of the nonsurgical ASD closure device for the VSD.

septal defects (Fig. 5). Shunt flow may be evaluated by comparing aortic flow to pulmonary artery flow. RF tagging provides CMR with a unique ability to more precisely evaluate regional myocardial function *(11)*. By using the appropriate perpendicular saturation band pulse sequence, dark lines in a regular crisscross pattern can be applied to the myocardium at the time of the ECG R wave. Since these lines move with the myocardium, intrinsic motion can be visualized to assess true function without the confounding effect of myocardial through-plane motion *(12)* or remote muscle influences (tethering). Furthermore, changes in distance between intersections of RF grid lines can be tracked and regional strains, indices of rotation, and translation amounts calculated. Unlike tracking of material markers, RF tagging does not impede or influence myocardial dynamics and it is completely noninvasive. CMR is the most reliable means for assessing right and left ventricular function.

CT Techniques

A number of studies have described the use of EBCT and MDCT to assess right and left ventricular function. After intravenous administration of radiopaque contrast medium, serial images depict the cardiac chambers with good contrast between ventricular wall and ventricular blood pool. From such an acquisition, left and right ventricular volume and ejection fraction can accurately be determined. Like CMR, EBCT provides a means of evaluating heart function, including chamber volumes, ejection fraction, and myocardial mass. Of course, it is essential to use radiopaque contrast medium to define the inner borders of the cardiac chambers. High-resolution images can be generated that allow precise measurement of regional and global ventricular function. As with CMR, a series of short-axis ventricular tomographs less than 1 cm thick are acquired. These slices can sample 10 to 20 or more images throughout the cardiac cycle. With a modification of Simpson's rule, ventricular volume and mass can be determined. Studies in both laboratory animals

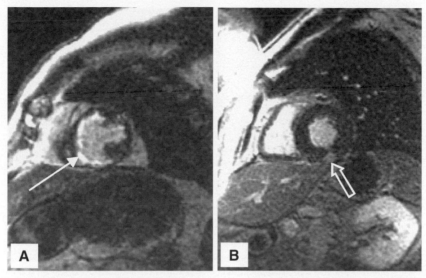

Fig. 6. A paramagnetic agent (gadolinium DTPA) was infused and the delayed enhancement image seen here acquired after a delay of 15 min. The accumulation of gadolinium is seen (arrows) indicating distribution of necrotic myocardium. (**A**) A large region is affected. (**B**) A small region is affected in a patient with equivocal troponin I (7 ng/dL). The latter patient underwent cardiac catheterization, demonstrating a left circumflex distal marginal occlusion.

and humans demonstrate the reliability of left ventricular volume and mass determination using EBCT. Similar results have been demonstrated recently using MDCT.

Coronary Artery Disease

Since CMR and MDCT can reliably evaluate the function of both ventricles by examining volumetric changes and changes in myocardial thickness during systole and diastole, they can be used to demonstrate regional wall motion abnormalities *(13)*. Using gadolinium MR contrast agents, one can see delayed hyperenhancement of the infarcted myocardium (Fig. 6) *(14,15)*. Unlike nuclear or echocardiographic techniques, this seems to be a unique phenomenon of CMR and presently is the subject of intense research.

Myocardial *ischemia* can be diagnosed by comparing resting cardiac images to images acquired after stressing by means of handgrip, infusion of a stressing agent such as dobutamine, or even more vigorous exercise using specialized equipment *(16)*. Coronary vasodilator agents such as persantine or adenosine may be infused during contrast-enhanced CMR perfusion studies to demonstrate reduced dynamic enhancement in territories served by stenotic coronary arteries (Fig. 7) *(17)*. The principles are similar to the other imaging techniques such as nuclear stress testing or echocardiographic stress testing *(18,19)*.

Using CMR cine, one sees deterioration in left ventricular myocardial contraction with higher doses of dobutamine in otherwise normally or nearly normally contracting segments supplied by a coronary artery with significant stenosis. Myocardial *viability* can also be assessed in poorly contracting myocardial segments, using dobutamine stress CMR. One would see improvement in wall motion with low-dose dobutamine but deterioration of the same segments at higher doses; i.e., the binary response, in the presence of viable but hypocontractile myocardium.

CT approaches to myocardial perfusion can be applied to semiquantitatively assess perfusion levels *(20)*. By analyzing the myocardium as the contrast agents perfuse it, it is possible to calculate a regional perfusion index via relative perfusion software evaluation of myocardial segments.

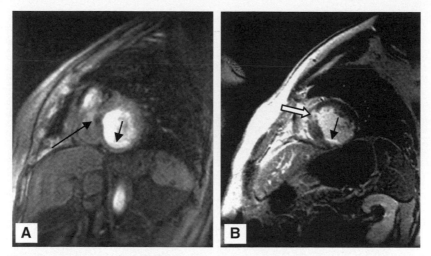

Fig. 7. (A) FSGRE image of a short-axis slice demonstrating the concept of first-pass perfusion using gadolinium. The large arrow indicates a focal hypoenhanced near-transmural anteroseptal lesion, representing the relative lack of gadolinium's T1 effect in poorly perfused myocardium (low signal) as compared to the otherwise normally perfused myocardium (higher signal). The small arrow points to a small endocardial lesion missed by nuclear imaging due to its 1–2 mm thickness, well below the 10–13 mm resolution required for radionuclide-based techniques. **(B)** A unique property of CMR, using this technique, is the relative late (5–20 min) effect that contrast provides to highlight necrotic (scarred) myocardium, outlined arrow. As shown in the small arrow, an even smaller endocardial scar can be seen, partially encircling the inferior/inferior lateral wall. This technique, referred to as "delayed hyperenhancement," is now demonstrated to be the reference standard for interrogation of myocardial viability.

CORONARY ARTERY IMAGING

In many instances, visualization of the coronary arteries is required, and substantial progress has been made toward this goal during the past decade. Using the latest instrumentation and MR techniques, imaging the proximal trunks and some more distal segments of the coronary arteries is feasible. It has already been shown to be more accurate for the delineation of anomalous coronary arteries than X-ray angiography (Fig. 8). More investigation is needed to refine coronary MRA. Such additions as the use of a blood pool contrast agent might improve the sensitivity and specificity as compared with catheter coronary angiography. A few investigators have even evaluated the potential for CMR to characterize arterial plaque. Clinical determination of plaque vulnerability may be within the realm of possibility for this versatile technology.

Currently, MDCT is able to routinely visualize normal coronary arteries using 1, 32, 40, and recently 64 slice detectors. However, serial 16-slice and over 32-slice detection is optional. Contrast requirements are still present and β-blockade to reduce the heart rate to near 60 beats per minute is still required, but improvements in spatial resolution may allow reductions in contrast dosage (Fig. 9B) *(21)*.

CORONARY CALCIUM

At present, cardiac CT's most common and unique cardiovascular application is for the detection of coronary artery calcification, as direct evidence of coronary atherosclerosis *(22)*. In view of the high speed of EBCT acquisition, the coronary arteries are virtually "frozen" in space, and the extent of calcification can be accurately assessed (Fig. 10). MDCT also can provide relatively fast (subsecond) imaging, but with 50–200 ms acquisitions the blurring effect due to cardiac motion could be problematic, although less so with the 16- or 32-slice systems (Fig. 11). Because of the widespread availability of MDCT scanners, in contrast to EBCT scanners, it is important to note that MDCT provides coronary artery calcification scoring comparable to that of EBCT. Use of coronary artery calcification as a predictor of functionally significant coronary artery disease

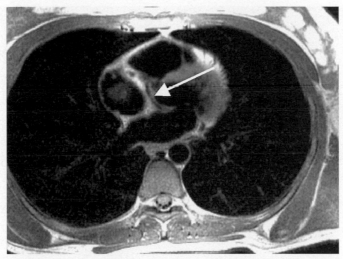

Fig. 8. This 45-yr-old patient presented with chest pain, underwent X-ray coronary angiography, and was found to have an anomalous left circumflex arising off the right coronary sinus. Regarding the question as to trajectory, the catheterization results were equivocal, prompting a cardiac MRI. This double-inversion recovery image was acquired in a breath-hold manner without administration of contrast, clearly demonstrating the benign nature of this anomaly. The vessel travels posterior to the aortic root as the great majority, if not all, of anomalous left circumflex vessels do.

remains controversial *(23)*. It clearly indicates the presence of atherosclerosis but not its physiologic significance. Proponents of the application of EBCT maintain that it should become a routine study for coronary risk assessment *(24)*. Meta-analysis suggests that calcium scoring may be no better than the much less expensive ECG exercise test or cholesterol screening. Others suggest that plaque rupture, a common cause of coronary occlusion, is related to the lipid constituents of plaque (invisible to X-rays), but not to the amount of calcium. At present, the value of the EBCT coronary calcium score is uncertain and it does not supplant current clinical methodologies, although it does provide another, albeit expensive, means for risk assessment. This position is supported by the American Heart Association *(25)*. Further data will be required to determine its actual utility. Several approaches to acquire coronary angiography by EBCT and MDCT have been reported. While the image quality is impressive, there is little anatomic and physiologic validation to support its use in current clinical practice *(26,27)*. Moreover, injection of contrast medium and β-blockade is required, and for MDCT, high-dose X-ray equivalent to a minimum of three times the dosage of a diagnostic catheterization.

Cardiomyopathies

With dilated and valvular cardiomyopathy (either acquired or of congenital origin), one might expect to find both left and right ventricular involvement and homogeneously depressed left ventricular wall motion (Fig. 12). Hemochromatosis, an infiltrative cardiomyopathy whereby iron accumulates in the myocardium, can be readily diagnosed by CMR. The iron that is localized in the myocardium and the liver generates a characteristic signal dropout pattern so that the liver and, in part, the myocardium, demonstrate very low signal. In *sarcoidosis*, one can visualize the granulomatous infiltrates that may lead to ventricular dysfunction as well as local inflammation.

One cardiomyopathy that may be well characterized by CMR is arrhythmogenic myocardial dysplasia. In this condition, which is associated with life-threatening ventricular arrhythmias, the right ventricle is involved with fat infiltration and myocardial thinning. The fatty infiltrate shows up as a bright signal on black-blood spin-echo CMR (in about half of these patients) and regional wall motion dysfunction (in most patients) on gradient-echo or SSFP images, combined with sig-

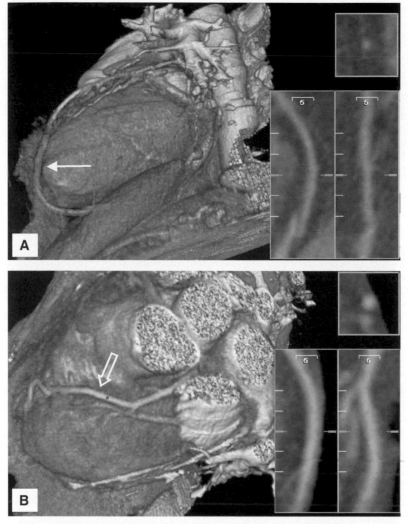

Fig. 9. Images obtained using MDCT processed to highlight the LAD and epicardium. (**A**) Distal view and (**B**) the proximal section. Inserted views depict orthogonal views of the highlighted sections.

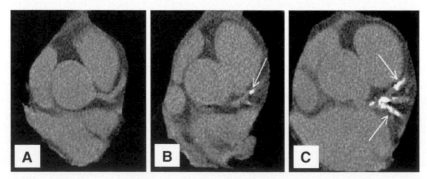

Fig. 10. Examples of progressive coronary artery calcification (**A–C**) depicting increasing signal as the intraluminal calcium burden rises. Formal calcium scores can be derived using the Agaston algorithm from the scans quantifying the signal from the calcium. Although calcium is a well-accepted marker for atherosclerosis, the direct relation between calcium and prediction of clinical events is less well established. (Courtesy of GE Imatron.)

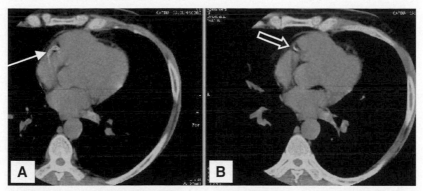

Fig. 11. Examples of low levels of coronary artery calcification (**A–B**) visualized as increased signal as the intraluminal calcium burden rises.

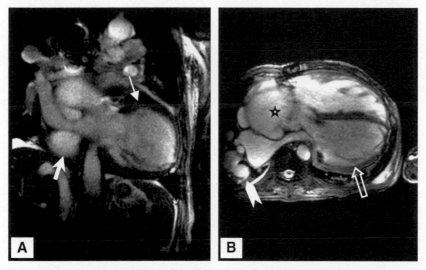

Fig. 12. A 32-yr-old female presented 25 yr after repair of tetralogy of Fallot. (**A**) The LV was dilated (small arrow), measuring 100 mm × 53 mm with a markedly compressed LA (large arrow). (**B**) Note the enlarged right ventricle, left ventricle (open arrow), and the RA/LA as well as small aortobronchiolar communications to augment pulmonic flow (chevron). The enlarged aortic root (star) is probably related to late correction and high early childhood systemic flow due to redirection of pulmonic flow. Poor migration of neural crest cells with their elastin, forming progenitor cells, has been implicated in the aortic root and ascending aortic dilation, as seen in this patient who was shown to have a small contained aortic dissection (not shown).

nal nulling on T2 weighted images, confirming the presence of intramyocardial fat deposits (or transformation) (Fig. 13). Morphologic imaging can also be accomplished with CT *(28)*.

Aortic and Peripheral Vascular Imaging

MRA offers excellent noninvasive imaging of the aorta, pulmonary arteries and veins, cerebral vasculature, and the iliofemoral arterial system. Satisfactory visualization of the lower extremity runoff vessels is routinely achievable. Because signal can be generated through the motion of blood, MRA may not require any contrast agent administration for many of these examinations. MR contrast agents have an excellent safety profile and are safe to use in patients with renal failure. The osmotic load is less than that of iodinated contrast agents. Intravenous contrast-enhanced MRA is routinely used for examinations of the aorta, pulmonary vessels, carotid arteries, renal arteries,

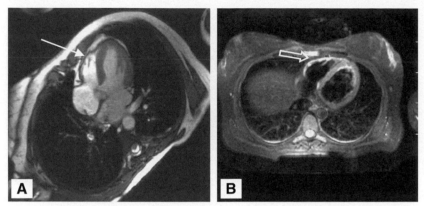

Fig. 13. A 34-yr-old female presented with several episodes of syncope and near-syncope. Prior to an invasive electrophysiological study, the patient was risk-stratified with CMR. (**A**) A 4-chamber view with arrow pointing to a mid-systolic asynergic, tardykinetic zone of the right ventricle free wall with thinning, meeting two major working group classifications for arrythmogenic right ventricular dysplasia (ARVD). The third classification (out of four) is met in (**B**) as shown by the triple-inversion recovery sequence, a unique sequence to magnetic resonance, that takes advantages of the faster relaxation of fat compared to protein. This T2 weighted image provides insight into specific tissue characteristics, which is another important property of CMR. Note the subtle but pathogomonic evidence of fat within the myocardium corresponding to the asynergic zone. The fat signal of the breast tissue is similar to that within the affected RV free wall. The patient was referred to the NIH-sponsored ARVD trial and likely for defibrillator placement, the current standard for treatment.

and arteries of the lower extremity but can be performed in their entirety without contrast through time-of-flight approaches.

MRA of the aorta is considered to have equivalent sensitivity but superior specificity to transesophageal echocardiography or multislice contrast-enhanced CT for the evaluation of aortic aneurysms and aortic dissection. In dissection, intimal flaps and entry site can be identified, allowing for identification of the true and false lumen, differentiation between blood flow and clot in the false-lumen, and involvement of branch vessels (Fig. 14). The critical distinction between DeBakey dissection type 1 or 2 and type 3 lesions is readily made with MR. Congenital anomalies of the aorta can also be identified, such as coarctation, arch interruption, and transposition. Imaging the cerebral arterial supply, including the carotid and vertebral arteries has become routine in clinical practice, supplanting X-ray angiography.

The thoracic and abdominal aorta can readily be evaluated using MDCT after a bolus injection of radiopaque contrast medium. Aortic aneurysms and dissections are detected and assessed. Where CMR is not available, MDCT, EBCT, or TEE are preferred for diagnostic assessment. Like CMR, CT methods are useful for visualizing the intimal flap and for determining the extent of branch vessel involvement. CMR and CT are useful for differentiating between aortic aneurysm with mural thrombus and dissection with thrombus in the false lumen.

Both MDCT and EBCT have been used to visualize the renal arteries in the evaluation of hypertensive patients with suspected renal artery stenosis. Using contrast enhancement patterns, kidney volumes (both cortical and medullary) can be determined. High-speed CT provides a means of examining renal blood flow and excretion. Branch vessels from the aorta can also be well visualized, including the carotids and vertebral arteries, the trifurcation, the celiac, the superior and inferior mesenteric, the brachiocephalic, the ileofemoral, and the popliteal arteries. CMR is the preferred technique in the majority of patients, especially if there is evidence for renal compromise.

Pulmonary Arteries

Pulmonary emboli have been reliably identified using MDCT, which requires breath holding for optimal imaging of the pulmonary arteries. For patients with possible pulmonary embolism,

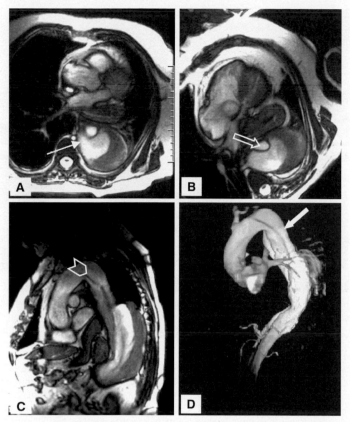

Fig. 14. Dissection and thrombus in the false lumen. Multiple views of a Type B descending aortic dissection are shown. (**A**) A SSFP axial slice depicts flow in the false lumen (arrow). (**B**) The partially thrombosed false lumen is seen to the right (dark) and the true lumen is seen to the left (arrow). (**C**) The high descending aortic origination of intimal flap is seen (chevron). (**D**) A 3-D surface rendering of an MRA acquired in 22 s with gadolinium demonstrates the intimal flap (arrow indicates false lumen). Note the tiny true lumen in the abdominal aorta. The dissection cleanly dissects the aorta with one lumen supplying the right renal artery and the false lumen perfusing the left renal artery.

breath-holding is a very difficult challenge. EBCT, however, requires no breath holding. Both breath-hold MDCT and non-breath-hold EBCT have been reported to have sensitivity on the order of 85% and specificity in the low 90% range, in a select group of patients with intermediate probability of pulmonary embolism by radionuclide ventilation-perfusion scanning. Generally, the combination of ventilation-perfusion scanning followed by CT is the optimal strategy for detecting pulmonary embolism in a minimally invasive way. CT, like MR, is also very useful for the evaluation of pulmonary veins for anomalies and thrombosis. MRI has been used in limited manner for pulmonary embolism evaluation, although is ideal for pulmonary arteriovenous malformations (Fig. 15).

Valvular Disease

CMR can demonstrate valve anatomy, leaflet motion, and blood flow. Regurgitant or stenotic valves appear as regions of signal loss, due to the dephasing of spins within the jet of disturbed flow, on bright-blood cine MR images (Fig. 16). Regurgitant lesions may be evaluated by the size of the signal void (for a given TE), the volume of the accepting chamber, the time over which the signal void persists, and the size and duration of persistence of the zone of proximal convergence (i.e., the region where blood converges radially toward the valve orifice) *(29)*.

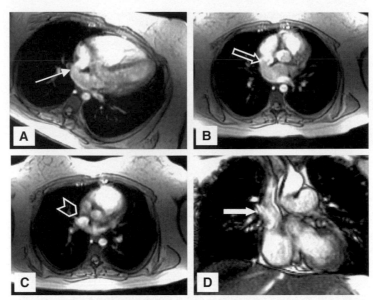

Fig. 15. A 24-yr-old female presented to the internal medicine clinic for establishment of routine care. A murmur was heard and an echo performed, demonstrating normal LV/RV size, no intracardiac shunt, and an atypical posterior RA signal by color Doppler, prompting a cardiac MRI. (**A**) Demonstrates an absent posterior inner atrial septum with flow saddling between the RA and LA. The 'broken ring sign" is present in **B** (arrow) demonstrating the classic sinus venosum defect as a defect between junction of the low SVC and high RA, a les common form of an ASD with an obligate anomalous right upper pulmonary vein. (**C**) Demonstrates the defect in the posterior RA. (**D**) Demonstrates the anomalous entry of the right upper pulmonary vein into the SVC/RA junction, confirming, on a second oblique, the presence of the congenital defect. Phase velocity mapping was performed demonstrating a Qp:Qs of 1.7 and a top normal RV size (115 mL) indicating a hemodynamically significant intracardiac shunt, worthy of repair, which was successfully conducted noninvasively.

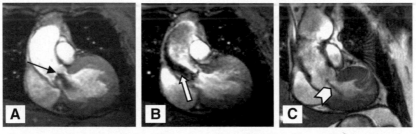

Fig. 16. Aortic regurgitation and aortic insufficiency. A 65-yr-old male with combined aortic valvular lesions. (**A**) Central aortic regurgitation and (**B**) the dephasing jet of an aortic stenosis. A moderately thickened, calcified, and restricted aortic leaflet is seen by SSFP imaging. Phase velocity mapping (not shown) quantified mean and peak gradient of 45 and 87 mmHg, respectively, confirming the diagnosis of severe aortic stenosis with moderate aortic regurgitation. (**C**) A mild jet of aortic regurgitation in another patient with an interposed tube graft (chevron).

The severity of valve disease may also be quantitatively evaluated with *phase velocity mapping*. This is similar to Doppler echocardiography. Phase velocity images are related to the velocity of spins passing through a given plane. Phase velocity mapping can be used to quantitate the flow rate volume and velocity of the blood. Stenotic valvular lesions are frequently characterized by phase image velocities as high as or even higher than 8 m/s (i.e., any velocity encountered in human valvular heart disease). Using a modified Bernoulli approach, pressure drop in mmHg may be estimated from phase contrast measured velocities:

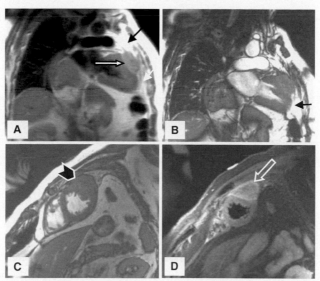

Fig. 17. A 73-yr-old male who presented with several months of progressive chest discomfort was eventually diagnosed with small-cell carcinoma and underwent resection. He returned 8 mo later for follow-up. A CT scan demonstrated a mass adjacent to the heart but was unable to distinguish invasion. (**A**) Demonstrates the large anterior oval mass (large arrow). The pericardium is clearly breached (small arrows **A–B**). (**C**) SSFP imaging demonstrated a loss of epicardial/mass continuity with penetration through the pericardium observed. (**D**) Late enhancement of the lesion and the LV epicardial effacement. The CMR images demonstrated pericardial breaching and loss of epicardial border, and other images (not shown) depicted clear epicardial invasion, including tagged images portraying dissynchronous motion of the tumor with impairment of the epicardial fibers, confirming lack of a separating surgical plane. The patient was deemed not a surgical candidate due to invasion, the high complexity, and risk of surgical resection.

$$\text{Pressure drop} = 4 \times \text{velocity}^2$$

Thus, CMR can be used to assess both regurgitant and stenotic valvular disease. However, its ability to directly visualize normal valve tissue and associated abnormalities, such as endocarditis, while improving, may be somewhat limited compared with echocardiography. It is possible, however, to make excellent images of a bicuspid or tricuspid aortic valve.

Cardiac Masses

Clearly, intracardiac masses such as atrial myxomas and atrial and ventricular thrombi can be detected and evaluated by CMR, EBCT, or MDCT. In fact, ventricular thrombi have been shown to be detected with higher sensitivity and specificity by CMR than by TEE. Virtually any tumor within the heart or that compromises atrial or ventricular function can be assessed. Unfortunately, rhabdomyomas and fibromas may not be distinguished from myocardium on CT, since their density is equivalent to that of myocardium. Differential dynamic contrast enhancement may be useful here. However, because of its sensitivity to T1 and T2 parameters, CMR can frequently differentiate tumors from myocardium (Figs. 17–21).

Pericardial Disease

CMR can readily visualize, measure, and characterize (i.e., distinguish transudate from exudate) pericardial effusions. The problem of differentiating between constrictive pericarditis and restrictive cardiomyopathies is made easier by using MR methods, since the pericardium can be visualized and its thickness measured (*see* Fig. 20) *(30)*. Adherence between the visceral and parietal pericardium, the equivalent of surgical visualization of adhesions, is possible employing RF tissue

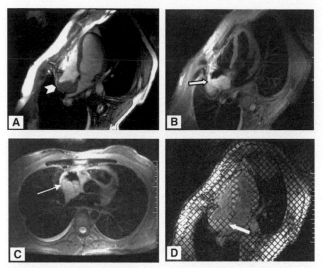

Fig. 18. A 39-yr-old with chronic cough and fullness in the upper airway for several months presented after a CT scan revealed a medastinal mass. Medastinoscopy/biopsy revealed a small-cell carcinoma, but the proximity to the cardiac structures was unclear. The CMR data show that the mediastinal mass has invaded through the pericardium and deep into the right atrium (arrows). (**A**) Demonstrates SSFP (**B**) and (**C**) T2 weighting shows the extra cardiac mass and (**C**) shows the multilobed nature of the invading mass. (**D**) RF tissue-tagging demonstrates the mechanical properties of the mass and the interrelationship to the myocardium.

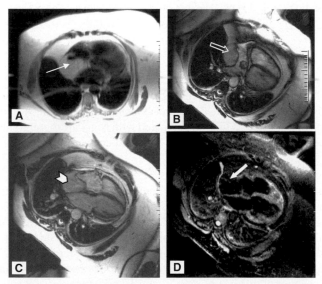

Fig. 19. A 65-yr-old female presented with shortness of breath and mild SVC syndrome and was shown to have a mass on CT involving the right atrium and confirmed by TEE. For further evaluation, the patient underwent CVMRI. (**A**) and (**B**) demonstrate a large homogeneous mass occupying a large segment of the RA as well as considerable anterior mediastinal extrapericardial tissue, all bright on spin-echo imaging (proton density weighted). (**C**) An SSFP sequence demonstrated the obliteration of the posterior RA. Not shown is the near obliteration of the SVC. (**D**) The benign pathology of this presentation in this obese patient is confirmed by the T2-weighted image demonstrating uniform nulling of the tissue, which is diagnostic of a large fatty lipoma. Note the capsule surrounding the mass, which is a characteristic feature, differentiating it from lipomatous inner atrial hypertrophy. Diet and weight loss with exercise were recommended as an interim solution to forestall surgical resection for this otherwise benign lipoma with nonneoplastic but "malignant" features.

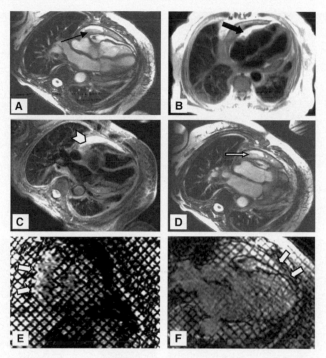

Fig. 20. A diagnosis of restrictive cardiomyopathy. (**A**) Demonstrates a pericardial effusion, which when combined with **B–D**, is better described as an effusive-constrictive pericarditis, as evidenced by fibrinous stranding and the densely adherent fibrous nature intermixed with the effusion. Radiofrequency tissue tagging (**E,F**) demonstrates the adherence between the visceral and parietal pericardium, as evidenced by the absence of slippage and deformation of the tag lines, confirming the finding of a constrictive anatomy and physiology that was confirmed at surgery.

tagging. Under normal circumstances pericardial thickness should not exceed 3 mm. Restrictive left ventricular filling can be demonstrated by volumetric analysis using CMR or by phase velocity mapping.

The pericardium can be visualized by CT techniques as a line, from 1 to 2 mm thick, surrounded with radio density similar to that of myocardium. As with CMR, pericardial thickening can readily be visualized by MDCT and EBCT, although the contrast between pericardium and myocardium may be better on CMR. While pericardial disease should be evaluated initially by two-dimensional echocardiography and Doppler, both CMR and CT methods are useful for more comprehensive evaluation of patients with possible pericardial disease. CT is clearly the optimal technique to detect pericardial calcification.

FUTURE APPLICATIONS

We are far from exhausting the potential of MR methods in applications to the cardiovascular system. As noted, it is now possible to obtain reasonable-quality images of the proximal coronary arteries. There is substantial work in progress to generate myocardial perfusion images using a bolus injection of gadolinium chelate at rest and with vasodilator stress under persantine or adenosine. This has provided accuracies similar to those obtained with the radiopharmaceuticals thallium-201 chloride and technetium-99m sestamibi or similar technetium-labeled compounds. CMR gadolinium perfusion may also have a role in identifying myocarditis or pericarditis and is the reference standard now for myocardial viability. Another unique application is the assessment of myocardial energy metabolism using MR spectroscopy (MRS). MRS allows assessment of the biochemical character of the myocardium by generating spectra from proton or phosphorus nuclei.

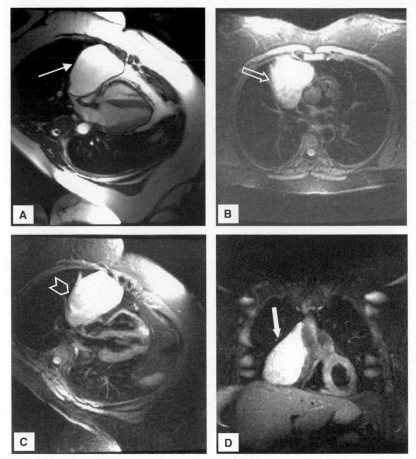

Fig. 21. A 45-yr-old female was followed for several years by CT and TEE for this right-sided homogeneous, well-circumscribed and encapsulated mass. (**A**) The bright signal characteristic on T1 imaging is seen and in (**B**) the lack of nulling on T2 imaging, consistent with its cystic nature (**C** and **D**). In (**C**) and (**D**) note the proper nulling of epicardial fat adjacent to mass (chevron). Tissue characteristics, as well as the anatomic position, makes this mass pathognomonic for a pericardial cyst, which is large but benign.

Phosphorus spectroscopy can show the relative concentrations of the two high-energy phosphates, ATP and PCr. A relative decrease in PCr relative to ATP indicates a myocardial insult such as ischemia. As MR contrast techniques (e.g., intravascular) evolve, and MR tracer (e.g., nanoparticles) and potentially use of higher field systems (e.g., 3T) progress, the opportunity for further creative utilization of CMR will abound.

CONCLUSIONS

Cardiac MR and CT (Table 1) have been available for clinical use since the early 1980s. Advances in both have been achieved throughout the years. CMR has proven to be the more versatile, owing to its ability to use a number of contrast mechanisms, whereas CT methods rely only on X-ray attenuation. Both technologies have substantial clinical utility, however, and can often be used for similar diagnostic applications. When a facility has only CMR or CT, it may be possible to use that modality as the primary diagnostic study. If the advances of the past decade are any indication, both techniques are poised for substantial breakthroughs in cardiovascular imaging for improving speed, resolution, and diagnostic accuracy.

REFERENCES

1. Pohost GM, O'Rourke RA, eds. Basic Principles of Magnetic Resonance. Principles and Practice of Cardiovascular Imaging. Little, Brown Boston, 1990.
2. Schroeder S, Kopp AF, Kuettner A, et al. Influence of heart rate on vessel visibility in noninvasive coronary angiography using new multislice computed tomography: experience in 94 patients. Clin Imaging 2002;26:106–111.
3. Fayad ZA, Fuster V, Nikolaou K, Becker C. Computed tomography and magnetic resonance imaging for noninvasive coronary angiography and plaque imaging: current and potential future concepts. Circulation 2002;106:2026–2034.
4. Morin RL, Gerber TC, McCollough CH. Radiation dose in computed tomography of the heart. Circulation 2003; 107:917–922.
5. Becker CR, Knez A, Ohnesorge B, et al. Imaging of noncalcified coronary plaques using helical CT with retrospective ECG gating. AJR Am J Roentgenol 2000;175:423–424.
6. Cranney GB, Lotan CS, Dean L, et al. Left ventricular volume measurements using cardiac axis nuclear magnetic imaging: validation by calibrated ventricular angiography. Circulation 1990;52:154–163.
7. Dell'Italia LI, Blackwell GC, Pearce WI, Pohost GM. Assessment of ventricular volumes using cine magnetic resonance in the intact dog. A comparison of measurement methods. Invest Radiol 1994;2:162–166.
8. Benjelloun H, Cranney GB, Kirk KA, et al. Interstudy reproducibility of biplane cine nuclear magnetic resonance measurements of left ventricular function. Am J Cardiol 1991;67:1413–1419.
9. Nagel E, Schneider U, Schalla S, et al. Magnetic resonance real-time imaging for the evaluation of left ventricular function. J Cardiovasc Magn Reson 2000;2:7–14.
10. Bottini PB, Can AA, Prisant LM, et al. Magnetic resonance imaging compared to echocardiography to assess left ventricular mass in the hypertensive patient. Am J Hypertens 1995;8:221–228.
11. Young AA, Kramer CM, Ferrari VA, et al. Three-dimensional left ventricular deformation in hypertrophic cardiomyopathy. Circulation 1994;90:854–867.
12. Marcus JT, Gotte LW, DeWaal LK, et al. The influence of through-plane motion on left ventricular volumes measured by magnetic resonance imaging: implications for image acquisition and analysis. J Cardiol Magn Reson 1999; 1:1–6.
13. Fujita N, Duerinckx AJ, Higgins CB. Variation in left ventricular wall stress with cine magnetic resonance imaging: normal subjects versus dilated cardiomyopathy. Am Heart J 1993;125(5 Pt. 1):1337–1344.
14. Wu E, Judd RM, Vargas JD, et al. Visualisation of presence, location, and transmural extent of healed Q-wave and non-Q-wave myocardial infarction. Lancet 2001;357:21–28.
15. Kim RJ, Wu E, Rafael A, et al. The use of contrast-enhanced magnetic resonance imaging to identify reversible myocardial dysfunction. N Engl J Med 2000;343:1445–1453.
16. van Rugge FP, van der Wall EE, Spanjersberg SJ, et al. Magnetic resonance imaging during dobutamine stress for detection and localization of coronary artery disease. Quantitative wall motion analysis using a modification of the centerline method. Circulation 1994;90:127–138.
17. Chiu CW, So NMC, Lam WWM, et al. Combined first-pass perfusion and viability study at mr imaging in patients with non-st segment- elevation acute coronary syndromes: feasibility study. Radiology 2003;226:717–722.
18. Baer FM, Voth E, Theissen P, et al. Gradient-echo magnetic resonance imaging during incremental dobutamine infusion for the localization of coronary artery stenoses. Eur Heart J 1994;15:218–225.
19. Wilke N, Jerosch-Herold M, Stillman AE, et al. Concepts of myocardial perfusion imaging in magnetic resonance imaging. Magn Reson Quart 1994;10:249–286.
20. Schmermund A, Beli MR, Lerman LO, et al. Quantitative evaluation of regional myocardial perfusion using fast x-ray computed tomography. Herz 1997;22:29–39.
21. Kopp AF, Schroeder S, Kuettner A, et al. Non-invasive coronary angiography with high resolution multi-detector-row computed tomography. Eur Heart J 2002;23:1714–1725.
22. Schmermund A, Bailey KR, Rumberger JA, et al. An algorithm for noninvasive identification of angiographic three-vessel and/or left main coronary artery disease in symptomatic patients on the basis of cardiac risk and electron-beam computed tomographic calcium scores. J Am Coll Cardiol 1999;33:444–452.
23. Callister TQ, Raggi P, Cooil B, et al. Effect of HMG-CoA reductase inhibitors on coronary artery disease as assessed by electron-beam computed tomography. N Engl J Med 1998;339:1972–1978.
24. Woo P, Mao S, Wang S, Detrano RC. Left ventricular size determined by electron beam computed tomography predicts significant coronary artery disease and events. Am J Cardiol 1997;79:1236–1238.
25. O'Rourke RA, Brungate BH, Froelicher VF, et al. American College of Cardiology/American Heart Association expert consensus document on electron-beam computed tomography for the diagnosis and prognosis of coronary artery disease. J Am Coll Cardiol 2000;36:326–340.
26. Rumberger JA, Brundage BH, Rader DJ, Kondos G. Electron beam computed tomographic coronary calcium scanning: a review and guidelines for use in asymptomatic persons. Mayo Clinic Proc 1999;74:243–252.
27. Detrano RC, Wong ND, Doherty TM, et al. Coronary calcium does not accurately predict near-term future coronary events in high-risk adults. Circulation 1999;99:2633–2638.
28. Budoff MI, Shavelle DM, Lamont DH, et al. Usefulness of electron beam computed tomography scanning for distinguishing ischemic from nonischemic cardiomyopathy. J Am Coll Cardiol 1998;32:1173–1178.

29. Fujita N, Chazoulliers AE, Hartialia JJ. Quantification of mitral regurgitation by velocity encoding cine nuclear magnetic resonance imaging. J Am Coll Cardiol 1994;23:951–952.
30. Friedrich MG, Strohm O, Schuiz-Menger I, et al. Contrast media-enhanced magnetic resonance imaging visualizes myocardial changes in the course of viral myocarditis. Circulation 1998;97:1802–1509.

RECOMMENDED READING

Detrano RC, Wong ND, Doherty TM, et al. Coronary calcium does not accurately predict near-term future coronary events in high risk adults. Circulation 1999;99(20):2633–2638.
O'Rourke RA, Brundage BH, Froelicher VF, et al. American College of Cardiology/American Heart Association Expert Consensus Document on Electron-Beam Computed Tomography for the Diagnosis and Prognosis of Coronary Artery Disease. J Am Coll Cardiol 2000;36:326–340.
Manning WJ, Li W, Edelman RR. A preliminary report comparing magnetic resonance coronary angiography with conventional angiography. N Engl J Med 1993;328:828–832.
Martin ET, Fuisz AR, Pohost GM. Imaging cardiac structure and pump function. Cardiol Clin 1998;16:135–160.
Pohost GM, O'Rourke RA. Basic Principles of Magnetic Resonance. Principles and Practice of Cardiovascular Imaging. Little, Brown, Boston, 1990.
Forder JR, Pohost GM. Cardiovascular nuclear magnetic resonance: basic and clinical applications. J Clin Invest 2003; 111:1630–1639.
Pohost GM, Hung L, Doyle M. Clinical use of cardiovascular magnetic resonance; special review, clinician update. Circulation 2003;108:647–653.
Manning WJ, Pennell DJ. Cardiovascular Magnetic Resonance. Churchill Livingstone, New York, 2002.
Ohnesorge BM, Becker CR, Flohr TG, Reiser MF. Multislice CT Cardiac Imaging. Springer-Verlag, Berlin, 2002.

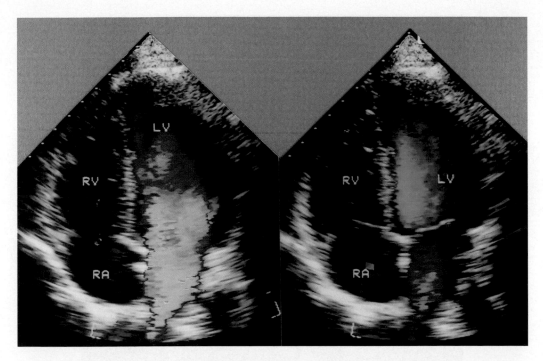

Color Plate 1. Apical four-chamber images with color-flow Doppler during diastole and systole. (Chapter 9, Fig. 5; *see* full caption and discussion on pp. 143–144.)

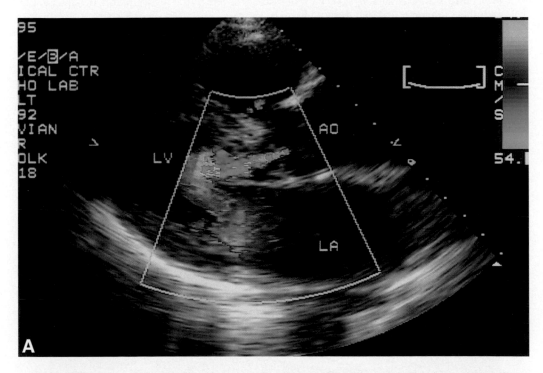

Color Plate 2. Parasternal long-axis image showing a multicolored jet (indicating turbulent flow) of aortic regurgitation in the left ventricular outflow tract. The jet is narrow in width, suggesting mild regurgitation. (Chapter 9, Fig. 11A; *see* complete figure and caption on p. 151 and discussion on pp. 150–151.)

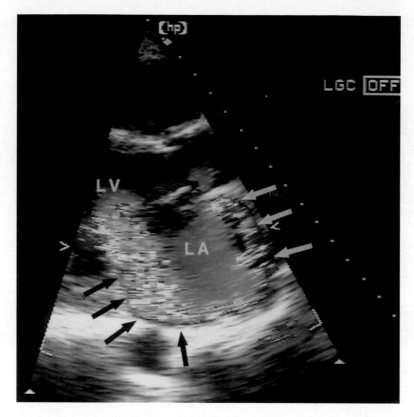

Color Plate 3. Parasternal long-axis view in a case of severe mitral regurgitation. (Chapter 9, Fig. 13; *see* full caption on p. 154 and discussion on p. 152.)

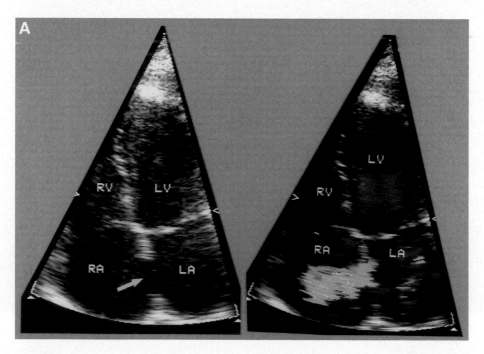

Color Plate 4. Apical four-chamber view of an ostium secundum atrial septal defect. (Chapter 9, Fig. 22A; *see* complete figure and caption on p. 164 and discussion on pp. 162–163.)

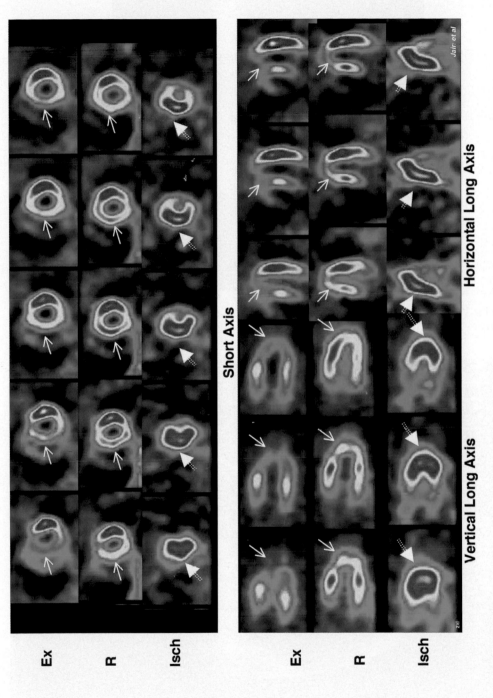

Short Axis

Vertical Long Axis

Horizontal Long Axis

Ex

R

Isch

Ex

R

Isch

Color Plate 5. Exercise (Ex) and rest (R) ^{99m}Tc-sestamibi and exercise ^{18}FDG (Isch) images of a 67-yr-old man with angina and no prior myocardial infarction. (Chapter 13, Fig. 10; *see* full caption on p. 239 and discussion on p. 238.)

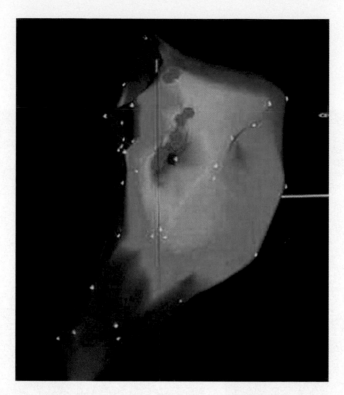

Color Plate 6. Right atrial electroanatomical mapping of automatic atrial tachycardia. (Chapter 17, Figure 2; *see* full caption on p. 311 and discussion on p. 310.)

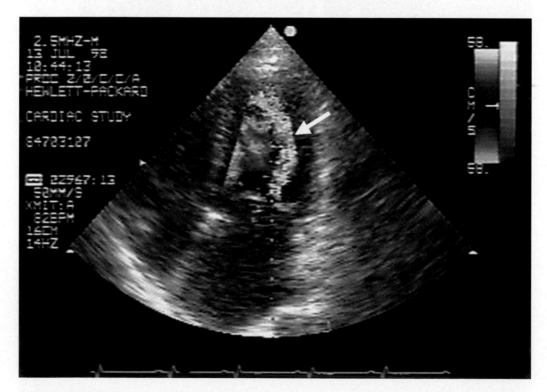

Color Plate 7. Color-flow Doppler echocardiography demonstrates the high-velocity jet entering the left ventricle (arrow). (Chapter 30, Fig. 4; *see* full caption on p. 551 and discussion on p. 550.)

15 Choosing Appropriate Imaging Techniques

Jonathan E. E. Fisher, MD
and Martin E. Goldman, MD

INTRODUCTION

In this chapter, a logical approach to choosing among the various cardiac imaging techniques is proposed. Imaging modalities most commonly employed in the evaluation of cardiac disease are chest roentgenography, cardiac angiography, radionuclide imaging, ultrasonography, computed tomography, and magnetic resonance imaging. Electrocardiography and electrophysiologic studies, though crucial in the evaluation of cardiac electrical abnormalities, are technically not imaging modalities. The decision algorithm requires a basic knowledge of the imaging modalities themselves, including their indications and contraindications, which have been described in the preceding chapters. Most important, however, the treating physician should formulate a clear clinical question which will guide selecting an appropriate imaging test. Most cardiac clinical scenarios can be thought of in terms of questions of structure, function, or both.

Coronary Artery Disease

The stepwise approach to imaging in coronary artery disease (CAD) syndromes depends on whether the symptoms reflect chronic or acute pathophysiology and whether the CAD is suspected or confirmed.

Imaging modalities in CAD either directly image the coronary arteries or allow indirect assessment of coronary stenoses based on inferences from rest and stress myocardial perfusion and/or function in territories supplied by a stenosed artery. Knowledge of left ventricular systolic function and ejection fraction is a key part of the evaluation of patients with suspected or confirmed CAD. Clinical decision algorithms for the treatment of CAD, especially in its chronic phase, are often guided by the left ventricular ejection fraction (LVEF). Therefore, an ideal imaging test for CAD would provide an accurate assessment of LVEF as well. Myocardial perfusion imaging with gated single-photon emission computed tomography (SPECT) and stress echocardiography allow simultaneous accurate noninvasive assessment of coronary stenoses and LVEF.

A Paradigm Shift

Direct imaging of coronary arteries previously focused exclusively on the detection of lumenal stenosis of greater than 50 to 70%, so-called "flow-limiting" stenoses. These lesions were thought to be the most significant culprits leading to acute myocardial infarction and its sequelae. However, there has been a critical paradigm shift in recent years: Possibly precipitated by an inflammatory process, most acute coronary syndromes result from rupture of nonstenotic soft lipid-laden plaques rather than typically fibrocalcific stenotic lesions. These high-risk plaques, if they are not flow-

From: *Essential Cardiology: Principles and Practice, 2nd Ed.*
Edited by: C. Rosendorff © Humana Press Inc., Totowa, NJ

limiting are undetectable by traditional coronary arterial imaging techniques—i.e., X-ray angiography, radionuclide myocardial perfusion imaging, and stress echocardiography—which rely on either visible lumenal encroachment by a stenotic plaques or their hemodynamic impact. For assessment of "global plaque burden" and extent of atherosclerotic disease that can develop into these high-risk nonstenotic plaques, other modalities, including measurement of serum inflammatory markers (i.e., C-reactive protein), brachial artery reactivity, carotid intimal medial thickness (IMT), ankle-brachial index (ABI), and plaque tissue characterization with cardiac magnetic resonance imaging (CMR) have been advocated. The ultimate utility of these newer tests for diagnosing atherosclerosis will be judged according to their ability to provide the clinician with incremental risk-stratifying information above and beyond existing standard clinical risk assessment tools (e.g., the Framingham risk score).

Thus, the clinician confronting a patient with suspected CAD must be clear whether the clinical question is "Does my patient have flow-limiting stenoses that may be accounting for the symptoms?" or "Is my patient at risk for acute myocardial infarction because of the development of nonstenotic lipid-rich plaques that are prone to rupture?" These two questions are not mutually exclusive. Ideally an imaging test would answer both, because acute intervention on one or several stenotic lesions may leave other potential at-risk lesions.

Chronic CAD

Suspected Chronic CAD

The suspicion of the presence of chronic atherosclerosis is raised either by symptoms (i.e., chest pain and/or dyspnea with exertion) or in a patient with multiple traditional coronary risk factors but no symptoms. In the case of a symptomatic patient, a search for flow-limiting endolumenal stenoses begins with history and physical examination accompanied by a 12-lead ECG with special attention for the presence or absence of pathologic Q waves or ST segment deviation.

According to Bayes' theorem, the clinician's pretest suspicion for the presence or absence of a disease will determine the posttest likelihood, and will only be affected by a test result in proportion to that test's sensitivity and specificity. Thus, in patients with pretest likelihood of CAD at the two ends of the likelihood spectrum, low (i.e., 0–20% chance of CAD), or high (80–100% likelihood), cardiac imaging is unlikely to add significantly to the clinical suspicion or lead to a conclusive diagnosis. Therefore, if the clinical suspicion for obstructive CAD is low based on a patient's profile, extensive testing beyond history, physical, and ECG is rarely warranted. Conversely, in a patient with multiple typical cardiac risk factors and a history of typical angina, proceeding directly to the "gold standard" test of X-ray angiography is sensible and cost-effective.

The algorithm for evaluating patients in the intermediate likelihood category is often the most challenging. One must decide whether to proceed with standard treadmill stress 12-lead electrocardiography or to pursue true imaging with either a radionuclide perfusion study or stress echocardiography. Coronary CT and MRI have the potential to provide accurate detail of coronary anatomy though they are costly and provide no information about the patient's functional status, which is perhaps the most relevant clinical information.

Because of its reliance on the insensitive phenomenon of surface ECG ST segment deviations for detection of myocardial ischemia, treadmill ECG should be reserved for patients in whom pretest suspicion is low to assess functional capacity, or to clarify atypical symptoms. False-positive and false-negative tests are relatively common. However, in a patient in whom the question of CAD is raised by exercise-induced chest pain or dyspnea, a treadmill ECG can reproduce the symptoms and assess overall functional capacity and anginal threshold in tandem with diagnostic ECG changes.

When the pretest suspicion is intermediate or high-intermediate, an accurate test for obstructive CAD is appropriate. The two most common modalities are indirect assessments: myocardial perfusion imaging yielding information on relative coronary flow based on regional uptake of a radionuclide-labeled perfusion agent, and stress echocardiography, which requires induction of

Table 1
Risk-Based Approach to Suspected CAD Based on Results
of ^{99m}Tc-Sestamibi Myocardial Perfusion With Gated SPECT or Stress Echo *(1)*

Normal: Very low risk for cardiac death, low risk for MI
  Reassurance
  Risk factor (RFM) modification
Mildly abnormal: low risk for cardiac death, intermediate risk for MI
  Antianginal therapy
  Aggressive risk factor modification (RFM)
  Catheterization if symptoms refractory to therapy
Moderately–severely abnormal: Intermediate to high risk for cardiac death or MI
  Cardiac catheterization
  RFM

myocardial ischemia and consequent regional ventricular systolic dysfunction to provide inferences about the presence and location of obstructive CAD.

RADIONUCLIDE PERFUSION IMAGING AND STRESS ECHOCARDIOGRAPHY

Some fundamental principles guide the decision to pursue either radionuclide perfusion imaging or stress echocardiography and whether these tests should accompany either exercise or pharmacologic "stress" (with dobutamine) or by pharmacologic vasodilation (with adenosine or persantine).

In general, any patient capable of walking on a treadmill should undergo exercise stress testing, typically with the Bruce or modified Bruce protocol. Exercise testing provides important prognostic information which relates directly to patient functional capacity. There are well-validated nomograms and criteria (i.e., the Duke treadmill score) that help the clinician accurately predict subsequent cardiac morbidity and mortality. In special circumstances, bicycle exercise can substitute for treadmill exercise.

However, if the 12-lead ECG ST segment is uninterpretable for ischemia (i.e., due to LVH, LBBB, pacemaker, digoxin therapy, or hormone therapy) and thus cannot be used as a guide for cessation of the treadmill exercise, pharmacologic stress with true myocardial or perfusion imaging is preferred.

For patients who are not able to exercise, pharmacologic stress with dobutamine or pharmacologic vasodilation with adenosine or persantine are indicated. For nuclear testing, adenosine or persantine are the preferred agents except in patients with bronchospastic airway disease, AV nodal conduction disease, or who have consumed caffeine or methylxanthine-containing medications (e.g., theophylline) within 4 to 6 h prior to testing. Dobutamine is preferred in these scenarios.

Whether stress echo or nuclear perfusion is utilized is determined primarily by the relative documented expertise of those performing either technique; while both echo and nuclear require expertise and experience in interpretation, acquisition of accurate stress echo is more technically challenging.

The two commonly used radiopharmaceuticals are thallium (Tl-201) and ^{99m}Tc-sestamibi. Tl-201 has a relatively long half-life with rapid extraction throughout the body in proportion to the cardial output. Tl-201 has a higher myocardial and hepatic uptake and slower washout than ^{99m}Tc-sestamibi (*see* Table 1).

COMPUTED TOMOGRAPHY AND CARDIAC MAGNETIC RESONANCE

Noninvasive imaging of chronic atheromatous plaque at risk for rupture but not hemodynamically significant is currently under investigation, with MRI and CT on the forefront. Imaging of the coronary artery, and particularly the endothelium, has been limited by artifacts resulting from patient motion, respiration, and cardiac motion. Current gating techniques, faster imaging sequences com-

Table 2
Comparison of Various Diagnostic Tests for CAD Accuracy (1)

Test	Dx	Prog	Avail	Function	Time	Cost
ETT ECG	+	+	+++	−	30 m	+
Stress echo	++	++	++	++	30–60 min	++
Stress MPI	++	+++	++	++	2–4 h	+++
EBCT	+	+/−	+	+/−	15 min	++++
PET	+++	++	+/−	++	1–2 h	++++

Avail, availability; DX, for diagnostic purposes; ETT ECG, exercise tolerance test electrocardiography; MPI, myocardial perfusion imaging; EBCT, electron beam computed tomography; PET, positron emission tomography; Prog, provides prognostic information.

bined with breath-holding, are permitting assessment of coronary plaque morphology by CT and MRI in several academic institutions; however, these techniques are not yet ready or available for widespread clinical application.

Detection of calcium deposits within the coronary arteries with either ECG-gated electron beam computed tomography (EBCT) or helical CT has been shown to correlate with risk of future CAD events. Compared with autopsy studies, both imaging tests have been shown to accurately detect the presence of coronary calcium (2–4).

Limitations of these techniques include high cost (>$1 million per scanner), radiation exposure (<200 mrem or approx 10 to 15 standard chest radiographs) (5), high frequency of incidental chest or abdominal findings (up to 50% in the elderly) (6), and significant variability (10 to 50%) (7–9).

Finally, although EBCT may be useful in further risk-stratifying patients in the intermediate–risk category by clinical criteria, its use will not become routine until studies demonstrate its cost-effectiveness and its superiority to existing risk-stratification methods (9).

Imaging for the purpose of plaque and tissue characterization remains a research tool and is typically achieved with a combination of cardiac magnetic resonance (CMR) and coronary CT. However, before plaque morphology determination becomes clinically useful, the benefits of targeting individual high-risk asymptomatic plaques must be proven. At that time, a scoring system for "vulnerable plaques" will likely be developed, incorporating variables determining plaque stability such as fibrous cap thickness, necrotic core size, and degree of macrophage infiltration (9). Global vulnerable plaque scores could then be followed in response to risk (see Table 2).

Confirmed Chronic CAD

When a patient is known to have coronary atherosclerosis on the basis of prior testing, there are a few specific principles to guide selection of subsequent imaging. Testing in this setting is done either because of a change in patient symptoms (e.g., worsening angina, dyspnea, or functional capacity), or to guide decisions about possible percutaneous or surgical coronary revascularization. "Routine" imaging with MPI or stress echocardiography is generally not recommended for the asymptomatic patient in the absence of worsening ventricular dysfunction because there are no data to support coronary revascularization in the asymptomatic patient with normal ventricular systolic function. Therefore, test results would not alter patient management; medical therapy for risk reduction and reduction in oxygen demand and "secondary prevention" measures are the only interventions proven to improve mortality in this patient group.

Knowledge of the extent and severity of obstructive coronary artery disease is occasionally insufficient. In cases of apparent myocardial scarring or regional dysfunction, the physician seeks to assess whether a previously injured segment or infarcted myocardium would regain function if blood flow were restored or improved to that segment. The detection of such "viable" myocardium within hypocontractile, hypokinetic, or akinetic segments might persuade a physician that coronary revascularization for the purpose of symptom relief or mortality benefit (in the case of

Table 3
Recommendations for Use of Radionuclide Techniques to Assess Myocardial Viability *(11)*

Indication	Test	Class	Level of evidence
1. Predicting improvement in regional and global LV function after revascularization	Stress/redistribution/reinjection Tl-201	I	B
	Rest-redistribution imaging	I	B
	Perfusion plus PET FDG imaging	I	B
	Resting sestamibi imaging	I	B
	Gated SPECT sestamibi imaging	IIa	B
	Late Tl-201 redistribution imaging (after stress)	IIb	B
	Dobutamine RNA	IIb	C
	Postexercise RNA	IIb	C
	Postnitroglycerin RNA	IIb	C
2. Predicting improvement in heart failure symptoms after revascularization	Perfusion plus PET FDG imaging	IIa	B
3. Predicting improvement in natural historyafter revascularization	Tl-201 imaging (rest-redistribution and stress/redistribution/reinjection)	I	B
	Perfusion plus PET FDG imaging	I	B

FDG, flurodeoxyglucose; PET, positron emission tomography; RNA, radionuclide angiography; SPECT, single-photon emission computed tomography; T1-201, thallium-201.

multivessel disease with impaired left ventricular systolic function) is warranted even though prior stress testing failed to demonstrate reversible perfusion defects.

Currently positron emission tomography (PET) is the gold standard for viability detection; regions of hypokinetic or akinetic myocardium with impaired radionuclide tracer uptake that display metabolic activity (i.e., glucose-labeled tracer uptake) are considered viable. Because of the expense and limited availability of PET, thallium-201 SPECT is a more commonly utilized to detect viability. Unlike technetium-99m, which is extracted on its way through the coronary vascular bed and is fixed in place in the myocardial mitochondria, thallium-201 rapidly redistributes to all segments of perfused myocardium and thus has the ability to percolate into regions of apparent scarring and be taken up by any living cardiac myocytes. Thus, for the purpose of viability detection, thallium is preferred over technetium-based agents. Dobutamine stress echocardiography has proven utility in detecting regions of viability as well through the "biphasic" response; a hypo- or noncontractile wall segment that augments systolic function with administration of low-dose dobutamine is distinguished from a scar that does not augment. MRI protocols using gadolinium contrast have been developed that accurately detect viability as well, though they are not used widely for clinical decision-making *(10)*.

Comparing modalities is difficult because they have different endpoints suited to the individual modality; dobutamine echo uses wall motion as an endpoint, while perfusion imaging techniques look at residual flow. Thus, PET or radionuclear viability may not translate into recovery of function if not enough myocardium is salvaged *(see* Table 3).

The ACC/AHA classifications I, II, and III are used to summarize indications as follows:

Class I: Conditions for which there is evidence and/or general agreement that a given procedure or treatment is useful and effective.

Class II: Conditions for which there is conflicting evidence and/or a divergence of opinion about the usefulness/efficacy of a procedure or treatment.

Class IIa: Weight of evidence/opinion is in favor of usefulness/efficacy.

Class IIb: Usefulness/efficacy is less well established by evidence/opinion.

Class III: Conditions for which there is evidence and/or general agreement that the procedure/treatment is not useful/effective and in some cases may be harmful.

Levels of evidence for individual class assignments are designated as follows:

A: Data derived from multiple randomized clinical trials.
B: Data derived from a single randomized trial or from nonrandomized studies.
C: Consensus opinion of experts.

Acute Coronary Syndromes

Acute coronary syndromes (unstable angina, non-ST elevation, and ST elevation myocardial infarction) typically result from rupture of a lipid-rich coronary plaque. The degree of myocardial ischemia and necrosis relates to the balance between impaired supply of oxygenated blood (i.e., the degree of intracoronary thrombosis, presence of collateral vasculature, ischemic preconditioning) and demand (relating especially to heart rate, blood pressure, wall stress, and systemic oxygenation).

SUSPECTED ACS

Acute syndromes should be described as either suspected or definite. A syndrome is not definite until some conclusive evidence of myocardial ischemia or necrosis is present. These typically are either an elevated level of a blood marker of myocardial necrosis (e.g., CK-MB or troponin) or documentation of a new or worsening coronary arterial occlusion. The absence of both typical ECG changes consistent with ischemia and serologic evidence of myocardial injury does not necessarily exclude the diagnosis of an ACS. For this reason, these routine initial steps are followed by more elaborate testing if clinical suspicion for an acute coronary syndrome remains high.

In cases of a suspected ACS, attention focuses on risk-stratification and attempts to classify the patient as low-, intermediate-, or high-risk. The 7-point Thrombolysis in Myocardial Infarction (TIMI) risk score is one favored algorithm for risk stratification *(12)*. In the so-called "aggressive" approach to high-intermediate- or high-risk patients with ACS, appropriate medical therapy is initiated and the patient should be brought for direct angiography with possible percutaneous or surgical intervention as indicated.

However, if there are sufficient relative contraindications for cardiac catheterization or if the patient is deemed intermediate- to low-risk by clinical criteria or TIMI scoring, some noninvasive indirect assessment of myocardial perfusion should be pursued to help the clinician predict the patient's risk of subsequent cardiac events and guide therapy.

There is scant evidence regarding the safety of early exercise or pharmacologic stress testing with dobutamine in patients with unstable angina *(13,14)*. According to the updated 2002 ACC/AHA guidelines for the use of stress testing, class I indications for treadmill stress testing are those patients with low-risk clinical features 8 to 12 h after presentation or those with intermediate-risk features 2 to 3 d after presentation; stress testing may be reasonably performed in the absence of any evidence of active ischemia (i.e., by ECG or serum markers) or of heart failure *(15)*.

In contrast, numerous studies have confirmed the safety and utility of pharmacologic vasodilator administration with myocardial perfusion imaging in the acute setting; this proven safety follows from the fact that these agents do not induce ischemia but merely exaggerate existing heterogeneity of coronary blood flow (*see* Table 4).

CONFIRMED ACS

When clinical history, physical examination, ECG, and serum markers confirm the diagnosis of ACS, testing may elucidate the extent and severity of atherosclerosis.

According to the 2002 updated ACC/AHA guidelines, any patient with high-risk indicators presenting with unstable angina or acute non-ST elevation MI will likely benefit from an early invasive strategy of aggressive antiplatelet and antithrombotic therapy and cardiac catheterization with an eye toward percutaneous or surgical revascularization as indicated. These high-risk features

Table 4
Recommendations for Emergency Department Imaging for Suspected ACS

Indication	Test	Class	Level of evidence
1. Assessment of myocardial risk in possible ACS patients with nondiagnostic ECG and initial serum markers and enzymes, if available	Rest MPI	I	A
2. Diagnosis of CAD in possible ACS patients with chest pain with nondiagnostic ECG and negative serum markers and enzymes or normal resting scan	Same day rest/stress perfusion imaging	I	B
3. Routine imaging of patients with myocardial ischemia/necrosis already documented clinically, by ECG and/or serum markers or enzymes	Rest MPI	III	C

See Fig. 6 of ACC/AHA 2002 Guideline Update for the Management of Patients With Unstable Angina and Non–ST-Segment Elevation Myocardial Infarction at http://www.acc.org/clinical/guidelines/unstable/incorporated/figure6.htm and Fig. 1 of ACC/AHA Guidelines for the Management of Patients with Acute Myocardial Infarction at www.acc.org/clinical/guidelines/nov96/1999/jac1716f01.htm.

ACS, acute coronary syndromes; CAD, coronary artery disease; ECG, electrocardiogram; MPI, myocardial perfusion imaging.

include recurrent ischemia or chest pain, elevated troponin T or I, ST segment depression, CHF, presumed new MR, high-risk noninvasive testing result, left ventricular ejection fraction less than 40%, hemodynamic instability, sustained ventricular tachycardia, or prior coronary artery bypass grafting *(16)*. Patients without any of these high-risk features may be treated with a more conservative approach focused on further risk stratification.

IMAGING ACUTE COMPLICATIONS OF ACS

For assessment of complications of the acute ischemic event (e.g., ischemic mitral regurgitation, congestive heart failure, ventricular septal defect, pericardial effusion) echocardiography is the first test of choice because it provides immediate information on valvular, myocardial, and pericardial function and structure; moreover, directed Doppler interrogation can provide extensive hemodynamic information, including estimations of right atrial, right ventricular, pulmonary arterial, left atrial, and left ventricular end-diastolic pressures. The speed and accuracy of 2-D echo and Doppler interrogation have relegated LV angiography and right heart catheterization to a supportive, confirmatory role in most cases. Transthoracic—and, if needed, transesophageal—echocardiography supersede other structural imaging techniques (i.e., MRI, CT, multigated acquisition [MUGA]) for the evaluation of acute complications of MI because of echo's portability for bedside use, accuracy, extent of information provided, and relatively low cost.

VALVULAR AND CONGENITAL HEART DISEASE

The test of choice for diagnosing and following cardiac valvular and congenital structural (i.e., ASD, VSD, coarctation of the aorta, PDA) lesions is transthoracic echocardiography (TTE). When higher-resolution images are needed, or when metallic valvular prostheses or body habitus preclude adequate visualization of intracardiac structures, transesophageal echocardiography (TEE) frequently provides better definition. TEE is frequently performed during valvular surgery to help guide the operation as well. A combination of M-mode, 2-D gray scale, Doppler, and color flow mapping provides virtually all necessary information to make definitive clinical decisions regarding medical management and the timing and utility of percutaneous or surgical intervention in valvular disease. In those cases (estimated as 10–15% of all echo studies) when body habitus or breast tissue make ultrasonographic images uninterpretable, the addition of IV echo contrast agents (i.e., precision gas containing microspheres of albumin, lipid, or polymer) sufficiently improves the quality of the study. Cardiac catheterization, including right heart catheterization and LV angiography, allows for accurate visual semiquantitative assessment of valvular regurgitant lesions and accurate measurement of transvalvular gradients in the case of valvular stenoses. In cases of congenital heart disease, intracardiac shunts can be visualized with either color flow mapping or IV contrast and accurately quantified with standard Doppler techniques.

MRI has assumed an important supporting role in the evaluation of complex valvular disease when echocardiography or right heart catheterization are suboptimal or conflicting. Flow-sensitive MRI techniques provide useful information on valvular pathophysiology as well as perhaps the most accurate assessment of ventricular systolic function *(10)*. For evaluation of complex congenital heart disease, MRI helps further delineate extracardiac conduits and intracardiac flow patterns as well as 3-D rendering of cardiac anatomy *(17)*. Radionuclide studies such as first-pass angiography allow accurate quantification of intracardiac shunts in congenital heart disease *(18)*.

More recently, the development of a portable hand-carried ultrasound (HCU) machine has proved a useful adjunct to the physical examination in cases of suspected valvular disease. The so-called "echo-stethoscope" has the potential for widespread use given its portability, ease of use, and ability to provide immediate critical information on both myocardial and valvular structure and function at the point of care in the office or ER or in the field. 3-D echo offers promise for anatomical definition rivaling MRI, but currently is not a routine clinical tool.

Infective Endocarditis

The prudent selection of either TTE or TEE echocardiography will confirm the diagnosis of infective endocarditis in the majority of cases and will guide decisions about medical versus surgical management *(19)*. In addition to identifying and localizing the vegetation, echocardiography readily detects any complications of endocarditis, including valvular regurgitation, chordal rupture, leaflet perforation, abscess, and fistula formation. TTE is a coarse screening test for endocarditis because its resolution may not differentiate between thickened or redundant valves and a vegetation. Unless the clinical suspicion is low or the valves are pristine by TTE, TEE should be the procedure of choice to exclude the presence of endocarditis and its complications. Additionally, intracardiac devices and intravenous catheters need to be imaged if endocarditis is suspected. Proceeding directly to TEE in cases of intermediate or high clinical suspicion is a more cost-effective approach.

PERICARDIAL DISEASE

When a patient is suspected of having pericardial disease on the basis of either history (typical pericardial chest pain), physical examination (pulsus paradoxicus, pericardial friction rub, diminished heart sounds, Kussmaul's sign), ECG (diffuse ST elevations suggestive of pericarditis, electrical alternans suggesting the heart showing the presence of a very large effusion), or X-ray (enlarged cardiac silhouette), further imaging of the pericardium is warranted.

Transthoracic echocardiography is the initial test of choice. It allows for detection and estimation of the amount of pericardial fluid, if present, and can detect pericardial thickening or nodularity, which may suggest inflammation, infection, or metastatic disease. The echocardiographic feature most supportive of a clinical diagnosis of cardiac tamponade is demonstration of >25% variability in transvalvular flow with inspiration; we Doppler across the aortic valve or in the LV outflow tract to detect changes in stroke volume due to respiratory changes in ventricular filling. Other less sensitive and specific features include early diastolic collapse of the right ventricle or right atrium.

Constriction is characterized by pericardial thickening, possible calcification, and respiratory variations in ventricular dimensions that are readily detected by M-mode and two-dimensional echocardiography. Hatle et al. *(20)* differentiated constrictive pericarditis from restrictive cardiomyopathy using pulsed Doppler echocardiography by respiratory-dependent changes in inflow velocity filling patterns across the mitral and tricuspid valves present in constriction but not restriction. Doppler tissue imaging can also differentiate between the two entities.

Direct measurement of right heart pressures by Swan-Ganz catheterization is an inevitable second step in cases of suspected restriction or constriction. CT and MRI provide supplemental information, including detection of pericardial calcification and accurate measurement of pericardial thickness, respectively *(21,22)*.

Percutaneous drainage of a significant pericardial effusion is often facilitated by echocardiographic guidance at the bedside in the cath lab using "contrast bubbles" generated by reinjection of aspirated fluid to confirm needle/catheter location.

CARDIOMYOPATHIES AND VENTRICULAR MYOCARDIAL DYSFUNCTION

The key clinical questions to be addressed in cases of cardiomyopathy are those of etiology and severity. Echocardiography not only establishes a diagnosis of dilated, hypertrophic, or restrictive cardiomyopathy, but also can often provide clues as to the specific etiology of each subtype. While endomyocardial biopsy is the definitive method to differentiate restriction from constriction and other causes of heart failure, echocardiography is the first imaging test of choice *(23)*. Abnormal patterns of thickening of the ventricular walls (e.g., HCM, muscular dystrophies), unusual myocardial echogenicity (e.g., amyloid, HCM), and the presence of nodules (e.g., sarcoid) can be important clues to diagnosis. In cases where echo data are suboptimal or incomplete, MRI can also accurately assess left and right ventricular systolic function and aid in tissue characterization in cases of cardiomyopathy. MUGA radionuclide imaging will also provide accurate quantification of both RV and LV function; the accuracy of MUGA ejection fraction assessment is due to the fact that volumetric measurements are made based on actual photon density arising from within the ventricular cavity during diastole and systole rather than on geometric assumptions about ventricular shape (as in echocardiography) or by edge-detection techniques (used in standard gated SPECT imaging) *(23)*. However, due to overlying chambers or septal position, a first-pass nuclear study will separate the ventricles better than standard MUGA.

Right Ventricular Dysfunction

Because of difficulties in assessing right ventricular morphology and systolic function with standard echocardiography due to the irregular geometry of the right ventricle, contrast echo and 3-D echo have improved echo assessment of RV size and function. MRI has an important role in providing accurate assessment of RV structure and function *(25)*, and CT *(26)* has been used as well, though their use is limited by cost and availability.

Diastolic Dysfunction

Up to 40% of patients presenting with dyspnea and symptoms of CHF may have normal LV systolic function. The same techniques used to diagnose and characterize the degree of impairment of ventricular relaxation in restrictive cardiomyopathies are those used in cases of suspected diastolic dysfunction. Restrictive cardiomyopathies are typically characterized by normal left and right ventricular size as well as valvular function on M-mode and two-dimensional echocardiography, features that help exclude a diagnosis of hypertrophic or valvular heart disease. The atria, pulmonary veins, vena cavae, and hepatic veins are all typically dilated, because of increased filling pressures *(27)*.

Four Doppler methods are used to assess LV diastolic compliance: transmitral E/A, pulmonary vein flow, Doppler tissue imaging (DTI), and strain imaging. Recently, Doppler tissue imaging of mitral annular motion has been advocated for assessment of restrictive diastolic filling (and diastolic dysfunction) because it is relatively independent of preload conditions. Elevated LV filling pressures (i.e., left atrial pressures) are inferred when E' (tissue Doppler velocity of the mitral annulus during early diastole) is less than 8 ms and E (i.e., early transmitral flow duration)/E' is greater than 15 ms *(28)*. Numerous echocardiographic criteria for stratifying the severity of diastolic dysfunction have been described.

MRI indices of diastolic function have been validated by comparison with echocardiographic Doppler criteria *(29)*.

AORTIC DISEASE

Any imaging modality performed in cases of suspected acute aortic dissection must be rapidly accessible and performed, and must be sufficiently sensitive to avoid false-negative test results in this life-threatening condition. To triage appropriately, the physician needs to determine the tear site, antegrade or retrograde extension, involvement of the coronary arteries, and the presence or absence of aortic regurgitation, pericardial effusion, or hemopericardium. Though TTE can occasionally diagnosis proximal ascending aortic dissections, TEE is the procedure of choice in an unstable patient; however, MRA has a higher sensitivity and specificity, and is the procedure of choice (when available) for the stable patient.

The major limitation of TEE is its "blind spot," where acoustic shadowing from the interposed trachea precludes imaging of a portion of the proximal aortic arch. In addition, TEE does not provide adequate imaging of the aorta below the level of the diaphragm. CT may yield false positives from calcific atherosclerotic plaques, which MRA and TEE should be able to discern. Intramural hematomas can be detected by all three methods. Cases of aortic aneurysm may be followed serially by any one of these three modalities, also depending on availability, local expertise, and cost concerns. In cases of suspected aortitis, CT and MRI both provide detailed imaging of the entire aorta, can be used to generate 3-D reconstructions, and permit characterization of aortic wall morphology. Local experience, available technologies, and patient stability will dictate the procedure of choice.

PULMONARY EMBOLISM

The ventilation perfusion (V/Q) scan was previously the first test of choice for diagnosing suspected pulmonary embolism. However, 73% of all V/Q scans performed are indeterminate, and there is significant interobserver variability in scan interpretation, facts that have driven the search for an updated clinical diagnostic algorithm *(30–32)*.

In addition, though X-ray pulmonary angiography is the "gold standard" for diagnosis, the inherent risks of this invasive test (i.e., vascular complications and contrast nephropathy) as well as significant interobserver variability (45–66%) for diagnosing subsegmental emboli have called the role of this test into question *(33,34)*.

The D-dimer ELISA assay is highly sensitive for diagnosing PE, though nonspecific *(35–38)*, and is thus helpful only for ruling out the diagnosis when negative.

Transthoracic and/or transesophageal echo can be used to quickly detect RV dilation and hypocontractility and even detect a large saddle or proximal pulmonary embolism *in situ*.

Multi-detector row CT angiography *(39,40)* holds promise as the new "gold standard" for diagnosing clinically important pulmonary emboli. With this modality, images of the entire chest with submillimeter resolution can be obtained during a single breath-hold of 10 s or less. The value of CTA lies not only in its sensitivity and specificity for diagnosing PE but also in its ability to rapidly provide an alternate diagnosis for a patient's symptoms. (e.g., pneumonia, pneumothorax, aortic dissection, lung cancer) *(31,41)* *(see* Table 5).

CONCLUSION

There is no single algorithm for choosing among myriad cardiac imaging tests. However, the clinician can narrow the selection by pairing a working knowledge of the strengths and weaknesses

Table 5
Relative Utility of Imaging Methods for Specific Cardiac Disorders

Disorder	CXR	Echo	Angio	Radionuclide	CT	MRI
Ischemic	+	+++	++++	+++	++	++
Valvular	+	++++	+++1	+	++	+++
Congenital	++	++++	++++	++	++	++++
Traumatic	++	++++	+++	++	++	+++
Myopathic	+	++++	+++	++	+++	+++
Pericardial	++	++++	++	0	+++	++++
Endocarditis	+	++++	++	0	++	+++
Masses	0	++++	+++	+	++++	++++

Modified after ref. *42*.

of each test with a narrowly focused clinical question regarding a particular cardiac structure, function, or clinical scenario. Before any imaging is performed, the clinician should consider how the results are likely to affect patient management and whether the benefits of testing outweigh any potential risks, cost, or inconvenience. As in all fields of medicine, a stepwise approach to cardiac diagnosis is followed, from least to most invasive modality.

Suspected or confirmed epicardial coronary artery stenoses are typically evaluated directly by X-ray angiography in settings where revascularization is under consideration or when the pretest likelihood of disease is sufficiently high to warrant bypassing less invasive indirect testing of coronary perfusion (i.e., treadmill stress electrocardiography, stress echocardiography, or myocardial perfusion imaging.) As the pathophysiologic model of acute coronary syndromes continues to evolve, more attention will focus on early detection of nonstenotic but high-risk "vulnerable" atheromatous plaques. CT, cardiac MRI, intravascular ultrasound, and nuclear imaging techniques will continue to evolve for the purpose of coronary plaque characterization and risk stratification.

Myocardial and valvular disorders, including myocardial tissue abnormalities and systolic and diastolic dysfunction, are best imaged by techniques that provide both structural and functional (i.e., hemodynamic) information. While 2-D echocardiography with Doppler imaging is currently the standard for assessing myocardial and valvular function, cardiac MR techniques may develop into a new "gold standard" for measuring systolic function. Invasive measurement of intracardiac pressures by right heart catheterization is reserved for cases in which noninvasive testing yields inconclusive results or results discrepant with clinical findings.

Clinicians should develop their own cost-effective and time-efficient algorithms based on their facilities' technical resources as well as local expertise in acquisition and interpretation of the various techniques.

REFERENCES

1. Gibbons RJ, Chatterjee K, Daley J, et al. ACC/AHA/ACP-ASIM guidelines for the management of patients with chronic stable angina: executive summary and recommendations. A report of the American College of Cardiology/American Heart Association Task Force on Practice Guidelines (Committee on Management of Patients with Chronic Stable Angina). Circulation 1999;99:2829–2848.
2. Janowitz WR. CT imaging of coronary artery calcium as an indicator of atherosclerotic disease: an overview. J Thorac Imaging 2001;16:2–7.
3. Guthrie RB, Vlodaver Z, Nicoloff DM, Edwards JE. Pathology of stable and unstable angina pectoris. Circulation 1975;51:1059–1063.
4. Burke AP, Farb A, Malcom GT, et al. Coronary risk factors and plaque morphology in men with coronary disease who died suddenly. N Engl J Med 1997;336:1276–1282.
5. Falk E, Shah PK, Fuster V. Coronary plaque disruption. Circulation 1995;92:657–671.
6. Burke AP, Farb A, Pestaner J, et al. Traditional risk factors and the incidence of sudden coronary death with and without coronary thrombosis in blacks. Circulation 2002;105:419–424.
7. Gertz SD, Malekzadeh S, Dollar AL, et al. Composition of atherosclerotic plaques in the four major epicardial coronary arteries in patients greater than or equal to 90 years of age. Am J Cardiol 1991;67:1228–1233.

8. Stary HC, Chandler AB, Dinsmore RE, et al. A definition of advanced types of atherosclerotic lesions and a histological classification of atherosclerosis. A report from the Committee on Vascular Lesions of the Council on Arteriosclerosis, American Heart Association. Circulation 1995;92:1355–1374.
9. Taylor AJ, Merz CN, Udelson JE. 34th Bethesda Conference: Executive summary—can atherosclerosis imaging techniques improve the detection of patients at risk for ischemic heart disease? J Am Coll Cardiol 2003;41: 1860–1862.
10. Ramani K, Judd RM, Holly TA, et al. Contrast magnetic resonance imaging in the assessment of myocardial viability in patients with stable coronary artery disease and left ventricular dysfunction. Circulation 1998;98:2687–2694.
11. Klocke FJ, Baird MG, Lorell BH, et al. ACC/AHA/ASNC guidelines for the clinical use of cardiac radionuclide imaging—executive summary: a report of the American College of Cardiology/American Heart Association Task Force on Practice Guidelines (ACC/AHA/ASNC Committee to Revise the 1995 Guidelines for the Clinical Use of Cardiac Radionuclide Imaging). J Am Coll Cardiol 2003;42:1318–1333.
12. Antman EM, Cohen M, Bernink PJ, et al. The TIMI risk score for unstable angina/non-ST elevation MI: a method for prognostication and therapeutic decision making. JAMA 2000;284:835–842.
13. Butman SM, Olson HG, Gardin JM, et al. Submaximal exercise testing after stabilization of unstable angina pectoris. J Am Coll Cardiol 1984;4:667–673.
14. Stein RA, Chaitman BR, Balady GJ, et al. Safety and utility of exercise testing in emergency room chest pain centers: an advisory from the Committee on Exercise, Rehabilitation, and Prevention, Council on Clinical Cardiology, American Heart Association. Circulation 2000;102:1463–1467.
15. Gibbons RJ, Balady GJ, Bricker JT, et al. ACC/AHA 2002 guideline update for exercise testing: summary article: a report of the American College of Cardiology/American Heart Association Task Force on Practice Guidelines (Committee to Update the 1997 Exercise Testing Guidelines). Circulation 2002;106:1883–1892.
16. Braunwald E, Antman EM, Beasley JW, et al. ACC/AHA 2002 guideline update for the management of patients with unstable angina and non-ST-segment elevation myocardial infarction—summary article: a report of the American College of Cardiology/American Heart Association task force on practice guidelines (Committee on the Management of Patients With Unstable Angina). J Am Coll Cardiol 2002;40:1366–1374.
17. Martinez JE, Mohiaddin RH, Kilner PJ, et al. Obstruction in extracardiac ventriculopulmonary conduits: value of nuclear magnetic resonance imaging with velocity mapping and Doppler echocardiography. J Am Coll Cardiol 1992; 20:338–344.
18. Askenazi J, Ahnberg DS, Korngold E, et al. Quantitative radionuclide angiocardiography: detection and quantitation of left to right shunts. Am J Cardiol 1976;37:382–387.
19. Lowry RW, Zoghbi WA, Baker WB, et al. Clinical impact of transesophageal echocardiography in the diagnosis and management of infective endocarditis. Am J Cardiol 1994;73:1089–1091.
20. Hatle LK, Appleton CP, Popp RL. Differentiation of constrictive pericarditis and restrictive cardiomyopathy by Doppler echocardiography. Circulation 1989;79:357–370.
21. Sechtem U, Higgins CB, Sommerhoff BA, et al. Magnetic resonance imaging of restrictive cardiomyopathy. Am J Cardiol 1987;59:480–482.
22. Sutton FJ, Whitley NO, Applefeld MM. The role of echocardiography and computed tomography in the evaluation of constrictive pericarditis. Am Heart J 1985;109:350–355.
23. Schoenfeld MH, Supple EW, Dec GW Jr, et al. Restrictive cardiomyopathy versus constrictive pericarditis: role of endomyocardial biopsy in avoiding unnecessary thoracotomy. Circulation 1987;75:1012–1017.
24. Rezai K, Weiss R, Stanford W, et al. Relative accuracy of three scintigraphic methods for determination of right ventricular ejection fraction: a correlative study with ultrafast computed tomography. J Nucl Med 1991;32:429–435.
25. Pattynama PM, Lamb HJ, Van der Velde EA, et al. Reproducibility of MRI-derived measurements of right ventricular volumes and myocardial mass. Magn Reson Imaging 1995;13:53–63.
26. Reiter SJ, Rumberger JA, Feiring AJ, Stanford W, Marcus ML. Precision of measurements of right and left ventricular volume by cine computed tomography. Circulation 1986;74:890–900.
27. Tam JW, Shaikh N, Sutherland E. Echocardiographic assessment of patients with hypertrophic and restrictive cardiomyopathy: imaging and echocardiography. Curr Opin Cardiol 2002;17:470–477.
28. Garcia MJ, Thomas JD, Klein AL. New Doppler echocardiographic applications for the study of diastolic function. J Am Coll Cardiol 1998;32:865–875.
29. Paelinck BP, Lamb HJ, Bax JJ, et al. Assessment of diastolic function by cardiovascular magnetic resonance. Am Heart J 2002;144:198–205.
30. The PIOPED Investigators. Value of the ventilation/perfusion scan in acute pulmonary embolism. Results of the prospective investigation of pulmonary embolism diagnosis (PIOPED). JAMA 1990;263:2753–2759.
31. Garg K, Welsh CH, Feyerabend AJ, et al. Pulmonary embolism: diagnosis with spiral CT and ventilation-perfusion scanning—correlation with pulmonary angiographic results or clinical outcome. Radiology 1998;208:201–208.
32. Schoepf UJ, Costello P. CT angiography for diagnosis of pulmonary embolism: state of the art. Radiology 2004;230: 329–337.
33. Diffin DC, Leyendecker JR, Johnson SP, et al. Effect of anatomic distribution of pulmonary emboli on interobserver agreement in the interpretation of pulmonary angiography. AJR Am J Roentgenol 1998;171:1085–1089.
34. Stein PD, Henry JW, Gottschalk A. Reassessment of pulmonary angiography for the diagnosis of pulmonary embolism: relation of interpreter agreement to the order of the involved pulmonary arterial branch. Radiology 1999; 210:689–691.

35. Wells PS, Anderson DR, Rodger M, et al. Excluding pulmonary embolism at the bedside without diagnostic imaging: management of patients with suspected pulmonary embolism presenting to the emergency department by using a simple clinical model and d-dimer. Ann Intern Med 2001;135:98–107.
36. Kruip MJ, Slob MJ, Schijen JH, et al. Use of a clinical decision rule in combination with D-dimer concentration in diagnostic workup of patients with suspected pulmonary embolism: a prospective management study. Arch Intern Med 2002;162:1631–1635.
37. Dunn KL, Wolf JP, Dorfman DM, et al. Normal D-dimer levels in emergency department patients suspected of acute pulmonary embolism. J Am Coll Cardiol 2002;40:1475–1478.
38. Brown MD, Rowe BH, Reeves MJ, et al. The accuracy of the enzyme-linked immunosorbent assay D-dimer test in the diagnosis of pulmonary embolism: a meta-analysis. Ann Emerg Med 2002;40:133–144.
39. McCollough CH, Zink FE. Performance evaluation of a multi-slice CT system. Med Phys 1999;26:2223–2230.
40. Hu H, He HD, Foley WD, Fox SH. Four multidetector-row helical CT: image quality and volume coverage speed. Radiology 2000;215:55–62.
41. Hull RD, Raskob GE, Ginsberg JS, et al. A noninvasive strategy for the treatment of patients with suspected pulmonary embolism. Arch Intern Med 1994;154:289–297.
42. Skorton DJ, Brundage BH, Schelbert HR, Wolf GL. Relative merits of technical imaging techniques. In: Braunwald E. Heart Disease. W. B. Saunders, Philadelphia, 1997, pp. 354, table 11–15.

RECOMMENDED READINGS

Antman EM, Cohen M, Bernink PJ, et al. The TIMI risk score for unstable angina/non-ST elevation MI: a method for prognostication and therapeutic decision making. JAMA 2000;284:835–842.
Gibbons RJ, Balady GJ, Bricker JT, et al. ACC/AHA 2002 guideline update for exercise testing: summary article: a report of the American College of Cardiology/American Heart Association Task Force on Practice Guidelines (Committee to Update the 1997 Exercise Testing Guidelines). Circulation 2002;106:1883–1892.
Gibbons RJ, Chatterjee K, Daley J, et al. ACC/AHA/ACP-ASIM guidelines for the management of patients with chronic stable angina: executive summary and recommendations. A Report of the American College of Cardiology/American Heart Association Task Force on Practice Guidelines (Committee on Management of Patients with Chronic Stable Angina). Circulation 1999;99:2829–2848.
Klocke FJ, Baird MG, Lorell BH, et al. ACC/AHA/ASNC guidelines for the clinical use of cardiac radionuclide imaging—executive summary: a report of the American College of Cardiology/American Heart Association Task Force on Practice Guidelines (ACC/AHA/ASNC Committee to Revise the 1995 Guidelines for the Clinical Use of Cardiac Radionuclide Imaging). J Am Coll Cardiol 2003;42:1318–1333.

IV   DISORDERS OF RHYTHM
AND CONDUCTION

16 Electrophysiology of Cardiac Arrhythmias

Sei Iwai, MD, *Steven M. Markowitz* MD,
Suneet Mittal, MD, *Kenneth M. Stein,* MD,
and Bruce B. Lerman, MD

INTRODUCTION

The normal cardiac cycle is initiated by electrical events that precede cardiac contraction. Abnormalities in the initiation and propagation of cardiac impulses may result in a variety of arrhythmias. The purpose of this chapter is to highlight the cellular mechanisms responsible for normal impulse formation and conduction, and to review the clinical consequences when these mechanisms are perturbed.

CELLULAR ELECTROPHYSIOLOGY: CARDIAC ACTION POTENTIAL

The cardiac action potential consists of five phases that are determined by channels that allow ions to flow passively down their electrochemical gradients, as well as by a series of energy-dependent ion pumps. Ion channels are protein tunnels that span the cell lipid membrane. By selectively permitting the passage of specific ions, they maintain the electrochemical cell membrane potential. Flow of a specific ion through a channel is dependent on gating of the channel as well as the electrical and chemical concentration gradients of that particular ion. Ions will flow passively down a chemical gradient if the channel is gated open, and will also be drawn toward their opposite charge.

Na^+ and Ca^{2+} channels consist of a single α-subunit that contains six hydrophobic transmembrane regions (Fig. 1) *(1)*. The voltage-gated K^+ channel consists of four identical subunits each containing a six-transmembrane-spanning unit similar to Na^+ and Ca^{2+} channels. The six transmembrane units, S1–S6, form the core of the sodium, calcium, and most potassium channels.

Na^+, K^+, Ca^{2+}, and Cl^- are principally responsible for the membrane potential (Fig. 2). It is helpful to recall the equilibrium potential of these ions when considering the cardiac action potential (Table 1). The positive and negative values reflect the intracellular potential relative to a reference electrode. When a single type of ion channel opens, the membrane potential will approach the equilibrium potential of that ion. Thus, during diastole (phase 4), the cell membrane is impermeable to Na^+. However, K^+ diffuses freely out of the cell until the concentration gradient is balanced by the negative intracellular potential that attracts K^+. This balance represents the potassium electrochemical equilibrium potential (E_K). During phase 0, when the cell membrane is freely permeable to Na^+, the membrane potential approaches +50 mV (Fig. 3) *(2)*. Typically, more than one channel type is open at a time. The resulting membrane potential is determined by the balance of the competing currents.

From: *Essential Cardiology: Principles and Practice, 2nd Ed.*
Edited by: C. Rosendorff © Humana Press Inc., Totowa, NJ

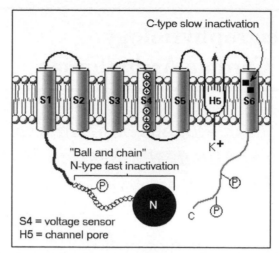

Fig. 1. Diagram of a subunit containing six transmembrane-spanning motifs, S1 through S6, that forms the core structure of sodium, calcium, and potassium channels. The "ball and chain" structure at the N-terminal of the protein is the region of a potassium channel that participates in N-type "fast inactivation," occluding the permeation pathway. The circles containing plus signs in S4, the voltage sensor, are positively charged lysine and arginine residues. Key residues lining the channel pore (H5) are found between S5 and S6. (Modified and used with permission from ref. *1*.)

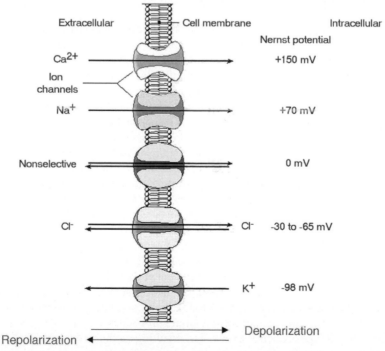

Fig. 2. Physiology of ion channels. Five major types of ion channels determine the transmembrane potential of a cell. The ionic gradients across the membrane establish the Nernst potentials (E_{rev}) of the ion-selective channels (approximate values are shown). Under physiologic conditions, calcium and sodium ions flow into the cell and *depolarize* the membrane potential (i.e, they drive the potential toward the values shown for E_{Ca} and E_{Na}), whereas potassium ions flow outward to *repolarize* the cell toward E_K. Nonselective channels and chloride channels drive the potential to intermediate voltages (0 mV and −30 to −65 mV, respectively). (Modified and used with permission from ref. *1*.)

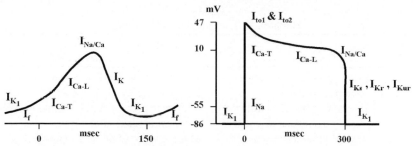

Fig. 3. The human cardiac action potential. Principal currents responsible for the sinoatrial nodal (left) and ventricular (right) action potential. (Modified and used with permission from ref. *2*.)

Phase 0 marks the initiation of the action potential. Nodal cells are characterized by an influx of Ca^{2+}, while atrial, ventricular, and His-Purkinje cells depend on an influx of Na^+. Initiation of each cardiac cycle is dependent on membrane depolarization initiated at the sinus node. In nodal cells, the pacemaker current, I_f, initiates each cycle. I_f is activated by the polarization of phase 4 and carries a nonselective inward current composed primarily of Na^+ and K^+ ions as well as a small Ca^{2+} current. I_f causes slow depolarization of the nodal cell membranes during diastole until a threshold for firing is achieved. Following initial local membrane depolarization by I_f, the upstroke of the nodal action potential is completed by a slow inward calcium current. Two types of calcium currents are present: the predominant slowly inactivating, dihydropyridine-sensitive L current (I_{Ca-L}) and the rapidly inactivating T current (I_{Ca-T}; *see* Fig. 3 and Table 1). Local membrane depolarization is propagated to neighboring cells via gap-junction channels.

In "nonpacemaker" tissue, I_f is absent. In these cells, phase 0 is triggered when the cell membrane is depolarized by adjacent cells. Once a sufficient proportion of a cell surface is depolarized and the cell reaches its activation threshold, the permeability of the cell surface membrane to I_{Na} is markedly increased, allowing Na^+ to enter the cell and complete phase 0 depolarization. Blocking this inward current decreases the rate of change of the upstroke of the action potential (*dV/dt*) and slows conduction velocity.

Phase 1 consists of rapid membrane repolarization. This is achieved by inactivation of the inward Na^+ current and activation of I_{to}, which is comprised of two currents. I_{to1} is a voltage-activated outward potassium current and I_{to2} is a calcium-activated chloride current. Phase 2, the plateau phase, may last as long as 100 ms and is characterized by a small change in membrane potential generated by I_{Ca-L}.

Rapid repolarization of the cell occurs during phase 3. I_{Ca-L} is inactivated in a time-dependent fashion, thus decreasing the flow of cations into the cell. Simultaneously, several outward potassium currents, known as the delayed slow (I_{Ks}), rapid (I_{Kr}), and ultra-rapid (I_{Kur}) currents become active. This results in a net outward positive current and a negative transmembrane potential.

MECHANISMS OF ARRHYTHMIAS

Automaticity

Rhythmic (pacemaker) activity is an inherent property of different cell types. There is a normal hierarchy in the frequency of the initiated action potentials, with the sinus node being the dominant pacemaker. Automaticity in the distal conduction system (or working myocardium) may compete with that in the sinus node on the basis of enhanced normal or abnormal automaticity.

Under pathologic conditions, a decrease in the resting membrane potential may occur, which can lead to spontaneous phase 4 depolarization in all cardiac cells *(3)*. Abnormal automaticity is defined as spontaneous impulse initiation in cells that are not fully polarized. The disturbances in the normal ionic balance leading to abnormal automaticity may result from perturbations in various

Table 1
Summary of Transmembrane Currents

Ion (Nernst Potential)	Currents	Role in AP
Potassium (−98 mV)	I_f—Inward "pacemaker" current (also carried by Na^+)	Activated in nodal tissue polarization of membrane during phase 4
	I_{K1}—Inward rectifier responsible for resting membrane potential	Maintains phase 4 resting membrane potential; absent in sinus node
	I_{Kur}—Inward ultrarapid rectifier	Minor current of phase 1 repolarization
	I_{Kr}—Inward rapid rectifier repolarization	Primary current of rapid phase 3
	I_{Ks}—Inward slow rectifier	Contributes to late phase 3 repolarization
	I_{to1} ($=I_{Kto1}$)—Transient voltage-sensitive outward current	Activated (by voltage) briefly during phase 1 rapid repolarization
	$I_{K(ACh)}$—Outward current	Activated by muscarinic (M_2) receptors via GTP; important in nodal and atrial cells where it may cause hyperpolarization and shortening of action potential duration
	$I_{K(Ado)}$—Outward current	Appears identical in function to $I_{K(ACh)}$, but activated by adenosine
	$I_{K(ATP)}$—Outward current	Blocked by ATP; activated during hypoxia (when ATP concentration low); shortens action potential during ischemia
Sodium (+70 mV)	I_{Na}—Fast inward current carried by Na^+ through a voltage-gated channel	Phase 0
	I_{Ti}—Transient inward current	Activated during phase 4 by release of Ca^{2+} from the sarcoplasmic reticulum; contributes to DADs
	$I_{Na-K\ pump}$—Bidirectional current	Pumps 3 Na^+ out for 2 K^+ in producing small rectifier current; when this channel is blocked by digoxin the Na/Ca exchanger $I_{Na/Ca}$ takes over, resulting in intracellular Ca^{2+} overload
	$I_{Na/Ca}$—Outward current	Exchanges 1 Ca^{2+} (into the cell) for 1 Na^+ (out of the cell) during intracellular Na^+ overload; during digoxin toxicity this may result in intracellular Ca^{2+} overload and triggered arrhythmias
Calcium (+150 mV)	I_{Ca-L}—Slow inward calcium current, blocked by dihydropyridines	Active during phase 0 in nodal cells, phase 2 of atrial, ventricular and His-Purkinje cells
	I_{Ca-T}—Transient inward current	May contribute to phase 4 depolarization in sinus and His-Purkinje cells
	$I_{Na/Ca}$—Inward current	Exchanges 1 Ca^{2+} (out of the cell) for 3 Na^+ (into the cell) during phase 2; during digoxin toxicity this may result in intracellular Ca^{2+} overload and triggered arrhythmias
Chloride (−30 mV)	I_{Cl}—Outward current	Contributes to phase 3 repolarization; activated by adrenergic stimulation
	I_{to2} ($= I_{Cl.Ca}$)—Transient (Ca^{2+} activated) outward chloride current	Activated briefly during phase 1 rapid repolarization

Table 2
Electropharmacologic Matrix

	Reentry	Automaticity	cAMP-triggered activity
Catecholamine stimulation	Facilitates/no effect	Facilitates	Facilitates
Induction with rapid pacing	Facilitates/no effect	No effect	Facilitates
Overdrive pacing	Terminates/accelerates	Transiently suppresses	Terminates/accelerates
β-blockade	No effect/rarely terminates	Terminates	Terminates
Vagal maneuvers	No effect	Transiently suppresses	Terminates
Calcium channel blockade	No effect*	No effect	Terminates
Adenosine	No effect	Transiently suppresses	Terminates

Automaticity refers to arrhythmias that arise from spontaneous phase 4 depolarization from nearly fully repolarized cells. Abnormal automaticity (which occurs in cells with resting membrane potentials ≤–60 mV) is not included in this table because it has not conclusively been shown to be a cause of clinical arrhythmias.

*An exception is intrafascicular reentry, which is sensitive to verapamil. (Used with permission from ref. *4*.)

currents, e.g., reduction in I_{K1}. During the subacute phase (24–72 h following coronary occlusion), automatic arrhythmias arise from the borders of the infarction.

CLINICAL CORRELATES

A representative clinical example of an automatic arrhythmia is atrial or ventricular tachycardia that is precipitated by exercise in patients without structural heart disease. These forms of tachycardia are thought to represent adrenergically mediated automaticity because programmed stimulation cannot initiate or terminate the arrhythmia, whereas the tachycardia is induced with catecholamine stimulation and is sensitive to β-blockade (Table 2) *(4,5)*.

The cellular mechanism governing automatic arrhythmias and their anatomic substrate is poorly delineated. Catecholamines modulate the rate in automatic cells by increasing cyclic AMP synthesis and alter the kinetics of I_f such that it is activated at less negative membrane potentials *(6)*. Adenosine appears to attenuate I_f through an inhibition of cAMP synthesis, an antiadrenergic mechanism similar to that mediated by vagal stimulation *(7)*.

Triggered Activity

In cardiac cells, oscillations of membrane potential that occur during or after the action potential are referred to as *afterdepolarizations*. They are generally divided into two subtypes: early and delayed afterdepolarizations (EADs and DADs, respectively; Fig. 4) *(8)*. When an afterdepolarization achieves a sufficient amplitude and the threshold potential is reached, a new action potential is evoked, known as a triggered response. Under appropriate circumstances, this process may become iterative, resulting in a sustained triggered rhythm (Fig. 5). Triggered activity differs fundamentally from abnormal automaticity in that abnormal automaticity occurs during phase 4 of the action potential and it depends on partial depolarization of the resting membrane potential.

EARLY AFTERDEPOLARIZATIONS AND ARRHYTHMOGENESIS

An EAD can appear during the plateau phase (phase 2) and/or repolarization (phase 3) of the action potential (Fig. 4). Distinction between phase 2 and phase 3 EADs is often based on the take-off potential of the EAD, e.g., above –35 mV for the phase 2 and below –35 mV for the phase 3 EADs. Sometimes both forms of EADs appear during the same action potential. A critical prolongation of

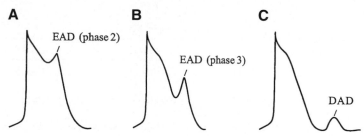

Fig. 4. Examples of (**A**) phase 2 early afterdepolarization (EAD); (**B**) phase 3 EAD; and (**C**) delayed after-depolarization (DAD). (Used with permission from ref. *8*.)

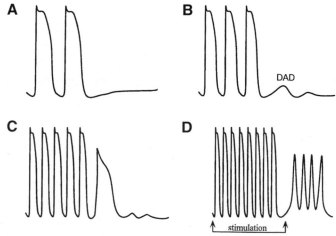

Fig. 5. Delayed afterdepolarizations (DADs) and triggered activity resulting from inhibition of the Na⁺-K⁺ pump. (**A**) No DADs following a rapid pacing. (**B**) Single DADs, but no sustained triggered activity, following rapid pacing. (**C**) One triggered beat following rapid pacing. (**D**) Repetitive triggered activity following very rapid pacing. (Used with permission from ref. *8*.)

repolarization either by a reduction in outward currents, an increase in inward currents or a combination of the two, is normally required for the manifestation of EAD-induced ectopic activity (Fig. 6) *(9)*. EADs are often potentiated by bradycardia or a pause, which further prolongs repolarization.

Clinical Correlates. A wide variety of medications can produce EADs, EAD-related triggered activity, or even a form of polymorphic ventricular tachycardia known as *torsade de pointes* (Fig. 7). These agents excessively prolong repolarization and include the Vaughn-Williams class Ia (e.g., quinidine and procainamide) and class III (e.g., sotalol and ibutilide) antiarrhythmic agents, and a variety of noncardiac drugs including antibiotics, (e.g., erythromycin), pentamidine, and nonsedating antihistamines (e.g., terfenadine and astemizole).

One of the most extensively studied EAD-related arrhythmias is that found in patients with congenital long-QT syndrome. While this is a rare disease (1 per 10,000 births) it provides an opportunity to examine the effects of ion-channel mutations on structure and function of these channels.

Two distinct phenotypes of congenital long-QT syndrome were initially recognized. In 1957 Jervell and Lange-Nielsen described the autosomal recessive pattern of the congenital long-QT syndrome associated with congenital sensorineural hearing loss and recurrent syncope *(10)*, and in 1963, an autosomal dominant form of the disease manifesting only as QT prolongation was described separately by Romano et al. and Ward *(11,12)*. Molecular genetics have now revealed at least seven forms of the long-QT syndrome (LQT1–LQT7) *(13)*.

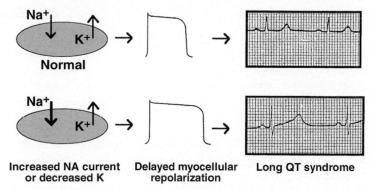

Normal

Increased NA current   Delayed myocellular   Long QT syndrome
or decreased K   repolarization

Fig. 6. Molecular and cellular mechanisms of early afterdepolarization (EAD)-induced arrhythmias, such as that observed in long-QT syndrome. "Gain of function" mutations in cardiac sodium channel genes, or "loss of function" mutations in cardiac potassium channel genes, lead to prolongation of the cardiac action potential. Abnormal myocellular repolarization and inhomogeneity of cardiac repolarization lead to QT prolongation. (Used with permission from ref. *9*.)

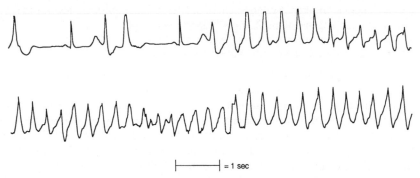

⊢————⊣ = 1 sec

Fig. 7. Initiation of torsade de pointes following a "long-short" interval in a patient with long-QT syndrome.

Certain clinical features appear to be common to most forms of the congenital long-QT syndrome. Most patients will have a corrected QT interval (QTc) of 460 ms or greater *(14)*. The standard heart rate correction, according to Bazett's formula, is $QTc = QT/RR^{1/2}$, where RR is the R–R interval expressed in seconds. A scoring system has been developed to assist in the diagnosis of the long-QT syndrome, and takes into account factors including the QT interval, patient symptoms, and family history *(15)*. The syndrome appears to be equally distributed between men and women.

Known mutations account for about 50% of those diagnosed with LQTS. LQT1 accounts for approx 45% of genotyped cases. The responsible gene is located on the short arm of chromosome 11 and encodes the pore forming the α-subunit (one of the two proteins) that comprise I_{Ks}, the slowly activating delayed rectifier current. The defective I_{Ks} is inactive, thus prolonging repolarization and predisposing to EADs.

Mutations in the gene encoding I_{Kr} (HERG) on chromosome 7, which result in prolonged phase 3 repolarization, appear to be responsible for another autosomal recessive form of the long-QT syndrome, LQT2, and accounts for another 45% of patients.

LQT3 has been linked to SCN5A, a gene on chromosome 3 that encodes I_{Na}, the current responsible for phase 0 rapid depolarization. LQT3 results from a sodium channel that fails to inactivate appropriately. This causes continued inward sodium current (beyond phase 0) throughout the action potential, thereby prolonging the action potential duration. Mexiletine, a selective Na^+ channel blocker, has been demonstrated to shorten the QTc in affected patients and may therefore have a therapeutic role.

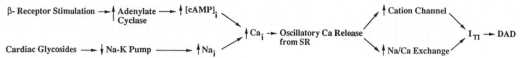

Fig. 8. Mechanism of DADs related to catecholamines and digoxin toxicity. Intracellular Ca^{2+} overload triggers I_{Ti}, a depolarizing inward Na^+ current. Ca_i, inward Ca^{2+} current; Na_i, increased intracellular Na^+ concentration; I_{TI}, depolarizing inward Na^+ current; SR, sarcoplasmic reticulum.

Less common mutations include LQT4 (ankyrin B), located on chromosome 4, which causes disruption in the cellular organization of the Na^+ pump, the Na^+/Ca^{2+} exchanger, and the inositol triphosphate receptor; extrasystoles are caused by altered Ca^{2+} signaling. In addition, the β-subunit of I_{Ks} and I_{Kr} are encoded by KCNE1 and KCNE2 (both on chromosome 21), and mutations in these genes can also result in prolonged QTc due to delayed repolarization (LQT5 and LQT6, respectively). Finally, LQT7 is caused by the mutant gene KCNJ2, which decreases inwardly rectifying K^+ current ($I_{Kir2.1}$).

Mutations in one allele of either the α- or β-subunit of I_{Ks} appear to be phenotypically expressed as the Romano-Ward syndrome. Both subunits have been demonstrated to be present in the stria vascularis of the inner ear in mice. Mutations in both alleles (i.e., homozygotes) for the α- or β-subunit are associated with the Jervell and Lange-Nielsen phenotype.

DELAYED AFTERDEPOLARIZATIONS AND ARRHYTHMOGENESIS

Delayed afterdepolarizations (DADs) are oscillations in membrane potential that occur after repolarization and during phase 4 of the action potential. In contrast to automatic rhythms that originate *de novo* during spontaneous diastolic depolarization, DADs are dependent on the preceding action potential. By definition they do not occur in the absence of a previous action potential.

During the plateau phase of the normal action potential, Ca^{2+} enters the cell. The increase in intracellular Ca^{2+} triggers release of Ca^{2+} from the sarcoplasmic reticulum (SR); this, in turn, further elevates intracellular calcium and initiates contraction. Relaxation occurs through sequestration of Ca^{2+} by the SR. DADs arise when the cytosol becomes overloaded with Ca^{2+} and triggers I_{Ti}, a transient inward current (Fig. 8). I_{Ti} is generated by the Na^+-Ca^{2+} exchanger (I_{NaCa}) and/or a nonspecific Ca^{2+}-activated current *(16,17)*. DADs can originate from Purkinje fibers, as well as from myocardial, mitral valve, and coronary sinus tissues. Rapid pacing potentiates DADs because more Na^+ (and Ca^{2+}) enters the cell during rapid depolarization, furthering Ca^{2+} loading the cell. Most experimental studies on triggered activity were performed under conditions of digoxin excess. By blocking the Na^+/K^+ pump, digoxin causes increased concentration of intracellular Na^+. The high concentration of Na^+ stimulates the Na^+/Ca^{2+} exchanger that moves Na^+ out of the cell in exchange for allowing Ca^{2+} entry into the cytosol. This results in intracellular Ca^{2+} overload and DADs. β-adrenergic stimulation, which is mediated by an increase in intracellular cAMP, also provokes delayed afterdepolarizations by increasing the inward Ca^{2+} current.

Clinical Correlates. The prototypical clinical arrhythmia due to cAMP-mediated triggered activity (DAD-dependent) is idiopathic ventricular tachycardia arising from the right ventricular outflow tract (RVOT) *(18)*, which segregates into two phenotypes: paroxysmal stress-induced VT and repetitive monomorphic VT (RMVT). These forms of arrhythmia represent polar ends of the spectrum of clinical VT due to cAMP-mediated triggered activity *(19)*. RMVT occurs during rest and is characterized by frequent ventricular extrasystoles, ventricular couplets, and salvos of nonsustained VT with intervening sinus rhythm. In contrast, paroxysmal stress-induced VT usually occurs during exercise or emotional stress and is a sustained arrhythmia. Common to both groups is the absence of structural heart disease, similar tachycardia morphology (left bundle branch block, inferior axis), and similar site of origin (RVOT), although the tachycardia can occasionally originate from other right ventricular sites as well as the left ventricle *(20)*. Overlap between these two subtypes of VT can be considerable.

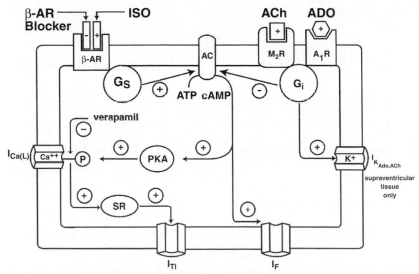

Fig. 9. Schematic representation of the cellular model for adenosine. AC, adenylyl cyclase; ACh, acetylcholine; ADO, adenosine; A_1R, adenosine A_1 receptor; β-AR, β-adrenergic receptor; G_i, inhibitory G protein; G_s, stimulatory G protein; ISO, isoproterenol; M_2R, muscarinic cholinergic receptor; PKA, protein kinase A; SR, sarcoplasmic reticulum. (Used with permission from ref. *21*.)

Since activation of adenylyl cyclase and I_{Ca-L} is critical for the development of cAMP-mediated triggered activity, the triggered arrhythmia would be expected to be sensitive to many electrical and pharmacological stimuli, including β-blockade, calcium-channel blockade (verapamil), vagal maneuvers, and adenosine (Table 2; Fig. 9) *(21)*. Termination of VT with adenosine is thought to be a specific response for identifying cAMP-mediated triggered activity due to DADs, since adenosine has no electrophysiologic effect in the absence of β-adrenergic stimulation, and has no effect on digoxin-induced DADs or quinidine-induced EADs. Furthermore, adenosine has no effect on catecholamine-facilitated reentry that is due to structural heart disease *(22)*. The clinical effects of adenosine and verapamil in a patient with VT attributed to cAMP-mediated triggered activity are shown in Fig. 10. While calcium blockers may be helpful in the cardiac electrophysiology laboratory in determining the mechanism of a specific arrhythmia (Table 2), their use is *contraindicated* in the treatment of most clinical forms of ventricular tachycardia.

Another arrhythmia that is possibly due to triggered activity related to delayed after-depolarizations is *catecholaminergic polymorphic ventricular tachycardia* (CPVT). CPVT also occurs in patients with no evidence of structural heart disease, who present with a distinctive pattern of stress-related, bidirectional VT, or polymorphic VT. Mutations in the cardiac ryanodine receptor gene (RyR2), and polymorphisms in calsequestrin 2 have been linked to CPVT *(23–25)*. RyR2 is responsible for calcium release from the sarcoplasmic reticulum, in response to calcium entry from the voltage-dependent L-type calcium channels (i.e., calcium-induced calcium release). Calsequestrin provides a calcium reservoir in the sarcoplasmic reticulum, and possibly serves as a luminal Ca^{2+} sensor for the ryanodine receptor. Malfunction of either of these molecules can result in calcium overload.

Reentry

The normal cardiac impulse follows a predetermined path. It is initiated at the sinus node and is extinguished after it has activated the ventricles. Reentrant arrhythmias arise when the cardiac impulse circulates around an anatomic or functional obstacle initiating an independent, repetitive rhythm. Reentry may be broadly classified as being either *anatomic* or *functional*.

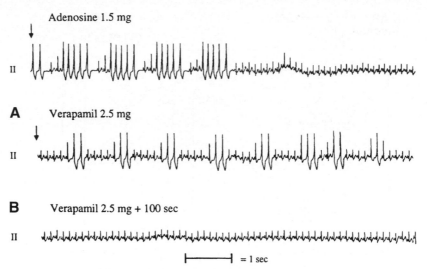

Fig. 10. (A) ECG recording showing termination of incessant repetitive monomorphic ventricular tachycardia (VT) by adenosine. The vertical arrow indicates the completion of adenosine administration and saline flush. **(B)** Administration of verapamil during incessant repetitive monomorphic VT. Vertical arrow indicates completion of verapamil infusion. **(C)** Termination of VT 100 s after verapamil administration. Surface lead II is shown. (Used with permission from ref. *19*.)

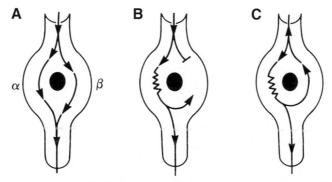

Fig. 11. Model of anatomic reentry. **(A)** The impulse passes through a hypothetical conduit via two pathways, α and β, which meet at a common exit point. **(B)** Since α and β have distinct refractory properties, a hypothetical extrastimulus could be blocked in β pathway and conduct slowly over α pathway and reenter β pathway retrogradely. **(C)** This could result in sustained circus movement. (Used with permission from ref. *26*.)

ANATOMIC REENTRY

In the anatomic model of reentrant arrhythmias, four prerequisites must be met to initiate reentry (Fig. 11): (1) a predetermined anatomic circuit must exist; (2) unidirectional block (e.g., due to an extrastimulus) must occur in one limb of the reentrant circuit; with (3) slow conduction in a contiguous pathway of the circuit, allowing recovery of excitability of the previously refractory limb; and (4) the wavelength of the impulse must be shorter than the length of the circuit *(8,26)*.

The concept of wavelength is inherent in the anatomical model of reentry. The leading edge of the wave must encounter excitable tissue in which to propagate. Therefore, the rotation *time* around the reentrant circuit must be longer than the recovery period of all segments of the circuit and the *length* of the circuit must exceed the product of the conduction velocity and the recovery period of the tissue (Fig. 12A). Interruption of the anatomical circuit at any point interrupts reentry.

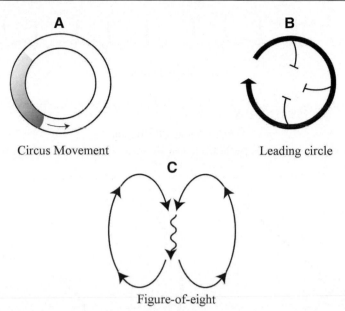

Fig. 12. (A) Circus movement reentry. The impulse (gray region) must be shorter than the entire length of the circuit (circle) and travel at a rate slow enough to allow separation of the impulse from its own refractory tail. This interval (depicted as white) is called the *excitable gap*. Reentry will be extinguished if the leading edge of the impulse (black) impinges on its tail (gray). (B) Model of leading circle reentry. Reentry follows the smallest possible circuit with tissue at the vortex remaining inexcitable. No anatomical barrier is present. (C) Figure eight reentry in anisotropic cardiac muscle. Two reentrant circuits rotate in opposite directions sharing a central common pathway.

FUNCTIONAL REENTRY

The mechanisms of most reentrant arrhythmias confined to the atria or ventricles appear to be more complex than anatomical reentry. It has become apparent that reentry may be sustained even in the absence of a specific anatomical circuit and in the absence of abnormal myocardium. This type of reentry is termed *functional*.

The *leading circle* hypothesis of reentry accounts for reentry in the absence of an anatomic obstacle. Reentry follows the smallest possible circuit with tissue at the vortex remaining inexcitable (Fig. 12B) *(8)*. The propagating wave must penetrate tissue that remains relatively refractory. Thus, the circuit is much smaller than the circuit in anatomical reentry and no portion of the circuit is ever fully recovered (i.e., there is no *excitable gap*). It is unclear whether leading circle reentry is responsible for clinical arrhythmias.

Propagation of impulses in cardiac tissue is dependent on myocyte fiber orientation. Cell-to-cell communication depends primarily on gap junction proteins that are unequally distributed along the cell surface. The greater density of gap junction proteins along the longitudinal axis (as compared with the transverse axis) accounts for more rapid conduction in this direction. However, the longitudinal axis is associated with a lower safety factor of conduction (i.e., longer refractory period). The differential conduction properties in the longitudinal and transverse directions provide a substrate for *anisotropic* reentry. Anisotropy may account for arrhythmias in the atria, AV node, and the peri-infarct regions of myocardium *(27)*.

Figure-eight reentry may be considered an "extension" of leading circle reentry (that also incorporates anatomic reentry), in which two reentrant circuits rotate in opposite directions in close proximity to one another utilizing a central common pathway (Fig. 12C). This mechanism may underlie sustained monomorphic ventricular tachycardia observed in patients with ischemic heart

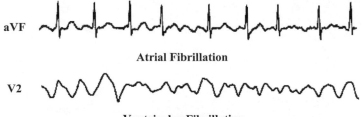

aVF

Atrial Fibrillation

V2

Ventricular Fibrillation

Fig. 13. Atrial fibrillation and ventricular fibrillation are examples of clinical arrhythmias that can be caused by spiral wave reentry.

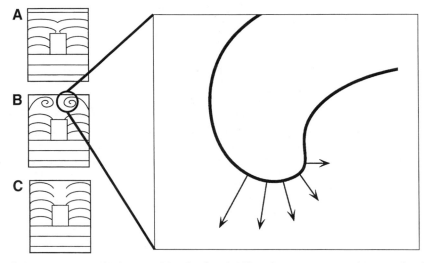

Fig. 14. Spiral wave reentry. (**A**) At normal levels of excitability, the wave separates into two daughter waves that circumnavigate the borders of the obstacle and fuse again at the opposite side. No wave-break occurs. (**B**) At lower levels of excitability, the broken wavefront curves and initiates a pair of counter-rotating spiral waves. The inset depicts propagation velocity along the curved wavefront of a spiral wave. The more pronounced the curvature, the slower the conduction velocity (small arrows). Toward the periphery, conduction velocity reaches the maximum (large arrows). (**C**) Finally, at lower levels of excitability, the broken wavefronts are unable to rotate, propagating decrementally until they disappear. (Used with permission from ref. *8*.)

disease. Unlike other forms of functional reentry, figure-of-eight reentry depends on a central common pathway between the rotating reentrant waves that is delimited by unexcitable tissue. Disruption of this central pathway effectively terminates reentry.

Spiral waves represent the most complex form of functional reentry and are believed to be a possible underlying mechanism for some forms of atrial and ventricular fibrillation (Fig. 13). In its simplest form, spiral wave reentry may be depicted as a broken wave front that curls at its broken end and begins to rotate (Fig. 14) *(8)*. The wave propagates through cardiac muscle but is interrupted by an obstacle such as a scar. When the obstacle causes a break in the wavefront, several outcomes are possible depending on the excitability of the tissue. When excitability is high after passing the obstacle, the broken ends will fuse rapidly. When excitability is lower, the broken ends cannot fuse but begin to spiral. The trajectory of each point on the wave varies according to the curvature of the wave: the greater the curvature, the slower the conduction velocity. The variable excitability of cardiac muscle compounds the complexity of propagation. When excitability of the tissue is further reduced, propagation of the wavefront is extinguished.

Finally, reentry may occur in a linear circuit in the absence of even a functional loop (Fig. 15). An example of this form of reentry, termed *reflection*, may be seen when local injury occurs over

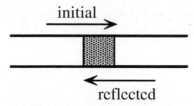

initial

reflected

Fig. 15. Model of reflection. *See* text for explanation. Used with permission from ref. *8*.

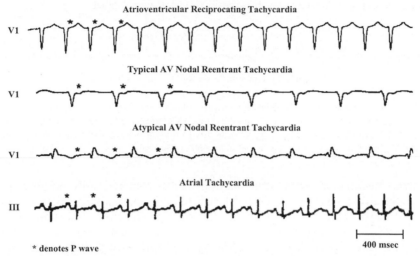

Fig. 16. Typical AV nodal reentrant tachycardia demonstrates a short RP' interval on the surface ECG. Similarly, orthodromic atrioventricular reciprocating tachycardia is characterized by a short RP' interval. Atrial tachycardias and atypical AV nodal reentrant tachycardia are characterized by a long RP' interval.

a short portion of the His-Purkinje fibers. In this model, reentry occurs over a single pathway and depends on the presence of a region of severely impaired (but not blocked) conduction *(8)*. The impulse propagates toward the region of depressed conduction, but the damaged cells are incapable of being excited and the action potential is unable to propagate further. However, a small current is generated across these cells, and if the distance across the gap is relatively small, current may reach the distal segment and bring those cells to threshold, where propagation of an action potential can be initiated. If there is sufficient delay in propagation of the current to the distal side of the gap, the distal action potential may be reflected backward across the gap, reinitiating (or reflecting) an action potential.

Clinical Correlates. Most clinical supraventricular and ventricular arrhythmias are due to reentry. In this section we describe the most common reentrant arrhythmias. The surface electrocardiogram (ECG) provides important clues to the mechanism of reentrant tachycardias (Fig. 16). Supraventricular tachycardias due to AV node reentry or an accessory AV pathway will typically have a short RP' interval (i.e., the interval between the P wave on surface ECG and the preceding R wave, denoted as the RP' interval <50% of the RR interval). Conversely, supraventricular tachycardias such as atrial tachycardias, the atypical form of AV node reentry (discussed below), and the permanent form of junctional reciprocating tachycardia (a reentrant SVT due to a slowly conducting retrograde accessory pathway) typically demonstrate a long RP' interval (≤50% of the RR interval). When evaluating wide complex tachycardia, dissociation of the surface ECG P waves from the QRS complexes supports the diagnosis of ventricular tachycardia (Fig. 17). However, a 1:1 relationship between the P waves and QRS complexes may be observed in ventricular tachycardia or supraventricular tachycardia conducted with a wide QRS complex.

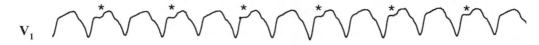

Ventricular Tachycardia with 2:1 Retrograde Conduction

Fig. 17. Dissociation of the P waves from the QRS complexes, or variable retrograde conduction to the atria, strongly supports the diagnostic of ventricular tachycardia. This is demonstrated in the figure. However, a 1:1 relationship of P waves to QRS complexes during a wide complex tachycardia may be due to either ventricular tachycardia with 1:1 retrograde conduction to the atria, *or* a supraventricular tachycardia with 1:1 anterograde conduction to the ventricles in a patient with a preexisting bundle branch block.

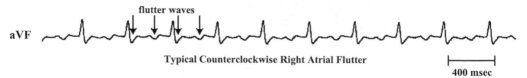

Typical Counterclockwise Right Atrial Flutter

Fig. 18. Typical counterclockwise right atrial flutter is often characterized by 2:1 ventricular response and a ventricular rate of 150 beats/min. Flutter waves on the surface ECG are usually negative in the inferior leads (II, III, aVF), as atrial activation proceeds down the right atrial free-wall and up the interatrial septum, activating the interatrial septum and left atrium in a caudal to cranial sequence.

Intraatrial Reentry. Intraatrial reentrant tachycardias comprise a diverse group of arrhythmias. Reentrant arrhythmias may occur anywhere in the atria, and may affect persons with or without structural heart disease. Because areas of scar tissue typically provide the substrate for reentry, these tachycardias have been called *incisional reentrant tachycardias (28)*. Another common form of intraatrial reentry is atrial flutter (Fig. 18). The "typical" form of atrial flutter occurs at a remarkably consistent rate of 250 to 300 beats/min with propagation proceeding counterclockwise around the tricuspid valve annulus, down the free wall of the right atrium, and up the interatrial septum. When conduction proceeds up the interatrial septum, the caudal–cranial activation inscribes the superiorly directed flutter waves (i.e., negative in the inferior leads) observed on the surface ECG. Clockwise, or "atypical," right atrial flutter (in the opposite direction) is less common.

Most intraatrial reentrant tachycardias are not responsive to adenosine, β-blockers, or calcium-channel blockers *(5)*. Over the past decade, electrophysiologists have made substantial progress in mapping and ablating reentrant atrial tachycardias. As with all reentrant arrhythmias, disruption of any part of the circuit will terminate tachycardia. For example, both the typical and atypical forms of flutter depend on a critical isthmus of slow conduction at the base of the right atrium. Creating a linear ablation lesion extending from the tricuspid valve annulus to the inferior vena cava blocks conduction across this isthmus and effectively eliminates tachycardia.

AV Nodal Reentrant Tachycardia. Excluding atrial flutter and fibrillation, typical AV nodal reentrant tachycardia is the single most common form of supraventricular tachycardia and accounts for nearly 50 to 60% of all sustained SVTs in adults *(29,30)*. Usually, it presents before age 40, and SVT rates typically range from 160 to 200 beats/min but may vary greatly (from 100 to 300 beats/min). The reentrant circuit is limited to the peri-AV nodal region, with anterograde conduction proceeding over a "slow" pathway and retrograde conduction traversing a "fast" pathway (Fig. 19) *(31)*. In the usual case, the fast pathway has a longer refractory period than the slow pathway. Therefore, initiation of reentry occurs when a premature atrial beat blocks in the fast pathway and is conducted over the slow pathway. By the time the impulse reaches the distal portion of the slow pathway, the retrograde fast pathway has regained excitability and is able to conduct the impulse to the atrium, perpetuating the arrhythmia by engaging and activating the slow anterograde pathway. The atypical form of AV nodal reentry activates these limbs in the opposite direction; anterograde conduction proceeds over the fast pathway and retrograde conduction across the slow pathway. As one would predict, the typical form of AV nodal reentry (with retrograde conduction up the fast pathway) is characterized by a short RP' interval on the surface ECG while atypical AV nodal reentry inscribes

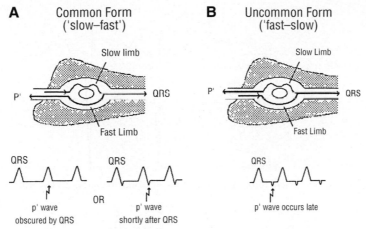

Fig. 19. Schematic drawing of AV nodal reentrant tachycardia. Illustrations depict two forms of supraventricular tachycardia due to reentry within the AV node. *See* text for details. (Used with permission from ref. *31*.)

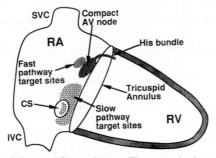

Fig. 20. Anatomical positions of slow and fast pathways. The posterior location of the "slow" pathway, remote from the compact AV node, makes it the target of choice for radiofrequency catheter ablation. (Used with permission from ref. *35*.)

a long RP' interval (Fig. 19). An electrophysiologic hallmark of AV nodal reentry is that neither the atria nor ventricles are necessary parts of the reentrant circuit.

Adenosine is effective in terminating reentrant tachycardias that involve the AV node, and is mediated by activation of the outward potassium current $I_{K(Ado, ACh)}$, which hyperpolarizes the AV node to about −90 mV and abbreviates the action potential. Adenosine can terminate tachycardia in either limb, but it occurs most often in the slow pathway (*32,33*). Vagal maneuvers (carotid sinus massage or Valsalva) also terminate AV nodal-dependent reentry by activating the same outward potassium current $I_{K(Ado, ACh)}$.

The slow pathway is located in the region of the posteroseptal space of the interatrial septum and is readily amenable to ablation (>95% success rate; Fig. 20) (*34,35*). This location, remote from the compact AV node, minimizes the chance of AV node damage during ablation. Ablation of the fast pathway also effectively treats AV nodal reentry but carries a relatively high risk of complete heart block.

Atrioventricular Reciprocating Tachycardia. Reentrant arrhythmias utilizing an accessory AV connection comprise the second most common form of regular narrow complex tachycardias (approx 35% of SVTs). Accessory pathways are composed of muscular bridges along the tricuspid and mitral valve annuli that provide an abnormal electrical connection between the atria and ventricles. The electrophysiologic properties of most accessory pathways resemble those of normal atrial tissue. Because the resting membrane potential is approx −90 mV, typically, accessory pathways are insensitive to vagal maneuvers, adenosine, and Ca^{2+} channel blockers.

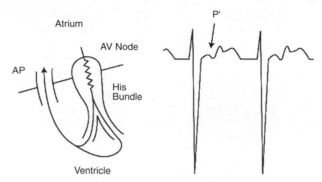

Fig. 21. Schematic of orthodromic atrioventricular reentrant tachycardia.

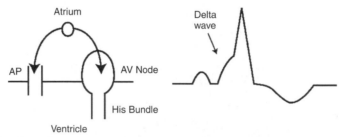

Fig. 22. Schematic of Wolff-Parkinson-White syndrome during normal sinus rhythm. Conduction over the accessory pathway (AP) activates the ventricle simultaneously with conduction over the AV node. Preexcitation of the ventricles by the accessory pathway creates the delta wave visible on the surface ECG.

Most accessory pathways conduct only in one direction—retrogradely from the ventricles to the atria—and are therefore concealed during sinus rhythm (Fig. 21). Conversely, accessory pathways with anterograde conduction properties usually result in ventricular preexcitation (known as Wolff-Parkinson-White syndrome). During sinus rhythm, conduction proceeds simultaneously down the AV node and accessory pathway (Fig. 22). Preexcitation of the ventricles by the accessory pathway inscribes a delta wave visible on the surface ECG that prolongs the QRS complex. Typically, the PR interval is abbreviated (<120 ms) owing to rapid conduction over the accessory pathway. Orthodromic reciprocating tachycardia (anterograde conduction over the AV node and retrograde conduction across the accessory pathway) accounts for 90% of reentrant arrhythmias in patients with Wolff-Parkinson-White syndrome. This arrhythmia may degenerate into atrial fibrillation; then conduction would proceed anterogradely over the accessory pathway. Atrial fibrillation in patients with Wolff-Parkinson-White syndrome may precipitate ventricular fibrillation because of rapid conduction over the accessory pathway. A less common arrhythmia, antidromic reciprocating tachycardia (the anterograde limb being the accessory pathway and the retrograde limb being the AV node), inscribes a wide QRS complex on the surface ECG.

Reentry utilizing an accessory pathway is initiated by an atrial or ventricular premature beat. For example, a premature atrial beat may encounter an accessory pathway that has not recovered excitability from the previous beat and thus can conduct only over the AV node and through the His-Purkinje system. When the impulse reaches the ventricular input of the accessory pathway it may engage the pathway, with conduction proceeding to the atrium, thus completing the reentrant circuit.

Ventricular Reentrant Arrhythmias. Most ventricular arrhythmias occur in patients with a prior history of myocardial infarction. Experimental evidence suggests that mechanism of the tachycardia may be dependent upon the time of the infarct. Within the first 30 to 60 min (early phase) following an acute myocardial infarction, the intracellular and extracellular milieus appear to favor reentrant ventricular arrhythmias, as does autonomic tone *(36)*. Automatic idioventricular

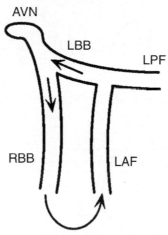

Fig. 23. Bundle branch reentry circuit, utilizing the left anterior fascicle (LAF) as the retrograde limb of the circuit, and the right bundle branch (RBB) as the anterograde limb. AVN, atrioventricular node; LBB, left bundle branch; LPF, left posteror fascicle. (Used with permission from ref. 8.)

rhythms, with rates typically between 60 and 120 bpm, are usually observed within the first 6 to 10 h (delayed phase). After the relatively quiescent second phase, the third and final stage of ventricular arrhythmias (late phase) begins within 48 to 72 h after infarct and is characterized by rapid monomorphic tachycardias, owing to reentry arising in the peri-infarct border zone. Inhomogeneous conduction properties of the peri-infarction tissue create regions of slow and rapid conduction, causing anisotropic and figure eight reentry. The risk of reentrant late-phase ventricular arrhythmias persists indefinitely following myocardial infarction and is thought to account for at least half of all deaths among myocardial infarction survivors. Electrophysiologic studies and endocardial mapping in humans have demonstrated that monomorphic VT that occurs late after a myocardial infarction is caused by areas of slow conduction and diastolic activation. These arrhythmias may be induced or terminated with pacing maneuvers, supporting the idea that reentry originating from the border zone of the infarcted myocardium is the mechanism of tachycardia.

Another example of reentrant ventricular tachycardia occurring in patients with heart disease is bundle branch reentrant VT. This example of anatomic reentry is usually observed in patients with diseased His-Purkinje system function, complete or incomplete left bundle branch block during sinus rhythm, and a nonischemic dilated cardiomyopathy. The incidence of bundle branch reentry as the cause of sustained monomorphic ventricular tachycardia ranges from less than 1% to 6% *(37)*; this form of VT most often has a left bundle branch block, left superior axis morphology. It is typically initiated by a ventricular premature beat that follows a pause. The premature impulse blocks in the retrograde direction within the right bundle but conducts retrogradely up the left bundle. When it reaches the His bundle it is able to engage the right bundle in the anterograde direction and then continues back to the left bundle (Fig. 23). It is important to recognize this form of tachycardia since it is readily curable by radiofrequency catheter ablation of the right bundle.

Functional reentry is responsible for the initiation of ventricular arrhythmias in patients with Brugada syndrome. These patients, first described in 1992 *(38)*, present with an ECG pattern of right bundle branch block, right precordial downsloping ST segment elevation (leads V1–V3) with a normal QTc interval, and have no evidence of structural heart disease. ST segment elevation is due to relatively early epicardial repolarization with respect to the endocardium, and results from greater expression I_{to} and I_{ks} in the epicardium. There is evidence that Brugada syndrome is a primary electrical disease, and in some families it has been linked to mutations causing loss of function in a sodium channel (SCN5A) *(39)*. This results in a outward shift of the balance of current at the end of phase 1 of the action potential, leading to the loss of the action potential dome. The subsequent abbreviation

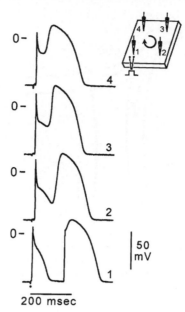

Fig. 24. Phase 2 reentry in a canine epicardial preparation exposed to simulated ischemia. The action potential develops a normal dome (phase 2) only at site 4. The dome then propagates in a clockwise direction, reexciting sites 3, 2, and 1 with progressive delays, generating a reentrant extrasystole. (Used with permission from ref. *40*.)

of the action potential at some epicardial sites (but not others) leads to the substrate for phase 2 reentry. Phase 2 reentry has been studied in a canine model of simulated ischemia (Fig. 24) *(40)*.

REFERENCES

1. Ackerman MJ, Clapham DE. Ion channels—basic science and clinical disease. N Engl J Med 1997;336:1575–1586.
2. Ackerman MJ, Clapham DE. Normal cardiac electrophysiology. In: Chien K, ed. Molecular Basis of Cardiovascular Disease. W. B. Saunders, Philadelphia, 1999, pp. 281–301.
3. Surawicz B. Normal and abnormal automaticity. In: Rosen MR, Janse MJ, Wit AL, eds. Cardiac Electrophysiology: A Textbook. Futura Publishing, Mount Kisco, NY, 1990, pp. 159–173.
4. Lerman BB, Stein KM, Markowitz SM. Adenosine-sensitive ventricular tachycardia: a conceptual approach. J Cardiovasc Electrophysiol 1996;7:559–569.
5. Markowitz SM, Stein KM, Mittal S, et al. Differential effects of adenosine on focal and macroreentrant atrial tachycardia. J Cardiovasc Electrophysiol 1999;10:489–502.
6. DiFrancesco D, Angoni M, Maccaferri G. The pacemaker current in cardiac cells. In: Zipes DP, Jalife J, eds. Cardiac Electrophysiology: From Cell to Bedside. W. B. Saunders, Philadelphia, 1995, pp. 96–103.
7. Lerman BB. Response of nonreentrant catecholamine-mediated ventricular tachycardia to endogenous adenosine and acetylcholine. Evidence for myocardial receptor-mediated effects. Circulation 1993;87:382–390.
8. Jalife J, Delmar M, Davidenko J, et al. Basic Cardiac Electrophysiology for the Clinician. Futura Publishing, Armonk, NY, 1999.
9. Curran ME, Sanguinetti MC, Keating MT. Molecular basis of inherited cardiac arrhythmias. In: Chien K, ed. Molecular Basis of Cardiovascular Disease. W. B. Saunders, Philadelphia, 1999, pp. 302–311.
10. Jervell A, Lange-Nielsen F. Congenital deaf-mutism, functional heart disease with prolongation of the QT interval, and sudden death. Am Heart J 1957;54:59–68.
11. Romano C, Gemme G, Pongiglione R. Aritmie cardiache rare dell'eta'pediatrica. II. Accessi sincopali per fibrillazione ventricolare parossistica. Clin Pediatr (Bologna) 1963;45:656–683.
12. Ward OC. A new familial cardiac syndrome in children. J Ir Med Assoc 1964;54:103–106.
13. Glaaser IW, Kass RS, Clancy CE. Mechanisms of genetic arrhythmias: from DNA to ECG. Prog Cardiovasc Dis 2003; 46:259–270.
14. Keating MT. The long QT syndrome: a review of recent molecular genetic and physiologic discoveries. Medicine 1996;75:1–5.
15. Schwartz PJ, Moss AJ, Vincent GM, et al. Diagnostic criteria for the long QT syndrome. An update. Circulation 1993; 88:782–784.

16. Luo CH, Rudy Y. A dynamic model of the cardiac ventricular action potential. II. Afterdepolarizations, triggered activity, and potentiation. Circ Res 1994;74:1097–1113.

17. Han X, Ferrier GR. Contribution of Na^+-Ca^{2+} exchange to stimulation of transient inward current by isoproterenol in rabbit cardiac Purkinje fibers. Circ Res 1995;76:664–674.

18. Lerman BB, Belardinelli L, West GA, et al. Adenosine-sensitive ventricular tachycardia: evidence suggesting cyclic AMP-mediated triggered activity. Circulation 1986;74:270–280.

19. Lerman BB, Stein K, Engelstein ED, et al. Mechanism of repetitive monomorphic ventricular tachycardia. Circulation 1995;92:421–429.

20. Lerman BB, Stein KM, Markowitz SM. Mechanisms of idiopathic left ventricular tachycardia. J Cardiovasc Electrophysiol 1997;8:571–583.

21. Cheung JW, Lerman BB. CVT-510: a selective A1 adenosine receptor agonist. Cardiovasc Drug Rev 2003;21:277–292.

22. Lerman BB, Stein KM, Markowitz SM, et al. Catecholamine-facilitated reentrant ventricular tachycardia: uncoupling of adenosine's antiadrenergic effects. J Cardiovasc Electrophysiol 1999;10:17–26.

23. Priori SG, Napolitano CN, Tiso N, et al. Mutations in the cardiac ryanodine receptor gene (hRyR2) underlie catecholaminergic polymorphic ventricular tachycardia. Circulation 2001;103:196–200.

24. Laitinen PJ, Brown DM, Piippo K, et al. Mutations of the cardiac ryanodine receptor (RyR2) gene in familial polymorphic ventricular tachycardia. Circulation 2001;103:485–490.

25. Laitinen PJ, Swan H, Kontula K. Molecular genetics of exercise-induced polymorphic ventricular tachycardia: identification of three novel cardiac ryanodine receptor mutations and two common calsequestrin 2 amino-acid polymorphisms. Eur J Hum Genet 2003;11:888–891.

26. Prystowsky EN, Klein GJ. Mechanism of tachycardia. In: Prystowsky E, Klein G, eds. Cardiac Arrhythmias: An Integrated Approach for the Clinician. McGraw-Hill, New York, 1994, pp. 81–95.

27. Spach MS, Dolber PC, Heidlage JF. Influence of the passive anisotropic properties on directional differences in propagation following modification of the sodium conductance in human atrial muscle. A model of reentry based on anisotropic discontinuous propagation. Circ Res 1988;62:811–832.

28. Lesh MD, Kalman JM. To fumble flutter or tackle "tach"? Toward updated classifiers for atrial tachyarrhythmias. J Cardiovasc Electrophysiol 1996;7:460–466.

29. Josephson ME, Kastor JA. Supraventricular tachycardia: mechanisms and management. Ann Intern Med 1977;87:346–358.

30. Wu D, Denes P. Mechanisms of paroxysmal supraventricular tachycardia. Arch Intern Med 1975;135:437–442.

31. Benditt D, Reyes W, Gornick C, et al. Supraventricular tachycardias: recognition and treatment. In: Naccarelli G, ed. Cardiac Arrhythmias: A Practical Approach. Futura, Mount Kisco, NY, 1991, pp. 135–176.

32. DiMarco JP, Sellers TD, Lerman BB, et al. Diagnostic and therapeutic use of adenosine in patients with supraventricular tachyarrhythmias. J Am Coll Cardiol 1985;6:417–425.

33. Lerman BB, Greenberg M, Overholt ED, et al. Differential electrophysiologic properties of decremental retrograde pathways in long RP' tachycardia. Circulation 1987;76:21–31.

34. Calkins H, Yong P, Miller JM, et al. Catheter ablation of accessory pathways, atrioventricular nodal reentrant tachycardia, and the atrioventricular junction: final results of a prospective, multicenter clinical trial. Circulation 1999;99:262–270.

35. Kalbfleisch SJ, Morady F. Catheter ablation of atrioventricular nodal reentrant tachycardia. In: Zipes D, Jalife J, eds. Cardiac Electrophysiology: From Cell to Bedside. W. B. Saunders, Philadelphia, 1995, pp. 1477.

36. Scherlag BJ, el-Sherif N, Hope R, et al. Characterization and localization of ventricular arrhythmias resulting from myocardial ischemia and infarction. Circ Res 1974;35:372–383.

37. Caceres J, Jazayeri M, McKinnie J, et al. Sustained bundle branch reentry as a mechanism of clinical tachycardia. Circulation 1989;79:256–270.

38. Brugada P, Brugada J. Right bundle branch block, persistent ST segment elevation and sudden cardiac death: a distinct clinical and electrocardiographic syndrome. J Am Coll Cardiol 1992;20:1391–1396.

39. Chen Q, Kirsch G, Zhang D, et al. Genetic basis and molecular mechanism for idiopathic ventricular fibrillation. Nature 1998;392:293–296.

40. Lukas A, Antzelevitch C. Phase 2 reentry as a mechanism of initiation of circus movement reentry in canine epicardium exposed to simulated ischemia. Cardiovasc Res 1996;32:593–603.

RECOMMENDED READING

Ackerman MJ, Clapham DE. Ion channels—basic science and clinical disease. N Engl J Med 1997;336:1575–1586.

Lerman BB, Stein KM, Markowitz SM, et al. Ventricular arrhythmias in normal hearts. Cardiol Clin 2000;18:265–291.

Glaaser IW, Kass RS, Clancy CE. Mechanisms of genetic arrhythmias: from DNA to ECG. Prog Cardiovasc Dis 2003; 46:259–270.

Zipes DP, Jalife F, eds. Cardiac Electrophysiology: From Cell to Bedside, 3rd ed. W. B. Saunders, Philadelphia, 2000, chapters 40, 70, 72, and 94.

Jalife J, Delmar M, Davidenko J, et al. Basic Cardiac Electrophysiology for the Clinician. Futura Publishing, Armonk, NY, 1999.

17   Treatment of Cardiac Arrhythmias

Davendra Mehta, MD, PhD

TACHYARRHYTHMIAS

The management of cardiac arrhythmias has been revolutionized by the use of new diagnostic and therapeutic modalities. The development and advancement of both pharmacologic and nonpharmacologic therapies, particularly radiofrequency catheter ablation and new implantable devices, have resulted in better treatment, suppression, and frequently cure of otherwise recalcitrant and life-threatening cardiac arrhythmias. Furthermore, catheter ablation has also helped to better elucidate the pathophysiology of these arrhythmias. For the purpose of this chapter, the management of cardiac arrhythmias is divided into that of tachyarrhythmias and bradyarrhythmias. Tachyarrhythmias are managed by antiarrhythmic drugs, radiofrequency catheter ablation, and implantable devices. Bradyarrhythmias are treated mainly by pacemakers.

SUPRAVENTRICULAR ARRHYTHMIAS

Sinus Tachycardia

Pathological sinus tachycardia is caused by extracardiac stresses such as fever, hypotension, anemia, thyrotoxicosis, hypovolemia, pulmonary emboli, shock, or increased cardiac demands related to myocardial infarction or congestive heart failure. Drugs such as atropine, caffeine, nicotine, isoproterenol, thyroid hormones, and aminophylline can cause sinus tachycardia. Inappropriate sinus tachycardia is defined as sinus tachycardia without any obvious cause (1). It is a nonparoxysmal condition and usually presents as an inappropriate high resting sinus rate and a marked increase in rate with minimal activity. It is often accompanied by an anxiety disorder and mitral valve prolapse syndrome. Although the mechanism remains undefined, imbalance between sympathetic and parasympathetic controls are thought to be one of the contributing factors (1).

The therapy for appropriate sinus tachycardia involves treatment of the primary condition such as infections by antibiotics, hypotension with fluid replacement, and thyrotoxicosis by β-blockers and antithyroid drugs. Management of inappropriate sinus tachycardia is more difficult. β-Blocker therapy is the first line of therapy and often results in control of sinus rate and associated symptoms. In patients with contraindications for the use of β-blockers, calcium-channel blockers such as verapamil or diltiazem are useful. In patients who are nonresponsive to β-blockers and calcium-channel blockers, modification of the sinoatrial node with radiofrequency catheter ablation results in slowing of the sinus node. Catheter ablation for sinus node modification is associated with a small risk of patients requiring permanent pacemakers. Although sinus node modification has high initial success rate, there is a high incidence of recurrence.

Sinus Node Reentry Tachycardia

Sinus node reentry accounts for less than 5% of patients with supraventricular tachycardias. It is usually associated with structural heart disease, and at times with AV nodal reentry tachycardia. The

From: *Essential Cardiology: Principles and Practice, 2nd Ed.*
Edited by: C. Rosendorff © Humana Press Inc., Totowa, NJ

diagnosis is suggested when the P waves during tachycardia are identical to the P waves in sinus rhythm and have similar relationship to QRS complex, and further by an abrupt termination of the tachycardia. The diagnosis is firmly established at electrophysiology study *(2)*. Sinus node reentry tachycardia can be terminated by intravenous adenosine, verapamil, or β-blockers. Oral therapy with calcium-channel blockers and β-blockers can be used to prevent recurrent episodes. Radio-frequency catheter ablation is highly effective in treating sinus node reentry *(3)*. A permanent pacemaker is usually not required, as lesions in the area of the sinus node result in modification of the node without loss of sinus node automaticity. The risk of complete loss of sinus node function with radiofrequency catheter ablation is indeed minimal.

Atrial Tachycardia

Atrial tachycardias can be related to automaticity, reentry, or triggered activity *(4)*. The atrial rate of these tachycardias is usually between 150 and 200 beats/min *(5)*. The morphology of the P wave is dependent on the site of origin of tachycardia and is usually located in the second half of the RR interval (long RP interval). These tachycardias are often associated with structural heart disease such as cardiomyopathy, cor pulmonale, or previous myocardial infarction. It is important to realize that persistent atrial tachycardia can lead to tachycardia-induced cardiomyopathy, and should be considered in any patient with atrial tachycardia and dilated cardiomyopathy *(6)*. Treatment of tachycardia leads to complete recovery of left ventricular function. Digitalis intoxication should always be considered as the diagnosis in patients with atrial tachycardia and AV block *(7)*.

Management involves treatment of the underlying condition, such as heart failure, cor pulmonale, or digoxin intoxication. In patients with persistent tachycardia and fast ventricular rate, β-blockers or calcium-channel blockers can be used to decrease ventricular response. Class Ia, Ic, or III drugs can be used in an attempt to terminate the tachycardia (Table 1). The choice of drugs is based on left ventricular function; in patients with impaired left ventricular function, class Ia and Ic antiarrhythmic drugs should be avoided because of a high risk of proarrhythmia. Sotalol is used if left ventricular function is normal or only mildly impaired. Amiodarone is the drug of choice in the presence of moderate to severe left ventricular dysfunction. Dofetilide, a newer antiarrhythmic agent (class III), is also an alternative and can be used in patients with heart failure *(8)*. If no reversible etiology is identifiable, radiofrequency catheter ablation is the treatment of choice for recurrent atrial tachycardias.

Junctional Tachycardia (AV Nodal and AV Reentry Tachycardia)

The two important causes of junctional tachycardia are AV nodal reentry and AV bypass tracts. These are the most frequent etiologies for regular narrow complex tachycardia; others include atrial tachycardia and atril flutter. Atrial flutter with 2:1 block should also be considered when the ventricular rate is 140 to 160 beats/min.

Acute Management

Acute management initially involves a trial with a vagal maneuver, the Valsalva maneuver being the most effective. Attempted in supine position soon after the onset of supraventricular tachycardia, 70% of supraventricular tachycardias terminate with the Valsalva maneuver *(9)*. Drugs used for acute termination include intravenous adenosine, verapamil, and diltiazem. As adenosine has a half-life of 3 to 5 s, it has become the treatment of choice *(10)*. It is given as a rapid bolus of 6 mg; if this is unsuccessful, 12 mg can be given. Lower doses should be used in younger patients or those on dipyridamole therapy, as dipyradamole inhibits its breakdown. Higher doses are needed in patients with a slow circulation time, left-to-right shunting of blood, and those who are on therapy with methylxanthines. Transient side effects include flushing, chest discomfort, difficulty in breathing, and AV block. Adenosine should be avoided in patients with bronchial asthma because of the risk of bronchospasm. Instead, intravenous verapamil or diltiazem should be used. Adenosine can be used safely in patients on other cardiac medications such as digoxin, β-blockers, calcium-channel

Table 1
Vaughan-Williams Classification of Antiarrhythmic Drugs

Table 1
Vaughan-Williams Classification of Antiarrhythmic Drugs

Class I (drugs that predominantly inhibit the fast sodium channel)
Ia
Procainamide
Quinidine
Ib
Lidocaine
Mexeletine
Ic
Flecainide
Propafenone

Class II (β-adrenergic antagonists)
Cardioselective
Metoprolol
Atenolol
Acebutalol
Nonselective
Propranolol
Nadolol
Pindolol
Timolol

Class III (primarily act on potassium channels and prolong repolarization)
Used intravenously
Ibutalide
Used orally
Sotalol (also has class II action)
Amiodarone (also has class I, II and IV action)
Dofetilide

Class IV (calcium-channel antagonists)
Diltiazem
Verapamil

blockers, and ACE inhibitors. It is effective in terminating 98% of supraventricular tachycardias caused by AV nodal reentry and AV bypass tracts. Use of adenosine in atrial tachcyardias typically leads to atrioventricular block with persistent tachycardia; however about 40% of atrial tachy-cardias are also terminated with adenosine. In patients in whom atrial flutter is suspected, adenosine is useful in confirming the diagnosis as it increases AV block and thus flutter waves can be distinctly identified.

Chronic Suppression

Table 2 lists the drugs used for chronic suppression of supraventricular tachycardias (11). Digoxin by itself has a limited role. In patients in whom the AV node is part of the reentrant circuit (AV nodal reentry, AV reentry tachycardia with accessory pathway) the initial therapy should be an AV nodal blocking agent such as a β-blocker or calcium-channel blocker. Class I and II antiarrhyth-mic drugs are used only in patients who fail to respond to AV nodal blocking agents. For supraven-tricular tachycardias not involving the AV node, AV nodal blocking agents may slow the ventricular response, but are not suppressive. In such patients procainamide (class Ib), flecainide (class Ic), propafenone (class Ic), amiodarone (class III), dofetilide (class III), or sotalol (class III) can be used for arrhythmia suppression. The choice of appropriate therapeutic approach is made after a detailed assessment of the clinical condition relative to the mechanism of arrhythmia and the pres-ence or absence of heart disease. A class Ic agent such as flecainide is the treatment of choice in

Table 2
Medical Treatment of Supraventricular Tachycardia

	Dose	Efficacy	Precautions/side effects
Acute conversion (used intravenously)			
1. Verapamil	5–12 mg	>85%	Avoid in wide complex tachycardia
2. Diltiazem	17–25 mg	>85%	Avoid in wide complex tachycardia
3. Adenosine	6–18 mg	95%	Less in patients on dipyridamole
4. ATP	6–30 mg	>90%	Similar to adenosine
5. Esmolol	35–50 mg	50%	Caution in bronchial asthma and hypotension
6. Propranolol	4–16 mg	50%	Similar to esmolol
7. Amiodarone	300 mg	80%	Delayed onset of action
Chronic suppression (oral therapy)			
1. Verapamil	240–480 mg	>70%	Bradycardia and hypotension
2. Diltiazem	90–270 mg	60%	Bradycardia and hypotension
3. Nadolol	80–160 mg	>60%	β-Blocker side effects
4. Procainamide	1–2 g	>60%	Proarrhythmic, causes hypotension
5. Flecainide	200–300 mg	>70%	Highly proarrhythmic
6. Propafenone	450–900 mg	>75%	Proarrhythmic and has β-blocker effects
7. Sotalol	240–320 mg	>70%	β-Blocker effects and prolongs QT interval
8. Amiodarone	200–600 mg	75%	Cumulative action

patients with resistant supraventricular tachycardia due to an accessory pathway. Their sodium channel properties serve to selectively block conduction in accessory pathways. Class III drugs, with their potassium channel blocking action that prolongs the atrial refractory period, are also highly effective for suppression of atrial arrhythmias such as atrial tachycardia, atrial flutter, and fibrillation *(11)*.

The Cardiac Arrhythmia Suppression Trial (CAST) and other antiarrhythmic trials have shown an increased risk of ventricular proarrhythmia with the use of class I antiarrhythmic drugs in patients with prior myocardial infarction *(12)*. Thus the use of class I antiarrhythmic agents for the treatment of supraventricular arrhythmias should be restricted to patients without a history of myocardial infarction or left ventricular dysfunction. In patients with a history of coronary artery disease, myocardial infarction, left ventricular dysfunction, or ventricular hypertrophy, supraventricular tachycardia is treated with the class III agents sotalol or amiodarone, as they are less likely to lead to ventricular proarrhythmia and increase mortality in these high-risk populations. As catheter ablation is a safe and effective therapy, when given the choice of long-term drug therapy and its potential toxicity compared with catheter ablation, the majority of the patients prefer the latter.

Radiofrequency Catheter Ablation

Radiofrequency catheter ablation is the treatment of choice for long-term management of supraventricular tachycardias. Most supraventricular tachycardias including AV nodal reentry tachycardia, AV reentry tachycardia due to accessory pathway, all types of atrial flutter, intraatrial reentry tachycardia, sinoatrial reentry, and automatic atrial tachycardias are potentially curable by radiofrequency catheter ablation technique (Table 3). It is the first line of therapy and is offered to all patients with supraventricular tachycardia as it is safe, cost-effective and results in elimination of the underlying arrhythmia mechanism with minimal risk of complications.

The technique involves application of radiofrequency current from an external generator via a catheter at the site of the accessory pathway, the slow AV nodal pathway, or the mapped site of atrial tachycardia, producing coagulation necrosis by controlled heat production. Catheter ablation is performed during the electrophysiology procedure after the mechanism of supraventricular tachycardia has been determined and the optimal site for ablation identified. As the application

Table 3
Indications for Catheter Ablation of Supraventricular Tachcyardia (SVT)

Conventional
 Drug refractory
 WPW syndrome with recurrent SVT
 High risk WPW syndrome (short refractory period)
 Women of childbearing potential

Newer
 Any patient having an electrophysiology study for SVT
 Young patients
 SVT in high-risk occupation (e.g., bus drivers and airline pilots)
 Patient preference over medication

WPW, Wolff-Parkinson-White.

of radiofrequency energy to heart leads to very little discomfort, general anesthesia is not necessary. The majority (95%) of patients go home on the day after catheter ablation. In AV nodal reentry tachycardias and AV reentry tachycardias the success rate of radiofrequency catheter ablation is 95 to 98%, and in atrial tachycardias and atrial flutter it is 80 to 90%. Use of three-dimensional mapping techniques has further increased the success of catheter ablation, as it helps to precisely localize arrhythmia substrate. The incidence of complications with catheter ablation is less than 2 to 3%. Complications include right- or left-sided thrombus, thromboembolic events, cardiac tamponade, AV block, vascular events (bleeding or hematoma), and coronary artery spasm (13).

CATHETER ABLATION OF SPECIFIC TACHYCARDIAS

AV Nodal Reentry Tachycardia. Catheter ablation is highly successful in curing AV nodal reentry tachycardia, the most common form of supraventricular tachycardia. The preferred technique for modification of AV nodal function for cure of AV nodal reentry tachycardia is ablation of the slow pathway (14). Ablation is guided anatomically between the ostium of the coronary sinus and the AV node. Application of radiofrequency current at the slow pathway location results in transient junctional rhythm. Successful ablation of the slow pathway does not alter the PR interval or retrograde VA conduction. The risk of complete heart block is less than 3%, significantly lower than that with fast pathway ablation; also, there is superior long-term success with slow pathway ablation. Fast pathway ablation is performed at the site of the AV node-His bundle region in the anterosuperior portion of the tricuspid annulus. Fast pathway ablation results in prolongation of the PR interval and loss of retrograde conduction. There is a 5% risk of AV block. It is only undertaken in a small proportion of patients who have failed slow pathway ablation.

Accessory Pathways. Accessory pathways can lead to orthodromic tachycardias or antidromic tachycardias, and atrial fibrillation with preexcitation. Preexcited atrial fibrillation is associated with a significant risk of ventricular arrhythmias. Ablation of accessory pathways is curative for all associated arrhythmias and is one of the most gratifying procedures in invasive cardiac electrophysiology (Fig. 1) (15). After mapping of the atrioventricular ring, the catheter is positioned at the site of the pathway and radiofrequency current applied to selectively cauterize the pathway. Ablation for left-sided accessory pathways can be performed via the femoral arterial access by advancing the catheter across the aortic valve and then to the AV ring or by the transseptal route. Use of a particular approach is based on operator preference; however, the transseptal access is preferred in very young and elderly patients who have a higher risk of complications with the retrograde arterial cannulation (16). Right-sided accessory pathways can be ablated via the femoral vein or right internal jugular vein approach. Success rate for accessory pathway ablation is 95 to 98% with a 2 to 5% risk of recurrence. Because of the success and the ease of the procedure, catheter ablation should be offered to all patients with Wolff-Parkinson-White syndrome who are symptomatic or undergoing electrophysiology procedures for other reasons.

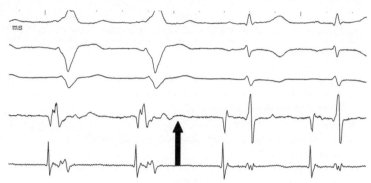

Fig. 1. Surface ECG and intracardiac electrograms in a patient with Wolff-Parkinson-White (WPW) syndrome. Onset of radiofrequency current (RF) at site of accessory pathway (indicated by arrow) leads to normalization of QRS. Delta wave disappears and PR interval becomes normal.

Atrial Tachycardia and Sinus Node Reentry. Focal atrial tachycardias are less common forms of SVT. In 70 to 80% of patients the atrial focus can be mapped and successfully ablated in the electrophysiology laboratory. The location for ablation is identified as the site of earliest atrial activation during the tachycardia. Ablation is also successful in the majority of patients with reentrant atrial tachycardias *(17)*. Reentant circuits and areas of slow conduction are identified by mid-diastolic potentials and entrainment mapping. Ablation of the areas of slow conduction is successful in curing reentrant atrial tachycardias. Newer three-dimensional mapping techniques are particularly useful in accurately mapping atrial tachycardias (Fig. 2; *see* Color Plate 6, following p. 268). For some patients with atrial tachycardia who cannot be cured by ablation of the atrial focus, palliative ablation of the AV node and permanent pacemaker implantation is successful in controlling symptoms. Control of rapid ventricular response by AV nodal ablation and pacemaker implantation also restores ventricular function in patients with tachycardia-induced cardiomyopathy.

Catheter ablation is highly successful in patients with sinus node reentry tachycardia. Lesions are given at the site of earliest atrial activation in the high right atrium presumably at the site of the sinus node. Interestingly, normal sinus node function is not affected by catheter ablation of sinus node reentry tachycardia *(2)*.

Atrial Flutter

Atrial flutter can be terminated by electrical or chemical cardioversion, or with overdrive atrial pacing *(18)*. Low-energy shocks of 50 to 100 J are often successful in terminating atrial flutter. Chemical cardioversion can be attempted with oral class I agents, or more rapid conversion with intravenous ibutalide, which is successful in converting 60% of patients with atrial flutter *(19)*. Typical or type 1 atrial flutter (defined by a 12-lead electrocardiogram as "saw-tooth" or "picket-fence" pattern P waves in the inferior leads and positive P waves in lead V1) can also be terminated by overdrive atrial pacing *(18)*. Overdrive pacing is particularly useful immediately following cardiac surgery, as postoperative patients have epicardial atrial wires in place. Atrial pacing can be performed using a transvenous pacing wire or an esophageal lead. Long-term medical therapy for atrial flutter is similar to that of atrial fibrillation and is discussed below. Patients with long-standing atrial flutter are at risk of thromboembolic complications, albeit lower than with atrial fibrillation. Despite this lower risk, guidelines for anticoagulation are identical to those for atrial fibrillation.

Type I (typical) atrial flutter is due to a macroreentrant circuit around the tricuspid valve ring *(20)*. Diagnosis is confirmed by 20-electrode catheter placement around the tricuspid ring. The circuit is activated in a counterclockwise direction with breakthrough anteriorly in the area of the His bundle, then proceeds along the lateral wall anteroposteriorly, followed by right-to-left acti-

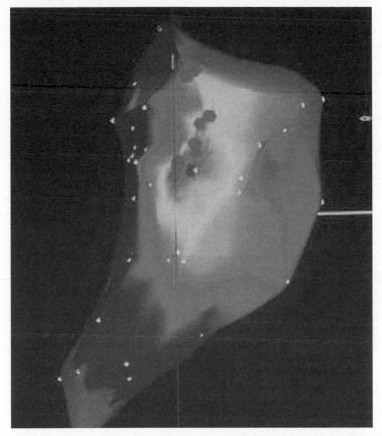

Fig. 2. Right atrial electroanatomical mapping of automatic atrial tachycardia. Timing of atrial electrograms is color-coded. Red areas represent sites of early activation. Application of radiofrequency current (blue dots) at the earliest site lead to termination of tachycardia. (*See* Color Plate 6, following p. 268.)

vation of the posterior tricuspid valve ring. The area of slow conduction in these patients is from the posterolateral right atrial free wall to the low posteromedial (septal) right atrium. Conduction block induced by radiofrequency catheter ablation between the low right atrium and the ostium of coronary sinus is associated with termination of atrial flutter and long-term cure *(20)*. Acute success with catheter ablation is achieved in approx 95% of patients with type I atrial flutter *(21)*. Atypical atrial flutter is either due to clockwise circuit with breakthrough at the upper end of crista terminalis or left atrial circuits, or related to multiple ill-defined circuits *(22,23)*. Electroanatomical mapping is particularly helpful in identifying the reentry pathway in atypical atrial flutters. Detailed activation and entrainment mapping of both left and right atria is required to identify the area of slow conduction. When identified, catheter ablation is often successful in these patients.

Atrial Fibrillation

Atrial fibrillation is the most common persistent arrhythmia seen in clinical practice. The prevalence increases dramatically with age. The overall prevalence in individuals over the age of 65 is approx 6%, and 85% of patients with atrial fibrillation are over the age of 65 *(22)*. In the elderly it results in substantial morbidity primarily related to the thromboembolic complications. Nonvalvular atrial fibrillation is associated with a four- to fivefold increase in the risk of stroke *(25)*. Although risks associated with atrial fibrillation have been identified, appropriate management of many aspects of atrial fibrillation is not clearly defined. The severity of symptoms with atrial fibrillation is determined by ventricular rate, nature and extent of underlying heart disease, ventricular function (both systolic and diastolic), and at times the precipitating cause. Symptoms include irregular palpitations, chest discomfort, lightheadedness, or fatigue. Severe symptoms can include heart failure, angina, and syncope. Stroke or systemic embolism may also be the initial presentation. At times it remains asymptomatic and is discovered when medical advice is sought for an unrelated problem. In a patient with new-onset atrial fibrillation careful clinical assessment is needed for detection of any associated cardiac conditions such as congestive heart failure, active myocardial ischemia, pericardial disease, significant valvular heart disease, hypertrophic cardiomyopathy, acute cor pulmonale, and preexcitation syndrome.

Management of atrial fibrillation involves control of ventricular rate, restoration of sinus rhythm, anticoagulation for the prevention of thromboembolic complications, and long-term treatment (26). Correction of the underlying cardiac abnormality, when feasible, should be undertaken. For example, if acute pulmonary embolism is the cause of atrial fibrillation, anticoagulation will lead to a decrease in pulmonary pressure, which will result in control of ventricular rate and very often spontaneous conversion to sinus rhythm. Although drugs continue to be the mainstay for long-term management of AF, devices (pacemakers and defibrillators) and especially catheter-based interventions are proving to be increasingly valuable.

CONTROL OF VENTRICULAR RATE

Patients with hemodynamic compromise should undergo immediate electrical cardioversion (26). Cardioversion is life-saving in patients with Wolff-Parkinson-White syndrome with pre-excited atrial fibrillation who are at risk of ventricular fibrillation from rapid ventricular rates. Use of AV nodal blocking drugs in these patients can be detrimental. Verapamil results in shortening in the refractory period of the accessory pathway and thus rapid ventricular rate and ventricular fibrillation.

If reasonably stable, initial treatment is directed at relieving symptoms by slowing the ventricular rate with AV nodal blocking agents such as diltiazem, verapamil, β-blockers, or digoxin. All of these drugs can be administered intravenously. The choice of an agent is determined by the clinical situation; in patients with mild symptoms, β-blockers might be adequate, while in patients with chronic lung disease and moderate symptoms, intravenous diltiazem is the drug of choice. In patients with heart failure, calcium-channel blockers and β-blockers should be used cautiously because of the risk of hypotension. Concomitant treatment of heart failure, lung disease, and chest infection, if present, are very important for the control of ventricular rate. Prolonged periods of fast ventricular rate can lead to tachycardia-induced cardiomyopathy. This diagnosis should always be considered in patients with dilated cardiomyopathy and chronic atrial fibrillation (27). When medical treatment fails to control ventricular rate, radiofrequency catheter ablation of the AV node and implantation of a rate-adaptive ventricular pacemaker (VVIR) should be undertaken. Dual-chamber pacemakers with capabilities for mode switching to ventricular mode when a patient goes into atrial fibrillation are used following catheter ablation of AV node in a patient with paroxysmal atrial fibrillation. In patients with tachycardia-induced cardiomyopathy, ablation of the AV node and pacemaker implantation restores left ventricular function. Following ablation of the AV node, as atrial fibrillation is still present, lifelong anti-coagulation is continued to prevent thromboembolic complications.

RESTORATION OF SINUS RHYTHM

Restoration of sinus rhythm, in nonanticoagulated patients, should be considered for patients with recent-onset (less than 48 h) atrial fibrillation, especially when it is associated with moderate symptoms. If performed within 48 h, the risk of thromboembolic complications is minimal. Both electrical and chemical cardioversion can be used. DC cardioversion is successful in 90 to 95% of patients. It is a safe procedure; however, it does require intravenous sedation. Use of a biphasic shock waveform has increased the success rate of external cardioversion; most patients can be cardioverted with lower-energy shocks of 100 J. Chemical cardioversion is attempted with intravenous ibutalide

Table 4
Risk Factors for Thromoembolic Complications in Atrial Fibrillation

1. Rheumatic valvular disease
2. History or presence of heart failure
3. History of prior stroke or transient ischemic attack
4. Echocardiographic systolic dysfunction
5. Diabetes
6. Hypertrophic cardiomyopathy
7. Hypertension

| | Recommendations for antithrombotic therapy | |
	No risk factors	One or more risk factors present
Age <65 yr	Aspirin/no therapy	Warfarin
Age 65–75 yr	Aspirin	Warfarin
Age >75 yr	Warfarin	Warfarin

(Corvert™) *(19).* This is a short-acting class III agent that prolongs the QT interval by acting on the potassium channels. It is successful in 60 to 70% of patients with atrial arrhythmias of recent onset, and also more successful in atrial flutter than in atrial fibrillation. Intravenous ibutalide is associated with a 3 to 5% risk of torsade de pointes, especially in patients with left ventricular dysfunction and relative hypokalemia and/or hypomagnesemia. Close monitoring for 3 to 4 h following administration of ibutalide is essential *(19).*

ANTITHROMBOTIC THERAPY

Persistant Atrial Fibrillation. Multivariate analysis of five large randomized controlled trials in patients with nonvalvular atrial fibrillation has shown that six independent predictors of stroke are previous history of stroke or transient ischemic attacks, history of diabetes, history of hypertension, age greater than 75, history of congestive heart failure, and a history of myocardial infarction (Table 4) *(28).* In patients less than 60 yr of age with none of the above risk factors, the risk of bleeding from long-term anticoagulation (0.5% per year) outweighs the risk of stroke. In patients above age 65 and with associated risk factors, the risk of stroke outweighs the risk of bleeding and thus oral anticoagulation with warfarin should be undertaken. The presence of an enlarged left atrium has also been shown to be a risk factor *(28).* All patients with valvular heart disease and atrial fibrillation should be anticoagulated, however. Dose-adjusted warfarin is highly effective for prophylaxis against ischemic strokes in patients with atrial fibrillation, but requires frequent blood monitoring. Recent data show that the oral direct thrombin inhibitor Ximelagatran™, used in fixed dosages, is as effective as dose-adjusted warfarin *(29).* Its use does not require monitoring for the anticoagulant intensity. It might soon prove to be an effective and convenient agent for anticoagulation in patients with atrial fibrillation who are at risk of thromboembolism.

Paroxysmal Atrial Fibrillation. In patients with short episodes of paroxysmal atrial fibrillation (less than 24 h in duration) the risk of thromboembolic complications is lower than with chronic atrial fibrillation. In this group the decision to anticoagulate is also based on the presence or absence of risk factors. In the absence of risk factors (hypertension, mitral stenosis, prior transient ischemic attacks or stroke, heart failure, and age over 75 yr), aspirin alone can be used. In the presence of risk factors, warfarin should be used, as longer episodes of atrial fibrillation, particularly those associated with a relatively slow ventricular rate, may be asymptomatic.

Pericardioversion. There is substantial risk of thromboembolic complications following chemical or electrical cardioversion. All patients with atrial fibrillation of longer than 48 h should be anticoagulated for 3 to 4 wk prior to and for 2 to 3 wk following cardioversion. However, patients in whom the left atrial appendage can be clearly visualized at transesophageal echocardiography, are free of thrombi, and have no risk factors for thromboembolism can be cardioverted without prior

Table 5
Comparative Efficacy of Antiarrhythmic Drugs in AF to Maintain Sinus Rhythm

Drug	Efficacy in AF	Proarrhythmic potential
Quinidine	+++	+++
Procainaminde	++	++
Disopyramide	++	+
Tocainide	–	–
Mexiletine	–	–
Flecainide	++++	++
Propafenone	+++	++
Amiodarone	++++	+ (mainly bradycardia)
Sotalol	+++	+
Ibutilide	++	++
Dofetilide	+++[a]	++
Beta-blockers	+	0
Verapamil	0	0
Digoxin	0	+

AF, atrial fibrillation.
[a]Has recently been approved by the FDA for treatment of atrial fibrillation.

anticoagulation *(30)*. In the presence of risk factors, even these patients should be treated with anticoagulation therapy for 3 to 4 wk prior to cardioversion.

Maintenance of Sinus Rhythm. Atrial fibrillation begets atrial fibrillation. The longer the patient has been in atrial fibrillation, the greater is the likelihood that he or she will remain in atrial fibrillation. In patients in whom sinus rhythm is restored, only 30 to 50% remain in sinus rhythm at 12-mo follow-up. Maintenance of sinus rhythm is influenced by the duration of atrial fibrillation and the size of the left atrium *(31)*. Patients with atrial fibrillation of less than 12-mo duration have a greater chance of maintaining sinus rhythm. The larger the left atrial size, the lesser are the chances of maintaining sinus rhythm after cardioversion.

Present pharmacologic therapy used to maintain sinus rhythm is far from ideal. Class Ia, Ic, and III drugs are used to maintain sinus rhythm (Table 5) *(32)*. Proarrhythmia continues to be a major concern with all of these drugs, more so in patients with left ventricular dysfunction *(33)*. It is difficult to compare the efficacy of these drugs as clinical trials have involved heterogenous groups of patients with variable left atrial sizes and duration of AF. Relative efficacy of these agents is shown in Table 5. The choice of drug is dependent on the side effect profile and the risk of proarrhythmia. A substudy of the Atrial Fibrillation Follow-up Investigation in Rhythm Management (AFFIRM) trial showed that amiodarone is better than sotalol or class I drugs for the maintenance of sinus rhythm without cardioversion *(34)*. The class Ic agents propafenone and flecainide are also very effective in maintaining sinus rhythm but their use should be restricted to patients with normal left ventricular function and no coronary artery disease. Like amiodarone, dofetilide, a relatively new Class III agent, can be used in patients with left ventricular dysfunction *(35)*. Therapy can be initiated only in a monitored setting as it can lead to prolongation of the QT interval and torsade de pointes. The dose of dofetilide has to be adjusted with renal function.

A large NIH multicenter trial (AFFIRM) and multiple smaller studies have compared mortality and morbidity with rate versus rhythm control in patients with atrial fibrillation. Results of these trials indicate a similar mortality with rate and rhythm control. Higher rates of thromboembolic complications were seen in the rhythm control arm. This was mostly in patients in whom anticoagulation was discontinued once they were maintained on antiarrhytmic agents *(36)*. Thus, it is recommended that long-term anticoagulation should be continued in all patients with atrial fibrillation who have risk factors for thromboembolism.

Several nonpharmacologic approaches have also been used. In patients with drug-resistant atrial fibrillation, catheter ablation has been found to be increasingly successful. Findings indicate that triggers for atrial fibrillation are in the pulmonary veins *(37)*. Electrical isolation of pulmonary veins by circumferential lesions around pulmonary vein attachments in left atria has become a preferred approach. Long-term success with these approaches has been as high as 80%. A recent trial has shown improved mortality and quality of life after catheter ablation of atrial fibrillation *(38)*. The major complication with ablation of these foci in and around pulmonary veins is late pulmonary vein stenosis. The risk of this is reduced by ablation farther away from the pulmonary veins. Surgical procedures such as maze and corridor operations have been shown to be successful in 70 to 80% of patients *(39)*. These involve creating multiple areas of block in the atria by surgical incisions and resuturing. Implantable atrial defibrillators have proven to be useful only in a small select group of patients with atrial fibrillation with infrequent but hemodynamically unstable episodes.

VENTRICULAR ARRHYTHMIAS

The management of ventricular arrhythmias has also changed radically over the last 15 yr. This is related to better understanding of the proarrhythmic effect of antiarrhythmic drugs, large multicenter trials showing the mortality benefits of implantable cardioverter-defibrillators (ICD), and the success of radiofrequency catheter ablation in certain forms of monomorphic ventricular tachycardias. The management of symptomatic ventricular premature beats and nonsustained ventricular tachycardia is less aggressive but is significantly affected by the presence of associated heart disease.

Ventricular Premature Complexes

Asymptomatic ventricular premature beats in the absence of an underlying cardiac abnormality do not need treatment. In patients with recent onset of frequent ventricular premature beats, every effort should be made to identify the etiology *(40)*. Electrolyte disturbances, especially hypokalemia or hypomagnesemia; excessive caffeine intake; and cardiac causes such as mitral valve prolapse, myocardial ischemia or infarction, cardiomyopathy, hypertensive heart disease, or persistent bradycardia are some of the important etiologies. Treatment of the reversible etiology, if identifiable, should be first attempted before using antiarrhythmic agents. In the presence of mitral valve prolapse, symptomatic ventricular premature beats are best treated with β-blocker therapy. If β-blockers are contraindicated or ineffective, class I antiarrhythmic agents such as mexiletine, procainamide, flecainide, or propafenone are very effective but should be avoided in the presence of left ventricular dysfunction. In patients with recent myocardial infarction, lidocaine is used only for frequent premature beats that result in hemodynamic compromise. Procainamide is used if lidocaine fails. Long-term suppression of asymptomatic ventricular premature beats with oral antiarrhythmic agents has not been associated with improved survival. In the Cardiac Arrhythmia Suppression Trial (CAST), postmyocardial-infarction suppression of asymptomatic ventricular arrhythmias with Type I antiarrhythmic agents was associated with increased mortality *(12)*. Similar results were seen with the pure class III agent d-sotalol *(41)*. Amiodarone, a class III agent with β-blocking and calcium-channel blocking properties, is highly effective in suppressing ventricular ectopy and has been shown not to increase mortality because of proarrhythmia. It has been associated with improved survival from arrhythmic death as shown in the European and Canadian Myocardial Infarction Amiodarone Trials (EMIAT and CAMIAT, respectively) but did not alter cardiac mortality *(42,43)*.

In patients with heart failure, the presence of ventricular premature beats is associated with a higher total mortality but not with an increased arrhythmic mortality. Again, class I antiarrhythmic agents should not be used to suppress ectopy, as patients with decreased left ventricular function have an associated risk of proarrhythmia. There is some evidence that amiodarone might be beneficial. The Grupo de Estudio de la Sobrevida en la Insuficiencia Cardiaca en Argentina trial (GESICA) showed improved survival in heart failure patients treated with low-dose amiodarone while in the Amiodarone in Patients with Congestive Heart Failure and Asymptomatic Ventricular

Arrhyhmias (CHF-STAT) trial use of amiodarone offered no benefit *(44,45)*. Thus the role of amiodarone in primary prevention of sudden death in patients with heart failure is not established.

Nonsustained Ventricular Tachycardia

Nonsustained ventricular tachycardia is defined as three consecutive ventricular beats at a rate of ≥120 beats/min lasting <30 s and that does not lead to hemodynamic compromise. Class I antiarrhythmic drugs have no role in the management of nonsustained ventricular tachycardia. As shown by the CAST study, they may lead to an increase in mortality because of their proarrhythmic effects *(12)*. Asymptomatic nonsustained VT in patients with normal left ventricular function is not associated with adverse long-term prognosis and thus does not warrant treatment. In post-myocardial-infarction patients with nonsustained VT and good left ventricular function, β-blockers should be used. In the presence of presyncope or syncope, patients with nonsustained ventricular tachycardia should undergo an electrophysiology study to see if sustained ventricular tachycardia can be induced. Inducible sustained ventricular tachycardia is a risk factor for sudden death. Patients with left ventricular dysfunction, nonsustained ventricular tachycardia, and coronary artery disease have an increased mortality primarily due to arrhythmic deaths *(46,47)*. In these patients further risk stratification is indicated by an electrophysiology study. The Multicenter Automatic Defibrillator Implant Trial (MADIT) has shown that in patients with nonsustained ventricular tachycardia, a past history of myocardial infarction, left ventricular ejection fraction of ≤35%, and inducible sustained ventricular tachycardia that is not suppressed with procainamide at electrophysiology study, implantation of a cardioverter-defibrillator was associated with significantly improved long-term survival when compared with conventional therapy *(47)*. In this trial, mortality in the control group of patients who had poor left ventricular function and were noninducible was also high. The issue of cardioverter-defibrillators in patients with prior myocardial infarction, poor left ventricular function, and no prior ventricular arrhythmia was further investigated in the MADIT 2 study. Patients with left ventricular ejection fraction of ≤30% were included. The trial was terminated prematurely as patients randomized to the implantable defibrillator had a 30% reduction in overall mortality compared with optimized medical therapy with high use of β-blockers. The benefit was highest in patients with prolonged QRS duration (≥120 ms). Thus, implantable defibrillator therapy is now recommended in all patients with ischemic cardiomypathy who have ejection fraction of <30% and no evidence of active myocardial ischemia *(48)*.

The prognostic significance of nonsustained ventricular tachycardia in patients with nonischemic cardiomyopathy is not established. In the absence of symptoms, no intervention is presently recommended. Ventricular tachycardia is usually not inducible at electrophysiology study so its use is limited in these patients and symptomatic nonsustained ventricular tachycardia may be treated with amiodarone alone. Ongoing large prospective studies are designed to determine the benefit of an implantable defibrillator vs amiodarone in patients with nonsustained ventricular tachycardia and cardiomyopathy. Recently published smaller studies suggest it may not have a benefit.

Sustained Ventricular Tachycardia

IMPLANTABLE CARDIOVERTER-DEFIBRILLATORS

The implantable cardioverter-defibrillator is the first line therapy for patients presenting with ventricular tachycardia and fibrillation, according to the joint guidelines of the American College of Cardiology and the American Heart Association *(52)*. This is based on three large multicenter trials. The Antiarrhythmic Versus Implantable Defibrillator (AVID) trial compared an implantable defibrillator with antiarrhythmic drugs (amiodarone or sotalol), the Cardiac Arrest Study, Hamburg (CASH) compared a defibrillator with amiodarone and metoprolol, and the Canadian Implantable Defibrillator Study (CIDS) compared a defibrillator to amiodarone. All three studies showed improved survival in patients with implantable defibrillators when compared to medical therapy. Current indications for the use of an implantable defibrillator are shown in Table 6.

Table 6
Indications for ICD Therapy
(American College of Cardiology /American Heart Association/
North American Society of Pacing and Electrophysiology Guidelines)

Class I (there is evidence and/or general agreement that a given procedure or treatment is useful and effective)
1. Cardiac arrest due to VF or VT not due to a transient or reversible cause.
2. Spontaneous sustained VT in association with structural heart disease.
3. Syncope of undetermined origin with clinically relevant, hemodynamically significant sustained VT or VF induced at electrophysiology study when drug therapy is ineffective, not tolerated, or not preferred.
4. Nonsustained VT in patients with coronary disease, prior myocardial infarction, left ventricular dysfunction, and inducible VF or sustained VT at electrophysiology study that is not suppressible by a class I antiarrhythmic drug.
5. Spontaneous sustained VT in patients who do not have structural heart disease that is not amenable to other treatments.

Class II (there is conflicting evidence and /or a divergence of opinion about the useful/efficacy of a procedure or treatment)

Class IIa (weight of evidence/opinion is in favor of usefulness/efficacy)
1. Patients with LV ejection fraction of less than or equal to 30%, at least 1 mo postmyocardial infarction and 3 mo post-coronary artery revascularization surgery.

Class IIb (usefulness/efficacy is less well established by evidence/opinion)
1. Cardiac arrest presumed to be due to VF when electrophysiology testing is precluded by other medical conditions.
2. Severe symptoms (e.g., syncope) attributable to ventricular tachyarrhythmias while awaiting cardiac transplantation.
3. Familial or inherited condition with a high risk for life-threatening ventricular tachyarrhythmias such as long-QT syndrome or hypertrophic cardiomyopathy.
4. Nonsustained VT with coronary artery disease, prior myocardial infarction, and left ventricular dysfunction, and inducible sustained VT or VF at electrophysiological study.
5. Recurrent syncope of undetermined etiology in the presence of ventricular dysfunction and inducible ventricular arrhythmias at electrophysiological study when other causes of syncope have been excluded.
6. Syncope of unexplained etiology or family history of sudden cardiac death in association with typical or atypical right bundle-branch block and ST segment elevation (Brugada syndrome).
7. Syncope in patients with advanced structural heart disease for which thorough invasive and noninvasive investigation have failed to define a cause.

Class III (there is evidence and/or general agreement that the procedure/treatment is not useful/effective and in some cases may be harmful)
1. Syncope of undetermined cause in a patient without inducible VT/VF and without structural heart disease.
2. Incessant VT or VF.
3. VF or VT resulting from arrhythmias amenable to surgical or catheter ablation; e.g., atrial arrhythmias associated with Wolff-Parkinson-White syndrome, right ventricular outflow tract VT, idiopathic left ventricular VT, or fascicular VT.
4. Ventricular tachyarrhythmias due to transient or structural disorder (acute myocardial infarction, electrolyte imbalance, drugs, or trauma) when correction of the disorder is considered feasible and likely to substantially reduce the risk of recurrent arrhythmia.
5. Significant psychiatric illnesses that may be aggravated by ICD implantation or may preclude systemic follow-up.
6. Terminal illness with projected life expectancy ≤6 mo.
7. Patients with coronary artery disease with LV dysfunction and prolonged QRS duration in the absence of spontaneous or inducible sustained or nonsustained VT who are undergoing coronary bypass surgery.
8. NYHA class IV drug-refractory congestive heart failure in patients who are not candidates for cardiac transplantation.

VT, ventricular tachycardia; VF, ventricular fibrillation; ICD, ischemic heart disease.

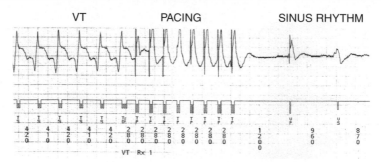

Fig. 3. Termination of sustained ventricular tachycardia by overdrive pacing from implantable defibrillator. Overdrive pacing is indicated by pacing spikes. Rate of VT was 160 beats/min. Post-pacing heart rate was 60 beats/min.

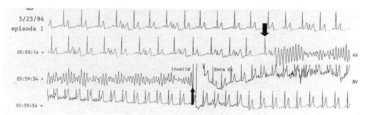

Fig. 4. Termination of spontaneous ventricular fibrillation by ICD shock. Trace was obtained while patient was being monitored on telemetery ward.

Like pacemakers, defibrillators are implanted under local anesthesia using a transvenous approach to place endocardial leads. Because of their relatively small size, all defibrillators are implanted subcutaneously in the pectoral region. Perioperative mortality, even in high-risk patients with left ventricular dysfunction and heart failure, is less than 1%.

All implantable defibrillators currently in use have complex discriminating algorithms and multiple programmable therapies. Ventricular tachycardia can be terminated by antitachycardia pacing (Fig. 3) or low-energy shocks. High-energy shocks are programmed for ventricular fibrillation therapy (Fig. 4). All defibrillators have backup single- or dual-chamber pacing capabilities and keep records of events, thus allowing complete analysis of previous arrhythmic events. Ventricular arrhythmias are diagnosed based on complex programmable discriminating algorithms that take into account the rate of tachycardia, relationship of atrial and ventricular electrograms, and morphology of intracardiac electrograms. Inappropriate shocks for supraventricular tachycardias are less frequent with the newer generation of implantable defibrillators.

There has been an exponential increase in the number of patients with implantable cardioverter defibrillators, and frequent shocks from an implantable defibrillator is a not uncommon cause for admissions in emergency rooms. Management of these patients requires close cooperation among emergency room physicians, cardiologists, and electrophysiologists. The history of symptoms prior to shock together with stored electrograms from the defibrillator memory is used to differentiate appropriate and inappropriate shocks.

ANTIARRHYTHMIC MEDICATIONS

Antiarrhythmic drugs are the first-line therapy only for the acute management of ventricular arrhythmias. Lidocaine, procainamide, bretylium, and amiodarone are available in intravenous forms. The use of amiodarone for acute management has increased as it is less proarrhythmic and intravenous therapy can easily be converted to oral therapy. Class I antiarrhythmics are no longer the first line of therapy for the long-term management of sustained ventricular tachycardia because their proarrhythmic effects have led to an increase in mortality. Both amiodarone (Cardiac Arrest in Seattle: Conventional Versus Amiodarone Drug Evaluation [CASCADE]) and sotalol (the Electro-

Table 7
Ventricular Tachycardia: Indications for Catheter Ablation

1. Catheter ablation is suggested as the first line of therapy
Idiopathic VT—right ventricular outflow tract tachycardia
                        —fascicular tachycardias
Bundle branch reentry in patients with cardiomyopathy
(VT has left bundle branch blocklike morphology)

2. Catheter ablation should be considered
VT with coronary artery disease with multiple ICD shocks
Slow incessant VT resistant to multiple medications

3. No data to suggest its efficacy, should not be performed
Arrhythmogenic right ventricular dysplasia
Dilated nonischemic cardiomyopathy

physiologic Versus Electrocardiographic Monitoring study [ESVEM]), class III antiarrhythmics, result in significantly better survival in patients with life-threatening ventricular arrhythmias compared with class I antiarrhythmic drugs (49,50). Use of sotalol is limited by its β-blocking properties and thus it cannot be used in patients with heart failure or significantly reduced left ventricular function. Amiodarone is the drug of choice in patients with sustained ventricular arrhythmias and reduced left ventricular function. Class I antiarrhythmic drugs are added in case of partial efficacy of amiodarone. Long-term therapy with amiodarone is associated with a significant incidence of side effects and thus requires close monitoring of thyroid, liver, and pulmonary functions. Approximately 40% of patients with ventricular arrhythmias with implantable cardioverter-defibrillators also need antiarrhythmic drugs for recurrent ventricular tachycardia (51).

RADIOFREQUENCY CATHETER ABLATION FOR VENTRICULAR TACHYCARDIA

Catheter ablation is useful in the management of selected cases of ventricular tachycardia (Table 7). It is the treatment of choice in patients with idiopathic ventricular tachycardia where there is no other evidence of structural heart disease. The prerequisite for catheter ablation of ventricular tachycardia is the ability to locate areas essential for initiating and sustaining ventricular tachycardia (53,54). These can be areas of slow conduction in a reentrant circuit or focal areas of abnormal automaticity or triggered activity. Ventricular tachycardia due to bundle branch reentry, which is usually seen in patients with dilated cardiomyopathy and valvular heart disease, is also amenable to catheter ablation. The right bundle forms an essential part of the reentrant circuit and ablation of the right bundle is curative. In patients with structural heart disease, such as coronary artery disease and cardiomyopathy, the substrate for reentrant ventricular tachycardia is less well defined because of large areas of scarring and fibrosis, and thus cannot always be eliminated by radiofrequency catheter lesions (54). Catheter ablation is undertaken if the patient has recurrent episodes of monomorphic ventricular tachycardia that lead to defibrillator shocks and are not responsive to medical therapy (Fig. 5).

Specific Forms of Ventricular Tachycardia

IDIOPATHIC VENTRICULAR TACHYCARDIA

Ventricular fibrillation and ventricular tachycardia can present without any underlying cardiac abnormality. In patients presenting with ventricular fibrillation, a detailed cardiac evaluation should be undertaken to rule out any underlying cardiac abnormality such as right ventricular dysplasia, hypertrophic cardiomyopathy, and long-QT and Brugada syndromes. In the majority of patients with idiopathic ventricular tachycardia and fibrillation, electrophysiologic study is normal. The risk of recurrence of idiopathic ventricular fibrillation is not firmly established and implantable defibrillator therapy is the treatment of choice as drug efficacy cannot be confirmed.

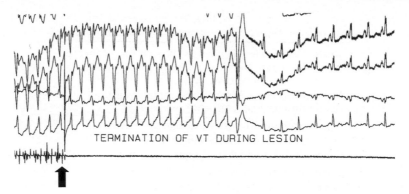

Fig. 5. Catheter ablation of ventricular tachycardia in a patient with recurrent shocks from implantable defibrillator. Left ventricle was mapped during ventricular tachycardia. Ablation catheter was placed at the site of slow conduction. Onset of radiofrequency current (arrow) led to termination of tachycardia with resumption of sinus rhythm.

Ventricular tachycardia without underlying heart disease is a diagnosis of exclusion. Two morphologies of idiopathic ventricular tachycardias are usually identified. A large proportion of ventricular tachycardias seen in patients with apparently normal hearts have left bundle branch blocklike morphology with an inferior frontal plane axis. The tachycardia originates form the right ventricular outflow tract, and the underlying mechanism for this tachycardia is thought to be triggered activity. It responds to adenosine, β-blockers and calcium-channel blockers. Radiofrequency catheter ablation is curative in this form of ventricular tachycardia, and is performed by mapping the focus of arrhythmia in the right ventricular outflow tract. The second form of idiopathic ventricular tachycardia, also known as "fascicular" tachycardia, originates from the left posterior septum in the region of the posterior fascicle of the left bundle branch. Electrophysiologic features of this tachycardia suggest a reentrant mechanism. This form of ventricular tachycardia can be terminated by intravenous verapamil. Medical therapy with calcium-channel and β-blocker therapy is successful in suppressing the arrhythmia. Catheter ablation at the site of Purkinje potential (P potential) found in the posteroinferior part of the left ventricle is curative. As catheter ablation is safe and curative, it is the treatment of choice for all symptomatic patients with idiopathic ventricular tachycardia (53).

ARRHYTHMOGENIC RIGHT VENTRICULAR DYSPLASIA

Arrhythmogenic right ventricular dysplasia leads to ventricular tachycardias with a right ventricular origin, identified by left bundle branch blocklike morphology. This condition can run in families. Diagnosis is suspected by the morphology of ventricular tachycardia and right ventricular abnormalities on echocardiography. Signal-averaged electrocardiograms are also grossly abnormal in this condition. The diagnosis is confirmed by MRI of the heart showing fat deposition in the right ventricular wall. This is an important cause of potentially fatal arrhythmias in young adults and children with an apparently normal left ventricle. The implantable defibrillator is the treatment of choice (55), with antiarrhythmic drug therapy reserved for those with recurrent defibrillator shocks.

HYPERTROPHIC CARDIOMYOPATHY

Ventricular arrhythmias account for significant mortality in patients with hypertrophic cardiomyopathy. The risk of sudden death is higher in patients with a history of syncope or "sudden cardiac death" in first-degree relatives. A history of syncope is very specific. In those without such history, electrophysiology study can be used to identify risk of sudden cardiac death. Amiodarone has been shown to reduce nonsustained ventricular tachycardia; however, its role in decreasing sudden death is not well established in these patients. Those with documented sustained ventricular tachycardia or with positive electrophysiologic study should have an implantable defibrillator

(56). Prophylactic use of an implantable defibrillator is recommended in patients with hypertrophic cardiomyopathy and risk of sudden death. The most specific risk factor is family history of sudden death at young age.

TORSADE DE POINTES

This term is used to describe polymorphic ventricular tachycardia with QRS complexes that progressively change in amplitude and morphology, with appearance of a twisting axis of depolarization and is usually associated with long-QT syndrome. In patients with acquired long-QT syndrome every effort must be made to identify and treat the underlying cause. A complete drug history is essential and any suspected drug should be eliminated. Intravenous magnesium is the initial treatment, followed by atrial or ventricular pacing at a rapid rate. In patients with torsades who have a normal QT interval, antiarrhythmic drugs might be needed for recurrent arrhythmia. Lidocaine, mexiletine, phenytoin, and potassium-channel openers have been tried. Antiarrhythmic drugs that prolong the QT interval, such as class IA (procainamide), and III (sotalol and amiodarone) drugs, may worsen the arrhythmia. In patients with congenital long-QT syndrome, β-blockers, stellate ganglionectomy, pacemakers, and implantable defibrillators have been used. Many different types of long-QT syndrome and channels involved have been identified. In patients with long-QT syndrome due to a defect in the sodium channel (LQT3), the sodium channel blocker mexiletine has been shown to normalize the QT interval *(57)*. Recently potassium has been found to reduce QT interval and possible sudden death in patients with LQT2. However, at present, the role of drugs on mortality in patients with long QT is still not established, and in symptomatic patients an implantable defibrillator should be used. Screening of asymptomatic family members should be undertaken.

BRUGADA SYNDROME

Brugada syndrome is a hereditary condition that has been shown to be an important cause of sudden cardiac death in patients with structurally normal hearts *(58)*. Electrocardiograms in sinus rhythm are typical and show ST elevation in leads V1 to V3 with a right bundle branch block pattern. ST changes might be intermittent and, if not present at rest, can be unmasked by administration of class I antiarrhythmic agents (sodium-channel blocking agents). These individuals are at risk of polymorphic ventricular tachycardia that can present with syncope when self-terminating, and sudden cardiac death when it does not terminate spontaneously. Occurrence is familial in 50 to 60% of patients with an autosomal mode of inheritance. The underlying basis for this syndrome has been shown to be a mutation in the gene SCNA5A that encodes for a human cardiac sodium channel. Left untreated patients with Brugada syndrome and symptoms have high mortality (10% per year). Implantable defibrillators are the only effective treatment to prevent sudden death, with antiarrhytmic drugs playing no role. Management of asymptomatic individuals with Brugada-like electrocardiographic features remains unclear. It is suggested that these patients should have an implantable defibrillator if sustained ventricular arrhythmias can be induced by programmed stimulation.

BRADYARRHYTHMIAS

Management of bradyarrhythmias involves critical decisions about the placement of temporary or permanent pacemakers. Indications for the placement of pacemaker are based on the etiology of the bradyarrhythmia.

Temporary Cardiac Pacing

Transvenous or transcutaneous pacing is performed for the immediate management of patients with life-threatening bradycardia. In the presence of syncope, hypotension, or heart failure, and when the underlying cause for bradycardia cannot immediately be corrected, a temporary pacemaker should be inserted. At times persistent bradycardia can lead to ventricular arrhythmias; the placement of a pacemaker in these patients can lead to suppression of these arrhythmias.

In acute myocardial infarction, the decision to insert a temporary pacemaker depends on the location of the myocardial infarction and the presence of preexisting conduction system disease. AV block in patients with inferior myocardial infarction is usually located above the His bundle, is associated with a narrow QRS complex and no hemodynamic compromise, responds to intravenous atropine, and is transient. A temporary pacemaker is inserted only if the heart rate is below 40 beats/min or if there are symptoms of low cardiac output, associated angina, or ventricular irritability. The presence of a stable escape rhythm usually precludes the need for temporary pacing. Atrioventricular conduction resumes in the majority of these patients, although the recovery might take up to 2 wk. In patients with anterior myocardial infarction, AV block is usually due to a block below the level of the His bundle. The resultant QRS complex is usually wide, and escape rhythms are slow and do not respond to atropine. These patients often have large myocardial infarctions and associated pump failure. As progression to complete heart block contributes independently to morbidity and mortality, temporary pacing should be performed promptly (59).

The availability of transcutaneous pacing systems have allowed both an increase in the indications for standby pacing and a decline in the need for transvenous pacing. Indications for the use of transcutaneous patches are shown in Table 8. Transcutaneous pacemaker systems are suitable for providing standby pacing in acute myocardial infarction, especially for those not requiring immediate pacing, who are at only moderate risk of progression to AV block. However, transcutaneous pacing may be uncomfortable, especially when prolonged, and it is intended to be only prophylactic and temporary. A transvenous pacing electrode should be placed in patients who require ongoing pacing and in those with a 30 to 40% probability of requiring prolonged pacing (60).

Antiarrhythmic drugs, β-blockers, calcium-channel blockers, digoxin, reserpine, and parasympathomimetic agents can lead to bradycardia, more so in patients with idiosyncratic reactions and conduction system disease. Bradycardia with these drugs may even occur at low blood levels. Temporary pacing may be required for the duration of the drug action or until the drug effect is counteracted. If long-term therapy with these agents is needed, as is the case with antiarrhythmic agents for ventricular arrhythmias, permanent pacing is indicated.

Prophylactic temporary pacing is needed in the cardiac catheterization laboratory when there is risk of complete heart block during the procedure. It should be inserted during right heart catheterization in patients with preexisting left bundle-branch block. It is also used during certain interventions to the right coronary artery where there is risk of prolonged ischemia. Temporary dual-chamber pacing is preferred for patients with bradycardia and noncompliant ventricles, e.g., those with hypertrophic cardiomyopathy, heart failure, or sizable myocardial infarctions and for hemodynamic compromise following cardiac surgery (61).

Permanent Cardiac Pacing

Table 9 shows the indications for the insertion of permanent pacemakers in patients *with heart block and sinus node disease*, per the 2002 update of the ACC/AHA/NASPE practice guidelines for implantation of antiarrhythmic devices (52). Despite these guidelines the decision regarding insertion of a pacemaker is influenced by several additional factors. Prior to implantation of a pacemaker, reversible causes for bradycardia must be excluded (e.g., Lyme disease, hypervagotonia, drugs, and metabolic and electrolyte imbalances). As a general principle, permanent pacing is performed for even asymptomatic patients with complete heart block, alternating bundle branch block, and second-degree AV block associated with bundle branch block.

Isolated first-degree AV block is usually due to delay in AV nodal conduction as a result of enhanced vagal tone or drug therapy. Patients with a very long PR interval may develop symptoms due to delayed opening of the AV valves and thus benefit from dual-chamber pacing with physiological AV delay. *First-degree AV block* with left or right bundle branch block, especially of recent onset, reflects the presence of infra-His conduction delay. This is an indication for placement of a permanent pacemaker as there is often progress to higher degrees of AV block (62).

Table 8
Indications for Placement of Transcutaneous Patches and Active (Demand)
Transcutaneous Pacing Patches in Acute Myocardial Infarction (ACC/AHA Recommendations)

Class I (Conditions for which there is evidence and/or general agreement that a given procedure or treatment is beneficial, useful, and effective)
1. Sinus bradycardia (rate less than 50 beats/min) with symptoms of hypotension (systolic blood pressure less than 80 mmHg) unresponsive to drug therapy.
2. Mobitz type II second-degree AV block.
3. Third-degree heart block.
4. Bilateral BBB (alternating BBB, or RBBB and alternating left anterior fascicular block [LAFB], left posterior fascicular block [LPFB]) (irrespective of time of onset).
5. Newly acquired or age indeterminate LBBB, LBBB and LAFBa, RBBB and LPFBa.
6. RBBB or LBBB and first-degree AV block.

Class II (Conditions for which there is conflicting evidence and/or a divergence of opinion about the usefulness/efficacy of a procedure or treatment)

Class IIa (Weight of evidence/opinion is in favor of usefulness/efficacy)
1. Stable bradycardia (systolic blood pressure greater than 90 mmHg, no hemodynamic compromise, or compromise responsive to initial drug therapy).
2. Newly acquired or age-indeterminate RBBB.

Class IIb (Usefulness/efficacy is less well-established by evidence/opinion)
1. Newly acquired or age-indeterminate first-degree AV block.

Class III (general agreement that a procedure/treatment is not useful/effective and in some cases may be harmful)
1. Uncomplicated acute MI without evidence of conduction system disease.

Recommendations for Temporary Transvenous Pacing in Acute Myocardial Infarction

Class I (Conditions for which there is evidence and/or general agreement that a given procedure or treatment is beneficial, useful, and effective)
1. Asystole.
2. Symptomatic bradycardia (includes sinus bradycardia with hypotension and type I second-degree AV block with hypotension not responsive to atropine).
3. Bilateral BBB (alternating BBB or RBBB with alternating LAFB/LPFB) (any age).
4. New or indeterminate age bifascicular block (RBBB with LAFB or LPFB, or LBBB) with first-degree AV block.
5. Mobitz type II second-degree AV block.

Class II (Conditions for which there is conflicting evidence and/or a divergence of opinion about the usefulness/efficacy of a procedure or treatment)

Class IIa (Weight of evidence/opinion is in favor of usefulness/efficacy)
1. RBBB and LAFB or LPFB (new or indeterminate).
2. RBBB with first-degree AV block.
3. LBBB, new or indeterminate.
4. Incessant VT, for atrial or ventricular overdrive pacing.
5. Recurrent sinus pauses (greater than 3 s) not responsive to atropine.

Class IIb (Usefulness/efficacy is less well established by evidence/opinion)
1. Bifascicular block of indeterminate age.
2. New or age-indeterminate isolated RBBB.

Class III
1. First-degree heart block.
2. Type I second-degree AV block with normal hemodynamics.
3. Accelerated idioventricular rhythm.
4. Bundle branch block or fascicular block known to exist before acute MI.

AV, atrio-ventricular; LAFB, left anterior fascicular block; LBBB, left bundle branch block; LPFB, left posterior fascicular block; RBBB, right bundle branch block.

Table 9
Indications for Placement of Permanent Pacemaker

A. *Indications for permanent pacing in acquired atrioventricular block in adults*
   (see definitions of classes in Table 8)

Class I

1. Third-degree and advanced second-degree AV block at any anatomic level, associated with any one of the following conditions:
   a. Bradycardia with symptoms presumed to be due to AV block.
   b. Arrhythmias and other medical conditions that require drugs that result in symptomatic bradycardia.
   c. Documented periods of asystole greater than or equal to 3 s or any escape rate less than 40 beats/min in awake, symptom-free patients.
   d. After catheter ablation of the AV junction. There are no trials that assess outcomes without pacing and pacing is virtually always planned in this situation unless operative procedure is AV junction modification.
   e. Postoperative AV block that is not expected to resolve after cardiac surgery.
   f. Neuromuscular diseases with AV block such as myotonic muscular dystrophy, Kearns-Sayre syndrome, Erb's dystrophy (limb-girdle), and peroneal muscular atrophy with or without symptoms, because there might be unpredictable progression of AV conduction disease.
2. Second-degree AV block regardless of type or site of block, with associated symptomatic bradycardia.

Class IIa

1. Asymptomatic third-degree AV block at any anatomic site with average awake ventricular rates of 40 beats/min or faster if especially cardiomegaly of LV dysfunction is present.
2. Asymptomatic type II second-degree AV block with narrow QRS. When type II second-degree AV block occurs with wide QRS, pacing becomes a class I indication.
3. Asymptomatic type I second-degree AV block at intra- or infra-His levels found at electrophysiological study performed for other indications.
4. First-degree AV block with symptoms suggestive of pacemaker syndrome.

Class IIb

1. Marked first-degree AV block (>0.30 s) in patients with LV dysfunction and symptoms of congestive heart failure in whom a shorter AV interval results in hemodynamic improvement, presumably by decreasing left atrial filling pressure.
2. Neuromuscular disease such as myotonic muscular dystrophy, Kearns-Sayre syndrome, Erb's dystrophy (limb-girdle), and peroneal muscular atrophy with any degree AV block (including first-degree AV block) with or without symptoms, because there may be unpredictable progression of AV conduction disease.

Class III

1. Asymptomatic first-degree AV block.
2. Asymptomatic type I second-degree AV block at the supra-His (AV node) level or not known to be intra-or infra-Hisian.
3. AV block expected to resolve and/or unlikely to recur (e.g., drug toxicity, Lyme disease, or during hypoxia in sleep apnea syndrome in absence of symptoms).

B. *Indications for permanent pacing in chronic bifascicular and trifascicular block*

Class I

1. Intermittent third-degree AV block.
2. Type II second-degree AV block.
3. Alternating bundle branch block.

Class IIa

1. Syncope not demonstrated to be due to AV block when other likely causes have been excluded, specifically ventricular tachycardia.
2. Incidental finding at electrophysiological study of markedly prolonged HV interval (100 ms) in asymptomatic patients.
3. Incidental finding at electrophysiological study of pacing-induced infra-His block that is not physiological.

(continued)

Table 9 (Continued)

Class IIb
1. Neuromuscular disease such as myotonic muscular dystrophy, Kearns-Sayre syndrome, Erb's dystrophy (limb-girdle), and peroneal muscular atrophy with any degree of fascicular block with or without symptoms, because there may be unpredictable progression of AV conduction disease.

Class III
1. Fascicular block without AV block or symptoms.
2. Fascicular block with first-degree AV block without symptoms.

C. Indications of pacing in patients with sinus node disease

Class I
1. Sinus node dysfunction with documented symptomatic bradycardia, including frequent sinus pauses that produce symptoms. In some patients, bradycardia is iatrogenic and will occur as a consequence of essential long-term drug therapy of a type and dose for which there are no acceptable alternatives.
2. Symptomatic chronotropic incompetence.

Class IIa
1. Sinus node dysfunction occurring spontaneously or as a result of necessary drug therapy, with heart rate of less than 40 beats/min when a clear association between significant symptoms consistent with bradycardia and the actual presence of bradycardia has not been documented.
2. Syncope of unexplained origin when major abnormalities of sinus node function are discovered or provoked in elelctrophysiologic studies.

Class IIb
1. In minimally symptomatic patients, chronic heart rate less than 40 beats/min while awake.

Class III
1. Sinus node dysfunction in asymptomatic patients, including those in whom substantial sinus bradycardia (heart rate <40 beats/min) is a consequence of long-term drug treatment.
2. Sinus node dysfunction in patients with symptoms suggestive of bradycardia that are clearly documented as not associated with a slow heart rate.
3. Sinus node dysfunction with symptomatic bradycardia due to nonessential drug therapy.

In *second-degree AV block* the level of block cannot be determined by ECG. However, in type I second-degree AV block with a normal QRS complex, the block is usually in the AV node and is not an indication for a pacemaker. Type II second-degree AV block, especially when associated with widening of the QRS complex, is usually infra-Hisan and associated with conduction system disease, and is thus an indication for implantation of a permanent pacemaker *(52)*.

Symptoms in patients with *sinus node disease* can be due to tachycardia, bradycardia, or both. Patients might present with palpitations, weakness, dizziness, or syncope. About one third of patients with sick sinus syndrome have an associated AV conduction abnormality. A permanent pacemaker should be implanted only in the presence of a causal relationship between bradycardia and symptoms. Asymptomatic *sinoatrial exit block*, *sinus bradycardia*, and *sinus pauses* do not constitute indication for pacing. In *tachycardia-bradycardia syndrome*, drugs might worsen bradycardia. These patients are best managed with a permanent pacemaker and antiarrhythmic drugs.

Electrophysiologic evaluation of sinus node function can be performed in patients who are asymptomatic during detailed noninvasive monitoring, but it has a low sensitivity. Dual-chamber pacing is being increasingly used for sick sinus syndrome as newer generations of pacemakers have the function of automatic mode switching, whereby the pacemaker changes pacing mode from dual-chamber to ventricular with the onset of an atrial arrhythmia *(63)*. In North America about 46% of permanent pacemakers are implanted for sinus node disease. Indications for the use of permanent pacing in the management of patients with sick sinus syndrome are shown in Table 9.

Neurally mediated syncope is a form of vasovagal syncope that is reproduced by tilt-table testing. Symptoms can be very disabling. Therapy with β-blockers, disopyramide, or mineralocorticoids alone or in various combinations should be tried initially. In patients with drug-refractory symptoms with a significant bradycardia component during syncope, permanent dual-chamber pacemakers are used. Use of permanent pacemakers has been shown to reduce the incidence of syncope, although it cannot prevent all the symptoms, especially in patients with a prominent vasodepressor component. In patients with the cardioinhibitory type of carotid sinus hypersensitivity, permanent dual-chamber pacemakers reduce the incidence of syncopal episodes.

REFERENCES

1. Krahn AD, Yee R, Klein GJ, Morillo C. Inappropriate sinus tachycardia: evaluation and therapy. J Cardiovasc Electrophysiol 1995;6:1124–1128.
2. Gomes JA, Mehta D, Langan MN. Sinus node reentrant tachycardia. Pacing-Clin-Electrophysiol 1995;18:1045–1057.
3. Sanders WE Jr, Sorrentino RA, Greenfield RA, et al. Catheter ablation of sinoatrial node reentrant tachycardia. J Am Coll Cardiol 1994;23:926–934.
4. Wellens HJJ, Brugada P. Mechanism of supraventricular tachycardia. Am J Cardiol 1988;62:10D–15D.
5. Haines DE, DiMarco JP. Sustained intra-atrial reentry tachycardia: clinical, electrocardiographic and electrophysiologic characteristics and long-term follow-up. J Am Coll Cardiol 1990;15:1345–1354.
6. Gillette PC, Smith RT, Garson A, et al. Chronic supraventricular tachycardia: a curable cause of congestive cardiomyopathy. JAMA 1985;253:391–392.
7. Lown B, Marcus F, Levin HD. Digitalis and atrial tachycardias with block. N Engl J Med 1959;260:301–309.
8. Singh S, Zobel RG, Brodsky MA, et al. Efficacy and safety of oral dofetilide in converting to and maintaining sinus rhythm in patients with chronic atrial fibrillation or atrial flutter: the symptomatic atrial fibrillation investigative research on dofetilidethe (SAFIRE-D) study. Circulation 2000;102;2385–2390.
9. Mehta D, Wafa S, Ward DE, Camm AJ. Relative efficacy of various physical manoeuvres in the termination of junctional tachycardia. Lancet 1988;28:1181–1185.
10. Malcolm AD, Garratt CJ, Camm AJ. The therapeutic and diagnostic cardiac electrophysiological uses of adenosine. Cardiovasc Drugs Ther 1993;7:139–147.
11. Basta M, Klein GJ, Yee R, et al. Current role of pharmacologic therapy for patients with paroxysmal supraventricular tachycardia. Cardiol Clin 1997;15:587–597.
12. Echt DS, Liebson PR, Mitchell LB, et al., and the CAST investigators. Mortality and morbidity in patients receiving encainide, flecainide or placebo. The Cardiac Arrhythmia Suppression Trial. N Engl J Med 1991;324:781–788.
13. Hindricks G. The Multicentre European Radiofrequency Survey (MERFS): complications of radiofrequency catheter ablation of arrhythmias. The Multicentre European Radiofrequency Survey (MERFS) investigators of the Working Group on Arrhythmias of the European Society of Cardiology. Eur Heart J 1993;14:1644–1653.
14. Jackman WM, Beckman KJ, McClelland JH, et al. Treatment of supraventricular tachycardia due to atrioventricular nodal reentry, by radiofrequency catheter ablation of slow-pathway conduction. N Engl J Med 1992;327:313–318.
15. Jackman WM, Wang XZ, Friday KJ, et al. Catheter ablation of accessory atrioventricular pathways (Wolff-Parkinson-White syndrome) by radiofrequency current. N Engl J Med 1991;324:1605–1611.
16. Saul JP, Hulse JE, De W, et al. Catheter ablation of accessory atrioventricular pathways in young patients: use of long vascular sheaths, the transseptal approach and a retrograde left posterior parallel approach. J Am Coll Cardiol 1993;21:571–583.
17. Chen SA, Chiang CE, Yang CJ, et al. Sustained atrial tachycardia in adult patients: electrophysiological characteristics, pharmacological response, possible mechanisms and effects of radiofrequency ablation. Circulation 1994;90:1262–1278.
18. Tucker KJ, Wilson C. A comparison of transesophageal atrial pacing and direct current cardioversion for the termination of atrial flutter: a prospective randomized clinical trial. Br Heart J 1993;69:530–538.
19. Ellenbogen KA, Stambler BS, Wood MA, et al. Efficacy of intravenous ibutilide for rapid termination of atrial fibrillation and atrial flutter: a dose-response study. J Am Coll Cardiol 1996;28:130–136.
20. Cosio FG, Arribas F, Lopez-Gil M, Palacios J. Atrial flutter mapping and ablation. I Studying atrial flutter mechanisms by mapping and entrainment. Pacing Clin Electrophysiol 1996;19:641–653.
21. Schwartzman D, Callans DJ, Gottlieb CD, et al. Conduction block in the inferior vena caval-tricuspid valve isthmus: association with outcome of radiofrequency ablation of type I atrial flutter. J Am Coll Cardiol 1996;28:1519–1531.
22. Cosio FG, Martin-Penaato A, Pastor A, et al. Atypical atrial flutter: a review. Pacing Clin Electrphysiol 2003;26:2157–2169.
23. Gomes JA, Santoni-Rugiu F, Mehta D, et al. Uncommon atrial flutter: characteristics, mechanisms, and results of ablative therapy. Pacing Clin Electrophysiol 1998;21:2029–2042.
24. Kannel W, Abbott R, Savage D, McNamara P. Epidemiologic features of chronic atrial fibrillation: the Framingham Study. N Engl J Med 1982;17:1018–1022.
25. Wipf JE, Lipsky BA. Atrial fibrillation. Thromboembolic risk and indications for anticoagulation. Arch Intern Med 1990;150:1598–1603.
26. Morris JJ Jr, Peter RH, McIntosh HD. Electrical cardioversion of atrial fibrillation. Immediate and long-term results and selection of patients. Ann Intern Med 1966;65:216–231.

27. Geelen P, Goethals M, de Bruyne B, Brugada P. A prospective hemodynamic evaluation of patients with chronic atrial fibrillation undergoing radiofrequency catheter ablation of the atrioventricular junction. Am J Cardiol 1997;80: 1606–1609.

28. Investigators of five atrial fibrillation studies. Risk factors for stroke and efficacy of antithrombotic therapy in atrial fibrillation: analysis of pooled data from five randomized controlled trials. Arch Intern Med 1994;154:1449–1457.

29. Olsson SB; Executive Steering Committee on behalf of the SPORTIF III Investigators. Stroke prevention with the oral direct thrombin inhibitor ximelagtran compared with warfarin in patients with non-valvular atrial fibrillation (SPORTIF III): randomized controlled trail. Lancet 2003;362:1691–1698.

30. Manning WJ, Silverman DI, Keighley CS, et al. Transesophageal echocardiographically facilitated early cardioversion from atrial fibrillation using short-term anticoagulation: final results of a prospective 4.5-year study. J Am Coll Cardiol 1995;25:1354–1361.

31. Van Gelder IC, Crijns HJ, Van Gilst WH, et al. Prediction of uneventful cardioversion and maintenance of sinus rhythm from direct current electrical cardioversion of chronic atrial fibrillation and flutter. Am J Cardiol 1991;68: 41–46.

32. Bolognesi R. The pharmacologic treatment of atrial fibrillation. Cardiovasc Drug Ther 1991;5:617–628.

33. Falk RH. Proarrhythmia in patients treated for atrial fibrillation or flutter. Ann Intern Med 1992;11:529–535.

34. AFFIRM First Antiarrhythmic Drug Substudy Investigators. Maintenance of sinus rhythm in patients with atrial fibrillation: an AFFIRM substudy of the first antiarrhythmic drug. J Am Coll Cardiol 2003;42:20–29.

35. Singh S, Zoble RG, Yellen L, et al. Efficacy and safety of oral dofetilide in converting to and sinus rhythm in patients with chronic atrial fibrillation or atrial flutter: the symptomatic atrial fibrillation investigative research on dofetilide (SAFIRE-D) study. Circulation 2000;102:2385–2390.

36. Wyse DG, Waldo AL, DiMarco JP, et al., Atrial Fibrillation Follow-up Investigation of Rhythm Management (AFFIRM) Investigators. A comparison of rate control and rhythm control in patients with atrial fibrillation. N Engl J Med 2002;347:1825–1833.

37. Haissaguerre M, Jais P, Shah DC, et al. Spontaneous initiation of atrial fibrillation by ectopic beats originating in the pulmonary veins. N Engl J Med 1998;339:659–666.

38. Pappone C, Rosanio S, Augello G, et al. Mortality, morbidity, and quality of life after circumferential pulmonary vein ablation for atrial fibrillation: outcome from a controlled non-randomized long-term study. J Am Coll Cardiol 2003;42(2):185–197.

39. Wellens HJ, Sie HT, Smeets JL, et al. Surgical treatment of atrial fibrillation. J Cardiovasc Electrophysiol 1998;9: S151–S154.

40. Wang K, Hodges M. The premature ventricular complex as a diagnostic aid. Ann Intern Med 1992;117:766–770.

41. Waldo AL, Camm AJ, deRuyter H, et al. Effect of d-sotalol on mortality in patients with left ventricular dysfunction after recent and remote myocardial infarction. The SWORD Investigators. Survival With Oral d-Sotalol. Lancet 1996; 348:7–12.

42. Cairns JA, Connolly SJ, Roberts R, Gent M. Randomised trial of outcome after myocardial infarction in patients with frequent or repetitive ventricular premature depolarisations: CAMIAT. Canadian Amiodarone Myocardial Infarction Arrhythmia Trial Investigators. Lancet 1997;349:675–682.

43. Julian DG, Camm AJ, Frangin G, et al. Randomised trial of effect of amiodarone on mortality in patients with left-ventricular dysfunction after recent myocardial infarction: EMIAT. European Myocardial Infarct Amiodarone Trial Investigators. Lancet 1997;349:667–674.

44. Doval HC, Nul DR, Grancelli HO, et al. GESICA, Capital Federal, Argentina randomised trial of low-dose amiodarone in severe congestive heart failure. Lancet 1994;344:493–498.

45. Singh SN, Fletcher RD, Fisher S, et al. Veterans Affairs congestive heart failure antiarrhythmic trial. CHF STAT Investigators. Am J Cardiol 1993;72:99F–102F.

46. Buxton AE, Lee KL, DiCarlo L, et al. Nonsustained ventricular tachycardia in coronary artery disease: relation to inducible sustained ventricular tachycardia. MUSTT Investigators. Ann Intern Med 1996;125:35–39.

47. Moss AJ, Hall WJ, Cannom DS, et al. Improved survival with an implanted defibrillator in patients with prior myocardial infarction, low, ejection fraction and asymptomatic non-sustained ventricular tachycardia. N Engl J Med 1996;335:1933–1940.

48. Moss AJ, Zareba W, Hall WJ, et al., Multicenter Automatic Defibrillator Implantation Trial II Investigators. Prophylactic implantation of a defibrillator in patients with myocardial infarction and reduced ejection fraction. N Engl J Med 2002;346:877–883.

49. Cardiac Arrest in Seattle: Conventional Versus Amiodarone Drug Evaluation (the CASCADE study). Am J Cardiol 1991;67:578–584.

50. The ESVEM investigators. Determinants of predicted efficacy of antiarrhythmic drugs in the electrophysiologic study versus electrocardiographic monitoring trial. Circulation 1993;87:323–329.

51. The AVID investigators. A comparison of antiarrhythmic drug therapy with implantable defibrillators in patients resuscitated from near fatal ventricular arrhythmias. N Engl J Med 1997;337:1576–1583.

52. Gregoratos G, Abrams J, Epstein AE, et al. ACC/AHA/NASPE 2002 Guideline Update for Implantation of Cardiac Pacemakers and Antiarrhythmia Devices: Summary Article—A Report of the American College of Cardiology/ American Heart Association Task Force on Practice Guidelines (ACC/AHA/NASPE Committee to update the 1988 Pacemaker Implantation). Circulation 2002;106:2145–2161.

53. Klein LS, Shih HT, Hackett FK, et al. Radiofrequency catheter ablation of ventricular tachycardia in patients without structural heart disease. Circulation 1992;85:1666–1674.

54. Stevenson WG, Khan H, Sager P, et al. Identification of reentry circuit sites during catheter mapping and radiofrequency ablation of ventricular tachycardia late after myocardial infarction. Circulation 1993;88:1647–1670.
55. Breithardt G, Wichter T, Haverkamp W, et al. Implantable cardioverter defibrillator therapy in patients with arrhythmogenic right ventricular cardiomyopathy, long QT syndrome, or no structural heart disease. Am Heart J 1994;127:1151–1158.
56. Almendral JM, Ormaetxe J, Martinez-Alday JD, et al. Treatment of ventricular arrhythmias in patients with hypertrophic cardiomyopathy. Eur Heart J 1993;14 Suppl J:71–72.
57. Splawski I, Timothy KW, Vincent GM, et al. Molecular basis of the long-QT syndrome associated with deafness. N Engl J Med 1997;336:1562–1567.
58. Brugada P, Brugada J, Brugada R. The Brugada syndrome. Card Electrophysiol Rev 2002;6:49–53.
59. Goldberg RJ, Zevallos JC, Yarzebski J, et al. Prognosis of acute myocardial infarction complicated by complete heart block (the Worcester Heart Attack Study). Am J Cardiol 1992;69:1135–1141.
60. Klein LS, Miles WM, Heger JJ, Zipes DP. Transcutaneous pacing: patient tolerance, strength interval relations and feasibility for programmed stimulation. Am J Cardiol 1988;62:1126–1131.
61. Shinbane JS, Chu E, DeMarco T, et al. Evaluation of acute dual-chamber pacing with a range of atrioventricular delays on cardiac performance in refractory heart failure. J Am Coll Cardiol 1997;30:1295–1300.
62. Barold SS. Indications for permanent cardiac pacing in first-degree AV block: class I, II, or III? Pacing Clin Electrophysiol 1996;19:747–751.
63. Connolly SJ, Kerr C, Gent M, Yusuf S. Dual-chamber versus ventricular pacing: critical appraisal of current data. Circulation 1996;94:578–583.

RECOMMENDED READING

Almendral JM, Ormaetxe J, Martinez-Alday JD, et al. Treatment of ventricular arrhythmias in patients with hypertrophic cardiomyopathy. Eur Heart J 1993;14(Suppl J):71–72.
Basta M, Klein GJ, Yee R, et al. Current role of pharmacologic therapy for patients with paroxysmal supraventricular tachycardia. Cardiol Clin 1997;15:587–597.
Barold SS. Indications for permanent cardiac pacing in first-degree AV block: class I, II, or III? Pacing Clin Electrophysiol 1996;19:747–751.
Bolognesi R. The pharmacologic treatment of atrial fibrillation. Cardiovasc Drug Ther 1991;5:617–628.
Camm AJ, Obel OA. Epidemiology and mechanism of atrial fibrillation and atrial flutter. Am J Cardiol 1996;78:3–11.
Connolly SJ, Kerr C, Gent M, Yusuf S. Dual-chamber versus ventricular pacing: critical appraisal of current data. Circulation 1996;94:578–583.
Falk RH. Proarrhythmia in patients treated for atrial fibrillation or flutter. Ann Intern Med 1992;11:529–535.
Gregoratos G, Cheitlin MD, Conill A, et al. ACC/AHA Guidelines for Implantation of Cardiac Pacemakers and Antiarrhythmia Devices: Executive Summary—a report of the American College of Cardiology/American Heart Association Task Force on Practice Guidelines (Committee on Pacemaker Implantation). Circulation 1998;97:1325–1335.
Hammill SC, Packer DL. Amiodarone in congestive heart failure: unravelling the GESICA and CHF-STAT differences [editorial]. Heart 1996;75:6–7.
Hohnloser SH, Woosley RL. Sotalol. N Engl J Med 1994;331:31–38.
Krahn AD, Yee R, Klein GJ, Morillo C. Inappropriate sinus tachycardia: evaluation and therapy. J Cardiovasc Electrophysiol 1995;6:1124–1132.
Malcolm AD, Garratt CJ, Camm AJ. The therapeutic and diagnostic cardiac electrophysiological uses of adenosine. Cardiovasc Drugs Ther 1993;7:139–147.
Mymin D, Mathewson FA, Tate RB, Manfreda J. The natural history of primary first-degree atrioventricular heart block. N Engl J Med 1986;315:1183–1187.
Roden DM. Risks and benefits of antiarrhythmic therapy. N Engl J Med 1994;331:785–792.
Sarter BH, Callans DJ, Gottlieb GD, et al. Implantable defibrillator diagnostic storage capabilities: evolution, current status, and future utilization. Pacing Clin Electrophysiol 1998;21:1287–1298.
Sopher SM, Camm AJ. New trials in atrial fibrillation. J Cardiovasc Electrophysiol 1998;9(8 Suppl):S211–S215.
Wellens HJJ, Brugada P. Mechanism of supraventricular tachycardia. Am J Cardiol 1988;62:10D–15D.
Wipf JE, Lipsky BA. Atrial fibrillation. Thromboembolic risk and indications for anticoagulation. Arch Intern Med 1990;150:1598–1603.

18 Syncope

Fei Lü, MD, PhD,
Scott Sakaguchi, MD,
and David G. Benditt, MD

INTRODUCTION

Syncope is a syndrome consisting of a relatively short period of temporary and self-limited loss of consciousness caused by transient diminution of blood flow to the brain *(1,2)*. In the absence of complete loss of consciousness, the individual is considered to have experienced a near-faint or near-syncope, or presyncope.

True syncope may be considered to fall within a larger set of conditions in which the loss of consciousness is transient and spontaneously reversible. Thus, syncope must be distinguished from other symptoms that are not true faints, but are often incorrectly classified as such (e.g., seizures, sleep disorders). Furthermore, an episode of loss of consciousness should not be considered syncope in the absence of spontaneous reversal. Similarly, if cerebral dysfunction is not due to insufficient cerebral nutrient flow, the loss of consciousness or apparent loss of consciousness should not be termed syncope. Finally, many patients complain of less-specific symptoms such as "dizziness" or "lightheadedness." More often than not, these latter symptoms are not related to syncope either clinically or pathophysiologically.

CLASSIFICATION AND ETIOLOGY

Establishing the cause (or causes) of syncope is crucial in order to assess prognosis and provide an effective treatment strategy. Unfortunately, however, the diagnostic evaluation of these patients continues to prove challenging. Often, syncope patients are admitted to the hospital and undergo expensive investigations, many of which are unnecessary and ultimately do not provide a definite diagnosis. The development of specialized syncope evaluation clinics and the publication of diagnosis and treatment guidelines may play an important role in improving care of these patients *(1)*.

Table 1 summarizes the most important causes of syncope, and a brief overview of the principal diagnostic categories is provided here.

1. *Neurally mediated syncope* comprises a number of related clinical conditions (Table 1), the best known of which is the common or vasovagal syncope. Other forms of neural reflex syncope include carotid sinus syndrome, or syncope triggered by micturition or defecation. Swallowing or emptying the bladder may also trigger a reflex syncope. Coughing may trigger reflex hypotension, but in this case hypotension induced by cough-related mechanics may also contribute to the faint.
2. *Orthostatic (postural) syncope* is very common. It is usually associated with movement from lying or sitting to a standing position. Most often, postural faints tend to occur a few moments after arising, especially if the affected individual has walked a short distance. Many healthy individuals experience a minor form of this syncope when they need to support themselves momentarily just

From: *Essential Cardiology: Principles and Practice, 2nd Ed.*
Edited by: C. Rosendorff © Humana Press Inc., Totowa, NJ

Table 1
Classification of Syncope

Neurally mediated reflex syncopal syndromes
   Vasovagal syncope (common faint)
   Carotid sinus syncope
   Situational syncope
      Acute hemorrhage
      Cough, sneeze
      Gastrointestinal stimulation (e.g., swallow, defecation, and visceral pain)
      Micturition (postmicturition)
      Post-exercise
      Other (e.g., brass instrument playing, weightlifting, and postprandial)
   Glossopharyngeal and trigeminal neuralgia
Orthostatic syncope
   Primary autonomic failure syndromes (e.g., pure autonomic failure, multiple system atrophy,
     Parkinson's disease with autonomic failure)
   Secondary autonomic failure syndromes (e.g., diabetic neuropathy, amyloid neuropathy, drugs, alcohol)
   Volume depletion (e.g., hemorrhage, diarrhea, Addison's disease)
Cardiac arrhythmias as primary cause
   Sinus node dysfunction (including bradycardia/tachycardia syndrome)
   Atrioventricular conduction system disease
   Paroxysmal supraventricular and ventricular tachycardias
   Inherited syndromes (e.g., long-QT syndrome and Brugada syndrome)
   Implanted device (pacemaker and ICD) malfunction
   Drug-induced proarrhythmias
Structural cardiac or cardiopulmonary disease
   Cardiac valvular disease
   Acute myocardial infarction/ischemia
   Obstructive hypertrophic cardiomyopathy
   Atrial myxoma
   Acute aortic dissection
   Pericardial disease/tamponade
   Pulmonary embolus/pulmonary hypertension
Cerebrovascular
   Vascular steal syndromes

after standing up. The most dramatic postural syncope occurs in older frail individuals, particularly in the presence of autonomic failure (e.g., diabetes or certain nervous system diseases) or persons who are dehydrated (e.g., from hot environments or inadequate fluid intake). Certain commonly prescribed medications that inhibit the autonomic nervous system and/or reduce blood volume (e.g., β-adrenergic blockers, diuretics, antihypertensives, or vasodilators) may predispose to postural syncope.

3. *Cardiac arrhythmias* may cause syncope if the heart rate is either too slow or too fast to permit maintenance of an adequate systemic arterial pressure. Bradycardia, such as sinus pauses or high-grade AV block, or asystole at the termination of an atrial tachyarrhythmia, is the most common cause of syncope in this section. Occasionally, however, syncope of this type also occurs at the onset of an episode of paroxysmal ventricular or supraventricular tachycardias. Neurally mediated hypotension plays an important role in these patients. Individuals with underlying heart disease (e.g., previous myocardial infarction or valvular heart disease) or disturbances of autonomic nervous system responsiveness are at greatest risk for arrhythmia-related syncope. Patients suspected of ventricular tachycardia-induced syncope should receive prompt referral for cardiac electrophysiological evaluation due to high risk of sudden cardiac death *(3)*.

Table 2
Causes of Conditions Commonly Misdiagnosed as Syncope

Disorders with impairment or loss of consciousness
    Metabolic disorders, (e.g., hypoglycemia, hypoxia, and hyperventilation with hypocapnia)
    Epilepsy
    Intoxication (drugs and alcohol)
    Vertebrobasilar transient ischemic attack
Disorders resembling syncope without loss of consciousness
    Cataplexy
    Drop attacks
    Psychogenic pseudosyncope
    Transient ischemic attacks of carotid artery origin

4. *Structural cardiopulmonary diseases* (such as acute myocardial infarction or pulmonary embolism) are relatively infrequent causes of syncope. Neurally mediated reflexes as well as the direct hemodynamic impact of the acute disease process are the important underlying mechanisms.

5. *Cerebrovascular disease* is almost never the cause of a true syncope *(1,2,4)*. A rare exception may be vertebrobasilar transient ischemic attack (TIA), but this condition is rare and is usually accompanied by other symptoms such as vertigo. Subclavian steal (evidenced by blood pressure difference of >20 mmHg between arms) is another example in this class.

6. *Conditions that mimic syncope* (Table 2) are included here only due to the fact that they often are mislabeled as syncope and thereby cause diagnostic confusion. In the absence of the essential mechanism of syncope (transient global cerebral hypoperfusion), a real or apparent episode of loss of consciousness should not be diagnosed as syncope. The most common conditions in this category include seizures, sleep disturbances, cataplexy, accidental falls, and some psychiatric conditions (e.g., anxiety attacks and hysterical reactions).

EPIDEMIOLOGY AND PROGNOSIS

The reported prevalence of syncope varies from 15% to 25% in different populations. The highest frequency of syncope occurs in patients with cardiovascular comorbidity and older patients in institutional care settings. Recent surveys indicate that syncope accounts for approximately 1% of emergency department visits in Europe *(5,6)*.

One third of syncope patients have symptom recurrences by 3 yr of follow-up *(1,7)*. The majority of these recurrences occur within the first 2 yr. Predictors of recurrence include a history of recurrent syncope at the time of presentation (i.e., recurrences lead to more future recurrences), age less than 45 yr, or a psychiatric diagnosis. After positive tilt-table testing, patients with more than six syncopal spells have a risk of recurrence of >50% over 2 yr.

Many syncopal patients, especially young healthy individuals with a normal ECG and without heart disease, have an excellent prognosis. Most of these individuals have one of the neurally mediated syndromes. However, the prognosis of syncope is not completely benign, especially in the presence of cardiac diseases. The 1-yr mortality of patients with cardiac syncope is consistently higher (18–33%) than patients with noncardiac causes (0–12%) or unexplained syncope (6%). The 1-yr sudden death rate is 24% in patients with a cardiac cause compared with 3% in the other two groups *(6–9)*.

The presence and severity of structural heart disease are the most important predictors of mortality risk in syncope patients. It had been thought that patients with cardiac causes of syncope have similar mortality to matched controls with comparable degrees of heart disease. However, recent data suggest that implantation of an implantable cardioverter defibrillator (ICD) may be associated with better prognosis in unexplained syncope in certain clinical settings, such as idiopathic dilated cardiomyopathy *(10)*.

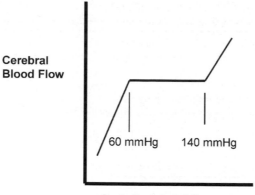

Fig. 1. Graph illustrating the manner in which cerebral blood flow is autoregulated over a wide range of systemic pressures under normal conditions. On this graph, cerebral blood flow (y-axis) remains relatively constant over the arterial pressure range (x-axis) 60 mmHg to 140 mmHg. Only at lower or higher pressures is flow pressure-dependent. Disease states, such as diabetes or hypertension, may move the "autoregulated" zone to higher pressures. In such cases, affected individuals may be even more predisposed to faints.

Four risk factors favoring cardiac arrhythmias as a cause of syncope or death are age >45 yr, history of congestive heart failure, history of ventricular arrhythmias, and abnormal ECG (other than nonspecific ST changes). Arrhythmias or death within 1 yr occurred in 4 to 7% of patients without any risk factors and progressively increased to 58 to 80% in patients with three or more factors.

PATHOPHYSIOLOGY AND CLINICAL PRESENTATION

Transient global cerebral hypoperfusion is the sine qua non of syncope pathophysiology *(1,2)*. In the vast majority of cases, diminished cerebral perfusion is due to a transient fall in systemic blood pressure. Cerebral blood flow is normally autoregulated within a range of systemic blood pressures. A decrease in systolic blood pressure to 60 mmHg or less usually leads to syncope (Fig. 1).

The integrity of cerebral nutrient flow is dependent on mechanisms that maintain systemic pressure. The most important of these factors are:

- Baroreflexes and autonomic adjustment in blood pressure, cardiac contractility, and heart rate;
- Intravascular volume regulation, incorporating renal and hormonal influences to maintain central blood volume; and
- Cerebrovascular autoregulation, which permits constant cerebral blood flow to be maintained over a relatively wide range of perfusion pressures.

Transient failure of protective mechanisms may be due to various factors, such as those that occur with autonomic failure, vasodilator drugs, diuretics, dehydration, or hemorrhage, may reduce systemic blood pressure below the autoregulatory range and can induce a syncopal episode.

Orthostatic blood pressure adjustment plays an important role in syncope. On moving from the supine to the erect posture there is a large gravitational shift of blood away from the chest to the venous capacitance system below the diaphragm *(1,11)*. This shift is estimated to total 500 to 1000 mL of blood, and largely occurs in the first 10 s of standing. With prolonged standing (within 10 min), the high capillary transmural pressure in dependent parts of the body causes a filtration of protein-free fluid into the interstitial spaces. As a consequence of this gravitationally induced blood pooling and superimposed decline in plasma volume, the return of venous blood to the heart is reduced, resulting in rapid diminution of cardiac filling pressure and decrease in stroke volume. Reflex-induced increase in heart rate is the immediate response to maintain cardiac output. However, vasoconstriction and subsequent neuroendocrine system adjustment are important to compensate for reduced effective blood volume.

In many forms of syncope, impaired vasoconstriction is a key factor leading to systemic hypotension. Similarly, reduced skeletal muscle pump activity due to prolonged quiet up-right posture is a frequent contributor as well. On the other hand, certain physiological maneuvers may help prevent hypotension. Physical movement and leg crossing enhance muscle pump activity, supine posture reduces gravitational demands on vascular constriction, and increased "respiratory pump" activity may increase venous return. In fact, enhancement of respiratory pump activity appears to be a promising means for reducing susceptibility to excessive orthostatic hypotension.

Loss of postural tone is an inevitable consequence of loss of consciousness. If the affected individual is not restrained, he or she will slump to a gravitationally neutral position (e.g., fall to the ground). Sometimes, nonskeletal muscles may be affected, resulting in loss of bladder (common) or bowel (rare) control. On occasion, patients may have jerky movements after onset of loss of consciousness; because of these muscle movements, true syncope may be mistaken for a seizure disorder or "fit" by untrained witnesses.

STRATEGY FOR SYNCOPE EVALUATION

The crucial first step in syncope evaluation is to ascertain whether the reported loss-of-consciousness episode(s) was in fact true syncope. In order to achieve this goal in a cost-effective manner, the assessment of these patients must be both well-organized and thorough, and at the same time avoid excessive application of inappropriate tests. The crux of the initial evaluation (and often, all that is really needed) is a detailed medical history and careful physical examination.

Initial Evaluation—The History

The story provided by the patient and witnesses very often reveals the most likely cause of the loss of consciousness, and provides a means of guiding any necessary subsequent evaluation. Three key questions are: (1) Is loss of consciousness attributable to syncope or other causes, including accidental falls? (2) Is heart disease present or absent? (3) Are there important clinical features in the history that suggest the diagnosis?

The details surrounding syncope events must be documented carefully. Witnesses can be valuable for filling in items that the patient may not recall. Key features to consider include:

Characterize situations in which syncope tends to occur.
Position (supine, sitting, or standing), activity (at rest, exercise, or postprandial period), abrupt neck movements, voiding or defecation, cough or swallowing; crowded or warm places, prolonged standing, or psychological stress (fear, intense pain, or emotional upset).
Define prodromal symptoms.
Are symptoms associated with nausea, vomiting, feeling of cold, sweating, visual aura, pain in neck or shoulders, blurred vision, or palpitations?
Document eyewitness observations.
Manner of fall (abrupt fall with possibility of injury or purposeful avoidance of injury), skin color changes, duration of syncope, breathing pattern, physical movements (e.g., tonic-clonic or myoclonic movements); incontinence, or tongue biting.
Document symptoms after syncope.
Fatigue, confusion, palpitations, headache, nausea, vomiting, sweating, feeling of cold, muscle aches, skin color, injury, or chest pain. Inability to stand up without triggering another episode may suggest neurally mediated reflex syncope.
Characterize risk for syncope recurrence and/or life-threatening consequences.
Family history of syncope, sudden death, or known genetically transmitted conditions (e.g., long-QT syndrome, Brugada syndrome, arrhythmogenic ventricular dysplasia). Fainter's medical history of structural cardiac disease (e.g., prior myocardial infarction, valvular heart disease, congenital conditions, and previous cardiac surgery), neurological conditions (e.g., Parkinson's disease, epilepsy, migraine), metabolic/intoxication disorders (e.g., diabetes and alcoholism), or drug abuse (e.g., cocaine).

Identify prescribed medications predisposing to syncope.

Drugs known to predispose to syncope include antihypertensives, antianginal drugs, antidepressant agents, antiarrhythmics, diuretics, or any QT-prolonging agents. Has there been any recent dosing change? Have any new drugs been added?

Initial Evaluation—Physical Findings

Physical findings that may help to establish a basis for syncope include orthostatic blood pressure changes, cardiovascular abnormalities, response to carotid sinus message, and (less frequently) neurological signs. Carotid sinus massage is a recommended diagnostic step during the physical examination, especially in the elderly (>60 yr). ECG, echocardiogram, chest X-ray, and blood count may also be reasonably incorporated.

Important cardiovascular findings that may lead to a suspected cause of syncope include differences in blood pressure in each arm, pathological cardiac and vascular murmurs, signs of pulmonary embolism, aortic stenosis, hypertrophic cardiomyopathy, myxoma, or aortic dissection. Signs of focal neurological lesions, such as hemiparesis, dysarthria, diplopia, and vertigo or signs of parkinsonism are suggestive of, but not diagnostic of, a neurological cause of impairment of consciousness. In most cases, these patients did not suffer from a true syncope, and as such should be referred for neurological evaluation.

Outcomes of Initial Evaluation

The outcome of the initial evaluation may be identification of a "certain" basis for symptoms, or perhaps a "suspected" (i.e., less confident) basis for symptoms, or symptoms may remain of an entirely unexplained cause.

CERTAIN DIAGNOSIS

A number of conditions can be sufficiently clearly identified by careful initial evaluation alone that no further testing is required. Examples include:

- "Classic" vasovagal syncope in which precipitating events such as fear, blood draw, severe pain, or emotional distress are associated with typical prodromal symptoms.
- Situational syncope that occurs during or immediately after certain circumstances, such as emptying the bladder, coughing, or swallowing.
- Postural ("orthostatic") syncope in which there is documentation of orthostatic hypotension associated with syncope or presyncope.
- Presence on routine ECG of a severe abnormality, such as asystolic pauses >3 s, Mobitz II second-degree AV block, or complete or high-grade AV block, although such findings are usually obtained only during longer-term monitoring.

SUSPECTED DIAGNOSIS

For patients with a suspected diagnosis after initial evaluation, carefully selected "confirmatory" testing (such as long-term ECG monitoring, tilt-table testing, and/or electrophysiological study) is necessary. In these cases, diagnostic testing should first be restricted to evaluation of the suspected diagnosis, and expanded only if that diagnosis does not prove to be satisfactory.

UNEXPLAINED DIAGNOSIS

In these cases, the strategy for subsequent assessment varies according to the severity and frequency of the episodes and the presence or absence of heart disease.

- *Patients without evidence of structural heart disease*: The majority of patients with single or rare syncope episodes in this category probably have neurally mediated syncope. In such cases, tilt-table testing and carotid sinus massage should be undertaken if not already done. Psychiatric illness should be considered for patients without structural heart disease and with a normal ECG, especially if the history suggests numerous syncope episodes (e.g., many episodes each week).

- *Patients with structural heart disease*: In patients with structural heart disease or who have an abnormal ECG, cardiac evaluation is recommended at this stage. This should consist of echocardiogram, stress testing, and if appropriate, prolonged ambulatory ECG monitoring (including use of implantable loop recorders [ILRs]) and invasive electrophysiological study. For patients with palpitations associated with syncope, ambulatory ECG monitoring (including ILRs) is especially valuable. In almost every case, these patients should be referred to a specialist in the evaluation of syncope or a syncope diagnostic center.

SPECIFIC CAUSES OF SYNCOPE

Neurally Mediated Reflex Syncope

The best known and most frequently occurring forms of the neurally mediated reflex faints are vasovagal syncope and carotid sinus syndrome. Situational syncope (e.g., postmicturition syncope and cough syncope) is also encountered relatively frequently.

VASOVAGAL SYNCOPE

Vasovagal syncope may be triggered by a variety of factors, including unpleasant sights, pain, extreme emotion, and prolonged standing. Autonomic activation (e.g., flushing and sweating) in the premonitory phase suggests a vasovagal origin. Typical presentations occur in about 40% of presumed vasovagal syncope. A head-up tilt-table test is often used to confirm the diagnosis, and is the only laboratory test deemed useful in diagnosing vasovagal syncope.

As a rule, the first step of the head-up tilt-table test is a "passive" head-up tilt at 70 degrees during which the patient is supported by a footplate and gently applied body straps for a period of 20 to 45 min *(12)*. If needed, tilt-testing in conjunction with a drug challenge (e.g., isoproterenol or nitroglycerin) may be employed. This is particularly pertinent if a short passive phase is used (i.e., 20–30 min). Until recently, the most frequently used provocative drug was isoproterenol, usually given in escalating doses from 1 to 3 µg/min. However, nitroglycerin intravenously or sublingually has gained favor, in part because it expedites the procedure without adversely affecting diagnostic utility.

The head-up tilt table test in a drug-free state appears to discriminate well between symptomatic patients and asymptomatic control subjects. The false-positive rate of the tilt test is approx 10%. Test sensitivity appears to be increased with the use of pharmacologic provocation (isoproterenol or nitroglycerin), but at the cost of reduced specificity. For patients without severe structural heart disease, a positive tilt-table test (especially if it reproduces the patient's spontaneous symptoms) can be considered diagnostic. On the other hand, for patients with significant structural heart disease, other more serious causes of syncope must be excluded prior to relying on a positive tilt-test result. For the most part, the head-up tilt test is not to be relied on for predicting treatment outcomes. Clinical follow-up is far better.

The Valsalva maneuver, active standing test, cold pressor test, and cough test are occasionally used for syncope evaluations in the autonomic-function testing laboratory, but their clinical value is unclear and they play little role in evaluation of the suspected vasovagal fainter. The previously used eyeball compression test is now strongly discouraged. Neurological studies (head MRI or CT scans, as well as electroencephalograms [EEGs]) are often ordered by physicians for syncope evaluation, but usually contribute little to the diagnosis, especially in the case of neural reflex syncope. The ATP test remains a controversial topic, but it is generally not undertaken in the vasovagal syncope patient. It may have a role to play in the older fainter, where neural reflex mechanisms may be relevant but are as yet undiagnosed. ATP-induced pauses >6–10 s, even if interrupted by escape beats, are defined as abnormal. The ATP test is contraindicated in patients with asthma.

In the vast majority of cases of vasovagal syncope, patients principally require reassurance and education regarding the nature of the condition. In patients with multiple recurrent syncopes, initial advice should include review of the types of environments in which syncope is more common (e.g., hot, crowded, and emotionally upsetting situations) and provide insight into the typical warning symptoms (e.g., hot/cold feeling, sweaty, clammy, nauseated), which may permit many individuals to recognize and respond to an impending episode and thereby avert the faint. Thus, avoiding venipunture may be desirable when possible, but psychological deconditioning may be necessary. Additional commonsense measures, such as keeping well hydrated and avoiding prolonged exposure to upright posture and/or hot confining environments, should also be discussed.

"Volume expanders" or moderate exercise training appear to be among the safest initial approaches (1,13). "Tilt-training" (progressively lengthening periods of enforced up-right posture) and certain physical maneuvers (leg crossing and arm tugging) upon onset of premonitory symptoms may be helpful (14).

Many drugs have been used in the treatment of vasovagal syncope (such as β-blockers, disopyramide, scopolamine, clonidine, theophylline, fludrocortisone, ephedrine, etilephrine, midodrine, clonidine, and serotonin inhibitors). While the results have often been satisfactory in uncontrolled trials, placebo-controlled prospective trials have been unable to show a benefit for most of these drugs (1). The principal exception is midodrine, a vasoconstrictor agent (15,16). The ultimate role of cardiac pacing for vasovagal syncope remains controversial. Cardiac pacing may be useful in selected older patients in whom a prolonged asystole has been documented.

CAROTID SINUS SYNDROME

Spontaneous carotid sinus syndrome (accounting for approx 1% of all causes of syncope) may be defined as syncope that seems to occur in close relationship with accidental mechanical manipulation of the neck (presumably mediated through the carotid sinuses) and can be reproduced by carotid sinus massage (CSM). *Induced* carotid sinus syndrome is diagnosed when patients are found to have an abnormal response to carotid sinus massage and an otherwise negative workup for syncope. Thus, diagnosis of the induced form does not require the "classic" history. Regarded in this way, carotid sinus syndrome is much more frequent, up to 26% to 60% of patients affected by unexplained syncope.

Carotid sinus syndrome may be diagnosed when CSM reproduces symptoms in conjunction with a period of asystole, paroxysmal AV block, and/or a marked drop (usually >50 mmHg systolic) in systemic arterial pressure. In many instances, the most convincing results from carotid sinus massage are obtained when massage is undertaken in the upright position. In the absence of a history of spontaneous syncope, the exaggerated response, which is defined as carotid sinus hypersensitivity, must be distinguished from carotid sinus syndrome. The main complications of CSM are neurological (0.01 to 0.14%) (17,18). CSM should not be performed in patients with TIAs or strokes within the past 3 mo or in patients with carotid bruits (unless carotid Doppler studies convincingly exclude significant carotid artery narrowing) (1).

Two approaches to CSM have been advocated. The first method is probably the most widely used. CSM is performed for no more than 5 s in the supine position. A positive response is defined as a ventricular pause ≥3 s and/or a fall of systolic blood pressure ≥50 mmHg. The estimated positive rate is 35%. Abnormal responses can also be observed in subjects without syncope. The diagnosis may be missed in about one third of cases if only supine massage is performed (19). The second method requires reproduction of spontaneous symptoms during CSM for 10 s in both supine and upright positions. A positive response was observed in 49% of patients with syncope of uncertain origin and in 60% of elderly patients with syncope and sinus bradycardia, but only in 4% of patients without syncope. The eliciting of symptoms is probably the more useful endpoint for evaluation of carotid sinus syndrome.

Treatment of carotid sinus syndrome is guided by the results of carotid sinus massage (i.e., relative importance of cardioinhibitory versus vasodepressor responses). Cardiac pacing appears to be beneficial in carotid sinus syndrome and is acknowledged to be the treatment of choice when bradycardia has been documented. Judicious use of vasoconstrictors (e.g., midodrine) may be needed for patients in whom the vasodepressor aspect of the reflex is prominent.

SITUATIONAL FAINTS

Situational faints encompass a wide range of clinical scenarios. Each is characterized by the specific clinical circumstances surrounding (and presumably triggering) the event. Thus, cough syncope, micturition syncope, and swallow syncope are examples of situational faints (Table 1). Recognition of these conditions clearly depends on the careful taking of the medical history. Thereafter, treatment relies heavily on avoidance of triggering circumstances, or at least reducing the risk associated with the circumstance. By way of example, males are encouraged to sit while voiding, especially if the bladder is very full or if they have recently consumed a significant amount of alcohol.

Orthostatic Hypotension

Orthostatic syncope can be diagnosed when there is documentation of posturally induced hypotension associated with syncope or presyncope. For the diagnosis of orthostatic hypotension, arterial blood pressure must be measured when the patient adopts the standing position after at least 5 min of lying supine. For practical purposes, orthostatic hypotension is often defined as a decline in systolic blood pressure of at least 30 mmHg within 3 min of assuming a standing posture, regardless of whether or not symptoms occur. If the patient cannot tolerate standing for this period, the lowest systolic blood pressure during the upright position should be recorded.

Identification of the underlying cardiovascular, neurological, or pharmacological etiology is of particular importance for patients with orthostatic hypotension. At the outset, it is important to identify nonneurogenic reversible causes of orthostatic hypotension, such as volume depletion, effect of medications (common), and effect of comorbidities (e.g., diabetes and alcohol, and more rarely adrenal insufficiency). The most frequent drugs associated with orthostatic syncope are vasodilators and diuretics. Alcohol can be associated with orthostatic syncope, because it not only causes orthostatic intolerance but also can induce autonomic and somatic neuropathy. Elimination of the responsible drug or offending agent is usually sufficient to improve symptoms.

The initial treatment for patients with orthostatic syncope includes education regarding factors that can aggravate or provoke hypotension upon assuming the upright posture. These include avoiding sudden head-up postural change, especially in the morning after being in bed all night, or standing still for a prolonged period of time. Other important considerations that may predispose to orthostatic hypotension are high environmental temperature (including hot baths, showers, and saunas leading to vasodilation), large meals (especially with refined carbohydrates), and severe exertion.

Patients with orthostatic hypotension should be encouraged to increase dietary salt and volume intake if there are no contraindications (i.e., hypertension). In some cases, head-up sleeping (elevating the head of the bed by 8–10 in. or 20–25 cm) may improve symptoms. Certain physical countermaneuvers, such as leg crossing, squatting, bending forward, arm tugging, and other measures, may be useful to combat orthostatic hypotension. The use of an inspiratory impedance device to facilitate respiratory "blood pump" activity is currently under investigation (Advanced Circulatory Systems Inc., Eden Prairie, MN).

When physical maneuvers alone are not sufficiently effective, pharmacological interventions may be warranted. Fludrocortisone and midodrine are probably the most commonly used drugs for orthostatic hypotension. Fludrocortisone is a synthetic mineralocorticoid with minimal glucocorticoid effect for expansion of intravascular and extravascular body fluid. The starting dose is usually 0.1 mg once a day, and then increased by 0.1 mg at 1–2-wk intervals up to 0.3 mg daily, if needed. The pressor action is not immediate and takes some days to be manifest, and the full effect requires a high dietary salt intake. A weight gain of 2–3 kg is a reasonably good clue for adequate volume expansion. Mild dependent edema can be expected. Patients on fludrocortisone may develop hypokalemia within 2 wk, and potassium supplements are advised. Midodrine is a prodrug that is converted to its active metabolite, desglymidodrine, after absorption. It acts on α-adrenore-

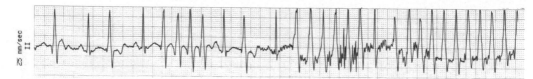

Fig. 2. Recordings from a 28-yr-old female without significant past medical history who presented to the emergency room with recurrent syncope. Recurrent episodes of wide QRS complex tachycardia associated presyncope/syncope were documented by telemetry. Orthodromic AV reentry tachycardia was easily induced during electrophysiological study. This tachycardia tended to degenerate into atrial fibrillation with a rapid ventricular response and ultimately on one occasion into ventricular fibrillation. A left anterior lateral accessory pathway was successfully ablated. The patient has remained symptom-free thereafter.

ceptors to cause constriction of both arterial resistance and venous capacitance vessels. Midodrine is administered in doses of 2.5 to 10 mg, three times daily. Midodrine is of particular value in patients with severe postural hypotension and in those with autonomic failure *(20)*. For patients with hypertension, supine hypertension is a potential problem during treatment of orthostatic hypotension. Better control of hypertension may improve orthostatic hypotension in some patients. In others, it may be necessary to accept higher resting blood pressures than would normally be considered desirable.

Cardiac Arrhythmias as Primary Cause of Syncope

Both bradycardias and tachycardias can cause syncope. Patients with syncope associated with cardiac arrhythmias or who are thought to be at increased risk of sudden cardiac death (e.g., severe underlying structural heart disease) are most appropriately evaluated by a cardiac electrophysiologist.

BRADYARRHYTHMIAS

Sinus node dysfunction leading to syncope is best established when symptoms are clearly correlated with sinoatrial bradycardia (occasionally a long pause following termination of an atrial tachycardia) using an event recorder or an implanted loop recorder. In absence of such correlation, severe sinus bradycardia lower than 40 beats/min or sinus pauses longer than 3 s are highly suggestive of symptomatic sinus node disease. Aggravation of bradycardia by drug treatment often unmasks sick sinus syndrome. A pacemaker, preferably an atrial-based pacing system with a rate-adaptive sensor, is usually required for treatment.

Chronic or paroxysmal atrioventricular (AV) block can be the cause of syncopal episodes. Bradycardia due to intermittent AV block is among the more important causes of syncope during prolonged monitoring. The presence of Mobitz II type second-degree AV block, third-degree AV block, or alternating left and right bundle branch block can reasonably be considered as being diagnostic of a bradycardic cause of syncope. In unsure cases, event monitor, electrophysiological assessment AV conduction with and without pharmacological challenge, and induction tachycardias may be warranted. A prolonged recording periods (5–10 mo duration is often needed using an insertable loop recorder) is sometimes required to detect correlation between arrhythmia (often paroxysmal AV block) and syncope in difficult cases.

TACHYARRHYTHMIAS

Supraventricular tachycardias (SVT) are not often the cause of syncope (Fig. 2). However, light-headed-ness and syncope may occur at the onset of episodes of tachycardia before vascular compensation occurs, or as the result of prolonged bradycardia at the termination of an episode. Patients with preexcitation syndrome (e.g., Wolff-Parkinson-White [WPW] syndrome) may also be at risk of sudden cardiac death. Radiofrequency catheter ablation is the treatment of choice for SVTs in most patients. Atrial flutter and fibrillation may cause syncope in patients with structural heart

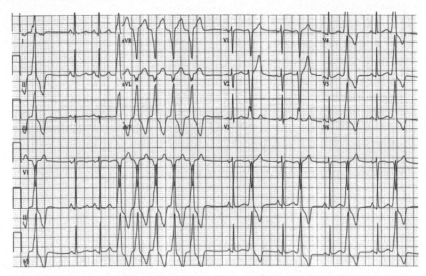

Fig. 3. Findings from a 52-yr-old male with a history of myocardial infarction and angina who presented for evaluation of recurrent syncope. Echocardiogram showed essentially normal left ventricular function. Telemetry recordings in-hospital revealed multiple episodes of ventricular tachycardia. The arrhythmia was associated with syncope, but without any other symptoms, such as palpitations. The ventricular tachycardia was successfully ablated. The patient has remained symptom-free thereafter.

disease or dehydration. A pacemaker may be needed for syncope associated with asystolic pause at termination of supraventricular tachyarrhythmias.

Ventricular tachycardias (VT) most often occur in patients with structural heart disease, especially ischemic heart disease and dilated cardiomyopathies. However, approx 10–15% of VT patients have no overt structural heart disease.

VT Associated With Ischemic Heart Disease or Dilated Cardiomyopathies. Ventricular tachyarrhythmias have been reported to be responsible for syncope in up to 20% of patients referred for electrophysiologic assessment (Fig. 3). Tachycardia rate, status of left ventricular function, and the efficiency of peripheral vascular constriction determine whether the arrhythmia will induce syncopal symptoms. ICDs are the mainstay of treatment of VT associated with structural heart diseases. Currently, pharmacological therapy and transcatheter ablation are considered principally as adjunctive measures. Treatment of nonsustained VT in the presence of syncope is a controversial topic. In essence, syncope associated with nonsustained VT and diminished LV function warrants ICD therapy. However, ICD might not prevent faints due to the delay in detection and charge of the ICD capacitor. Antiarrhythmic drugs and/or ablation may be considered in this setting when indicated.

Idiopathic Ventricular Tachycardias and Syncope. Idiopathic right ventricular outflow tract tachycardia (RVOT) is the most frequent type of idiopathic VT (Fig. 4). It represents approx 80% of all idiopathic VTs, and about 10% of all patients who are evaluated for VTs. Syncope is not an uncommon presentation (23–58%). Some patients with a clinically normal heart may present with idiopathic left ventricular VTs. These may come from the left ventricular outflow tract or of presumed fascicular origin. These idiopathic VTs can be easily ablated in most cases. Pharmacological treatment, including class I and III drugs, β-blockers, calcium-channel blockers, and adenosine, may be effective in these patients.

Less Common Arrhythmic Causes. Other, less common, arrhythmic causes of syncope include arrhythmogenic right ventricular dysplasia, long-QT syndromes, Brugada syndrome, and hypertrophic cardiomyopathy. These conditions are crucial to recognize and are best referred to specialized centers for management, as they are often associated with increased risk of sudden cardiac death.

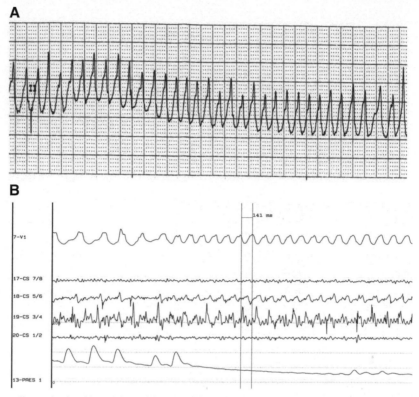

Fig. 4. Recordings obtained in a 36-yr-old male with a clinically normal heart who presented for evaluation of recurrent syncope. A Holter monitor recording showed frequent ventricular ectopic beats and nonsustained ventricular tachycardia, which correlated well with his symptoms. The morphology of these ventricular ectopic beats on 12-lead ECG was consistent with RVOT origin. He underwent electrophysiological study and his ventricular arrhythmias were successfully ablated.

Structural Cardiac and Cardiopulmonary Causes of Syncope

The most common causes of syncope as a result of structural cardiac and pulmonary disease are listed in Table 1. In these cases, syncope occurs as either a direct result of the structural disturbance or as a consequence of a neural-reflex disturbance triggered by the heart condition. Thus, syncope in acute myocardial infarction or severe aortic stenosis may be due to a diminution of cardiac output in some cases. Alternatively, neural-reflex vasodilation may be triggered and cause hypotension. Probably both mechanisms most often participate. In any event, treatment is best directed at amelioration of the specific structural lesion and its consequences.

Cerebrovascular Causes of Syncope

In general, cerebrovascular diseases are rarely the cause of true syncope. Neurological causes are even less frequent. As a result, tests looking for these diseases are hardly ever of value in the early assessment of the syncope patient. Conditions that may reasonably be considered include (1) subclavian steal, (2) migraine, (3) primary autonomic failure, and (4) Parkinson's disease. On the other hand, TIAs and epilepsy are not part of the differential diagnosis. TIAs do not cause loss of consciousness as a rule, with an exceedingly rare exception being vertebral-basilar TIAs. Epilepsy is not a form of syncope, but must be considered in the differential diagnosis of transient loss of consciousness (*see* next section).

Table 3
Clinical Features Distinguishing Syncope From Seizures

Clinical findings that suggest the diagnosis	Seizure likely	Syncope likely
Findings during loss of consciousness (as observed by an eyewitness)	Tonic-clonic movements are usually prolonged and their onset coincides with loss of consciousness Hemilateral clonic movement Clear automatisms such as chewing or lip-smacking or frothing at the mouth Tongue-biting	Jerky movements are always of short duration (<15 s) and start after loss of consciousness
Symptoms before the event	Blue face Aura (such as funny smell) "Pins and needles"	Nausea, vomiting, abdominal discomfort, feeling of cold, sweating (neurally mediated)
Symptoms after the event	Prolonged confusion Aching muscles Incontinence Injury Headache Sleepiness	Usually short duration Nausea, vomiting, and pallor (neurally mediated) Usually no confusion Fatigue (vasovagal faint)

Conditions That Mimic Syncope

Certain medical conditions (Table 2) may cause a real or apparent loss of consciousness that might appear to be syncope, but that is in fact not true syncope. Whether conditions listed below actually "mimic" syncope depends largely on the quality of the account of the events obtained by the physician.

EPILEPSY

Table 3 summarizes the main differences between syncope and epilepsy. Perhaps the aspect of greatest importance is abnormal motor activity. In syncope, it is not uncommon for patients to exhibit jerky movements of the arms and legs for a brief period of time. Not infrequently, nonexpert bystanders misinterpret these movements as being indicative of a "seizure." However, the jerky movements during syncope differ from those accompanying a grand mal epileptic seizure: (1) they are briefer in syncope patients; (2) they occur *after* the loss of consciousness has set in; (3) they are less coarse; and (4) they do not have the "tonic-clonic" features of a true grand mal epileptic seizure.

CATAPLEXY

Cataplexy refers to loss of muscle tone, often associated with emotional lability. In contrast to vasovagal syncope, triggers such as pain, fear, and anxiety are not important. Startle or laughing may provoke cataplexy. Partial attacks are more common (dropping of the jaw and sagging or nodding of the head). Complete attacks look like syncope in that the victim is unable to respond at all, although he or she is completely conscious and aware of what is going on. Narcolepsy is diagnosed based on the narcolepsy tetrad: (1) excessive daytime somnolence; (2) cataplexy; (3) hypnogogic hallucination; and (4) sleep paralysis.

PSYCHOGENIC PSEUDOSYNCOPE

The diagnosis of a psychiatric origin for an apparent (not "true") episode of loss of consciousness relies on careful exclusion of other causes of syncope. In psychogenic pseudosyncope, there is no change in blood pressure or heart rate. Further, psychogenic pseudosyncope is often characterized by a frequency of symptoms far in excess of what might be expected for a "true" fainter. Indeed, there are "too many" episodes to be believable. Psychiatric assessment is especially recommended for patients with frequent pseudosyncope and recurrences in conjunction with multiple other somatic complaints and medical concern for stress, anxiety, and possibly other psychiatric disorders. However, a specific neurological diagnosis should be made if any signs of autonomic failure or neurological disease are detected. An implantable loop recorder may be needed to rule out arrhythmias in some patients.

HYPERVENTILATION

Hyperventilation simply refers to breathing more than metabolic requirements demand. This leads to a series of physiological events, including hypocapnia, constriction of cerebral vessels, and reduced cerebral blood flow. As such, the act of hyperventilation could lead to syncope. However, this is probably exceedingly rare. Lightheadedness and tingling fingers or toes may, with good reason, be seen as physiological manifestations of overbreathing and are the more common manifestation of hyperventilation syndrome.

SYNCOPE IN PSYCHIATRIC PATIENTS

Nonpsychiatrists may tend to label complaints of patients with a psychiatric history as "psychogenic." The three psychiatric disorders most likely to lead to symptoms mimicking syncope are conversion reactions, factitious disorders, and malingering. However, other psychiatry patients with "major" psychiatric conditions such as bipolar disorder, depression, and schizophrenia take medications that can cause autonomic failure leading to syncope, or other syncope-prone conditions such as long-QT syndrome. The main culprits are phenothiazines, tricyclic antidepressives, and monoamine oxidase inhibitors.

DROP ATTACKS

The term "drop attack" refers to a phenomenon in which there is a very short-lasting spell in which the affected individual suddenly falls without any warning. These attacks tend to occur in middle-aged people, especially women. Usually the events are too brief for patients to be certain whether there was any loss of consciousness, but most likely there was none. Commonly, the victim remembers hitting the ground, often experiencing some degree of minor physical injury. History-taking is crucial, particularly in terms of documenting that the patient recalls falling and usually denies any loss of consciousness.

IN-HOSPITAL VERSUS OUT-OF-HOSPITAL EVALUATION OF SYNCOPE

In-hospital evaluation of patients with syncope may be a necessity in certain cases. Unfortunately most hospital facilities are inadequately equipped and organized to manage these patients optimally. The development of an organized multidisciplinary group of physicians (e.g., cardiologists, neurologists, and psychiatrists) may be warranted in order to provide a more efficient approach to the problem. In certain hospitals, this type of organized approach is incorporated within a "syncope clinic" or "syncope unit." Syncope units offer the potential for improving the accuracy and cost-effectiveness of syncope evaluation and treatment.

Hospitalization is strongly recommended for patients suspected of cardiac syncope or at risk of sudden cardiac death (e.g., ischemic heart disease with reduced ejection fraction). These patients often have syncope associated with significant physical injury or traffic accident. The presence of underlying structural heart disease and/or abnormalities of the baseline ECG are important indicators suggesting cardiac syncope. A less frequent, but crucial, prognostic marker is the family history of sudden death, as certain malignant ventricular arrhythmias can have a genetic basis (e.g., long-QT syndrome, Brugada syndrome, familial cardiomyopathies). Suspected neurally mediated syncope, especially in patients without evidence of cardiac disease, does not usually need in-hospital evaluation. In essence, for those cases in whom risk of death is thought to be low and when there is low likelihood of a near-term recurrence precipitating injury or harm to the public health, there is little need for hospitalization. However, cautionary advice regarding avoidance of unnecessary driving and risky occupational and/or avocational exposure should be provided, as further outpatient evaluation is needed before a final diagnosis can be established.

SUMMARY

Syncope is a very common problem in daily practice. In order to provide the syncope patient with appropriate advice regarding treatment and prognosis, it is essential to establish a diagnosis of the cause of the symptoms. In order to accomplish this task, it is important to develop an organized approach to the assessment of the syncope patient, keeping in mind which of the many possible causes is most likely in a given clinical setting. The initial patient evaluation, particularly a detailed medical history, is the key to finding the most likely diagnosis. Based on findings from this initial step, subsequent carefully selected diagnostic tests can be chosen to confirm the clinical suspicion. Unselected random screening tests for syncope are not cost-effective and should be avoided.

It has been the goal of this chapter to provide an evaluation and treatment pathway that minimizes waste of resources and focuses attention on the most efficient means for making an accurate diagnosis of syncope.

ACKNOWLEDGMENT

The authors would like to express their appreciation to Wendy Markuson and Barry L. S. Detloff for assistance with preparation of the manuscript.

REFERENCES

1. Brignole M, Alboni P, Benditt D, et al. Guidelines on management (diagnosis and treatment) of syncope. Europace 2004;6:467–537.
2. Blanc JJ, Benditt DG. Syncope: definition, classification, and multiple potential causes. In: Benditt DG, Blanc JJ, Brignole M, Sutton RS, eds. The Evaluation and Treatment of Syncope. A Handbook for Clinical Practice. Futura Blackwell, Elmsford, NY, 2003, pp. 3–10.
3. Lü F, Bergfeldt L. Role of electrophysiological testing in the evaluation of syncope. In: Benditt DG, Blanc JJ, Brignole M, Sutton RS, eds. The Evaluation and Treatment of Syncope. A Handbook for Clinical Practice. Futura Blackwell, Elmsford, NY, 2003, pp. 80–95.
4. Kapoor WN. Evaluation and outcome of patients with syncope. Medicine (Baltimore) 1990;69:160–175.
5. Disertori M, Brignole M, Menozzi C, et al. Management of patients with syncope referred urgently to general hospitals. Europace 2003;5:283–291.
6. Blanc JJ, L'Her C, Touiza A, Garo B, et al. Prospective evaluation and outcome of patients admitted for syncope over a 1 year period. Eur Heart J 2002;23:815–820.
7. Soteriades ES, Evans JC, Larson MG, et al. Incidence and prognosis of syncope. N Engl J Med 2002;347:878–885.
8. Sarasin FP, Louis-Simonet M, Carballo D, et al. Prospective evaluation of patients with syncope: a population-based study. Am J Med 2001;111:177–184.
9. Martin GJ, Adams SL, Martin HG, et al. Prospective evaluation of syncope. Ann Emerg Med 1984;13:499–504.
10. Gregoratos G, Abrams J, Epstein AE, et al. ACC/AHA/NASPE 2002 Guideline Update for Implantation of Cardiac Pacemakers and Antiarrhythmia Devices—summary article: a report of the American College of Cardiology/ American Heart Association Task Force on Practice Guidelines (ACC/AHA/NASPE Committee to Update the 1998 Pacemaker Guidelines). J Am Coll Cardiol 2002;40:1703–1719.
11. Smit AA, Halliwill JR, Low PA, Wieling W. Pathophysiological basis of orthostatic hypotension in autonomic failure. J Physiol 1999;519:1–10.
12. Benditt DG, Ermis C, Lü F. Head-up tilt table testing. In: Zipes DP, Jalife J, eds. Cardiac Electrophysiology. From Cell to Bedside. W. B. Saunders, Philadelphia, 2004, pp. 812–822.
13. Younoszai AK, Franklin WH, Chan DP, et al. Oral fluid therapy. A promising treatment for vasodepressor syncope. Arch Pediatr Adolesc Med 1998;152:165–168.
14. Krediet CT, van Dijk N, Linzer M, et al. Management of vasovagal syncope: controlling or aborting faints by leg crossing and muscle tensing. Circulation 2002;106:1684–1689.

15. Samniah N, Sakaguchi S, Lurie KG, et al. Efficacy and safety of midodrine hydrochloride in patients with refractory vasovagal syncope. Am J Cardiol 2001;88:A80–A83.
16. Perez-Lugones A, Schweikert R, Pavia S, et al. Usefulness of midodrine in patients with severely symptomatic neurocardiogenic syncope: a randomized control study. J Cardiovasc Electrophysiol 2001;12:935–938.
17. Davies AJ, Kenny RA. Frequency of neurologic complications following carotid sinus massage. Am J Cardiol 1998; 81:1256–1257.
18. Munro NC, McIntosh S, Lawson J, et al. Incidence of complications after carotid sinus massage in older patients with syncope. J Am Geriatr Soc 1994;42:1248–1251.
19. Menozzi C, Brignole M, Garcia-Civera R, et al. Mechanism of syncope in patients with heart disease and negative electrophysiologic test. Circulation 2002;105:2741–2745.
20. McTavish D, Goa KL. Midodrine. A review of its pharmacological properties and therapeutic use in orthostatic hypotension and secondary hypotensive disorders. Drugs 1989;38:757–777.

RECOMMENDED READING

Brignole M, Alboni P, Benditt D, et al. Guidelines on management (diagnosis and treatment) of syncope. Europace 2004;6:467–537.
Kapoor WN. Evaluation and outcome of patients with syncope. Medicine (Baltimore) 1990;69:160–175.
Blanc JJ, L'Her C, Touiza A, Garo B, et al. Prospective evaluation and outcome of patients admitted for syncope over a 1 year period. Eur Heart J 2002;23:815–820.
Krediet CT, van Dijk N, Linzer M, et al. Management of vasovagal syncope: controlling or aborting faints by leg crossing and muscle tensing. Circulation 2002;106:1684–1689.

V HEART FAILURE

19 Pathophysiology of Heart Failure

Mark Scoote, MB BS, BSc, Ian F. Purcell, MD, and Philip A. Poole-Wilson, MD

INTRODUCTION

Heart failure is a clinical syndrome initiated by abnormal function of the heart. Until recently our understanding of this condition has centered on various pathological insults to the heart that lead to abnormal function, usually in the form of contractile dysfunction. One of the earliest terms used to describe heart failure syndrome was "hydrops," which has its origins in the observation that salt and water retention was a common feature of the condition. Despite this obvious systemic manifestation, heart failure was still considered primarily a disease of the heart. In recent years advances have been made in our understanding of the pathophysiology of heart failure; key to these has been the realization that heart failure is a multisystem disorder in which abnormalities of the heart, vasculature, skeletal muscle, and kidneys all combine with various neurohormonal derangements to produce the heart failure syndrome. Of particular importance has been the emerging concept that many of the compensatory mechanisms designed to overcome the initial insult to the heart are the very same processes that paradoxically set in motion a variety of detrimental consequences for cardiac function, gradually worsening the heart failure syndrome further. Our increasing understanding of these concepts has resulted in a rapid advancement in drug development and many new therapeutic targets continue to emerge. In this chapter we summarize the pathophysiology of heart failure, beginning with the specific insults that initiate heart failure and continuing with a discussion of the body's responses to such insults, and how compensatory mechanisms ultimately cause further deterioration in cardiac function.

DEFINITIONS AND TERMINOLOGY

Various attempts at defining and classifying heart failure have been proposed; these are summarized in Tables 1 and 2, respectively. Many definitions are unsatisfactory because they emphasize particular pathological or clinical features. Definitions based on clinical criteria are limited as observations can vary over time, with the level of exercise or with transient comorbidity, and in response to treatment. Likewise our emerging understanding of heart failure pathophysiology indicates that specific biochemical, anatomical, or physiological features do not occur in isolation and cannot fully explain heart failure syndrome on their own. The definition "a clinical syndrome caused by an abnormality of the heart and recognized by a characteristic pattern of hemodynamic, renal, neural, and hormonal responses" *(1)* is a useful one, as it recognizes that an abnormality of the heart is the origin of heart failure but that systemic responses to cardiac dysfunction are important in further defining its pathophysiology and clinical manifestations. Nevertheless this definition would have limitations in epidemiological data collection where more objective and measurable criteria are needed to define heart failure. In this respect the European Society of Cardiology guidelines *(2)* are more useful, as they require heart failure to be based on a clinical diagnosis whereby symptoms

From: *Essential Cardiology: Principles and Practice, 2nd Ed.*
Edited by: C. Rosendorff © Humana Press Inc., Totowa, NJ

Table 1
Some Definitions of Heart Failure

Lewis 1933	A condition in which the heart fails to discharge its contents adequately.
Wood 1950	A state in which the heart fails to maintain an adequate circulation for the needs of the body despite a satisfactory filling pressure.
Braunwald 1980	A pathophysiological state in which an abnormality of cardiac function is responsible for the failure of the heart to pump blood at a rate commensurate with the requirements of the metabolising tissues.
Poole-Wilson 1985	A clinical syndrome caused by an abnormality of the heart and recognised by a characteristic pattern of haemodynamic, renal, neural and hormonal responses.
Harris 1987	A syndrome which arises when the heart is chronically unable to maintain an appropriately high blood pressure without support.
Cohn 1988	A syndrome in which cardiac dysfunction is associated with reduced exercise tolerance, a high incidence of ventricular arrhythmias and shortened life expectancy.
Denolin 1993	Heart failure is the state of any heart disease in which, despite adequate ventricular filling, the heart's output is decreased or in which the heart is unable to pump blood at a rate adequate for satisfying the requirements of the tissues with function parameters remaining within normal limits.
Lenfant 1994	The principal functions of the heart are to accept blood from the venous system, deliver it to the lungs where it is oxygenated (aerated), and pump the oxygenated blood to all body tissues. Heart failure occurs when these functions are disturbed substantially.
Jackson 2000	A multisystem disorder characterized by abnormalities of cardiac, skeletal muscle, and renal function, stimulation of the sympathetic nervous system and a complex pattern of neurohormonal changes.
Jessup & Brozena 2003	A clinical syndrome…the final pathway for myriad diseases that affect the heart.

and signs of heart failure have been observed, where a demonstrable abnormality of the heart is present, and where, preferably, there is a favorable response to treatment. Terms such as forward vs backward failure and right-sided vs left-sided failure have confused generations of students and although they may be useful clinical shorthand they are often misleading or based on outdated concepts.

Diastolic vs Systolic Dysfunction

Diastolic heart failure has recently emerged as a distinct clinical entity and is characterized by clinical features suggestive of heart failure but with mininimal or no systolic dysfunction. Diastolic heart failure may occur in up to 50% of patients with heart failure and is associated with the elderly, women, hypertension, obesity, diabetes mellitus, and the presence of concentric left ventricular hypertrophy (3). It can be defined as heart failure due to increased resistance in diastolic filling of the heart and is usually given as a diagnosis of exclusion when clinical features are suggestive and other pathology and systolic dysfunction have been excluded (4). Although evidence-based data are lacking on the application of standard heart failure therapy to lone diastolic dysfunction, its identification is still important as an appreciation of its underlying pathology would suggest specific treatment options that reduce ventricular load, slow heart rate, and increase ventricular filling time are most likely to be of benefit. Due to the overlap between diastolic and systolic heart failure in terms of etiology and pathophysiology, we will not consider diastolic heart failure separately at this stage; rather, throughout this chapter we will highlight particular pathophysiological aspects that are of relevance to diastolic dysfunction.

Table 2
Classification Schemes for Heart Failure

Acute vs Chronic
   Clinical classification based on the duration of symptoms and speed of onset.
High Output vs Low Output
   Pathophysiological classification based on whether increased circulatory or metabolic demands exceed
   the capacity of a normal functioning heart (high-output failure) or whether a poorly functioning heart
   is unable to meet the normal circulatory and metabolic demands of the body (low-output failure).
Forward vs Backward
   Clinical classification based on whether the predominant features are those directly relating to a poor
   cardiac output, such as hypotension and poor peripheral perfusion (forward failure), or those of
   systemic and pulmonary venous congestion (backward failure).
Right-Sided vs Left-Sided
   A clinical classification that recognizes that specific causes have an impact primarily on either the
   left- or right-sided cardiac chambers and produce a characteristic cluster of clinical features, namely
   abdominal discomfort and peripheral edema (right-sided failure) and dyspnea, hypotension, and poor
   peripheral perfusion (left-sided failure).
Diastolic vs Systolic
   Pathophysiological classification based on whether the primary cardiac abnormality is reduced
   ventricular contractile force generation during systole or impaired chamber filling resistance and
   ventricular relaxation during diastole.

ETIOLOGY

The etiology of heart failure represents the specific underlying insult to the heart that initiates a decline in cardiac performance. Many of the pathological and clinical features of heart failure occur whatever the specific underlying etiology. Nevertheless the underlying etiology is still important, as it may influence the nature and speed of heart failure progression over time, and if still active may suggest particular therapeutic options in the overall management strategies of patients. For these reasons the diagnosis of heart failure on its own is always inadequate without a further search to identify the underlying cause (2). Diagnosis may be aided by a pattern of clinical and investigative findings that are particular to a specific etiology. In contrast, the initial pathological insult may have been a transient event many months or years before, in which case the search for its identification may prove extremely difficult. This highlights the concept that heart failure can persist and indeed worsen long after the initial insult to the heart has occurred as a result of various compensatory mechanisms that are designed to overcome the initial insult in the first place but eventually become harmful and disadvantageous if chronically activated. When considering causes it is also important to bear in mind the nature of the population in question; for example, hypertension and coronary artery disease are responsible for most heart failure in Western society today, whereas valvular disease and the manifestations of infection or nutritional deficiency are much more important causes worldwide due to their higher relative prevalence in the developing world. The general causes of heart failure are listed in Table 3.

Coronary Artery Disease

Coronary artery disease is the cause of heart failure in up to 75% of patients in industrialized countries (5). However, many of the risk factors for coronary artery disease, such as hypertension and diabetes, are also independent risk factors for the development of heart failure, irrespective of whether coronary artery disease is present or not. Myocardial ischemia may produce altered functional states within the myocardium known as hibernation, stunning, and ischemic preconditioning. However, it is primarily within the context of myocardial ischaemia and infarction that coronary artery disease manifests as heart failure. The outcomes of coronary artery disease on the myocardium are summarized in Table 4.

Table 3
Causes of Heart Failure: General Classification

Coronary artery disease
Intrinsic myocardial disease
   Dilated cardiomyopathy
   Hypertrophic cardiomyopathy
   Restrictive cardiomyopathy
Valvular heart disease
   Congenital
   Age-related/calcific
   Infective endocarditis
   Immunological (e.g., rheumatic fever)
   Collagen disease (e.g., Marfan's syndrome)
   Neoplastic (metastases, carcinoid syndrome)
Congenital heart disease
Hypertension
   Systemic and pulmonary
Arrhythmias and cardiac conduction disturbances
   Tachyarrhythmias
   Bradyarrhythmias
   Intraventricular conduction disturbance
High-output cardiac failure
   Anemia
   Thyrotoxicosis
   Pregnancy
   Arteriovenous fistula
   Liver cirrhosis
   Paget's disease
   Renal cell carcinoma
Pericardial disease
   Constrictive pericarditis
   Pericardial effusion with tamponade

Hypertension

Hypertension is the second major cause of heart failure in Western society and often coexists with coronary artery disease. Indeed there is still no consensus on which of these is the most important etiological factor for heart failure. Hypertension is particularly associated with heart failure in specific populations, including women, diabetics, and people of African origin (5). Furthermore, its causal role in the development of left ventricular hypertrophy makes it a very important etiologic factor in the development of diastolic heart failure.

Cardiomyopathy

The term *cardiomyopathy* is widely used in the context of heart failure and, at its most basic level, can be defined as a disease process involving cardiac muscle. It is traditionally reserved for intrinsic cardiac muscle disease in the absence of coronary artery disease, hypertension, valvular, congenital, and pericardial heart disease. Cardiomyopathy can be divided on descriptive terms into three functional categories: dilated, hypertrophic, and restrictive.

Dilated cardiomyopathy (Table 5) can be defined as heart muscle disease in which the predominant abnormality is dilation of the left ventricle (with or without right ventricular dilation). It is the end result of numerous pathological insults on the heart, although in many cases it is idiopathic. It is the most common form of cardiomyopathy, highlighting the fact that the final response of the heart to sustained injury is a global chamber remodeling resulting in a globular heart with thinned walls, decreased systolic function, and functional valvular regurgitation.

Table 4
Outcomes of Coronary Artery Disease on Myocardial Function

Acute ischemia
  Atheromatous plaque rupture and thrombosis formation
  Impaired resting and exercise myocardial contractility
Chronic ischemia
  Stable atheromatous plaque disease with flow limitation on exercise/stress
  Impaired contractility during exacerbations
  Potential to initiate ischemic preconditioning
Myocardial infarction
  Prolonged vessel occlusion with irreversible myocardial damage
  Impaired contractility due to replacement of muscle with scar tissue
  Cardiogenic shock, ventricular septal rupture, and acute mitral regurgitation cause life threatening
    left-ventricular dysfunction
Stunning
  Transient and reversible contractile dysfunction following ischemia, despite restored coronary flow
Hibernation
  Persistent but potentially reversible contractile dysfunction due to episodes of reduced coronary
    perfusion and/or limited coronary reserve
Ischemic preconditioning
  Resistance of myocardium to sustained ischemia, conferred by transient sublethal periods of ischemia
  Potential for subsequent infarct size reduction
  Reduced demand for ATP under ischemic conditions

Hypertrophic cardiomyopathy is characterized by hypertrophy of a nondilated left and/or right ventricle. It is a term usually applied to situations in which hypertrophy of the ventricles occurs in the absence of an identified systemic or cardiac stimulus such as hypertension or aortic stenosis. As a result it tends to be either idiopathic in nature or a familial disorder with an underlying genetic basis. The classic form of familial hypertrophic cardiomyopathy is an autosomal dominant disorder characterized by asymmetrical septal hypertrophy and, in severe cases, symptoms of aortic outflow tract obstruction. Various genetic defects within sarcomeric proteins, such as β-myosin heavy chain, troponin, and tropomyosin, have been identified in familial hypertrophic cardiomyopathy (6). Restrictive cardiomyopathy is characterized by a stiff, noncompliant ventricle with abnormal ventricular filling. It is especially associated with diastolic dysfunction and is caused by a diverse range of conditions associated with fibrosis or infiltration of the heart such as endomyocardial fibrosis, hypereosinophilic syndromes, sarcoidosis, amyloidosis, radiation, and neoplastic disease. Restrictive cardiomyopathy is rare in Western societies and is seen more commonly in the developing world, primarily due to its association with tropical parasitic infection and eosinophilia.

THE FAILING HEART: FROM ORGAN TO MOLECULE

In response to cardiac injury, mechanisms are activated that compensate for depressed cardiac performance and these attempt to restore both cardiac output and tissue perfusion to normal. Many of these responses take place within the heart; these intrinsic cardiac responses to injury occur at the gross anatomical, cellular, molecular, and genetic levels. Although these responses to injury occur initially as a mechanism to augment cardiac function many subsequently become detrimental to ongoing cardiac function if allowed to continue (Table 6). This concept of secondary injury mechanisms, distinct from the initial insult to the heart, is outlined in Fig. 1, which summarizes our current understanding of the major pathophysiological processes involved in heart failure syndrome.

Ventricular Chamber Size, Shape, and Remodeling

All four cardiac chambers possess the capacity to alter their size and shape in response to acute or chronic injury and changes in hemodynamic load and wall stress. Changes in chamber geometry

Table 5
Causes of Dilated Cardiomyopathy

Genetic
    Genetic basis unknown
    Chromosomal loci identified (e.g., chromosome 1q32, 3p22–25)
    Specific genetic defect identified (e.g., cardiac actin)
    Mitochondrial myopathies
    Arrhythmogenic right ventricular dysplasia
Infection
    Viral (e.g., coxsackievirus, HIV)
    Bacterial (e.g., *Clostridium diphtheriae* exotoxin)
    Protozoal (e.g., trypanosomiasis)
    Parasitic (e.g., schistosomiasis, trichinosis)
    Rickettsiae (e.g., epidemic typhus-induced myocarditis)
    Spirochetes (e.g., Lyme disease)
Drugs and toxins
    Heavy metal (e.g., cobalt, mercury, lead)
    Alcohol & recreational drugs (e.g., cocaine)
    Carbon monoxide poisoning
    Cytotoxic drugs (e.g., bleomycin, doxorubicin, busulfan, adriamycin)
    Antimicrobial drugs (e.g., chloroquine, zidovudine)
    Antipsychotic drugs (e.g., clozapine, haloperidol, risperidone)
Pregnancy (peripartum cardiomyopathy)
Nutritional deficiency
    Keshan disease (selenium)
    Beri-beri (thiamine)
    Pellagra (niacin)
    Kwashiorkor (generalized protein/energy malnutrition)
Storage disease
    Hemochromatosis
    Refsum's disease
    Fabry's disease
Autoimmune/vasculitides
    Systemic lupus erythematosus
    Polyarteritis nodosa
    Rheumatoid arthritis
    Churg-Strauss disease
Endocrine
    Diabetes mellitus
    Myxoedema and thyrotoxicosis
    Acromegaly
    Pheochromocytoma

may occur rapidly over a period of hours and days, for example following myocardial infarction. Alternatively they may occur gradually over many months by a process known as remodeling *(7)*. Remodeling is influenced, at least initially, by the underlying etiology of the primary cardiac injury process, although ultimately a grossly dilated spherical heart chamber phenotype occurs if resolution or death does not intervene in the interim period. Remodeling is associated with worsening cardiac function, yet it occurs initially as an adaptive response that counteracts abnormal wall stresses and hemodynamic load forces placed on the heart chambers. It is an important clinical process, as it is readily identifiable with cardiac imaging techniques and is associated with an increased mortality secondary to end-stage contractile failure or complications such as myocardial rupture and intracardiac thrombus formation. Several patterns of remodeling are recognised; these are summarized in Fig. 2. The most common pattern of remodeling in the context of chronic heart

Table 6
Abnormalities of the Failing Heart

Macroscopic
    Loss of muscle mass
    Alteration in chamber size and shape (dilation and/or hypertrophy)
    In-coordinate contraction and abnormal timing of contraction
Microscopic
    Myocyte changes (cell thinning, lengthening, hypertrophy, necrosis, apoptosis)
    Disorganized muscle fiber orientation and myocyte slippage
    Extracellular matrix inflammatory cell infiltrate, fibroblast expansion, and fibrosis
Intracellular
    Disorganized cytoskeleton
    Impaired cell-to-cell communication (gap junctions)
    Contractile protein structural and functional derangements
    Deranged excitation–contraction coupling and calcium homeostasis
    Reduced efficiency of intracellular signal-transduction pathways
    Altered energy metabolism
    Regression to de-differentiated "fetal" gene expression pattern

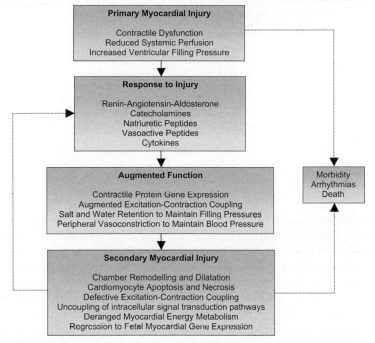

Fig. 1. Primary and secondary injury mechanisms in heart failure pathophysiology. Primary injury to the myocardium occurs and is followed by various responses that augment cardiac performance. Subsequent detrimental responses eventually predominate which themselves worsen cardiac function, even if the initial cause of injury has resolved, resulting in an ever-worsening cycle of deterioration. Once critical thresholds of damage are exceeded, either as a result of primary or secondary injury mechanisms, heart failure becomes clinically apparent.

failure is the dilated cardiomyopathy phenotype, either occurring *de novo* due to intrinsic myocardial disease, secondary to chronic volume overload on the ventricles, or finally as the ultimate outcome of other remodeling patterns when end-stage heart failure approaches. At the macroscopic level there is an increase in chamber size and a thinning of the ventricular wall dimensions,

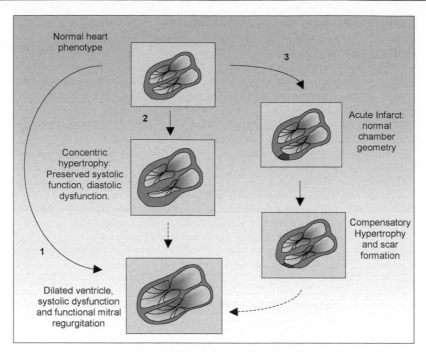

Fig. 2. Patterns of ventricular remodeling. (1) Intrinsic myocardial disease leads to a dilated ventricle, systolic dysfunction, and disruption of the mitral/tricuspid valve apparatus. (2) Concentric left ventricular hypertrophy leads to initially preserved systolic function, diastolic dysfunction, and left ventricular outflow tract obstruction. Progression may eventually lead to chamber dilation and systolic dysfunction. (3) Myocardial infarction leads to scar formation and wall thinning, with compensatory hypertrophy in remaining viable muscle as an attempt to alleviate abnormal loading on chamber and elevated wall stress. Progression may eventually lead to chamber dilation and systolic dysfunction.

resulting in an enlarged globular heart. This phenotype is associated with reduced systolic function and functional mitral/tricuspid regurgitation and often coexists with intraventricular conduction abnormalities such as bundle branch block. A second pattern of remodeling is concentric hypertrophy caused by pressure overload on the ventricles. This produces a stiff noncompliant ventricle with impaired relaxation as the primary problem, with systolic function initially preserved. This remodeling response is common in diastolic heart failure and is most commonly associated with hypertensive heart disease and other causes of pressure overload. Progressive dilation may eventually follow and although this will ultimately lead to thinning of the ventricular wall the presence of chamber dilation and myocardial wall hypertrophy are not mutually exclusive and often coexist. A third pattern is focal myocardial injury, most commonly encountered in acute myocardial infarction. This results in an initial remodeling process at the site of injury and its boundaries, which takes the form of a destruction of normal myocardial architecture and its eventual replacement by scar tissue. It may also initiate changes in ventricular wall stress and loading throughout the affected heart chamber, resulting in compensatory hypertrophy and a progressive global dilation if the initial infarct insult was of sufficient magnitude. The appearance of the remodeling phenomenon and its partial reversal with modern treatment is useful in the clinical management of patients as it can readily be observed on serial noninvasive imaging. At the pathological level, however, it simply represents the phenotypic manifestation of underlying processes occurring within the myocardium at the cellular, molecular, and genetic levels.

Cardiomyocyte Plasticity in Heart Failure

Individual myocyte responses seen in heart failure comprise alterations in cell size, shape, and number. Increases in myocyte number were previously thought to be impossible, with cardiomyocytes believed to be terminally differentiated cells, incapable of reentering the cell cycle and undergoing further division. In fact there is now a growing body of evidence that indicates that cardiomyocyte cell division does occur in the heart but is not common (8). It is estimated that without this phenomenon the observed rates of cell death in the normal heart are such that by early adult life the myocardium and myocyte population present at birth would have totally disappeared (9). Mitosis has long been observed in cardiomyocytes but without subsequent cytokinesis, suggesting that cardiomyocyte mitosis simply resulted in the development of polyploidy and multinucleated cells rather than an expansion in total cell number. Evidence that cardiomyocytes can regenerate and actually do undergo division has now been widely published. One hypothesis is that whereas the majority of cardiomyocytes are terminally differentiated and possess no regenerative capacity, a small number of precursor cells do exist and these retain the ability to divide and form mature cardiomyocytes. It is unclear whether these cells are a specific population of myocytes present within the myocardium from birth or whether they represent a population of circulating stem cells capable of differentiating into numerous specialized tissue types upon appropriate stimulus. Evidence for the latter is supported by observations in male patients who receive a female donor heart at transplantation. Subsequent analysis of these hearts reveals the presence of numerous myocytes possessing the Y chromosome, raising the possibility that a circulating male stem cell migrates into the female donor myocardium and differentiates into a mature functioning myocyte. Some time after bone marrow transplants from male donors, female recipients have Y-chromosome-positive mature cardiomyocytes, suggesting that the circulating stem cells originate in the bone marrow. What remains to be established is the functional significance of such observations; at present the widely held consensus is that any compensatory response to augment cardiac performance is primarily via hypertrophy of preexisting cells rather than by division and expansion of the cell population.

Cardiomyocyte hypertrophy represents an increase in intracellular volume, enlarging the cell primarily in its transverse diameter. It is most readily demonstrated in response to situations of pressure overload, such as hypertension, and occurs without any significant increase in cell length along the longitudinal axis. Cellular hypertrophy occurs to a certain extent in most remodeling processes, including dilated cardiomyopathy. The most obvious change in cardiomyocyte hypertrophy is an increase in contractile protein content and sarcomere number, but nuclear polyploidy also occurs and hypertrophied cardiomyocytes may be heavily multinucleated. In familial hypertrophic cardiomyopathy there is considerable loss of normal cellular architecture, termed myocyte disarray. When hypertrophy occurs as a secondary phenomenon, however, the underlying cellular architecture is, in comparison, relatively well maintained. The mechanisms underlying the cardiomyocyte hypertrophy response involve a complex interaction between extrinsic stimuli and growth factors, intracellular amplification cascades, and transcription factors (Fig. 3).

Cellular elongation along the longitudinal axis is the primary response in dilated cardiomyopathy. This response is also mediated at a cellular level by altered gene expression that affects both the cytoskeleton and contractile protein components of the cell. Extrinsic factors such as changes in the cellular and matrix components of the myocardial interstitium may also contribute to cardiomyocyte shape change and elongation. In fact, myocyte elongation alone cannot in itself account for the macroscopic increase in chamber size seen in dilated cardiomyopathy. This state of affairs can be accommodated only if there is a degree of myocyte slippage between adjacent muscle fibers that are normally closely apposed.

In addition to the structural changes in cellular architecture described above, there is also evidence that functional connections between adjacent cardiomyocytes are defective in heart failure. Adjacent cardiomyocytes are functionally connected with one another at the level of the gap junction, a set of transmembrane channels that link adjoining myocytes and mediate electrical coupling

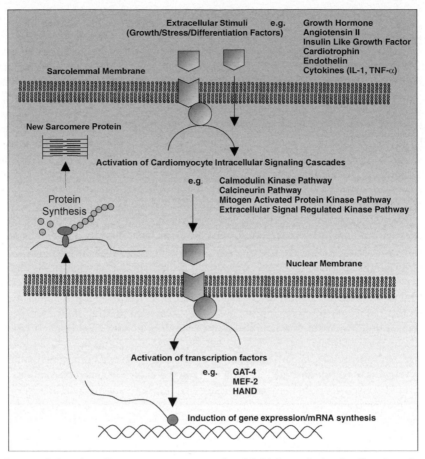

Fig. 3. Pathways of altered cardiomyocyte gene expression. Multiple extrinsic stimuli activate intracellular pathways that induce cardiomyocyte gene expression and protein synthesis. Early gene expression comprises specific regulator genes that control cell growth and differentiation, such as *c-myc*, *c-fos*, and *c-jun*. Increased sarcomere protein synthesis can be detected within 6 h of expression induction. Within 24 h increases in sarcomere number and cell size are demonstrable.

and communication. Individual gap junction proteins are called *connexins*; these are assembled in a hexamer configuration termed a *connexon*. In addition to alterations in the absolute number and distribution of connexons in heart failure, the expression pattern of individual connexin isoforms is also altered by heart failure *(10)*. Connexin-43 is the most widely expressed and important connexin in normal human hearts but in heart failure its expression is significantly reduced relative to other isoforms. This may disrupt the electrical coupling that facilitates synchronized contraction and may predispose to the electrical instability that precipitates arrhythmias.

Cardiac cell loss is a key feature of both primary and secondary injury mechanisms in the failing heart and occurs via necrosis or apoptosis. Necrosis is most commonly seen in Western society in the context of myocardial infarction. Such acute necrosis allows no time for the development of compensatory hypertrophy in remaining viable cells, and if a critical mass of myocardium is lost (~40% or above), cardiogenic shock and death will quickly ensue. Gradual cell loss through necrosis is much better tolerated and is seen throughout the heart at the microscopic level in most underlying conditions causing chronic heart failure. It is an unregulated process characterized by cell swelling and its eventual fragmentation in response to oxidative stress and the actions of destructive enzymes. Necrotic cells also initiate an inflammatory response and eventually lead to fibrosis,

Table 7
Composition and Function of Myocardial Interstitium

Cellular
    Fibroblasts, mast cells, macrophages, plasma cells
Extracellular matrix
    Proteins (e.g., collagen, elastin, reticulin)
    Ground substance (e.g., glycosaminoglycans, glycoproteins)
    Tissue fluid
Blood vessels
Nerve endings
Lymphatics
Function
    Transmit force
    Maintain alignment of myocytes and muscle fibers
    Prevent overdistension of myocardium
    Support and attachment to intracellular cytoskeleton
    Store energy in systole (contribute to relaxation)
    Repair of myocardial damage
    Vehicle for movement and migration of immunocompetent cells
    Medium for exchange of nutrients, signaling molecules, and metabolic wastes

features not seen in myocyte apoptosis. Apoptosis is characterized by cell shrinkage, the condensation of nuclear chromatin, and the disintegration of cytoplasmic and nuclear contents into discrete vesicles that are phagocytosed by neighboring cells without associated inflammation or any change in the microscopic morphology of the myocardium. It is a normal physiological process during cardiac development but is now recognized as a phenomenon induced by ischemia, infarction, and various systemic responses in heart failure *(11)*. Apoptosis depends on the activation of intracellular enzymatic cascades, such as the caspase pathway, which eventually leads to the fragmentation of cytoplasmic proteins and nuclear material. Cardiomyocyte apoptosis may sometimes be cut short by inhibition of the activated caspase pathways at the point where nuclear fragmentation begins. These cells retain their nuclear integrity and survive but will have suffered irreversible damage to cytoplasmic metabolic pathways and contractile proteins such that they can no longer function as a competent cardiomyocytes. This process has been called "apoptosis interruptus" and the nonfunctioning cells that remain are appropriately named "zombie myocytes" *(12)*. Many factors have been shown to initiate apoptosis in heart failure, such as hypoxia, nitric oxide, cytokines, angiotensin II, and catecholaminergic signaling pathways. However, the functional relevance of apoptosis in heart failure and whether it represents a beneficial or harmful aspect of the remodeling process remains unclear. To date experimental caspase blockade and inhibition of apoptosis in animal models of heart failure has not yielded dramatic improvements in myocardial function.

Interstitium and Myocardial Fibrosis in Heart Failure

The myocardial interstitium is made up of various components and has an important structural and supportive role in the normal heart, as outlined in Table 7. Ventricular remodeling is facilitated by changes in the composition and function of various interstitial components. Ultimately these changes manifest as an increase in myocardial fibrosis if they are allowed to continue unopposed for any length of time; indeed, in certain disease states such as arrhythmogenic right ventricular dysplasia, fibrosis may be the most prominent microscopic abnormality. The increased myocardial fibrosis in heart failure is associated with an increase of the interstitial fibroblast population. These cells proliferate and undergo differentiation into an active phenotype known as a myofibroblast. Myofibroblasts produce various extracellular matrix proteins, along with a variety of autocrine and paracrine signalling molecules, cytokines, and enzymes. The proportion of total ventricular weight that is due to collagen fibers can increase from insignificant levels in the normal heart to anything approaching 25% in established heart failure. Excess collagen deposition initially leads to an impairment of diastolic relaxation and increased stiffness of ventricular chambers. As deposition continues, systolic function is also eventually compromised. The turnover of collagen in the heart is governed by the activity of extracellular matrix metalloproteinases (MMPs), a family of proteolytic enzymes responsible for the degradation of various extracellular matrix proteins. In various models of heart failure the activity of MMPs has been shown to be dysregulated. Isoforms such as MMP-13 are expressed at very low levels in normal hearts and substantially upregulated in heart failure, whereas MMPs expressed in the normal heart are downregulated in heart failure *(13)*. Furthermore the normal regulators of MMP activity, known as the tissue inhibitors of the MMPs, are upregulated in heart failure, and these MMP inhibitors contribute to the overall defective turnover and accumulation of collagen seen in the failing heart. Increased MMP activity is associated with a weakening of the interstitial support network and a net loss of collagen. Paradoxically a reduction in activity of specific MMP isoforms also weakens the interstitial support network because without the normal physiological repair and reabsorption of damaged collagen fibrils, the strength and structural integrity of the extracellular matrix will gradually worsen over time despite an absolute increase in content. Weakened extracellular matrix support and increased fibrosis results in myocyte slippage and ventricular chamber dilation but hypertrophied myocardium also demonstrates increased fibrosis tissue deposition between muscle fibers on specific staining. Many stimulants of collagen synthesis and turnover (and ultimately increased myocardial fibrosis) are known, including cytokines, catecholamines, oxidative stress, angiotensin II, and aldosterone. The importance of myocardial fibrosis in heart failure pathophysiology is demonstrated by the observation that much of the beneficial effect of aldosterone antagonist drug therapy in heart failure appears to be secondary to an inhibitory effect on its fibrosis-inducing properties.

Excitation–Contraction Coupling in Heart Failure

Cardiac excitation–contraction (EC) coupling is the process whereby myocyte electrical depolarization acts as the stimulus for a coordinated movement of Ca^{2+} in the cell to bring about contraction. It is a highly efficient amplification system and its modulation is one of the primary mechanisms where by the inotropic state of the heart can be increased in response to injury. The major components of cardiac EC coupling are outlined in Fig. 4A. When the myocyte depolarizes, extracellular Ca^{2+} enters the cell through the L-type, voltage-dependent (dihydropyridine [DHPR] sensitive) Ca^{2+} channel, a phenomenon represented by the phase 2 plateau of the cardiac action potential. This inward Ca^{2+} current is, on its own, insufficient to bring about the required conformational change in troponin needed for contraction to occur. Additional Ca^{2+} is required; this is obtained from a pool of stored Ca^{2+} within the myocyte sarcoplasmic reticulum (SR). The initial inward movement of Ca^{2+} acts as an amplification signal for the release of this storage pool of Ca^{2+}, through an SR membrane ion channel known as the cardiac ryanodine receptor (RyR-isoform 2). Individual populations of RyR2 localize in areas of the SR membrane that are adjacent to DHPR channels deep within the t-tubule invaginations of the outer sarcolemma membrane. Influx of Ca^{2+} through the DHPR activates its associated local RyR2 population causing a synchronized release of Ca^{2+} known as a Ca^{2+} spark. The synchronized release of Ca^{2+} from RyR2 is facilitated by the coupled gating of adjacent RyR2 channels, a property mediated by the RyR2-associated regulatory protein FKBP 12.6 *(14)*. The synchronized release of multiple Ca^{2+} sparks throughout the cell following depolarization creates a global intracellular Ca^{2+} transient of sufficient magnitude to bring about contraction. Conversely, diastole and myocyte relaxation results from closure of RyR2 and the rapid removal of cytosolic Ca^{2+}, either by reuptake into the SR through the SR Ca^{2+}/ATPase pump (SERCA) or by its efflux out of the cell through the sarcolemmal Na^{+}/Ca^{2+} exchanger (NCX).

As an early response in heart failure β-adrenergic receptor-mediated intracellular signaling pathways mediate phosphorylation of individual EC coupling components, which increases the efficiency of both systolic and diastolic components of the process. Despite these initial beneficial

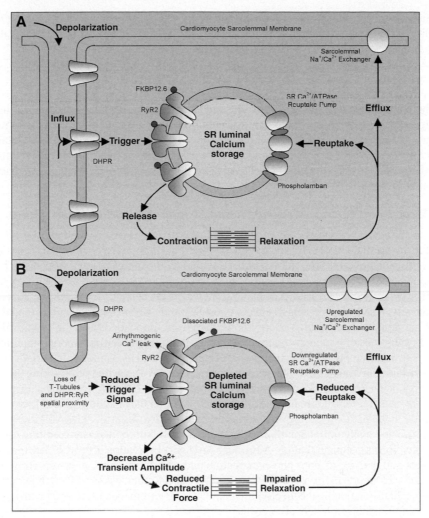

Fig. 4. Cardiac excitation–contraction coupling. Cardiac EC coupling and intracellular calcium movement. (**A**) Normal cardiac EC coupling; (**B**) Abnormalities of cardiac EC coupling in heart failure. The movement of calcium is shown in bold text/arrows. *See* text for further description and abbreviations.

improvements in EC coupling efficiency, ongoing intracellular signaling eventually leads to a blunting of β-adrenergic mediated compensatory mechanisms. Downregulation of β-adrenergic receptors contributes to this but specific molecular targets such as RyR2, NCX, and DHPR become "hyperphosphorylated." Not only does this render these components incapable of further augmentation in function, but it is also now apparent that hyperphosphorylation of EC coupling molecular targets has detrimental effects. The consequences of RyR2 hyperphosphorylation are the most extensively studied *(15)* and include dissociation of FKBP12.6, a loss of coupled RyR2 gating, and a diastolic release of SR Ca^{2+}. These effects may in turn lower SR Ca^{2+} stores and precipitate proarrhythmogenic delayed afterdepolarizations. Interestingly, β-blockers in heart failure reverse RyR2 hyperphosphorylation and their action on RyR2 may be one mechanism by which their beneficial effects in heart failure are mediated *(16)*.

Studies of EC coupling in heart failure have consistently demonstrated a reduction in the SR storage pool of Ca^{2+}. This leads to a reduced amplitude of the systolic intracellular Ca^{2+} transient that initiates contraction. As a result, contractile force is reduced. SERCA is significantly downregulated in heart failure, and this will prevent adequate loading and replenishment of SR Ca^{2+} stores *(17)*. Ca^{2+} availability may also be worsened by an upregulation of NCX, which leads to the removal of Ca^{2+} from the cell. Downregulation of SERCA, preventing the removal of cytosolic Ca^{2+} back into the SR at the end of systole, impairs relaxation as it leads to a prolongation of the systolic Ca^{2+} transient duration and is likely to contribute to the specific pathophysiology of diastolic dysfunction *(4)*. The close structural and functional relationship between DHPR and RyR2 at the base of sarcolemmal t-tubule invaginations may also be disrupted in heart failure. T-tubules run deep within the cell and bring the outer depolarizing sarcolemmal membrane into close contact with the intracellular machinery of EC coupling. Isolated cardiomyocytes from failing hearts consistently demonstrate a loss of the t-tubule network, which would also be expected to impair efficient EC coupling and contribute to contractile dysfunction *(18)*. Detrimental consequences of EC coupling in heart failure are outlined in Fig. 4B.

Myocardial Energy Metabolism and Oxidative Stress in Heart Failure

Normal cardiac function depends on the adequate delivery of oxygen and energy substrate to the cell for the production of ATP via aerobic respiration. Under normal circumstances the delivery of energy substrate into the mitochondrial oxidative phosphorylation pathways is preferentially through the β-oxidation of fatty acids (>60%) with glucose utilization via the glycolysis pathway less important (<40%). A further important pathway in the heart is the phosphocreatine/creatine kinase pathway, which provides a high-energy phosphate store within the myocardium and is responsible for the translocation of high-energy phosphate from mitochondria to the myofibril myosin ATPase. In situations of ischemia and tissue hypoxia, glycolysis becomes a more important source of energy substrate supply, a phenomenon that can precipitate lactic acidosis. In various models of heart failure numerous qualitative and quantitative changes have been identified within the enzymes and cofactors of the myocardial energy metabolism pathways *(19)*. The importance of many of these observations is unclear and it remains speculative as to whether they have a causal role or contribute significantly to the pathophysiology of heart failure. In specific diseases that involve some of these components, such as the mitochondrial myopathies and Refsum's disease, cardiomyopathy can certainly develop as a clinical feature. A further consistent observation in heart failure is a reduction in the levels and activity of both phosphocreatine and creatine kinase, an observation that may contribute to a reduction in myocardial energy reserve *(20)*. Rather less consistent, however, are the experimental data concerning the levels of myocardial ATP within the failing heart with reductions, increases, and unchanged levels all reported.

Free radicals, such as the superoxide anion and hydroxyl radical, are transiently generated within the heart during normal myocardial energy metabolism. Fortunately any potential for these to cause significant damage is offset by the presence of highly efficient free-radical scavengers such as superoxide dismutase and catalase. In heart failure free-radical generation is increased via several mechanisms leading to damage and impairment of cardiac structure and function, a phenomenon termed *oxidative stress (21)*. Furthermore, scavenger systems may become downregulated and less efficient at removing harmful free radicals before damage occurs. This may also be of importance and has been shown to cause dilated cardiomyopathy in experimental models *(22)*. A summary of the important mediators and effects of myocardial oxidative stress is outlined in Table 8. The possible role of oxidative stress in heart failure has led to the development of various antioxidant therapies as potential treatment strategies. Unfortunately initial trials to date have not shown large-scale benefit; nevertheless, several drugs used successfully in heart failure, such as angiotensin-converting enzyme inhibitors and the β-blocker carvedilol, are known to have antioxidant properties, which may in part contribute to their beneficial actions.

Contractile Protein Dysfunction in Heart Failure

The molecular and cellular physiology of cardiac contraction and the various sarcomere proteins is outlined in Chapter 2. The importance of contractile proteins in cardiac function is demonstrated

Table 8
Oxidative Stress in Heart Failure

Initiating mechanisms of oxidative stress
    Tissue hypoxia and reperfusion injury
    Angiotensin II and aldosterone
    Cytokines
    Catecholamines
    Prostaglandins
    Endothelin
Manifestations of oxidative stress
    Biological membrane damage (lipid peroxidation)
    "Uncoupling" of excitation–contraction coupling pathways
    Activation of matrix metalloproteinases and collagen/elastin fiber damage
    Induced apoptosis
    Induced fetal gene expression pattern
    Direct mitochondrial DNA damage
    Reduced high-energy phosphate availability
Consequences
    Contractile dysfunction
    Endothelial dysfunction
    Chamber remodeling

by the observation that mutations in both myosin and actin have been identified in many of the familial cardiomyopathy syndromes; for example, classical autosomal dominant hypertrophic cardiomyopathy commonly occurs secondary to mutations in the β-myosin heavy chain (MHC) gene. In all forms of heart failure, however, altered expression of completely normal contractile protein genes and other proteins involved in their regulation also occurs and may contribute to contractile dysfunction in heart failure. Expression of fetal isoforms of troponin T and myosin light change (MLC) I have been demonstrated in heart failure; however, one of the most consistent and important abnormalities in heart failure is an upregulation of β-MHC expression and a reduction in α-MHC expression, confirmed at both the mRNA and protein levels. This altered MHC isoform expression pattern is detected in failing myocardium before chamber remodeling occurs; the consequences of it are an absolute reduction in total myosin levels and a reduction in myosin ATPase activity, both of which will lead to systolic dysfunction *(23)*.

SYSTEMIC RESPONSES TO HEART FAILURE

A variety of systemic responses occur within the body as a result of impaired cardiac function. It is our emerging understanding of these that has lead to recent advances in heart failure therapeutics. The majority of systemic responses to heart failure occur as compensatory mechanisms and produce short-term improvements in various parameters of cardiac performance. This situation cannot be maintained indefinitely, though, and their continued activation eventually results in further cardiac damage.

Activation of the Sympathetic Nervous System

The release of norepinephrine from sympathetic nerves and epinephrine from the adrenal medulla is one of the first responses to worsening cardiac function. This is largely because one of the most rapid and effective mechanisms to improve contractile performance is via catecholamine-mediated intracellular signal transduction pathways that improve the efficiency of myocardial excitation–contraction coupling and contractile protein function. Increased sympathetic nervous system (SNS) activity is initiated by low- and high-pressure sensory baroreceptors within the vasculature, which respond

Table 9
Short- and Long-Term Effects of Catecholamines in Heart Failure

Cardiac:	*Short-term*:
	Increased intrinsic inotropic properties
	Increased chronotropic response
	Induced gene expression to initiate hypertrophy phenotype
	Long-term:
	Increased energy expenditure and oxygen consumption
	Ischemia and reactive oxygen species generation (oxidative stress)
	Deranged excitation–contraction coupling and calcium homeostasis
	Myocyte apoptosis and necrosis
	Interstitial fibrosis induction
	Chamber remodeling
Renal:	*Short-term*:
	Increased tubular reabsorption of sodium and water (independently and via induction of renin-angiotensin-aldosterone system), which augments preload and maintains ventricular filling pressures
	Long-term:
	Ventricular chamber remodeling in response to chronic increases in hemodynamic load
Vasculature:	*Short-term*:
	Vasoconstriction to maintain peripheral blood pressure and organ perfusion
	Long-term:
	Smooth muscle hypertrophy and reduced vessel compliance

to falling cardiac output and blood pressure. As an early compensatory mechanism this activity produces numerous positive benefits within the heart, kidneys, and vasculature that improve cardiac output. Ongoing activation eventually produces a drop-off in beneficial effect because of adrenergic receptor downregulation and a maximizing of intracellular signaling pathway effecter mechanisms. Continued activation sees the appearance of additional deleterious responses that actually begin to worsen cardiac performance. These contrasting short- and long-term actions of catecholamines in the heart are summarized in Table 9. Cardiomyocytes contain various classes of adrenergic receptors, the number and function of which is known to change in heart failure. The properties of human cardiac adrenergic receptors in both the normal and failing heart are summarized in Table 10. In addition to changes in receptor expression, myocardial catecholamine responses in heart failure are modified by various mechanisms *(23)*. Upregulation of β-adrenergic receptor kinase-1 (β-ARK-1) activity results in receptor phosphorylation, a primary mechanism to uncouple the receptor from its intracellular signal transduction pathway. There is also increased activity of inhibitor G proteins (G_i), decreased catalytic activity of adenylate cyclase, and reduced availability of intracellular cyclic AMP, all of which will curtail the activity of β-adrenergic intracellular signaling pathways. A summary of myocardial responses to β-adrenergic receptors in heart failure is outlined in Fig. 5. The initial beneficial and subsequent harmful responses of the SNS and catecholamines in heart failure are clearly demonstrated by our own experiences with the use of catecholaminergic-based positive inotropic drugs and β-blockers in heart failure. In acute heart failure positive inotropic drugs produce short-term improvements in various hemodynamic parameters. Their long-term use and ongoing β-adrenergic receptor activation lead to ever-decreasing beneficial effects and an eventual increase in morbidity and mortality. Conversely, whereas β-blocking drugs have a deleterious effect on cardiac contraction in acute heart failure, they have been shown to bring dramatic improvement in chronic heart failure, where it is the harmful adrenergic responses that predominate.

Activation of the Renin-Angiotensin-Aldosterone System

Activation of the renin-angiotensin-aldosterone system (RAAS), as outlined in Fig. 6, is a key feature of the systemic response to heart failure. The initial effects of RAAS activation help maintain

Table 10
Adrenergic Receptors in the Heart

Alpha-1

Postsynaptic G protein-coupled receptor, secondary messenger effects via phospholipase C and inositol-1,4,5-triphosphate

15% of total adrenoceptor population in normal heart, but up to 50% of total population in heart failure

Activates sarcolemmal voltage-dependent Ca^{2+} channels, Na^{2+}/H^+ exchanger, Na^{2+}/K^+/ATPase and delayed rectifier K^+ current. Also induces hypertrophic phenotype and increase myofilament calcium sensitivity

Alpha-2

Presynaptic receptor that regulates postsynaptic norephedrine release during enhanced sympathetic activity. Small population in human heart

Beta-1

Most abundant cardiac adrenoceptor, 70% of total β-adrenoceptor population in normal heart, down-regulated and uncoupled from signal transduction pathways in heart failure

Postsynaptic G protein-coupled receptor, secondary messenger effects via adenylate cyclase, cAMP, and protein kinase A mediated phosphorylation

Augments myocardial inotropy and chronotropic response

Beta-2

30% of total β-adrenoceptor population in normal human heart

Postsynaptic G protein-coupled receptor, secondary messenger effects as β1

Augments myocardial inotropy and chronotropic response

Downregulated to a lesser extent than β1 receptors in heart failure

Uncoupled from signal transduction pathways in heart failure

Beta-3

Postsynaptic receptor, coupled to inhibitory G proteins that have negatively inotropic properties

Not downregulated in heart failure

Beta-4

Increasing evidence for existence, cardiostimulatory effects similar to β1/β2

Significance in normal and failing heart unknown

systemic blood pressure (through peripheral vasoconstriction) and cardiac output (through salt and water retention and maintained ventricular filling pressures). Unfortunately efforts to maintain ventricular filling pressure will eventually become more and more ineffective at supporting cardiac output (classical Starling's law of the heart). Angiotensin II, in addition to being a potent vasoconstrictor and activator of the SNS, has many other direct effects on both the heart and vasculature. It is known to contribute directly to cardiac chamber remodeling through inducing defective collagen deposition, myocyte hypertrophy, and apoptosis. It also acts as the primary stimulus for aldosterone release from the adrenal cortex, a potent mineralocorticoid hormone that induces sodium retention within the renal distal tubule at the expense of potassium and hydrogen ions. It has been observed, however, that the beneficial effects of aldosterone blockade in heart failure are much greater than could be explained by inhibition of this effect alone; recent work has revealed aldosterone to be an important mediator of numerous harmful responses in heart failure. Aldosterone is a potent inducer of both vascular and myocardial inflammation and is known to promote the recruitment of inflammatory mediator cells from the circulation to vascular and myocardial tissue *(24)*. Cyclooxygenase 2 and osteopontin are two of the main cited proinflammatory mediators released in response to aldosterone *(25)*; it also directly induces NADPH oxidase within the vasculature, which in turn is a major source of superoxide anions and a cause of oxidative stress-induced inflammation *(26)*. Animal model experiments designed to look at the specific actions of aldosterone show inflammatory cell infiltrates, ischemia, and patchy necrosis throughout the heart and vasculature, effects that are removed by the addition of specific aldosterone-antagonist agents. In addition aldosterone has a direct effect on the turnover and composition of extracellular matrix proteins such

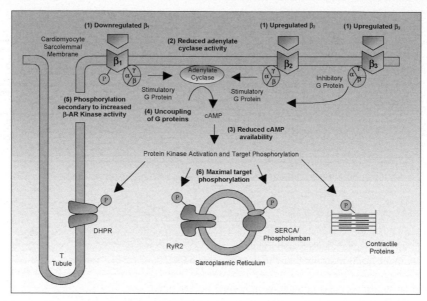

Fig. 5. β-Adrenergic receptor activation in heart failure. Normal β-adrenergic receptor signal transduction pathways activate protein kinase A and cause target protein phosphorylation, which enhances contractile function. Alterations in heart failure (1–6) are shown in bold (for abbreviations *see* main text): (1) Reduction in β1 receptor expression leading to a relative increase in β2 and the inhibitory β3 receptor as a proportion of total β-adrenergic receptor numbers. (2) Reduced adenylate cyclase activity. (3) Reduced cAMP availability. (4) Uncoupling of stimulatory G proteins. (5) Increased phosphorylation of β-adrenergic receptors uncouples receptor from signal transduction pathway. (6) Target molecules are phosphorylated to full stoichiometry with no further augmentation of function possible.

as collagen *(27)*; this effect, in conjunction with its proinflammatory action, makes aldosterone a potent cause of fibrosis in the vasculature and heart of individuals with chronic heart failure *(28)*. The actions of aldosterone and their sequelae are outlined in Table 11.

Peripheral Vascular Responses to Heart Failure

The vasculature is an important organ for modifying the response to worsening cardiac function; indeed, increased systemic vascular resistance is a cardinal feature of heart failure. This is an initial beneficial response maintaining left ventricular afterload, peripheral blood pressure, and organ perfusion. Persistent systemic vascular resistance also eventually becomes a maladaptive response and contributes to a decrease in cardiac performance. SNS activation on vascular α_1-adrenoceptors and the direct actions of angiotensin II are one component of vasoconstriction. The vasculature also exerts local control over smooth muscle tone through the relative production of endothelin (a potent vasoconstrictor peptide) and nitric oxide (a potent vasodilator). In heart failure the balance is tipped firmly in the direction of endothelin and subsequent vasoconstriction. Indeed, plasma endothelin levels are elevated in heart failure and correlate closely to prognosis and reduced cardiac performance *(21)*. This mismatch is caused partly by increased production of vascular endothelin but also by a reduced bioavailability of nitric oxide, which is rapidly scavenged by reactive oxygen anions produced under mechanisms of oxidative stress. Endothelin has also been shown to promote fibrosis and collagen accumulation in the heart *(29)* and promotes the retention of sodium within the kidney. Vascular remodeling, such as smooth muscle hypertrophy and hyperplasia, secondary to the effects of various mediators also adversely affects vascular function by reducing vessel wall compliance.

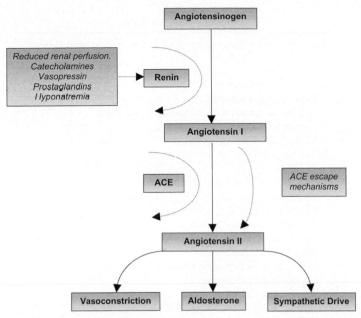

Fig. 6. The renin-angiotensin-aldosterone system. In heart failure the kidneys release renin in response to various stimuli. Circulating angiotensinogen (produced in the liver, vasculature, and CNS) is converted into angiotensin I by renin and subsequently into angiotensin II via angiotensin-converting enzyme in the lungs and vasculature. Angiotensin II has diverse actions throughout the body (*see* text). Note the presence of angiotensin-converting enzyme escape mechanisms, alternative pathways for the production of angiotensin II that become significant in the presence of ACE inhibitor treatment.

Table 11
The Actions and Consequences of Aldosterone

Distal tubule sodium and water retention in exchange for potassium and hydrogen ions
    Increased ventricular filling pressures and peripheral edema
    Hypokalemia, hypomagnesemia, alkalosis, and arrhythmias
Deranged collagen and extracellular matrix turnover in vasculature and heart
    Reduced ventricular and vascular compliance
    Chamber remodeling and dilation secondary to fibrosis
Blunted baroreceptor responses and reduced vagal tone
    Loss of normal heart rate variability
Reactive oxygen-derived free-radical generation
    Necrosis, inflammation, and eventual fibrosis
Recruitment of inflammatory mediator cells
    Release of various proinflammatory mediator and cytokines, eventual fibrosis
    Proatherosclerotic effect in vasculature
Endothelial vasomotor dysfunction
    Reduced nitric oxide availability
    Impaired vessel relaxation

Cytokine Activation in Heart Failure

Cytokines are a diverse group of proinflammatory peptides secreted by various tissues and cell types. Cytokine activation is a well-recognized feature of chronic heart failure and increased levels of inflammatory markers, such as C-reactive protein, are correlated closely to severity of heart failure and prognosis. Indeed, activation of cytokine responses is detectable prior to the onset

Table 12
Cytokines in Heart Failure

Inflammatory mediators known to be elevated in heart failure
    Interleukin-1, 6, 8, 10
    Interferon-γ
    Tumor necrosis factor α
    Soluble CD14 receptor
    Soluble tumor necrosis factor receptors 1 and 2
    Intracellular adhesion molecule 1
    Leukocyte adhesion molecule 1
Effects of cytokine activation
    Reactive oxygen-derived free-radical generation
    Induction of fetal gene expression pattern
    Hypertrophy and contractile protein synthesis
    Chamber remodeling and dilation
    Left ventricular dysfunction
    Pulmonary edema
    Anorexia and cachexia
    Reduced skeletal muscle blood flow
    Endothelial dysfunction
    Cardiomyocyte apoptosis

of symptomatic heart failure and predicts subsequent development of clinical heart failure *(30)*. A diverse range of cytokines are activated in heart failure, including TNF-α, interleukin-1, and interleukin-6 *(31)*. Peripheral blood leukocytes are known to migrate into the myocardium during heart failure, where they take on an enhanced cytokine production capacity. Furthermore, cardiomyocytes and myocardial fibroblasts are themselves induced to synthesize specific cytokines in heart failure through altered gene expression *(32)*. Cytokines are released locally within the heart in response to ventricular wall stress and from various other tissues in response to hypoperfusion, hypoxia, and oxidative stress. They have various local effects on the heart as outlined in Table 12. In addition they have a range of systemic metabolic and immunological actions, particularly on skeletal muscle, where they induce wasting and impaired contraction. The systemic action of cytokines may underlie the cardiac cachexia syndrome in severe chronic heart failure, similar to their causative role in cancer cachexia syndrome *(33)*.

Natriuretic Peptide Response in Heart Failure

The natriuretic peptides are a group of small peptides released by the heart in response to wall stretch when there is circulatory volume expansion in heart failure. Atrial natriuretic peptide (ANP) is secreted from both the atria and ventricles. It is secreted at low levels in normal hearts but levels rise dramatically in heart failure. Even more sensitive as a marker of myocardial dysfunction is its counterpart, brain natriuretic peptide (BNP), confusingly named as it was first identified within the central nervous system. Its sensitivity stems from the fact that BNP gene expression and ultimate secretion from the ventricle is initiated only in heart failure and does not occur under normal circumstances. Natriuretic peptides act on the kidney tubule, where they promote a natriuresis, and also on the peripheral vasculature, where they produce vasodilation. In this way they are seen as direct antagonists of the actions of angiotensin II, aldosterone, and catecholamines. Natriuretic peptides also inhibit endothelin secretion and may also protect against collagen accumulation, fibrosis, and ventricular remodeling *(34)*. Unfortunately the characteristic progressive decline in heart failure suggests that their beneficial actions fail to compensate for RAAS activation. Indeed it has been suggested that this failure of natriuretic activity is itself a manifestation of heart failure in that poorly functioning myocytes are unable to release biologically active peptides due to a failure of intracellular enzymatic cleavage of the expressed propeptide *(35)*. Increasing attention is being

Table 13
Clinical Manifestations of Heart Failure

Symptoms
  Fatigue
  Dyspnea (exertional, orthopnea, paroxysmal nocturnal)
  Swelling (limbs, abdomen)
Signs
  Tachycardia
  Hypotension
  Jugular venous elevation
  Abnormal hepatojugular reflex
  Abnormal apex beat (displaced, sustained, dyskinetic)
  Third heart sound
  Inspiratory crepitations on lung auscultation
  Edema (peripheral and peritoneal)
  Cold peripheries and poor pulses

given to the role of natriuretic peptides as diagnostic tools in heart failure, as BNP and its precursors (pro-BNP/N-pro-BNP) have good sensitivity, specificity, and predictive accuracy for heart failure (both systolic and diastolic). Furthermore, in view of the above beneficial effects, research is also focusing on their role as a therapeutic target, either by enzymatic inhibition to prevent their breakdown or via the use of exogenous natriuretic agents.

SKELETAL MUSCLE DYSFUNCTION IN HEART FAILURE

A consistent finding of established heart failure is fatigue and reduced exercise tolerance in excess of that expected from cardiac pump dysfunction alone. It is known that exercise capacity correlates poorly with left ventricular function in chronic heart failure. Furthermore, skeletal muscle wasting is a key feature of cardiac cachexia syndrome in heart failure, of which the above symptoms are a key component. In view of these observations attention has recently been given to identifying specific aspects of skeletal muscle dysfunction in heart failure. Activation of immunological cells and the increased levels of circulating cytokines are believed to play an important role in much the same way as they are implicated in cancer cachexia *(33)*. The improvements in skeletal muscle performance seen from exercise training schemes in heart failure patients are associated with a reduction in skeletal muscle cytokine content and attenuation of reactive oxygen species generation, both of which appear to contribute to a skeletal muscle chronic inflammatory process in heart failure *(36)*. More recently defects in the skeletal muscle ryanodine receptor (RyR1) have also been identified in heart failure, similar to those present in the cardiac ryanodine receptor (RyR2) *(37)*. Hyperphosphorylation of RyR1 in heart failure impairs contraction as it reduces the overall efficiency of EC coupling, suggesting that heart failure induces a generalized EC coupling myopathy that impairs both cardiac and skeletal muscle function.

PATHOLOGIC AND CLINICAL DECLINE IN HEART FAILURE: A FINAL INTEGRATED VIEWPOINT

The pathophysiological changes outlined in this chapter underlie our current understanding of the syndrome of heart failure and the rationale behind many of the currently available therapeutic strategies. It is always important to remember, however, that every case of heart failure, regardless of the specific cause, represents an individual patient whose functional capacity and quality of life are impaired. It is usual to think of the clinical manifestations of heart failure, outlined in Table 13, as simply reflective of an impaired ventricular ejection fraction. Objective cardiac measurements, however, often correlate poorly with the clinical manifestations of heart failure syndrome and often fail to take into account the impact of secondary consequences and complications such as increased infection risk, anemia, hypoalbuminemia, atrial fibrillation, thromboembolism, and depression. Furthermore, clinical features of heart failure may only indirectly reflect contractile dysfunction. For example, dyspnea may be secondary to both diaphragmatic weakness (skeletal muscle myopathy) and reduced lung compliance (lymphatic distension) secondary to lymphatic distention. In general the syndrome of heart failure comprises a gradual decline in cardiac function, which may be asymptomatic for a considerable period until a critical threshold is passed at which clinical manifestations occur. This may be relatively late in the overall decline of cardiac function and usually represents the beginning of a more rapid decline manifest by worsening symptoms and eventually resulting in death. Depending on etiology this decline may be stepwise, as in myocardial infarction, or progressive, as in hypertensive heart disease. Furthermore, at any stage sudden cardiac death may occur secondary to arrhythmia generation.

Heart failure remains one of the most pressing medical problems and significant consumers of health care resources in developed countries, and its incidence is also increasing in the developing world. The initial adaptive responses to provide short-term improvements in cardiac performance were ideally suited to our previous hunter-gatherer lifestyles, where the fight-or- flight response either would result in swift evasion of a life-threatening situation or would be insufficient, resulting in death. The fact that they would result in maladaptive responses if made to continue for any length of time was largely irrelevant. There has been little time on an evolutionary scale for physiological mechanisms to develop that can offer a more sustained and long-term compensation for impaired cardiac performance, yet this is what our extended life spans and partial successes in therapeutics are now demanding. Our increasing understanding of heart failure pathophysiology and recent therapeutic advances have allowed us to address this imbalance to a certain extent and partially overcome the maladaptive consequences of our responses to heart failure. Despite this, further improvements are still needed if we are to adequately tackle the increasing burden of heart failure in society and reduce mortality rates, which are still worse than those of many common cancers. Whatever the next major advance in heart failure therapeutics is, there is no doubt that its development will stem from our increasing understanding of the complex heart failure syndrome and its underlying pathophysiology.

REFERENCES

1. Poole-Wilson PA. Heart failure. Med Int 1985;2:866–871.
2. Task Force for the Diagnosis and Treatment of Chronic Heart Failure of the European Society of Cardiology. Guidelines for the diagnosis and treatment of chronic heart failure. Eur Heart J 2001;22:1527–1560.
3. Jessup M, Brozena S. Heart failure. N Engl J Med 2003;348:2007–2018.
4. Angeja BG, Grossman W. Evaluation and management of diastolic heart failure. Circulation 2003;107:659–663.
5. Krum H, Gilbert RE. Demographics and concomitant disorders in heart failure. Lancet 2003;362:147–158.
6. Bonne G, Carrier L, Richard P, et al. Familial hypertrophic cardiomyopathy: from mutations to functional defects. Circ Res 1998;83:580–593.
7. Gaballa MA, Goldman S. Ventricular remodelling in heart failure. J Card Fail 2002;8(Suppl):S476–S486.
8. Leri A, Kajstura J, Anversa P. Myocyte proliferation and ventricular remodelling. J Card Fail 2002;8(Suppl):S518–S525.
9. Nadal-Ginard B, Kajstura J, Leri A, et al. Myocyte death, growth, and regeneration in cardiac hypertrophy and failure. Circ Res 2003;92:139–150.
10. Severs NJ. Gap junction remodelling in heart failure. J Card Fail 2002;8(Suppl):S293–S299.
11. Haider N, Narula N, Narula J. Apoptosis in heart failure represents programmed cell survival, not death, of cardiomyocytes and likelihood of reverse remodelling. J Card Fail 2002;8(Suppl):S512–S517.
12. Narula J, Arbustini E, Chandrashekhar Y, et al. Apoptosis and the systolic dysfunction in congestive heart failure. story of apoptosis interruptus and zombie myocytes. Cardiol Clin 2001;19:113–126.
13. Spinale FG. Matrix metalloproteinases: regulation and dysregulation in the failing heart. Circ Res 2002;90:520–530.
14. Marx S, Gaburjakova J, Gaburjakova M, et al. Coupled gating between cardiac calcium release channels (ryanodine receptors). Circ Res 2001;88:1151–1158.
15. Marx SO, Reiken S, Hisamatsu Y, et al. PKA phosphorylation dissociates FKBP12.6 from the calcium release channel (ryanodine receptor): defective regulation in failing hearts. Cell 2000;101:365–376.

16. Reiken S, Wehrens XHT, Vest JA, et al. β-Blockers restore cardiac calcium release channel function and improve cardiac muscle performance in human heart failure. Circulation 2003;107:2459–2466.
17. Hasenfuss G. Alterations of calcium regulatory proteins in heart failure. Cardiovas Res 1998;37:279–289.
18. Brette F, Orchard CT. Tubule function in mammalian cardiac myocytes. Circ Res 2003;92:1182–1192.
19. Carvajal K, Moreno-Sanchez R. Heart metabolic disturbances in cardiovascular diseases. Arch Med Res 2003;34: 89–99.
20. Ingwall JS, Kramer MF, Fifer MA, et al. The creatine kinase system in normal and diseased human myocardium. N Engl J Med 1985;313:1050–1054.
21. Givertz MM, Colucci WS. New targets for heart failure: endothelin, inflammatory cytokines and oxidative stress. Lancet 1998;352(Suppl I):34–38.
22. Lebovitz RM, Zhang H, Vogel H, et al. Neurodegeneration, myocardial injury, and perinatal death in mitochondrial superoxide dismutase-deficient mice. Proc Natl Acad Sci USA 1996;93:9782–9787.
23. Bristow MR. Why does the myocardium fail? Insights from basic science. Lancet 1998;352(Suppl I):8–14.
24. Rocha R, Rudolph AE, Frierdich GE, et al. Aldosterone induces a vascular inflammatory phenotype in the rat heart. Am J Physiol Heart Circ Physiol 2002;283:H1802–H1810.
25. Rocha R, Martin-Berger CL, Yang P, et al. Selective aldosterone blockade prevents angiotensin II/salt-induced vascular inflammation in the rat heart. Endocrinology 2002;143:4828–4836.
26. Sun Y, Zhang J, Lu L, et al. Aldosterone induced inflammation in the rat heart: role of oxidative stress. Am J Pathol 2002;161:1773–1781.
27. Qin W, Rudolph AE, Bond BR, et al. Transgenic model of aldosterone driven cardiac hypertrophy and heart failure. Circ Res 2003;93:69–76.
28. Suzuki G, Morita H, Mishima T, et al. Effects of long term monotherapy with eplerenone, a novel aldosterone blocker, on progression of left ventricular dysfunction and remodelling in dogs with heart failure. Circulation 2002;106:2967–2972.
29. Fraccarollo D, Galuppo P, Bauersachs J, et al. Collagen accumulation after myocardial infarction: effects of endothelin a receptor blockade and implications for early remodelling. Cardiovasc Res 2002;54:559–567.
30. Vasan RS, Sullivan LM, Roubenoff R, et al. Inflammatory markers and risk of heart failure in elderly subjects without prior myocardial infarction. Circulation 2003;107:1486–1491.
31. Mann DL. Inflammatory mediators and the failing heart. Circ Res 2002;91:988–998.
32. Paulus WJ. Cytokines and heart failure. Heart Fail Monit 2000;1:50–56.
33. Anker SD, Sharma R. The syndrome of cardiac cachexia. Int J Card 2002;85:51–66.
34. Tamura N, Ogawa Y, Chusho H, et al. Cardiac fibrosis in mice lacking brain natriuretic peptide. Proc Natl Acad Sci USA 2000;97:4239–4444.
35. Goetze JP, Kastrup J, Rehfeld JF. The paradox of increased natriuretic hormones in congestive heart failure patients: does the endocrine heart also fail in heart failure. Eur Heart J 2003;24:1471–1472.
36. Mann DL, Reid MB. Exercise training and skeletal muscle inflammation in chronic heart failure: feeling better about fatigue. J Am Coll Cardiol 2003;42:869–872.
37. Reiken S, Lacampagne A, Zhou H, et al. PKA phosphorylation activates the calcium release channel (ryanodine receptor) in skeletal muscle: defective regulation in heart failure. J Cell Biol 2003;160:919–928.

20 Treatment of Congestive Heart Failure

Stephen S. Gottlieb, MD

INTRODUCTION

The goals of heart failure treatment include both symptomatic improvement and prolongation of life. These goals are not necessarily concordant. Related to this problem is the observation that the acute actions of an intervention may be very different from the chronic effects. When treating heart failure, therefore, one must understand the immediate and long-term desires of a particular patient and the immediate and long-term consequences of one's therapy. The result is an uncomfortable use of acute treatments known to have adverse consequences when given for a prolonged period and chronic treatments that are counterintuitive. Fortunately, however, congestive heart failure has been well investigated, with multiple large studies demonstrating the multiple consequences of many of our standard interventions.

INITIAL WORKUP

The terms *systolic dysfunction* and *congestive heart failure* (CHF) are often inappropriately used interchangeably; half of patients with heart failure do not have systolic dysfunction. Since treatment of systolic dysfunction is different from treatment of other causes of heart failure, an assessment of left ventricular function is essential when a patient presents with heart failure. If systolic dysfunction is the cause of the heart failure, proper treatment can be tailored based on the results of well-controlled studies (most studies of heart failure limit themselves to this defined group of patients). For patients with heart failure without systolic dysfunction, however, few studies provide guidance. The rest of this chapter refers to patients with systolic dysfunction unless stated otherwise.

Determining Whether Dyspnea is CHF

The initial diagnostic dilemma in many patients with dyspnea is whether the symptoms are of cardiac or pulmonary causes. If pulmonary function tests are abnormal and there is left ventricular dysfunction, it may be difficult to determine the etiology of the symptoms. Physical findings, such as wheezing, may be nonspecific. Certainly, rales, orthopnea, and paroxysmal nocturnal dyspnea suggest a cardiac origin and chronic hypoxia suggests a pulmonary cause, but fluid overload could be secondary to either right- or left-sided failure. Even experienced clinicians are often fooled.

Measurement of brain natriuretic peptide (BNP) may be helpful in determining whether dyspnea is from heart failure. Indeed, in a large study it more accurately diagnosed CHF than emergency room physicians (1). However, BNP concentrations may be elevated in right-sided failure from pulmonary emboli or other sources of pulmonary hypertension, and should never be relied on alone to make the diagnosis. A right heart catheterization may be needed in patients in whom questions remain.

From: *Essential Cardiology: Principles and Practice, 2nd Ed.*
Edited by: C. Rosendorff © Humana Press Inc., Totowa, NJ

Similarly, it may be difficult to determine if dyspnea in a patient with heart failure is secondary to deconditioning or continued volume overload and poor cardiac function. The role of BNP in these patients is not well defined. Proper treatment may depend on the results of a right heart catheterization. Often it is felt that such intervention is needed only for patients with severe symptoms. However, it is more likely to affect treatment when there is a question as to the cause of the patient's symptoms.

Reversible Causes of Systolic Dysfunction

In addition to assessing cardiac function, initial evaluation includes eliminating the possibility of reversible causes of systolic dysfunction. Ischemic heart disease is always a possibility to be considered, and the perceived risk of atherosclerosis should determine which tests, if any, are needed to rule out coronary artery disease. Although many cardiologists perform a cardiac catheterization on every patient with heart failure, a young patient without risk factors or clinical suggestion of ischemia can probably be assessed by an exercise tolerance test. This is especially true if another cause, such as alcohol abuse, can be identified. Similarly, a patient without ischemic symptoms who is not a surgical candidate need not undergo a catheterization. It should be noted, though, that assessment of myocardial viability and exercise-induced ischemia may be useful even in some patients with very poor contractility at rest.

An echocardiogram should be helpful for ascertaining some causes of heart failure, such as valvular disease. The importance of mitral regurgitation, however, may be difficult to evaluate. Mitral regurgitation is common in patients with dilated ventricles, and it may be impossible to determine whether the valvular disease is primary or secondary. In the setting of poor contractility, however, surgical correction of either primary or secondary mitral regurgitation is accompanied by high risk. While there are increasing numbers of surgeons willing to undertake mitral valve repair or replacement in such patients, the proper role of mitral valve surgery in patients with poor systolic function remains uncertain.

The possibility that nonischemic cardiomyopathy is caused by thyroid abnormalities, hemochromatosis, or complications of HIV infection can usually be eliminated simply by blood tests. Treatment of these disorders is straightforward, but resultant cardiomyopathies may persist despite treatment of the underlying problem. Nutritional abnormalities and alcohol abuse should also be considered as potential causes of a reversible cardiomyopathy.

There are increasing data that sleep apnea can lead to cardiac dysfunction and worsening heart failure. Conversely, heart failure can cause disturbances in sleep patterns. While the interaction is complicated and incompletely understood, physicians should consider sleep apnea as a possible cause of chronic dyspnea in patients with heart failure.

Myocardial Biopsies

The detection of myocarditis rarely affects treatment. Since there is no randomized support for the use of immunosuppressive therapy and this treatment entails considerable risk, immunosuppressive therapy is controversial and not prescribed by most clinicians. Thus, a diagnosis of myocarditis usually does not affect treatment. However, a diagnosis of myocarditis might have prognostic implications by suggesting potential rapid changes (either positive or negative) in condition. If a patient's expected prognosis will affect the clinical management, a myocardial biopsy might be indicated.

When a clinical suspicion exists for a reversible disease that can be diagnosed by a myocardial biopsy (such as sarcoidosis, hemochromatosis, or amyloidosis) and treatment would be affected, a biopsy is indicated. A biopsy may also diagnose giant-cell myocarditis, a rare entity that is generally felt to have a poor prognosis. Since immunosuppression may be considered for these patients, a biopsy could be appropriate in a patient with recent onset of symptoms, a rapid downhill course, and no obvious cause of heart failure.

Follow-Up Assessments of Cardiac Function

Once the etiology of the heart failure is determined, further assessments are needed only when there are questions as to the patient's status. Thus, repeat echocardiograms or gated blood pool scans are rarely needed if a patient has known systolic dysfunction and continued symptoms. A slight increase or decrease in ejection fraction will add little to a physician's clinical judgment and should not be the basis of a change in therapy. Occasionally, a repeat assessment is needed to rule out the possibility of normalization of cardiac function (at which point treatment might be cautiously withdrawn) or a marked deterioration in function.

DIURETICS

Diuretic medications (Table 1) remain the primary treatment for the acute symptomatic relief of patients with congestive heart failure. They lead to rapid and dramatic improvements in patients with exacerbations or newly diagnosed disease. In addition, they are needed for relief of chronic symptoms. However, potential long-term adverse consequences mandate that they not be the only treatment for patients with systolic dysfunction.

Fluid Restriction

The best means of keeping patients euvolemic would be the avoidance of the causes of fluid and sodium retention. Reducing sodium intake can decrease the need for high doses of diuretics, and should be encouraged in all patients, but fluid restriction is rarely beneficial. While the hyponatremia and fluid overload associated with congestive heart failure makes fluid restriction appealing, such an approach is rarely successful. First, the drive to drink water is strong, and it is virtually impossible to successfully fluid-restrict a patient. Second, diuresis can be successful without fluid restriction. Third, chronic hyponatremia rarely causes problems, and excessive hyponatremia can be successfully treated by modifying the diuretic regimen. In patients with congestive heart failure, only the combination of diuresis and angiotensin-converting enzyme (ACE) inhibition has been demonstrated to reverse hyponatremia. It is therefore not surprising that the overwhelming majority of patients with heart failure need diuretic medications.

Extent of Diuresis

The most common clinical problem related to diuretics is underutilization of the drugs. Hospitalized patients who are treated for pulmonary edema are often discharged with marked fluid overload and prescribed doses of diuretics inadequate to continue diuresis. Such patients frequently return to the hospital because of repeat exacerbations. The absence of rales should therefore not be taken as evidence of adequate diuresis. Rather, assessment of total body fluid (using peripheral edema, ascites, and sacral edema as guides) is easy and can indicate the need for more diuresis. While it is still controversial whether treatment should be guided by using a pulmonary artery catheter to determine an optimal pulmonary capillary wedge pressure, it is clear that adequate diuresis is essential and should be guided by clinical endpoints.

Another common problem preventing the proper utilization of diuretic medications is fear of using elevated doses. Patients with severe heart failure and evidence of renal dysfunction often need doses perceived as extremely high; daily dosing with 200 mg of furosemide is not uncommon. Despite the frequent need for high concentrations of diuretics, intravenous administration of furosemide is not necessarily needed in order to achieve a clinically important diuresis. Oral regimens may be successful even in markedly fluid-overloaded individuals. This is important, as successful outpatient diuresis can save money, prevent iatrogenic complications, and improve a patient's quality of life. However, outpatient diuresis mandates close follow-up to ensure success and prevent deadly electrolyte abnormalities. Although the data suggest that a trial of oral diuretics should be given in most edematous patients, there are patients in whom intravenous administration

Table 1
Comparison of Diuretic Medications, Listed According to Site of Action

Diuretic	FENa$^+$ (max) (%)	Dosage (mg/d)	Onset of action		Action duration		Peak oral effect (h)	Comments
			oral (h)	IV (min)	oral (h)	IV (h)		
Ascending loop of Henle								
Furosemide	20–25	40–400	1	5	6	2–3	1–3	
Bumetanide	20–25	1–5	0.5	5	6	2–3	1–3	
Torsemide	20–25	10–200	1	10	6–8	6–8	1–3	
Ethacrynic acid	20–25	50–100	0.5	5	6–8	3	2	High ototoxicity risk, but (unlike other loop diuretics) can use in sulfa allergic pts
Early distal tubule								
Metolazone	5–8	2.5–20	1	—	12–24	—	2–4	Greatest potential for potassium loss; also slight actions in proximal tubule
Chlorthalidone	5–10	25–200	2	—	24–48	—	6	Ineffective when GFR < 30
Hydrochlorothiazide	5–8	25–100	2	—	12	—	4	Ineffective when GFR <30
Chlorothiazide	5–8	500–1000	1	15–30	8	—	4	Ineffective when GFR <30
Late distal tubule								
Spironolactone	2	50–400	48–72	—	48–72	—	1–2 d	Efficacy dependent upon aldosterone presence
Triamterene	2	75–300	2	—	12–16	—	6–8	
Amiloride	2	5–10	2	—	24	—	6–16	
Proximal tubule								
Acetazolamide	4	250–375	1	30–60	8	3–4	2–4	Efficacy limited by metabolic acidosis it causes

FENa$^+$ (Max, %), maximal natriuretic effect (maximum fractional excretion of filtered sodium). (Adapted from ref. 45.)

will be necessary. When immediate diuresis is necessary because of severe decompensation and pulmonary edema, the more rapid onset of intravenous diuretics may be essential.

Diuretic Combinations

It is often difficult to get effective diuresis in patients with severe heart failure. The physiologic stimulus to retain fluid may be strong enough to overwhelm the diuretic actions of any single agent. Thus, potent diuretics (such as loop diuretics) may be rendered ineffective by distal reabsorption. In contrast, agents that act distally, such as the potassium-sparing agents, may not be potent enough to yield the desired results. In such patients, the synergistic effects of combining diuretics can have many beneficial consequences.

The combination of loop diuretics and metolazone has proven to be particularly potent *(2)*. With the combined use of these agents, effective diuresis may be produced in patients who have been resistant to other interventions. However, it may take days to see the results of the addition of metolazone because of the pharmacokinetics of the drug. It is also important to realize that the hypokalemia that results from the combined use of loop diuretics and metolazone may be severe; serum potassium concentrations need to be watched especially carefully in these patients. The other useful method of combining diuretics is to add a potassium-sparing agent to the diuretic regimen. Not only does this potentiate the diuretic actions of the original regimen, but it also prevents extreme potassium loss and simplifies electrolyte management.

Spironolactone is not a potent diuretic, but the Randomized Aldactone Evaluation Study (RALES) showed improvement in survival in patients who received relatively small doses of the drug *(3)*. The reason for the result of the RALES study is uncertain. Spironolactone conserves potassium and magnesium and can be synergistic when combined with other diuretic medications. However, other effects of spironolactone may be even more important and need further investigation. For example, spironolactone may affect fibrosis formation in hearts of patients with cardiomyopathy and may exert direct effects on the sodium-potassium pump. Eplerenone, a more selective aldosterone antagonist without the side effect of gynecomastia, has been shown to be effective in patients with heart failure and an acute myocardial infarction and can be used when spironolactone has been found to cause gynecomastia.

Refractory Patients

In some patients, inotropic therapy may be required to produce acute diuresis. Agents such as dobutamine and milrinone often lead to diuresis in patients with worsening renal function secondary to cardiac dysfunction. Routine use of inotropic therapy in hospitalized patients, however, was not shown to be beneficial *(4)*. Anecdotes continue to support the use of low dose dopamine in patients whose renal function is limited by severe heart failure. While, there are few studies documenting increased renal perfusion and urine output with low doses of dopamine (2–3 µg/kg/min) *(5)*, its use is commonplace.

Nesiritide is a vasodilator that is approved for the acute treatment of congestive heart failure *(6)*. It lowers cardiac filling pressures and can improve symptoms. However, it is expensive and it is still unclear whether it leads to better outcomes than more conventional treatment. Its renal effects in sick heart failure patients are uncertain *(7)*.

When all else fails, ultrafiltration may improve the fluid status of a patient. The result can be long-lasting in some patients, with no need to continue the treatment once euvolemia is reached. Perhaps the many actions of diuresis upon cardiac performance and neurohormones explain the reports of the chronic benefits of this intervention *(8)*.

Since improving the volume status is so important for treating the symptoms of congestive heart failure, chronic dialysis can be considered for volume control, not just for renal failure. Some patients will develop renal failure when euvolemic, with renal function maintained only with fluid overload. Since dialysis can lead to marked improvements in quality of life in such patients, its use is appropriate if agreed to by the patient.

Adverse Effects

There is no doubt that diuretics, though essential for symptomatic relief and decreasing cardiac distension, exert adverse consequences; electrolyte depletion, neurohormonal activation, and renal failure can ensue. While potentially harmful, these side effects can be overcome with other interventions. For example, the use of ACE inhibitors and spironolactone can prevent potassium and magnesium depletion. In the rare instances when it is necessary, potassium replacements can also be given.

Diuretics lead to activation of the renin-angiotensin, sympathetic, and other neurohormonal systems, with potential immediate and long-term repercussions that are discussed below. However, these problems should not prevent adequate use of diuretic medications; these actions can generally be blocked with ACE inhibitors, β-blockers, and aldosterone antagonists.

The physician must always be alert when combining agents with opposing actions. Treatment of congestive heart failure usually includes both potassium-wasting and potassium-sparing agents. The results may be unpredictable, and patients need to be followed carefully to ensure neither hypokalemia nor hyperkalemia.

A slight increase in serum creatinine and blood urea nitrogen (BUN) concentrations should be expected (and tolerated) in order to achieve adequate diuresis. Diuretic-induced increases in serum creatinine concentrations can be worrisome, but can usually be resolved by a slower rate of diuresis. It may also be advisable to limit the use of ACE inhibitors while aggressively diuresing a patient. Patients who develop renal failure with ACE inhibition are usually sodium and volume intravascularly deplete *(9)*. Initiation of ACE inhibitors after the patient is euvolemic may prevent the renal failure that occasionally occurs when ACE inhibitors are prescribed while the patient is being actively diuresed.

ACE INHIBITORS AND OTHER VASODILATORS

The long-term effects of ACE inhibitors on both symptoms and mortality are clear (Table 2). Not only has their survival benefit been consistently demonstrated in patients with systolic dysfunction *(10,11)*, but the use of ACE inhibitors results in increased exercise tolerance, decreased hospitalization rates, and improvements in other indices reflective of symptoms. This information has been well disseminated and the utilization of ACE inhibition is now appropriately widespread. However, concerns remain as to whether these agents are being used in a manner that provides the most benefit.

Dosing

The commonly used dosages of ACE inhibitors (Table 3) are lower than those studied and that demonstrated benefit. Patients in SOLVD reached mean daily enalapril doses of 16.6 mg and the severely ill Cooperative North Scandinavian Enalapril Survival Study (CONSENSUS) patients received a mean dose of 18.4 mg of this drug. Nevertheless, enalapril and lisinopril (both have equivalent daily dosing) are frequently prescribed at 2.5 or 5 mg daily.

The doses with demonstrated efficacy are also doses that were tolerated in multiple studies of patients who ranged from being severely ill to being relatively asymptomatic. It is therefore important to explore the reasons physicians frequently are reluctant to prescribe these doses. Understanding the effects of ACE inhibition and the ways to prevent adverse consequences should lead to more effective use of these agents.

Adverse Effects

Patients with heart failure often have low blood pressures, but the evidence seems clear that asymptomatic hypotension should not limit the use of these agents. Indeed, ACE inhibitors will often not decrease (and may even increase) the blood pressure of patients with heart failure. It should be remembered, however, that blood pressure will decrease when ACE inhibition is combined with intravascular depletion. Thus, patients who do not tolerate these agents when they are being actively diuresed may tolerate them after they have stabilized. A slight liberalization of fluid status might also help patients with symptomatic hypotension when receiving ACE inhibitors.

Table 2
Major Heart Failure Survival Trials

Acronym	Drug	n	Dose goal	% Improvement
Renin-angiotensin-aldosterone axis and vasodilators				
CONSENSUS (11)	Enalapril vs placebo in advanced disease	253	40 mg	27%
SOLVD-treatment (10)	Enalapril vs placebo	2569	20 mg	16%
SOLVD-prevention (42)	Enalapril vs placebo	4228	20 mg	No effect on mortality, hospitalizations decreased
V-HeFT-II (17)	Hydralazine/isosorbide dinitrate vs enalapril	804	enal: 20 mg hydral: 300 mg nitrates: 160 mg	28% improvement with enalapril
VHeFT-III (43)	Felodipine vs placebo	450	10 mg	No effect
V-HeFT (16)	Hydralazine/nitrates vs prazosin vs placebo	642	hydral: 300 mg nitrates: 160 mg prazosin: 20 mg	Improvement with hydralazine/nitrates
CHARM (44)	Candesartan vs placebo	7599	32 mg	12% in combined patient groups: low EF with and without ACE-I, normal EF
RALES (3)	Spironolactone vs placebo	1663	25 mg	30%
Inotropes				
PROMISE (27)	Milrinone vs placebo	1088	40 mg	Increased mortality
DIG (25)	Digoxin vs placebo	6800	varied	No effect on mortality, hospitalizations decreased
Beta-blockers				
CIBIS-II (19)	Bisoprolol vs placebo	2647	10 mg	34%
MERIT-HF (20)	Long-acting metoprolol vs placebo	3991	200 mg	34%
COPERNICUS (21)	Carvedilol vs placebo	2289	25 mg bid	35%
COMET (24)	Carvedilol vs metoprolol tartrate	3029	Carv: 25 bid Metop: 50 bid	17% improvement with carvedilol
Amiodarone				
GESICA (30)	Amiodarone vs placebo	516	300 mg	28%
CHF-STAT (31)	Amiodarone vs placebo	674	300 mg	No effect

377

Table 3
Therapeutic Doses of ACE Inhibitors

Captopril	25–50 mg tid
Enalapril	10–20 mg bid
Lisinopril	20–40 mg qd
Monopril	20–40 mg qd
Ramipril	5–10 mg bid
Quinapril	20 mg bid

These are recommendations for final doses,
based on the doses used in heart failure studies.

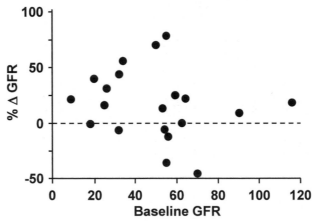

Fig. 1. The baseline glomerular filtration rate (GFR) as related to the percentage change in GFR after ACE inhibition. There was no relation between baseline renal function and the change in GFR. (From ref. *12*. Copyright 1992, with permission from Elsevier.)

The other factor which often limits dosing of ACE inhibition is renal dysfunction. Contrary to many physicians' assumptions, preexisting kidney disease does not increase the risk of renal deterioration *(12)* (Fig. 1). ACE inhibitors may cause renal dysfunction in a small percentage of people with any baseline kidney function (especially those with renal artery stenosis), and this complication should be carefully looked for in any patient during initiation of ACE inhibition. However, a worsening serum creatinine is usually the result of intravascular depletion, and a change in fluid status will usually permit initiation and upward titration of these agents in patients who at first appear intolerant. Effective ACE inhibition can be achieved in the overwhelming majority of patients.

Hyperkalemia may occur with ACE inhibition. Often this is because of continued potassium supplementation, either by prescription or by ingestion of potassium through salt substitutes or foods rich in potassium. Before blaming and discontinuing the drug, therefore, a careful dietary history must be taken.

Angioedema, neutropenia, and other clear contraindications to ACE inhibitors are infrequent. Other side effects, such as cough and rash, are often ascribed to these agents, even though it may be difficult to differentiate a side effect from a concomitant condition. Furthermore, these conditions are often well tolerated and need not necessarily lead to discontinuation of medications known to be effective. Nevertheless, there are times when these side effects will be severe enough to warrant discontinuation of an ACE inhibitor. At that time other agents can be tried.

Angiotensin II Blockers

Angiotensin II receptor blockers (ARBs) have been studied in heart failure and, while not better than ACE inhibitors, they appear to be effective *(13)*. In contrast to ACE inhibitors, which lead to increased bradykinin concentrations in addition to preventing angiotensin II production, the angiotensin II receptor blockers work only on a single system. Bradykinin presumably causes some of the adverse side effects related to ACE inhibitors, such as cough, but may also provide some of the benefits. Thus an ARB should be prescribed to patients intolerant of the cheaper ACE inhibitors.

The use of ARBs as additive therapy has also been evaluated. While one study showed a statistically significant, but modest, benefit *(14)*, a study in patients with a myocardial infarction showed additional adverse effects with no added efficacy *(15)*. If used, it is important to carefully look for hyperkalemia or harmful renal effects.

Hydralazine and Nitrates

The other treatment choice for ACE-intolerant patients is the combination of hydralazine and nitrates. This combination appeared to improve survival in the Vasodilator-Heart Failure Trial (V-HeFT) *(16)*. While clearly not as good as ACE inhibitors *(17)*, these drugs may also improve symptoms and exercise tolerance. Daily doses up to 300 mg have been prescribed, but nausea often limits how much a patient will tolerate. Long-term side effects, such as lupus syndrome, are much less frequent. Unfortunately, hydralazine has a short half-life and needs to be given three to four times daily in order to be effective. For this reason, its utility has been limited.

In patients with severe disease, however, hydralazine may be effective when given in addition to ACE inhibitors. This has not been widely investigated, but the decreased afterload induced by hydralazine may be particularly beneficial in patients with mitral regurgitation. Furthermore, patients with advanced disease may be more willing to take this medicine as frequently as it needs to be administered.

Nitrates can also be effective for symptomatic relief of patients. The medication should always be prescribed with an appreciation of the tolerance that may develop with its use. Thus, patients should receive nitrates to prevent the most important symptoms. In some patients, a single dose of isosorbide nitrate (10–40 mg) prior to sleep may prevent orthopnea and paroxysmal nocturnal dyspnea. Others will benefit from longer-acting preparations for use prior to activities during the day. Sublingual nitroglycerin can also be helpful prior to unusual exertion. When tailored to the individual patient, nitrates can improve the quality of life.

There are data to suggest that African-Americans, in particular, might benefit from the combination of hydralazine and nitrates *(18)*. The best evidence for the use of these agents is as adjunctive therapy in African-Americans.

Calcium-Channel Blockers

Most calcium-channel blockers have negative inotropic properties and have been shown to have adverse consequences when given to patients with congestive heart failure. The use of these drugs is appealing because of their benefit in treating anginal symptoms, a common condition in patients with heart failure. However, their use in studies following myocardial infarction consistently show that patients with poor ventricular function have worse survival when given calcium-channel blockers. Similarly, studies in patients with heart failure suggest that the older calcium-channel blocking agents, such as nifedipine, diltiazem, and verapamil, produce a worse outcome. If needed for treatment of hypertension, amlodipine and felodipine do not have negative inotropic actions, and appear safe when used in heart failure patients.

β-BLOCKERS

Studies conclusively support the concept that chronic β-blockade can improve cardiac function, decrease symptoms, and prolong survival *(19–21)* (Fig. 2; Table 2). The large survival studies have included patients with a wide-ranging severity of illness, and have demonstrated very consistent improvements in survival of more than 30%. They are very well tolerated, even in the sickest patients *(22,23)*. However, there are still many misconceptions about their actions and it is important to understand their proper use in patients with heart failure. If used incorrectly, there is no doubt that they can lead to exacerbations of heart failure and death. If used properly, they can have long-lasting benefit (Table 4).

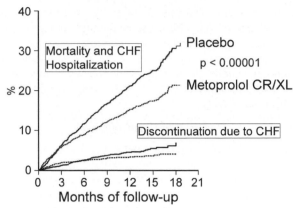

Fig. 2. Cumulative percentages for the combined endpoint of total mortality or heart failure hospitalization (time to first event) from MERIT-HF. Patients who received β-blockade had a 31% improvement in hospitalization and mortality rates and less frequent withdrawal from study the drug. (From ref. *40*. Copyright 2003, American Medical Association.)

β-Blockers should be given only to patients who are euvolemic, optimally treated with other medications, and stable. These agents are properly initiated with slow titration. They are started at minuscule doses (hence the misconception that low-dose β-blockade is given), but the evidence suggests that the final dose should be higher. Indeed, the Metoprolol, CR/XL Randomized Intervention Trial (MERIT) trial gave a final daily dose of 200 mg of metoprolol XL to patients, while initiating treatment with either 12.5 or 25 mg and doubling the dose at weekly or biweekly intervals. Similarly, the carvedilol and bisoprolol studies started treatment with extremely low doses and slowly titrated to effective β-blocking doses.

The titration of β-blocking agents should be performed cautiously and carefully. With each increase in dose, patients must be evaluated to ensure safety. For approximately the first month, one is not looking for a positive effect. Rather, the physician is acting to prevent deterioration. Fluid retention may occur, and increased diuretic doses may be temporarily needed. If there is clinical deterioration and evidence of worsening cardiac function, the usual weekly or biweekly titration should be lengthened. Bradycardia or heart block may limit dosing in some patients and pacemaker placement may be considered.

If the patient deteriorates with initiation of β-blockade, the dose may have to be decreased. Slower titration can be considered for patients with an initial adverse effect. These caveats refer to all β-blockers, including carvedilol, metoprolol, and bisoprolol, used in patients with heart failure.

The consequences of the differences among β-blockers are controversial. There have been theoretical concerns about beta selectivity, other vasodilatory properties, and even antioxidant effects. Carvedilol, in particular, has vasodilating properties that may be beneficial (for initiation) or harmful (if hypotension is a problem). One study reported improved survival with carvedilol 25 mg bid as compared to short acting metoprolol at 50 mg bid *(24)*. However, there are questions about using the unproven short-acting metoprolol (at a relatively low dose) in this study. The only drugs that have been proven to be beneficial are bisoprolol, long-acting metoprolol succinate, and carvedilol. It seems reasonable to use these drugs when possible (financial considerations might lead to the use of short-acting metoprolol when that is the only option). While it may be possible that one drug has more of an effect than another, it is clearly far more important to make sure that patients receive β-blockade at a proven dose than to worry about which drug to give.

DIGOXIN

The frequency of the use of digoxin varies from nation to nation because of conflicting data as to its efficacy. However, the consequences of using digoxin were recently clarified by the Digitalis

Table 4
Initiation of β-Blockade in CHF

Stabilize patient with:
    Diuretics
    Maximize ACE inhibition
    Digoxin
Evaluate
    Euvolemic
    No bradycardia without pacemaker
    No heart block without pacemaker
Step 1

Carvedilol	3.125 mg bid
Metoprolol XL	12.5 mg qd (can start with step 2 in NYHA class II)
Metoprolol	6.25 mg bid (can start with step 2 in NYHA class II)
Bisoprolol	1.25 mg qd

Step 2

Carvedilol	6.25 mg bid
Metoprolol XL	25 mg qd
Metoprolol	12.5 mg bid
Bisoprolol	2.5 mg qd

Step 3

Carvedilol	12.5 mg bid
Metoprolol XL	50 mg qd
Metoprolol	25 mg bid
Bisoprolol	3.75 mg qd

Step 4

Carvedilol	25 mg bid
Metoprolol XL	100 mg qd
Metoprolol	50 mg bid
Bisoprolol	5 mg qd

Step 5

Carvedilol	If weight >85 kg: 50 mg bid
Metoprolol XL	150 mg qd (can skip to step 6 if very stable)
Metoprolol	75 mg bid
Bisoprolol	7.5 mg qd

Step 6

Metoprolol XL	200 mg qd
Metoprolol	100 mg bid
Bisoprolol	10 mg qd

Cautions:
Between steps (every 1–2 wk):
    If no increased CHF symptoms and no increased weight, proceed to next step.
    If no increased symptoms but increased fluid weight, increase diuretics and check patient in 1 wk. When
        back to baseline, proceed to next step.
    If increased symptoms and weight, increase diuretics and check patient in 1 wk. When back to baseline,
        proceed to next step.
    If slight increase in symptoms and no weight gain, make no change and check patient in 1 wk. When
        back to baseline, proceed to next step.
    If marked increase in symptoms, stop drug.
    If symptomatic bradycardia, decrease dose of β-blocker.
    If heart block, decrease dose of β-blocker.

Doses are based on clinical CHF experience with each drug.

Investigation Group (DIG) in a Veterans Administration study of 6800 patients with an ejection fraction less than 45% *(25)*. There was no effect on mortality in this study, with identical survival curves seen in patients receiving digoxin and those receiving placebo.

Despite the lack of an effect on mortality, the use of digoxin in DIG decreased the hospitalization rate by 6% and the rate of hospitalizations for heart failure by 28%. This improvement is consistent with previous studies that showed that patients withdrawn from digoxin had more exacerbations of heart failure *(26)*. The use of digoxin to improve symptoms therefore appears appropriate. Furthermore, as opposed to other positive inotropic agents, digoxin can be given for symptom relief without concern that it will have long-term adverse effects. There are some questions about differences in response between men and women, but these may be related to differences in serum concentration.

The narrow therapeutic window of digoxin unfortunately leads to frequent toxicity. For example, worsening renal function might lead to digoxin accumulation in a patient who has tolerated a particular dose without any problem. The result might be bradyarrhythmias, tachyarrhythmias, nausea, or visual disturbances. One reason for the high prevalence of digoxin toxicity is the lack of correlation between serum concentration and toxicity. Adverse effects of digoxin occur at different concentrations in different individuals, often within the "therapeutic range." This obviously decreases the utility of following the serum digoxin concentration.

Obtaining routine digoxin concentrations is also not indicated because of a lack of a clear optimal concentration. Furthermore, it is not even known whether high or low concentrations are preferable. Numerous studies demonstrate that low digoxin concentrations exert beneficial neurohormonal actions. The chronic symptomatic benefit observed with digoxin might be secondary to these effects rather than the positive inotropic effects which occur at higher "therapeutic" concentrations. For this reason, the dose for patients with heart failure and normal renal function and without atrial fibrillation is usually 0.125 mg daily.

While elevated serum digoxin concentrations can support the diagnosis of digoxin toxicity, the routine monitoring of the concentration is expensive and not necessary. It appears wiser to treat patients with doses unlikely to cause toxicity and to check concentrations only when there is a clinical question.

POSITIVE INOTROPES

Chronic Use

There are no controlled studies supporting the use of positive inotropes for the chronic treatment of congestive heart failure. Although anecdotal uncontrolled studies suggest that intermittent use of dobutamine or milrinone may be beneficial, controlled studies are lacking or are negative. Furthermore, trials of oral inotropes, such as milrinone *(27)* and vesnarinone *(28)*, have demonstrated increased mortality, especially in the sickest patients. While inotropic therapy is beneficial acutely for patients with decompensated heart failure, its chronic use cannot be justified except in very rare patients with absolutely no other alternative.

The analogy with β-blockers strongly supports the conclusion that inotropic therapy should be used only acutely. Just as β-blockers initially have adverse consequences, it is not surprising that catecholamines (such as dobutamine) and phosphodiesterase inhibitors (such as milrinone) may be useful acutely to improve symptoms, increase renal perfusion (and diuresis), and permit time for other treatments to be effective. However, the long-term improvement in contractility and survival seen with beta-blockers suggests that chronic inotropic therapy will lead to decreased contractility, more rapid progression of the disease, and increased mortality. The studies of oral inotropes confirm this conclusion.

At present, the use of chronic or intermittent infusion therapy of positive inotropes is inappropriate and not supported by data. It is conceivable that these agents are suitable for occasional patients who are willing to accept long-term risks because of the inability of any other intervention to improve debilitating symptoms. Chronic therapy with inotropic drugs should only be used if both the doctor and patient understand that refractory symptoms might be treated at the cost of more rapid progression of the disease.

SUDDEN DEATH

Despite recent improvements in treatment of congestive heart failure, the mortality rate of these patients remains high. Unexpected deaths in patients who appear to be doing well are frequently targeted as tragic and preventable. Although these deaths are frequently assumed to reflect primary ventricular arrhythmias, other causes, such as pulmonary embolus, ischemia, and infarction, undoubtedly also contribute to mortality. Furthermore, bradyarrhythmias may be the cause of a substantial number of electrical deaths (29). Nevertheless, ventricular arrhythmias are often seen in patients with congestive heart failure and clearly cause sudden death in some patients. This has led to a search for treatments to prevent arrhythmic deaths.

Amiodarone

The adverse consequences of conventional antiarrhythmic agents have led to a marked decrease in their use. When an antiarrhythmic is needed for atrial or symptomatic ventricular arrhythmias, amiodarone is the most commonly prescribed agent. It is clearly an excellent drug for the treatment of atrial arrhythmias, and is increasingly used as the safest and most reliable antiarrhythmic for the maintenance of sinus rhythm in patients with heart failure.

While amiodarone may be used to prevent ventricular arrhythmias and sudden death, controlled studies have not been as positive as once hoped. Two large, randomized, and high-quality studies came to opposite conclusions about amiodarone. The Grupo de Estudio de la Sobrevida en la Insuficiencia Cardiaca en Argentina (GESICA) study found a 28% reduction in mortality (30) while the Veterans Administration-sponsored Survival Trial of Antiarrhythmic Therapy in Congestive Heart Failure (CHF-STAT) found a trend toward worse survival (31). There have been many attempts to explain the conflicting results, but the reasons remain uncertain. However, with the Sudden Cardiac Death in Heart Failure Trial (SCD-HeFT) showing no benefit of amiodarone, it should not be used routinely (32).

The side effects of amiodarone can be clinically important, difficult to diagnose, and a possible (partial) explanation of the worse outcome seen in some studies. Particularly problematic is pulmonary toxicity, both acute and chronic. This may go undiagnosed in patients with heart failure who complain of dyspnea, with devastating results. Pulmonary function tests should be followed at least yearly in patients placed on amiodarone and the diagnosis of pulmonary toxicity should be considered in any patient with worsening symptoms. The physician must also remember to search for other side effects, such as thyroid and dermatologic abnormalities.

Implantable Defibrillators

There are increasing data supporting the use of implantable defibrillators in patients with heart failure. The data are strongest for patients with ischemic heart disease, previous infarction, and a low ejection fraction. Ideally, identification of patients at high risk, in whom defibrillators will prolong life, not dying, will permit cost-effective use of this technology. The Sudden Cardiac Death in Heart Failure Trial (SCD-HeFT) showed that both ischemic and nonischemic patients with an ejection fraction less than 35% benefit when given defibrillators (32).

ANTICOAGULATION

Warfarin

The use of warfarin, aspirin, and other antiplatelet agents in patients with heart failure has been debated. Clots can form in large poorly contracting ventricles, and there is concern that these clots may embolize, causing cerebrovascular accidents. Unfortunately, the use of anticoagulants in heart failure patients is supported only by retrospective studies. These studies, while suggesting that anticoagulation might be beneficial, are limited by the realistic concern that patients who are prescribed anticoagulants in uncontrolled reports are healthier. This would then explain their better outcome. Controlled studies have not shown benefit.

Since the side effects of warfarin are not negligible, many physicians are very concerned about prescribing an agent that might cause harm when the benefit is not clear. At present, there are no accepted recommendations regarding anticoagulation in patients with poor cardiac function and normal sinus rhythm.

There are other groups of patients in whom anticoagulation is clearly indicated. Patients with atrial fibrillation and cardiac disease, for example, experience decreased events when prescribed effective therapeutic doses of warfarin (33). Since atrial fibrillation patients with congestive heart failure are at particularly high risk of embolism, they should be given warfarin unless strong contra-indications exist. The warfarin dose should be adjusted so that the International Normalized Ratio (INR) remains between 2.0 and 3.0.

Aspirin

Even more problematic is the use of aspirin in patients with heart failure. The benefits of aspirin in ischemic heart disease are well documented, and many patients with heart failure receive these agents following myocardial infarctions and other ischemic episodes.

There are suggestions, however, that aspirin might negate some of the beneficial effects of ACE inhibitors. Aspirin can decrease kidney function in heart failure patients in whom renal perfusion may be dependent on prostaglandins. Other adverse hemodynamic actions can occur because of vasoconstriction. Aspirin also inhibits bradykinin production, antagonizing the effects of ACE inhibitors on bradykinin. The impact of bradykinin in patients with heart failure (and whether it contributes to the beneficial actions of ACE inhibitors) is not known. Thus, whether the actions of aspirin are detrimental in patients with heart failure or patients receiving ACE inhibitors are uncertain.

It is possible that clopidogrel or ticlopidine will prove to have useful antiplatelet actions without adversely affecting prostaglandins or bradykinin. However, such benefit remains theoretical and the cost of these agents mandates proof prior to their widespread use. Until such a study is completed, patients with a clear indication for aspirin should be placed on aspirin. Theoretical concerns cannot overpower the known marked benefit in patients with previous bypass surgery or myocardial infarction. However, the prophylactic use of aspirin in patients with heart failure but without known ischemic heart disease is inappropriate.

TRANSPLANTATION

Cardiac transplantation is now a routine and accepted option for patients with severe heart failure refractory to medical therapy (Table 5). One-year survival in many programs approaches 90%, far superior to the expected prognosis in patients with severe disease. Furthermore, patients can symptomatically improve, returning to work and functioning independently.

The clinical outcome of patients who survive transplantation suggests important clinical benefit (34). Four fifths of patients who survive the initial hospitalization have no activity limitations at 1 yr. Considering that these patients were generally New York Heart Association class III and IV prior to transplant, this is a dramatic benefit. These same patients continue to be impacted by their disease, however; only 27% have returned to work full-time.

The reason for low employment rates are many, but can be explained in large part by complications of the transplant. Despite improving survival rates, the risks of transplantation remain considerable, with rejection and infectious complications most worrisome for the first year, and coronary artery disease and neoplasms becoming more prevalent with time. Indeed, 42% of patients who survive the initial hospitalization are rehospitalized in the first year. Furthermore, important chronic diseases, such as renal failure, hypertension, and diabetes, commonly develop. It is not easy for a patient to undergo a cardiac transplantation.

Considering both the risks and the limited availability of hearts for transplantation, patients with both a very poor prognosis and severe symptoms should be selected for transplantation. While any

Table 5
Indications for Transplantation

Definite
1. Volume of oxygen use <10 mL/kg/min
2. NYHA class IV
3. History of recurrent hospitalization for congestive heart failure
4. Refractory ischemia with inoperable coronary artery disease and left ventricular ejection fraction <20%
5. Recurrent symptomatic ventricular arrhythmias
Probable
1. Volume of oxygen use <14 mL/kg/min
2. NYHA class III–IV
3. Recent hospitalizations for congestive heart failure
4. Recurrent "high-grade" VEA with family history of sudden death
5. Unstable angina not amenable to coronary artery bypass grafting, percutaneous transluminal coronary angioplasty with left ventricular ejection fraction <30%
Inadequate
1. Volume of oxygen use >14 mL/kg/min
2. NYHA class I–II
3. Left ventricular ejection fraction <20%
4. Stable, exertional angina with left ventricular ejection fraction >20%.

Adapted from ref. 35.

patient with congestive heart failure is at increased risk of dying, the severity of the disease is directly related to the risk of mortality. For this reason, mortality benefits can be assumed only in the sickest patients. Since a low ejection fraction itself does not portend a particularly poor prognosis, patients with minimal symptoms may not experience an improved chance of survival when transplanted.

It is apparent that only patients with severe symptoms can improve their quality of life with a cardiac transplant. With the morbidity associated with transplantation, some assurance that the patient will benefit is mandatory. Partially for this reason, it is common to objectively evaluate symptoms by performing an exercise test with metabolic monitoring. Peak oxygen consumption gives an excellent documentation of limitation of activity; with low peak oxygen consumption (below approx 14 mL/kg/min) indicating marked limitation of function. When evaluating a patient with heart failure, the physician must also remember that deconditioning can lead to continued symptoms of dyspnea and fatigue. Differentiation of symptoms of heart failure and deconditioning can be extremely difficult, and often only time will make the diagnosis evident.

One needs to continually assess patients with heart failure. Patients who have substantially improved need to be removed from transplant lists, and patients who initially appeared too healthy may have deteriorated. While it may be psychologically difficult to inform a patient that a transplant is no longer needed, transplanting a heart into a healthy patient is of no benefit to anyone.

It is also unwise to transplant patients with a high risk of complications from the procedure (35). Patients with end organ damage, such as fixed pulmonary hypertension, hepatic failure, renal failure, and peripheral vascular disease, are at high risk. Similarly, because brief episodes of noncompliance can have devastating effects, patients without the social support and ability to carefully follow medical regimens should not be transplanted. Transplantation is miraculous for some patients, but can cause irrevocable harm if used inappropriately.

MECHANICAL INTERVENTIONS

Left Ventricular Assist Devices (Fig. 3)

A mechanical heart substitute that could be permanently implanted (as destination therapy) would be an ideal solution for patients with end-stage heart disease; the small supply of hearts available

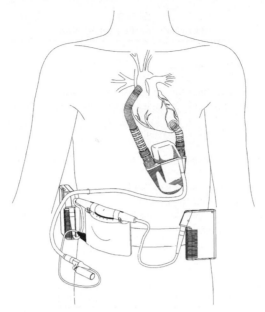

Fig. 3. The placement of the inflow and outflow cannulae, the pumping chamber, and the external controls in a wearable left ventricular assist device. (Adapted from ref. *41*.)

for transplantation and the complications inherent with immunosuppression severely limit the number of patients who can benefit from transplantation. Recent advances in technology, including thrombosis prevention and miniaturization, have brought the possibility of widespread use of ventricular-assist devices closer to reality. Indeed, in an extremely high-risk patient population, the outcome of patients who received left ventricular assist devices (LVADs) as destination therapy was better than those who received optimal medical care *(36)*. However, the complication rate remains high and the benefit is proven only with patients likely to die imminently.

LVADs are placed with an outflow conduit sewn into the apex of the left ventricle after removal of an adequate-size plug. The inflow conduit is then placed into the ascending aorta and the LVAD implanted in the abdomen outside the peritoneum. Ventricular assist devices can permit end-organ perfusion in patients whose own hearts are unable to perform adequately.

At present, most assist devices have been placed as a bridge to transplantation. First used in hospitals, patients can now be sent home until a transplant becomes available. With the long waiting lists for transplantation and the consequent prolonged time that even very ill hospitalized patients experience before receiving hearts, mechanical support has become essential as a means of maintaining life until a transplant is available. Furthermore, the normal cardiac output provided by the device can reverse chronic problems (such as organ failure, anorexia, and muscular weakness) and improve the outcome of transplant surgery when it is ultimately performed.

Ultimately, it is possible that these devices will be alternatives to transplantation rather than mere bridges. In some patients they provide the opportunity for cardiac remodeling, and after enough time might be able to be removed. In a larger number of patients unable to receive a transplant because of medical reasons or the small number available, however, their permanent use would be life-saving. At present, only the sickest patients receive LVADs as permanent destination therapy.

Mitral Valve Repair

Patients with severe heart failure often have marked mitral regurgitation, caused by annular dilation. The regurgitation can severely exacerbate the underlying problem, causing increased pulmonary pressures and decreased forward flow. If a patient can tolerate the operation, the benefits of surgically decreasing backward flow are obvious.

Such surgery was previously felt to be too high-risk in patients with left ventricular dysfunction. Indeed, because the ejection fraction can be markedly increased by mitral regurgitation, the true extent of myocardial dysfunction is difficult to assess in patients with mitral regurgitation, and patients with extremely poor myocardial function have increased risk of not surviving the surgery or not substantially improving their cardiac performance. However, a few surgeons are now reporting excellent outcomes by correcting mitral regurgitation with mitral annuloplasty, even in patients with severe congestive heart failure and left ventricular dysfunction *(37)*. The factors that portend a better outcome with this surgery need to be understood before accepting the role of mitral annuloplasty in patients with severe heart failure.

Resynchronization

The idea that the nature of the wave of contraction of each beat might affect cardiac efficiency and output prompted investigation of techniques to initiate contraction more physiologically in heart failure patients with prolonged QRS duration. Large-scale studies suggest that at least some patients may benefit *(38)*. While difficulty in blinding such studies and surrogate endpoints have left it unclear which patients will benefit, the data suggest that patients with very prolonged QRS durations are more likely to benefit. At present, therefore, symptomatic patients with QRS durations greater than 140 ms are generally considered the best candidates for resynchronization (biventricular pacing). Usually, resynchronization is considered in combination with implantable defibrillators. One study, Comparison of Medical Therapy, Pacing and Defibrillation in Heart Failure (COMPANION) looked at the impact of both defibrillators and resynchronization in a mortality study. Resynchronization improved survival, and most physicians believe that this is additive to the effects of a defibrillator.

NURSING INTERVENTIONS

One of the most important interventions that can be used to treat patients with heart failure is close follow-up and treatment of problems before major decompensations. This is the philosophy behind many nursing interventions being used. Managed care has realized that the prevention of hospitalization by close follow-up can both save money and make patients feel better.

The optimal means of close follow-up is not known. Many studies report the benefit of combined interventions: frequent nursing visits, ready access to knowledgeable physicians, education, diet modification, and social work help are often tried in combination *(39)*. Close follow-up with frequent home nursing visits, transtelephonic monitoring, and heart failure clinics have all been tried and appear to be successful (usually in uncontrolled trials). Personnel used have ranged from qualified nurses with heart failure expertise to lesser-trained individuals asking a few scripted key questions.

However it is done, addressing fluid overload before it leads to pulmonary edema and ensuring that patients are prescribed medications proven to be beneficial (and are taking these medications) will prevent heart failure exacerbations and hospitalizations. Expenditures on outpatient care will inevitably lead to lower overall costs.

EXERCISE

Exercise intolerance is often the result of decreased muscular tone, the result of deconditioning, anorexia, and malnutrition. While decreased cardiac output and increased ventricular and pulmonary pressures initially limit exercise in patients with heart failure, improvement in cardiac performance does not lead to immediate return of normal capabilities. Indeed, the old philosophy that patients with heart failure should not exercise led to the inability of medically treated patients to improve their functional status. Presently, it is clear that steady exercise will improve muscular (and perhaps vascular) function, leading to a better quality of life.

Many studies have shown that formalized exercise programs lead to increased oxygen consumption and exercise tolerance. Unfortunately, the applicability of these reports is suspect. Motivated young patients are often studied, and compliance of sicker and elderly patients may be different.

Furthermore, it is unclear if the cost associated with these programs is necessary. Formal cardiac programs with monitoring instill confidence, but are expensive. In addition, it has never been demonstrated that they improve the safety of exercising.

Another unanswered question is whether exercise must be aerobic. Traditionally, isometric exercise was said to be prohibited for heart failure patients. Physicians were concerned that the increased afterload induced by the exercise would be detrimental. However, this has not been tested. At present, one must conclude that aerobic exercise should be encouraged in whatever setting is possible.

METABOLIC INTERVENTIONS

Coenzyme Q_{10}

The hypotheses behind the use of coenzyme Q_{10} in patients with congestive heart failure are varied. It is reputedly an antioxidant, with supplementation preventing lipid peroxidation. Perhaps more interesting is its role in the electron transfer within the respiratory chain, with the potential to affect oxidative phosphorylation. It has captured the imagination of many patients and, despite is expense, is being used widely.

However, there are few controlled trials, and those that do exist have had conflicting results. The studies are small, however, and it is possible that there are groups of patients who benefit. At the present time, the risks of using coenzyme Q_{10} appear few, but its benefit is questionable. Physicians and patients should be aware that the high doses that have been used in the trials are expensive for such an unproven therapy.

Nutrition

Functional capacity is dependent on the nutritional status of patients, with cachexia reflective of increased mortality and morbidity. For example, patients with lower muscle mass have a worse functional capacity. However, whether cachexia causes the poor outcome or merely reflects the severity of disease is not clear. A number of investigational approaches are addressing this issue by attempting to improve nutrition and prevent the effects of cachexia.

The simplest means of improving nutrition would be to provide supplements. Good nutrition should be encouraged in all patients, but there is no evidence that this can have a major impact in patients with heart failure. Other interventions, such as anabolic hormones, are therefore being investigated. Growth hormone and other anabolic steroids could theoretically improve both cardiac and peripheral muscular function. Another approach to improve nutritional status would be to prevent cachexia. Since cytokines, such as tumor necrosis factor-α (TNF-α), can cause anorexia as well as other potential adverse effects, their antagonism might improve nutrition. However, studies of TNF-binding proteins have not improved outcome. While the importance of nutrition is clear, it is not clear whether addressing it as a primary problem will improve the status of patients with heart failure.

CONCLUSION (TABLE 6)

The treatment of congestive heart failure demands close follow-up, attention to detail, and listening to the patient. Fortunately, careful studies have guided us to effective treatment of these patients, and the questions that remain can and must also be addressed in ways leading to evidence-based medicine. Physicians should learn from these studies, treating patients with medicines proven to be effective at doses that are appropriate. The treatments can affect symptoms or mortality, but the physician should understand the impact of any treatment on both.

REFERENCES

1. Maisel AS, Krishnaswamy P, Nowak RM, et al. Measurement of B-type natriuretic peptide in the emergency diagnosis of heart failure. N Engl J Med 2002;347:161–167.
2. Channer KS, McLean KA, Lawson-Matthew P, Richardson M. Combination diuretic treatment in severe heart failure: a randomized controlled trial. Br Heart J 1994;71:146–150.

Table 6
Routine Treatment of CHF in 2004

Proven therapy:	
ACE inhibitors	Lisinopril 20–40 mg, captopril 25–50 mg tid, enalapril 10–40 mg bid, or equivalent
Diuretics	Furosemide as needed, or other diuretics
β-blockers	Metoprolol XL, carvedilol, or bisoprolol
Spironolactone	25 mg
May be beneficial in select patients:	
Digoxin	0.125–0.25 mg
ARBs	
Warfarin	
Amiodarone	
Aspirin	
Resynchronization	
ICD	

All the above should be considered for all patients with heart failure.

3. Pitt B, Zannad F, Remme WJ, et al. The effect of spironolactone on morbidity and mortality in patients with severe heart failure. N Engl J Med 1999;341:709–717.
4. Cuffe MS, Califf RM, Adams KF Jr, et al. Short-term intravenous milrinone for acute exacerbation of chronic heart failure: a randomized controlled trial. JAMA 2002;287:1541–1547.
5. Vargo DL, Brater DC, Rudy DW, Swan SK. Dopamine does not enhance furosemide-indiced natriuresis in patients with congestive heart failure. J Am Soc Nephrol 1996;7:1032–1037.
6. Colucci WS, Elkayam U, Horton DP, et al. Intravenous nesiritide, a natriuretic peptide, in the treatment of decompensated congestive heart failure. N Engl J Med 2000;343:246–253.
7. Wang DJ, Dowling TC, Meadows D, et al. Nesiritide does not improve renal function in patients with chronic heart failure and worsening serum creatinine. Circulation 2004;110:1620–1625.
8. L'Abbate A, Emdin M, Piacenti M, et al. Ultrafiltration: a rational treatment for heart failure. Cardiology 1989;76: 384–390.
9. Hricik DE. Captopril-induced renal insufficiency and the role of sodium balance. Ann Int Med 1985;103:222–223.
10. The SOLVD Investigators. Effect of enalapril on survival in patients with reduced left ventricular ejection fractions and congestive heart failure. N Engl J Med 1991;325:293–302.
11. The CONSENSUS Trial Study Group. Effects of enalapril on mortality in severe congestive heart failure: results of the Cooperative North Scandanavian Enalapril Survival Study (CONSENSUS). N Engl J Med 1987;316:1429–1434.
12. Gottlieb SS, Robinson S, Weir MR, et al. Determinants of the renal response to ACE inhibition in patients with congestive heart failure. Am Heart J 1992;124:131–136.
13. Granger CB, McMurray JJV, Yusuf S, et al. Effects of candesartan in patients with chronic heart failure and reduced left ventricular systolic function and intolerant to ACE inhibitors: the CHARM-Alternative Trial. Lancet 2003;362: 772–776.
14. McMurray JJV, Östergren J, Swedberg K, et al. Effects of candesartan in patients with chronic heart failure and reduced left ventricular systolic function treated with an ACE inhibitor: the CHARM-Added trial. Lancet 2003;362: 767–771.
15. Pfeffer MA, McMurray JJV, Velazquez EJ, et al. Valsartan, captopril, or both in myocardial infarction complicated by heart failure, left ventricular dysfunction, or both. N Engl J Med 2003;349:1893–1906.
16. Cohn JN, Archibald DG, Ziesche S, et al. Effect of vasodilator therapy on mortality in chronic congestive heart failure. Results of a Veterans Administration Cooperative Study. N Engl J Med 1986;314:1547–1552.
17. Cohn JN, Johnson G, Ziesche S, et al. A comparison of enalapril with hydralazine-isosorbide dinitrate in the treatment of chronic congestive heart failure. N Engl J Med 1991;325:303–310.
18. Taylor AL, Ziesche S, Yancy C, et al. Combination of isosorbide dinitrate and hydralazine in blacks with heart failure. N Engl J Med 2004;351:2049–2057.
19. CIBIS II Investigators and Committees. The cardiac insufficiency bisoprolol study II (CIBIS-II): a randomized trial. Lancet 1999;353:9–13.
20. MERIT-HF Study Group. Effect of metoprolol CR/XL in chronic heart failure: metoprolol CR/XL Randomized Intervention Trial in Congestive Heart Failure (MERIT-HF). Lancet 1999;353:2001–2007.
21. Packer M, Fowler MB, Roecker EB, et al. Effect of carvedilol on the morbidity of patients with severe chronic heart failure: results of the carvedilol prospective randomized cumulative survival (COPERNICUS) study. Circulation 2002;106:2194–2199.
22. Gottlieb SS, Fisher ML, Kjekshus J, et al. Tolerability of beta-blocker initiation and titration in the Metoprolol CR/XL Randomized Intervention Trial in Congestive Heart Failure (MERIT-HF). Circulation 2002;105:1182–1188.

23. Krum H, Roecker EB, Mohacsi P, et al. Effects of initiating carvedilol in patients with severe chronic heart failure: results from the COPERNICUS Study. JAMA 2003;289:712–718.

24. Poole-Wilson PA, Swedberg K, Cleland JG, et al. Comparison of carvedilol and metoprolol on clinical outcomes in patients with chronic heart failure in the Carvedilol or Metoprolol European Trial (COMET): randomised controlled trial. Lancet 2003;362:7–13.

25. The Digitalis Investigation Group. The effect of digoxin on mortality and morbidity in patients with heart failure. N Engl J Med 1997;336:525–533.

26. Packer M, Gheorghiade M, Young JB, et al. Withdrawal of digoxin from patients with chronic heart failure treated with angiotensin-converting-enzyme inhibitors. RADIANCE Study N Engl J Med 1993;329:1–7.

27. Packer M, Carver JR, Rodeheffer RJ, et al. Effect of oral milrinone on mortality in severe chronic heart failure. N Engl J Med 1991;325:1468–1475.

28. Cohn JN, Goldstein SO, Greenberg BH, et al. A dose-dependent increase in mortality with vesnarinone among patients with severe heart failure. Vesnarinone Trial Investigators. N Engl J Med 1998;339:1810–1816.

29. Luu M, Stevenson W, Stevenson L, et al. Diverse mechanisms of unexpected cardiac arrest in advanced heart failure. Circulation 1989;80:1675–1680.

30. Doval HC, Nul DR, Grancelli HO, et al. Randomised trial of low-dose amiodarone in severe congestive heart failure. Grupo de Estudio de la Sobrevida en la Insuficiencia Cardiaca en Argentina (GESICA). Lancet 1994;344:493–498.

31. Singh SN, Fletcher RD, Fisher SG, et al. Amiodarone in patients with congestive heart failure abd asymptomatic ventricular arrhythmia: Survival Trial of Antiarrhythmic Therapy in Congestive Heart Failure. N Engl J Med 1995; 333:77–82.

32. Bardy GH, Lee KL, Mark DB, et al. Amiodarone or an implantable defibrillator for congestive heart failure. N Engl J Med 2005;352:225–237.

33. Adjusted-dose warfarin versus low-intensity, fixed-dose warfarin plus aspirin for high-risk patients with atrial fibrillation: Stroke Prevention in Atrial Fibrillation III randomised clinical trial. Lancet 1996;348:633–638.

34. Brann WB, Bennett LE, Keck BM, Hosenpud JD. Morbidity, functional status, and immunosuppressive therapy after heart transplantation: an analysis of the Joint International Society for Heart and Lung Transplantation/United Network for Organ Sharing Thoracic Registry. J Heart Lung Transplant 1998;17:374–382.

35. Miller LW, Kubo SH, Young JB, et al. Report of the Consensus Conference on Candidate Selection for Heart Transplantation—1993. J Heart Lung Transplant 1995;14:562–571.

36. Rose EA, Gelijns AC, Moskowitz AJ, et al. Long-term use of a left ventricular assist device for end-stage heart failure. N Engl J Med 2001;345:1435–1443.

37. Bach DS, Bolling SF. Improvement following correction of secondary mitral regurgitation in end-stage cardiomyopathy with mitral annuloplasty. Am J Cardiol 1996;78:966–969.

38. Abraham WT, Fisher WG, Smith AL, et al. Cardiac resynchronization in chronic heart failure. N Engl J Med 2002; 346:1845–1853.

39. Rich MW Beckham V, Wittenberg C, et al. A multidisciplinary intervention to prevent the readmission of elderly patients with congestive heart failure. N Engl J Med 1995;333:1190–1195.

40. Hjalmarson Å, Goldstein S, Fagerberg B, et al. Effects of controlled-release metoprolol on total mortality, hospitalizations, and well-being in patients with heart failure: the Metoprolol CR/XL Randomized Intervention Trial in Congestive Heart Failure (MERIT-HF). JAMA 2003;283:1295–1302.

41. Hirsch DJ, Cooper JR. Cardiac failure and left ventricular assist devices. Anesthesiol Clin N Am 2003;21:625–638.

42. The SOLVD Investigators. Effect of enalapril on mortality and the development of heart failure in asymptomatic patients with reduced left ventricular ejection fractions. N Engl J Med 1992;327:685–691.

43. Cohn JN, Ziesche S, Smith R, et al. Effect of the calcium antagonist felodipine as supplementary vasodilator therapy in patients with chronic heart failure treated treated with enalapril: V-HeFT III. Circulation 1997;96:856–863.

44. Pfeffer MA, Swedberg K, Granger CB, et al. Effects of candesartan on mortality and morbidity in patients with chronic heart failure: the CHARM-Overall programme. Lancet 2003;362:759–766.

45. Gottlieb SS. Diuretics. In: Hosepud JD, Greenberg B, eds. Congestive Heart Failure, 2nd ed. Pathophysiology, Differential Diagnosis, and Comprehensive Approach to Management. Lippincott Williams & Wilkins, 2000, pp. 421–433.

RECOMMENDED READING

Hunt SA, Baker DW, Chin MH, et al. ACC/AHA Guidelines for the evaluation and management of chronic heart failure in the adult: executive summary. A report of the American College of Cardiology/American Heart Association Task Force on Practice Guidelines. Circulation 2001;104:2996–3007.

VI CONGENITAL HEART DISEASE

21 Congenital Heart Disease

Julien I. E. Hoffman, MD

INTRODUCTION

Major chromosomal abnormalities account for 5 to 8% of congenital heart disease (CHD). A few congenital anomalies are due to teratogens such as alcohol, lithium, or retinoic acid, or to single gene defects. Most, however, are due to the interplay of genetic abnormalities with environmental factors or chance.

At birth, about 3% of infants have a tiny muscular ventricular septal defect (VSD); these usually close spontaneously by 1 yr of age and pose few clinical problems. Another 1% have a bicuspid but not stenotic aortic valve that seldom causes problems in childhood, but may calcify or degenerate later in life. About 1% of live-born children have various classical types of CHD: left-to-right shunts in 60 to 70%, obstructive lesions in about 15 to 20%, and 20 to 25% with right-to left shunts and cyanosis *(1)*. A fourth smaller group has congenital lesions of the coronary arterial origins (Table 1).

Not all these patients reach adult life, despite improved treatment available today. Even those with successful repair may have late complications that need medical attention. Details of survival at different ages and thus the numbers who survive to adulthood are given by Hoffman et al *(2)*.

LEFT-TO-RIGHT SHUNT LESIONS

Pretricuspid Shunts

Left-to-right shunting occurs across an atrial septal defect (ASD) or through anomalous pulmonary veins when the right ventricle becomes more distensible than the left ventricle a few weeks after birth. When pulmonary blood flow is more than twice systemic blood flow, the right atrium and ventricle are enlarged and hyperactive, with prominent pulsation over the lower left sternal border, and cardiomegaly and increased pulmonary arterial markings on chest X-ray. No murmur occurs across the atrial defect, but the large pulmonary blood flow causes a moderately loud systolic pulmonic ejection murmur; a tricuspid mid-diastolic rumble may also be heard. In large adults with thick chests these physical signs may be absent. Pulmonary arterial pressures are usually normal, so pulmonic closure is soft. However, there is always a wide fixed split-second heart sound. In ostium primum (partial AVSD) defects there may also be a murmur of mitral incompetence and sometimes of a small VSD.

Children with a secundum ASD or partial anomalous pulmonary veins are usually asymptomatic, and form one of the largest groups of patients with untreated CHD seen in adult clinics. If a large atrial shunt is not closed, the patients may develop congestive heart failure or pulmonary vascular disease, usually after 20 yr of age *(3)*. Late-onset mitral incompetence can occur, as can thrombosis of large pulmonary arteries. These patients often have severe atrial arrhythmias, and some have strokes from paradoxical embolism. Therefore any patient with a large shunt (one with right ventricular dilation) needs prophylactic closure by surgery or catheter-inserted closure devices.

From: *Essential Cardiology: Principles and Practice, 2nd Ed.*
Edited by: C. Rosendorff © Humana Press Inc., Totowa, NJ

Table 1
Incidence of Congenital Heart Disease

| Lesion | Incidence per million live births (% of all CHD) | | Relative frequency in adults |
	Median (%)	75th percentile (%)	
A. Left-to-right shunts			
1. Pretricuspid			
Atrial septal defect	564 (7)	1059 (10)	Common
Atrioventricular septal defect (partial)	84 (1)		Uncommon
Partial anomalous pulmonary venous connection	?		Rare
2. Postricuspid			
Ventricular septal defect	2829 (37)	4482 (42)	Common
Patent ductus arteriosus	567 (7)	782 (7)	Common
Atrioventricular septal defect (complete)	242 (3)	340 (3)	Rare
B. Pure obstructive lesions			
Pulmonic stenosis	532 (7)	836 (8)	Common
Aortic stenosis	256 (3)	388 (4)	Common
Coarctation of the aorta	356 (5)	492 (5)	Common
C. Right-to-left shunts (cyanotic)			
Transposition of the great arteries	303 (4)	388 (4)	Rare
Tetralogy of Fallot	356 (5)	577 (5)	Rare+
Persistent truncus arteriosus	94 (1)	136 (1)	Rare
Hypoplastic left heart (aortic, mitral atresia)	226 (3)	279 (3)	Very Rare
Hypoplastic right heart (tricuspid, pulmonary atresia)	160 (2)	224 (2)	Rare
Double-inlet left ventricle (single ventricle)	85 (1)	136 (1)	Rare+
Double-outlet right ventricle	127 (2)	245 (2)	Rare
Total anomalous pulmonary venous connection	91 (1)	120 (1)	Rare
D. Coronary artery anomalies			
Left main coronary artery from pulmonary artery			Rare
Left main coronary artery from right sinus of Valsalva			Rare
Right main coronary artery from left sinus of Valsalva			Rare
All CHD	7669	10567	
Bicuspid nonstenotic aortic valves	9244	13817	

Median and 75th percentile incidence from ref. *1*.
Excludes miscellaneous lesions, and combinations of several lesions.
Figures in parentheses are percentages of the lesions shown in the table.
Rare+: rare in adults but seen more often than are other rare forms of congenital heart disease.

A patient with a small ASD is at risk only from paradoxical embolism. Catheter closure may become the recommended treatment for this.

Patients with a partial AVSD usually develop severe arrhythmias or congestive heart failure in early adult life, and need surgical repair that has low operative mortality and fairly good long-term results. Late reoperations for mitral valve repair or subaortic stenosis may be needed.

Posttricuspid Shunts

GENERAL PATHOPHYSIOLOGY

The degree of shunting and its effect on heart and lungs depend on the size of the defect between the two circulations and the pulmonary vascular resistance. A small VSD or patent ductus arteriosus (PDA) <3 mm in diameter has only a small left-to-right shunt. The patient has no symptoms. Apart from the distinctive murmur, the heart and lungs are normal on clinical, radiological, and electrocardiographic examination. Echocardiography confirms the small shunt, normal right ventricular and pulmonary arterial systolic pressures, and normal chamber sizes.

A large defect has a large left-to-right shunt once pulmonary vascular resistance decreases, and right ventricular and pulmonary arterial systolic pressures are systemic. With complete atrioventricular septal defect (AVSDc), also termed endocardial cushion defect or common atrioventricular canal, because of the associated left-to-right atrial shunt there is often a mid-diastolic rumble at the tricuspid valve as well, and the second heart sound has a wide fixed split characteristic of an atrial septal defect. Severe congestive heart failure in early infancy is the rule with these large lesions, and without surgical treatment these patients either die or develop pulmonary vascular disease.

Intermediate-sized defects give moderate left-to-right shunts and pulmonary arterial systolic pressures less than half systemic levels. Symptoms vary from mild fatigue and dyspnea on exertion to moderate congestive heart failure. The left ventricle is moderately hyperactive, dilated, and hypertrophied. The right ventricle not dilated in a PDA because the shunt does not pass through the right ventricle, but is hyperactive and moderately dilated in the VSD or AVSDc because the shunt goes from left to right ventricle; it is forceful and moderately hypertrophied in all these lesions. The second heart sound may be loud, and there may be a soft mid-diastolic murmur at the apex. Pulmonary vascular markings are moderately increased.

If pulmonary vascular resistance is high, there is a small or even no left-to-right shunt, no matter how large the defect; there may even be right-to-left shunting. The left ventricle is normal, but the right ventricle has a forceful lift due to right ventricular systolic hypertension. Pulmonic closure is very loud, and there may be an early systolic ejection click. In early diastole there may be a high-pitched blowing murmur of pulmonic incompetence along the left sternal border (Graham Steell murmur). The chest X-ray shows a rounded and enlarged right ventricle, and large central pulmonary arteries with sparse narrow peripheral arteries ("tree in winter" appearance). The electrocardiogram shows pure right ventricular hypertrophy. The site of the defect is shown by echocardiography.

These features are common to all post-tricuspid shunts. Each lesion, however, has distinctive differences.

Ventricular Septal Defect

After infancy, 85% of VSDs are perimembranous (in the region of the membranous septum below the aortic and tricuspid valves), and another 5 to 10% are in the muscular septum; at both sites, spontaneous closure is common. A few inlet VSDs under the tricuspid valve are always large, never close spontaneously, and need surgical closure early in infancy. Others in the outflow tract below the pulmonary valves are called *supracristal* or doubly committed subarterial defects. These defects leave the aortic valve cusp (noncoronary or sometimes right coronary cusp) unsupported; the cusp prolapses into the defect and partly occludes it so that the left-to-right shunt is small even if the VSD is large. Progressive prolapse of the valve cusp is the rule, and aortic insufficiency follows; the cusp may be damaged and need replacement. This site for the VSD occurs in about 5% of Caucasians and African-Americans, but in about 35% of Chinese and Japanese. Because of the risk of aortic valve damage, it is essential to locate the site of the defect by careful echocardiography in every patient with a VSD.

A tiny VSD, <2 mm diameter, has a soft, high-pitched systolic murmur localized to the lower left sternal border. A small or medium-sized VSD has a typical harsh loud systolic murmur, usually pansystolic, obscuring the first heart sound, and heard best at the left lower sternal border. It may be heard at the upper left sternal border with an outflow tract VSD, but this sign is not reliable. The size of the VSD and the amount of shunting must be judged not on the murmur but on the activity of the heart and precordium. With a large VSD and a high pulmonary vascular resistance, the systolic murmur becomes soft and short because there is little left-to-right shunt across a large defect, and a right-to-left shunt across the VSD causes little or no murmur.

Because 70 to 80% of VSDs close spontaneously, initial treatment is conservative. Small defects need only prophylaxis against infective endocarditis. Larger symptomatic defects usually respond to digoxin, diuretics, afterload reduction, and maintaining normal hemoglobin concentration. The few who fail therapy have surgical closure of the VSD with very low operative mortality and excellent outcome. Often at about 1 yr of age the patients improve clinically. This change may be due either to decrease in VSD size or else early pulmonary vascular disease, and is a reason for concern and investigation. A few patients have large shunts and low pulmonary arterial pressures, with no or minimal symptoms. If they do not close their defects spontaneously in a few years, the VSD should be closed surgically to preserve optimal ventricular function.

PATENT DUCTUS ARTERIOSUS

There is a continuous "machinery" or "train in a tunnel" murmur heard best below the left clavicle. The size of the PDA and the amount of shunting are diagnosed not from the murmur but from associated features: a big ductus has a loud second heart sound, bounding pulses, and left ventricular dilation and hypertrophy on clinical, radiological, electrocardiographic, and echocardiographic examination. The defects are closed to prevent heart failure and pulmonary vascular disease with big shunts, and infective endocarditis with small shunts. Defects less than 5 mm in diameter are closed at cardiac catheterization by coils or other devices, or sometimes by thoracoscopic procedures. Large defects are closed surgically by open thoracotomy but occasionally by catheter-introduced devices. Outcome after surgery is essentially normal.

COMPLETE ATRIOVENTRICULAR SEPTAL DEFECT

These patients have huge volume loads early in life, and develop congestive heart failure and pulmonary vascular disease by a few months after birth. Survival without surgery is short. Surgery involves closing the atrial and ventricular defects, and repairing the cleft atrioventricular valves. Late valve problems and even reoperation are relatively common, and complete atrioventricular block may occur.

PULMONARY VASCULAR DISEASE

Any large left-to-right shunt (alone, or plus a right-to-left shunt) may cause pulmonary vascular disease. With a high pulmonary arterial pressure, small pulmonary arteries thicken due to increased smooth medial muscle that extends farther down the vascular tree than is normal for children (4,5). The high pulmonary blood flow produces abnormal shear forces on the endothelial cells. A local elastase is activated and damages the internal elastic lamina of the small pulmonary arteries (6). Endothelial dysfunction causes aggregation of platelets and macrophages, with release of cytokines that enter the media and induce smooth muscle cells to transform into fibroblastlike cells and migrate into and thicken the intima, thus narrowing the lumen. These cells secrete a hyalinized, collagenlike material that eventually replaces them. Finally the small arteries become occluded. In addition, the growth of new pulmonary arteries after birth is inhibited, so that not only are the small arteries narrowed or occluded, but eventually there may also be as few as one third of the normal number.

These changes begin under 1 yr of age except in ASD, in which they are rare under 20 yr of age. Once the changes start, they are progressive, although surgical closure of the defect under 2 yr of age may prevent newly formed vessels from being damaged.

With progressive disease, pulmonary vascular resistance increases, and the left-to-right shunt decreases and finally becomes a right-to-left shunt (Eisenmenger's syndrome). At this stage closure of the defect is dangerous. Even if the patient survives surgery, the high fixed pulmonary vascular resistance limits increased flow out of the right ventricle with an increased venous return (as in exercise), so that acute right ventricular hypertension, heart failure, or fatal arrhythmias can occur. Furthermore, the increased right ventricular muscle mass demands a high myocardial blood flow, and any decrease in aortic pressure may cause acute right ventricular failure and arrhythmias. A few patients improve after an atrial opening is created, but for most only lung transplantation avails. These patients are cyanotic, but often do well until the third or fourth decades (7). Death is either sudden (presumably arrhythmic) or from congestive heart failure in the majority, but from hemoptysis or brain abscess in a few. Death during pregnancy is common (8,9).

OBSTRUCTIVE LESIONS

Valvar Pulmonic Stenosis

Most patients have moderate valvar pulmonic stenosis (PS) and are asymptomatic. They have varying degrees of right ventricular hypertrophy with a forceful lift at the left lower sternal border and typical changes in the electrocardiogram and chest X-ray. The pulmonic component of the second heart sound is soft and delayed (wide split second heart sound), but the split varies during respiration. At the upper left sternal border there is usually an early systolic ejection click that may vary with respiration and is due to post-stenotic dilation of the pulmonary artery. There is a characteristic harsh long ejection murmur. As the stenosis becomes more severe, the right ventricle takes longer to eject its stroke volume, splitting of the second heart sound widens, the murmur gets longer and its peak shifts toward the second sound, and the frequency of the murmur rises because a higher velocity of flow is needed for the normal stroke volume to flow through a narrower orifice. These changes give reliable estimates of severity that are confirmed by echocardiography. Sometimes secondary infundibular hypertrophy increases the obstruction. Those with substantial RVH can have the valve opened by balloon valvotomy, which is as effective as surgery and has replaced it unless the valve is dysplastic. Long-term results are excellent, except in a few adults with persistent ventricular dysfunction.

Valvar Aortic Stenosis

Most patients have mild or moderate valvar aortic stenosis when young, and are usually asymptomatic. They have an ejection murmur maximal anywhere between the apex and the upper right sternal border, and in the same region an early systolic ejection click that does not vary with respiration. The second heart sound is normal, but the first heart sound is soft with severe stenosis. Left ventricular hypertrophy may be palpable or shown on the electrocardiogram, but palpation, murmur, and the electrocardiogram are unreliable in diagnosing severity. Inversion of T waves in left chest leads with exercise predicts severity, but false negatives occur. The only effective noninvasive test is the echocardiogram, which should be done at least yearly; annual exercise testing may also be needed.

Balloon valvotomy is effective if there is not much aortic incompetence, and can be repeated easily. Unfortunately, the aortic valve is usually bicuspid or monocuspid, and recurrent obstruction is common. Eventually the valve may have to be replaced because of calcification or severe incompetence. Replacement is usually by an aortic homograft, sometimes by a mechanical valve, and with increasing frequency by the Ross procedure, in which the native pulmonary valve is moved to the aorta and a homograft is used in the pulmonary position. Early surgical results for all these are good, but fewer than 25% of patients will go for 25 yr without having repeat valvotomy, valve replacement, congestive heart failure, or infective endocarditis that is more common after than before valvotomy.

Bicuspid aortic valves without stenosis, the most common congenital heart lesion, may be asymptomatic for many decades, but are at risk of infective endocarditis. Most eventually calcify and become obstructive, often over 1 to 2 yr, or deteriorate and produce aortic incompetence.

Subaortic Stenosis

Occasionally just below the aortic valve there is a membranous, fibrous, or fibromuscular ring that is either isolated or associated with other lesions, especially a VSD. There may be aortic incompetence, perhaps due to valve damage from the high-velocity jet through the stenosis. Clinically these lesions resemble valvar aortic stenosis, and echocardiography is needed to distinguish them. Balloon valvotomy is less useful than in valvar stenosis, and surgical excision may be needed. Complete removal of the obstruction is difficult because the stenosis involves the septal leaflet of the mitral valve, and recurrences are common.

Supravalvar Aortic Stenosis

This is rare, and often associated with Williams' syndrome (infantile hypercalcemia, mental retardation, elfin facies). The stenosis may be localized or be long and diffuse; it can narrow coronary ostia. The features resemble those for valvar aortic stenosis, but with no ejection click. Frequently, systolic blood pressure is about 15 mmHg higher in the right than in the left arm because of the direction of the jet coming through the stenosis. When severe, surgical repair is indicated. Stenoses of other arteries may occur.

Coarctation of the Aorta

This is a localized narrowing of the aorta just beyond the left subclavian artery. Most patients are asymptomatic, although a few have congestive heart failure; intermittent leg claudication is rare. The main features are hypertension in the upper body with decreased pulses and pressures in the legs; diastolic pressures are often similar in arms and legs, but systolic pressures differ markedly. Most have palpable collateral arteries around the scapula. There is left ventricular hypertrophy clinically and on electrocardiogram, but no T-wave inversion. A systolic or continuous murmur is heard best in the mid-back, and sometimes there is a mid-diastolic rumble at the apex even though there is no mitral stenosis. On chest X-ray, the ascending aorta is dilated, as is the descending aorta below the constricted site of the coarctation; the hourglass pattern shows a "3" sign on plain X-ray. Confirmation by echocardiography should include demonstration of delayed acceleration of flow in the descending aorta by Doppler study. MRI shows the lesion well.

This lesion is frequently missed in childhood, and forms a large proportion of the patients with CHD seen by adult cardiologists. If untreated, patients die prematurely from consequences of hypertension: congestive heart failure, cerebral vascular accidents (especially subarachnoid hemorrhage), infective endocarditis, rupture of the aorta, or premature coronary artery disease) (10). Some experts treat the coarctation by balloon dilation and stenting, but others, concerned about the small risks of early aortic rupture or late aneurysm formation, resect the narrowed region surgically.

About 50% of these patients have a bicuspid aortic valve, and need prophylaxis against infective endocarditis even after successful repair of the coarctation. Even after adequate repair, systemic hypertension is common.

RIGHT-TO-LEFT SHUNTS (CYANOTIC HEART DISEASE)

The most common of these are transposition of the great arteries (d-TGA) and tetralogy of Fallot (with or without pulmonary atresia), each accounting for 4 to 5% of classical CHD. Others are double-outlet right ventricle (DORV), tricuspid atresia, pulmonary atresia with intact ventricular septum, truncus arteriosus, total anomalous pulmonary venous connection (TAPVC), single ventricle, hypoplastic left heart syndromes, and a collection of rarities. The relative frequency of these lesions is shown in Table 1, and the main ones are diagrammed in Fig. 1.

Principles of Treatment

Medical treatment is never curative. Most infants with serious congenital heart disease can have early "corrective" surgery within the first few weeks or months after birth. Waiting too long (more than 2 to 3 mo) in those with a large pulmonary blood flow risks severe pulmonary vascular disease.

For the few inoperable cyanotic patients, it is important to prevent iron-deficiency anemia that can lead to cerebral thrombosis because of the increased rigidity of iron-deficient red blood cells. On the other hand, if the hematocrit rises over 65%, the increased viscosity of blood not only predisposes to thromboses but also reduces oxygen delivery to tissues (11). Some patients need periodic phlebotomy with volume replaced by saline or albumin solution (12). Apart from being at risk for thromboses, these patients are at risk for brain abscess because not all bacteria in the blood stream are filtered in the lungs. Unexplained fever and headache, even without neurological signs, are indications for a CT scan of the head. Bleeding problems, especially nosebleeds, may follow thrombo-

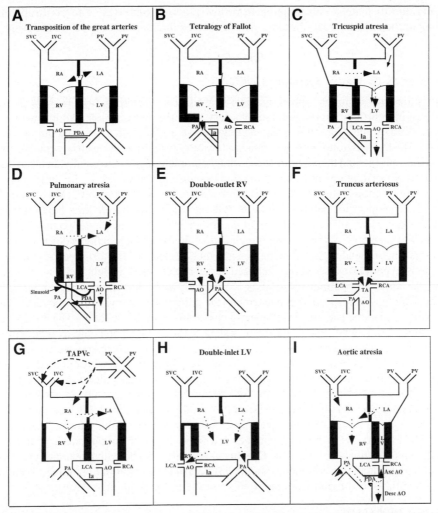

Fig. 1. Forms of cyanotic heart disease. (**A**) d-Transposition of the great arteries with small bidirectional atrial shunt and closing ductus arteriosus. (**B**) Tetralogy of Fallot, with severe infundibular pulmonary stenosis and small pulmonary annulus and arteries. The overriding aorta is shown. (**C**) Tricuspid atresia with small right ventricle. Small solid arrows show that pulmonary blood flow is lower than systemic flow (dotted arrows). These arrows do not indicate the saturations of the bloodstreams. (**D**) Pulmonary atresia with intact ventricular septum. Right ventricle is small but hypertrophied (due to suprasystemic systolic pressure). About half of these patients have sinusoids conducting blood from the right ventricle to coronary arteries. Pulmonary blood flow comes via the ductus arteriosus. (**E**) One form of double-outlet right ventricle (DORV) with pulmonary artery related to the VSD. Only one coronary artery is shown for clarity. (**F**) Truncus arteriosus, in which aorta, pulmonary arteries, and coronary arteries all come off a single great artery at the base of the heart. All have a VSD. (**G**) Total anomalous pulmonary venous connection, with all the pulmonary veins joining to form a single venous trunk that enters the heart via the superior vena cava, or inferior vena cava (usually via the portal vein), or the right atrium directly or via the coronary sinus. All systemic flow must pass from RA to LA through the foramen ovale. (**H**) The most common form of single ventricle, a double-inlet left ventricle. There is no true right ventricle, only a rudimentary outflow tract chamber that gets blood from the single ventricle through a bulboventricular foramen and conducts it to an l-transposed aorta. (**I**) Hypoplastic left heart with aortic atresia. The left ventricle is tiny or even absent. All systemic blood comes via the ductus arteriosus, including coronary arterial blood that flows retrograde through a very hypoplastic ascending aorta. Abbreviations: SVC, superior vena cava; IVC, inferior vena cava; PV, pulmonary veins; RA, LA, right and left atria; RV, LV, right and left ventricles; PA, pulmonary artery; AO, aorta; la, ligamentum arteriosum; RCA, LCA, right and left coronary arteries; PDA, patent ductus arteriosus; TA, truncus arteriosus; Asc AO, Desc AO, ascending and descending aorta.

cytopenia due to platelet consumption from low-grade thromboses or to erythropoietic over-crowding of the bone marrow. Precautions against bleeding may need to be taken during surgery.

Specific Lesions

TRANSPOSITION OF GREAT ARTERIES (D-TGA)

This is the most common type of cyanotic heart disease (Table 1). In d-TGA the aorta comes from the right ventricle and the pulmonary artery from the left ventricle. About two thirds have only a small PDA and a foramen ovale; the others have a VSD with or without pulmonic stenosis (Fig. 1A). The former group is treated immediately after birth by balloon atrial septostomy to open up the atrial septum, and then within 1 to 6 wk by complete repair. Originally an atrial baffle was placed to direct systemic venous blood to the left ventricle and thence to the lungs, and to direct the pulmonary venous return to the right ventricle and thence to the aorta (Mustard or Senning procedure). The operation had low mortality, but extensive atrial suture lines led to atrial arrhythmias, often severe atrial flutter or fibrillation, or damaged the sinus node, so that by 10 yr after surgery fewer than 50% of the patients were in sinus rhythm. Many patients developed right ventricular dysfunction and tricuspid incompetence that, because of the atrial baffle, caused pulmonary venous hypertension. Surgeons therefore began to treat these patients with an arterial switch. Moving the aorta and pulmonary arteries is relatively easy, but the coronary arteries must be detached from the aortic root and implanted into the pulmonic root (the new aortic root). This is not always easy, and some patients develop early or late myocardial ischemia. The 10–15-yr follow-up after the arterial switch shows excellent results, with an occasional supravalvar pulmonic or aortic stenosis at the suture line and with a few patients needing coronary artery bypass surgery.

Those with d-TGA and VSD have early congestive heart failure with minimal cyanosis, and develop irreversible pulmonary vascular disease unless pulmonary blood flow and pressure are lowered before 3 mo of age. They can be repaired with low risk by an arterial switch.

A few patients with d-TGA have a VSD and PS (usually subpulmonic). Because pulmonary flows and pressures are not high, patients get neither congestive heart failure nor pulmonary vascular disease. The PS may not be resectable and an arterial switch is unsuitable because these patients would then have "subaortic" stenosis. Options are an atrial baffle with closure of the VSD, or an intraventricular tunnel to lead blood from the left ventricle to the aorta, combined with an extracardiac conduit to lead blood from the right ventricle to the pulmonary artery.

TETRALOGY OF FALLOT

This has the best natural history of any cyanotic heart disease and is the most common form of untreated cyanotic heart disease seen in adult clinics. The abnormality includes a large VSD, right ventricular outflow tract obstruction from infundibular and sometimes valvar PS, an over-riding aorta, and right ventricular hypertrophy (Fig. 1B). The right ventricular outflow tract is narrowed, and sometimes the main obstruction is a small pulmonary annulus and small peripheral pulmonary arteries, often with peripheral stenoses. The severity of obstruction varies.

Definitive treatment is resecting the hypertrophied infundibular muscle, opening stenotic valvar commissures, cutting across and patching a small annulus, and closing the VSD; a preliminary palliative systemic artery–pulmonary shunt is seldom needed. Results of surgery are good but not perfect. A small residual VSD in 5 to 10% or mild residual stenosis is more a nuisance than a severe problem, and demands prophylaxis against infective endocarditis. However, many patients with annular patches have marked pulmonic incompetence, with resulting right ventricular dilation. When severe, or producing congestive heart failure, a homograft or prosthetic pulmonary valve needs to be inserted.

Some patients develop complete atrioventricular block after surgery, and then need a pacemaker. Of more concern are those with ventricular tachycardias and the occasional patient who suffers sudden death. Prediction of the risk of sudden death is poor; the best predictor is a QRS duration over 0.18 s plus marked pulmonic incompetence, but many without these abnormalities die suddenly. Prophylactic antiarrhythmic agents have not been useful.

One variant of tetralogy has pulmonary atresia. Pulmonary blood flow is initially maintained through a ductus arteriosus, but soon needs an aortopulmonary shunt for better flow. Later a conduit from RV to pulmonary artery replaces the shunt. The main problem is that the pulmonary arteries are usually small and may supply only part of the lungs, the remainder being supplied by large collaterals from the aorta. Often the surgeon can detach these collaterals from the aorta and anastomose them to the native pulmonary arteries, a procedure termed *unifocalization*. These collaterals often have stenoses, and postoperative balloon dilation with stent placement is often needed.

A second variant has an absent pulmonary valve, and these patients have a classical to-and-fro "sawing wood" murmur at the base. Because the infundibular stenosis is usually not severe, they are only mildly cyanotic. Some infants have massively dilated main and branch pulmonary arteries that obstruct airways and cause early death. Surgical repair involves closing the VSD, resecting the infundibular stenosis, and usually inserting a pulmonary valve.

TRICUSPID ATRESIA

Systemic venous return passes from right to left atrium across a foramen ovale and then into the left ventricle. In most patients blood then passes into the aorta and across a VSD into the hypoplastic right ventricle and to the lungs (Fig. 1C). There is usually a decreased pulmonary blood flow because of restriction to flow through the VSD, and often neonates depend on the ductus arteriosus for their main pulmonary blood flow. Even if the VSD is initially big, it may become smaller with time, or the patient may develop infundibular PS, so that the trend is for increasing cyanosis. The electrocardiogram shows a large right atrial P wave, short PR interval, and left superior axis QRS deviation, a chest X-ray has decreased pulmonary vascular markings and a small heart like an apple on a stalk, and the echocardiogram is definitive.

Treatment is initially to relieve severe hypoxemia by dilating the ductus arteriosus with PGE_1 to increase pulmonary blood flow and then doing a systemic-pulmonary shunt. Because this increases the already elevated left ventricular volume, it will eventually produce dilated cardiomyopathy. Therefore the shunt is closed and replaced with a bidirectional Glenn shunt (superior vena cava connected to both pulmonary arteries) at about 6 mo of age. At 2–4 yr of age, or later, the inferior vena caval return is directed to the pulmonary arteries, usually by an intra- or extraatrial conduit, so that all the systemic venous drainage bypasses the right ventricle and drains by gravity into the pulmonary vascular bed. This complete repair is termed the Fontan or Fontan–Kreuzer procedure. Because of gravity drainage, pulmonary vascular resistance must be low and left ventricular and mitral valve function must be normal. Similar repairs are done for a variety of cardiac lesions with only one ventricle: single ventricle, aortic, or mitral atresia and hypoplastic left ventricle, atrioventricular septal defect with a hypoplastic ventricle, and the like. This type of repair, in which only one pumping ventricle exists, is termed a single ventricle repair.

A few patients with tricuspid atresia have transposition of the great arteries; most left ventricular blood goes directly to the lungs, and aortic blood comes indirectly from the left ventricle via the VSD and the right ventricle. Early congestive heart failure with minimal cyanosis and pulmonary vascular disease are the rule. Banding the pulmonary artery under 3 mo of age protects the pulmonary vessels so that a Glenn shunt can be done a few months later.

Problems After Bidirectional Glenn and Fontan-Kreuzer Procedures. The bidirectional Glenn shunt improves saturation but there is still some cyanosis and possible problems from chronic cyanosis (*see* above). The shunt may be effective for many years, but eventually oxygen saturations decrease because, as children grow, a greater proportion of total venous return comes from the lower body and bypasses the lungs. A more serious problem is that some of these patients develop arteriovenous fistulae in the lungs, so that an increasing amount of pulmonary blood flow bypasses the alveoli. Shunting the IVC blood into the lungs causes regression of these fistulae, and cyanosis disappears. Even in the best Fontan-Kreuzer procedures, however, deterioration may occur after 10–20 yr, with atrial arrhythmias, progressive mitral valve incompetence, and the development of protein-losing enteropathy. At times, the only effective therapy for these problems may be cardiac transplantation.

Pulmonary Atresia With Intact Ventricular Septum

This is an extreme form of pulmonic stenosis, and all lung blood flow comes via the ductus arteriosus. The right ventricle is hypoplastic, despite suprasystemic systolic pressures, and there are often large sinusoids that go from RV to coronary arteries (Fig. 1D); at times, all the coronary flow comes from these sinusoids. Multiple coronary arterial stenoses develop. Treatment consists of valvotomy, an aortopulmonary shunt, or both. With sinusoid-dependent coronary blood flow, reduction of right ventricular pressure must be avoided. Sometimes a bidirectional Glenn followed by a Fontan-Kreuzer procedure is done, but the results are frequently poor.

Double-Outlet Right Ventricle

This is a group of lesions in which both great arteries arise from the right ventricle, and the obligatory VSD may be at various sites. If the aorta arises from the right ventricle near the VSD, the patient resembles one with a large VSD and is acyanotic. Treatment is by closing the VSD so that left ventricular blood passes into the aorta. If the VSD is below the pulmonary artery (Fig. 1E) or remote from both arteries, a variety of procedures can be done, depending on the anatomy. Sometimes a long intracardiac tunnel can be placed to connect the left ventricle to the aorta without obstructing the outflow from the right ventricle to the pulmonary artery. At other times, the VSD is closed so that the left ventricle ejects into the pulmonary artery, as in transposition of the great arteries, and an atrial baffle restores the direction of the circulation. In others, various forms of intracardiac tunnels and extracardiac conduits are placed.

Truncus Arteriosus

In this lesion, the base of the heart gives off a large arterial trunk from which the aorta, coronary arteries, and pulmonary arteries arise (Fig. 1F). There is a large VSD. These children have early and severe congestive heart failure, and may develop pulmonary vascular disease by 3 mo of age. Treatment is to remove the pulmonary arteries from the aorta, patch the resulting aortic hole, close the VSD, and put a conduit from the RV to the pulmonary arteries. Because the pulmonary arteries are big the conduit can be quite large, but will have to be replaced as the child grows, and several times thereafter.

Total Anomalous Pulmonary Venous Connection

Here the pulmonary veins join behind the heart to form a common pulmonary venous trunk that connects either to the SVC (supracardiac: 55%), the coronary sinus or right atrium (cardiac: 25%), or the portal vein (infracardiac: 20%) (Fig. 1G). There may be obstruction to the common pulmonary venous drainage in the supracardiac or cardiac types, but it always occurs in the infracardiac type. Those with obstructed drainage present soon after birth with intense cyanosis and pulmonary edema, and need early surgical repair; the left atrium is anastomosed to the common pulmonary vein. The procedure is usually successful, but some infants develop stenoses of the pulmonary veins that are difficult to treat. Those without obstruction behave like ASDs with a large shunt and minimal cyanosis. They often have congestive heart failure in the first year of life, and can develop pulmonary vascular disease if left untreated. Surgical repair at time of diagnosis is usually successful.

Single Ventricle

A group of lesions falls under this heading. Most common is the double-inlet single left ventricle from which the pulmonary artery arises (Fig. 1H). The aorta comes off a rudimentary right ventricle that receives blood through a bulboventricular foramen. There may or may not be PS. Without PS, early congestive heart failure develops, and early pulmonary arterial banding is needed to prevent pulmonary vascular disease and prepare the child for a staged single ventricle repair. With PS, there is often marked cyanosis, and a small systemic-pulmonary shunt is needed until the child is old enough to undergo a single ventricle repair. A few patients have only moderate PS and moderate cyanosis. These are seen quite often in adult clinics.

HYPOPLASTIC LEFT HEART SYNDROMES

These have a hypoplastic left ventricle, most commonly with aortic (± mitral) atresia (Fig. 1I). Flow to the aorta comes from the right ventricle via the pulmonary artery and ductus arteriosus. Without treatment, most die under 1 mo of age. Surgical treatment is by cardiac transplantation or the Norwood procedure, in which the diminutive ascending aorta is anastomosed to the main pulmonary artery, in effect creating a truncus arteriosus. The peripheral pulmonary arteries are disconnected from the main pulmonary artery and connected to the aorta or right ventricle by a conduit. A few months later, a staged single ventricle repair is carried out.

CORRECTED TRANSPOSITION OF THE GREAT ARTERIES (L-TGA)

Abnormal looping of the cardiac tube connects the right atrium to the mitral valve and anatomic left ventricle, and the latter to the pulmonary artery. The left atrium is connected by a tricuspid valve to the anatomic right ventricle that ejects blood into the aorta. The aorta is anterior and to the left, producing a characteristic straight segment at the left upper heart border on chest X-ray; hence the term l-TGA, where *l* refers to *levo*. Because both atrioventricular and ventriculo arterial connections are discordant, systemic venous blood enters the lungs and oxygenated blood enters the aorta; hence the term *physiologically corrected transposition*. Most patients have a VSD, many have PS as well, and impaired atrioventricular conduction is common; some have an Ebstein deformity of the tricuspid valve. They may present like patients with a simple VSD or a tetralogy of Fallot. The pulmonic stenosis is often due to accessory mitral valve tissue, and the RV outflow tract is posterior, so that surgical repair is difficult. Many of these patients with balanced shunts attend adult clinics. Characteristically they have a loud aortic second sound heard best at the upper left sternal border because of the abnormal aortic position, and their electrocardiograms show prominent Q waves in the right chest leads, leading often to the mistaken diagnosis of anterior myocardial infarction. About 2% of them develop complete atrioventricular block each year.

EBSTEIN ANOMALY

The septal leaflet of the tricuspid valve arises from the ventricular septum below the tricuspid annulus, so that part of the right ventricle is included in the right atrium. With deep displacement of the valve there is tricuspid incompetence and a right-to-left atrial shunt. These patients often have a gigantic right atrium on chest X-ray, and may have severe atrial arrhythmias. Those with mild lesions are asymptomatic, but when severe the lesion shortens life. Surgical procedures involve repair or replacement of the tricuspid valve, resection of the redundant part of the right atrium, and sometimes procedures to ablate arrhythmogenic foci.

Coronary Arterial Anomalies

Although rare, these are potentially fatal but treatable if diagnosed. There are many variations, but three are of the most importance *(13)*.

Anomalous Origin of Left Coronary Artery From Pulmonary Artery

The right coronary artery arises in the right sinus of Valsalva, but the left comes from the pulmonary artery. After birth, when pulmonary vascular resistance decreases, the left ventricle cannot be perfused from the low-pressure left coronary artery, but gets blood via collaterals from the right coronary artery. The low pulmonary arterial pressure diverts some of the collateral flow into the pulmonary artery (coronary steal). Perfusion of the left ventricle becomes inadequate, and an anterolateral infarction occurs after a few weeks of age. These patients usually present with congestive heart failure in infancy, but some are asymptomatic until adult life. If diagnosed as adults after investigation of ischemic symptoms or accidentally, they should be treated, because sudden death is frequent. Treatment is best done by surgical implantation of the anomalous artery into the aortic root.

Table 2
Types of CHD in Adults

Without prior surgery
1. Asymptomatic
   a. Potentially unimportant: small VSD, PDA, mild PS
   b. Potentially important: ASD, bicuspid aortic valve, coarctation of the aorta
2. Symptomatic (all serious)
   a. Moderately large left-to-right shunts in patients from underdeveloped countries
   b. Cyanotic heart disease: e.g., tetralogy of Fallot, single ventricle with PS, d-TGA with VSD and PS, Ebstein anomaly, tetralogy of Fallot with absent pulmonary valve.
   c. Eisenmenger's syndrome (pulmonary vascular disease)
With prior surgery
A. Potentially minor
   1. Small residual lesions: small VSD, minor PS, mild mitral, pulmonic, aortic or tricuspid incompetence
B. Potentially serious
   2. Major residual lesions, including marked pulmonic, aortic, and mitral incompetence, significant RV or LV outflow tract obstruction
   3. Prosthetic valves, conduits
   4. Single-ventricle repair: tricuspid atresia, single ventricle, aortic atresia
   5. Two-ventricle repair with systemic right ventricle: d-TGA with atrial baffle, l-TGA
   6. Coronary artery problems in those after an arterial switch for TGA

Anomalous Origin of Left Coronary Artery From Right Sinus of Valsalva

The left coronary artery may reach the left ventricle by passing through the ventricular septum, behind the aorta, anterior to the right ventricular outflow tract, or between the aorta and the main pulmonary artery. The last pathway often leads to sudden death. The subjects at risk are almost always adolescent athletes who may have warning episodes of ischemic pain, faintness, or syncope during or just after strenuous exercise; however, the first episode may be sudden death. Not only is the distal course of the artery abnormal, but also the artery may be acutely angulated at its origin and have a flap of tissue over the orifice; its proximal intramural course through the aortic wall may be narrowed. There are usually no distinguishing physical findings or electrocardiographic changes. Echocardiography may show the abnormal course of the artery, but false negatives occur. The safest diagnostic test is imaging by ultrafast CT or magnetic resonance imaging, although coronary angiography by experienced cardiologists is useful. If diagnosed, treatment by surgical implantation into the left sinus of Valsalva is curative.

Anomalous Origin of Right Coronary Artery From Left Sinus of Valsalva

These right coronary arteries usually run between the two great vessels, and also may have narrowing of their aortic intramural portion, acute angulation of the take off, and a flap over the ostium. Signs and symptoms and diagnosis are as described above. Surgical treatment to reimplant the artery is warranted.

PRESENTATION IN ADULT LIFE

Patients seen in adult clinics may be divided into those without and with previous surgery (Table 2). How do they differ from children with similar forms of CHD? Children with severe forms of CHD will either have been operated on in early life or will have died. If they become adults with minor lesions, whether or not they have had previous surgery, their outcomes are likely to be almost normal, and other than appropriate prophylaxis against infective endocarditis, including good dental hygiene, they need little specialized attention. Those with more major lesions have problems specific to those lesions, but there are certain problems that they all share.

Atrial arrhythmias become more frequent with age, particularly in those with a large right atrium (previous ASD, Ebstein anomaly) or with atrial surgery, e.g., atrial baffle in d-TGA. Atrial flutter and fibrillation are common, and restoration of sinus rhythm, if necessary with anticoagulation, may be necessary. It is difficult to prevent recurrences, and many medications or even surgical procedures may need to be explored.

Ventricular arrhythmias occur with previous ventriculotomy, or even just with chronic ventricular hypertrophy. These may be difficult to treat. Sudden death is assumed to be due to such arrhythmias, but we have little ability to prevent it other than to use an implantable defibrillator.

Chronic ventricular hypertrophy is associated with myocardial scarring and biochemical changes that add to the risks of surgery and often prevent the expected improvement after a volume or pressure load has been removed by surgery.

Infective endocarditis is rare after surgery in those with complete repairs and no residua, but in most lesions is low. Morris et al. observed a cumulative incidence of endocarditis of below 2.5% over 30 yr in most major treated forms of CHD (14). The notable exception was aortic stenosis, with a 30-yr cumulative risk of 20%.

Pregnancy is usually well tolerated after successful cardiac surgery or with mild or moderate lesions (9,15,16). Patients with severe obstructive lesions should have these treated before pregnancy, but some have needed emergency valvotomy during pregnancy. This can usually be done with balloon catheterization, avoiding surgery and anesthesia with their effects on the fetus. Cyanotic patients have reduced fertility. If they become pregnant the mothers are usually at little increased risk, but there is a higher-than-normal fetal mortality. Those at greatest risk during pregnancy are patients with pulmonary vascular disease; most series have found a high death rate in these mothers, so that avoidance of pregnancy and, if necessary, sterilization are recommended. Most women with CHD can take usual contraceptive measures, although estrogenic preparations with the risk of thrombosis are contraindicated for women with pulmonary vascular disease and after single ventricle repairs where thrombosis in the slow-flowing venous channels is a risk. Intrauterine devices, not popular today, should be avoided in those with artificial valves because of the risk of bacteremia and infective endocarditis.

Socioeconomic problems are important in adults with CHD. Employers often discriminate against them, especially if issues of health insurance are at stake. Even if they are not, employers may be unwilling to risk frequent absences or sick leave. Exercise for most of these subjects can be done at a level that they are comfortable with. Several recent publications give some guidance about the levels of exercise that can safely be undertaken (17,18).

Many of these subjects are denied life insurance, or can obtain it only with greatly increased premiums. Some insurance companies will give certain patients with adequately corrected defects or minor lesions life insurance with little increased premium. There are big differences between the policies of different companies, and it is worthwhile having the applicants explore several companies (19–21).

A more serious problem is health insurance. This problem varies with each country, but is most serious in the United States. Children are usually covered by some form of Medicare, Medicaid, or Children's Medical Services, but these may not cover them after childhood. Many people get their health insurance from their work, a problem alluded to above. Short of a comprehensive insurance plan, it is difficult to know what to do for many of these patients.

REFERENCES

1. Hoffman JIE, Kaplan S. The incidence of congenital heart disease. J Am Coll Cardiol 2002;39:1890–1900.
2. Hoffman JIE, Kaplan S, Liberthson R. Prevalence of congenital heart disease. Am Heart J 2004;147:425–429.
3. Shah D, Azhar M, Oakley CM, et al. Natural history of secundum atrial septal defect in adults after medical or surgical treatment: historical prospective study. Br Heart J 1994;71:224–228.
4. Heath D, Edwards JE. The pathology of pulmonary hypertensive disease. A description of six grades of structural changes in the pulmonary artery with special reference to congenital cardiac septal defects. Circulation 1958;18: 533–547.

 5. Reid LM. Structure and function in pulmonary hypertension. New perceptions. Chest 1986;89:279–288.
 6. Rabinovitch M. It all begins with EVE (endogenous vascular elastase). Isr J Med Sci 1996;30:803–808.
 7. Saha A, Balakrishnan KG, Jaiswal PK, et al. Prognosis for patients with Eisenmenger syndrome of various aetiology. Int J Cardiol 1994;45:199–207.
 8. Bitsch M, Johansen C, Wennevold A, et al. Eisenmenger's syndrome and pregnancy. Eur J Obst Gynec Rep Biol 1988;28:69–74.
 9. Perloff J, Koos B. Pregnancy and congenital heart disease: the mother and the fetus. In: Perloff J, Child J, eds. Congenital Heart Disease in Adults. W. B. Saunders, Philadelphia, 1998, pp. 144–164.
10. Reifenstein GH, Levine SA, Gross RE. Coarctation of the aorta. A review of 104 autopsied cases of the "adult type," 2 years of age or older. Am Heart J 1947;33:146–168.
11. Rosenthal A, Nathan DG, Marty AT, et al. Acute hemodynamic effects of red cell volume reduction in polycythemia of cyanotic congenital heart disease. Circulation 1970;42:297–308.
12. Perloff JK, Rosove MH, Sietsema KE, et al. Cyanotic heart disease: a multisystem disorder. In: Perloff JK, Child JS, eds. Congenital Heart Disease in Adults. W. B. Saunders, Philadelphia, 1998, pp. 199–226.
13. Hoffman JIE. Congenital anomalies of the coronary vessels and the aortic root. In: Emmanouilides GC, Allen HD, Riemenschneider TA, Gutgesell HP, eds. Moss and Adams Heart Disease in Infants, Children and Adolescents, Williams & Wilkins, Philadelphia, 1995, pp. 769–790.
14. Morris CD, Reller MD, Menashe VD. Thirty-year incidence of infective endocarditis after surgery for congenital heart defect. JAMA 1998;279:599–603.
15. Pitkin RM, Perloff JK, Koos BJ, et al. Pregnancy and congenital heart disease. Ann Int Med 1990;112:445–454.
16. Mendelson MA. Congenital heart disease and pregnancy. Clin Perinat 1997;24:467–482.
17. Mitchell JH, Haskell WL, Raven PB. Classification of sports. 26th Bethesda Conference. Recommendations for determining eligibility for competition in athletes with cardiovascular abnormalities. J Am Coll Cardiol 1994;24: 864–866.
18. Kaplan S, Perloff JK. Exercise and athletics before and after cardiac surgery or interventional catheterization. In: Perloff JK, Child JS, eds. Congenital Heart Disease in Adults. W. B. Saunders, Philadelphia, 1998, pp. 189–198.
19. Truesdell SC, Skorton DJ, Lauer RM. Life insurance for children with cardiovascular disease. Pediatrics 1986;77: 687–691.
20. Allen HD, Gersony WM, Taubert KA. Insurability of the adolescent and young adult with heart disease. Report from the fifth conference on insurability, October 3–4, 1991, Columbus, Ohio. Circulation 1992;86:703–710.
21. Celermajer DS, Deanfield JD. Employment and insurance for young adults with congenital heart disease. Br Heart J 1992;69:539–543.

RECOMMENDED READING

Perloff JK, Child JS. Congenital Heart Disease in Adults. W. B. Saunders Philadelphia, 1998.

Emmanouilides GC, Allen HD, Riemenschneider TA, Gutgesell HP. Moss and Adams' Heart Disease in Infants, Children and Adolescents. Williams & Wilkins, Baltimore, 1995 (2 vol.).

VII CORONARY ARTERY DISEASE

22 Pathogenesis of Atherosclerosis

Prediman K. Shah, MD

INTRODUCTION

Atherosclerotic vascular disease is the leading cause of death in the United States and much of the industrialized world and is rapidly gaining the same dubious distinction in the developing world *(1)*. Atherosclerosis involves the development of a plaque composed of variable amounts of connective tissue matrix (collagen, proteoglycans, glycoseaminoglycans), vascular smooth muscle cells, lipoproteins, calcium, inflammatory cells (chiefly monocyte-derived macrophages, T lymphocytes, and mast cells) and new blood vessels (neoangiogenesis). The precise etiology and pathogenesis of atherosclerosis are incompletely understood but an emerging paradigm suggests that atherosclerosis may reflect a chronic inflammatory response to vascular injury caused by a variety of agents that activate or injure endothelium, or promote lipoprotein infiltration, lipoprotein retention, and lipoprotein oxidation *(2)*.

SITES OF PREDILECTION FOR ATHEROSCLEROSIS

Atherosclerosis involves the aorta and the large and medium-sized elastic and muscular arteries of the heart, brain, kidneys, and extremities, predisposing such organs to ischemic injury. The sites of predilection for atherosclerosis (Table 1 and Fig. 1) appear to be characterized by increased influx and or prolonged retention of lipoproteins, evidence of endothelial activation with expression of leukocyte adhesion molecules, and low shear stress. Changes in flow alter the expression of genes that have elements in their promoter regions that respond to shear stress. For example, the genes for intercellular adhesion molecule 1, platelet-derived growth factor B chain, and tissue factor in endothelial cells have these elements, and their expression is increased by reduced shear stress *(2–4)*. Alterations in blood flow appear to be critical in determining which arterial sites are prone to developing lesions *(4)*. Specific arterial sites, such as branches, bifurcations, and curvatures, cause characteristic alterations in the flow of blood, including decreased shear stress and increased turbulence. Rolling and adherence of monocytes and T cells occur at these sites as a result of the upregulation of adhesion molecules on both the endothelium and the leukocytes. At these sites, specific molecules form on the endothelium that are responsible for the adherence, migration, and accumulation of monocytes and T cells. Such adhesion molecules, which act as receptors for glycoconjugates and integrins present on monocytes and T cells, include several selectins, intercellular adhesion molecules, and vascular-cell adhesion molecules *(2–4)*. Molecules associated with the migration of leukocytes across the endothelium, such as platelet-endothelial-cell adhesion molecules, act in conjunction with chemoattractant molecules generated by the endothelium, smooth muscle, and monocytes—such as monocyte chemotactic protein 1, osteopontin, and modified LDL—to attract monocytes and T cells into the artery *(2–4)*. Flow-mediated upregulation of various adhesion molecules and inflammatory genes is regulated through shear stress responsive elements that are present in the promoter regions of genes like ICAM-1, PDGF-B, and tissue factor *(2–5)*. Chemokines may be involved in the chemotaxis and accumulation of macrophages in fatty streaks *(6)*. Activation

From: *Essential Cardiology: Principles and Practice, 2nd Ed.*
Edited by: C. Rosendorff © Humana Press Inc., Totowa, NJ

Table 1
Key Steps in Atherogenesis

Endothelial injury with increased Infiltration of atherogenic lipoproteins at sites of low or oscillating
  shear stress
Subendothelial retention and modification of atherogenic lipoproteins (LDL/VLDL)
LDL oxidation, glycation, aggregation
Endothelial activation with increased mononuclear leukocyte (inflammatory cell) adhesion, chemotaxis,
  and subendothelial recruitment
Subendothelial inflammatory cell activation with lipid ingestion through monocyte scavenger receptor
  expression resulting in foam cell formation
Inflammatory cell (monocyte-macrophage) proliferation
Migration to intima and proliferation of medial/adventitial smooth muscle cells/myofibroblasts in response
  to growth factors released by activated monocytes with matrix production and formation of fibrous
  plaque and fibrous cap
Abluminal plaque growth with positive (outward) arterial adventitial remodeling preserving lumen size
  in early stages; later plaque growth or negative remodeling results in luminal narrowing
Neoangiogenesis due to angiogenic stimuli produced by macrophages and other arterial wall cells
  (VEGF, IL-8)
Plaque hemorrhage and expansion of lipid core
Death of foam cells by necrosis/apoptosis leading to necrotic lipid-core formation
Rupture of fibrous cap or endothelial erosion, exposure of thrombogenic substrate, and arterial thrombosis

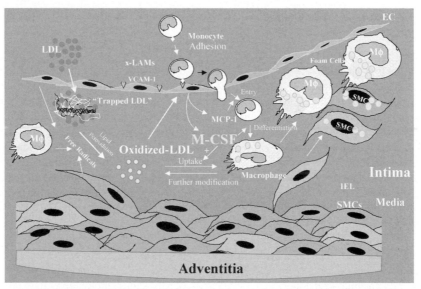

Fig. 1. This schematic describes the various postulated steps in the initiation and progression of an atherosclerotic plaque (*see* Table 1 and text for details). LDL, low-density lipoprotein; VCAM, vascular cell adhesion molecule; x LAMs, leukocyte adhesion molecules; M-CSF, macrophage colony-stimulating factor; MCP-1, monocyte chemotactic protein; Mϕ, monocyte-derived macrophages; EC, endothelial cell; SMC, smooth muscle cell; IEL, internal elastic lamina.

of monocytes and T cells leads to upregulation of receptors on their surfaces, such as the mucin-like molecules that bind selectins, integrins that bind adhesion molecules of the immunoglobulin superfamily, and receptors that bind chemoattractant molecules. These ligand-receptor interactions further activate mononuclear cells, induce cell proliferation, and help define and localize the inflammatory response at the sites of lesions.

Table 2
Endothelial Dysfunction in Atherosclerosis: Phenotypic Features

Reduced vasodilator and increased vasoconstrictor capacity
   Enhanced oxidant stress with increased inactivation of nitric oxide
   Increased expression of endothelin
Enhanced leukocyte (inflammatory cell) adhesion and recruitment
   Increased adhesion molecule expression (ICAM,VCAM)
   Increased chemotactic molecule expression (MCP-1,IL-8, osteopontin)
Increased prothrombotic and reduced fibrinolytic phenotype
   Increased tissue factor expression and reduced nitric oxide bioavailability
   Increased plasminogen activator inhibitor (PAI-1) expression
Increased growth-promoting phenotype
   Reduced nitric oxide bioavailability
   Increased endothelin expression

Table 3
Factors Contributing to Endothelial Dysfunction

Dyslipidemia and atherogenic lipoprotein modification
   Elevated LDL, VLDL, LP(a)
   LDL modification (oxidation, glycation)
   Reduced HDL
Increased oxidant stress
   Hypertension, excess angiotensin II, diabetes, smoking
Obesity and insulin resistance
Estrogen deficiency
Hyperhomocysteinemia
Advancing age
Genetic factors
Infections?

In genetically modified mice that are deficient in apolipoprotein E (and have hypercholesterolemia), intercellular adhesion molecule-1 (ICAM-1) is constitutively increased at lesion-prone sites long before the lesions develop *(4)*. In contrast, vascular-cell adhesion molecule 1 (VCAM-1) is absent in normal mice but is present at the same sites as ICAM-1 in mice with apolipoprotein E deficiency *(4)*. Mice that are completely deficient in ICAM-1, P-selectin, CD18, or combinations of these molecules have reduced atherosclerosis in response to lipid feeding. Proteolytic enzymes may cleave adhesion molecules such that in situations of chronic inflammation it may be possible to measure the "shed" molecules in plasma as markers of a sustained inflammatory response to help identify patients at risk for atherosclerosis or other inflammatory diseases *(2,7)*.

KEY ROLE OF ENDOTHELIAL ACTIVATION/DYSFUNCTION AND INJURY IN ATHEROGENESIS

Several studies have suggested that one of the earliest steps in atherogenesis is endothelial activation or injury/dysfunction with infiltration and retention of atherogenic lipoproteins (predominantly the apo B-containing lipoproteins) in the subendothelial space of the vessel wall (Tables 2 and 3) *(8)*.

Various factors that may contribute to endothelial activation or the development of endothelial injury/dysfunction predisposing to atherosclerosis include risk factors such as elevated and modified LDL /VLDL cholesterol; reduced HDL cholesterol, oxidant stress caused by cigarette smoking, hypertension, excess angiotensin II, obesity, insulin resistance, and diabetes mellitus; genetic alterations; elevated plasma homocysteine concentrations; infectious microorganisms such as herpesviruses or *Chlamydia pneumoniae*; and estrogen deficiency and advancing age *(9)*. Endothelial activation and injury/dysfunction may manifest in (1) increased adhesiveness of the endothelium to leukocytes or platelets; (2) increased permeability; (3) change from an anticoagulant to a procoagulant phenotype; (4) change from a vasodilator to a vasoconstrictor phenotype; or (5) change from a growth-inhibiting to a growth-promoting phenotype through elaboration of cytokines. Abnormal vasomotor function has been one of the most well-studied manifestations of endothelial dysfunction in subjects with either established atherosclerosis or risk factors for atherosclerosis. Normal healthy endothelium produces nitric oxide from arginine through the action of a family of enzymes known as nitric oxide synthases *(9)*. Nitric oxide acts as a local vasodilator by increasing smooth muscle cell cyclic GMP levels while at the same time inhibiting platelet aggregation and smooth muscle cell proliferation *(9)*. In the presence of risk factors, a reduced vasodilator response to endothelium-dependent vasodilator stimuli or even paradoxical vasoconstrictor response to such stimuli have been observed in large vessels as well as in the microcirculation, even in absence of structural abnormalities in the vessel wall *(9)*. These abnormal vasomotor responses have been attributed to reduced bioavailability of endothelium-derived relaxing factor(s), specifically nitric oxide, due to rapid inactivation of nitric oxide by oxidant stress or excess generation of asymmetric dimethylarginine and or increased production of vasoconstrictors such as endothelin *(9,10)*.

HYPERCHOLESTEROLEMIA AND MODIFIED LDL (FIG. 1)

One of the major contributors to endothelial injury is LDL cholesterol. When LDL is modified by processes such as oxidation, glycation (in diabetes), aggregation, association with proteoglycans, or incorporation into immune complexes, it is able to induce endothelial dysfunction *(11)*. Subendothelial retention of LDL particles results in progressive oxidation and its subsequent internalization by macrophages through the scavenger receptors *(11,12)*. The ability of apo B-containing atherogenic lipoproteins to be retained within the subendothelium is dependent on their ability to bind to the vascular proteoglycans. Thus transgenic mice expressing modified forms of LDL that are defective in their binding to proteoglycans have substantially less atherosclerosis despite comparable degress of hyperlipidemia compared to wild-type mice *(13)*. These findings support the concept of the "response to retention" hypothesis of atherosclerosis. The internalization of modified LDL leads to the formation of lipid peroxides and facilitates the accumulation of cholesterol esters, resulting in the formation of foam cells. The degree to which LDL is modified can vary greatly *(11)*. Once modified and taken up by macrophages, LDL activates the foam cells. In addition to its ability to injure these cells, modified LDL is chemotactic for other monocytes and can upregulate the expression of genes for macrophage colony-stimulating factor and monocyte chemotactic protein derived from endothelial cells *(11–14)*. Thus, it may help expand the inflammatory response by stimulating the replication of monocyte-derived macrophages and the entry of new monocytes into lesions. Oxidized LDL is present in lesions of atherosclerosis in animals and in humans *(11)*. In animal models of hypercholesterolemia, antioxidants can reduce the size of atherosclerotic lesions *(11)*. Antioxidants increase the resistance of human LDL to oxidation ex vivo in proportion to the vitamin E content of the plasma. Vitamin E intake is inversely correlated with the incidence of myocardial infarction, and vitamin E supplementation reduced coronary events in a preliminary clinical trial, whereas β-carotene produced no benefit *(15,16)*. More recent clinical trials have failed to show cardiovascular benefits of vitamin E supplements.

Continued inflammatory response stimulates migration and proliferation of smooth-muscle cells that accumulate within the areas of inflammation to form an intermediate fibroproliferative lesion resulting in thickening of the artery wall.

VASCULAR REMODELING IN ATHEROSCLEROSIS

Several experimental as well as clinical studies have demonstrated that progressive accumulation of plaque in the vessel wall can lead to progressive enlargement of the entire vessel through expansion of the adventitia (positive remodeling) that helps to minimize luminal narrowing *(17)*. Eventually failure of further remodeling in the face of continued plaque growth can result in luminal narrowing; alternatively, luminal narrowing may result from adventitial constriction or contraction (negative remodeling) *(17)*. Several studies have further shown that medial thinning, loss of external elastic lamina, and outward vessel remodeling are more common in ruptured plaques and that plaques associated with outward remodeling tend to have a higher lipid content and more inflammatory cell infiltration *(18,19)* (Table 1).

INFLAMMATORY AND IMMUNE RESPONSE IN ATHEROSCLEROSIS

The inflammatory and immune response in atherosclerosis (Table 1 and Fig. 1) consists of accumulation of monocyte-derived macrophages and specific subtypes of T lymphocytes at every stage of the disease *(20,21)*. The fatty streak, the earliest type of lesion, is common in infants and young children and consists of monocyte-derived macrophages and T lymphocytes *(20,21)*.

Continued inflammation results in increased numbers of macrophages and lymphocytes, which both emigrate from the blood and multiply within the lesion. Activation of these cells leads to the release of proteolytic enzymes, cytokines, chemokines, and growth factors, which can induce further damage and eventually lead to focal necrosis *(22)*. Necrosis and/or apoptosis of foam cells results in the formation of the necrotic lipid core in the plaque. Recent experimental observations have highlighted the potential role of free cholesterol accumulation in foam cells activating an endoplasmic reticulum-dependent macrophage apoptotic program that is inhibited by heterozygous Niemann–Pick type-C gene mutation *(23)*. Thus, cycles of accumulation of mononuclear cells, migration and proliferation of smooth-muscle cells, and formation of fibrous tissue lead to further enlargement and restructuring of the lesion, so that it becomes covered by a fibrous cap that overlies a core of lipid and necrotic tissue, resulting in the formation of an advanced and complicated plaque.

The inflammatory response can also influence lipoprotein transfer within the vessel wall. Inflammatory mediators such as tumor necrosis factor α, interleukin-1 (IL-1), and macrophage colony-stimulating factor (MCSF) increase binding of LDL to endothelium and smooth muscle and increase the transcription of the LDL-receptor gene *(2)*. After binding to scavenger receptors in vitro, modified LDL initiates a series of intracellular events that include the induction of proteases and inflammatory cytokines *(2)*. Thus, a vicious circle of inflammation, modification of lipoproteins, and further inflammation can be maintained in the artery by the presence of these lipids.

Monocyte-derived macrophages are present in various stages of atherogenesis and act as scavenging and antigen-presenting cells. They produce cytokines, chemokines, growth-regulating molecules, metalloproteinases, and other hydrolytic enzymes. The continuing entry, survival, and replication of monocytes/macrophages in lesions depend in part on growth factors such as MCSF and granulocyte-macrophage colony-stimulating factor (GM-CSF), whereas interleukin-2 is involved in a similar manner for T lymphocytes.

Activated macrophages as well as lesional smooth muscle cells express class II histocompatibility antigens, such as HLA-DR, that allow them to present antigens to T lymphocytes *(2,24)*. Atherosclerotic lesions contain both CD4 and CD8 T cells, implicating the immune system in atherogenesis *(2,24)*. T-cell activation following antigen processing results in production of various cytokines such as interferon-γ and tumor necrosis factor α and β, which can further enhance the inflammatory response *(2)*. Among the antigens presented include oxidized LDL and heat shock protein 60, which may participate in the immune response *(25)*.

Macrophages, T cells, and endothelial and smooth muscle cells in the atherosclerotic lesions express CD40 ligand and its receptor, which may play a role in atherogenesis by regulating the function of inflammatory cells *(26,27)*. The antiatherogenic effect of CD40-blocking antibodies. In the murine model of atherosclerosis suggests that CD40 may play an important role in atherogenesis *(26,27)*. Recent experimental observations have also highlighted the involvement of innate immune signaling receptors in atherosclerosis with the demonstration of Toll-like receptor (TLR) expression in murine and human plaques and the inhibitory effects of disruption of MyD88, an adaptor molecule involved in TLR-signaling, on atherosclerosis *(28)*.

Platelet adhesion and mural thrombosis are ubiquitous in the initiation and generation of the lesions of atherosclerosis in animals and humans *(2)*. Platelets can adhere to dysfunctional endothelium, exposed collagen, and macrophages. When activated, platelets release their granules, which contain cytokines and growth factors that, together with thrombin, may contribute to the migration and proliferation of smooth-muscle cells and monocytes *(29)*. Activation of platelets leads to the formation of free arachidonic acid, which can be transformed into prostaglandins such as thromboxane A2, one of the most potent vasoconstricting and platelet-aggregating substances known, or into leukotrienes, which can amplify the inflammatory response.

Angiotensin II, a potent vasoconstrictor, may also contribute to atherogenesis by stimulating the growth of smooth muscle, increasing oxidant stress, inducing LDL oxidation and a proinflammatory response *(2,30)*.

Elevated plasma homocysteine concentrations, resulting from enzymatic defects or vitamin deficiency, may also facilitate atherothrombosis by inducing endothelial dysfunction with a reduction in vasodilator capacity and enhanced prothrombotic phenotype and smooth muscle cell replication *(31)*. Hyperhomocysteinemia is associated with an increased risk of atherosclerosis of the coronary, peripheral, and cerebral arteries *(31)*. Trials are under way to determine whether reduction of plasma homocysteine levels by vitamins such as folic acid or vitamins B6 and B12 can reduce atherothrombotic events in humans *(32)*.

POTENTIAL ROLE OF INFECTION IN ATHEROTHROMBOSIS

Several recent reports have suggested that certain infectious organisms such as cytomegalovirus (CMV), *Chlamydia pneumoniae*, or *Helicobacter pylori* may contribute to inflammation, thereby contributing to atherogenesis and/or plaque disruption and thrombosis in presence of preexisting atherosclerosis *(33–39)*. Increased titers of antibodies to these organisms have been used as a predictors of further adverse events in patients who have had a myocardial infarction. Organisms, particularly *C. pneumoniae*, have been identified in atheromatous lesions in coronary arteries and in other organs obtained at autopsy. The case for *C. pneumoniae* is of particular interest since in both hypercholesterolemic rabbits as well as genetically hyperlipidemic mice, acceleration of atherosclerosis with *C. pneumoniae* infection has been demonstrated. In addition, pilot clinical trials of antichlamydial macrolide antibiotics have raised the intriguing possibility that such therapy may reduce the risk of recurrent coronary events *(34,38)*. In vitro studies have suggested that *C. pneumoniae* can trigger proatherogenic events such as foam cell formation, procoagulant activity, and metalloproteinase activity in monocytes, probably mediated by its heat-shock protein 60 (HSP60) *(33,35)*. Molecular antigenic mimicry between certain chlamydia antigens and myosin have also raised the additional possibility that such antigenic mimicry may also be involved in an immune-mediated vascular and myocardial injury *(39)*. Although there is no direct evidence that these organisms can cause the lesions of atherosclerosis, it is nevertheless possible that infection, combined with other risk factors, may contribute to atherogenesis or destabilization of preexisting atherosclerotic lesions in some patients. Recent large-scale clinical trials of antichlamydial antibiotic therapy have failed to demonstrate clinical benefit *(40,41)* (Tables 4 and 5).

ANGIOGENESIS IN ATHEROSCLEROSIS

Angiogenesis or neovascularization is an essential process that results from inflammation and in turn supports chronic inflammation and fibroproliferation, processes that are involved in atherogenesis (Table 1). Several studies have demonstrated increased neoangiogenesis in atherosclerotic lesions and hypercholesterolemia has been shown to increase adventitial neovascularity in porcine arteries before the development of an atherosclerotic lesion *(42)*. Proinflammatory chemokines such as IL-8 and other angiogenic growth factors such as vascular endothelial growth factor (VEGF) have been demonstrated in atherosclerotic lesions, where they may contribute to angiogenesis *(42)*. Increased adventitial and plaque neovascularity may also predispose to intraplaque hemorrhage, which could contribute to expansion of lipid core through incorporation of red cell membrane-derived cholesterol, thereby leading to rapid plaque progression *(43)*. Recent data show

Table 4
Potential Role of Infection
in Atherosclerosis and Thrombosis

Infectious organisms implicated
Viruses
Herpes virus
CMV
Bacteria
Chlamydia pneumoniae
Helicobacter pylori
Porphyromonas gingivalis?

Table 5
Mechanism(s) by Which Infections May Contribute to Atherothrombosis

Direct infection of the vascular wall with endothelial injury, inflammatory cell recruitment and activation
  (*Chlamydia pneumoniae*, herpesvirus, CMV)
Immune-mediated vascular injury through molecular mimicry (*C. pneumoniae*)
Remote infections with systemic activation of the inflammatory response (*Helicobacter pylori*,
  Porphyromonas gingivalis)

Table 6
Determinants of Vulnerability to Plaque Disruption

Large lipid core
Thin fibrous cap
Increased number and activity of inflammatory cells
Macrophages, T cells, mast cells
Reduced collagen and smooth muscle cell content
Increased neovascularity

increased atherosclerosis with administration of VEGF and an inhibitory effect of angiostatin in murine models of atherosclerosis suggests the potential proatherogenic role for angiogenesis *(44,45)*.

Plaque Instability/Vulnerability, Plaque Rupture, Plaque Erosion, and Thrombosis (Table 6 and Fig. 2)

Thrombosis complicating atherosclerosis is the mechanism by which atherosclerosis leads to acute ischemic syndromes of unstable angina, non-Q and Q wave myocardial infarction, and many cases of sudden cardiac death *(46,47)*. In most cases coronary thrombosis occurs as a result of uneven thinning and rupture of the fibrous cap, often at the shoulders of a lipid-rich lesion where macrophages enter, accumulate, and are activated and where apoptosis may occur *(46,47)*. Thinning of the fibrous cap may result from (1) elaboration of metalloproteinases (MMP) such as collagenases, gelatinases, elastases, and stromelysins *(46,47)*, which in turn may be stimulated by oxidized LDL, cell-to-cell interaction such as activated T cells, mast cell-derived proteases, oxidant radicals, or infectious agents *(46,47)*; or (2) increased smooth muscle cell death and reduced matrix production *(46,47)*. These changes may also be accompanied by the production of tissue-factor procoagulant and other hemostatic factors, further increasing the possibility of thrombosis *(46,47)*. Thrombosis may also occur on a proteoglycan-rich matrix without a large lipid core; in such cases, evidence of superficial endothelial erosion is found *(48)*. This plaque erosion may account for thrombosis in a relatively higher proportion of young victims of sudden death, particularly in women and smokers *(48)*. The precise molecular basis for these plaque erosions is not

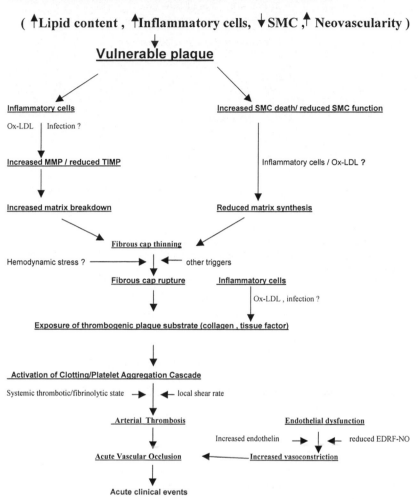

Fig. 2. This schematic describes the postulated key steps involved in plaque rupture and thrombosis.

clear although endothelial desquamation through activation of basement membrane-degrading MMP, increased circulating blood thrombogenicity, or endothelial cell apoptosis mediated local procoagualnt activity may be involved *(49).*

Plaques with a large lipid core, active inflammatory infiltration, and a thinned-out fibrous cap are therefore considered vulnerable or unstable plaques. Their identification may be particularly difficult because they may not produce symptoms because of lack of a flow-limiting stenosis and may thus escape detection by stress testing and even angiography *(46,47).* Macrophage accumulation may be associated with increased plasma concentrations of both fibrinogen and C-reactive protein (CRP), two markers of inflammation thought to be early signs of atherosclerosis *(50).* Elevated CRP levels have been shown to predict an increased risk of adverse cardiac events in patients with symptomatic vascular disease as well as in asymptomatic subjects at risk for vascular disease *(50).*

SUMMARY AND CONCLUSIONS

Atherosclerosis is a complex disease process that involves lipoprotein influx, lipoprotein modification, increased prooxidant stress, and inflammatory, angiogenic, and fibroproliferative responses intermingled with extracellular matrix and lipid accumulation resulting in the formation of an atherosclerotic plaque. Endothelial dysfunction is common in atherosclerosis and often manifests as a reduced vasodilator or enhanced vasoconstrictor phenotype, which contributes to luminal compromise. Thrombosis resulting from plaque rupture or superficial erosion complicates atherosclerosis, often resulting in abrupt luminal occlusion with resultant acute ischemic syndromes. Infectious agents may contribute to the inflammatory response and thus to destabilization of lesions. An improved understanding of the pathophysiology of atherosclerosis is providing novel directions for its prevention and treatment.

REFERENCES

1. Breslow JL. Cardiovascular disease burden increases, NIH funding decreases. Nat Med 1997;3:600–601.
2. Ross R. Atherosclerosis: an inflammatory disease. N Engl J Med 1999;340:115–126.
3. Nagel T, Resnick N, Atkinson WJ, et al. Shear stress selectively upregulates intercellular adhesion molecule-1 expression in cultured human vascular endothelial cells. J Clin Invest 1994;94:885–891.
4. Nakashima Y, Raines EW, Plump AS, et al. Upregulation of VCAM-1 and ICAM-1 at atherosclerosis-prone sites on the endothelium in the ApoE-deficient mouse. Arterioscler Thromb Vasc Biol 1998;18:842–851.
5. Springer TA, Cybulsky MI. Traffic signals on endothelium for leukocytes in health, Inflammation, and atherosclerosis. In: Fuster V, Ross R, Topol EJ, eds. Atherosclerosis and Coronary Artery Disease. Vol. 1. Lippincott-Raven, Philadelphia, 1996, pp. 511–538.
6. Boisvert WA, Santiago R, Curtiss LK, Terkeltaub RA. A leukocyte homologue of the IL-8 receptor CXCR-2 mediates the accumulation of macrophages in atherosclerotic lesions of LDL receptor-deficient mice. J Clin Invest 1998;101:353–363.
7. Hwang S-J, Ballantyne CM, Sharrett AR, et al. Circulating adhesion molecules VCAM-1, ICAM-1, and E-selectin in carotid atherosclerosis and incident coronary heart disease cases: the Atherosclerosis Risk in Communities (ARIC) study. Circulation 1997;96:4219–4225.
8. Napoli C, D'Armiento FP, Mancini FP, et al. Fatty streak formation occurs in human fetal aortas and is greatly enhanced by maternal hypercholesterolemia: intimal accumulation of low density lipoprotein and its oxidation precede monocyte recruitment into early atherosclerotic lesions. J Clin Invest 1997;100:2680–2690.
9. Kinlay S, Ganz P. Role of endothelial dysfunction in coronary artery disease and implications for therapy. Am J Cardiol 1997;80:111–161.
10. Lerman A, Edwards BS, Hallett JW, et al. Circulating and tissue endothelin immunoreactivity in advanced atherocslerosis. N Engl J Med 1991;325:997–1001.
11. Steinberg D. Low density lipoprotein oxidation and its pathobiological significance. J Biol Chem 1997;272:20,963–20,966.
12. Rajavashisth TB, Andalibi A, Territo MC, et al. Induction of endothelial cell expression of granulocyte and macrophage colony-stimulating factors by modified low-density lipoproteins. Nature 1990;344:254–257.
13. Skalen K, Gustafsson M, Rydberg EK, et al. Subendothelial retention of atherogenic lipoproteins in early atherosclerosis. Nature 2002;417:699–701.
14. Leonard EJ, Yoshimura T. Human monocyte chemoattractant protein-1 (MCP-1). Immunol Today 1990;11:97–101.
15. Stephens NG, Parsons A, Schofield PM, et al. Randomised controlled trial of vitamin E in patients with coronary disease: Cambridge Heart Antioxidant Study. Lancet 1996;347:781–786.
16. Omenn GS, Goodman GE, Thornquist MD, et al. Effects of a combination of beta carotene and vitamin A on lung cancer and cardiovascular disease. N Engl J Med 1996;334:1150–1155.
17. Gibbons GH, Dzau VJ. The emerging concept of vascular remodeling. N Engl J Med 1994;330:1431–1438.
18. Schoenhagen P, Ziada KM, Kapadia SR, et al. Extent and direction of arterial remodeling in stable versus unstable coronary syndromes: an intravascular ultrasound study. Circulation 2000;101:598–603.
19. Varnava AM, Mills PG, Davies MJ. Relationship between coronary artery remodeling and plaque vulnerability. Circulation 2002;105:939–943.
20. Jonasson L, Holm J, Skalli O, et al. Regional accumulations of T cells, macrophages, and smooth muscle cells in the human atherosclerotic plaque. Arteriosclerosis 1986;6:131–138.
21. van der Wal AC, Das PK, Bentz van de Berg D, et al. Atherosclerotic lesions in humans: in situ immunophenotypic analysis suggesting an immune mediated response. Lab Invest 1989;61:166–170.
22. Falk E, Shah PK, Fuster V. Pathogenesis of plaque disruption. In: Fuster V, Ross R, Topol EJ, eds. Atherosclerosis and Coronary Artery Disease. Vol. 2. Lippincott-Raven, Philadelphia, 1996, pp. 492–510.
23. Feng B, Yao PM, Li Y, et al. The endoplasmic reticulum is the site of cholesterol-induced cytotoxicity in macrophages. Nature Cell Biol 2003;5:781–792.
24. Hansson GK, Jonasson L, Seifert PS, Stemme S. Immune mechanisms in atherosclerosis. Arteriosclerosis 1989;9:567–578.
25. Wick G, Romen M, Amberger A, et al. Atherosclerosis, autoimmunity, and vascular-associated lymphoid tissue. FASEB J 1997;11:1199–1207.
26. Schonbeck U, Mach F, Sukhova GK, et al. Regulation of matrix metalloproteinase expression in human vascular smooth muscle cells by T lymphocytes: a role for CD40 signaling in plaque rupture? Circ Res 1997;81:448–454.

27. Mach F, Schonbeck U, Sukhova GK, et al. Reduction of atherosclerosis in mice by inhibition of CD40 signalling. Nature 1998;394:200–203.
28. Xu XH, Shah PK, Faure E, et al. Toll-like receptor-4 is expressed by macrophages in murine and human lipid-rich atherosclerotic plaques and upregulated by oxidized LDL. Circulation 2001;104:3103–3108.
29. Bombeli T, Schwartz BR, Harlan JM. Adhesion of activated platelets to endothelial cells: evidence for a GPIIbIIIa-dependent bridging mechanism and novel roles for endothelial intercellular adhesion molecule 1 (ICAM-1), $\alpha v \beta 3$ integrin, and GPIb$. J Exp Med 1998;187:329–339.
30. Chobanian AV, Dzau VJ. Renin angiotensin system and atherosclerotic vascular disease. In: Fuster V, Ross R, Topol EJ, eds. Atherosclerosis and Coronary Artery Disease. Vol. 1. Lippincott-Raven, Philadelphia, 1996, pp. 237–242.
31. Verhoef P, Stampfer MJ. Prospective studies of homocysteine and cardiovascular disease. Nutr Rev 1995;53:283–288.
32. Omenn GS, Beresford SAA, Motulsky AG. Preventing coronary heart disease: B vitamins and homocysteine. Circulation 1998;97:421–424.
33. Libby P, Egan D, Skarlatos S. Roles of infectious agents in atherosclerosis and restenosis: an assessment of the evidence and need for future research. Circulation 1997;96:4095–4103.
34. Gupta S, Leatham EW, Carrington D, et al. Elevated *Chlamydia pneumoniae* antibodies, cardiovascular events, and azithromycin in male survivors of myocardial infarction. Circulation 1997;96:404–407.
35. Shah PK. Plaque disruption and coronary thrombosis: new insight into pathogenesis and prevention. Clin Cardiol 1997;20:II-38–44.
36. Muhlestein JB, Anderson JL, Hammond EH, et al. Infection with *Chlamydia pneumoniae* accelerates the development of atherosclerosis and treatment with azithromycin prevents it in a rabbit model. Circulation 1998;97:633–636.
37. Hu H, Pierce GN, Zhong G. The atherogenic effects of chlamydia are dependent on serum cholesterol and specific to *Chlamydia pneumoniae*. J Clin Invest 1999;103:747–753.
38. Gurfinkel E, Bozovich G, Daroca A, et al. Randomised trial of roxithromycin in non-Q-wave coronary syndromes: ROXIS Pilot Study. ROXIS Study Group [see comments]. Lancet 1997;350:404–407.
39. Bachmaier K, Neu N, de la Maza LM, et al. Chlamydia infections and heart disease linked through antigenic mimicry. Science 1999;283:1335–1339.
40. Cercek B, Shah PK, Noc M, et al. AZACS Investigators. Effect of short-term treatment with azithromycin on recurrent ischaemic events in patients with acute coronary syndrome in the Azithromycin in Acute Coronary Syndrome (AZACS) trial: a randomised controlled trial. Lancet 2003;361:809–813.
41. O'Connor CM, Dunne MW, Pfeffer MA, et al. Investigators in the WIZARD Study. Azithromycin for the secondary prevention of coronary heart disease events: the WIZARD study: a randomized controlled trial. JAMA 2003;290:1459–1466.
42. Folkman J. Angiogenesis in cancer, vascular, rheumatoid and other diseases. Nature Med 1995;1:27–31.
43. Kolodgie FD, Gold HK, Burke AP, et al. Intraplaque hemorrhage and progression of atheroma. N Engl J Med 2003;349:2316–2325.
44. Moulton KS, Heller E, Konerding MA, et al. Angiogenesis inhibitor endostatin or TNP-470 reduces intimal neovascularization and plaque growth in apolipoprotein E deficient mice. Circulation 1999;99:1726–1732.
45. Celletti FL, Waugh JM, Amabile PG, et al. Vascular endothelial growth factor enhances atherosclerotic plaque progression. Nature Med 2001;7:425–429.
46. Lee RT, Libby P. The unstable atheroma. Arterioscler Thromb Vasc Biol 1997;17:1859–1867.
47. Shah PK. Pathophysiology of coronary thrombosis: role of plaque rupture and plaque erosion. Prog Cardiovasc Dis 2002;44:357–368.
48. Burke AP, Farb A, Malcom GT, et al. Coronary risk factors and plaque morphology in men with coronary disease who died suddenly. N Engl J Med 1997;336:1276–1282.
49. Rajavashisth TB, Xu XP, Jovinge S, et al. Membrane type 1 matrix metalloproteinase expression in human atherosclerotic plaques: evidence for activation by proinflammatory mediators. Circulation 1999;99:3103–3109.
50. Ridker PM, Cushman M, Stampfer MJ, et al. Inflammation, aspirin, and the risk of cardiovascular disease in apparently healthy men. N Engl J Med 1997;336:973–979.

RECOMMENDED READING

Ross R. Atherosclerosis: an inflammatory disease. N Engl J Med 1999;340:115–126.
Springer TA, Cybulsky MI. Traffic signals on endothelium for leukocytes in health, inflammation, and atherosclerosis. In: Fuster V, Ross R, Topol EJ, eds. Atherosclerosis and Coronary Artery Disease. Vol. 1. Lippincott-Raven, Philadelphia, 1996, pp. 511–538.
Kinlay S, Ganz P. Role of endothelial dysfunction in coronary artery disease and implications for therapy. Am J Cardiol 1997;80:111–161.
Steinberg D. Low density lipoprotein oxidation and its pathobiological significance. J Biol Chem 1997;272:20,963–20,966.
Gibbons GH, Dzau VJ. The emerging concept of vascular remodeling. N Engl J Med 1994;330:1431–1438.
Libby P. Inflammation in atherosclerosis. Nature 2002;420:868–874.
Shah PK. Mechanisms of plaque vulnerability and rupture. J Am Coll Cardiol 2003;41(4 Suppl):15s–22s.

23 Risk Factors and Prevention, Including Hyperlipidemias

Antonio M. Gotto, Jr., MD, DPhil
and John Farmer, MD

INTRODUCTION

Cardiovascular disease is the leading cause of death in the United States for both men and women *(1)*. However, great strides have been made in the field of preventive cardiology over the past decade, that, combined with the significant advances in revascularization technologies, have enhanced the clinician's ability to manage patients across the spectrum of atherosclerosis, from subclinical coronary heart disease (CHD) to congestive heart failure. Additionally, advances in noninvasive and invasive imaging have improved the capacity to diagnose the presence and vulnerability of the atherosclerotic plaque. Hypertension, smoking, and dyslipidemia remain the major remediable risk factors for the development and progression of atherosclerosis. This chapter will briefly review the major risk factors for CHD, then place a special emphasis on the management of lipid disorders based on the 2001 iteration of guidelines from the US National Cholesterol Education Program (NCEP), which stress the management of low-density lipoprotein cholesterol (LDL-C) as the primary target of lipid therapy *(2)*.

Nonmodifiable Risk Factors

Besides elevated LDL-C, the NCEP considers a number of other risk factors for CHD (Table 1) in its approach. Coronary risk factors fall into two broad categories: those that may be modified with treatment and those that may not. This latter category includes such factors as age, sex, and family history of premature heart disease. The general principles here are that CHD risk increases with age; men are at higher risk than women, up until menopause; and a patient who has a first-degree relative with a history of early heart disease is at risk as well. The first two are discussed later as issues for special populations, but a special point should be made about family history. Atherosclerosis tends to aggregate in families, and genetic factors may confer increased risk for the subsequent development of cardiovascular disease *(3)*. Obesity, hypertension, dyslipidemia, and diabetes also have a genetic component, and the family history should be carefully analyzed in an attempt to identify clustering of risk factors and to tailor lipid-modifying and antihypertensive therapy to minimize cardiac risk. Screening for family history is underappreciated in clinical practice, but represents an important opportunity to improve identification of a high-risk group of patients who may warrant an aggressive risk-reduction approach.

MODIFIABLE RISK FACTORS

For brevity, this chapter will consider the major modifiable CHD risk factors to be hypertension, tobacco use, and dyslipidemia. Other modifiable factors that influence risk, such as obesity, diabetes, or metabolic syndrome, or emerging risk factors, are discussed later.

From: *Essential Cardiology: Principles and Practice, 2nd Ed.*
Edited by: C. Rosendorff © Humana Press Inc., Totowa, NJ

Table 1
Other Risk Factors in Evaluating CHD Risk

Positive risk factors
  Age
  Family history of CHD
  Hypertension
  Current tobacco use
  Low HDL-C (<40 mg/dL [1.03 mmol/L])[a]
Negative risk factor
  HDL-C ≥ 60 mg/dL (1.55 mmol/L)[b]
CHD risk equivalents
  Multiple risk factors >20% risk for CHD in 10 yr
  Other cardiovascular disease (stroke, peripheral vascular disease, aortic aneurysm)
  Diabetes mellitus

[a]Confirmed by measurements on several occasions.
[b]If the HDL-C level is ≥60 mg/dL (1.55 mmol/L), subtract one risk factor (because high HDL-C levels decrease CHD risk).

Hypertension

Elevations of both systolic and diastolic blood pressure have been correlated with increased morbidity and mortality. The seventh report of the Joint National Committee on Prevention, Detection, Evaluation, and Treatment of High Blood Pressure (JNC VII) (4) identifies several other key messages related to hypertension control, including the following: (1) in persons older than 50 yr, systolic blood pressure (BP) of more than 140 mmHg is a much more important cardiovascular disease (CVD) risk factor than high diastolic BP; and (2) the risk of CVD, beginning at 115/75 mmHg, doubles with each increment of 20/10 mmHg; individuals who are normotensive at 55 years of age have a 90% lifetime risk for developing hypertension. JNC VII also identifies a category of "pre-hypertensive" patients who have a systolic BP of 120 to 139 mmHg or a diastolic BP of 80 to 89 mmHg and require health-promoting lifestyle modifications to prevent CVD.

The recent and controversial Antihypertensive and Lipid Lowering Treatment to Prevent Heart Attack Trial (ALLHAT) showed no difference in reduction of the primary endpoint of nonfatal myocardial infarction (MI) and CHD death when a thiazide diuretic, a dihydropyridine calcium-channel blocker, and an angiotensin-converting enzyme inhibitor were compared (5). Based in part on this finding, JNC VII recommends that thiazide-type diuretics should be used in drug treatment for most patients with uncomplicated hypertension, either alone or combined with drugs from other classes. For certain high-risk conditions, other antihypertensive drug classes may be indicated. Most patients with hypertension will require two or more antihypertensive medications to achieve goal BP (<140/90 mmHg, or <130/80 mmHg for patients with diabetes or chronic kidney disease). If BP is more than 20/10 mmHg above goal BP, JNC VII gives consideration to initiating therapy with two agents, one of which usually should be a thiazide-type diuretic. Management of blood pressure has clearly been demonstrated to decrease the risks for stroke, MI, and heart failure and should be a cornerstone of preventive measures.

Tobacco Use

The association between tobacco use and a number of health risks is incontrovertible. Although tobacco product consumption by adults has declined by 45% since 1965, 25.7% of men and 21% of women above the age of 18 are current smokers (6). Tobacco is associated with a number of pro-atherogenic abnormalities, including decreased high-density lipoprotein cholesterol (HDL-C), endothelial dysfunction, and heightened oxidation of LDL. Smoking may also adversely affect lipoprotein lipase activity and result in a deleterious effect on the lipid profile due to reduced catabolism of triglyceride-rich lipoproteins (7). Tobacco-mediated endothelial dysfunction also results in an imbalance between thrombogenic and fibrinolytic factors. The use of tobacco products has been demonstrated to reduce the production of tissue plasminogen activator (t-PA) and to increase levels of plasminogen activator inhibitor (PAI-I) and fibrinogen, resulting in a potential decreased ability to lyse a coronary thrombus *(8)*.

Smoking cessation reduces cardiovascular risk. Meta-analysis of mortality evaluations following smoking cessation demonstrated a 36% reduction in crude relative risk for total mortality in smokers with CHD *(9)*.

Dyslipidemia

Dyslipidemia is a major modifiable risk factor for coronary disease. However, an isolated serum total cholesterol has minimal predictive value in the individual patient because of a considerable overlap of values between patients with and without atherosclerosis *(10)*. Cholesterol is distributed in a number of lipoprotein fractions that have variable clinical impact on cardiovascular risk. The major circulating lipoproteins to be discussed are the triglyceride-rich lipoproteins, LDL, and HDL *(11)*. These are structurally complex, water-soluble particles responsible for the transport of lipids within the vascular compartment.

TRIGLYCERIDE-RICH LIPOPROTEINS

Chylomicrons are large triglyceride-rich particles that are generated in the intestine from dietary fat sources. The density of these particles is less than 0.95 g/mL for chylomicrons and 1.006 g/mL for chylomicron remnants *(11)*. Chylomicrons have a diameter ranging from 800 to 5000 Å and have no mobility when subjected to lipoprotein electrophoresis. Chylomicron remnants, which are normally rapidly cleared from the circulation, are incompletely hydrolyzed particles. Remnant particles have a diameter greater than 300 Å and also remain at the origin during electrophoretic studies. Hyperchylomicronemia is rare, predominantly seen in the pediatric population, and may be due to a congenital absence of lipoprotein lipase or its naturally occurring activator apolipoprotein (apo) C-II *(12)*. In the adult, hyperchylomicronemia may be seen in diabetes, multiple myeloma, systemic lupus erythematosus, or acute intermittent porphyria.

As opposed to chylomicrons, which are derived from exogenous sources, very-low-density lipoproteins (VLDL) carry endogenously produced triglycerides and have a density of less than 1.006 g/mL and a particle diameter ranging between 300 and 800 Å *(11)*. Genetically mediated overproduction of VLDL is a feature of familial hypercholesterolemia and of familial combined hyperlipidemia. Elevated triglycerides are also seen in a variety of acquired conditions, such as diabetes, obesity, and the use of a variety of medications, including noncardioselective β-blockers and estrogens. VLDL particles are produced by the liver and demonstrate electrophoretic mobility in the pre-beta region. Intermediate-density lipoproteins (IDL) are formed from incomplete catabolism of VLDL and are also triglyceride-rich particles. The density of these particles ranges from 1.006 to 1.019 g/mL with a diameter of 250 to 350 Å *(11)*. IDL particles migrate in the broad β-region. VLDL remnant particles may be atherogenic lipoproteins, especially when inefficiently cleared, as in diabetes *(13)*.

LOW-DENSITY LIPOPROTEIN

LDL carries the bulk of circulating cholesterol; its main component is cholesteryl ester. The density of this highly atherogenic particle ranges from 1.019 to 1.063 g/mL, with a diameter of 180 to 280 Å *(11)*. LDL migrates in the β-region in electrophoresis. LDL is the major atherogenic lipoprotein; elevations of LDL-C enhance the risk for CHD. Current guidelines consider LDL-C to be the primary target of lipid-modifying therapy.

HIGH-DENSITY LIPOPROTEIN

HDL carries mainly cholesteryl ester, and is a small particle that migrates in the alpha region, with a density ranging between 1.063 and 1.210 g/mL with a diameter of 50 to 90 Å *(11)*. Epidemiologic studies have shown a correlation between high levels of HDL cholesterol (HDL-C) and reduced risk

Table 2
Fredrickson Classification of Hyperlipidemias

Phenotype	Elevated lipoprotein(s)	Elevated lipid levels	Plasma TC	Plasma TG	Relative frequency (%)[a]
I	Chylomicrons	TG	N to ↑	—	<1
IIa	LDL-C	TC	↑↑	N	10
IIb	LDL-C and VLDL-C	TG, TC	↑↑	↑↑	40
III	IDL	TG, TC	↑↑	↑↑↑	<1
IV	VLDL-C	TG. TC	N to ↑	↑↑	45
V	VLDL-C and chylomicrons	TG, TC	↑ to ↑↑	↑↑↑↑	5

TC, total cholesterol; TG, triglyceride; N, normal; LDL-C, low-density lipoprotein cholesterol; VLDL-C, very-low-density lipoprotein cholesterol; IDL, intermediate-density lipoprotein.

[a]% of patients in the US patients with hyperlipidemia.

Adapted from International Lipid Information Bureau. The ILIB Lipid Handbook for Clinical Practice. New York City, 1995, p. 29.

for atherosclerosis *(14)*. The postulated mechanisms for this cardioprotection are complex and include reverse cholesterol transport, endothelial repair, antioxidant activity, and increased prostacyclin production. The major protein constituents of HDL are apo A-I and A-II, both of which may play a role in atherogenesis. A preliminary study of intravenous infusion with a mutant of apo A-I known as apo A-I milano demonstrated significant lesion regression, as assessed by intravascular ultra-sonography, and may prove a novel therapeutic approach *(15)*.

Additionally, HDL metabolism is intimately related to triglyceride catabolism and may therefore be a gauge of the efficiency of VLDL metabolism. Low HDL-C is often associated with physical inactivity, obesity, diabetes, hypertriglyceridemia, genetic conditions, and the use of tobacco products.

CLINICAL DYSLIPIDEMIA

The circulating lipoproteins may be quantified and subsequently classified by a variety of techniques, including density ultracentrifugation or electrophoretic mobility, or by the chemical constituents, such as apolipoproteins, on the surface of these particles. Although there are sophisticated molecular biologic and genetic classifications available, the traditional Fredrickson's phenotype system still has utility for the practicing physician, despite the fact that it does not differentiate between primary and secondary dyslipidemias and includes no consideration of HDL, the atherogenic particle lipoprotein(a), or lipoprotein subforms (Table 2).

Primary and Secondary Dyslipidemias

Primary dyslipidemias usually arise from an interaction of genetic and environmental influences. Table 3 highlights some of the major primary hyperlipidemias. The diagnosis of a primary genetic dyslipidemia requires a systematic exclusion of all secondary causes of dyslipidemia. Multiple clinical disorders express dyslipidemia as a secondary feature of a number of conditions (Table 4), and, in these cases, management of the primary underlying disease precedes management of the dyslipidemia itself.

NCEP Guidelines

The NCEP has established guidelines for the screening, diagnosis, and treatment of dyslipidemia. The guidelines specify desirable and undesirable levels of the various lipid fractions (Table 5). Because atherogenesis begins relatively early in life, the NCEP recommends that all adults above the age of 20 have a lipid profile performed at least once every 5 yr.

The most recent guidelines of the NCEP's third Adult Treatment Panel (ATP III) stress the assessment of patients' near-term (that is, within the next 10 yr) risk for CHD to determine the aggres-

Table 3
Selected Causes of Primary Dyslipidemia

Hypercholesterolemia
    Heterozygous familial hypercholesterolemia
    Homozygous familial hypercholesterolemia
    Familial defective apo B-100
    Polygenic hypercholesterolemia
Disorders of HDL metabolism
    Familial hypoalphalipoproteinemia
    Lecithin:cholesterol acyltransferase deficiency
    Familial apo A-I/C-III deficiency
    Tangier disease, fish-eye disease
    apo A-I$_{\text{Milano}}$ (A-I variant)
Primary combined hyperlipidemias
    Familial combined hyperlipidemia
    Type III hyperlipidemia
Primary hypertriglyceridemia
    Familial hypertriglyceridemia (Type IV or V hyperlipidemia)
    Familial chylomicronemia
    Lipoprotein lipase deficiency
    apo C-III deficiency

Table 4
Selected Causes of Secondary Dyslipidemia

↑LDL-C	Hypothyroidism	Cholestasis
	Nephrotic syndrome	Dysglobulinemia
	Chronic liver disease	Anorexia nervosa
↑TG	Excessive alcohol consumption	Diuretics
	Obesity	Exogenous estrogens
	Pregnancy	(oral administration)
	Diabetes mellitus	Isotretinoin
	Hypothyroidism	Cushing's syndrome
	Chronic renal failure	Oral contraceptives
	β-blockers	
↓HDL-C	Physical inactivity	Obesity
	Smoking	Hypertriglyceridemia
	Diabetes mellitus	

siveness of treatment. Patients may fall into one of three categories: those with CHD or with a risk factor profile equivalent to having CHD, or "CHD equivalent"; those with multiple risk factors (2 or more); and those with 0 to 1 risk factors. The identification of a "CHD-equivalent" group is an important modification from previous guidelines. Included in this category are patients who have other forms of atherosclerotic disease, those with diabetes, and those with a 10-yr CHD risk greater than 20%. This schema shows an appreciation for the continuum of cardiovascular risk that blurs the distinction between "primary" and "secondary" prevention.

GLOBAL RISK ASSESSMENT

Global risk is calculated using a modified version of the Framingham algorithm (Table 6). In patients with no history of CHD and two or more risk factors in addition to high LDL-C, global risk should be calculated to determine at what LDL-C level to initiate drug therapy. Because the modified Framingham score used by ATP III reflects the contributions of the traditional major risk factors (i.e., smoking, total cholesterol, HDL-C, age, blood pressure, and sex), they do not consider the risks associated with emerging risk factors, such as homocysteine, lipoprotein(a), or inflammatory

Table 5
ATP III Classification of Lipid Levels

Total cholesterol (mg/dL)	
<200	Desirable
200–239	Borderline high
≥240	High
LDL-C (mg/dL)	
<100	Optimal
100–129	Near optimal/above optimal
130–159	Borderline high
160–189	High
≥190	Very high
HDL-C (mg/dL)	
<40	Low
≥60	High
Triglycerides (mg/dL)	
<150	Normal
150–199	Borderline high
200–499	High
≥500	Very high

LDL-C, low-density lipoprotein cholesterol; HDL-C, high-density lipoprotein cholesterol.

To convert to mmol/L, multiply cholesterol by 0.02586 and triglycerides by 0.01129. (Adapted from ref. 2.)

markers. ATP III acknowledges that the presence of such factors may influence clinical judgment in favor of initiating more aggressive intervention, such as lipid-modifying drugs, and the American Heart Association and Centers for Disease Control and Prevention have issued a joint statement in favor of using measurement of the inflammatory marker C-reactive protein for this purpose (16). In addition, ATP III recognizes that some persons with high long-term risk are candidates for LDL-C-lowering drugs even though use of drugs may not be cost-effective by current standards.

In the initial patient assessment, physicians should establish a risk factor profile that consists of the level of LDL-C combined with six other positive and one negative risk factor (Table 1). Elevated HDL-C is generally associated with a decreased risk for premature atherosclerosis, and a level >60 mg/dL (1.55 mmol/L) is thus considered to be a negative risk factor and allows one risk factor to be subtracted from the total. High risk, defined as a net of two or more CHD risk factors, leads to more aggressive intervention in primary prevention in adults despite the lack of clinical evidence for CHD. Age (defined differently for men and women) is treated as a risk factor because the incidence and prevalence of CHD are higher in the elderly than in the young, and in men than in women of the same age until later in the postmenopausal period.

Because of the current health care environment, universal lipid screening of patients may be considered impractical or economically unfeasible. However, selective screening of high-risk individuals should be undertaken.

PRIMARY PREVENTION

The NCEP has established lipid goals for primary prevention and has designated a total cholesterol of <200 mg/dL (5.17 mmol/L) as being desirable. Cholesterol levels determined to be between 200 and 239 mg/dL (5.17–6.18 mmol/L) are classified as borderline high and above 240 mg/dL (6.21 mmol/L) are definitely elevated. The designation of the recommended lipid levels for risk stratification is somewhat arbitrary, as a definite clinical threshold below which lipid lowering is either ineffective or detrimental has not been determined in prospective trials.

Following the establishment of the patient's risk factor profile and lipid status, physicians should use the total risk factor score to decide on further interventions. Patients who are clinically free

Table 6
Framingham Risk Algorithm to Estimate 10-Yr Risk for CHD

1. Add Up Points by Risk Factor

Age (years)	Points Men	Points Women
20-34	-9	-7
35-39	-4	-3
40-44	0	0
45-49	3	3
50-54	6	6
55-59	8	8
60-64	10	10
65-69	11	12
70-74	12	14
75-79	13	16

TC (mg/dL)	Points by Age (years)									
	20-39		40-49		50-59		60-69		70-79	
	M	W	M	W	M	W	M	W	M	W
<160	0	0	0	0	0	0	0	0	0	0
160-199	4	4	3	3	2	2	1	1	0	1
200-239	7	8	5	6	3	4	1	2	0	1
240-279	9	11	6	8	4	5	2	3	1	2
≥280	11	13	8	10	5	7	3	4	1	2

	Points by Age (years)									
	20-39		40-49		50-59		60-69		70-79	
	M	W	M	W	M	W	M	W	M	W
Nonsmoker	0	0	0	0	0	0	0	0	0	0
Smoker	8	9	5	7	3	4	1	2	1	1

Systolic BP (mmHg)	If untreated M	If untreated W	If treated M	If treated W
<120	0	0	0	0
120-129	0	1	1	3
130-139	1	2	2	4
140-159	1	3	2	5
≥160	2	4	3	6

HDL-C (mg/dL)	Points Men	Points Women
≥60	-1	-1
50-59	0	0
40-49	1	1
<40	2	2

2. Estimate Risk

MEN Point Total	MEN 10-year Risk, %	WOMEN Point Total	WOMEN 10-year Risk, %
<0	<1	<9	<1
0	1	9	1
1	1	10	1
2	1	11	1
3	1	12	1
4	1	13	2
5	2	14	2
6	2	15	3
7	3	16	4
8	4	17	5
9	5	18	6
10	6	19	8
11	8	20	11
12	10	21	14
13	12	22	17
14	16	23	22
15	20	24	27
16	25	≥25	≥30
≥17	≥30		

M, men; W, women; TC, total cholesterol; BP, blood pressure; HDL-C, high-density lipoprotein cholesterol. (Adapted from ref. 2.)

of manifestations of atherosclerosis and have an acceptable risk factor profile, including a normal total cholesterol and HDL-C, require no specific intervention recommendation, although they should receive instruction in lifestyle changes such as increased physical activity and dietary approaches to risk reduction. The risk factor profile and cholesterol should be reassessed in 5 yr in low-risk patients. Patients whose cholesterol level falls in the borderline range but is associated with a normal HDL-C and fewer than two risk factors should also be instructed about dietary therapy and other measures (exercise, weight loss, etc.) as a means to reduce the risk for developing coronary atherosclerosis. However, increased scrutiny of these individuals should be implemented, and the risk factor and lipid profile should be reassessed in 1 to 2 yr.

A full lipid analysis with the determination of LDL-C is recommended in patients with low HDL-C plus two or more risk factors if the cholesterol falls in the high or borderline elevated levels. LDL-C is considered to be desirable if it falls below 130 mg/dL (3.36 mmol/L). LDL-C above 160 mg/dL (4.14 mmol/L) is considered to be elevated in primary prevention with a borderline level falling between 130 and 159 mg/dL (3.36–4.11 mmol/L). A desirable LDL-C should be managed with dietary measures similar to the general population. LDL-C that falls in the borderline elevated range but is accompanied by fewer than two other risk factors should also receive hygienic interventions utilizing diet and exercise, and the lipoprotein analysis should be repeated in 1 yr. Subjects in the borderline elevated LDL-C range who have two or more risk factors or with elevated LDL-C should have a repeat analysis within 2 mo coupled with an attempt to lower LDL-C to a more desirable range.

SECONDARY PREVENTION

Key among ATP III recommendations for patients following an acute coronary event is that therapy be started before or at the time of discharge. There are two perceived advantages with this approach: (1) patients are particularly motivated to undertake and adhere to risk-lowering interventions at that time, and (2) failure to initiate indicated therapy early contributes to a "treatment gap" characterized by potentially inconsistent and fragmented patient follow-up.

Table 7
Components of the TLC Diet

Nutrient	Recommended intake
Saturated fat	Less than 7% of total calories
Polyunsaturated fat	Up to 10% of total calories
Monounsaturated fat	Up to 20% of total calories
Total fat	25–35% of total calories
Carbohydrate	50–60% of total calories
Fiber	20–30 g per day
Protein	Approx 15% of total calories
Cholesterol	Less than 200 mg/d
Total calories (energy)	Balance energy intake and expenditure to maintain desirable body weight/prevent weight gain

TLC, therapeutic lifestyle changes.

Secondary prevention strategies are more aggressive because of the high risk for a recurrent event. Cholesterol levels fall during a number of acute illnesses, including MI, thereby potentially rendering a lipid determination obtained in the peri-infarction period to be clinically misleading. However, lipid values obtained within the first 24 h of an acute MI are generally reliable and may be utilized for risk-stratification purposes (17). Additionally, patients whose levels are elevated after 24 h may be presumed to have had significantly higher levels of LDL-C prior to the acute event and therefore are at increased risk because of the potential for an underlying genetic cause of dyslipidemia. In the presence of documented CHD, a therapeutic goal of LDL-C <100 mg/dL (2.59 mmol/L) has been recommended, and in the highest-risk patients an optional LDL-C goal <70 mg/dL (1.81 mmol/L) may be considered. However, subsequent clinical trial data have suggested that an even lower target may be reasonable (18). Pharmacologic therapy may be begun simultaneously with a diet and exercise program in high-risk subjects who would not be expected to achieve NCEP goals with hygienic measures as the sole intervention.

Secondary Targets of Treatment

The ATP III guidelines allow that once LDL-C is controlled, clinical attention may shift to other issues. In patients with triglycerides >200 mg/dL (2.26 mmol/L), physicians may use non-HDL-C as a secondary target of treatment. This measurement, intended to capture the cholesterol level of both LDL and the triglyceride-rich atherogenic lipoproteins, is calculated by subtracting the HDL-C value from the total cholesterol value. The goals for non-HDL-C may be established by adding 30 mg/dL (0.76 mmol/L) to the goals for LDL-C. Another secondary target of treatment is the cluster of proatherosclerotic risk factors known as metabolic syndrome (see below).

TREATMENT
Lifestyle Intervention

Therapeutic lifestyle changes (TLC) in all patients should always be the first line of preventive therapy and continued even with the subsequent initiation of pharmacologic therapy. Restrict dietary intake of calories and saturated fat as the primary means to maintain ideal body weight and to reduce circulating total and LDL-C. Dietary therapy should be coupled with a regular exercise program. Patients with known atherosclerosis may require close monitoring or additional guidance.

The NCEP has developed a TLC eating pattern for both primary and secondary prevention (Table 7). In primary prevention, when the subject has fewer than two risk factors, dietary intervention is recommended if the LDL-C is 160 mg/dL (4.14 mmol/L) or higher. The presence of two or more risk factors in primary prevention mandates a more aggressive approach, and TLC are initiated at an LDL-C of 130 mg/dL (3.36 mmol/L) or higher. Secondary prevention recommendations initiate dietary therapy in order to bring LDL-C levels below 100 mg/dL (2.59 mmol/L).

Table 8
Treatment Decisions Based on LDL-C

Risk category	LDL-C goal	TLC initiation level	Drug treatment initiation level
0–1 Other risk factors[a]	<160 mg/dL (4.14 mmol/L)	≥160 mg/dL	≥190 mg/dL (4.91 mmol/L) (160–189; LDL-C-lowering drug optional)
2+ Other risk factors (10-yr risk ≤20%)	<130 mg/dL (3.36 mmol/L)	≥130 mg/dL	10-yr risk 10–20%: ≥130 mg/dL 10-yr risk <10%: ≥160 mg/dL
CHD or CHD risk equivalents (10-yr risk >20%)	<100 mg/dL (2.59 mmol/L)	≥100 mg/dL	≥130 mg/dL (100–129; drug optional)[b]

LDL-C, low-density lipoprotein cholesterol; TLC, therapeutic lifestyle changes; CHD, coronary heart disease.

[a]Almost all people with 0–1 other risk factors have a 10-yr risk <10%: thus, 10-yr risk assessment in people with 0–1 risk factor is not necessary.

[b]Some authorities recommend use of LDL-C-lowering drugs in this category if an LDL-C level of <100 mg/dL (2.59 mmol/L) cannot be achieved by therapeutic lifestyle changes alone. Others prefer use of drugs that primarily modify triglyceride and HDL, e.g., nicotinic acid or fibrate. Clinical judgment also may call for deferring drug therapy in this subcategory.

Adapted from ref. 2.

Dietary therapy should be monitored for both compliance and achievement of body-weight or lipid goals. Dietary intervention generally requires at least a 3-mo evaluation period prior to considering pharmacologic therapy. However, because of the demonstrated efficacy of lipid modification in high-risk patients (i.e., secondary prevention or CHD risk equivalence) in prospective clinical trials, the simultaneous institution of pharmacologic therapy and TLC is permissible (19).

PHYSICAL ACTIVITY

Physical inactivity is not listed as a primary CHD risk factor, but it should be considered a target for intervention. Decreased physical activity frequently coexists with cardiac risk factors including dyslipidemia, obesity, and impaired glucose tolerance, whereas regular physical exercise correlates with a decreased rate of CHD in epidemiologic studies (20). The impact of exercise on cardiovascular risk factors is a function of both the duration and intensity of the level of activity. Physical exercise increases HDL-C, and the degree of increase appears to be more closely correlated with the cumulative distance run per week rather than with intense short bursts of speed. Long-distance runners have a significantly greater rise in HDL-C when compared with subjects who ran fewer than 16 km/wk (21). Leisure-time physical activity has been inversely correlated to the angiographic presence of coronary disease and inversely and independently associated with a variety of inflammatory markers, including C-reactive protein, serum amyloid-A, and intracellular adhesion molecule, thus implying that improvement in coronary risk achieved by increasing leisure-time physical activity is at least partially due to alteration of inflammation, which may be independent of the traditional effects of exercise on weight and lipid parameters (22). Physical activity should be encouraged in patients at risk for coronary atherosclerosis.

Drug Therapy

Failure to achieve NCEP goals on TLC alone may prompt the institution of pharmacologic therapy. However, the decision to initiate a lipid-modifying drug should consider cost and potential long-term adverse effects of drug monotherapy, as well as risks for drug–drug interactions with any other concomitant medications. In relatively low-risk primary prevention, dietary therapy is recommended for at least 3 mo before considering adding on a drug. However, in primary prevention patients at high risk due to a severe underlying genetic dyslipidemia or multiple CHD risk factors, or in secondary prevention or CHD-equivalent patients, an earlier institution of pharmacologic therapy may be warranted because of the beneficial risk–benefit ratio in those groups.

Table 9
Summary of Drug Choices for Diet-Resistant Dyslipidemia

Dyslipidemia (Fredrickson phenotype[s])	Drug therapy

Elevated LDL-C-C (Type II-A)[a]	First choice
	  Resin (cholestyramine, colestipol, colesevelam)
	  Statin (atorvastatin, rosuvastatin, fluvastatin, lovastatin, pravastatin, simvastatin)
	Second choice
	  Fibrate (clofibrate, gemfibrozil, fenofibrate, bezafibrate, ciprofibrate)

Elevated triglyceride (Types IV and V)[b]	Fibrate (clofibrate, gemfibrozil, fenofibrate, bezafibrate, ciprofibrate) Nicotinic acid
Elevated LDL-C-C and triglyceride (Types II-B and III)[c]	Nicotinic acid Fibrate (clofibrate, gemfibrozil, fenofibrate, bezafibrate, ciprofibrate) Statin (atorvastatin, rosuvastatin, fluvastatin, lovastatin, pravastatin, simvastatin)
Isolated low HDL-C[d]	Nicotinic acid

LDL-C, low-density lipoprotein cholesterol; HDL-C, high-density lipoprotein cholesterol.

[a]Nicotinic acid or higher-dose statin therapy may be of use in individuals with familial defective apoB-100.

[b]For individuals with Type I hyperlipidemia (hyperchylomicronemia), drug therapy is ineffective if lipoprotein lipase is absent.

[c]For individuals with Type II-B hyperlipidemia (elevated LDL-C and VLDL-triglyceride), combination therapy with fibrate and statin may be warranted, but is not approved by the Food and Drug Administration because of the 1–5% risk for muscle toxicity with this combination. Type III hyperlipidemia is managed by dietary fat restriction and fibrate therapy.

[d]Fibrates may also be used to raise HDL-C, but are more efficacious with associated hypertriglyceridemia. Some experts recommend lowering LDL-C with statin therapy in these patients in order to improve the LDL-C:HDL-C ratio.

ATP III established action limits based on LDL-C for drug therapy in both primary and secondary prevention that depend on the lipid level and associated risk factors (Table 8). However, since the publication of these guidelines, a number of studies using the 3-hydroxy-3-methylglutaryl coenzyme A (HMG-CoA) inhibitors, or statins, have reported robust results that have argued for wider use of these drugs in high-risk patients, regardless of the baseline LDL-C (18,19).

Choosing drugs whose lipid effects address a patient's main lipid abnormality (e.g., elevated total cholesterol and LDL-C or abnormalities predominantly involving triglycerides and HDL-C) may help optimize drug therapy. Table 9 summarizes available drug choices based on the dyslipidemia presented.

PHARMACOLOGIC AGENTS WITH A PREDOMINANT EFFECT ON LDL-C

Bile Acid Sequestrants. The bile acid sequestrants, or resins, are quaternary ammonium salts, and cholestyramine, colestipol, and colesevelam are the currently available agents. The efficacy, mechanism of action, and side effect profile of the three currently available resins are basically similar, although colesevelam has a unique polymeric structure that reduces gastrointestinal side effects and drug–drug interactions (23). The bile acid sequestrants interrupt the enterohepatic circulation of the cholesterol-rich bile acid pool by binding the negatively charged bile salts within the gastrointestinal tract, thus increasing fecal loss of cholesterol. Colesevelam may bind an equivalent amount of bile acids at a lower dose because of the structural modification of the molecule. The increased fecal loss results in a reduction in intrahepatic cholesterol, which stimulates the subsequent upregulation of the hepatic apo B/E receptor, also known as the LDL receptor, but which recognizes and binds lipoproteins containing apo B (e.g., LDL, VLDL) or apo E (e.g., chylomicrons). The increase in receptor activity results in an increased removal of LDL-C from the plasma compartment. The gastrointestinal loss of cholesterol generally exceeds the clearance of LDL-C from the plasma, resulting in a decrease in intrahepatic cholesterol and a secondary stimulus of HMG-CoA reductase which is the rate limiting enzyme in cholesterol synthesis. The secondary activation of HMG-CoA reductase blunts the long-term efficacy of bile acid resin monotherapy, because it stimulates increased cholesterol production.

Cholestyramine can be dosed up to a maximum of 24 g/d and colestipol may be dosed to a maximum of 30 g/d. The bile acid resins are poorly palatable and are generally mixed in various vehicles to improve compliance. Colesevelam is administered in caplet form at a dose of six tablets per day (625 mg of colesevelam per caplet), which improves compliance. Patients who are able to tolerate the maximum dose of the bile acid sequestrants may expect to achieve an LDL-C reduction of 15 to 30%. Resin therapy generally does not have major effects on HDL-C levels although an increase of 3 to 5% may be achieved in selected individuals. Plasma VLDL-C levels are generally not affected by the bile acid resins. However, in subjects with metabolic conditions prone to hypertriglyceridemia (e.g., diabetes, obesity, insulin resistance), resin therapy may result in an increase in circulating triglycerides.

The use of the bile acid resins as monotherapy has decreased over recent years because of the availability of more efficacious and palatable agents such as the statins. The major side effects of bile acid sequestrants relate to a variety of gastrointestinal complaints including constipation, nausea, and other nonspecific gastrointestinal symptoms. Because these agents are nonspecific binders of other drugs, resin therapy has the potential to interfere with the absorption of a number of commonly coadministered cardiovascular drugs, such as digoxin, β-blockers, thiazides, coumadin, and other agents. Colesevelam has a lower frequency of nonspecific binding and should be considered in subjects with multiple coadministered drugs.

HMG-CoA Reductase Inhibitors. Based on a substantial database of clinical trials that report significant coronary and other cardiovascular risk reductions with these drugs, the HMG-CoA reductase inhibitors, or statins, have emerged at the forefront of drug therapies for CVD prevention *(18,19,24–30)*. The currently available agents, in the order of their commercial release, are lovastatin, pravastatin, simvastatin, fluvastatin, atorvastatin, and rosuvastatin. Cerivastatin was removed from the market in 2001 because of an excess risk for fatal rhabdomyolysis that does not appear to be shared by other agents in this group *(31)*. The statins have differing structural characteristics and also may be differentiated on the basis of lipophilicity or metabolism. However, statins seem to share a common hypolipidemic mechanism of action, despite these differences, through their partial inhibition of HMG-CoA reductase, the rate-limiting enzyme in the production of cholesterol. The resulting reduction in intrahepatic cholesterol synthesis stimulates increased expression of the hepatic LDL receptor, thus increasing clearance of LDL from the circulation. The more lipophilic agents (e.g., atorvastatin or simvastatin) may have a direct intrahepatic effect on the synthesis or release of apo B-containing particles. Depending on the agent and dosage used, decreases in LDL-C ranging from 20 to 60% may be expected with the various agents. The major impact on LDL-C levels occurs with the initial dose, with an approximate 6 to 7% additional LDL-C lowering with each doubling of the statin dose *(32)*. Statins exert a modest effect on HDL-C (about 5–15% increase) and moderate triglyceride lowering.

The side effect profile of the statins is well documented, and overall, the potential risks of this class do not outweigh the potential benefits. The main side effects attributed to the statins relate to liver and muscle toxicity. Significant hepatic toxicity has been defined as elevations in transaminase enzymes which exceeded three times the upper limits of normal. The statin-induced elevation in transaminases has been generally determined to be reversible following discontinuation of the drug and the incidence of fatal hepatic necrosis is extremely rare. A definite pathogenetic link with statin therapy has not been made. The large-scale Extended Clinical Evaluation of Lovastatin (EXCEL) demonstrated that the incidence of significant elevations of transaminases was less than 1% when the usually clinically administered dose of lovastatin was employed *(33)*. Liver toxicity associated with statin therapy is relatively dose-dependent, but clinical trials have demonstrated this to be a relatively uncommon phenomenon with significant transaminitis generally occurring with less than a 3% incidence. However, it is recommended that liver enzymes be monitored early in the course following the initiation of statin therapy or in patients felt to be at increased risk due to the concomitant administration of potentially hepatic-toxic drugs or preexisting liver disease.

Statin therapy has been associated with muscle toxicity, which may be defined across a clinical spectrum that includes myalgia, myositis, and rhabdomyolysis. Although monitoring for abnormal elevations of creatine kinase levels is the standard method for evaluating muscle toxicity, some data have suggested evidence of statin-related myalgia in the absence of elevated creatine kinase levels. Biopsy studies performed in a small sample of individuals who experienced statin-associated myalgia have reported abnormal findings in histopathologic structure (e.g., lipid-filled vacuoles and cytochrome oxidase negative myocytes) coupled with reversible changes in muscle strength *(34)*. Myositis is defined as muscle symptoms which occur in concert with elevated muscle enzymes and both symptoms and creatine kinase levels return to normal following discontinuation of the medication.

The most serious statin-associated muscle toxicity is rhabdomyolysis. Rhabdomyolysis, as defined as creatine kinase elevations in excess of 1000 international units with a compatible clinical presentation, occurs in approx 0.1% of patients receiving statin monotherapy, although the risk is increased when statins are coadministered with fibric acid derivatives, nicotinic acid, cyclosporine, or erythromycin. The mechanism involved in statin-induced rhabdomyolysis has not been definitely determined, but may be at least partially related to drug metabolism involving interactions with the cytochrome P450 enzyme systems. However, P450-mediated metabolism does not totally explain statin-mediated myopathy, as cerivastatin has a dual (CYP 3A4 and 2C8) excretory pathway, which would theoretically reduce the risk for myopathy. Cotherapy with gemfibrozil may inhibit glucuronidation of statins, especially cerivastatin, and thereby increase plasma levels of active statin. Another mechanism may involve reduction of intracellular metabolic intermediate compounds such as ubiquinone, which are also generated utilizing the cholesterol biosynthetic pathway. Ubiquinone-deficient muscle cell mitochondria may impair normal cellular metabolism, thereby inducing myopathy. However, muscle biopsy findings in dyslipidemic patients treated with simvastatin revealed no alteration of the skeletal muscle concentration of high-energy phosphates or ubiquinone levels *(35)*.

Ezetimibe. Ezetimibe is the first of a new class of agents that are potent and selective inhibitors of cholesterol absorption *(36)*. The administration of ezetimibe results in binding of cholesterol within the gastrointestinal tract and decreases the delivery of cholesterol to the liver. The resultant decrease in intrahepatic cholesterol results in an upregulation of the LDL receptors and increased clearance of circulating lipoproteins that carry apo B or apo E on their surface. However, the precise mechanism by which ezetimibe reduces cholesterol absorption at the brush border is unclear. A specific transport molecule that facilitates the absorption of cholesterol from bile acid micelles into the brush border of the intestinal villi has been proposed but not isolated. Possibly, ezetimibe may increase cholesterol movement from the enterocyte utilizing the ABCG5/G8 transporter. Ezetimibe has a long half-life, which allows once-per-day dosing. Ezetimibe undergoes rapid and extensive glucuronidation within the intestinal wall and hepatic tissue. Systemic absorption does occur, although it is minimal, which at least partially explains the very low side profile of ezetimibe. Because the primary action of ezetimibe is within the liver, the drug is contraindicated in subjects with active liver disease until further clinical studies have been performed. As opposed to the bile acid resins, ezetimibe does not interact with coumadin, digoxin, glypizide, and oral contraceptives. However, it is typically bound by the resins. The major hypolipidemic effect of ezetimibe is a reduction in LDL-C in the range of 8 to 22%. In individuals who are hyperabsorbers of cholesterol, more dramatic reductions may be observed. Ezetimibe may be used in combination therapy with statins, thus allowing the use of lower statin doses and thereby potentially reducing the risk for side effects.

PHARMACOLOGIC AGENTS PREDOMINANTLY AFFECTING TRIGLYCERIDES AND HDL

Nicotinic Acid. Nicotinic acid is an essential B vitamin that acts as a cofactor in the intermediary metabolism of carbohydrates. When utilized at doses that far exceed those needed to prevent deficiency, nicotinic acid has a complex mechanism of action that favorably modifies all circulating lipoproteins, with the exception of chylomicrons. Nicotinic acid is the only commonly utilized pharmacologic agent that has been able consistently to demonstrate reductions in circulating levels of lipoprotein(a).

Nicotinic acid is generally utilized at a dosing range between 1.5 and 5 g/d and may be expected to reduce LDL-C by up to 25%. Triglyceride levels will fall between 20 and 50% and there is generally a significant rise in HDL-C levels of up to 35%. The use of nicotinic acid has been hampered by its side effect profile, which ranges from mild clinical irritants to life-threatening fulminant hepatic necrosis *(37)*. Cutaneous vasodilation results in the common flushing and pruritis, which is seen early in the administration of nicotinic acid. The flushing is prostaglandin-mediated and may be blunted by pretreatment with aspirin. Nicotinic acid is also associated with a number of gastrointestinal complaints including activation of peptic ulcer disease. Metabolic abnormalities associated with the administration of nicotinic acid include hyperuricemia, which may be associated with the precipitation of gouty arthritis and worsening of glucose tolerance. The most serious side effect associated with the use of nicotinic acid is fulminant hepatic necrosis. Mild elevations of liver enzymes may be seen in up to 5% of people who receive nicotinic acid, but transaminitis is not an absolute indication for cessation of therapy, although close clinical monitoring is warranted.

Fibric Acid Derivatives. The currently available fibric acid derivatives in the United States are clofibrate, gemfibrozil, and fenofibrate, although a number of other agents are available worldwide. The fibric acid derivatives, or fibrates, have a complex mechanism of action that involves agonism of the peroxisome-proliferator-activated receptor α (PPAR-α) that produces a number of lipid-modifying effects *(38)*.

Gemfibrozil has the largest clinical experience in the United States and the hypolipidemic efficacy at the generally utilized dose range of 1200 mg/d results in a decline in triglycerides of 20 to 50% with an associated increase in HDL-C of 10 to 15%. The effect of gemfibrozil on LDL-C is variable and is partially a function of preexisting triglyceride levels and the functional activity of the apo B/E receptor. LDL-C may fall by approx 10 to 15% if the receptor activity is normal. Gemfibrozil may beneficially alter the composition of LDL particles, with a shift from the more atherogenic small, dense LDL phenotype to a larger, buoyant, and presumably less atherogenic form. Fibric acids may also exert beneficial clinical effects by altering a number of hemostatic factors including PAI-I, platelet activity, and fibrinogen.

The adverse effects of the fibric acid derivatives are generally mild and do not require cessation of therapy. The most common side effects of the fibrates are a mild, nonspecific gastrointestinal symptom complex including dyspepsia and nausea. Fibrates have been associated with an increased prevalence of gallstones, although this has not been definitely correlated with other agents. Hepatic and muscle toxicity are uncommon with fibrate monotherapy, although it may be seen with increased incidence when combined with other agents such as the statins. Gemfibrozil, in particular, inhibits glucuronidation of statins, especially cerivastatin, and, therefore, may increase blood levels of active statin *(39)*. Fenofibrate does not appear to share this characteristic to the same degree and therefore may be a hypothetical better partner with statins in combination therapy.

Special Issues

AGE

Improved prevention and treatment of CHD have resulted in a marked decrease in age-adjusted morbidity and mortality for CHD. As a consequence, there has been a progressive shift in the incidence of the first cardiac event to an older age group *(1)*. The first coronary event now occurs in patients over age 65 in 80% of cases and the attributable risk for coronary atherosclerosis increases significantly with age. Clinical trials involving modification of hypertension or dyslipidemia in this group have demonstrated benefits of treatment *(40)*.

Subgroup analyses from the large statin trials reported comparable coronary benefits for subjects both above and below age 65, up to age 70 *(24–28)*. The large-scale Prospective Evaluation of Pravastatin in the Elderly at Risk (PROSPER) trial prospectively evaluated the effect of pravastatin, 40 mg/d, versus placebo on clinical cardiovascular endpoints in 5804 elderly men and women over a 3.2-yr follow-up period *(29)*. The subjects randomized in the PROSPER trial were required to be between 70 and 82 yr old at the time of initiation of therapy. Pravastatin significantly reduced LDL-C (34%) and resulted in a significant reduction in the composite endpoint of coronary death, nonfatal MI, and fatal or nonfatal stroke. The benefits in the PROSPER trial were primarily driven by a reduction in coronary events, which fell by 24%. In this trial, pravastatin did not significantly reduce the risk for stroke, perhaps because of its shorter duration compared with other trials that reported a cerebrovascular benefit with statins.

Patients should not be excluded from the institution of risk factor modification based purely on chronologic age. For older patients, prolonging good health in the remaining years of life may be as important as increasing longevity.

WOMEN

Premenopausal women have a lower incidence of acute MI when compared with age-matched male subjects. However, in the postmenopausal years, LDL-C begins to rise, accompanied by an increase in cardiac event rates. Women tend to have the same modifiable risk factors as men, although diabetes appears to confer a greater risk in women than men and diabetic young women lose the protection associated with their age and sex. Guidelines for hypertension, dyslipidemia, and diabetes management are generally similar for men and women. An expert writing group comprised of a number of US cardiovascular scientific and policy organizations has endorsed an evidence-based set of guidelines for CVD prevention in women *(41)*. Among those recommendations that met the standard of being useful and effective for all women were smoking cessation, a heart-healthy lifestyle, and control of individual risk factors, when present. Aspirin therapy may be useful in intermediate- or high-risk women, but is not recommended for low-risk women. Clinical trials of statins have reported comparable clinical coronary benefits of treatment in women and men and, therefore, may be used in high-risk women regardless of their baseline LDL-C values, unless otherwise contraindicated. Other agents may be used to control LDL-C as well. Based on negative trial findings, hormone replacement therapy cannot be recommended for primary or secondary prevention of CHD in women *(42,43)*.

OBESITY AND METABOLIC SYNDROME

The prevalence of obesity in the US has reached epidemic proportions, and its clinical consequences will have a broad impact on morbidity and mortality rates in the coming decades *(44)*. In ATP III, obesity is not listed as a primary CHD risk factor, because it is not clearly independent and may operate through other risk factors that are included, such as hypertension, hyperlipidemia, decreased HDL-C, and diabetes mellitus. However, obesity should be considered a definite target for intervention, and weight should be optimized.

Adults who are overweight (defined as a body mass index of 25–29.9 kg/m^2) or obese (defined as a body mass index of 30 kg/m^2 or greater) have enhanced cardiovascular risk and an increased prevalence of impaired glucose tolerance, hypertension, dyslipidemia, and clotting abnormalities. More importantly, prospective clinical trials have demonstrated that achievement of ideal body weight may improve the lipid profile, blood pressure, and glucose tolerance *(45)*.

Localization of fat may be a major determinant of the subsequent risk for developing atherosclerosis *(46)*. The male pattern of obesity is characterized by truncal or central adiposity and may be either estimated by the waist-hip circumference ratio or quantitated by computerized tomography. The waist-to-hip ratio is associated with increased cardiovascular risk when it is in excess of 0.95 in men and 0.8 in women. Peripheral fat localization, characteristic of women, appears to be associated with reduced atherosclerotic risk compared with a central fat mass *(47)*.

Obesity is a central feature of metabolic syndrome, which is a common and increasing problem in the United States *(48)*. The diagnosis of metabolic syndrome is controversial and definite clinical criteria have not been universally accepted. However, the majority of individuals with metabolic syndrome are significantly overweight and a variety of clinical studies have documented a high statistical correlation between the characteristics of metabolic syndrome and abdominal obesity.

Table 10
Characteristics of Metabolic Syndrome

Abdominal obesity	Truncal obesity has been recognized as a major defining characteristic of metabolic syndrome and may be characterized by a waist circumference exceeding 40 in. in men and 35 in. in women. Male subjects may manifest multiple risk factors even when the waist circumference is only marginally increased, presumably because of a strong genetically mediated predisposition to insulin resistance. The mechanism by which truncal obesity conveys increased cardiovascular risk is complex but is clearly associated with interrelated metabolic abnormalities including dyslipidemia, hypertension, and hyperinsulinemia. In addition to the abnormal metabolic profile associated with truncal obesity, hemostatic abnormalities have been correlated with increased truncal adiposity, including elevated fibrinogen and PAI-I in combination with reduced t-PA activators.
Hypertriglyceridemia	The defining level for hypertriglyceridemia associated with the metabolic syndrome is in excess or equal to 150 mg/dL (1.69 mmol/L). The hypertriglyceridemia associated with the metabolic syndrome is generally associated with an endogenous overproduction of VLDL by the liver, partially due to increased free fatty acid flux from the peripheral adipocyte. The hypertriglyceridemia in the metabolic syndrome is a combination of over-production coupled with impaired catabolism due to impaired activity of lipoprotein lipase and is phenotypically represented by the lipid triad (elevated triglycerides, low HDL-C, and small, dense LDL particles).
HDL-C	HDL-C is generally decreased in metabolic syndrome. The defining limits are <40 mg/dL (1.03 mmol/L) in men and <50 mg/dL (1.29 mmol/L) in women. The degree of low HDL-C is magnified in individuals with a higher triglyceride concentration. Hypertriglyceridemia and low HDL-C are markers for the presence of small, dense LDL, which is relatively atherogenic because of its increased endothelial permeability, susceptibility to oxidation, and potential cytotoxic effects on the endothelial lining.
Hypertension	Mild hypertension is common in obesity-related metabolic syndrome, and the qualifying level is generally defined as being ≥130 mmHg systolic blood pressure in combination with a ≥85 mmHg diastolic blood pressure.
Fasting glucose	Fasting glucose levels in the range of 110–125 mg/dL is a clinically relevant marker of insulin resistance and is frequently associated with the presence of other metabolic risk factors. Subjects with impaired glucose tolerance frequently develop type 2 diabetes, a CHD risk equivalent.

On clinical grounds, metabolic syndrome may be marked by five major and easily identifiable clinical characteristics (Table 10) (49,50).

A variety of other clinical markers have been associated with the metabolic syndrome but are not routinely clinically evaluated. Metabolic syndrome has been demonstrated to be a proinflammatory state and serum C-reactive protein has been shown to be increased (51). Additionally, the metabolic syndrome is prothrombotic and abnormalities in fibrinogen and PAI-I have also been associated with metabolic syndrome.

In ATP III, metabolic syndrome is diagnosed by the presence of three of the five major clinical criteria (Table 10). Metabolic syndrome is considered an important secondary target of therapy, after control of LDL-C abnormalities. Lifestyle measures such as weight loss and exercise will frequently improve the metabolic parameters and should be vigorously employed. Increased physical activity is associated with improvements in fatty acid oxidation and insulin-stimulated glucose disposal (52). The combination of increased physical activity and weight loss improves metabolic parameters in obese individuals who qualify for insulin resistance syndrome (53). Highly restrictive or ketogenic diets for weight loss in morbidly obese subjects should generally be monitored by an obesity specialist, because of a variety of metabolic and electrolyte problems that may be induced.

Although TLC and increased physical activity are the primary recommended modes for obesity management, surgery and pharmacologic therapies have gained attention. Both are controversial. Dexfenfluramine hydrochloride and fenfluramine hydrochloride were voluntarily withdrawn from the market because of their potential association with the induction of cardiac valvular abnormalities. Meta-analysis of 11 orlistat trials and three sibutramine trials reported attrition rates of 33% and 48%, respectively *(54)*. Both treatments were associated with reduced weight after 1 yr of follow-up, with 12% of orlistat and 15% of sibutramine patients achieving a 10% or greater weight loss. Orlistat caused gastrointestinal side effects while sibutramine therapy was associated with an increase in both blood pressure and pulse rate. Conclusive and methodologically rigorous studies that evaluate clinical endpoints such as cardiovascular morbidity and mortality have not been performed with the anorectic drugs.

DIABETES

Both Type I and Type II diabetes are associated with increased cardiovascular risk and a number of epidemiologic trials have demonstrated vascular disease to be the major cause of morbidity and mortality in diabetic subjects. Diabetic subjects who suffer an acute MI have a significant peri-infarction morbidity and mortality when compared with nondiabetic controls. Women with diabetes lose the protection from CHD conferred by their sex and also have a higher post-MI complication rate compared with men. Based on these kinds of data, diabetes falls into the CHD-equivalent risk category and therefore, patients with this disorder should receive as aggressive risk reduction as those with preexisting CHD.

In addition to the abnormal carbohydrate metabolism (which correlates with microvascular disease such as retinopathy and neuropathy), other risk factors including obesity, dyslipidemia, and hypertension frequently cluster in patients with diabetes. In the United States, diabetes is an increasingly prevalent condition with 29 million individuals (14.4% of the population) having either diagnosed diabetes, undiagnosed diabetes, or impaired glucose tolerance *(55)*. Moreover, a number of individuals may not satisfy strict criteria for the diagnosis of diabetes, but demonstrate peripheral insulin resistance with either normal or minimally elevated glucose levels and associated hyperinsulinemia. Elevated insulin levels have been determined to be an independent cardiac risk factor for vascular disease and also may be involved in the pathogenesis of hypertension, because of stimulation of vascular smooth muscle cell growth, and sympathetic activation and increased sodium reabsorption by the renal tubules.

Dyslipidemia characterized by borderline elevations of triglycerides associated with low levels of HDL-C and increased levels of small, dense LDL is common in diabetic individuals. While weight loss, exercise, and glycemic control may improve the lipid abnormalities in diabetics, metabolic parameters may not normalize. Although treatment of the carbohydrate abnormality in diabetes has been shown to decrease the risk for microvascular complications, glucose control does not decrease macrovascular atherosclerotic events. On the other hand, subgroup analyses from the large trials of lipid modification have suggested no heterogeneity of benefit between diabetic and nondiabetic participants. The Medical Research Clinic/British Heart Foundation Heart Protection Study (HPS) was a large-scale trial of 20,536 subjects who were considered to be at high risk for atherosclerosis, but who fell into categories that lacked definitive clinical trial evidence of benefit. The HPS study prospectively evaluated the role of lipid lowering in 5963 diabetic subjects between the ages of 40 and 80 yr. Subjects who fit standard criteria for diabetes were randomized to receive 40 mg of simvastatin versus a matching placebo. Simvastatin therapy achieved an LDL-C difference between the diabetic and control populations of 39 mg/dL (1.01 mmol/L), despite the fact that a progressively increasing number of subjects randomized to placebo began lipid-lowering therapy during the trial. Simvastatin therapy resulted in a significant reduction in the incidence of first major ischemic event and provided definite clinical evidence of the benefits of lipid lowering in the diabetic subjects *(58)*.

On the basis of both prospective and *post hoc* analysis of clinical trials, experts recommend aggressive LDL-C lowering (to <100 mg/dL [2.59 mmol/L]) in diabetic patients with or without

CHD, in concert with optimization of blood glucose, blood pressure, body weight, and exercise levels in an attempt to decrease subsequent risk for coronary atherosclerosis. Based on HPS, the American Diabetes Association recommends that statin therapy to achieve an LDL-C reduction of approx 30% regardless of baseline LDL levels may be appropriate *(59)*. For diabetic patients with hypertriglyceridemia, glycemic control will help normalize undesirable levels, although a fibrate or niacin may be considered if the abnormality persists after optimal glycemic control. Doctors should exercise their clinical judgment. Besides behavioral interventions, low doses of nicotinic acid (≤ 2 g nicotinic acid/d) to minimize the risk for worsened glucose tolerance or fibrates may be used to increase HDL-C levels.

SUMMARY

Major advances have been made over the past decade in the identification and management of patients who have or are at risk for atherosclerosis, and CVD prevention has become a major theme in clinical practice. Despite the progress made, much more can be done to promote the serious application of preventive strategies to all at-risk patients. Approaches to risk factor modification are continually being refined, particularly in the pharmacologic ability to alter blood pressure, dyslipidemia, and other factors felt to be involved in atherogenesis. The promise of the growing pharmacopoeia of cardiovascular drugs, however, does not negate the need to emphasize greater adoption of a heart-healthy lifestyle at both the individual and population-wide levels. Physicians must consider themselves at the front line of this kind of advocacy. Epidemiological data from the National Health and Nutrition Examination Surveys have demonstrated progressive declines in total cholesterol values in US birth cohorts across several decades, across the distribution of subjects' cholesterol values. At the higher end of the distribution, the decline is probably associated with improvements in acute interventions to lower cholesterol, while at the lower end of the distribution, the decline may reflect the impact of population-wide preventive efforts *(60)*. These successes suggest that the current approach to risk management is in the right direction and should prompt further action toward improvement.

REFERENCES

1. American Heart Association. Heart and stroke facts: 2004 statistical supplement. Dallas: American Heart Association, 2003.
2. Expert Panel on Detection, Evaluation and Treatment of High Blood Cholesterol in Adults: Executive summary of the third report of the National Cholesterol Education Program (NCEP). Expert Panel on the Detection, Evaluation and Treatment of High Blood Cholesterol in Adults (Adult Treatment Panel III). JAMA 2001;285:2486–2497.
3. Swanson JR, Pearson TA. Screening family members at high risk for coronary disease. Why isn't it done? Am J Prev Med 2001;20:50–55.
4. Chobanian AV, Bakris GL, Black HR, et al., and the National High Blood Pressure Education Program Coordinating Committee. The Seventh Report of the Joint National Committee on Prevention, Detection, Evaluation, and Treatment of High Blood Pressure: The JNC 7 Report. JAMA 2003;289:2560–2571.
5. ALLHAT Officers and Coordinators for the ALLHAT Collaborative Research Group. The Antihypertensive and Lipid Lowering Treatment to Prevent Heart Attack Trial. Major outcomes in high-risk hypertensive patients randomized to angiotensin converting enzyme inhibitor or calcium channel blocker versus diuretic. The Antihypertensive and Lipid Lowering Treatment to Prevent Heart Attack Trial (ALLHAT). JAMA 2002;288:2981–2997.
6. Giovino GA. Epidemiology of tobacco use in the United States. Oncogene 2002;21:7326–7340.
7. Senti M, Elosua R, Tomas M, et al. Physical activity modulates the combined effect of a common variant of the lipoprotein lipase gene and smoking on serum triglyceride levels and high density lipoprotein cholesterol in men. Hum Genet 2001;109:385–392.
8. Jastrzebska M, Goracy I, Naruszewicz M. Relationships between fibrinogen, plasminogen activator inhibitor-1, and their gene polymorphisms in current smokers with essential hypertension. Thromb Res 2003;110:339–344.
9. Critchley JA, Capewell S. Mortality risk reduction associated with smoking cessation in patients with CHD: a systematic review. JAMA 2003;290:86–97.
10. Kannel WB. Range of serum cholesterol values in the population developing CHD. Am J Cardiol 1995;76(9 Suppl):69C–77C.
11. Gotto A, Pownall H. The Manual of Lipid Disorders: Reducing the Risk for Coronary Heart Disease, 3rd ed. Lippincott Williams & Wilkins, New York, 2003.

12. Fojo SS, Brewer HB. Hypertriglyceridaemia due to genetic defects in lipoprotein lipase and apolipoprotein C-II. J Intern Med 1992;231:669–677.
13. Segrest JT. The role of non-LDL-C:non-HDL particles in atherosclerosis. Current Diabetes Reports 2002;2:282–288.
14. Gotto AM Jr, Brinton EA. Assessing low levels of high-density lipoprotein cholesterol as a risk factor in coronary heart disease: a working group report and update. J Am Coll Cardiol 2004;3:717–724.
15. Nissen SE, Tsunoda T, Tuzcu EM, et al. Effect of recombinant ApoA-I Milano on coronary atherosclerosis in patients with acute coronary syndromes: a randomized controlled trial. JAMA 2003;290:2292–2300.
16. Pearson TA, Mensah GA, Alexander RW, et al. AHA/CDC scientific statement markers of inflammation and cardiovascular disease application to clinical and public health practice: a statement for healthcare professionals from the centers for disease control and prevention and the american heart association. Circulation 2003;107:499–511.
17. Ryan TJ, Antman EM, Brooks NH, et al. 1999 Update: ACC/AHA guidelines for the management of patients with acute MI. A report of the American College of Cardiology/American Heart Association Task Force on Practice Guidelines (Committee on Management of Acute Myocardial Infarction). Circulation 1999;100:1016–1030.
18. Grundy SM, Cleeman JI, Merz CN, et al. Implications of recent clinical trials for the National Cholesterol Education Program Adult Treatment Panel III guidelines. Circulation 2004;110:227–239.
19. Heart Protection Study Collaborative Group. MRC/BHF Heart Protection Study of cholesterol lowering with simvastatin in 2,536 high risk individuals: a randomized placebo-controlled trial. Lancet 2002;360:7–22.
20. Thompson PD, Lim D. Physical activity in the prevention of atherosclerotic CHD. Curr Treat Options Cardiovasc Med 2003;5:279–285.
21. Williams PT. The relationship of heart disease risk factors to exercise quantity and intensities. Arch Int Med 1998;158:237–245.
22. Rothenbacher D, Hoffmeister A, Brenner H, Koenig W. Physical activity, coronary heart disease and inflammatory response. Arch Int Med 2003;163:1200–1205.
23. Bays H, Dujovne C. Colesevelam: a nonsystemic lipid altering drug. Expert Opin Pharmaco Ther 2003;4:779–790.
24. Downs JR, Clearfield M, Weis S, et al., for the AFCAPS/TexCAPS Research Group. Primary prevention of acute coronary events with lovastatin in men and women with average cholesterol levels. Results of AFCAPS/TexCAPS. JAMA 1998;279:1615–1622.
25. Sacks FM, Pfeffer MA, Moye LA, et al., for the Cholesterol and Recurrent Events Trial Investigators. The effect of pravastatin on coronary events after MI in patients with average cholesterol levels. N Engl J Med 1996;335:1001–1009.
26. Shepherd J, Cobbe SM, Ford I, et al., for the West of Scotland Coronary Prevention Study Group. Prevention of CHD with pravastatin in men with hypercholesterolemia. N Engl J Med 1995;333:1301–1307.
27. Scandinavian Simvastatin Survival Study Group. Randomised trial of cholesterol lowering in 4444 patients with CHD: the Scandinavian Simvastatin Survival Study (4S). Lancet 1994;344:1383–1389.
28. The Long-Term Intervention with Pravastatin in Ischaemic Disease (LIPID) Study Group. Prevention of cardiovascular events and death with pravastatin in patients with CHD and a broad range of initial cholesterol levels. N Engl J Med 1998;339:1349–1357.
29. Shepherd J, Blauw JG, Murphy MD, et al. The PROSPER Study Group. Pravastatin in elderly subjects at risk of vascular disease (PROSPER): a randomized controlled trial. Lancet 2002;360:1623–1630.
30. Sever PS, Dahlof B, Poulter NR, et al., for the ASCOT investigators. Prevention of coronary and stroke events with atorvastatin in hypertensive patients who have average or lower-than-average cholesterol concentrations, in the Anglo-Scandinavian Cardiac Outcomes Trial—Lipid Lowering Arm (ASCOT-LLA): a multicentre randomised controlled trial. Lancet 2003;361:1149–1158.
31. Thompson PD, Clarkson P, Karas RH. Statin-associated myopathy. JAMA 2003;289:1682–1690.
32. Roberts WC. The rule of 5 and the rule of 7 in lipid-lowering by statin drugs. Am J Cardiol 1997;80:106–107.
33. Bradford RH, Schear CL, Chremos AN. Expanded Clinical Evaluation of Lovastatin (EXCEL) study results. I. Efficacy in modified plasma lipoproteins and adverse event profile in 8,245 patients with moderate hypercholesterolemia. Arch Int Med 1991;151:43–50.
34. Phillips PS, Haas RH, Bannykh S, et al. Statin associated myopathy with normal creatine kinase levels. Ann Intern Med 2002;137:581–585.
35. Laaksonen R. The effect of simvastatin treatment on natural antioxidants in low-density lipoproteins and high-energy phosphates and ubiquinone in skeletal muscle. Am J Cardiol 1996;77:851–854.
36. Bruckert E, Giral P, Tellier P. Perspectives in cholesterol lowering therapy: the role of ezetimibe, a new selective inhibitor of intestinal cholesterol absorption. Circulation 2003;107:3124–3128.
37. Rader JI, Calvert RJ, Habcock JN. Hepatic toxicity of unmodified and time-released preparations of niacin. Am J Med 1992;92:77–81.
38. Lee CH, Olson T, Evans RM. Lipid metabolism, metabolic diseases and peroxisome proliferator-activated receptors. Endocrinology 2003;144:2001–2007.
39. Prueksaritanont T, Tang C, Qiu Y, et al. Effects of fibrates on metabolism of statins in human hepatocytes. Drug Metab Dispos 2002;30:1280–1287.
40. SHEP Cooperative Research Group. Prevention of stroke by antihypertensive drug therapy in older persons with isolated systolic hypertension: final results of the Systolic Hypertension in the Elderly Program (SHEP). JAMA 1991;265:3255–3261.
41. Mosca L. Summary of the American Heart Association's Evidence-Based Guidelines for Cardiovascular Disease Prevention in Women. Arterioscler Thromb Vasc Biol 2004;24:394–396.

42. Hulley S, Grady D, Bush T, et al. Randomized trial of estrogen plus progestin for secondary prevention of coronary heart disease in post menopausal women. Heart and Estrogen/Progestin Replacement Study (HERS Research Group). JAMA 1998;280:605–613.
43. Writing Group for the Women's Health Initiative Investigators. Risks and benefit of estrogen plus progestin in healthy post menopausal women: principal results from the Women's Health Initiative randomized controlled trial. JAMA 2002;288:321–333.
44. Ford ES, Mokdad AH, Giles WH. Trends in waist circumference among US adults. Obes Res 2003;11:1223–1231.
45. Pasanisi F, Contaldo F, de Simone G, Mancini M. Benefits of sustained moderate weight loss in obesity. Nutr Metab Cardiovasc Dis 2001;11:401–406.
46. Bonora E, Zenere M, Branzi P, et al. Influence of body fat and its regional localization on risk factors for atherosclerosis in young men. Am J Epidemiol 1992;135:1271–1278.
47. Tanko LB, Bagger YZ, Alexandersen P, et al. Peripheral adiposity exhibits an independent dominant antiatherogenic effect in elderly women. Circulation 2003;107:1626–1631.
48. Ford ES, Giles WH, Dietz WH. Prevalence of the metabolic syndrome among US adults: findings from the third National Health and Nutrition Examination Survey. JAMA 2002;287:356–359.
49. Grundy SM, Hansen B, Smith SC Jr, et al. American Heart Association; National Heart, Lung, and Blood Institute; American Diabetes Association. Clinical management of metabolic syndrome: report of the American Heart Association/National Heart, Lung, and Blood Institute/American Diabetes Association conference on scientific issues related to management. Circulation 2004;109:551–556.
50. Grundy SM, Brewer HB Jr, Cleeman JI, et al. American Heart Association; National Heart, Lung, and Blood Institute. Definition of metabolic syndrome: report of the National Heart, Lung, and Blood Institute/American Heart Association conference on scientific issues related to definition. Circulation 2004;109:433–438.
51. Grundy SM. Inflammation, metabolic syndrome, and diet responsiveness. Circulation 2003;108:126–128.
52. Goodpaster BH, Katsiaras A, Kelley DE. Enhanced fat oxidation through physical activity is associated with improvement in insulin sensitivity and obesity. Diabetes 2003;52:2191–2197.
53. Hamdy O, Ledbury S, Mullooly C, et al. Lifestyle modification improves endothelial function in obese subjects with the insulin resistance syndrome. Diabetes Care 2003;26:2119–2125.
54. Padwal R, Li SK, Lau DC. Long-term pharmacotherapy for overweight and obesity: a systematic review and meta-analysis of randomized controlled trials. Int J Obes 2003;27:1437–1446.
55. Morbidity and Mortality Weekly Report. Prevalence of diabetes and impaired glucose tolerance in adults—United States, 1999–2003;52:833–837.
56. Pyorala K, Pedersen TR, Kjekshus J, et al. Cholesterol lowering with simvastatin improves prognosis of diabetic patients with CHD. A subgroup analysis of the 4S study. Diabetes Care 1997;20:614–620.
57. Sacks FM, Tonkin AM, Craven T, et al. CHD in patients with low LDL-C: benefits of pravastatin in diabetics and enhanced role for HDL-C and triglycerides as risk factors. Circulation 2002;105:1424–1428.
58. Collins R, Armitage J, Parish S, et al. Heart Protection Study Collaborative Group. MRC/BHF Heart Protection Study of cholesterol lowering with simvastatin in 5,963 people with diabetes: a randomized, placebo-controlled trial. Lancet 2003;361:205–216.
59. American Diabetes Association. Dyslipidemia management in adults with diabetes. Diabetes Care 2004;27:S68–S71.
60. Goff DC Jr, Labarthe DR, Howard G, Russell GB. Primary prevention of high blood cholesterol concentrations in the United States. Arch Intern Med 2002;162:913–919.

RECOMMENDED READING

Expert Panel on Detection, Evaluation and Treatment of High Blood Cholesterol in Adults: Executive summary of the third report of the National Cholesterol Education Program (NCEP). Expert Panel on the Detection, Evaluation and Treatment of High Blood Cholesterol in Adults (Adult Treatment Panel III). JAMA 2001;285:2486–2497.

Chobanian AV, Bakris GL, Black HR, et al., and the National High Blood Pressure Education Program Coordinating Committee. The Seventh Report of the Joint National Committee on Prevention, Detection, Evaluation, and Treatment of High Blood Pressure: The JNC 7 Report. JAMA 2003;289:2560–2571.

Gotto A, Pownall H. The manual of lipid disorders: reducing the risk for coronary heart disease (3rd ed.). Lippincott Williams & Wilkins, New York, 2003.

Pearson TA, Mensah GA, Alexander RW, et al. AHA/CDC Scientific Statement Markers of Inflammation and Cardiovascular Disease Application to Clinical and Public Health Practice: A Statement for Healthcare Professionals From the Centers for Disease Control and Prevention and the American Heart Association. Circulation 2003;107:499–511.

Grundy SM, Hansen B, Smith SC Jr, Cleeman JI, Kahn RA. American Heart Association; National Heart, Lung, and Blood Institute; American Diabetes Association. Clinical management of metabolic syndrome: report of the American Heart Association/National Heart, Lung, and Blood Institute/American Diabetes Association conference on scientific issues related to management. Circulation 2004;109:551–556.

24 Coronary Blood Flow and Myocardial Ischemia

Robert J. Henning, MD *and Ray A. Olsson,* MD

INTRODUCTION

Technical advances over the past few years now enable clinicians to measure coronary blood flow velocity *(1)* and myocardial perfusion *(2)*. Such measurements confirm in humans the concepts of coronary physiology developed through animal investigations. This chapter summarizes important coronary physiological principles as the basis for discussing myocardial ischemia.

PHASIC CORONARY FLOW *(3)*

Instantaneous flow through epicardial coronary arteries varies throughout the cardiac cycle in a way that reflects the interaction of aortic perfusion pressure and the massaging action of the myocardium as an intramyocardial pump. Under basal conditions flow to the left ventricle is antegrade throughout the cardiac cycle, but flow in diastole is substantially greater than in systole. Sixty to 80% of left coronary inflow is during ventricular diastole. This unique feature of the coronary circulation is exploited by the inflation of an intraaortic balloon during ventricular diastole in patients with cardiac pump failure due to myocardial infarction or heart failure in order to augment diastolic coronary perfusion. Conversely, increases in heart rate decrease the duration of diastole and increase myocardial oxygen requirements and can lead to myocardial ischemia in patients with occlusive coronary artery disease.

The lower left coronary flow rate in systole, when perfusion pressure is higher than in diastole, is due to the massaging action of the myocardium. Cardiac contraction does not simply hinder forward blood flow; rather, it actively pumps blood backward, reducing antegrade systolic flow through the intramural coronary arteries. Increasing cardiac contractility—for example, by cardiac β-adrenergic receptor stimulation—can reverse systolic flow, which provides evidence of an intramyocardial pump rather than a throttle mechanism, which would only lower flow to zero. Studies that employ intracoronary Doppler wires also show reversal of systolic flow with microvascular obstruction after myocardial infarction *(4)*. Here the intramyocardial pump can only eject blood back into the arterial side of the circulation. The effect of systole is especially important in patients with severe aortic valvular or subvalvular stenosis and in patients with severe aortic regurgitation, where systolic intramyocardial pressure can exceed coronary perfusion pressure.

Phasic flow in epicardial coronary arteries supplying the right ventricle differs from flow in arteries supplying the left ventricle, again reflecting an interaction between perfusion pressure and myocardial pumping. Wall stress in the right ventricle is much lower than in the left ventricle and, consequently, mean flow rate in the right coronary artery in systole is higher than in diastole. Diseases that increase right ventricular wall stress—for example, pulmonic stenosis or pulmonary hypertension—alter the phasic flow pattern such that coronary flow during systole is low or even retrograde, resembling that in arteries supplying the left ventricle.

From: *Essential Cardiology: Principles and Practice, 2nd Ed.*
Edited by: C. Rosendorff © Humana Press Inc., Totowa, NJ

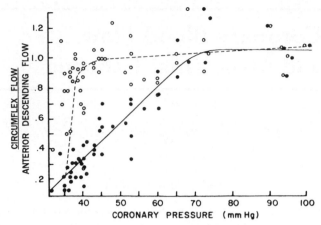

Fig. 1. Coronary autoregulation and autoregulatory reserve. Radiomicrosphere measurements of regional myocardial perfusion in the subendocardial (*closed circles*) and subepicardial (*open* circles) layers of left ventricle
supplied by the left circumflex coronary artery of a dog, normalized by reference to perfusion in the corresponding layers of myocardium supplied by the left anterior descending coronary artery. Controlled constriction of
the circumflex branch lowered perfusion pressure. Autoregulatory reserve is high in the epicardium, flow being
independent of pressure above 40 mmHg. By contrast, autoregulatory reserve in the subepicardium is lower,
perfusion becoming pressure-dependent below about 70 mmHg.

Coronary blood flow is regulated by vascular myogenic mechanisms that constrict coronary
smooth muscle in response to increases in perfusion pressure and dilate vascular muscle in response
to decreases in coronary perfusion pressure. The basal resistance is higher in the coronary circulation than in any other vascular bed. The relatively low coronary perfusion rate is the consequence
of high basal coronary tone. Basal coronary flow rate, 50 to 100 mL/min/100 g, is much lower than
flow to the kidney, which is approx 400 mL/min/100 g. Myogenic tone is the basis for coronary
artery autoregulation, the tendency for coronary perfusion to remain constant over perfusion pressures between about 45 and 150 mmHg (Fig. 1). Below or above the autoregulatory range coronary
perfusion is pressure-dependent. There is a transmural gradient of autoregulatory capacity in the
coronary circulation that diminishes from the epicardium, where autoregulation begins to fail at
a perfusion pressure of approx 40 mmHg, to the endocardium, where failure begins at approx 70
mmHg *(5)*. This gradient explains the vulnerability of the subendocardium to ischemia at reduced
perfusion pressures.

MYOCARDIAL PERFUSION AND METABOLISM

The major determinants of myocardial oxygen demand are myocardial tension, which is determined by left ventricular systolic pressure and ventricular radius, myocardial contractility, and
heart rate. The constant activity of the beating heart demands an oxygen consumption of 5 to 10 mL
O_2/min/100 g under basal conditions, which is significantly higher than in the brain, ~4 mL/min/
100 g, or skeletal muscle, ~0.2 mL/min/100 g. Although the heart can use carbohydrates and
amino acids as fuels, the oxidation of fatty acids accounts for at least two thirds of cardiac oxygen
consumption.

In the normal heart, an increase in myocardial tension, contractility, or heart rate results in an
increase in oxygen demand that is matched by an increase in coronary artery blood flow and oxygen delivery. The relationship between coronary blood flow and myocardial oxygen demand in
the normal heart is linear over a broad range of coronary blood flows from approx 10 to 600 mL/
min/100 g of myocardial tissue. Under normal conditions, coronary flow per gram in the subendocardium is 10 to 30% greater than flow in the subepicardium because the subendocardium utilizes
more oxygen than the subepicardium. The close coupling between myocardial oxygen consump-

tion and coronary blood flow is adjusted on a second-by-second basis in the normal heart. This relationship is the dominant mechanism that regulates coronary blood flow.

The combination of a high oxygen demand and high basal coronary resistance causes a high transcoronary oxygen extraction, which is usually 65 to 80%, and a low coronary venous PO_2, of ~ 20 mmHg, which is at an inflection point in the oxyhemoglobin saturation curve. Consequently, the increase in thermodynamic work required to deoxygenate oxyhemoglobin limits further oxygen extraction, so that increasing coronary flow is the predominant response to increased myocardial oxygen demand.

Measurement of Myocardial Perfusion

Although measurements of flow in epicardial arteries provide some information about the status of myocardial perfusion, they are of limited use in defining the regional distribution of flow and identifying areas of underperfusion. Owing to rapid recirculation of indicator that obscures the latter portion of an indicator dilution curve, the Stuart-Hamilton technique is inapplicable to measurements of coronary flow. However, this measurement is accomplished by another method based on the Fick principle. In brief, an indicator injected into the circulation will deposit in tissue in proportion to local flow rate. The first studies of this sort used ^{40}K or its surrogate ^{81}Rb and depended on cellular uptake of those isotopes. Today, myocardial perfusion imaging (Chapter 13), a descendant of this technique, uses another potassium surrogate, ^{201}Tl, or alternatively ^{99m}Tc-sestamibi.

Heterogeneity of Coronary Flow and Myocardial Metabolism

Under normal physiological conditions there is a transmural gradient of regional perfusion and oxygen consumption. In the subepicardium, perfusion rate and oxygen consumption are ~55 mL/min/100 g and ~6.4 mL/min/100 g, respectively. Because wall stress is higher in the subendocardium, both perfusion and oxygen consumption are higher, ~70 mL/100 g/min and ~10 mL/min/100 g. Consequently, the subendocardium is more vulnerable to myocardial ischemia due to coronary obstructive disease. A reduction of coronary flow by 40% can decrease the endocardial to epicardial flow ratio by as much as 60 to 70%. Left ventricular hypertrophy or left heart failure can further reduce the endocardial to epicardial flow ratio due to increases in left ventricular end-diastolic and intramyocardial pressure. The effects of left ventricular hypertrophy are especially significant in patients with severe aortic stenosis, where intramyocardial pressure and intraventricular pressure are much higher than aortic and coronary perfusion pressures. In these patients, the restriction of nutrient coronary flow to the endocardium can produce symptoms of myocardial ischemia in the absence of any significant occlusive coronary artery disease. In patients with acute myocardial infarction, raising aortic diastolic pressure by intraaortic balloon counterpulsation can increase subendocardial blood flow.

The regional differences described above reflect averages over the perfusion fields supplied by large numbers of resistance vessels. Nevertheless, myocardial metabolism parallels regional perfusion and perfusion–metabolism matching occurs despite regional differences in myocardial perfusion.

Coronary Flow Reserve

Coronary flow reserve (CFR), the capacity to increase coronary flow over basal levels, is normally about threefold in sedentary adults but can be sixfold in world-class endurance athletes. CFR is a useful way to assess the physiological impact of coronary stenosis and the outcome of revascularization by coronary angioplasty or coronary artery bypass surgery. With either a pressure-monitoring or Doppler flow velocity wire one can measure the maximum pressure or coronary flow in comparison with the aortic response to the systemic administration of a vasodilator such as adenosine. Obstructions reducing coronary luminal diameter by less than 40% do not affect CFR, but reductions of >80% exhaust vasodilatory reserve *(6)*. Coronary lesions less than 80% may show a poor vasodilatory reserve response and therefore are candidates for angioplasty. Although the pressure and flow methods appear to have equivalent clinical value, the pressure measurements give additional

Table 1
Mechanisms of Coronary Flow Regulation

Mechanism	Definition	Target coronary vessel
Endothelial	Vasoactivity of nitric oxide, endothelin, prostaglandins	Arteries; arterioles 80–150 μm
Metabolic	Vasoactivity of metabolites such as adenosine	Arterioles 25–100 μm
Myogenic	Vascular smooth muscle contraction and relaxation in response to rises and falls in intraluminal pressure	Arterioles 50–100 μm
Neurohumoral	Vasoactivity of neurotransmitters released from autonomic nerves, receptors, or circulating in the blood	Arterioles 140–300 μm arteries

(From Feliciano L and Henning RJ. Clin Cardiol 1999;22:775–786; with permission from Clinical Cardiology Publishing Company, Inc., Mahwah, NJ.)

information. Coronary artery "wedge" pressure distal to an inflated angioplasty balloon is normally less than 25% of aortic pressure; higher pressures reflect coronary collateral development *(7)*.

REGULATION OF CORONARY FLOW

Coronary blood flow is regulated by myogenic vascular tone and endogenous vasoactive drugs (Table 1). Myogenic tone, the contraction of vascular smooth muscle in response to the distending force of intraluminal pressure, is due to the activation of a vascular smooth muscle cell volume-activated cation current *(8)* and, secondarily, a Ca^{2+}-activated K^+ current *(9)*. Although the two currents have opposite effects on contractile state, the predominance of the cation current at physiological membrane potentials results in vascular smooth muscle contraction. Important modifiers of coronary artery basal tone include endothelium-generated nitric oxide (NO) and endogenous metabolites such as adenosine.

The shear stress exerted on endothelial cells by flowing blood is the preponderant stimulus for the release of calcium from internal stores that initiates production of the endogenous vasodilator nitric oxide (Fig. 2). Several G protein-coupled receptors also activate endothelial nitric oxide synthase (eNOS). NO-initiated vasodilation is an important target for drug therapy; indeed, the activity of nitrovasodilators depends on the release of NO. Phosphodiesterase (PDE) inhibitors such as sildenafil (Viagra) act by preserving cGMP, thus prolonging NO signaling and vasodilation. Conversely, NOS inhibitors raise vascular resistance and provide additional evidence that NO participates in setting basal coronary tone.

When myocardial oxygen demand exceeds oxygen supply, there is a net breakdown of ATP in myocardial cells and the release of adenosine into the interstitial space, where it produces coronary arteriolar dilation. Adenosine is generated by three hydrolytic processes *(10)*: (1) intracellular AMP by a cytosolic 5'-nucleotidase, (2) intracellular *S*-adenosylhomocysteine by the action of a specific hydrolase, and (3) from the action of an *ecto*-phosphatase cascade on ATP extruded from cells. Adenosine also comes from ATP in adrenergic nerve terminals, where it is copackaged with neurotransmitter in secretory granules. Coronary endothelial cells take up adenosine avidly and incorporate it into the cellular adenylate pool, thus acting as an "endothelial barrier" to the loss of purines. This salvage pathway is important in the heart, which has a very limited capacity for *de novo* purine synthesis. Adenosine produces coronary artery dilation through stimulation of vascular muscle adenosine A_2 receptors. Stimulation of these receptors activates adenylyl cyclase to produce cAMP. Increases in cAMP decrease intracellular calcium and the affinity of vascular muscle myosin light chain kinase for calcium, thereby relaxing vascular muscle.

The activation of outward potassium currents in coronary smooth muscle cells appears to be a key event in coronary vasodilation initiated by nitric oxide, adenosine, and other vasodilators that act through G protein-coupled receptors. These currents hyperpolarize the myocyte cell membrane, raising the threshold for the calcium current (I_{Ca}) that contributes to vasoconstrictor tone.

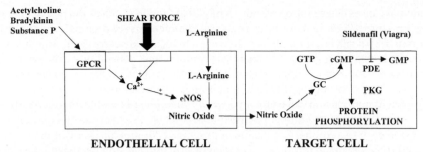

Fig. 2. Nitric oxide formation from L-arginine in endothelial cells. eNOS, endothelial (constitutive) nitric oxide synthase; GC, guanylate cyclase; GPCR, G protein-coupled receptor; cGMP, cyclic guanosine-3',5'-monophosphate; GMP, guanosine-5'-monophosphate; GTP, guanosine-5'-triphosphate; PDE, cyclic nucleotide phosphodiesterase; PKG, cGMP-dependent protein kinase.

Which of the several types of channel mediates vasodilation seems to depend on the stimulus. For example, nitric oxide acts through both the large conductance, Ca^{2+}-activated ($I_{K,Ca}$), and delayed rectifier (I_{Kdrf}) potassium channels, but adenosine acts primarily through the sulfonylurea-sensitive (K_{ATP}) channel.

Nitric oxide and adenosine act at different levels in the coronary microcirculation. Nitric oxide acts at larger pre-resistance vessels while adenosine acts at the level of the true resistance vessels with diameters of 100 μm or less. Small imbalances between oxygen supply and demand generate adenosine, which dilates the resistance vessels. The resulting increases of flow and pulsatile shear stress on the endothelium of preresistance vessels generates nitric oxide, thus amplifying the effect of adenosine. Disordered coronary regulation or "endothelial dysfunction" is important in patients with hyperlipidemias, atherosclerosis, and diabetes mellitus, where there is decreased responsiveness to endothelium-dependent vasodilation. Each of the several explanations advanced to account for decreased vasodilator reserve in these patients has partial support, and, indeed, the pathogenesis is probably multifactorial. Proposed mechanisms include destruction of nitric oxide through increased production of superoxide, interference with G protein-mediated signaling by lipid oxidation, decreased membrane fluidity, and depletion of the NOS cofactor tetrahydrobiopterin. In some clinical trials of patients with coronary endothelial dysfunction, dietary supplementation with L-arginine, the precursor of nitric oxide, improved coronary endothelium-dependent responses.

The coronary arteries are richly innervated with autonomic fibers, and both sympathetic and parasympathetic nerves participate in flow regulation. Whereas α-adrenergic receptors mediate vasoconstriction, muscarinic and α-adrenergic receptors initiate vasodilation. However, coronary vasodilation caused by stimulation of sympathetic efferent nerves is principally a consequence of increased cardiac contractility and metabolism rather than a direct effect on the coronary vessels. Similarly, the blockade of coronary α-adrenergic receptors has no effect on basal coronary flow, indicating that these receptors do not participate in setting basal tone. However, stimuli such as exercise do not usually cause maximum coronary vasodilation because exercise evokes coronary α-adrenergic vasoconstrictor tone. The increase in adrenergic tone during exercise is not transmural. Rather, because coronary sympathetic fibers extend only partway into the ventricular wall, vasoconstriction is subepicardial and shunts blood preferentially to subendocardium.

In addition to classical neurotransmitters released during nerve stimulation, cotransmitters such as vasoactive intestinal peptide and ATP probably also contribute to coronary vasomotion.

MYOCARDIAL ISCHEMIA

The heart's high workload and dependence on oxidative metabolism makes the myocardium extremely vulnerable to ischemia. For example, the occlusion of a major coronary artery in an experimental animal causes deterioration of indices of global function such as the rate of change of left ventricular pressure (*dP/dt*) in 3 to 5 heart beats and complete loss of regional contractile function in about 1 min. Cell death is not immediate, however; myocardial necrosis requires at least 15 min of ischemia. The adaptive response to ischemia is complex and, depending on the *degree* and *duration* of hypoperfusion, can be either deleterious or cardioprotective. *Angina pectoris* is a clinical manifestation of transient myocardial ischemia. Either a coronary occlusion of short duration or transient global hypoperfusion can cause *myocardial stunning*, reversible contractile dysfunction lasting hours to days after restoration of perfusion. In contrast, brief periods of coronary occlusion and reperfusion prior to a coronary occlusion of prolonged duration markedly reduces infarct size and is termed *ischemic preconditioning*. Subtotal obstruction causing persistent and often insufficient coronary flow can produce chronic, reversible contractile dysfunction termed *myocardial hibernation*. In some patients chronic, progressive coronary narrowing serves as a stimulus for the development of *coronary collaterals* that preserve perfusion in potentially ischemic myocardium.

Angina Pectoris (11)

Adenosine release from underperfused myocardium formerly was thought to be a marker of myocardial ischemia but coincidental to the chest pain of angina pectoris. The observation that patients receiving adenosine for myocardial perfusion scans experience chest pain similar in character to angina suggested that adenosine might actually trigger the pain. Subsequent studies have shown that adenosine infused into peripheral arteries is algogenic, causing pain in the perfusion field of the recipient artery. The intracoronary administration of adenosine to patients with stable angina reproduces their pain, often without evoking electrocardiographic evidence of ischemia. Adenosine receptor blockade alleviates the chest pain and delays the onset of exercise angina. The activation of A_1 adenosine receptors on sympathetic fibers initiates the pain signal, which ultimately projects bilaterally to the cerebral cortex. The failure of intracoronary adenosine to cause pain in heart transplant patients is additional evidence of the importance of cardiac nerves. Similarly, patients with diabetic neuropathy are less sensitive to the algogenic effect of adenosine and have less severe angina.

The duration and severity of ischemia can separate patients who have ischemia without angina (silent ischemia) from those with angina. Electrocardiographic and hemodynamic monitoring of patients with obstructive coronary artery disease indicates that, in general, episodes of silent ischemia tend to be shorter and have a smaller hemodynamic impact than attacks of typical angina. Up to 75% of patients with stable angina have silent ischemia, and 40% with silent ischemia demonstrate ECG changes on ambulatory monitoring. Symptomatic ischemia often occurs with more severe and prolonged ischemia and is preceded by diastolic and then systolic dysfunction, abnormal lactate metabolism, and ECG changes. Myocardial ischemia resulting in infarction without chest pain is not rare, especially among patients with diabetes mellitus.

Cardiac Syndrome X

Approximately 10% of patients with typical angina pectoris and electrocardiographic evidence of ischemia have normal coronary angiograms, a condition termed cardiac syndrome X (CSX) *(12)*. Some patients with CSX have microvascular angina, characterized by a reduced capacity of the coronary circulation to augment flow in the presence of an increase in oxygen demand. Other patients with CSX have abnormal pain perception and sensitivity. Proposed causes of CSX include endothelial dysfunction, abnormal release of adenosine or potassium, and autonomic dysfunction. Mortality is low, but so is the quality of life.

Prinzmetal's Vasospastic Angina (13)

Prinzmetal's vasospastic angina classically occurs at rest and differs from classical angina in that increased oxygen demand is not the stimulus for pain, and there are characteristic transient elevations of the ST segments on the electrocardiogram. Coronary angiography shows focal spasm in one or more epicardial coronary arteries, and radionuclide imaging demonstrates reversible regional myocardial ischemia. The right coronary artery is the most frequent site for coronary spasm, followed by the left anterior descending coronary artery. On occasion, the site of spasm may fluctuate from one coronary artery to another. The severity of the coronary spasm may vary from subtotal occlusion to mild stenosis. In general, patients with vasospastic angina are younger than those with classical angina, and are more likely to be female. Many patients have a fixed coronary obstruction proximal to the site of spasm. Although angiography between attacks of spasm may show relatively normal coronary artery diameter; intravascular ultrasonography often shows some coronary atherosclerosis.

The trigger(s) for coronary vasospasm are unclear; indeed, the conflicting evidence raises the possibility of a different trigger from patient to patient. An association with smoking and, in a substantial number of patients, Raynaud's phenomenon or migraine, suggests that vasospastic angina may be one facet of a wider spastic vasculopathy. Intracoronary infusion of ergonovine, a stimulant of α-adrenergic and serotonin receptors, is a useful diagnostic tool. This does not point to an etiology, however, as α-adrenergic, serotonin, or thromboxane receptor antagonists are of no prophylactic value. However, nitrates and calcium-channel antagonists can be effective in both treatment and prophylaxis.

The risk of infarction can be as high as 5–20%, and sudden death 2–10%, especially in patients with left ventricular dysfunction or cardiac arrhythmias. However, the use of intensive nitrate regimens and calcium-channel antagonists has significantly reduced the frequency of these problems.

Myocardial Stunning

Myocardial stunning *(14)* is *mechanical systolic and diastolic ventricular dysfunction* that may persist for hours to weeks after *coronary artery occlusion and reperfusion* despite the absence of irreversible myocardial damage and the return of *normal or near-normal coronary perfusion*. The broad spectrum of myocardial stunning ranges from transient regional hypokinesis without infarction following a short coronary occlusion to a zone of dysfunctional myocardium surrounding a subendocardial infarct. Myocardial stunning may also occur as a functional manifestation of ischemia-reperfusion injury after thrombolytic therapy for coronary reperfusion, coronary angioplasty, or heart transplantation. Monocytes, polymorphonuclear leukocytes, and endothelial cells play key roles in the pathogenesis of myocardial stunning. Ischemia induces the production and release of reactive oxygen species in leukocytes, proinflammatory cytokines in monocytes, and the expression of cell adhesion molecules in endothelial cells, all of which contribute to myocardial stunning.

At the molecular level, two complementary hypotheses in combination, the oxyradical and calcium hypotheses, best account for myocardial stunning at this time (Fig. 3). The oxyradical hypothesis posits that reperfusion generates reactive oxygen species (ROS), such as hydroxyl radicals, that indiscriminately attack almost all proteins and lipids in the myocyte, including ion pumps and contractile proteins. This causes protein denaturation and enzyme inactivation and, ultimately, myocyte apoptosis. Decreased ventricular contractile function may be caused by free-radical activation of proteases that damage and/or digest contractile proteins, and impair ATPase activity. Administering antioxidants before or during the interval of myocardial ischemia—but not during coronary reperfusion—blunts stunning. The calcium hypothesis posits that myocardial stunning results from (1) myocyte calcium overload, (2) decreased responsiveness of the contractile proteins to calcium, and (3) excitation-contraction uncoupling due to sarcoplasmic reticulum dysfunction. Increased intracellular calcium results from open voltage-sensitive calcium channels in the sarcolemma and release of calcium from the sarcoplasmic reticulum. As a consequence, calcium may activate proteases that damage troponin and blunt the calcium sensitivity of the contractile proteins. This model provides the rationale of several therapeutic approaches for treating ischemia/reperfusion injury in general and stunning in particular. Agonist activation of A_{2A} adenosine receptors on polymorphonuclear leukocytes and monocytes curtails the oxidative burst and release of substances that initiate

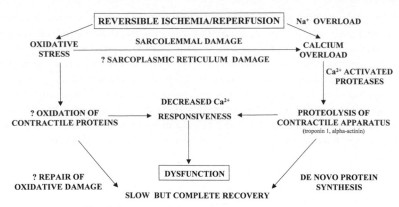

Fig. 3. Pathophysiology of myocardial stunning.

the inflammatory response. Antioxidants act at the next step, mopping up ROS, and calcium-channel antagonists lessen calcium overload in myocytes.

Myocardial Hibernation

Myocardial hibernation *(15)* is chronic, reversible myocardial contractile dysfunction in the setting of obstructive coronary artery disease that is due to an imbalance between myocardial oxygen supply and oxygen demand rather than a primary reduction in coronary blood flow. Hibernation may result from repetitive myocardial stunning as myocardial blood flow can be either normal or moderately reduced. In the short term, hibernation preserves cellular integrity by reducing contractile work to match oxygen delivery so that, strictly speaking, one cannot call hibernation a response to ischemia. In the long term, hibernating myocytes undergo morphologic changes, including vesiculation of the sarcolemma membrane, an increase in glycogen and the density of mitochondria, loss of an organized sarcoplasmic reticulum, and eventually loss of myofibrils. Immunohistological studies show that hibernating cardiomyocytes express contractile proteins specific to the fetal heart, such as α-smooth muscle actin, and cytoskeletal proteins such as titin and cardiotin. Ultimately, apoptosis may reduce myocyte number.

The importance of hibernation is that it is reversible by revascularization. Clinically, it may be difficult to differentiate hibernating myocardium from myocardium undergoing repeated stunning due to coronary obstruction that provides adequate flow during rest but not exercise. Accordingly, tests that discriminate between hibernating and scarred myocardium are important in planning management and determining prognosis. The capacity of hypokinetic or akinetic myocardium to increase contractility in response to a low dose of an inotropic drug such as dobutamine is an important test of hibernating myocardium. Hibernating myocardium contracts in response to 5 to 10 µg/kg dobutamine but myocardial function often deteriorates at higher doses because the reduced coronary flow reserve cannot meet the increase in myocardial metabolic demand. Other tests include imaging techniques such as the delayed uptake of ^{201}Tl, uptake of ^{99m}Tc-sestamibi that is >50 % of normally contracting myocardium measured by SPECT, and the uptake of [^{11}C]acetate or [^{18}F]2-fluorodeoxyglucose measured by positron emission tomography (PET). Increased uptake of [^{18}F]2-fluorodeoxyglucose in the presence of decreased myocardial perfusion, or metabolism-flow mismatch, indicates hibernating myocardium. Conversely, matching defects in flow and metabolism indicates scar tissue. The advantage of PET imaging is that it measures myocardial metabolism directly; it is widely used in Europe but is of limited availability in the United States.

Treatment of hibernating myocardium involves administration of β-adrenergic receptor antagonists to improve the ratio of myocardial oxygen supply to demand and coronary revascularization. Recovery of contractile function in hibernating myocardium may take weeks to months, depending on the severity of the histopathologic changes and the time necessary for cellular recovery.

Ischemic Cardiomyopathy

Ischemic cardiomyopathy is the term describing arteriosclerotic coronary vascular disease that produces severe myocardial dysfunction with multifocal wall motion abnormalities, a left ventricular ejection fraction less than 40% and clinical manifestations indistinguishable from those of primary dilated cardiomyopathy. Later refinements of the definition include previous myocardial infarction or coronary artery narrowing >70% and myocardial dysfunction out of proportion to the size of the infarct or degree of coronary stenosis. Myocardial stunning and hibernating myocardium contribute to this disparity. Patients with ischemic cardiomyopathy have increased activity of the sympathetic nervous and the renin-angiotensin-aldosterone systems. At the cellular level, there are changes in myocyte phenotype with expression of fetal proteins and myocyte hypertrophy, myocyte death due to necrosis and apoptosis and progressive fibrosis, and changes in the quantity and nature of the interstitial matrix. Histochemical studies reveal preservation of the enzymes of glycolysis but depletion of the enzymes of fatty acid metabolism. Consequently, glucose replaces fatty acids as the main fuel for ATP production in the myocardium.

These changes produce alternations not only in the structure of the ventricle but also in the function of the ventricle. Symptoms from low cardiac output and elevation of left ventricular diastolic pressure dominate the clinical picture. The prognosis for patients with ischemic cardiomyopathy is worse than for those with dilated cardiomyopathy because the risks of ischemic events and of the cardiomyopathy are additive. Different studies place mortality at between 5 and 50% per year, depending on the mass of myocardium involved, the degree of dysfunction, the age of the patient, and the presence of arrhythmias and hypertension. Treatment goals are (1) reduction of myocardial oxygen demand/supply imbalance with nitrates, (2) decreasing the activity of the renin-angiotensin systems with angiotensin converting enzyme inhibitors or angiotensin receptor blockers and (3) blunting sympathetic stimulation with β-adrenergic receptor antagonists. In patients with significant prolongation of ventricular depolarization as manifested by ECG QRS durations ≥130 ms and substantial left ventricular septal-lateral wall dysynchrony, biventricular pacing resynchronizes the ventricular activation sequence and increases coordination of atrial-ventricular filling, thereby increasing cardiac output and decreasing pulmonary congestion. Biventricular pacing does not increase myocardial oxygen consumption.

Ischemic Preconditioning

Studies in experimental animals show that an interval of coronary occlusion too brief to cause infarction reduces the size of the infarct caused by a subsequent prolonged coronary occlusion. This effect is termed *ischemic preconditioning (16)*. Cardioprotection is substantial; infarct size reductions of 75% are the rule. Adenosine released from ischemic tissue was one of the first preconditioning stimuli identified, but subsequent investigations showed that a number of G protein-coupled receptors (GPCRs) could initiate the response, as could physical stimuli such as stretch of cardiac muscle, mitogens such as fibroblast growth factors 1 and 2, or chemicals such as calcium or free radicals. The administration of α-adrenergic, muscarinic, opioid, bradykinin, or angiotensin-receptor agonists induces myocardial protection in the absence of ischemia and is termed *pharmacological preconditioning*. Preconditioning is not unique to the heart; this response also occurs in other organs—for example, skeletal muscle, brain, spinal cord, and pancreas. A reduction of infarct size is not the only index of cardioprotection that preconditioning offers; during reperfusion preconditioned hearts have fewer arrhythmias and recover contractility faster.

Preconditioning is a biphasic response (Fig. 4). "Classical" preconditioning protects the heart immediately but only lasts 2 to 4 h. "Delayed" preconditioning, sometimes referred to as the "second window" of protection, follows the preconditioning stimulus by a day and may persist for up to 3 to 4 d. Delayed preconditioning protects against both myocardial infarction and stunning and may represent a more generalized response of the heart to stress.

The molecular mechanisms involved in the two forms of preconditioning are different and incompletely understood (Fig. 4). Activation of any of the G protein-coupled receptors is a major

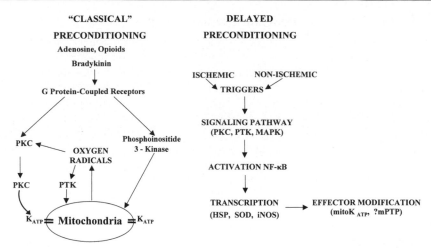

Fig. 4. Mechanisms proposed for classical and delayed preconditioning. GPCR, G protein-coupled receptor; K_{ATP}, mitochondrial ATP-sensitive potassium channel; MITO, mitochondrion; mPTP, mitochondrial permeability transition pore; PI 3 K, phosphoinositide-3 kinase; PKC, protein kinase C; PLC/D, phospholipases C and D; PTK, protein tyrosine kinase.

stimulus for classical preconditioning. Depending on the receptor, preconditioning follows parallel transduction pathways that include phospholipases C and D, one or more isoforms of protein kinase C (PKC) such as PKCε, phosphoinositide-3 kinase, and mitogen-activated protein kinases (MAPKs) that converge on the mitochondrial K_{ATP} channel. In this regard, drugs that open K_{ATP} channels, such as cromakalin and pinacidil, induce preconditioning. Conversely, drugs that block K_{ATP} channel opening, such as glibenclamide, can prevent preconditioning. The mechanism of mitochondrial K_{ATP} protection involves optimization of mitochondrial energy production and modulation of reactive oxygen species.

The same stimuli that cause classical preconditioning also initiate delayed preconditioning, as do nitric oxide, exercise, and heat stress. The signaling pathways for delayed preconditioning involve protein kinase C and MAPKs. The several transcription pathways converge on the transcriptional regulator NF-κB, which initiates cardiac gene expression to induce new proteins that promote cell repair and protect against subsequent ischemic insults. A number of investigations document increased expression of several heat shock proteins, oncogenes and enzymes of antioxidant systems. Strong evidence also implicates the mitochondrial K_{ATP} channel in delayed cardioprotection, but its precise role is unclear.

The importance of preconditioning lies in the evidence that human hearts undergo preconditioning during preinfarction angina and during coronary angioplasty and the hope that ways can be found to translate into patient care the dramatic cardioprotection demonstrated with pharmacological preconditioning in experimental animals.

Coronary Collaterals (17)

The coronary arteries are not end arteries. Rather, there are two types of coronary collateral vessels that differ in size, structure, and location. Ischemia is a powerful stimulus for collateral formation, and involves angiogenesis and arteriogenesis. Angiogenesis is the sprouting and enlargement of capillaries from preexisting vascular networks or endothelial tubes the size of capillaries that occur at all depths in the ventricular wall but are more numerous in the subendocardium, where they form a plexus. Arteriogenesis is the enlargement of existing epicardial collateral arterioles after total or subtotal occlusion of a major coronary artery. Collateral arterioles extend from one epicardial artery to another. Collateral formation is a dynamic response determined by physical factors such as wall stress, by the pressure gradient along the collateral vessel, and by an inflammatory response that elaborates chemical signals such as vascular endothelial growth factor, transforming growth factors α and β, basic fibroblast growth factor, and granulocyte-monocyte colony-stimulating factor. These chemical factors stimulate migration and proliferation of endothelial and smooth muscle cells and direct vascular remodeling. Clinical studies are currently in progress to induce angiogenesis in patients by either surgical or catheter delivery of growth factors or stem cells. However, these studies are hampered by the lack of accurate, inexpensive, and reproducible techniques for the measurement of collateral blood flow. Myocardial contrast echocardiography and radionuclide perfusion imaging are promising noninvasive techniques that are currently under investigation *(18)*.

REFERENCES

1. Doucette JW, Corl PD, Payne HM, et al. Validation of a Doppler guide wire for intravascular measurement of coronary artery flow velocity. Circulation 1992;85:1899–1911.
2. Wei K, Firoozan S, Jayaweera AR, et al. Quantification of myocardial blood flow with ultrasound-induced destruction of microbubbles administered as a continuous infusion. Circulation 1998;97:473–482.
3. Spaan JAE. Coronary Blood Flow. Mechanics, Distribution and Control. Kluwer Academic Publishers, Dordrecht, The Netherlands, 1991.
4. Yamamuro A, Akasaka T, Tamita K, et al. Coronary flow velocity pattern immediately after percutaneous coronary intervention as a predictor of complications and in-hospital survival after acute myocardial infarction. Circulation 2002;106:3051–3056.
5. Guyton RA, McClenathan JH, Newman GE, et al. Significance of subendocardial ST segment elevation caused by coronary stenosis in dog–epicardial ST segment depression, local ischemia and subsequent necrosis. Am J Cardiol 1977;40:373–380.
6. Uren NG, Melin JA, De Bruyne B, et al. Relation between myocardial blood flow and the severity of coronary-artery stenosis. N Engl J Med 1994;330:1782–1788.
7. Piek JJ, van Liebergen RAM, Koch KT, et al. Clinical, angiographic and hemodynamic predictors of recruitable collateral flow assessed during balloon angioplasty coronary occlusion. J Am Coll Cardiol 1997;29:275–282.
8. Wu X, Davis MJ. Characterization of stretch-activated cation current in coronary smooth muscle cells. Am J Physiol 2001;280:H1751–H1761.
9. Jaggar JH, Wellman GC, Hepner TJ, et al. Ca^{2+} channels, ryanodine receptors and Ca^{2+}-activated K^+ channels: a functional unit for regulating arterial tone. Acta Physiol Scand 1998;164:577–587.
10. Deussen A. Metabolic flux rates of adenosine in the heart. Naunyn-Schmiedeberg's Arch Pharmacol 2000;362:351–363.
11. Sylvén C, Crea F. Mechanisms of anginal pain: the key role of adenosine. In: Belardinelli L, Pelleg A, eds. Adenosine and Adenine Nucleotides: From Molecular Biology to Integrative Physiology. Kluwer Academic Press, Dordrecht, The Netherlands, 1995, pp. 315–325.
12. Kaski JC. Pathophysiology and management of patients with chest pain and normal coronary arteriograms (cardiac syndrome X). Circulation 2004;109:568–572.
13. Crea F, Kaski JC, Maseri A. Key references on coronary spasm. Circulation 1997;96:3766–3773.
14. Bolli R, Marban E. Molecular and cellular mechanisms of myocardial stunning. Physiol Rev 1999;79:609–634.
15. Wijns W, Vatner SE, Camici PG. Hibernating myocardium. N Engl J Med 1998;339:173–181.
16. Yellon DM, Downey JM. Preconditioning the myocardium: from cellular physiology to clinical cardiology. Physiol Rev 2003;83:1113–1151.
17. Koerselman J, van der Graaf Y, de Jaegere PPTh, Grobbee DE. Coronary collaterals. An important and underexposed aspect of coronary artery disease. Circulation 2003;107:2507–2511.
18. Kaul S, Ito H. Microvasculature in acute myocardial ischemia.II. Evolving concepts in pathophysiology, diagnosis and treatment. Circulation 2004;109:310–315.

RECOMMENDED READING

Feliciano L, Henning RJ. Coronary artery blood flow: physiologic and pathophysiologic regulation. Clin Cardiol 1999;22:775–786.
Weiss JN, Korge P, Honda HM, Ping P. Role of the mitochondrial permeability transition in myocardial disease. Circ Res 2003;93:292–301.
Murphy E. Primary and secondary signaling pathways in early preconditioning that converge on the mitochondria to produce cardioprotection. Circ Res 2004;94:7–16.
Bilton R, Booker GW. The subtle side to hypoxia inducible factor (HIFα) regulation. Eur J Biochem 2003;270:791–798.
Marcus M. The Coronary Circulation in Health and Disease. McGraw-Hill, New York, 1983.
Ganz P, Ganz W. Coronary blood flow and myocardial ischemia. In: Braunwald E, Zipes DP, Libby E, eds. Heart Disease, 6th ed. W. B. Saunders, Philadelphia, 2001, pp. 1087–1113.
Schaper W, ed. Arteriogenesis. Boston, Kluwer, 2005.

25 Stable Angina

Satya Reddy Atmakuri, MD,
Michael H. Gollob, MD,
and Neal S. Kleiman, MD

INTRODUCTION

As the 21st century progresses, the prevalence of coronary artery disease (CAD) will reach epidemic proportions in both the Western and the developing world. In the US alone, it is estimated that more than 11 million people have CAD *(1)*. As our population ages, and as the frequency of diabetes increases *(2)*, these numbers will be expected to increase exponentially. The associated morbidity and costs exceed those of any other chronic disease in modern society. While tremendous progress in diagnostic techniques as well as in medical and interventional management has occurred over recent decades, the impetus for more novel strategies remains.

This chapter will review the current approach to stable angina. Although a variety of etiologies of angina pectoris exists (Table 1), this discussion will assume the most common pathology manifesting this entity, coronary artery atherosclerosis.

CLINICAL HISTORY

As with other diseases, a careful history is essential in diagnosing angina pectoris accurately. Attention to specific details often allows the clinician to discern between other potential causes of chest discomfort and thus offset the expense and risk of unnecessary testing. Exploring the quality, location, duration, and relieving and exacerbating features of the symptoms often permits a correct diagnosis. Angina pectoris typically manifests as a "heavy," "squeezing" chest discomfort brought on by exertional stress. The discomfort generally has a retrosternal component, often described as "bandlike" in nature. Radiation to the throat, jaw, and left shoulder are common. Relief usually occurs within minutes of cessation of the precipitating stress. Under most circumstances, sublingual nitroglycerin also succeeds in providing rapid relief. Anginal symptoms are considered stable if there has been no change in the pattern of intensity, frequency, or duration over several weeks. Grading of the severity of angina pectoris is useful in monitoring progression of symptoms, conveying information to other clinicians, and assessing treatment strategies (Table 2). Symptoms that are described as fleeting, sharp, or pinpoint in location are not suggestive of angina pectoris. Similarly, the absence of characteristic precipitating and relieving features should lead the clinician to suspect other diagnoses.

Classical symptoms of myocardial ischemia may not always be present in patients with angina pectoris. Particularly in the elderly, and in patients with diabetes, symptoms of recurrent nausea or unexplained vomiting may be the first clinical clues. Shortness of breath on minimal exertion may be due to ischemia-induced left ventricular dysfunction (systolic, diastolic, or both) or mitral regurgitation. Rarely, syncope due to ischemia-mediated ventricular arrhythmia may be the first presenting symptom.

Independent "classical" risk factors for CAD must also be kept in mind during history-taking. These include hypertension, diabetes mellitus, hyperlipidemia, smoking, and a family history of

From: *Essential Cardiology: Principles and Practice, 2nd Ed.*
Edited by: C. Rosendorff © Humana Press Inc., Totowa, NJ

Table 1
Etiologies of Angina Pectoris

Pathology	Disease
Coronary artery obstruction	Atherosclerosis
	Vasospasm
	Vasculitis
	Dissection
	Myocardial bridge
	Anomalous coronary origin
	Kawasaki's disease
Left ventricular hypertrophy	Hypertension
	Aortic valvular/subvalvular stenosis
	Idiopathic/familial hypertrophic cardiomyopathy
Right ventricular hypertrophy	Pulmonary hypertension
	Pulmonary stenosis

Table 2
Canadian Cardiovascular Society Classification of Angina Pectoris

Class I   "Ordinary physical activity does not cause angina"
               such as walking or climbing stairs. Angina with strenuous or rapid or prolonged exertion at work
               or recreation.
Class II   "Slight limitation of ordinary activity"
               walking or climbing stairs rapidly, walking uphill, walking or stair climbing after meals, in cold,
               or in wind, or when under emotional stress, or only during the few hours after awakening.
               Walking more than two blocks (100–200 m) on the level and climbing more than one flight of
               stairs at a normal pace and in normal conditions.
Class III "Marked limitation of ordinary physical activity"
               walking one or two blocks on the level and climbing one flight of stairs in normal conditions and
               at normal pace.
Class IV   "Inability to carry on any physical activity without discomfort"
               anginal syndrome may be present at rest.

Reprinted with permission from ref. 3.

ischemic heart disease (in first-degree relatives with cardiovascular events when younger than 60 yr). In women over age 50, early menopause or a prolonged estrogen-deficient state should also be considered possible risk factors. Newer risk factors have been identified as well, and are gradually assuming roles similar to those identified during previous decades. These include such markers of inflammation as C-reactive protein (CRP) (4,5) as well as certain newly identified gene mutations (6).

PHYSICAL EXAMINATION

There are no clinical findings specific to CAD. However, since CAD is the most common heart disease of Western society, any abnormal cardiac findings should be viewed as possibly related to chronic ischemic disease. The physical examination should focus on the detection of general findings that may be relevant to diagnosis and management. For example, hyperlipidemic syndromes may first be discovered by observing the skin lesions of xanthelasma or tendinous xanthomata. Patients with diabetes may show signs of microvascular disease, such as retinopathy, prior to large-vessel atherosclerosis. Evidence of peripheral vascular disease may be detected by the presence of carotid or femoral bruits and diminished peripheral pulses. Palpation of the precordium may provide evidence of left ventricular dysfunction by revealing a laterally displaced and sustained apical impulse. Auscultation of the chest may reveal a fourth heart sound (S_4), indicating long-standing hypertension with left ventricular hypertrophy.

During an acute anginal attack, the presence of a fourth heart sound may be secondary to ischemic, noncompliant myocardium. Careful examination of the venous system will give an indication of the volume status of a patient as well as of ventricular compliance. Elevated jugular venous pressure and/or peripheral edema may be findings of right heart failure, with or without concomitant left ventricular dysfunction.

Certain physical findings may lead to a diagnosis other than angina. Palpation of a right ventricular heave at the left sternal border with a prominent pulmonic component of the second heart sound suggests right ventricular hypertrophy secondary to pulmonary hypertension. Characteristic murmurs of hypertrophic obstructive cardiomyopathy or aortic stenosis would implicate these etiologies as causes of angina, but do not exclude concomitant CAD.

DIAGNOSTIC TESTING

Rest Electrocardiography and Ambulatory Monitoring

A resting 12-lead electrocardiogram (ECG) should be obtained in all patients undergoing evaluation for symptoms of stable angina pectoris. However, with the exception of abnormal Q waves in contiguous leads suggesting prior myocardial infarction, there are no findings on the resting 12-lead ECG that are absolutely diagnostic of CAD. In fact, many patients with a normal rest ECG may subsequently be found to have severe coronary atherosclerosis. Conversely, repolarization abnormalities such as T-wave inversions or ST segment sloping are not uncommon in the general population found to have no evidence of CAD. Certain ECG abnormalities, namely left anterior fascicular block or left bundle branch block occurring in patients with classic angina pectoris, may identify a subset of patients at higher risk of death or myocardial infarction. However, it is important to remember that the variety of abnormal ECG findings has a low sensitivity and specificity to reach diagnostic conclusions.

The principle of ambulatory electrocardiographic (Holter) monitoring is to detect symptomatic or asymptomatic evidence of myocardial ischemia by evaluation of ST segment changes during routine daily activities. While this test may be useful in some individuals, and has been the subject of a good deal of research concerning asymptomatic or "silent" ischemia, ambulatory monitoring as a clinical tool rarely provides additional useful information in the diagnosis of angina pectoris beyond that revealed by standard exercise stress testing.

Exercise Treadmill Electrocardiography

Exercise treadmill electrocardiography is a frequently used test in the diagnostic workup for symptoms of stable angina. This is also discussed fully in Chapter 10. The test is readily available, easily performed, and low in cost. The goal is to correlate symptoms of angina with ST segment changes consistent with myocardial ischemia. Objective parameters assessed during testing include maximal heart rate achieved, blood pressure response, ST segment shifts, and workload capacity attained. Adequate sensitivity of the test is accomplished with target heart rates approx 85% of the age-predicted maximum ($\geq$220 – age). Inability to reach this target while remaining symptom-free is considered submaximal exercise and has a very low negative predictive value for coronary artery disease, as the stress conditions met may not have been adequate to produce myocardial ischemia. Blood pressure measurements at increasing workloads are expected to show incremental increases in systolic blood pressure. Failure to do so suggests left ventricular dysfunction secondary to ischemia. ST segment depression $\geq$1 mm with a horizontal or downsloping appearance is interpreted as indicative of myocardial ischemia, although other conditions, particularly increased left ventricular mass, may also produce this abnormality even in the absence of obstructive epicardial coronary artery disease. Workload capacity (or metabolic equivalents [METs]) achieved is best viewed as a prognostic marker. Treating patients empirically with antianginal medications prior to testing may be necessary, but will lower the sensitivity of the procedure. Therefore, clinicians should use their discretion in opting to discontinue medical therapy a few days before evaluation.

Exercise electrocardiography has an overall sensitivity and specificity of 68% and 77%, respectively. Sensitivity is greatest in patients with multivessel disease, noted to be 81% in an overview of 24,000 patients who eventually underwent coronary angiography *(7)*. Indicators of severity of disease include onset of symptoms or positive ST segment changes at low workload capacity (≤5 METs), a sustained drop of ≥10 mmHg in systolic blood pressure, or delayed recovery of ST segments after stopping exercise. In contrast, patients capable of achieving a workload capacity of 10 METs or more have an excellent prognosis, regardless of the extent of CAD *(3)*. Clearly, such information derived from the exercise study will guide further diagnostic and management decisions, as will be discussed in a later section.

Myocardial Perfusion Imaging

Myocardial perfusion or single photon emission computed tomography (SPECT) imaging by use of low dose radioactive-labeled perfusion agents is a valuable test in the evaluation of CAD (*see also* Chapter 13). This technique is most often used in conjunction with exercise electrocardiography. At peak exercise, where myocardial oxygen consumption and coronary blood flow are at their maximum, the perfusion tracer (thallium-201 or technetium-99m) is injected. If no obstructive coronary lesions are present, the tracer will be taken up equally in all territories of the myocardium. In any area of myocardium that is underperfused due to significant obstructive coronary lesions, impaired extraction of the tracer will produce a less-intense radioactive signal or "defect" on imaging. These stress images may then be compared to images at rest, where the defect may either "fill in" with signal, reflecting reversible ischemia in the territory, or remain unchanged, indicating a myocardial scar.

The sensitivity and specificity of SPECT imaging are in the range of 80% and 90%, respectively. Sensitivity is highest for single-vessel disease and falls to approx 70% for multivessel disease *(8)*. Additional information obtained from SPECT imaging includes identifying involved coronary arteries and the ischemic burden. Also, using the newer ECG-gated SPECT technology, assessment of stress and rest left ventricular ejection fraction may be acquired.

In patients unable to exercise, pharmacologic stress tests are available. Dipyridamole and adenosine are vasodilators that enhance blood flow to normally perfused myocardium, with a lower tracer uptake in underperfused areas. These agents are safe and also provide results with high sensitivity and specificity. Either agent may also precipitate angina in the absence of epicardial disease, but here scintigraphic findings are normal. Both drugs are contraindicated in patients with reactive airway disease, as they may precipitate acute bronchospasm. In this setting, a dobutamine stress test is a reasonable alternative.

Exercise Radionuclide Ventriculography

The value of radionuclide ventriculography in the detection of CAD is much diminished in light of more advanced techniques now utilized. It had been proposed that failure to increase ejection fraction more than 5% during peak exercise was diagnostic of CAD. However, this finding has poor specificity *(9)*. Perhaps the best use of this test is in deciding which patients may benefit from revascularization. The observation at high stress levels of wall motion abnormalities that recover at rest indicates myocardium that may be protected by a revascularization procedure.

Rest and Stress Echocardiography

Rest echocardiography alone is not sensitive for the detection of CAD, as many patients with disease have both a normal left ventricular ejection fraction and wall motion at rest. In rare cases, abnormal Doppler velocities in the aortic root may signal narrowing of the left main coronary artery. However, other pathologies responsible for nonspecific symptoms may be recognized—for example, hypertrophic cardiomyopathy or valvular disease.

Stress echocardiography used in combination with rest imaging offers a good opportunity to observe signs of myocardial ischemia. Stress may be performed with exercise or more commonly with dobutamine, adenosine, or dipyridamole. The preferred agent is dobutamine. At high infusion (10–40 µg/g/min), localized hypokinesis or impaired systolic wall thickening relative to rest images signals the presence of compromised myocardium. Transient LV dilation and impaired diastolic function as assessed by transmitral Doppler inflows may be other clues to ischemia. Additional benefits of this technique include accurate assessment of left ventricular mass and ejection fraction, assessment of concomitant valvular heart disease, and estimates of right and left heart filling pressures using Doppler techniques. Limitations include the inability to achieve adequate two-dimensional views in 5–15% of studies. Overall, relative to myocardial perfusion imaging, dobutamine stress echocardiography has been found to detect CAD with a comparable sensitivity and specificity in the hands of experienced operators *(10)*. It also has the additional advantage that technically difficult studies in which the presence or absence of an abnormal response cannot be discerned are easier to identify than they are with scintigraphic testing.

Invasive Testing

Although coronary angiography is the best test to define the anatomical severity of CAD, it is often not required as the first choice to establish the diagnosis of angina pectoris in patients with stable symptoms. Exceptions to this include patients presenting with a history of angina associated with malignant ventricular arrhythmias and patients for whom definitive diagnosis is required for occupational reasons, as in airline pilots. The optimal use of coronary angiography is for patients who are moderately or severely symptomatic or who have strongly positive noninvasive tests, and in whom knowledge of the degree of coronary disease may lead to decisions of appropriate revascularization procedures. Such scenarios include patients with myocardial ischemia at low exercise thresholds (≤5 METs) or a myocardial perfusion scan indicating moderate to severe (>15%) defect size. Angiographic lesions reducing the lumen by 70% are thought to be consistent with symptoms and signs of myocardial ischemia. Following evaluation of the coronary arteries, left ventriculography is usually performed for assessment of ejection fraction and wall motion abnormalities.

Although coronary angiography remains the "gold standard" in defining the anatomic appearance of CAD, visual interpretation of the severity of lesions varies between observers *(11)*. In addition, major discrepancies between angiographic and postmortem findings have been found to exist, usually showing underestimation of lesion severity by angiography *(12)*. These difficulties arise due to the limitations of angiographic imaging. A contrast-filled vessel lumen provides only a planar two-dimensional longitudinal view of a lesion, the severity of which may be misrepresented by the angiographic viewing angle. Obtaining multiple views may help resolve this issue; however, optimal imaging is often limited by radiographic foreshortening or overlapping vessels that obscure the arterial segment in question, particularly in patients in whom the vessels are tortuous. These limitations may be overcome by the use of intravascular ultrasound or by intracoronary pressure measurement. These techniques allow visualization of the entire circumference of the vessel wall in addition to characterization of deeper intramural structures or characterization of the physiologic significance of observed narrowings. Tomographic views may demonstrate eccentricity of lesions, diffusely diseased segments, and ostial disease, all of which may be underestimated by conventional angiography. Finally, by virtue of the ability of intravascular ultrasound to characterize intramural anatomy, insight into the pathophysiology of coronary lesions is often gained. Pressure ratios (mean aortic to distal coronary) exceeding 0.90 after intracoronary adenosine indicate functional limitation to coronary flow by the lesion *(13)*.

It is essential to keep in mind the imperfect sensitivity of noninvasive testing in diagnosing CAD. Therefore, in any patient where clinical suspicion is high despite a negative noninvasive test, coronary angiography should be performed.

Diagnostic Strategy

A thoughtful and systematic diagnostic approach is necessary to ensure cost-effective and accurate diagnoses. The value of a diagnostic test is related to the difference between the pretest probability of the diagnosis in question and the posttest probability using information derived from the diag-

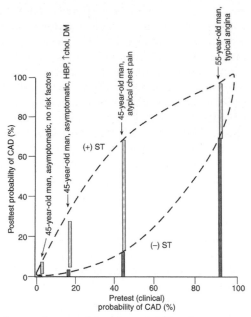

Fig. 1. Illustration of Bayes' theorem in ascertaining the probability of coronary artery disease by exercise electrocardiography. Four specific patient examples are shown along with pre- and posttest probabilities based on negative ("–" ST) or positive ("+" ST) test results. The value of the test is most useful for patients with intermediate pretest probability for coronary disease.

nostic procedure. This concept is the foundation of Bayesian theory, which utilizes the patient's clinical information to arrive at pre- and posttest probabilities for CAD. For example, the use of exercise electrocardiography alone as a diagnostic tool has varying diagnostic power depending on the prevalence of CAD in selected patient populations (Fig. 1). Thus, in patients with low pretest probability of CAD, positive results of the test minimally increase the posttest probability, primarily due to high false-positive rates. Conversely, in patients with a high pretest probability, minimal additional information is obtained about the likelihood of CAD. It is clear from Fig. 1 that the exercise treadmill is most powerful for predicting CAD in patients with an intermediate pretest probability (30–70%) for CAD (Table 3). It is also important to realize that the aim of exercise testing is not solely the detection of CAD, but also the integration of a larger picture including an objective measure of overall exercise performance, the ease of provocation of symptoms, and obtaining prognostic information. Figure 2 illustrates an algorithmic approach to diagnostic testing. Patients with a higher likelihood of CAD should receive adjunctive imaging that can provide further prognostic information and guide management decisions more precisely. While myocardial perfusion imaging and stress echocardiography may have comparable sensitivity for detecting CAD, a there is a larger body of data based on quantitative perfusion defect size *(14,15)*. Patients unable to exercise or with left bundle branch block or hypertrophic or infiltrative cardiomyopathies should undergo pharmacologic stress due to the poor specificity of stress ECG in these conditions.

MEDICAL THERAPY

Antiplatelet Agents

Aspirin, available since the 19th century for its pain-relieving effects, was not recognized as an antiplatelet drug until the 1970s. It has now become the mainstay of treatment for both chronic and acute coronary syndromes. The antiplatelet effect of aspirin is believed to arise predominantly from its ability to diminish platelet production of thromboxane A_2 (TXA_2), a vasoconstrictor and proaggregant. In an overview by the Antiplatelet Trialists of more than 300 studies involving

Table 3
Profiles of Low, Intermediate, and High Probability CAD

	Low probability (<30%)			Intermediate probability (30–70%)				High probability (>70%)	
				A. <40	>40	B. >40[b]	>40	>40	>55
Age	Any age[a]	<40	>45	Typical	Atypical	Asymptomatic	Typical	Typical	Typical
Symptoms	Asymptomatic	Atypical	Asymptomatic	0	≥2	≥2	≥2	≥2	0–5
Risks	0	≤2	≤2	Abnormal[c]	Abnormal	Normal or abnormal	Normal	Abnormal	Normal
ECG	Normal	Normal	Normal						

[a]Diagnostic testing not indicated.
[b]Patients considering onset of new vigorous exercise regimen or those with high-risk occupation (aviators, firefighters).
[c]"Abnormal ECG" refers to nonspecific abnormalities.

457

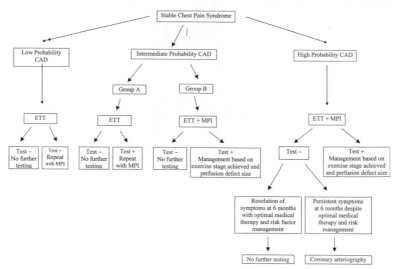

Fig. 2. Choice of diagnostic test.

140,000 patients with stable angina pectoris, previous myocardial infarction, prior stroke, and coronary bypass, aspirin was shown to significantly reduce the risk events of myocardial infarction and vascular death *(16)*. Doses ranging from 81 to 325 mg/d have been proven effective in smaller studies. There does not appear to be any additional benefit of higher doses. In fact, observational data indicate that the risk of bleeding is higher with 325 mg than with 81 mg *(17)*. Recent data also indicate that as many as 5 to 15% of patients may be resistant to the actions of aspirin. It is difficult to define aspirin resistance precisely. However, when patients are categorized as aspirin-resistant on the basis of adenosine diphosphate (ADP)-induced platelet aggregation *(18)* or by chronic urinary excretion of TXA_2 metabolites *(19)*, they have higher rates of myocardial infarction.

Aspirin is relatively ineffective in preventing platelet aggregation by physiologic agonists such as ADP. Clopidogrel, ticlopidine, and thienopyridines belong to a unique class of antiplatelet agents that interfere with ADP-mediated platelet activation. These drugs inhibit the action of ADP on one of the three purinergic receptors on the human platelet, P2Y12 *(20)*. Ligation of this receptor by ADP stimulates the platelet shape change reaction as well as conversion of GP IIb-IIIa to the active conformation, thus permitting platelet aggregation to occur *(21)*. Although this class of agents has not been studied specifically in patients with stable angina, evidence from a large trial in patients with atherosclerotic vascular disease has demonstrated a decreased incidence of myocardial infarction and vascular death, particularly in patients who also have peripheral vascular disease *(22)*. Clopidogrel lacks the risk of transient neutropenia present with ticlopidine, and may also be an effective secondary prevention agent *(22)*. For these reasons, ticlopidine or clopidogrel may be acceptable substitutes for aspirin in the rare instances of documented aspirin intolerance. In fact, the Clopidogrel versus Aspirin in Patients at Risk of Ischemic Events (CAPRIE) *(22)* trial suggested that clopidogrel was more effective than aspirin in preventing future myocardial infarctions. The superiority of aspirin in combination with a thienopyridine on secondary prevention in the setting of CAD is established following PCI or in patients with acute coronary syndromes *(23,24)* for up to 1 yr. The utility of this combination in patients with stable angina has not yet been established, and is currently the subject of a large clinical trial.

Nitrates

Sublingual nitroglycerin administered during an anginal attack is an effective means of aborting the episode within minutes. Smooth-muscle relaxation in vascular tissue mediated by nitric

Table 4
Commonly Used Drugs in Stable Coronary Artery Disease

Drug	Dose range
Anti-Platelets	
Aspirin	75–325 mg qd
Nitrates	
Sublingual NTG tablets	0.3–0.6 mg prn, maximum 3 doses in 15 min
Sublingual NTG spray	0.4 mg prn, maximum 3 doses in 15 min
NTG paste/ointment	½–2" 2% NTG q 8 h/off 8 h–10 h daily
NTG patch	0.1–0.8 mg/h, on 12 h/off 12 h
Isosorbide dinitrate	10–60 mg (7 AM, noon, 5 PM)
Isosorbide mononitrate	20 mg (8 AM and 3 PM)
Beta-blockers	
Cardioselective	
Metoprolol	25–150 mg bid
Atenolol	25–100 mg qd
Bisoprolol	5–10 mg bid
Noncardioselective	
Propranolol	20–80 mg qid
Nadolol	40–80 qd
Carvedilol	3.125–25 mg bid
Calcium-Channel Blockers	
Nondihydropyridines	
Diltiazem	30–90 mg qid
Verapamil	80–120 mg tid
Dihydropyridines	
Nifedipine	30–60 mg qd
Amlodipine	5–10 mg qd
Felodipine	5–20 mg qd
HMG CoA Reductase Inhibitors	
Rosuvastatin	5–40 mg q hs
Atorvastatin	10–80 mg q hs
Simvastatin	5–40 mg q hs
Pravastatin	10–40 mg q hs
Lovastatin	20–80 mg q hs
Fluvastatin	20–40 mg q hs

oxide (NO) and cyclic guanosine monophosphate (cGMP) results in venodilation and peripheral artery and coronary artery dilation *(25)*. The resulting decrease in preload and afterload reduces myocardial oxygen demand, while myocardial oxygen supply is improved. These effects may persist for up to 30 min.

A variety of nitrate formulations exist, ranging from short-acting to long-acting preparations (Table 4). Because of nitrate tolerance, longer-acting derivatives are best suited for patients with more frequent and severe symptoms. To avoid the development of tolerance, an 8–10-h nitrate-free interval is needed. Hence, patients should take nitrates only during periods when episodes most commonly occur.

Although nitrates clearly relieve anginal symptoms, no trials exist to demonstrate their effect on cardiovascular morbidity or mortality in stable angina pectoris. Nitrates are contraindicated in patients treated with phosphodiesterase-5 antagonists commonly prescribed for erectile dysfunction (sildenafil, vardenafil, tadalafil) *(26,27)*.

β-Adrenergic Blockers

β-Adrenergic blocking agents are essential components of the successful management of stable angina pectoris. Well recognized for their antihypertensive and antiarrhythmic properties, β-blockers exert a powerful antiischemic effect in CAD. β_1-Receptor blockade in the heart reduces myocardial oxygen demand by reducing heart rate and myocardial contractility. Also, increased diastolic perfusion time and reduced wall stress improve myocardial oxygen supply. Therapy is usually titrated to achieve a heart rate in the 50–60 beats/min range.

β-Blockers are generally well tolerated. Serious side effects include excessive bradycardia, heart block, hypotension, and bronchospasm. More common side effects are fatigue and impotence. Even with cardioselective β_1-blocking agents, some β_2-blockade occurs, making β-blockers contraindicated in patients with severe asthma or chronic obstructive pulmonary disease. Patients with mild reactive airway disease generally tolerate cardioselective (β_1-) blockers well, although dose titration should be done cautiously.

Although clinical trials have not evaluated clinical outcomes following β-blocker therapy in patients with chronic stable angina, abundant data exist indicating prolonged survival in patients following acute myocardial infarction, as well as in patients with hypertension (28–30). The favorable effects of these agents on ischemia and sudden death in these patient populations can probably be extrapolated to individuals with stable angina pectoris. For this reason, β-blocker therapy is a first-line agent in the management of chronic stable angina, unless absolutely contraindicated.

Calcium-Channel Antagonists

The calcium-channel antagonists are a heterogeneous group of compounds, which act through the common mechanism of decreasing calcium entry into smooth muscle cells and myocytes. The net effect is both coronary and peripheral vasodilation, an improvement in myocardial oxygen supply, and a reduction in oxygen consumption through afterload reduction. The nondihydropyridine classes, verapamil (a phenylalklyamine) and diltiazem (a benzothiazepine) have the additional effect of decreasing the heart rate. Conversely, abrupt lowering of the blood pressure with dihydropyridines such as nifedipine may produce a reflex tachycardia, though this unwanted effect is less of an issue with longer-acting formulations. Other side effects of these agents include ankle edema, headache, flushing, and hypotension. Profound bradycardia may occur with high doses of verapamil as a result of its AV node blocking ability. In addition, due to the potent negative inotropic effect of verapamil and, to a lesser degree, diltiazem, these drugs are relatively contraindicated in patients with depressed left ventricular function. However, in one study, amlodipine was well tolerated in patients with congestive heart failure (31).

All classes of calcium-channel antagonists have been shown to reduce exercise-induced angina. However, unlike β-blockers, these agents have not been shown to improve survival in patients with known CAD. Meta-analyses suggest that they may actually increase long-term mortality (32,33), but these were based mainly on studies using the short-acting dihydropyridines, which are very rarely used now. There is now good evidence that verapamil and diltiazem can reduce reinfarction rates when used for secondary prevention after myocardial infarction, provided that there is no evidence of left ventricular dysfunction (34,35). Therefore, they may be considered a reasonable alternative when β-blocker therapy is contraindicated, as in cases of severe reactive airway disease. β-Blockers and calcium-channel antagonists may be used in combination for patients requiring a more intensified medical regimen.

Lipid-Lowering Therapy

Numerous randomized studies of HMG CoA reductase inhibitors (statins) support their routine use in patients with CAD. Lowering total cholesterol and low-density cholesterol (LDL) levels in patients with hypercholesterolemia reduced the incidence of death and myocardial infarction in the primary prevention West of Scotland Trial (WOSCOPS) (36). The Air Force/Texas Coronary Atherosclerosis Prevention Trial (AFCAPS/TEXCAPS) evaluated men and women with average cholesterol levels and without CAD. This study was terminated prematurely due to the superior benefit shown with lovastatin in preventing acute coronary syndromes (37). The Scandinavian Simvastatin Survival Study (4S trial) of hypercholesterolemic patients with stable angina or previous myocardial infarction clearly established the secondary prevention benefit of cholesterol lowering in patients with known CAD *(38)*. The Cholesterol and Recurrent Events (CARE) trial provided strong evidence that treatment with 40 mg of simvastatin daily in postmyocardial infarction patients with average cholesterol levels prolonged survival and reduced recurrent cardiac events *(39)*. The Anglo-Scandinavian Cardiac Outcomes Trial (ASCOT) *(40)* studied primary prevention of CAD in hypertensive patients with low-dose atorvastatin and demonstrated significant reduction in cardiovascular events with 10 mg of atorvastatin that resulted in premature termination of the trial. The Heart Protection Study (HPS) *(41)* revealed that patients with total cholesterol greater than 135 mg/dL who were at high risk for coronary artery disease derived benefit from simvastatin 40 mg even when the enrollment LDL was less than 100. Within this study, the composite endpoint of death, stroke, or myocardial infarction was reduced by 35% at 3 yr. Finally, the Pravastatin or Atorvastatin Evaluation and Infection Therapy (PROVE-IT) *(42)* study demonstrated that intensive LDL lowering therapy with atorvastatin 80 mg daily (median LDL achieved was 62 mg/dL) compared with moderate LDL reduction achieved (median LDL 95 mg/dL) by using pravastatin 40 mg daily reduced cardiovascular endpoints significantly in patients presenting with acute coronary syndromes. On the basis of these overwhelming data, the National Cholesterol Education Program (NCEP) has recommended cholesterol lowering in all patients at high risk for CAD or extracardiac atherosclerosis to LDL levels to a goal of less than 100 mg/dL with an option of decreasing LDL to less than 70 at the discretion of the provider *(43)*. These recommendations may be changed further in the near future to lower LDL cholesterol to a goal of less than 70 in all patients with CAD or at high risk of developing CAD, as there are several large clinical trials evaluating the same question of aggressive LDL lowering.

An often-forgotten risk factor in CAD is serum triglyceride level. Although most epidemiological studies have demonstrated an association between triclyceride level and heart disease, the strength of the association often weakens when controlled for HDL levels. A recently completed 8-yr follow-up study in asymptomatic men with elevated triglyceride levels found an increased rate of cardiac events and all-cause mortality, independent of HDL levels *(44)*. Thus, patients with CAD receive should be aggressively treated to reduce their triglyceride levels as well as LDL cholesterol. Effective treatments include the use of fibric-acid derivatives, such as gemfibrozil or clofibrate. Niacin is also an effective triglyceride-lowering agent. In a recent small study of 164 patients, the addition of niacin (mean dose of 2.4 g/d) to low doses of simvastatin (mean dose 13 mg/d) led to regression of atherosclerosis and reduced clinical events by 60% when compared to placebo *(45)*. The use of combined therapies for mixed hyperlipidemia disorders raises concerns over increased risk of hepatic toxicity and skeletal myopathy. Combination therapy is not absolutely contraindicated. Patients should be monitored closely for laboratory indicators of these complications. Newer-generation HMG CoA reductase inhibitors have been shown to be useful in reducing borderline increases in triglyceride level and may obviate the need for combined therapies in some circumstances; however, data establishing their efficacy are not available at the time of this writing *(46)*.

Hormone Replacement Therapy

The controversy of hormone replacement therapy for primary and secondary prevention in CAD is has been resolved by the Women's Health Initiative (WHI) *(47)* and the Heart Estrogen/Progestin Replacement Study (HERS) *(48)*.

Although lack of estrogen has been implicated as a risk factor for CAD for more than three decades, only in recent years have well-designed trials been initiated to assess the efficacy of estrogen replacement. The beneficial effect of hormone replacement therapy on the lipid profile is less of an issue. Many studies have demonstrated the lowering of LDL and lipoprotein(a) levels, while elevating HDL *(49)*. The proposed efficacy of hormone replacement therapy was believed to arise from this enhanced lipid profile and to positive effects of estrogen-mediated endothelial vasomotor function.

The data suggesting the benefit of hormone replacement therapy in CAD have come from observational studies *(50,51)*. The Nurses Health Study found that a large cohort of women currently using hormone replacement therapy had a 50% reduction for myocardial infarction or all-cause mortality as compared to nonusers *(52)*. Observational studies such as these may be criticized for inherent selection biases. For example, individuals choosing to use hormone replacement therapy typically lead a healthier lifestyle, seek regular medical care, and follow exercise regimens. The Heart and Estrogen/Progestin Replacement Study (HERS) is a recently completed double-blind, randomized secondary prevention trial with hormone replacement therapy. Despite improved lipid profiles in the treatment arm, there was no significant benefit in preventing recurrent myocardial infarction or cardiac death during an average 4-yr follow-up. Thromboembolic events, including pulmonary embolism, occurred more frequently in the treated arm, particularly in the first year after beginning therapy *(48)*. The results of the Women's Health Initiative *(47)* showed an increased risk of adverse coronary events when estrogen and progesterone combination therapy was used for primary prevention. Based on these trials, hormonal therapy is not indicated for either primary or secondary prevention of coronary heart disease, although in patients at low risk for cardiac complications, hormone replacement therapy may still be indicated for treatment of symptoms resulting from estrogen deficiency.

Antioxidant Therapy

It is hypothesized that the oxidation of LDL cholesterol particles may play a pivotal role in the initiation and progression of atherosclerosis. There are observational study data to suggest that naturally occurring antioxidants may slow this process. However, as previously mentioned, selection biases of epidemiological studies render these data inconclusive.

To date, three randomized, double-blind, placebo-controlled trials have examined the effects of antioxidants on cardiovascular events. The Physicians Health Study was a primary prevention trial of 22,000 physicians over a 12-yr period. Supplementing the diet with the antioxidant β-carotene produced no reduction in cardiovascular morbidity or mortality *(53)*. Conflicting evidence exists in secondary prevention. A Finnish study failed to detect any benefit of vitamin E or β-carotene in limiting progression to severe symptomatic angina or myocardial infarction in men with established CAD *(54)*. In contrast, the Cambridge Heart Anti-Oxidant Study (CHAOS), using a higher dose of vitamin E (400–800 IU), demonstrated a 47% risk reduction in cardiovascular death and nonfatal myocardial infarction *(55)*. The Gruppo Italiano per lo Studio della Sopravvivenza nell'Infarcto miocardico (GISSI) Prevention study *(56)* and Heart Outcome Prevention Evaluation study *(57)* did not show any benefit from antioxidant therapy.

Based on the current data, the empiric use of antioxidant therapy for primary or secondary prevention of coronary atherosclerotic heart disease is not recommended.

REVASCULARIZATION: CATHETER-BASED METHODS

Percutaneous Transluminal Coronary Angioplasty

The concept of therapeutic percutaneous angioplasty was first introduced in 1964 by Dotter and Judkins *(58)*. However, their technique for the treatment of peripheral vascular stenosis was not widely accepted because of the frequent occurrence of local trauma and hemorrhage. The subsequent development by Andreas Gruentzig of a double-lumen balloon catheter pioneered the modern era of interventional cardiology. In September 1977 in Zurich, Gruentzig performed the first percutaneous transluminal coronary angioplasty (PTCA) procedure in humans, successfully dilating the proximal left anterior descending coronary artery of a 37-yr-old man with angina pectoris *(59)*. Repeat coronary angiography on the 10th and 20th anniversaries of the procedure revealed continued vessel patency.

Since this initial introduction in 1977, operator experience has expanded the selection of patients for whom PTCA may be appropriate, including those with stable multivessel disease and acute coronary syndromes. The ideal candidates for PTCA were originally described as patients with stable angina pectoris as a result of single-vessel CAD without complex angiographic characteristics. In such patients, procedural success rates exceeded 97% even before the widespread use of intracoronary stents and were associated with a low risk of early complications such as myocardial infarction or death. Clinical variables such as advanced age, history of congestive heart failure, or left ventricular dysfunction, as well as complex lesion features including calcification, presence of thrombus, eccentric morphology, and ostial location increased the periprocedural risk of PTCA. Experienced operators in high-volume catheterization laboratories have lower complication rates compared with low-volume medical centers.

Early complications of PTCA are most often the result of abrupt vessel closure, defined as the sudden occlusion of the target vessel during or shortly after the revascularization procedure. The incidence of this complication is in the range of 1 to 2%. Before the availability of intracoronary stents, the pathophysiology typically involved local vessel dissection with obstructive dissection flaps, accompanied by development of thrombus secondary to platelet activation from exposed subendothelial vascular wall components. Currently, stenting has allowed the achievement of widely patent coronary lumina with "sealing" of dissection flaps. Subacute stent thrombosis has replaced abrupt vessel closure as the bugbear of intracoronary intervention. Fortunately, it is now quite rare. Risk factors appear to include multiple stent placement, incomplete stent apposition to the arterial wall, incomplete expansion of the stent struts, and residual stenosis within the stent. Recently, resistance to the antiplatelet effects of clopidogrel and/or aspirin have also been suggested as etiologies. The clinical consequences of such an event may lead to acute myocardial infarction, the need for urgent surgical revascularization, or even death. The use of thienopyridine platelet glycoprotein IIb/IIIa antagonists and intracoronary stenting have successfully reduced the incidence and adverse outcomes of acute vessel closure *(60,61)* and have augmented the ability to approach patients with more complex lesions and multivessel disease. Placement of a bare metal intracoronary stent mandates a minimal 4-wk course of clopidogrel and continued aspirin to prevent subacute stent thrombosis. Clinical trials of drug-eluting stents have mandated 3 to 6 mo of therapy *(62–64)* with clopidogrel, and a recent trial of clopidogrel in patients undergoing balloon angioplasty alone or implantation of a bare metal stent has indicated that benefits continue to accrue when clopidogrel is continued through at least the first year after stenting *(65)*. Reports of late thrombosis of drug eluting stents, even after one year, are now emerging. These events appear related to cessation of antiplatelet therapy *(66,67)*.

The principal limitation of PTCA is restenosis, which has been reported in 30 to 40% of patients within 6 mo of the procedure *(68)*. The most common clinical presentation of restenosis is recurrence of stable anginal symptoms. Myocardial infarction as the initial presentation of restenosis is a rare occurrence. The pathogenesis of restenosis in response to mechanical injury induced by angioplasty is incompletely understood and is probably multifactorial. A number of pharmacological agents of various classes have been evaluated for the prevention of restenosis, including antiplatelet drugs, anticoagulants, calcium-channel blockers, and antiproliferative agents. The recent introduction of drug-eluting stents with sirolimus and paclitaxel have decreased the incidence of in-stent restenosis in discrete lesions to less than 8% and the incidence of target vessel revascularization to less than 5% in patients who undergo PCI of a lesion within a single vessel. Although reduced by drug-eluting stents, restenosis still occurs more commonly in patients with diabetes and small vessels *(62,63)*.

Over the years, methods adjunctive to angioplasty have been developed to assist in managing lesions with complex characteristics. As a result of the increasing frequency with which these newer techniques are used, the term *percutaneous transluminal coronary angioplasty* is gradually being replaced by the more accurate term, *percutaneous coronary intervention* (PCI). Directional coronary atherectomy employs a blade housed within a balloon catheter. Inflation of the balloon forces the blade's housing against the protruding portion of the plaque; the blade trims away the plaque and forces the debris into the housing, opening the lumen of the artery more widely. Evaluation of this technique versus balloon angioplasty has not shown conclusive improvement in 6-mo restenosis rates. Moreover, the use of directional atherectomy is associated with an increased rate of periprocedural non-Q-wave infarction *(69,70)*. Rotational atherectomy (Rotablator®) employs a rotary cone containing diamond chips at the end of a catheter that is capable of abrading rigid or calcified lesions. Observational data suggest that rotational atherectomy is useful in managing complex lesion subsets not suitable for balloon angioplasty alone. Direct comparison in a randomized trial against standard balloon angioplasty has shown superior procedural success rates for rotational atherectomy in complex lesions without an excess of periprocedural complications. However, restenosis rates at 6 mo were significantly higher in the rotational atherectomy group than in those patients who had balloon angioplasty (71).

ANGIOGENESIS

Percutaneous Transmyocardial Revascularization

A significant number of patients with chronic CAD and severe angina pectoris despite maximal medical therapy are not candidates for revascularization strategies because of their coronary anatomy. Until recently, no alternative therapy has been available to palliate these patients. In response to this need, a variety of angiogenic therapies have been proposed.

Transmyocardial revascularization is an innovative procedure whereby multiple channels 1 mm in width are created in ischemic myocardium. The mechanism by which myocardial channels lead to neovascularization has remained controversial. Initial conceptions of this technique suggested that the new channels would provide myocardial perfusion directly from the left ventricular cavity, as occurs in the reptilian heart. Perspectives on the mechanism have been obtained in animal models in which channels using lasers were compared with channels created by a hardware store power drill. After several weeks of followup, the histological appearances of the channels were identical and none were patent. However, all previous channels were surrounded by some degree of fibrosis and neovascularization (72). Thus, the laser channels are not the new vessels themselves, but their creation stimulates chemical signals that lead to new vessel growth. Furthermore, the neovascularization may be dependent not on laser therapy per se but rather on a nonspecific healing response to injury. Complications of these techniques are rare, though they may have serious consequences. These include ventricular fibrillation, pericardial tamponade, perforation of large arteries, and damage to the chordae tendinae or the Purkinje network. In the surgical approach, channels are generated via a carbon dioxide (CO_2) laser from the epicardial surface inward. Several studies that are either nonrandomized or unblinded indicate improved exercise treadmill time and subjective surveys have reported anginal relief (73). A catheter-based approach creates conduits from the left ventricular cavity into the myocardium, obviating the need for general anesthesia and thoracotomy. However, one of two randomized blinded trials did not support its efficacy, while another yielded equivocal results (74,75).

Gene-Related Therapy

Progress in the field of molecular biology and recombinant genetic technology has paved the way for novel strategies for the treatment of chronic ischemic disease (see also Chapter 42). The aim of gene therapy for vascular ischemia is to stimulate the growth of new blood vessels for individuals with advanced, nonreconstructable arterial disease. The development of high-yield gene transfer techniques has allowed for the introduction of known angiogenic factors to ischemic tissues. Modes of delivery have utilized various molecular packages or "vectors." Examples range from simple naked plasmid DNA encoding the desired protein to complex viral particles containing nucleic acid cores. More recent attention has been directed to "master genes," such as hypoxia inducible factor (HIF-1) that regulates a large family of genes that facilitate tissue accommodation to hypoxia and ischemia, and to stem cell transplantation or stimulation (76–78).

The two most extensively studied angiogenic growth factors to date in the context of tissue ischemia are vascular endothelial growth factor (VEGF) and fibroblast growth factor (FGF). VEGF-1 exists in four subtypes, alternative splicing products produced from the same gene. These proteins are secreted by smooth muscle cells and platelets and have high-affinity binding sites on the surface of endothelial cells. VEGF stimulates vascular permeability and endothelial cell migration, and accelerates the process of endothelialization (79). Fibroblast growth factors are members of a family of nearly 20 proteins. FGF-1 and FGF-2 are known to stimulate the proliferation of three principal vascular cell types: fibroblasts, endothelial cells, and smooth muscle cells (80).

Preliminary evidence now exists that intramuscular VEGF gene transfer in humans can achieve expression of VEGF protein, but can also lead to angiogenesis. Naked plasmid DNA encoding a VEGF isoform was administered into muscle of 10 ischemic limbs of 9 patients. Newly developed collateral vessels were demonstrated angiographically in 7 limbs. Ischemic ulcers were markedly improved in 4 of 7 limbs with salvage of limbs in 3 patients recommended for below-knee amputation *(81)*. Further promising data have come from a randomized, controlled study of genetically engineered fibroblast growth factor (FGF-1) in patients with CAD. At the time of coronary bypass, patients received an injection of active or denatured FGF-1 protein in close proximity to left anterior descending (LAD) artery distal anastomoses after revascularization. After 3 mo, coronary angiography revealed the presence of capillary networks sprouting from the LAD in all 20 patients receiving the active agent, as opposed to zero angiogenesis for controls *(82)*. A small pilot study of basic FGF-2 carried by an adenoviral vector and administered through the intracoronary route to patients with CAD and scintigaphic evidence of myocardial ischemia revealed a nonsignificant trend toward a reduction in quantitative measures of ischemic defect size *(83)*. Two large trials of this therapy in patients with exercise-induced ischemia were terminated prematurely due to futility.

Trials using catheter-based intramyocardial gene transfer are now under way. This exciting and revolutionary technology shows great hope for having an impact on the future of cardiovascular treatment in the new millennium.

CORONARY ARTERY BYPASS SURGERY

Coronary artery bypass grafting (CABG) has remained a very effective procedure for relief of angina pectoris since first used in 1964 as a "bailout" technique by Dr. Michael DeBakey *(84)* and further refinement by Dr. Rene Favoloro *(85,86)*. Symptoms of ischemia can be alleviated in more than 85% of patients *(87)*. Though initial costs are high compared to other strategies, particularly PCI, in selected patients the expenditure is comparable when repeated PCI and long-term. intensive post-PCI medical therapy may be needed.

Over the last 30 yr modifications of the procedure have continued to lead to high success rates in more complicated patients. The use of the internal thoracic artery (left internal mammary artery) to bypass the left anterior descending coronary artery (LAD) is superior to use of saphenous venous grafts. Patency rates for this graft are approx 90% at 10 yr compared with 30% for saphenous vein grafts *(88)*. Evidence suggests that the use of two arterial grafts rather than one may lead to improved long-term symptomatic relief in selected patients *(89)*. A beneficial effect on mortality rates of using two rather than one arterial conduit on reoperation remains unclear. The present-day practice of chronic aspirin and aggressive lipid-lowering therapy in patients beginning immediately after CABG may make the choice of a second conduit (in addition to an internal thoracic artery) less of an issue, particularly in elderly patients.

Complication rates are related to the extent of CAD, left ventricular dysfunction, and comorbid illnesses. Overall, the perioperative composite rates of mortality and myocardial infarction approximate 5%. Repeat operations are always associated with higher complication rates.

MANAGEMENT DECISION MAKING

The goals of the effective management of stable angina pectoris are to achieve symptom relief and improve long-term survival. Management decisions should be based on prognostic information derived from an appropriately chosen diagnostic test. The choice of medical therapy and/or revascularization should be made after consideration of the known comparative efficacies of the strategy options. However, it must be emphasized that all patients should be encouraged to adopt lifestyle changes known to improve prognosis, such as smoking cessation and a adoption of a low-cholesterol diet.

A management algorithm based on current available data is presented in Fig. 3. As mentioned previously, the diagnostic test shown to provide the most robust and objective prognostic value for risk of cardiac death or myocardial infarction is myocardial perfusion imaging (MPI) *(14,15)*. The

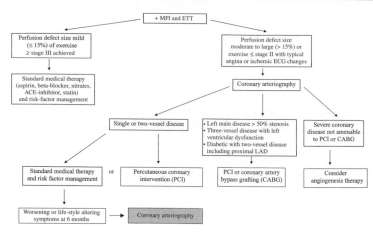

Fig. 3. Management strategy based on diagnostic test results.

predictive value is enhanced by computer-generated quantitation of ischemic defect size. Patients with stable angina who have mild perfusion defects (<15%) have been shown to be at low risk (<1% per year) for cardiac death or myocardial infarction *(14,15)*. Patients capable of achieving ≥10 METs (Stage III, Bruce Protocol) on exercise treadmill have a prognosis with medical therapy as good as revascularization and are considered to be at low risk for cardiac events *(90)*. In such patients, an initial approach of "standard medical therapy" is reasonable. Standard medical therapy consists of ASA, β-blockers, ACE inhibitors, short-acting nitrates, and lipid-lowering therapy if LDL levels exceed 100 mg/dL after diet modification. Randomized trial data support such an approach. The Angioplasty Compared to Medicine trial (ACME) for stable angina pectoris demonstrated that 48% of medically treated patients with stable angina may be rendered symptom-free by 6 mo *(91)*. The Second Randomized Intervention Treatment of Angina trial (RITA-II) randomized more than 1000 patients with stable angina pectoris to medical therapy or coronary angioplasty. After a median 2.7-yr follow-up, interventional management (largely balloon angioplasty without intracoronary stenting) conferred no benefit in terms of death or myocardial infarction *(92)*. Similarly, data from the Coronary Artery Surgery Study (CASS) registry showed no mortality difference over 10 yr between medical therapy and bypass grafting for single-vessel or two-vessel disease (excluding the proximal left anterior descending artery), in patients with normal left ventricular function *(93)*.

Although test results indicating low risk suggest medical therapy, there is no dispute that percutaneous interventions and coronary artery bypass grafting are effective in relieving symptoms of angina that persist despite adequate medical regimens. Therefore, patients with lifestyle-altering stable angina persisting after 6 mo of aggressive medical therapy should proceed to coronary angiography with the intent of revascularization. The interpretation of many studies of PCI is limited by the fact that they were performed before the widespread use of drug-eluting stents and aggressive lipid lowering. At least one large trial, the BARI 2D study, is now being performed to evaluate the effect of modern revascularization compared with medical therapy on mortality in patients with diabetes and moderate risk ischemia as demonstrated by functional testing *(94)*.

Coronary angiography should be carried out in patients with moderate to severe perfusion defect size (>15%) or poor treadmill exercise tolerance (≤5 METs). Cardiac event rates in these groups are in the range of 3 to 4% per year *(15)*. Following determination of the extent of CAD and the need for revascularization, the decision of percutaneous coronary intervention versus coronary artery bypass grafting arises. The Coronary Artery Surgery Study (CASS) registry has clearly shown survival benefit in patients with three-vessel or left main disease in excess of 50% stenosis *(93)*. There is little dispute that the symptomatic patient with significant disease in the left main coronary artery should proceed directly to bypass grafting. On the other hand, percutaneous intervention has proven to be successful in relieving anginal symptoms in the vast majority of patients who have single-vessel disease and therefore obviates the need for major surgery. The gray zone occurs for patients with two- or three-vessel disease whose anatomy appears amenable to either surgical or percutaneous revascularization.

To date, five major trials have compared percutaneous revascularization with bypass surgery in patients with stable angina pectoris *(95–99)*. The results of these trials are uniform and consistent in showing similar risks of death and nonfatal myocardial infarction in long-term follow-up for as long as 7 yr. However, an increase in the need for repeated revascularization procedures has been seen in percutaneous-treatment arms. In the Bypass Angioplasty Revascularization Investigation (BARI) trial, the largest of the studies, an 8% repeat revascularization rate for coronary artery bypass versus 54% for coronary angioplasty was seen *(99)*. It was also clear from this trial that the subgroup of patients with diabetes mellitus requiring glucose-lowering treatment benefited significantly more from bypass grafting than from angioplasty. In the Arterial Revascularization Therapy Study (ARTS), patients with diabetes and multivessel disease had a better mortality outcome at 1 yr with bypass grafting than with PCI, although the difference was not statistically significant *(100)*. Also, in the Stent of Surgery (SOS) trial, patients with diabetes needed fewer repeat revascularization procedures when they underwent coronary artery bypass surgery compared to PCI with stents *(101)*. While these data may provide general guidelines, decisions regarding revascularization must still be individualized with consideration of comorbidities and patient preference. It should also be kept in mind that percutaneous revascularization techniques have advanced dramatically since these studies have been performed. Intracoronary drug eluting stents have reduced the rate of restenosis from 40% to less than 5% in clinical trials *(62,63)*, and permitted much more aggressive use of multivessel angioplasty. The use of adjunctive platelet glycoprotein IIb-IIIa antagonists during percutaneous coronary interventions has reduced the periprocedure infarction rate and is associated with long-term reduction in mortality compared to balloon angioplasty alone *(61,102,103)*. There are clinical trials under way to compare PCI with drug-eluting stents versus coronary artery bypass surgery. Patients with severe disease not suitable for revascularization should be considered for one of the novel strategies now available, including gene-related therapy or transmyocardial revascularization.

REFERENCES

1. Centers for Disease Control and Prevention. National Center for Health Statistics, National Vital Statistics and The United States Bureau of the Census. Health, United States 1993, p. 31.
2. Prevalence of diabetes and impaired fasting glucose in adults—United States, 1999–2000, MMWR 2003;52:833–837.
3. Campeau L. Grading of angina pectoris. Circulation 1976;54:522–523.
4. Haverkate F, Thompson SG, Pyke SD, et al. Production of C-reactive protein and risk of coronary events in stable and unstable angina. European Concerted Action on Thrombosis and Disabilities Angina Pectoris Study Group. Lancet 1997;349:462–466.
5. Ridker PM, Rifai N, Pfeffer MA, et al. Inflammation, pravastatin, and the risk of coronary events after myocardial infarction in patients with average cholesterol levels. Cholesterol and Recurrent Events (CARE) Investigators. Circulation 1998;98:839–844.
6. Wang L, Fan C, Topol SE, et al. Mutation of MEF2A in an inherited disorder with features of coronary artery disease. Science 2003;302:1578–1581.
7. Gianrossi R, Detrano R, Mulvihill D, et al. Exercise-induced ST depression in the diagnosis of coronary artery disease: a meta-analysis. Circulation 1989;80:87–98.
8. Kaul S, Boucher CA, Newell JB, et al. Determination of the quantitative thallium imaging variables that optimize detection of coronary artery disease. J Am Coll Cardiol 1986;7:527.
9. Gibbons RJ, Fyke FE, Clements IP, et al. Noninvasive identification of severe coronary artery disease using exercise radionuclide angiography. J Am Coll Card 1988;11:28.
10. Quinones MA, Verani MS, Haichin RM, et al. Exercise echocardiography versus Tl-201 single photon emission computerized tomography in evaluation of coronary artery disease: analysis of 292 patients. Circulation 1992;85: 1026-1031.
11. Galbraith JE, Murphy ML, Desoyza N. Coronary angiogram interpretation: interobserver variability. JAMA 1981; 240:2053–2059.
12. Grodin CM, Dydra I, Pastgernac A, et al. Discrepancies between cineangiographic and post-mortem findings in patients with coronary artery disease and recent myocardial revascularization. Circulation 1974;49:703–709.
13. Pijls NH, De Bruyne B, Peels K, et al. Measurement of fractional flow reserve to assess the functional severity of coronary-artery stenosis. N Engl J Med 31996;34:1703–1708.
14. Iskandrian AS, Chae SC, Heo J, et al. Independent and incremental prognostic value of exercise single-photon emission computed tomographic (SPECT) thallium imaging in coronary artery disease. J Am Coll Cardiol 1993;22: 665–670.

15. Hachamovitch R, Berman DS, Shaw LJ, et al. Incremental prognostic value of myocardial perfusion single photon emission computed tomography for the prediction of cardiac death. Circulation 1998;97:535–543.
16. Antiplatelet Trialists' Collaboration. Collaborative overview of randomized trials of antiplatelet therapy. I: prevention of death, myocardial infarction, and stroke by prolonged anti platelet therapy in various categories of patients. Br Med J 1994;308:81–98.
17. Topol EJ, Easton D, Harrington RA. BRAVO Trial Investigators. Randomized, double-blind, placebo-controlled, international trial of the oral IIb/IIIa antagonist lotrafiban in coronary and cerebrovascular disease. Circulation 2003;108:399–406.
18. Gum PA, Kottke-Marchant K, Poggio ED, et al. Profile and prevalence of aspirin resistance in patients with cardiovascular disease. Am J Cardiol 2001;88:230–235.
19. Eikelboom JW, Hirsh J, Weitz JI, et al. Aspirin-resistant thromboxane biosynthesis and the risk of myocardial infarction, stroke, or cardiovascular death in patients at high risk for cardiovascular events. Circulation 2002;105: 1650–1655.
20. Conley PB, Delaney SM. Scientific and therapeutic insights into the role of the platelet P2Y12 receptor in thrombosis. Curr Opin Hematol 2003;10:333–338.
21. Dorsam RT, Kunapuli SP. Central role of the P2Y12 receptor in platelet activation. J Clin Invest 2004;113:340–345.
22. Cannon CP, CAPRIE Investigators. Clopidogrel versus Aspirin in Patients at Risk of Ischemic Events (CAPRIE). Am J Cardiol 2002;90:760–762.
23. Steinhubl SR, Berger PB, Mann JT III, et al. Clopidogrel for the reduction of events during observation. JAMA 2002;288:2411–2420.
24. CURE Trial Investigators. Clopidogrel in unstable angina to prevent recurrent events. N Engl J Med 2001;345: 494–502.
25. Abrams J, ed. Third North American conference on nitroglycerine therapy. Am J Cardiol 1992;70:1B–103B.
26. Cheitlin MD, Hutter AM Jr, Brindis RG, et al. Use of sildenafil (Viagra) in patients with cardiovascular disease: ACC/AHA Expert Consensus Document. Circulation 1999;99:168–177.
27. Kloner RA, Hutter AM, Emmick JT, et al. Time course of the interaction between tadalafil and nitrates. J Am Coll Cardiol 2003;42:1855–1860.
28. The BHAT Research Group. A randomized trial of propranolol in patients with acute myocardial infarction. The Beta-blocker Heart Attack Trial. JAMA 1982;247:1707–1714.
29. The MIAMI trial research group. Metoprolol in acute myocardial infarction (MIAMI). A randomized placebo-controlled international trial. Eur Heart J 1985;6:199–211.
30. The ISIS-1 Collaborative Group. Randomized trial of intravenous atenolol among 16027 cases of suspected acute myocardial infarction: ISIS-1. Lancet 1986;ii:57–66.
31. Packer M, O'Connor CM, Ghali JK, et al. Effect of amlodipine on morbidity and mortality in severe chronic heart failure. N Engl J Med 1996;335:1107–1114.
32. Psaty BM, Smith NL, Siscovick DS, et al. Health outcomes associated with antihypertensive therapies used as first-line agents. A systematic review and meta-analysis. JAMA 1997;277:739–745.
33. Pahor M, Psaty BM, Alderman MH, et al. Health outcomes associated with calcium antagonists compared with other first-line antihypertensive therapies: a meta-analysis of randomised controlled trials. Lancet 2000;356:1949–1954.
34. The MDPIT Research Group. The effect of diltiazem on mortality and reinfarction after myocardial infarction. N Engl J Med 1988;319:385–392.
35. The Danish Study Group on Verapamil in Myocardial Infarction. Effect of verapamil on mortality and major events after acute myocardial infarction (The Danish Verapamil Infarction Trial II-DAVIT II). Am J Cardiol 1990; 66:779–785.
36. The West of Scotland Coronary Prevention Study Group. Prevention of coronary heart disease with pravastatin in men with hypercholesterolemia. N Engl J Med 1995;333:1301–1307.
37. The Air Force/Texas Coronary Atherosclerosis Prevention Research Study Group. Primary prevention of acute coronary events with lovastatin in men and women with average cholesterol levels. JAMA 1998;279:1615–1622.
38. Scandinavian Simvastatin Survival Study Group. Randomized trial of cholesterol lowering in 4444 patients with coronary heart disease: the Scandinavian Simvastatin Survival Study (4S). Lancet 1994;344:1383–1389.
39. The Cholesterol and Recurrent Events Trial Investigators. The effect of pravastatin on coronary events after myocardial infarction inpatients with average cholesterol levels. N Engl J Med 1996;335:1001–1009.
40. ASCOT Investigators. Prevention of coronary and stroke events with atorvastatin in hypertensive patients who have average or lower-than-average cholesterol concentrations, in the Anglo-Scandinavian Cardiac Outcomes Trial —Lipid Lowering Arm (ASCOT-LLA): a multicentre randomised controlled trial. Lancet 2003;361:1149–1158.
41. Heart Protection Study Collaborative Group. MRC/BHF Heart Protection Study of cholesterol lowering with simvastatin in 20,536 high risk individuals: a randomised placebo-controlled trial. Lancet 2002;360:7–22.
42. Cannon CP, Braunwald E, McCabe CH, et al. Intensive versus moderate lipid lowering with statins after acute coronary syndromes (PROVE-IT). N Engl J Med 2004;350:1495–1504.
43. Grundy SM, Cleeman JI, Merz CN, et al. Implications of Recent Clinical Trials for the National Cholesterol Education Program Adult Treatment Panel III Guidelines. Circulation 2004;110:227–239.
44. Jeppesen J, Hein HO, Suadicani P, et al. Triglyceride concentration and ischemic heart disease: an eight-year follw-up in the Copenhagen male study. Circulation 1998;97:1029–1036.
45. Zhao XQ, Morse JS, Dowdy AA, et al. Safety and tolerability of simvastatin plus niacin in patients with coronary artery disease and low high-density lipoprotein cholesterol (The HDL Atherosclerosis Treatment Study). Am J Cardiol 2004;93:307–312.

46. McKenney JM, McCormick LS, Weiss S, et al. A randomized trial of the effects of atorvastatin and niacin in patients with combined hyperlipidemia or isolated hypertriglyceridemia. Am J Med 1998;104:137–143.
47. WHI Investigators. Risks and benefits of estrogen plus progestin in healthy postmenopausal women—principal results from the Women's Health Initiative randomized controlled trial. JAMA 2002;288:321–333.
48. The Heart and Estrogen/progestin Replacement Study (HERS) Group. Randomized trial of estrogen plus progestin for secondary prevention of coronary heart disease in postmenopausal women. JAMA 1998;280:605–613.
49. The Writing Group for the PEPI Trial. Effects of estrogen or estrogen/progestin regimens on heart disease risk factors in postmenopausal women: the postmenopausal estrogen/progestin interventions (PEPI) trial. JAMA 1995;273:199–208.
50. Belchetz PE. Hormonal treatment of postmenopausal women. N Engl J Med 1994;330:1062–1071.
51. Grady D, Rubin SM, Petitti DB, et al. Hormone therapy to prevent disease and prolong life in postmenopausal women. Ann Intern Med 1992;117:1016–1037.
52. Stampfer MJ, Colditz GA, Willett WC, et al. Postmenopausal estrogen therapy and cardiovascular disease. Ten-year follow-up from the Nurses' Health Study. N Engl J Med 1991;325:756.
53. Hennekens CH, Buring JE, Manson JE, et al. Lack of effect of long-term supplementation with beta-carotene on the incidence of malignant neoplasms and cardiovascular disease. N Engl J Med 1996;334:1145–1149.
54. Rapola JM, Virtamo J, Ripatti S, et al. Effects of alpha-tocopherol and beta-carotene supplements on symptoms, progression, and prognosis in angina pectoris. Heart 1998;79:454–458.
55. Stephens NG, Parsons A, Schofiled PM, et al. Randomized controlled trial of vitamin E in patients with coronary disease: Cambridge Heart Antioxidant Study (CHAOS). Lancet 1996;347:781–786.
56. GISSI Prevenzione Investigators. Dietary supplementation with n-3 polyunsaturated fatty acids and vitamin E after myocardial infarction: results of the GISSI Prevenzione trial. Lancet 1999;354:447–455.
57. The Heart Outcomes Prevention Evaluation Study Investigators. Effects of an angiotensin-converting enzyme inhibitor, ramipril, on cardiovascular events in high risk patients. N Engl J Med 2000;342:145–153.
58. Dotter CT, Judkins MP. Transluminal treatment of arteriosclerotic obstruction: description of a new technique and a preliminary report of its application. Circulation 1964;30:654–670.
59. King SB III. Angioplasty from bench to bedside to bench. Circulation 1996;93:1621–1629.
60. The EPILOG Investigators. Platelet glycoprotein IIb/IIIa blockade and low-dose heparin during percutaneous coronary revascularization. N Engl J Med 1997;336:1689–1696.
61. The EPISTENT Investigators. Randomized placebo-controlled and balloon-angioplasty-controlled trial to assess safety of coronary stenting with use of platelet glycoprotein-IIb/IIIa blockade. Lancet 1998;352:87–92.
62. The SIRIUS Investigators. Sirolimus-eluting stents versus standard stents in patients with stenosis in a native coronary artery. N Engl J Med 2003;349:1315–1323.
63. Colombo A, Drzewiecki J, Banning A, et al. Randomized study to assess the effectiveness of slow- and moderate-release polymer-based paclitaxel-eluting stents for coronary artery lesions. Circulation 2003;108:788–794.
64. RAVEL Study Group. Randomized comparison of a sirolimus-eluting stent with a standard stent for coronary revascularization. N Engl J Med 2002;346:1773–1780.
65. Mehta SR, Yusef S, Peters RJ, et al. Effects of pre-treatment with clopidogrel and aspirin followed by long-term therapy in patients undergoing percutaneous coronary intervention: the PCI-CURE study. Lancet 2001;358:527–533.
66. Iakovou I, Schmidt T, Bonizzoni E, et al. Incidence, predictors, and outcome of thrombosis after successful implantation of drug-eluting stents. JAMA 2005;293:2126–2130.
67. McFadden EP, Stabile E, Regar E, et al. Late thrombosis in drug-eluting coronary stents after discontinuation of antiplatelet therapy. Lancet 2004;364:1519–1521.
68. Kuntz RE, Baim DS. Defining coronary restenosis. Circulation 1993;88:1310.
69. Elliott JM, Berdan LG, Holmes DR, et al. One-year follow-up in the coronary angioplasty versus excisional atherectomy trial (CAVEAT I). Circulation 1995;91:2158.
70. Baim DS, Cutlip DE, Sharma SK, et al. Final results of the balloon versus optimal atherectomy trial. Circulation 1998;97:322–331.
71. Reifart N, Vandormael M, Krajcar M, et al. Randomized comparison of angioplasty of complex coronary lesions at a single center. Excimer Laser, Rotational Atherectomy, and Balloon Angioplasty Comparison (ERBAC) Study. Circulation 1997;96:91–98.
72. Malekan R, Reynolds C, Narula R, et al. Angiogenesis in transmyocardial laser revascularization: a nonspecific response to injury. Circulation 1998;98:II-62–II-66.
73. Horvath KA, Cohn LII, Cooley DA, et al. Transmyocardial laser revascularization: results of a multicenter trial with transmyocardial laser revascularization used as sole therapy for end-stage coronary artery disease. J Thorac Cardiovasc Surg 1997;113:645–654.
74. Stone GW, Teirstein PS, Rubenstein R, et al. RA prospective, multicenter, randomized trial of percutaneous transmyocardial laser revascularization in patients with nonrecanalizable chronic total occlusions. J Am Coll Cardiol 2002;39:1581–1587.
75. Salem M, Rotevatn S, Stavnes S, et al. Usefulness and safety of percutaneous myocardial laser revascularization for refractory angina pectoris. Am J Cardiol 2004;93:1086-1091.
76. Semenza GL, Agani F, Iyer N, et al. Hypoxia-inducible factor 1: from molecular biology to cardiopulmonary physiology. Chest 1998;114:40S–45S.
77. Lee SH, Wolf PL, Escudero R, et al. Early expression of angiogenesis factors in acute myocardial ischemia and infarction. [see comment]. N Engl J Med 2000;342:626–633.

78. Shyu KG, Wang MT, Wang BW, et al. Intramyocardial injection of naked DNA encoding HIF-1alpha/VP16 hybrid to enhance angiogenesis in an acute myocardial infarction model in the rat. Cardiovasc Res 2002;54:576–583.
79. Isner JM. Vascular endothelial growth factor: gene therapy and therapeutic angiogenesis. Am J Cardiol 1998;10A: 63S–64S.
80. Goncalves LM. Fibroblast growth factor-mediated angiogenesis for the treatment of ischemia. Lessons learned from experimental models and early human experience. Rev Port Cardiol 1998 199;2S:11–20.
81. Baumgartner I, Pieczek A, Manor O, et al. Constitutive expression of phVEGF after intramuscular gene transfer promotes collateral vessel development in patients with critical limb ischemia. Circulation 1998;97:1114–1123.
82. Schumacher B, Pecher P, von Specht, et al. Induction of neoangiogenesis in ischemic myocardium by human growth factors. Circulation 1998;97:645–650.
83. Grines CL, Watkins MW, Mahmarian JJ, et al. Angiogene GENe Therapy (AGENT-2) Study Group. A randomized, double-blind, placebo-controlled trial of Ad5FGF-4 gene therapy and its effect on myocardial perfusion in patients with stable angina. J Am Coll Cardiol 2003;42:1339–1347.
84. Garrett HE, Dennis EW, DeBakey ME, et al. Aortocoronary bypass with saphenous vein graft: seven-year follow-up. JAMA 1973;223:792–794.
85. Favaloro RG. Bilateral internal mammary artery implants: operative technique: a preliminary report. Cleve Clin Q 1967;34:61–66.
86. Favaloro RG. Landmarks in the development of coronary artery bypass surgery. Circulation 1998;98:466–478.
87. Cameron AAC, Davis KB, Rogers WJ, et al. Recurrence of angina after coronary bypass surgery. Predictors and prognosis (CASS Registry). J Am Coll Cardiol 1995;26:895–899.
88. Goldman S, Copeland J, Moritz T, et al. Internal mammary artery and saphenous vein graft patency. Effects of aspirin. Circulation 1990;82(Suppl IV):237–242.
89. Borger MA, Cohen G, Buth KJ, et al. Multiple arterial grafts. Radial versus right internal thoracic arteries. Circulation 1998;98:II-7–II-14.
90. Fletcher GF, Balady G, Froelicher VF, et al. Exercise standards: a statement for health professionals from the American Heart Association Writing Group. Circulation 1995;91:580–615.
91. Parisi AF, Folland ED, Hartigan P. Angioplasty compared to medicine. N Engl J Med 1992;326:10–16.
92. RITA-2 Trial Participants. Coronary angioplasty versus medical therapy for angina: the second Randomized Intervention Treatment of Angina (RITA-2) trial. Lancet 1997;350:461–468.
93. Yusuf S, Zucker D, Pedruzzi P, et al. Effect of coronary artery bypass graft surgery on survival: overview of 10-year results from randomized trials by the Coronary Artery Bypass Graft Surgery Trialists Collaboration. Lancet 1994;344:563–570.
94. Sobel BE, Frye R, Detre KM. Bypass Angioplasty Revascularization Investigation 2 Diabetes Trial. Burgeoning dilemmas in the management of diabetes and cardiovascular disease: rationale for the Bypass Angioplasty Revascularization Investigation 2 Diabetes (BARI 2D) Trial. Circulation 2003;107:636–642.
95. RITA Trialists. Coronary angioplasty versus coronary artery bypass surgery: the Randomized Intervention Treatment of Angina (RITA) trial. Lancet 1993;341:573–580.
96. Hamm CW, Reimers J, Ischinger T, et al. A randomized study of coronary angioplasty compared with bypass surgery in patients with symptomatic multivessel coronary disease. German Angioplasty Bypass Surgery Investigation (GABI). N Engl J Med 1994;331:1037–1043.
97. CABRI Trial Participants. First-year results of CABRI (Coronary Angioplasty versus Bypass Revascularization Investigation). Lancet 1995;346:1178–1184.
98. King SB, Lembo NJ, Weintraub WS, et al. A randomized trial comparing coronary angioplasty with coronary bypass surgery. Emory Angioplasty versus Surgery Trial (EAST). N Engl J Med 1994;331:1044–1050.
99. The BARI (Bypass Angioplasty Revascularization Investigation) Investigators. Comparison of coronary bypass surgery with angioplasty in patients with multi-vessel disease. N Engl J Med 1996;335:217–225.
100. Abizaid A, Costa MA, Centemero M, et al. Arterial Revascularization Therapy Study Group. Clinical and economic impact of diabetes mellitus on percutaneous and surgical treatment of multivessel coronary disease patients: insights from the Arterial Revascularization Therapy Study (ARTS) trial. Circulation 2001;104:553–558.
101. SoS Investigators. Coronary artery bypass surgery versus percutaneous coronary intervention with stent implantation in patients with multivessel coronary artery disease (the Stent or Surgery Trial): a randomised controlled trial. Lancet 360:965–970.
102. Kong DF, Hasselblad V, Harrington RA, et al. Meta-analysis of survival with platelet glycoprotein IIb/IIIa antagonists for percutaneous coronary interventions. Am J Cardiol 2003;92:651–655.
103. Boersma E, Harrington RA, Moliterno DJ. Platelet glycoprotein IIb/IIIa inhibitors in acute coronary syndromes: a meta-analysis of all major randomised clinical trials. Lancet 2002;359:189–198.

RECOMMENDED READING

The Heart Outcomes Prevention Evaluation Study Investigators. Effects of an angiotensin-converting enzyme inhibitor, ramipril, on cardiovascular events in high risk patients. N Engl J Med 2000;342:145–153.
Grundy SM, Cleeman JI, Merz CN, et al. Implications of recent clinical trials for the National Cholesterol Education Program Adult Treatment Panel III Guidelines. Circulation 2004;110:227–234.
O'Toole L, Grech ED. Chronic stable angina: treatment options. BMJ 2003;326:1185–1188.
Solomon AJ, Gersh BJ. Management of chronic stable angina: medical therapy, percutaneous transluminal coronary angioplasty, and coronary artery bypass graft surgery. Lessons from the randomized trials. Ann Intern Med 128:216–223.

26 Unstable Angina and Non-ST Segment Elevation Myocardial Infarction (Acute Coronary Syndromes)

Satya Reddy Atmakuri, MD
and Neal S. Kleiman, MD

INTRODUCTION

Approximately 8 million patients present annually to the emergency room with symptoms of acute chest pain. Of these, 2 million turn out to have a cardiac cause resulting in hospitalization. Fewer than 10% of these patients have ST segment elevation on the electrocardiogram *(1)*. Since the diagnostic sensitivity and specificity of the electrocardiogram are poor in this setting, there is a strong impetus for effective emergency room stratification. The spectrum of "acute coronary syndromes" includes unstable angina and non-ST segment elevation myocardial infarction as the clinical presentations. The distinction between these syndromes is usually made retrospectively based on biochemical markers, and hence, initial treatment strategies are identical. The diagnosis of *primary* unstable angina excludes external factors that may exacerbate the symptoms of coronary ischemia, such as severe anemia, thyrotoxicosis, and tachyarrhythmias.

Four clinical scenarios are consistent with a diagnosis of unstable angina (Table 1). Patients with acute chest pain represent a heterogeneous population. An approach to management must take into account the severity of symptoms, the circumstances in which they are occurring, and indicators of the risk of such catastrophic events as death or myocardial infarction. The Braunwald Classification of Unstable Angina *(2)* summarizes these important items and assists in early stratification of patients at higher risk for adverse clinical outcomes (Table 2). Clinical features to consider immediately when first evaluating the patient include history of coronary artery disease (CAD), the presence or absence of ST-segment depression, hemodynamic status, and signs of congestive heart failure. A number of different scoring systems to determine risk have been developed *(3–5)*. These scores were developed based on clinical characteristics of patients enrolled in large clinical trials of acute coronary syndromes, and are intended to allow rapid prognostication and triage to a variety of treatments based on the risk-benefit ratio (Tables 3 and 4, Figs. 1 and 2).

The term "unstable angina" is currently falling into disuse and is being replaced with the term "acute coronary syndrome without ST segment elevation" or, more simply, "acute coronary syndrome." This new nosology has developed for three reasons. First, the syndromes that do and do not cause ST segment elevation both have a common pathology, namely vascular inflammatory changes leading to disruption of a previously stable atherosclerotic plaque, and subsequent thrombosis. The second reason for the adoption of the new terminology reflects the development of increasingly "sensitive" markers of myocardial necrosis. Patients with small amounts of myonecrosis as

From: *Essential Cardiology: Principles and Practice, 2nd Ed.*
Edited by: C. Rosendorff © Humana Press Inc., Totowa, NJ

Table 1
Clinical Presentations of Unstable Angina

1. Rest angina
2. New onset angina of CCSC class III or IV within 4 wk of presentation
3. Increasing frequency and intensity of previously stable angina to CCSC class III or IV
4. Angina within 6 wk of myocardial infarction

CCSC, Canadian Cardiovascular Society Classification.

Table 2
Braunwald Classification of Unstable Angina

Severity
Class I   New-onset, severe, or accelerated angina
            Patients with angina of less than 2 mo duration, severe or occurring three or more times per day,
            or angina that is distinctly more frequent and precipitated by distinctly less exertion; no rest pain
            in the last 2 mo
Class II   Angina at rest; subacute
            Patients with one or more episodes of angina at rest during 3 preceding months but not within
            the preceding 48 h.
Class III   Angina at rest; acute
            Patients with one or more episodes at rest within the preceding 48 h

Clinical Circumstances

Class A   Secondary unstable angina
            A clearly identified condition extrinsic to the coronary vascular bed that has intensified
            myocardial ischemia, e.g., anemia, infection, fever, hypotension, tachyarrhythmia,
            thyrotoxicosis, hypoxemia secondary to respiratory failure
Class B   Primary unstable angina
Class C   Postinfarction unstable angina (within 2 wk of documented myocardial infarction)

Intensity of Treatment

1. Absence of treatment or minimal treatment
2. Occurring in presence of standard therapy for chronic stable angina (conventional doses of oral beta-
   blockers, nitrates, and calcium antagonists)
3. Occurring despite maximally tolerated doses of all three categories of oral therapy, including nitroglycerin

CCSC, Canadian Cardiovascular Society Classification.
Adapted from ref. 2.

Table 3
TIMI Risk Scores

TIMI risk score factors	TIMI score
Age	1
At least 3 risk factors for CAD	1
ST deviation	1
More than 2 anginal events in 24 h	1
Prior coronary stenosis >50%	1
Use of aspirin in last 7 d	1
Elevated serum cardiac markers	1

Adapted from ref. 3.

well as those with recent, rather than acute, episodes of necrosis who were previously classified as having "unstable angina" are now recognized as having myocardial infarction using the modern classification scheme espoused by the joint European Society of Cardiology/American College of Cardiology guidelines (6). Third, effective forms of therapy do not differ between patients with

Table 4
PURSUIT Risk Scores

PURSUIT risk variables		Mortality at 30 d (USA/NSTEMI)	Mortality/MI at 30 d (USA/NSTEMI)
Age	50	0	8/11
	60	2/3	9/12
	70	4/6	11/13
	80	6/9	12/14
Gender	Male	1	1
	Female	0	0
Worst CCS in last 6 wk	Class I–II		
	0	0	
	Class III–IV	2	2
Heart rate	80	0	0
	100	1/2	0
	120	2/5	0
Systolic BP	120	0	0
	100	1	0
	80	2	0
Heart failure	Yes	3	2
	No	0	0
ST depression	Yes	3	1
	No	0	0

Adapted from ref. 4.

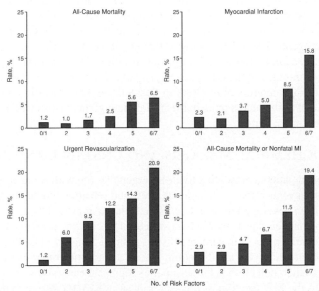

Fig. 1. Risk stratification by TIMI scores for clinical events at 14 d from Thrombolysis in Myocardial Infarction (TIMI) 11B trial. (Adapted from ref. 3.)

or without biochemical indications of necrosis, but rather are distinguished according to risk score and to the presence or absence of ST segment elevation on the surface electrocardiogram.

The majority of patients presenting with non-ST segment elevation acute coronary syndromes have multiple plaques in the coronary arteries (7). However, in most studies, approx 20% of patients with suspected acute coronary syndromes are found to have minimally obstructed or normal coronary arteries when coronary angiography is performed. This proportion is somewhat lower

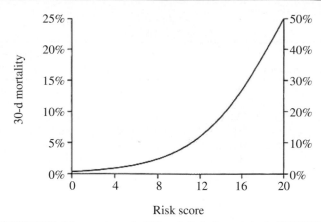

Fig. 2. Conversion of PURSUIT risk score to probability of clinical events in the PURSUIT trial. Adapted from Boersma E et al. Predictors of outcome in patients with acute coronary syndromes without persistent ST-segment elevation. Results from an international trial of 9461 patients; *see* ref. *4.*

in studies that use more stringent entry criteria. The precipitating event of myocardial ischemia is most commonly coronary plaque disruption or erosion *(8)*. Plaques vulnerable to this process tend to be relatively soft and lipid-rich, and have abundant extracellular matrix and smooth muscle cells. Following disruption of the fibrous cap, platelets are activated by local thrombogenic and inflammatory factors such as lipid and inflammatory mediators from lipid-laden macrophages. As a result thrombosis may occur *(9,10)*. The final component of arterial damage involves local vasoconstriction, most likely in response to secretion of platelet-derived serotonin and thromboxane A_2 (TXA_2).

Thrombolytic therapy has been shown to be ineffective, and potentially detrimental in non-ST segment elevation acute coronary syndromes *(11,12)*. Treatment is based primarily on antithrombotic and antiplatelet agents. The utility of most of these therapies has been codified and promulgated as sets of guidelines by a joint American College of Cardiology/American Heart Association committee *(13)* and by a committee of the European Society of Cardiology *(14)*. This chapter will review the diagnostic utility of biochemical markers in non-ST segment elevation acute coronary syndromes, and the role of traditional agents in the initial management of as well as more novel antithrombotic and antiplatelet drugs.

BIOCHEMICAL MARKERS AND UNSTABLE ANGINA

The identification of patients presenting to the emergency room with acute chest pain at high risk for subsequent cardiac events remains a challenge. New and sensitive biochemical markers of myocardial injury have been developed in recent years in the hope of providing early risk stratification.

Cardiac troponin T and cardiac troponin I are structural sarcomeric proteins that regulate the calcium-mediated contractile process in cardiac muscle. A small quantity of cardiac troponin remains free in the cytosol of cardiac myocytes. Troponin T and I are absent from the circulation under normal circumstances, so their detection in the serum may represent early signs of myocardial damage. This is in contrast to the MB fraction of creatine kinase (CK-MB) in which basal levels can be detected in the plasma of normal individuals. Therefore, serum troponins are useful markers of a range of ischemic myocardial damage from minor degrees of myocyte permeability to major myocardial necrosis. The timing of cell necrosis and biomarker release has been established for creatine kinase and its isoenzymes, but still remains controversial for the troponins. Blood levels may rise as early as 3 h after onset of symptoms, although a time frame of 6 to 12 h is more generally accepted. Normal or undetectable levels of troponin should not be viewed as excluding the presence of an acute coronary syndrome when the measurements are performed within the first 12 h of the onset of angina. Elevated levels of troponin T and troponin I may persist beyond 10 d *(15)*. The goal of measuring cardiac troponin in the emergency room is to assist in the early identification of patients presenting with acute chest pain without ST elevation who may have severe coronary ischemia and therefore be at increased risk of adverse clinical outcomes. Serial cardiac troponin determination has in many cases replaced creatine kinase in the diagnosis of myocardial infarction; both markers are measured in most medical centers.

Numerous studies have indeed demonstrated that "early" elevation of troponin in the emergency room does provide independent prognostic value for adverse outcomes, such as death, recurrent myocardial infarction, and need for revascularization in patients presenting with and without ST-elevation ischemic chest pain (16–20). However, these studies were performed in high-risk patients in whom the majority had documented coronary disease and abnormal ECGs on admission. Also, elevation of CK-MB subsequently occurred in more than 95% of patients developing myocardial infarction (17). Therefore, although "early" positive troponin may be a marker for adverse cardiac events, the negative predictive value of elevated troponin within the first 6 h after the onset of symptoms remains in question. Indeed, in a study assessing more than 10,000 patients admitted for acute chest pain, patients with a <1% likelihood of cardiac complications could be selected using the clinical features of admission ECG, description of chest discomfort, and hemodynamic status (21). The Diagnostic Marker Cooperative Study evaluated the sensitivity of biochemical markers for myocardial injury in 955 consecutive patients presenting to the emergency room with chest pain. The authors of this study concluded that the most sensitive and specific markers were CK-MB isoforms at 6 h (91% and 89%), CK-MB at 10 h (96% and 98%), followed by troponin I at 18 h (96% and 93%) (22).

The largest prospective trial to assess the value of cardiac troponin I included more than 1200 patients presenting to an emergency department with acute chest pain. Initial cardiac troponin I and CK-MB were collected (21,23). This patient population represented the "real-life" situation of a heterogeneous group of patients, without regard to admission electrocardiogram or CAD history. The positive predictive value for cardiac events up to 72 h for "early" positive cardiac troponin I (>0.4 ng/mL) in all patients was 19% vs 22% for CK-MB. In patients ruling out for acute myocardial infarction, cardiac troponin I had a positive predictive value for cardiac events of ventricular arrhythmia, hemodynamic collapse, or the need for semiurgent revascularization of only 8%. A similar study assessing initial emergency room troponin, CK-MB, and admission ECG has shown that only ST segment depression in the baseline electrocardiogram carried independent prognostic value to predict cardiac events at 30 d in acute chest pain patients without ST elevation (23).

The negative predictive value of serial troponin determination appears powerful. In patients with negative test results, the risk of major cardiac events appears very low. In a study by Hamm et al., negative troponin T or I within 12 h of chest pain and without ST segment elevation was associated with a 1.1% and 0.03% risk of myocardial infarction or death over 30 d, respectively (23).

The predictive value of troponin determination suggests that when the measurements are used injudiciously, their routine use may confuse the scenario when a good clinical history and benign electrocardiogram suggest a presentation not consistent with an acute coronary syndrome. Abnormal levels of troponin may occur in renal insufficiency, cancer, rhabdomyolysis, pulmonary embolism, and accelerated hypertension (22,24–26). Analysis of data from the Global Use of Strategies to Open Occlude Coronary Arteries IV trial reveals that serial troponin measurements provide good cardiac prognostic information across the spectrum of renal failure (27). Also, the availability of third-generation assays of troponin I has improved their diagnostic specificity, particularly in patients with renal insufficiency and heart failure. Perhaps the best use of the troponin is in patients with moderate probability of having an acute coronary syndrome and minimal electrocardiographic abnormalities. In patients with negative cardiac troponin measurements, triage may be handled in a more cost-effective manner given the low likelihood of a cardiac event. Consideration of discharge home, admission to a ward other than the intensive care unit, or early stress testing may be warranted.

Currently, other blood serum markers are being evaluated for their prognostic value. Myoglobin is released very rapidly after cell death, and is cleared rapidly. Thus, myoglobin levels rise and fall very quickly after cell necrosis. However, myoglobin is also released after skeletal muscle injury; therefore its specificity is limited. C-reactive protein (CRP) and interleukin-6 are acute-phase reactants associated with the presence of ongoing inflammation. Elevated levels of C-reactive protein have been correlated with adverse clinical outcomes at 14 d in patients presenting with acute coronary syndromes *(28)*. A rapid decline of C-reactive protein levels parallels resolution of clinical symptoms, but persistent elevation for up to 15 d is associated with an unfavorable outcome *(29)*. These studies strongly implicate inflammation as a key factor in the pathophysiology of the unstable phase of angina.

Heart fatty acid binding protein (H-FABP) is a member of a larger family of proteins found in a diverse array of tissues, and is involved in intracellular lipid transport. H-FABP is released within 90 min of myocardial sarcolemmal damage, and is currently being investigated as an early marker of myonecrosis *(14)*.

Two studies evaluated the utility of measuring myeloperoxidase (a leukocyte enzyme) in patients presenting with chest pain *(30)* and acute coronary syndromes *(31)*. Myeloperoxidase was an independent prognostic marker for cardiovascular morbidity and mortality at 30 d and 6 mo.

Brain natriuretic peptide (BNP) can be routinely measured in an emergency room setting and has been shown to predict mortality and the risk of congestive heart failure in patients presenting with acute coronary syndromes *(32)*. A recent meta-analysis of the measurement of both BNP and N-terminal BNP in patients with myocardial ischemia showed that these markers predicted short-term and long-term cardiovascular morbidity and mortality *(33)*.

Soluble CD40 ligand is a transmembrane protein of the tumor necrosis factor family that is present in platelets, is shed from the surface of the activated platelets, and the plasma level of which is elevated in patients with acute coronary syndromes, who are undergoing percutaneous coronary intervention (PCI) and cardiopulmonary bypass *(34,35)*. Also, it has been shown to have both independent and synergistic (combined with other markers such as troponin) prognostic value in patients with acute coronary syndromes *(36)*.

MEDICAL THERAPY
Antiischemic Therapy

Angina is often associated with inappropriate vasoconstriction and heart rate elevation due to excessive catecholamine drive. The aim of antiischemic therapy is to alter hemodynamics to improve the balance between myocardial oxygen supply and demand. Nitrates, β-blockers, and calcium-channel blockers are all known to improve this ratio.

The recommendation for nitrate therapy is based more on observational evidence and knowledge of its physiologic effect than on clinical trial data. Following administration of nitroglycerin, vascular smooth muscle cells convert nitrates to the nitric oxide (NO) radical. Nitric oxide, in turn, activates intracellular guanylate cyclase to produce cyclic guanosine monophosphate (cGMP), triggering smooth muscle relaxation and inhibiting platelet aggregation. Nitroglycerin decreases preload and afterload, and induces coronary vasodilation *(37)*.

The routine use of β-blocker therapy is based on data obtained in patients with myocardial infarction, where a beneficial effect on long-term mortality is clearly evident *(38–40)*. Ideally, the heart rate should be less than 60 beats/min; however, in patients with poorly compensated heart failure or reactive airways, less aggressive β-blockade is indicated. If β-blockers cannot be used at all, calcium-channel blockers are also effective in relieving chest pain. The combination of β-blockers and calcium-channel blockers is usually reserved for patients with refractory symptoms, or in whom effective control of the heart rate proves elusive.

Antiplatelet Agents

ASPIRIN

Aspirin is standard therapy in patients with acute coronary syndromes. The efficacy of aspirin in reducing early and long-term cardiac events has been well established in randomized trials *(41–44)*. Early event rates have been reduced up to 50% with a dose of 81 or 325 mg *(42)*. Long-term benefits extending to 2 yr are seen when daily administration is continued *(45)*.

Side effects with aspirin are relatively rare, dose-dependent, and usually present after long-term use. The only contraindication to immediate aspirin administration in the emergency room is prior aspirin allergy causing angioedema or anaphylaxis. It is recommended that a bolus of 160 mg to 325 mg in chewable form be given to rapidly achieve full inhibition of platelet aggregation and TXA_2 release. Maintenance therapy may range from 81 mg to 325 mg daily, although 81 mg is better tolerated.

THIENOPYRIDINES

Ticlopidine and clopidogrel are acceptable alternatives when aspirin can not be tolerated. These agents are prodrugs whose active metabolites interfere with ADP-mediated activation of the P2Y12 receptor (46). In a randomized trial of patients with unstable angina, ticlopidine as monotherapy was superior to aspirin in preventing death and myocardial infarction at 6 mo (47). The rate of fatal and nonfatal myocardial infarction was 5.1% in the ticlopidine group and 10.9% in the control group, a risk reduction of 53.2%. Clopidogrel, a new-generation thienopyridine, has a longer half-life and a much lower side-effect profile. Because it is better tolerated, clopidogrel can be administered as a loading dose of 300 to 600 mg. The superiority of clopidogrel to 325 mg aspirin for secondary prevention of recurrent ischemic events in patients with previous stroke, myocardial infarction more than 1 mo previously, or peripheral vascular disease has been shown in the CAPRIE study (48). The combination of clopidogrel with aspirin was demonstrated in a second trial, CURE (49). The use of clopidogrel (300 mg "loading dose" followed by 75 mg daily maintenance) on a background of aspirin led to a 20% relative reduction (CI = 0.72–0.90) in the combination of cardiovascular death, myocardial infarction, or stroke after 9 mo of therapy. Interestingly, the beneficial effect of clopidogrel became apparent within the first day after initiating treatment. Analysis of subgroups revealed that this benefit was present regardless of the concomitant use of GP IIb-IIIa antagonists and of coronary revascularization strategies. Major bleeding in patients treated with clopidogrel was 3.7%, higher ($p = 0.01$) than with aspirin (2.7%). The routine use of clopidogrel in patients presenting with acute coronary syndromes has remained controversial because of the perceived bleeding risk, particularly in patients who undergo coronary artery bypass surgery. Within the CURE study, patients who were to undergo coronary bypass by protocol had their clopidogrel held for 5 d. The trends, particularly within North America and Western Europe, toward earlier revascularization in patients with non-ST segment elevation acute coronary syndromes have created concern about the safety of clopidogrel administration before the coronary anatomy is determined. While observational data indicated that clopidogrel use is associated with increased bleeding at the time of coronary artery bypass surgery (50), it appears that referral of patients to coronary artery bypass within the first 48 h after presentation is relatively uncommon. Protocols for the use of clopidogrel in patients with non-ST segment elevation acute coronary syndromes vary considerably between institutions.

GLYCOPROTEIN IIB-IIIA ANTAGONISTS

Awareness of the role of platelet glycoprotein IIb-IIIa (GP IIb-IIIa) in platelet aggregation has resulted in a major pharmacologic breakthrough in antiplatelet therapy. Not since thrombolytic agents has a new class of drugs received such attention for its potential benefits in acute coronary syndromes. The value of GPIIb-IIIa blocker drugs is that blockade of the GPIIb-IIIa $\alpha_2\beta_3$ receptor inhibits platelet aggregation in response to all agonists, since ligation of this integrin by circulating macromolecules represents the ultimate step in the formation of firm platelet-platelet bonds.

The prototypic agent is c7E3 Fab or abciximab, a chimeric fragment of a monoclonal antibody, which binds avidly to GP IIb-IIIa. Since abciximab, synthetic peptide and nonpeptide intravenous and oral formulations have been developed, each mimicking the fibrinogen binding site allowing for highly specific and reversible inhibition of the GP IIb-IIIa receptor (Table 5). However, four trials that evaluated long-term efficacy of the oral GP IIb-IIIa inhibitors xemilofiban (51), orbofiban (52), sibrafiban (53), and lotrafiban (45) did not reveal any benefit and, in fact, were associated with increases rather than decreases in mortality (54). Therefore, current clinical use of GP

Table 5
Currently Available Platelet GPIIb/IIIa Receptor Antagonists

Drug	Indication	Dose
Abciximab (antibody)	Elective PCI	Bolus: 0.25 mg/kg
	Urgent PCI	Maintenance: 0.125 µg/kg/min
	Refractory unstable angina pending PCI	
Tirofiban (nonpeptide)	Acute coronary syndromes	Bolus: 0.4 µg/kg/min × 30 min
		Maintenance: 0.1 µg/kg/min × 48– 96 h
Eptifibatide (cyclic peptide)	Elective PCI	Bolus: 135 µg/kg
		Maintenance: 0.50 µg/kg/min × 24 h
	Acute coronary syndromes	Bolus: 180 µg/kg
		Maintenance: 2 µg/kg/min
	Urgent PCI	Bolus: 180 µg/kg, repeat in 10 min
		Maintenance: 2 µg/kg/min

IIb-IIIa inhibitors is limited to intravenous formulation of the monoclonal antibody abciximab, the peptide fragment eptifibatide, and the peptidomimetic tirofiban.

The clinical use of abciximab is limited to both elective and urgent percutaneous coronary interventions, where its protective effects have been clearly documented. Used with aspirin and heparin, abciximab results in a significant reduction in periprocedural myocardial infarction following the procedure (55,56). A long-term reduction in mortality has also been observed, particularly in patients receiving intracoronary stents (57).

In the Global Strategies to Open Occluded Coronary Arteries (GUSTO) IV trial (58), two regimens of abciximab were tested compared with a placebo, on a background of aspirin and heparin, in patients presenting with non-ST segment elevation acute coronary syndromes. The two abciximab regimens consisted of the standard 0.25 mg/kg bolus used during coronary interventions, but infusions were given for periods of either 24 or 48 h. The protocol for this study mandated that patients not undergo early coronary intervention except under circumstances of refractory myocardial ischemia. In this trial of 7800 patients abciximab had no benefit on the rates of death or myocardial infarction at 30 d, and in fact was associated with a trend toward higher mortality (0.7% for 24-h infusion, 0.9% for 48-h infusion vs 0.3% for the placebo group, $p = 0.008$).

The efficacy of nonmonoclonal antibody GP IIb-IIIa inhibitors in acute coronary syndromes has been evaluated in multiple trials (59–62). The inclusion criteria for these trials broadly included patients presenting with angina consistent with non-ST elevation acute coronary syndromes associated with electrocardiographic changes and/or presence of cardiac enzymes. The Platelet Receptor Inhibition for Ischemic Syndrome Management (PRISM) trial investigators randomized patients to receive intravenous tirofiban or heparin for 48 h in non-ST elevation ischemic chest pain. The composite endpoint of death, new myocardial infarction, or refractory ischemia at 2 d statistically favored tirofiban. This benefit was not evident at 30 d although there was a significant reduction in mortality (59). The PRISM-PLUS investigators evaluated tirofiban in a higher-risk population with documented electrocardiogram abnormalities or non-Q wave myocardial infarction. In contrast to PRISM, all patients received heparin and were randomized to tirofiban or placebo. Evaluation of the primary composite endpoint at 7 d revealed a 34% event relative risk reduction in favor of combined therapy, 12.9% vs 17.9% (CI = 0.53–0.88, $p = 0.004$). A tirofiban-only arm in this study was terminated prematurely due to an observed excess mortality. The continued advantage of combination therapy persisted to 6 mo, although most benefit was in the refractory ischemia component of the composite endpoint (60). It is important to note that all patients received mandatory angiography at 48 h and, if indicated, coronary angioplasty was performed.

The largest of the trials, the Platelet Glycoprotein IIb-IIIa in Unstable Angina: Receptor Suppression Using Integrilin (PURSUIT) study, evaluated eptifibatide or placebo with heparin in 10,948 patients. In this trial, all management decisions were left to the discretion of the physician in an attempt to mimic "real life." A significant reduction in the rate of death or myocardial infarction was present at 96 h, 7 d, and 30 d. The effect at 30 d was attenuated to a 10% relative reduction, although the absolute reduction in the number of events was maintained at 15 out of 1000 treated. Rates of blood transfusion (including perioperative bleeding after coronary bypass) were 11.8% and 9.3% in the eptifibatide and placebo groups, respectively *(62)*. Taken together, the above trials make a strong case for the use of GP IIb-IIIa antagonists in combination with heparin and aspirin, at least in patients with high risk features.

A meta-analysis of six trials with 31,402 patients to evaluate efficacy and safety of intravenous glycoprotein IIb-IIIa inhibitors with acute coronary syndromes revealed that the combined endpoint of death and MI were reduced by 16% at 5 d ($p = 0.0003$) and 30 d. There was more benefit in men (RR = 0.81, CI = 0.75–0.89) than women; however, there was benefit in both men and women who had elevated troponin measurements. Greater benefit was obtained in patients undergoing PCI than medical treatment; however, patients on GP IIb-IIIa inhibitors had reduced likelihood of undergoing PCI. However, this is a postrandomization analysis and the trials analyzed did not have a factorial design to evaluate the question of whether GP IIb-IIIa inhibitors are equally efficacious in patients managed conservatively as in those undergoing PCI. Major bleeding at 30 d was increased with an odds ratio of 1.62 (95% CI: 1.36–1.94) with no significant increase in intracranial hemorrhage *(63)*.

Antithrombotic Agents

Unfractionated Heparin

Heparin consists of an unfractionated mixture of glycosaminoglycans with molecular weights from 5000 to more than 30,000 Daltons. These molecules bind the serpin antithrombin. Subsequent binding of this complex to the enzyme factor Xa inhibits the soluble coagulation cascade by preventing factor Xa-induced amplification of the conversion of prothrombin (factor II) to thrombin (factor IIa). Heparin binding to antithrombin also inactivates this final enzyme in the coagulation cascade and prevents the cleavage of fibrinogen to fibrin.

The efficacy of intravenous heparin in unstable angina has been suggested by many moderate-sized trials and is supported by meta-analyses *(44,64)*. The relative risk of death and MI were reduced by 33% (CI = 0.44–1.02) *(64)*. A phenomenon of reactivation angina with risk of cardiac events following cessation of heparin has also been observed. This phenomenon is more likely to occur following prolonged administration of heparin exceeding 72 h. The use of concomitant aspirin may attenuate this effect *(65)*. Data that suggest prolonged unfractionated heparin infusion decreases antithrombin levels and increases thrombin generation and activity can be observed when a heparin infusion is stopped abruptly *(66)*. Therefore, when using unfractionated heparin, it may be prudent to wean heparin after long durations of therapy and to continue close observation for at least 12 h after cessation of unfractionated heparin infusion.

The therapeutic effect of unfractionated heparin is not linearly related to the activated partial thromboplastin time (aPTT) value. Clinical trial observations in patients presenting with acute coronary syndromes have shown no additional benefit when aPTTs were in excess of 2.0 times baseline aPTT. In fact, sustained anticoagulation beyond this value is associated with a tendency to increased adverse outcomes, including recurrent myocardial infarctions as well as hemorrhage *(66, 67)*. The mechanism of this paradoxical effect remains uncertain. In vivo and ex vivo studies have demonstrated platelet activation in the presence of unfractionated heparin in normal volunteers *(68)*. This effect may be more likely to occur when heparin blood levels are high *(69)*. Therapeutic dosing of unfractionated heparin should target an aPTT 1.5 to 2.0 times baseline value. In most laboratories, this range corresponds to an aPTT in the range of 45 to 60 s. Dose titration is easier to achieve by the use of weight-based dosing nomograms. Use of a bedside aPTT monitor also facilitates the monitoring of heparin infusions and reduces the time required to obtain an aPTT level from approx 90 min to less than 5 min. In one study, bedside aPTT monitoring was associated with reduced rates of hemorrhage compared with standard laboratory monitoring *(70)*.

The most common complication of continuous unfractionated heparin administration is bleeding. Heparin-induced thrombcytopenia has been reported in 1.0 to 2.4% of patients receiving therapeutic doses of unfractionated heparin, most commonly occurs with prolonged dosing, and is associated with a severalfold increase in hospital mortality. More rare complications include alopecia, skin necrosis, urticaria, and transient serum transaminase elevations *(71,72)*.

LOW-MOLECULAR-WEIGHT HEPARINS

The low-molecular-weight heparins (LMWHs) are derived by fractionation of standard heparin and retrieving molecules less than 8000 Daltons in size. Compared with unfractionated heparin, these products bind less avidly to plasma proteins, thereby allowing more predictable anticoagulation dosing. When administered subcutaneously they are highly bioavailable. Compared with unfractionated heparin, these agents have a much more pronounced effect on coagulation factor Xa than on thrombin. Therefore, the total antithrombotic action is not reflected by the aPTT. This antifactor Xa effect impairs thrombin generation from prothrombin *(73)*. Since anti-Xa activity resides predominantly in the lower-molecular-weight fractions, the anti-Xa activity is greater compared to unfractionated heparin and varies among the various LMWHs.

Many clinical trials evaluating LMWHs in acute coronary syndromes without ST elevation have been performed. The Fragmin during Instability in Coronary Artery Disease (FRISC) trial *(74)* randomized patients to receive subcutaneous dalteparin (Fragmin) or placebo. Although there was a significant reduction in death and myocardial infarction by 6 d, this effect disappeared at 5 mo despite continued once-daily administration of dalteparin for up to 45 d. This study did not incorporate standard heparin in the control group *(75)*. The related FRIC study used identical dosing and duration of dalteparin in a comparison with standard heparin. No benefit of dalteparin was observed. A negative feature of this trial was the slightly higher mortality observed in the dalteparin-treated patients, 1.5% vs 0.4% *(76)*.

Most data concerning LMWHs in acute coronary syndromes have been obtained using enoxaparin (Lovenox). Two early studies, the Efficacy and Safety of Subcutaneous Enoxaparin in Non-Q-wave Coronary Events (ESSENCE) and Thrombolysis in Myocardial Ischemia-11 (TIMI 11) trials, compared enoxaparin with standard heparin in patients managed with a predominantly conservative revascularization strategy *(77,78)*. When PCI was performed in these trials, unfractionated heparin was used as the foundation anticoagulant. ESSENCE showed a statistical benefit favoring enoxaparin. At 14 d, the composite endpoint of death, myocardial infarction, or recurrent ischemia occurred in 16.6% of patients randomized to enoxaparin vs 19.9% for the standard heparin group ($p = 0.019$). A statistically nonsignificant trend persisted to 30 d. Recurrent angina was responsible for approx 75% of all endpoints in this trial *(77)*. The TIMI 11 trial investigators evaluated an alternative dosing regimen of enoxaparin versus unfractionated heparin in 3910 patients presenting with non-ST segment elevation acute coronary syndromes. Enoxaparin was initially administered as an intravenous bolus of 30 mg/kg, followed by 1 mg/kg subcutaneous injections twice daily for 3 d. There was a statistically significant benefit of enoxaparin in the primary composite endpoint of death, myocardial infarction, or refractory ischemia at 8 d. The event rates were 12.4% vs 14.5% for enoxaparin and unfractionated heparin, respectively *(78)*. A planned meta-analysis of these two trials revealed that at 1 yr, the composite of death, myocardial infarction, and refractory ischemia was reduced from 25.8% to 23.3% ($p = 0.008$), while the composite of death and myocardial infarction was reduced from 13.7% to 12.7% ($p = 0.16$) *(79)*.

Two recent trials evaluated enoxaparin in the context of a modern management strategy utilizing glycoprotein IIb/IIIa inhibitors, but without early revascularization. The Integrilin and Enoxaparin Randomized Assessment of Acute Coronary Syndrome Treatment (INTERACT) trial compared enoxaparin with unfractionated heparin in 746 patients who were also treated with eptifibatide for non-ST segment elevation acute coronary syndromes and who were managed without mandatory early revascularization. The rates of major and minor bleeding were less with treatment with enoxaparin (1.8% vs 4.6%, $p = 0.03$), and there was also a significant reduction in the endpoint of death or myocardial infarction (5% vs 9%, $p = 0.031$) *(80)*. In the Antithrombotic Combination Using Tirofiban and Enoxaparin (ACUTE II) study, 525 patients were randomized to receive tirofiban with either unfractionated heparin or enoxaparin. The rates of bleeding were similar and there was a trend toward decreased urgent revascularization and rehospitalization with tirofiban/enoxaparin *(81)*.

The Superior Yield of the New Strategy of Enoxaparin Revascularization and Glycoprotein IIb/IIIa Inhibitors (SYNERGY) trial was designed to compare the two forms of heparin in a modern context of frequent use of GP IIb/IIIa antagonists and early coronary angiography and intervention. More than 10,000 patients with high-risk features (two of the following: age >65 yr, ST segment deviation, or elevated levels of troponin or CK) of non-ST segment elevation acute coronary syndromes were randomized to enoxaparin, given as a 30 mg/kg intravenous bolus followed by 1 mg/kg subcutaneously every 12 h, or unfractionated heparin. Early angiography was encouraged. Fifty-six percent of patients in this trial received a GP IIb/IIIa antagonist and more than 90% underwent early angiography. In patients receiving enoxaparin, a supplemental bolus of 0.3 mg/kg was given intravenously if the last dose of enoxaparin was given more than 8 h before the intervention. The composite endpoint of death or myocardial infarction occurred in 14% of patients assigned to enoxaparin and 14.5% of patients assigned to unfractionated heparin. Although there was not evidence that enoxaparin was a superior treatment, statistical requirements to demonstrate noninferiority were met. The risk of severe bleeding was increased in patients assigned to enoxaparin (2.9% vs 2.4%, $p = 0.106$), as was the risk of major hemorrhage using a modified TIMI definition (9.1% vs 7.6%, $p = 0.008$). This risk appeared to be increased predominantly in the elderly and in patients with renal insufficiency, suggesting accumulation of the drug. The risk of abrupt closure of the revascularized coronary artery was not different between the two groups (1.3% vs 1.6%). However, an important point to consider is that about three fourths of patients in the trial had received some form of antithrombin therapy (either unfractionated or low-molecular-weight heparin) prior to randomization, and about one seventh of patients assigned to enoxaparin also received unfractionated heparin at some point during the hospitalization, largely during coronary intervention. Thus, contamination with nonprotocol antithrombin therapies confounds interpretation of these results. Nonetheless, the data in aggregate do not present a strong case for selecting a low-molecular-weight heparin over unfractionated heparin if an aggressive invasive strategy is planned *(82)*.

DIRECT-THROMBIN INHIBITORS

The direct-thrombin inhibitors act independently of antithrombin and are unaffected by heparin-inactivating proteins. They are more capable than heparin of inhibiting clot-bound thrombin and can therefore theoretically more aggressively prevent the perpetuation of local coagulation *(83)*. These agents are administered intravenously. Prolongation of the aPTT occurs due to their direct effect on thrombin.

The prototype drug is hirudin, a naturally occurring anticoagulant found in the saliva of the medicinal leech. It is now produced through recombinant DNA technology. The clinical value of hirudin was assessed in the GUSTO-II trial. Patients with acute chest pain with or without ST elevation were randomized to receive intravenous hirudin (0.1 mg/kg bolus and 0.1 mg/kg/h infusion) or unfractionated heparin. The primary endpoint of death, nonfatal myocardial infarction, or reinfarction at 30 d occurred in 9.8% of the heparin group compared with 8.9% of the hirudin group, not reaching statistical significance *(84)*. The Canadian Organization to Assess Strategies for Ischemic Syndromes (OASIS-2) study evaluated a higher hirudin dose (0.4 mg/kg bolus and 0.15 mg/kg/h infusion) in patients with acute coronary syndromes without ST elevation. The primary endpoint, a composite of cardiovascular death or myocardial infarction at 7 d, occurred in 3.6% of hirudin-treated patients and 4.2% of heparin-treated patients. These results fell short of statistical significance. Major bleeding occurred more frequently with hirudin, 1.2% vs 0.7% for standard heparin *(85)*.

Bivalirudin is a synthetic 20-amino-acid analog of hirudin proposed to inhibit clot-bound thrombin more effectively due to its smaller size. It is has been shown to be superior to heparin in a nonurgent PCI setting and is currently being compared with heparin in a large trial of patients with non-ST segment elevation acute coronary syndromes (Acute Catheterization and Urgent Intervention Triage Strategy [ACUITY] trial).

Table 6
Early Stratification for Risk of Adverse Outcome
in Patients Presenting With Unstable Angina

	Low risk	Intermediate risk	High risk
Clinical history	Effort angina with little progression	Gradual evolution of anginal symptoms to CCSC class III or IV (>4 wk)	Rapid evolution of anginal symptoms to CCSC class III or II (<4 wk)
	<2 cardiac risk factors	2 cardiac risk factors	Advanced age (>60)
	Negative troponin T or I		Known CAD
			Postmyocardial infarction (<6 wk)
Physical Exam	No abnormal cardiovascular findings	Signs of peripheral vascular disease	Hemodynamic instability
		Carotid/femoral bruits	
		Diminished pulses	Signs of CHF "+" S_3 gallop Lung rales
ECG	Normal or minimal abnormality	Minimal ST or T wave abnormalities	ST-segment depression ≥1 mm

STATINS

There have been multiple clinical trials establishing the efficacy of statins in primary and secondary prevention of coronary artery disease. Also, statins have been shown to decrease C-reactive protein and hence are thought to reduce inflammation (86,87). This led to studies to evaluate the role of statins in acute coronary syndromes. In the Myocardial Ischemia Reduction with Aggressive Cholesterol Lowering (MIRACL) study, high-dose atorvastatin (80 mg/d) started within 24 to 96 h of admission for unstable angina or non-Q-wave myocardial infarction reduced recurrent ischemic events over a 16-wk treatment period compared with placebo (88). Recently, in the Pravastatin or Atorvastatin Evaluation and Infection Therapy (PROVE-IT) trial, intense LDL lowering to a mean level of 62 mg/dL with atorvastatin (80 mg/d) vs a mean level of 95 mg/dL with pravastatin (40 mg/d) in the context of acute coronary syndromes led to substantial reduction in cardiovascular morbidity and mortality (16% reduction in hazard ratio, CI = 5–26%) (89).

MANAGEMENT APPROACH

Since clinical presentations of acute chest pain will vary, the intensity of the management strategy will necessarily vary as well. The clinician must first assess the patient's risk for evolving further cardiac events based on the risk scores (Figs. 1 and 2; Table 6).

Although it would seem intuitively that revascularization procedures would confer protection against recurrent infarction and ischemia, the results of early randomized trials were inconclusive as to when, or even whether, a more aggressive approach with early coronary angiography should be pursued. Early coronary angiography may avoid the waiting period required until noninvasive testing can be performed safely, and may also aid in the identification of the 20% of patients without significant coronary arterial narrowing, in whom alternative diagnostic procedures may be needed (1). Based on the results of the TIMI IIIB (12) and Veterans Affairs Non-Q-Wave Infarction Strategies in Hospital (VANQWISH) (90) studies in the early 1990s, a routine early invasive strategy for all patients with non-ST elevation acute coronary syndromes conferred no benefit in terms of preventing death or myocardial infarction. The OASIS registry of more than 7900 consecutive patients with non-ST segment elevation acute coronary syndromes observed no difference in the rate of cardiovascular death or myocardial infarction in countries with the highest rate of invasive procedures (59%) versus the lowest (21%). This registry also pointed out that operators were more likely to

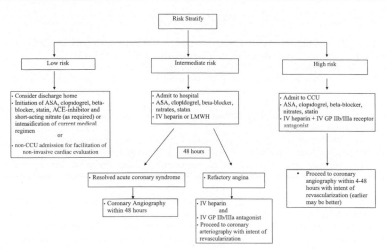

Fig. 3. Algorithm for the early management of acute coronary syndromes without ST segment elevation.

select patients with relatively low rather than high acuity for invasive procedures *(91)*. These data are no longer applicable, as there have been significant improvements in revascularization techniques.

Recent trials that evaluated early invasive strategy utilizing a modern strategy incorporating stents and glycoprotein IIb/IIIa inhibitors showed significant benefit in the reduction of cardiovascular endpoints. The Fragmin and Fast Revascularization during Instability in CAD (FRISC II) *(75)* study evaluated 2457 patients presenting with non-ST segment elevation acute coronary syndromes who underwent coronary angiography within 7 d, with backgound therapy of dalteparin or placebo. The combined endpoints of death and MI were significantly lower (9.4% vs 12.1%, $p = 0.031$) with dalteparin, and that continued at 1 yr follow-up analysis (10.4% vs 14.1%, $p = 0.005$). The Treat Angina with Aggrastat and Determine Cost of Therapy with an Invasive or Conservative Strategy (TACTICS-TIMI 18) *(92)* study evaluated early invasive strategy versus conservative treatment in 2220 patients with ACS. All patients received tirofiban at the time of study enrollment. In this study, patients underwent coronary angiography within 4 to 48 h in the invasive group (median 9 h to angiography, 23 h to PCI). In the conservative arm, patients had cardiac catheterization only if they developed objective evidence of recurrent ischemia. The patients in the invasive group had a significantly lower incidence of the combined endpoints of death, MI, and rehospitalization for ACS (15.9% vs 19.4%, $p = 0.025$). The absolute and relative benefits of the invasive strategy increased as the TIMI risk score increased from low to intermediate to high risk. The Randomized Intervention Trial of Unstable Angina (RITA-3) *(93)* study evaluated the use of early angiography and revascularization in 1810 patients with non-ST elevation ACS. Compared with patients assigned to the conservative management strategy, patients assigned to an invasive strategy had 34% reduction in the combined end point of death, MI, or refractory angina (9.6% vs 14.5%, $p = 0.01$). Finally, the Intracoronary Stenting With Antithrombotic Regimen Cooling-Off (ISAR-COOL) trial evaluated prolonged treatment with antithrombotic medications prior to coronary intervention. In this study, 410 patients with non-ST elevation ACS were randomized to an early invasive strategy (within 6 h) or coronary intervention after 3 to 5 d of contemporary antithrombotic therapy that included aspirin, clopidogrel, heparin, and tirofiban. The combined endpoint of death or MI at 30 d was significantly reduced in the early invasive strategy group (5.9% vs 11.6%, $p = 0.04$) *(94)*. Based on these contemporary trials, the American College of Cardiology and American Heart Association (ACC/AHA) guidelines recommend an early invasive strategy as Class I indication in patients with ACS and high risk features *(1,13)*.

Tailoring decision making to the dynamics of the individual clinical scenario is essential. The algorithm presented in Fig. 3 provides a decision-making guideline for patients presenting to the emergency room with non-ST elevation acute coronary syndromes.

REFERENCES

1. Chen MS, Bhatt DL. Highlights of the 2002 update to the 2000 American College of Cardiology/American Heart Association acute coronary syndrome guidelines. Cardiol Rev 2003;11:113–121.
2. Braunwald E. Unstable angina. A classification. Circulation 1989;80:410–414.
3. Antman EM, Cohen M, Bernink PJ, et al. The TIMI risk score for unstable angina/non-ST elevation MI: A method for prognostication and therapeutic decision making. JAMA 2000;284:835–842.
4. Boersma E, Pieper KS, Steyerberg EW, et al. Predictors of outcome in patients with acute coronary syndromes without persistent ST-segment elevation. Results from an international trial of 9461 patients. The PURSUIT Investigators. Circulation 2000;101:2557–2567.
5. Lindahl B. Noninvasive risk stratification in unstable coronary artery disease: excercise test and biochemical markers. FRISC Study Group. Andren B, ed. Am J Cardiol 2004;80:40–44.
6. Myocardial infarction redefined—a consensus document of The Joint European Society of Cardiology/American College of Cardiology Committee for the redefinition of myocardial infarction. Eur Heart J 2004;21:1502–1513.
7. Goldstein JA, Demetriou D, Grines CL, et al. Multiple complex coronary plaques in patients with acute myocardial infarction. N Engl J Med 2000;343:915–922.
8. Libby P. Molecular bases of the acute coronary syndromes. Circulation 1995;91:2844–2850.
9. Buffon A, Biasucci LM, Liuzzo G, et al. Widespread coronary inflammation in unstable angina. N Engl J Med 2002;347:5–12.
10. Lafont A. Basic aspects of plaque vulnerability. Heart 2003;89:1262–1267.
11. Bar FW, Verheugt FW, Col J, et al. Thrombolysis in patients with unstable angina improves the angiographic but not the clinical outcome. Results of UNASEM, a multicenter, randomized, placebo-controlled, clinical trial with anistreplase. Circulation 1992;86:131–137.
12. Effects of tissue plasminogen activator and a comparison of early invasive and conservative strategies in unstable angina and non-Q-wave myocardial infarction. Results of the TIMI IIIB Trial. Thrombolysis in Myocardial Ischemia. Circulation 1994;89:1545–1556.
13. Bertrand ME, Simoons ML, Fox KA, et al. Management of acute coronary syndromes in patients presenting without persistent ST-segment elevation. Eur Heart J 2002;23:1809–1840.
14. Alhadi HA, Fox KA. Do we need additional markers of myocyte necrosis: the potential value of heart fatty-acid-binding protein. QJM 2004;97:187–198.
15. de Winter RJ, Koster RW, Sturk A, Sanders GT. Value of myoglobin, troponin T, and CK-MBmass in ruling out an acute myocardial infarction in the emergency room. Circulation 1995;92:3401–3407.
16. Lindahl B, Venge P, Wallentin L. Relation between troponin T and the risk of subsequent cardiac events in unstable coronary artery disease. The FRISC study group. Circulation 1996;93:1651–1657.
17. Ohman EM, Armstrong PW, Christenson RH, et al. Cardiac troponin T levels for risk stratification in acute myocardial ischemia. GUSTO IIA Investigators. N Engl J Med 1996;335:1333–1341.
18. Newby LK, Christenson RH, Ohman EM, et al. Value of serial troponin T measures for early and late risk stratification in patients with acute coronary syndromes. The GUSTO-IIa Investigators. Circulation 1998;98:1853–1859.
19. Antman EM, Tanasijevic MJ, Thompson B, et al. Cardiac-specific troponin I levels to predict the risk of mortality in patients with acute coronary syndromes. N Engl J Med 1996;335:1342–1349.
20. Goldman L, Cook EF, Johnson PA, et al. Prediction of the need for intensive care in patients who come to the emergency departments with acute chest pain. N Engl J Med 1996;334:1498–1504.
21. Holmvang L, Luscher MS, Clemmensen P, et al. Very early risk stratification using combined ECG and biochemical assessment in patients with unstable coronary artery disease (A thrombin inhibition in myocardial ischemia [TRIM] substudy). The TRIM Study Group. Circulation 1998;98:2004–2009.
22. Konstantinides S, Geibel A, Olschewski M, et al. Importance of cardiac troponins I and T in risk stratification of patients with acute pulmonary embolism. Circulation 2002;106:1263–1268.
23. Hamm CW, Goldmann BU, Heeschen C, et al. Emergency room triage of patients with acute chest pain by means of rapid testing for cardiac troponin T or troponin I. N Engl J Med 1997;337:1648–1653.
24. Bodor GS, Porter S, Landt Y, Ladenson JH. Development of monoclonal antibodies for an assay of cardiac troponin-I and preliminary results in suspected cases of myocardial infarction. Clin Chem 1992;38:2203–2214.
25. Punukollu G, Gowda RM, Khan IA, et al. Elevated serum cardiac troponin I in rhabdomyolysis. Int J Cardiol 2004;96:35–40.
26. De Z, Jr. Cardiac troponins and renal disease. Nephrology (Carlton) 2004;9:83–88.
27. Aviles RJ, Askari AT, Lindahl B, et al. Troponin T levels in patients with acute coronary syndromes, with or without renal dysfunction. N Engl J Med 2002;346:2047–2052.
28. Morrow DA, Rifai N, Antman EM, et al. C-reactive protein is a potent predictor of mortality independently of and in combination with troponin T in acute coronary syndromes: a TIMI 11A substudy. Thrombolysis in Myocardial Infarction. J Am Coll Cardiol 1998;31:1460–1465.
29. Caligiuri G, Liuzzo G, Biasucci LM, Maseri A. Immune system activation follows inflammation in unstable angina: pathogenetic implications. J Am Coll Cardiol 1998;32:1295–1304.
30. Brennan ML, Penn MS, Van LF, et al. Prognostic value of myeloperoxidase in patients with chest pain. N Engl J Med 2003;349:1595–1604.

31. Baldus S, Heeschen C, Meinertz T, et al. Myeloperoxidase serum levels predict risk in patients with acute coronary syndromes. Circulation 2003;108:1440–1445.
32. Morrow DA, de Lemos JA, Sabatine MS, et al. Evaluation of B-type natriuretic peptide for risk assessment in unstable angina/non-ST-elevation myocardial infarction: B-type natriuretic peptide and prognosis in TACTICS-TIMI 18. J Am Coll Cardiol 2003;41:1264–1272.
33. Galvani M, Ferrini D, Ottani F. Natriuretic peptides for risk stratification of patients with acute coronary syndromes. Eur J Heart Fail 2004;6:327–333.
34. Aukrust P, Muller F, Ueland T, et al. Enhanced levels of soluble and membrane-bound CD40 ligand in patients with unstable angina. Possible reflection of T lymphocyte and platelet involvement in the pathogenesis of acute coronary syndromes. Circulation 1999;100:614–620.
35. Andre P, Nannizzi-Alaimo L, Prasad SK, Phillips DR. Platelet-derived CD40L: the switch-hitting player of cardiovascular disease. Circulation 2002;106:896–899.
36. Varo N, de Lemos JA, Libby P, et al. Soluble CD40L: risk prediction after acute coronary syndromes. Circulation 2003; 108:1049–1052.
37. Abrams J. Mechanisms of action of the organic nitrates in the treatment of myocardial ischemia. Am J Cardiol 1992; 70:30B–42B.
38. Beta-Blocker Heart Attack Study Group. A randomized trial of propanolol in patients with acute myocardial infarction. JAMA 1982;247:1707–1714.
39. Metoprolol in acute myocardial infarction (MIAMI). A randomised placebo-controlled international trial. The MIAMI Trial Research Group. Eur Heart J 1985;6:199–226.
40. Randomised trial of intravenous atenolol among 16 027 cases of suspected acute myocardial infarction: ISIS-1. First International Study of Infarct Survival Collaborative Group. Lancet 1986;2:57–66.
41. Lewis HD Jr, Davis JW, Archibald DG, et al. Protective effects of aspirin against acute myocardial infarction and death in men with unstable angina. Results of a Veterans Administration cooperative study. N Engl J Med 1983;309: 396–403.
42. Cairns JA, Gent M, Singer J, et al. Aspirin, sulfinpyrazone, or both in unstable angina. Results of a Canadian multicenter trial. N Engl J Med 1985;313:1369–1375.
43. Randomised trial of intravenous streptokinase, oral aspirin, both, or neither among 17,187 cases of suspected acute myocardial infarction: ISIS-2. ISIS-2 (Second International Study of Infarct Survival) Collaborative Group. Lancet 1988;2:349–360.
44. Theroux P, Ouimet H, McCans J, et al. Aspirin, heparin, or both to treat acute unstable angina. N Engl J Med 1988; 319:1105–1111.
45. Topol EJ, Easton D, Harrington RA, et al. Randomized, double-blind, placebo-controlled, international trial of the oral IIb/IIIa antagonist lotrafiban in coronary and cerebrovascular disease. Circulation 2003;108:399–406.
46. Conley PB, Delaney SM. Scientific and therapeutic insights into the role of the platelet P2Y12 receptor in thrombosis. Curr Opin Hematol 2003;10:333–338.
47. Balsano F, Rizzon P, Violi F, et al. Antiplatelet treatment with ticlopidine in unstable angina. A controlled multicenter clinical trial. The Studio della Ticlopidina nell'Angina Instabile Group. Circulation 1990;82:17–26.
48. A randomised, blinded, trial of clopidogrel versus aspirin in patients at risk of ischaemic events (CAPRIE). CAPRIE Steering Committee. Lancet 1996;348:1329–1339.
49. Yusuf S, Zhao F, Mehta SR, et al. Effects of clopidogrel in addition to aspirin in patients with acute coronary syndromes without ST-segment elevation. N Engl J Med 2001;345:494–502.
50. Steinhubl SR, Berger PB, Mann JT, III, et al. Early and sustained dual oral antiplatelet therapy following percutaneous coronary intervention: a randomized controlled trial. JAMA 2002;288:2411–2420.
51. O'Neill WW, Serruys P, Knudtson M, et al. Long-term treatment with a platelet glycoprotein-receptor antagonist after percutaneous coronary revascularization. EXCITE Trial Investigators. Evaluation of Oral Xemilofiban in Controlling Thrombotic Events. N Engl J Med 2000;342:1316–1324.
52. Cannon CP, McCabe CH, Wilcox RG, et al. Oral glycoprotein IIb/IIIa inhibition with orbofiban in patients with unstable coronary syndromes (OPUS-TIMI 16) trial. Circulation 2000;102:149–156.
53. Comparison of sibrafiban with aspirin for prevention of cardiovascular events after acute coronary syndromes: a randomised trial. The SYMPHONY Investigators. Sibrafiban versus Aspirin to Yield Maximum Protection from Ischemic Heart Events Post-acute Coronary Syndromes. Lancet 2000;355:337–345.
54. Quinn MJ, Plow EF, Topol EJ. Platelet glycoprotein IIb/IIIa inhibitors: recognition of a two-edged sword? Circulation 2002;106:379–385.
55. Platelet glycoprotein IIb/IIIa receptor blockade and low-dose heparin during percutaneous coronary revascularization. The EPILOG Investigators. N Engl J Med 1997;336:1689–1696.
56. Randomised placebo-controlled trial of abciximab before and during coronary intervention in refractory unstable angina: the CAPTURE Study. Lancet 1997;349:1429–1435.
57. Randomised placebo-controlled and balloon-angioplasty-controlled trial to assess safety of coronary stenting with use of platelet glycoprotein-IIb/IIIa blockade. The EPISTENT Investigators. Evaluation of Platelet IIb/IIIa Inhibitor for Stenting. Lancet 1998;352:87–92.
58. Cavallini C. [Effect of glycoprotein IIb/IIIa receptor blocker abciximab on outcome in patients with acute coronary syndromes without early coronary revascularization: the GUSTO IV-ACS randomised trial]. Ital Heart J Suppl 2001; 2:1124–1126.

59. A comparison of aspirin plus tirofiban with aspirin plus heparin for unstable angina. Platelet Receptor Inhibition in Ischemic Syndrome Management (PRISM) Study Investigators. N Engl J Med 1998;338:1498–1505.

60. Inhibition of the platelet glycoprotein IIb/IIIa receptor with tirofiban in unstable angina and non-Q-wave myocardial infarction. Platelet Receptor Inhibition in Ischemic Syndrome Management in Patients Limited by Unstable Signs and Symptoms (PRISM-PLUS) Study Investigators. N Engl J Med 1998;338:1488–1497.

61. International, randomized, controlled trial of lamifiban (a platelet glycoprotein IIb/IIIa inhibitor), heparin, or both in unstable angina. The PARAGON Investigators. Platelet IIb/IIIa Antagonism for the Reduction of Acute coronary syndrome events in a Global Organization Network. Circulation 199823;97:2386–2395.

62. Inhibition of platelet glycoprotein IIb/IIIa with eptifibatide in patients with acute coronary syndromes. The PURSUIT Trial Investigators. Platelet Glycoprotein IIb/IIIa in Unstable Angina: Receptor Suppression Using Integrilin Therapy. N Engl J Med 199813;339:436–443.

63. Boersma E, Harrington RA, Moliterno DJ, et al. Platelet glycoprotein IIb/IIIa inhibitors in acute coronary syndromes: a meta-analysis of all major randomised clinical trials. Lancet 2002;359:189–198.

64. Oler A, Whooley MA, Oler J, Grady D. Adding heparin to aspirin reduces the incidence of myocardial infarction and death in patients with unstable angina. A meta-analysis. JAMA 1996;276:811–815.

65. Theroux P, Waters D, Lam J, et al. Reactivation of unstable angina after the discontinuation of heparin. N Engl J Med 1992;327:141–145.

66. Granger CB, Miller JM, Bovill EG, et al. Rebound increase in thrombin generation and activity after cessation of intravenous heparin in patients with acute coronary syndromes. Circulation 1995;91:1929–1935.

67. Becker RC, Cannon CP, Tracy RP, et al. Relation between systemic anticoagulation as determined by activated partial thromboplastin time and heparin measurements and in-hospital clinical events in unstable angina and non-Q wave myocardiaL infarction. Thrombolysis in Myocardial Ischemia III B Investigators. Am Heart J 1996;131:421–433.

68. Xiao Z, Theroux P. Platelet activation with unfractionated heparin at therapeutic concentrations and comparisons with a low-molecular-weight heparin and with a direct thrombin inhibitor. Circulation 1998;97:251–256.

69. Mascelli MA, Kleiman NS, Marciniak SJ Jr, et al. Therapeutic heparin concentrations augment platelet reactivity: implications for the pharmacologic assessment of the glycoprotein IIb/IIIa antagonist abciximab. Am Heart J 2000; 139:696–703.

70. Zabel KM, Granger CB, Becker RC, et al. Use of bedside activated partial thromboplastin time monitor to adjust heparin dosing after thrombolysis for acute myocardial infarction: results of GUSTO-I. Global Utilization of Streptokinase and TPA for Occluded Coronary Arteries. Am Heart J 1998;136:868–876.

71. Hirsh J, Fuster V. Guide to anticoagulant therapy. Part 1: Heparin. American Heart Association. Circulation 1994;89: 1449–1468.

72. Hirsh J, Fuster V. Guide to anticoagulant therapy. Part 2: Oral anticoagulants. American Heart Association. Circulation 1994;89:1469–1480.

73. Boneu B. Low molecular weight heparin therapy: is monitoring needed? Thromb Haemost 1994;72:330–334.

74. Low-molecular-weight heparin during instability in coronary artery disease, Fragmin during Instability in Coronary Artery Disease (FRISC) study group. Lancet 1996;347:561–568.

75. Wallentin L, Husted S, Kontny F, Swahn E. Long-term low-molecular-weight heparin (Fragmin) and/or early revascularization during instability in coronary artery disease (the FRISC II Study). Am J Cardiol 1997;80:61E–63E.

76. Klein W, Buchwald A, Hillis SE, et al. Comparison of low-molecular-weight heparin with unfractionated heparin acutely and with placebo for 6 weeks in the management of unstable coronary artery disease. Fragmin in unstable coronary artery disease study (FRIC). Circulation 1997;96:61–68.

77. Cohen M, Demers C, Gurfinkel EP, et al. A comparison of low-molecular-weight heparin with unfractionated heparin for unstable coronary artery disease. Efficacy and Safety of Subcutaneous Enoxaparin in Non-Q-Wave Coronary Events Study Group. N Engl J Med 1997;337:447–452.

78. Antman EM, McCabe CH, Gurfinkel EP, et al. Enoxaparin prevents death and cardiac ischemic events in unstable angina/non-Q-wave myocardial infarction. Results of the thrombolysis in myocardial infarction (TIMI) 11B trial. Circulation 1999;100:1593–1601.

79. Antman EM, Cohen M, McCabe C, et al. Enoxaparin is superior to unfractionated heparin for preventing clinical events at 1-year follow-up of TIMI 11B and ESSENCE. Eur Heart J 2002;23:308–314.

80. Goodman SG, Fitchett D, Armstrong PW, et al. Randomized evaluation of the safety and efficacy of enoxaparin versus unfractionated heparin in high-risk patients with non-ST-segment elevation acute coronary syndromes receiving the glycoprotein IIb/IIIa inhibitor eptifibatide. Circulation 2003;107:238–244.

81. Cohen M, Theroux P, Borzak S, et al. Randomized double-blind safety study of enoxaparin versus unfractionated heparin in patients with non-ST-segment elevation acute coronary syndromes treated with tirofiban and aspirin: the ACUTE II study. The Antithrombotic Combination Using Tirofiban and Enoxaparin. Am Heart J 2002;144:470–477.

82. Ferguson JJ, Califf RM, Antman EM, et al. Enoxaparin vs unfractionated heparin in high-risk patients with non-ST-segment elevation acute coronary syndromes managed with an intended early invasive strategy: primary results of the SYNERGY randomized trial. JAMA 2004;292:45–54.

83. Johnson PH. Hirudin: clinical potential of a thrombin inhibitor. Annu Rev Med 1994;45:165–177.

84. A comparison of recombinant hirudin with heparin for the treatment of acute coronary syndromes. The Global Use of Strategies to Open Occluded Coronary Arteries (GUSTO) IIb investigators. N Engl J Med 1996;335:775–782.

85. Effects of recombinant hirudin (lepirudin) compared with heparin on death, myocardial infarction, refractory angina, and revascularisation procedures in patients with acute myocardial ischaemia without ST elevation: a

randomised trial. Organisation to Assess Strategies for Ischemic Syndromes (OASIS-2) Investigators. Lancet 1999; 353:429–438.

86. Ridker PM, Rifai N, Clearfield M, et al. Measurement of C-reactive protein for the targeting of statin therapy in the primary prevention of acute coronary events. N Engl J Med 2001;344:1959–1965.
87. Kinlay S, Timms T, Clark M, et al. Comparison of effect of intensive lipid lowering with atorvastatin to less intensive lowering with lovastatin on C-reactive protein in patients with stable angina pectoris and inducible myocardial ischemia. Am J Cardiol 2002;89:1205–1207.
88. Kinlay S, Schwartz GG, Olsson AG, et al. High-dose atorvastatin enhances the decline in inflammatory markers in patients with acute coronary syndromes in the MIRACL study. Circulation 2003;108:1560–1566.
89. Cannon CP, Braunwald E, McCabe CH, et al. Intensive versus moderate lipid lowering with statins after acute coronary syndromes. N Engl J Med 2004;350:1495–1504.
90. Boden WE, O'Rourke RA, Crawford MH, et al. Outcomes in patients with acute non-Q-wave myocardial infarction randomly assigned to an invasive as compared with a conservative management strategy. Veterans Affairs Non-Q-Wave Infarction Strategies in Hospital (VANQWISH) Trial Investigators. N Engl J Med 1998;338:1785–1792.
91. Yusuf S, Flather M, Pogue J, et al. Variations between countries in invasive cardiac procedures and outcomes in patients with suspected unstable angina or myocardial infarction without initial ST elevation. OASIS (Organisation to Assess Strategies for Ischaemic Syndromes) Registry Investigators. Lancet 1998;352:507–514.
92. Cannon CP, Weintraub WS, Demopoulos LA, et al. Comparison of early invasive and conservative strategies in patients with unstable coronary syndromes treated with the glycoprotein IIb/IIIa inhibitor tirofiban. N Engl J Med 2001;344:1879–1887.
93. Fox KA, Poole-Wilson PA, Henderson RA, et al. Interventional versus conservative treatment for patients with unstable angina or non-ST-elevation myocardial infarction: the British Heart Foundation RITA 3 randomised trial. Randomized Intervention Trial of unstable Angina. Lancet 2002;360:743–751.
94. Neumann FJ, Kastrati A, Pogatsa-Murray G, et al. Evaluation of prolonged antithrombotic pretreatment ("cooling-off" strategy) before intervention in patients with unstable coronary syndromes: a randomized controlled trial. JAMA 2003;290:1593–1599.

RECOMMENDED READING

Boersma E, Harrington RA, Moliterno DJ, et al. Platelet glycoprotein IIb/IIIa inhibitors in acute coronary syndromes: a meta-analysis of all major randomised clinical trials. Lancet 2002;359:189–198.
Buffon A, Biasucci LM, Liuzzo G, et al. Widespread coronary inflammation in unstable angina. N Engl J Med 2002;347: 5–12.
Chen MS, Bhatt DL. Highlights of the 2002 update to the 2000 American College of Cardiology/American Heart Association acute coronary syndrome guidelines. Cardiol Rev 2003;11:113–121.
Goldman L, Cook EF, Johnson PA, et al. Prediction of the need for intensive care in patients who come to the emergency departments with acute chest pain. N Engl J Med 1996;334:1498–1504.
Libby P. Molecular bases of the acute coronary syndromes. Circulation 1995;91:2844–2850.

27

ST Segment Elevation Myocardial Infarction

Rajat Deo, MD, Christopher P. Cannon, MD, and James A. de Lemos, MD

INTRODUCTION

Management of acute ST elevation myocardial infarction (STEMI) has been transformed in the last 20 yr by the results of large, prospective, randomized trials. Advances have been made in all components of acute myocardial infarction (AMI) management, from primary and secondary prevention to prehospital care, acute reperfusion therapy, adjunctive medical therapy, and management of complications. Despite this progress, however, acute MI remains the most common cause of death in industrialized nations; in addition, while mortality rates have been falling, the incidence of new infarction has not fallen in concert. The long-term consequences of myocardial infarction, congestive heart failure and ventricular arrhythmias, consume a large and growing proportion of health care resources. Thus, there is great need for continued progress in the prevention and treatment of acute MI.

OVERVIEW OF PATHOPHYSIOLOGIC MECHANISMS

The different acute coronary syndromes exist on a continuum of plaque rupture and thrombus formation (Fig. 1): the continuum ranges from a ruptured plaque with little or no thrombus (often asymptomatic), to a ruptured plaque with moderate thrombus leading to partial coronary occlusion (unstable angina and non-ST elevation MI), to a ruptured plaque with extensive thrombus and complete occlusion of the artery (ST segment elevation MI). In a minority of patients, superficial plaque erosion, rather than plaque rupture, may be the precipitating event.

Angiographic studies have consistently shown that MI more commonly develops from lesions associated with minor (<70%), rather than severe (≥70%) luminal narrowing. Atherosclerotic lesions that lead to acute MI tend to be associated with positive (eccentric) vessel remodeling, in which the entire vessel, including the external elastic lamina, is enlarged to accommodate the growing, lipid-rich plaque. Much work has been done to identify the factors that contribute to plaque erosion or rupture. The "vulnerable" atherosclerotic plaque has been characterized as having a dense lipid-rich core and a thin protective fibrous cap. The molecular factors that govern formation and breakdown of the extracellular matrix appear to regulate integrity of this protective fibrous cap. In vulnerable atherosclerotic lesions, inflammatory cells predominate at the shoulder region of the plaque; local release of cytokines from these inflammatory cells contributes to weakening of the fibrous cap at this critical site. When the plaque ruptures, platelets adhere and aggregate, thrombin is activated, and the fibrin clot forms, leading to myocardial ischemia or infarction.

In acute MI, thrombosis is composed of platelets, fibrin, erythrocytes, and leukocytes. Platelet activation leads to the release of specific mediators including thromboxane A_2, serotonin (5HT), adenosine diphosphate (ADP), platelet-activating factor (PAF), thrombin, tissue factor, and oxygen-

From: *Essential Cardiology: Principles and Practice, 2nd Ed.*
Edited by: C. Rosendorff © Humana Press Inc., Totowa, NJ

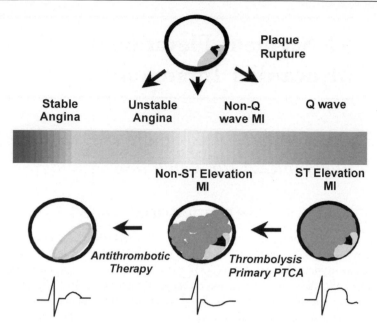

Fig. 1. The spectrum of acute coronary syndromes. The various clinical syndromes of coronary artery disease can be viewed as a spectrum, ranging from patients with stable angina to those with acute ST elevation MI. Across the spectrum of the acute coronary syndromes, atherosclerotic plaque rupture leads to coronary artery thrombosis: In acute ST elevation MI, complete coronary occlusion is present. In those with unstable angina or non-Q wave MI, a flow-limiting thrombus is usually present. In patients with stable angina, thrombus is rarely seen. (Adapted from Cannon CP, J Thrombolysis 1995;2:205–218.)

derived free radicals. The presence of these mediators in conjunction with the relative absence of prostacyclin (PGI_2), tissue plasminogen activator (t-PA), and endothelial nitric oxide at sites of vascular injury promotes platelet aggregation and obstruction of the narrowed coronary lumen. On the surface of the activated platelet, the coagulation cascade is propagated, leading to the deposition of thrombin and fibrin, obstructing arterial blood flow and leading to myocardial necrosis.

The process of thrombotic occlusion of an epicardial coronary artery is not a static one. Variation in vasomotor tone and in the balance of endogenous fibrinolytic and procoagulant factors can lead to cyclic occlusion and reperfusion of the occluded artery. Moreover, it has recently been appreciated that the coronary microcirculation plays a critical role in STEMI. Microvascular obstruction can occur due to embolization of platelet and platelet-thrombin aggregates, microvascular spasm, and *in situ* leukocyte plugging. Even among patients with successful reperfusion of the occluded epicardial artery, microvascular obstruction is associated with adverse clinical outcomes. Thus, the coronary microcirculation has emerged as an additional target for therapies in STEMI.

ST Elevation vs Non-ST Elevation MI

Experience with fibrinolytic therapy has identified important differences in the pathophysiologic mechanisms underlying different types of acute MI and has dramatically improved mortality in certain subsets of patients. Patients whose acute MI is manifested by ST segment elevation experience a substantial benefit from fibrinolytic therapy, while those whose MI is not associated with ST segment do not. Angiographic studies have shown that this difference is due to the initial status of the infarct-related artery: Patients with ST segment elevation exhibit 100% occlusion of the artery while patients without ST segment elevation exhibit a severely stenotic, but nevertheless patent, coronary artery (Fig. 1).

Q Wave MI vs Non-Q Wave MI

As opposed to the distinction of ST elevation versus non-ST elevation MI, the determination of Q wave versus non-Q wave MI can be made only retrospectively, and is a less useful classification in the early hours of patient management. Untreated, most patients with ST segment elevation MI usually evolve a transmural infarction and develop Q waves on the surface electrocardiogram. With successful reperfusion therapy, however, 25 to 30% of patients with ST elevation have necrosis limited to the subendocardial regions and do not develop Q waves. Patients without ST elevation at baseline generally do not develop Q waves since infarction is limited to subendocardial regions.

DIAGNOSIS OF ACUTE MYOCARDIAL INFARCTION

History

A careful history is the most important initial diagnostic step in a patient with suspected acute MI. Most patients complain of chest pain, which resembles classic angina pectoris, and describe a severe, pressure-type pain in the mid-sternum, often radiating to the left arm, neck, or jaw. The pain may be distinguished from angina by its intensity, duration (>30 min), and failure to resolve with nitroglycerin administration. The pain may be accompanied by dyspnea, diaphoresis, nausea, vomiting, and profound weakness.

In nearly half of the patients presenting with an acute MI, an inciting factor can be identified. Heavy exercise, particularly among individuals who are fatigued or emotionally stressed, may trigger plaque rupture and precipitate an acute MI.

Particular attention should be given to the quality of pain, its variation with respiration and position, and whether it is similar to prior anginal episodes in quality. Characterization of the pain may help to distinguish it from other conditions that also cause chest discomfort. Aortic dissection, for example, typically causes a "tearing" pain, radiating through to the back. Pulmonary embolism is usually accompanied by pleuritic pain, shortness of breath, and occasionally hemoptysis. Pericardial pain is also usually pleuritic, and frequently changes with position, such that the patient may feel better sitting forward. The pain of pericarditis may radiate to the left shoulder or trapezius ridge. Not infrequently, inferior-wall myocardial infarction (IMI) masquerades as indigestion or nausea, rather than chest pain. Differentiating this from cholecystitis, peptic ulcer, and mesenteric ischemia by history alone may be very difficult, and a high index of suspicion for myocardial infarction is necessary.

Many patients, particularly the elderly and women, present with "atypical" symptoms, which include dyspnea, indigestion, unusual locations of pain, agitation, altered mental status, profound weakness, and syncope. Furthermore, infarction may be silent in more than 25% of cases. This occurs more frequently in diabetic patients, as a result of the neuropathy that accompanies longstanding diabetes mellitus.

Physical Exam

The physical examination is usually unremarkable in patients with uncomplicated acute MI. Particularly in the modern era, where noninvasive imaging has supplanted the physical examination for confirmation of structural abnormalities, the examination should be performed efficiently, focusing on narrowing the differential diagnosis and assessing the stability of the patient. A focused examination can help to eliminate diagnoses such as pericarditis, pneumothorax, pulmonary embolus, and aortic dissection, which may mimic acute MI. It can also exclude aortic (or mitral) stenosis or regurgitation, which may complicate patient management. In addition, hemodynamic and mechanical complications of acute MI can often be detected by careful attention to physical findings.

Patients with acute MI often appear pale, cool, and clammy; in many cases they are in obvious distress. Elderly patients, in particular, may be agitated and incoherent. Patients with cardiogenic shock may be confused and listless. Blood pressure and pulses should be checked in both arms, since a pulse deficit or decreased blood pressure in the left arm would shift the focus of the diagnostic workup toward aortic dissection. Cardiac examination should focus on eliciting murmurs and rubs. A pericardial rub, although often difficult to appreciate, suggests that pericarditis may be the cause of a patient's chest discomfort.

A brief survey for signs of congestive heart failure should be performed. Cool extremities or impaired mental status suggest decreased tissue perfusion, while elevated jugular venous pressure, rales on chest exam, and peripheral edema suggest elevated cardiac filling pressures. A careful examination of the peripheral arterial pulses and temperature can detect peripheral or cerebral vascular disease, which in itself increases the likelihood of coronary disease.

ECG Findings

The 12-lead ECG remains the most important initial diagnostic step in patients with suspected MI (see Chapter 8). Patients reporting to the emergency room with chest pain should have a 12-lead ECG performed immediately. If ST segment elevation is seen, and there are no contraindications to nitrates, a single sublingual nitroglycerin tablet should be given while patient assessment continues. If chest pain and ST elevation resolve completely with sublingual nitroglycerin, a diagnosis of coronary vasospasm (Prinzmetal's variant angina) or possibly spontaneous reperfusion of a thrombotic coronary occlusion is likely. Persistent ST elevation is virtually diagnostic of occlusive thrombus, and immediate reperfusion therapy should be administered to all patients who are candidates. ST segment elevation suggestive of MI should be distinguished from that of pericarditis and the normal early repolarization variant. In pericarditis, ST elevation is usually diffuse, and may be associated with depression of the PR segment. In the early repolarization variant, the contour of the elevated ST segment is concave rather than convex. Patients with prior transmural infarction and aneurysm formation may have persistent ST elevation, but this is generally associated with the presence of Q waves.

The presence of a new, or presumed new, left bundle branch block (LBBB) in the setting of chest pain is suggestive of a large anterior infarction; these patients should be considered for reperfusion therapy as well. Patients with LBBB of undetermined age present a diagnostic dilemma, and either emergency echocardiography (to look for an anterior wall motion abnormality) or cardiac catheterization should be considered. In patients with a preexisting LBBB, alternative methods are needed to make the diagnosis of acute MI, as ECG findings are not sufficiently reliable to guide therapy.

Cardiac Biomarkers

In recent years, many new serum markers for myocardial necrosis have been developed. Measurements of cardiac troponin T (cTNT) and I have become routine, and rapid whole blood assays for myoglobin, creatinine kinase (CK), its myocardial isoform (CKMB), and cTNT are now available. The advent of more sensitive and specific cardiac biomarkers has facilitated the diagnosis of non-ST elevation MI; however, patients with STEMI are identified primarily on their clinical syndrome and presenting ECG. As a result, interventions to facilitate reperfusion are implemented before the measurement of cardiac biomarkers has been completed. For patients with ST elevation MI, cardiac marker measurements are used to confirm the diagnosis in patients with equivocal electrocardiographic changes or a paced rhythm, to help gauge prognosis, and sometimes to estimate the likelihood of successful reperfusion therapy. The time course of rise and fall of the most commonly measured cardiac enzymes is shown in Fig. 2.

While cardiac markers have little role in the emergent diagnosis of STEMI, they remain valuable for prognostic assessment. For example, patients with evidence of myoglobin or troponin elevation prior to the administration of reperfusion therapy are at increased risk for failure of fibrinolytic therapy or primary percutaneous coronary intervention (PCI), and are at increased risk for death, independent of the success or failure of reperfusion therapy. Interestingly, this association with outcomes is also independent of infarct location and time to treatment, suggesting that measuring cardiac markers at the time of emergency room presentation provides an objective assessment of the amount of irreversible myocyte injury that has occurred prior to the initiation of therapy. In

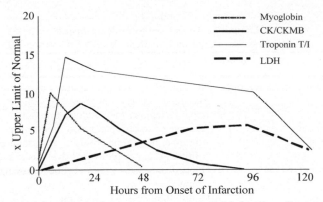

Fig. 2. Time course of serum marker release in acute myocardial infarction. *See* text for details. (From Antman, EM. General hospital management. In: Julian DG, Braunwald E, eds. Management of Acute Myocardial Infarction. W. B. Saunders, Ltd., London, 1994, p. 63, reprinted with permission.)

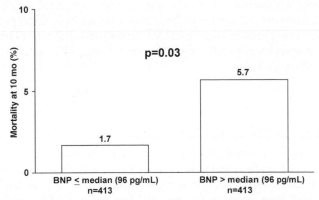

Fig. 3. BNP levels greater than the median were associated with a higher 10-mo mortality among patients with STEMI. (Adapted from ref. 2.)

addition, the rate of rise of cardiac biomarkers can be used to help determine which patients have had successful or unsuccessful reperfusion, and may help to select appropriate patients for coronary angiography. Myoglobin appears to be the most useful for this purpose, due to its smaller size, cytosolic location, and rapid renal clearance *(1)*.

B-type natriuretic peptide (BNP) is a cardiac hormone that is released in response to increases in wall stress. Levels of circulating BNP are in wide clinical use for diagnosis and prognostic assessment in patients with suspected heart failure. BNP levels also appear to be useful in ST elevation MI. Following STEMI, BNP levels rise and peak at approximately day 2. A second peak may occur several days later as the ventricular remodeling process begins. Higher levels of BNP, measured several days after MI, have been associated with a greater likelihood of death, CHF, and ventricular remodeling after STEMI *(2)* and have a role for assessing prognosis (Fig. 3). Whether specific therapies should be applied to those with increased BNP is being investigated in clinical trials.

Echocardiography

Portable echocardiography can help to confirm myocardial ischemia or infarction in patients with nondiagnostic electrocardiograms, particularly in situations where rapid assays for serum markers are not available. In our experience, this is particularly useful when left bundle branch block of undetermined duration is present, or when it is necessary to distinguish pericarditis or early repolari-

Table 1
Diagnostic Tools Used to Evaluate Tissue
and Microvascular Perfusion in Patients With ST Elevation MI[a]

Technique	Finding suggestive of microvascular injury
Myocardial contrast echocardiography	Absence of microbubble contrast uptake in the infarct zone
Doppler flow wire	Abnormal coronary flow reserve; systolic reversal of coronary flow
PET scanning	Impaired regional myocardial blood flow as measured with $^{13}NH_3$
Nuclear SPECT imaging	Absence of tracer uptake into infarct zone
Contrast angiography	Abnormal myocardial "blush," with failure to opacify myocardium or prolonged dye washout from myocardium
MRI	Hypoenhancement of infarct zone following gadolinium contrast injection
ECG	Failure to resolve ST elevation

[a]Assumes that the epicardial infarct artery is patent. These techniques can be presumed to reflect microvascular and tissue perfusion only when the infarct artery has been successfully recanalized.

zation from acute MI. Transmural ischemia is almost always associated with hypokinesis or akinesis of the subtended myocardial segments. Therefore, absence of regional or global wall motion abnormalities argues strongly against transmural MI. Transesophageal echo (TEE) should be considered when suspicion arises for aortic dissection. In expert hands, TEE has >90% sensitivity for the diagnosis of aortic dissection.

THERAPY FOR ACUTE MI

Reperfusion Therapy

EVOLVING DEFINITION OF "OPTIMAL" REPERFUSION

Early, successful coronary reperfusion limits infarct size, and improves left ventricular dysfunction and survival. These benefits are due at least in part to the early restoration of antegrade flow in the infarct-related artery (IRA). In a retrospective analysis of six angiographic trials of different fibrinolytic regimens, patients who achieved normal (Thrombolysis in Myocardial Infarction [TIMI] grade 3) flow in the IRA had a 30-d mortality rate of 3.6%, vs 6.6% in patients with slow (TIMI grade 2) flow, and 9.5% in patients with an occluded artery (TIMI grade 0 or 1 flow) (3).

Even among patients who achieve normal (TIMI grade 3) epicardial blood flow in the IRA after reperfusion therapy, tissue-level perfusion may be inadequate. Using a number of different diagnostic tools (Table 1), investigators have demonstrated that measures of tissue and microvascular perfusion provide prognostic information that is independent of TIMI flow grade (Fig. 4) (4). For example, Ito and colleagues, using myocardial contrast echocardiography, found impaired tissue and microvascular perfusion in approximately one third of patients with TIMI grade 3 flow after primary PCI (5). These patients were at increased risk for the development of CHF and death. Microvascular dysfunction is thought to occur in the setting of myocardial infarction as a result of distal embolization of microthrombi, tissue inflammation from myocyte necrosis, and arteriolar spasm caused by tissue injury.

Perhaps the most clinically relevant measure of tissue perfusion is a simple bedside assessment of the degree of resolution of ST segment elevation on the 12-lead electrocardiogram. Greater degrees of ST resolution are associated with a higher probability of achieving a patent IRA and TIMI grade 3 flow (4). Furthermore, patients who have normal epicardial blood flow, but persistence of ST elevation on the 12-lead ECG, have been shown to have abnormal tissue and microvascular perfusion using myocardial contrast echocardiography. In addition, persistent ST elevation has been shown to predict poor recovery of infarct zone wall motion and the clinical endpoints of death and heart failure (4). In summary, ST resolution appears to integrate epicardial and myocardial (microvascular) reperfusion. As a result, it may actually provide a more clinically useful assessment of reperfusion than coronary angiography.

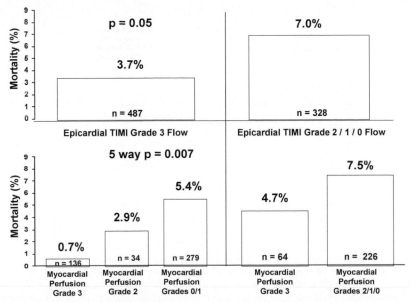

Fig. 4. Relationship between epicardial perfusion, myocardial perfusion, and mortality after fibrinolytic admin-istration in the TIMI 10B trial. TIMI Myocardial Perfusion Grade measures the degree of microvascular flow during routine coronary angiogram. Findings from this study revealed that myocardial perfusion was significantly associated with mortality independent of epicardial blood flow. (Adapted from Gibson CM, Cannon CP, Murphy SA, et al., for the TIMI Study Group. The relationship of the TIMI Myocardial Perfusion Grade to mortality after thrombolytic administration. Circulation 2000;101:125–130.)

Pharmacologic Reperfusion

FIBRINOLYTIC THERAPY

Time is a critical determinant in the success of any fibrinolytic regimen. Patients who are treated within 1 h from the onset of chest pain have an ~50% reduction in mortality, while those presenting more than 12 h after onset of symptoms derive little, if any, benefit from fibrinolysis. For each hour earlier that a patient is treated, there is an approximately absolute 1% decrease in mortality, which translates into an additional 10 lives saved per 1000 treated. Figure 5 illustrates the crucial time-dependence of administration of fibrinolytic therapy.

Fibrinolysis has been shown to reduce mortality in numerous placebo-controlled trials using streptokinase, anistreplase (APSAC), and tissue plasminogen activator (t-PA). These benefits have been shown to persist through at least 10 yr of follow up. The Fibrinolytic Therapy Trialists' overview of all the large placebo-controlled studies showed a 2.6% absolute reduction in mortality for patients with ST-segment elevation MI treated within the first 12 h after the onset of symptoms *(6)*. Patients presenting with left bundle branch block and a strong clinical history for acute MI also derive a large benefit from fibrinolysis. However, those without ST segment elevation or left bundle branch block do not benefit from fibrinolysis, and indeed may be harmed by it.

COMPARISON OF DIFFERENT FIBRINOLYTIC AGENTS

All the fibrinolytic agents currently available and under investigation are plasminogen activators. They all work enzymatically, directly or indirectly, to convert the single-chain plasminogen molecule to the double-chain plasmin, which has potent intrinsic fibrinolytic activity.

The initial description of fibrinolytic therapy for STEMI involved intracoronary administration of streptokinase (SK), a nonenzymatic protein produced by β-hemolytic streptococci. SK forms an activator complex with plasminogen that results in its cleavage and the subsequent formation of plasmin. Plasmin degrades fibrin and fibrinogen as well as procoagulant factors V and VIII. The

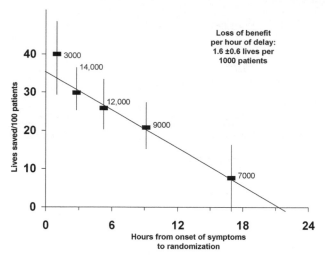

Fig. 5. Absolute reduction in 35-d mortality versus delay from symptom onset to randomisation and treatment among 45,000 patients with ST segment elevation or LBBB. (From Fibrinolytic Therapy Trialists' (FTT) Collaborative Group. Indications for fibrinolytic therapy in suspected acute myocardial infarction: collaborative overview of early mortality and major morbidity results from all randomised trials of more than 1000 patients. Lancet 1994;343:311–322. Reprinted with permission from Elsevier.)

Gruppo Italiano per lo Studio della Streptochinasi nell'Infarto Miocardico (GISSI) trial and the Second International Study on Infarct Survival (ISIS)-2 demonstrated that the administration of SK for evolving MI reduced mortality when compared to standard (no reperfusion) therapy. Readministration of streptokinase to patients should be avoided for at least 4 yr (preferably indefinitely) because of a high prevalence of potentially neutralizing antibodies, and because there is a risk for anaphylaxis upon reexposure to these drugs.

The potential for improved survival with more specific fibrinolytic agents such as alteplase (t-PA) was suggested by the first TIMI trial, which demonstrated infarct-related artery patency in nearly twice as many patients randomly allocated to receive t-PA vs SK. In addition, the effect of early and sustained infarct-vessel patency on mortality was evaluated in the Global Utilization of Streptokinase and Tissue Plasminogen Activator for Occluded Coronary Arteries (GUSTO) trial, conceived in 1989. The GUSTO trial *(7)* directly compared four thrombolytic regimens: "accelerated" or "front-loaded" t-PA and concomitant IV heparin, streptokinase with IV heparin, streptokinase with subcutaneous heparin, and a combination of t-PA and streptokinase with IV heparin. The accelerated t-PA and heparin regimen achieved the highest 90-min infarct-related artery patency, and was associated with the lowest mortality. The 14% mortality reduction associated with tPA versus streptokinase was highly significant ($p = 0.001$), although there was a significant excess of hemorrhagic stroke for tPA compared with streptokinase (0.7% of patients treated with tPA vs 0.5% of patients treated with streptokinase). When comparing the net clinical benefit (death or disabling stroke) between the different regimens, t-PA was still clearly beneficial compared to the other three regimens (9 fewer deaths or disabling strokes per 1000 patients treated with t-PA). Other complications of acute MI were less frequent with t-PA as well, including allergic reactions, CHF, cardiogenic shock, and atrial and ventricular arrhythmias.

Given the importance of rapid reperfusion, one would expect that a more aggressive fibrinolytic regimen, which achieves a higher rate of early infarct-related patency, would be associated with a lower mortality. Traditional fibrinolytic regimens, however, fail to induce early and sustained reperfusion in nearly half the patients (Fig. 6). In addition, reocclusion occurs in another 10 to 30% of patients. As a result, recent efforts have concentrated on the development of newer fibrinolytics, anticoagulants, and antiplatelet therapies to improve early and sustained reperfusion.

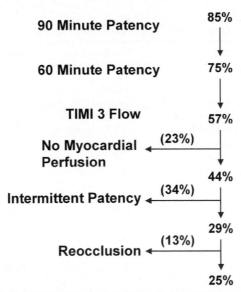

Fig. 6. Limitations of current fibrinolytic regimens. (From Lincoff AM, Topol EJ. Illusion of reperfusion. Does anyone achieve optimal reperfusion during acute myocardial infarction? Circulation 1993;87:1792–1805.)

Molecular modification of the recombinant tissue plasminogen activator (rt-PA) structure has provided agents such as reteplase and tenecteplase (TNK) with longer plasma half-lives that allow a simplified single or double bolus administration regimen (Table 2). Despite these more favorable pharmacologic characteristics, however, improvements in 30-d mortality rates have not been observed in phase III clinical trials. Reteplase is a double bolus agent with limited fibrin specificity that was shown to have similar efficacy and risk to accelerated t-PA in the GUSTO III trial *(8)*. Reteplase, however, is easier to administer than t-PA, a factor that could prevent dosing errors and possibly decrease "door to needle" time. ASSENT II *(9)* demonstrated that the single bolus agent TNK is equivalent to tPA in terms of efficacy. TNK was also equivalent in terms of ICH. One potential advantage of TNK over other agents is its fibrin specificity, which appears to result in a 20% reduction in non-ICH bleeding when compared to tPA.

Overall, the benefits of tenecteplase or reteplase over tPA are modest and mostly related to a more convenient dosing regimen; the failure of these agents to improve outcomes over the accelerated regimen of alteplase (Fig. 7) suggests that we have reached a therapeutic plateau with fibrinolytic monotherapy and demonstrate the importance of continued evaluation of novel adjunctive anticoagulant and antiplatelet or interventional reperfusion strategies for STEMI.

COMBINATION THERAPY WITH GLYCOPROTEIN IIB/IIIA INHIBITORS AND REDUCED-DOSE LYTICS

The recognition of the pivotal role of platelets in the pathophysiology of STEMI has further improved our understanding of the limitations of fibrinolytic monotherapy. Fibrinolytic agents are believed to act on only one component of the clot and lead to platelet activation. Platelets induce release of PAI-1, α-2 antiplasmin, and thromboxane A_2, which lead to prothrombosis and vasoconstriction. Fibrinolytics also enhance fibrin activation by exposure of clot-bound thrombin *(10)*. The glycoprotein IIb/IIIa receptor is the final common pathway for platelet aggregation. By blocking the final common pathway of platelet aggregation, fibrinogen-mediated cross-linkage, GP IIb/IIIa receptor inhibition may contribute to disaggregation of platelet-rich thrombus *(10)*.

Preclinical studies have suggested that the use of GP IIb/IIIa receptor inhibitors with thrombolytic agents may accelerate reperfusion and reduce the risk of reocclusion. The combination of a

Table 2
Thrombolytic Agents in Current Clinical Use

	Alteplase	Reteplase	Tenecteplase	Streptokinase
Fibrin-selective	+++	++	++++	–
Half-life	5 min	14 min	17 min	20 min
Dose	15 mg bolus; then 0.75 mg/kg over 30 min; then 0.5 mg/kg over 60 min (max 100 mg total dose)	Two 10 unit bolus doses given 30 min apart	0.53 mg/kg as a single bolus	1.5 million units over 30–60 min
Weight-adjusted	Partial	No	Yes	No
Adjunctive heparin	Yes	Yes	Yes	No
Possible allergy	No	No	No	Yes
TIMI 2/3 flow (90 min)	80%	80%	80%	60%
TIMI 3 flow (90 min)	55–60%	60%	55–65%	32%
Efficacy vs tPA	NA	Similar	Equivalent	1% ↑ mortality
Safety	NA	Similar	Similar ICH ↓ non-ICH bleeding	↓ ICH ↓ overall bleeding
Cost	+++	+++	+++	+

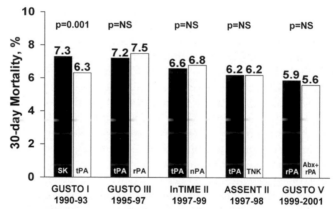

Fig. 7. Results from major clinical trials comparing different fibrinolytic regimens. Note the steady decline in mortality over the decade, and the absence of improvement in mortality with newer fibrinolytic agents. (Abx, abciximab; SK, streptokinase; tPA, alteplase; rPA, reteplase; TNK, tenecteplase.)

reduced-dose thrombolytic agent and a GP IIb/IIIa inhibitor was evaluated in the TIMI 14 trial, a phase II dose-ranging and confirmation trial. The rate of TIMI 3 flow was significantly higher at both 60 and 90 min in patients receiving half-dose tPA and abciximab (72% and 77%, respectively) (11). In addition, ST segment resolution was improved, even among those with TIMI grade 3 flow, suggesting an additional benefit of combination therapy in improving microvascular perfusion. Major hemorrhage and intracranical hemorrhage (ICH) were similar between the combination tPA and abciximab and t-PA control groups. In follow-up trials only nonsignificant trends toward increased TIMI 3 flow were observed with half-dose reteplase (TIMI 14 and SPEED) and TNK in the ENTIRE-TIMI 23, INTEGRITI-TIMI 20, and FASTER-TIMI 24 trials.

Despite only modest increase in TIMI 3 flow in these follow-up trials, larger clinical endpoint trials were already under way. GUSTO-V examined mortality in patients with STEMI who were randomly allocated to receive either conventional dose reteplase and heparin or a combination of

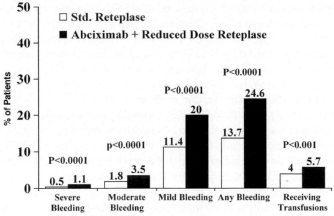

Fig. 8. Combination therapy with reduced dose reteplase and abciximab in GUSTO-V led to increased rates of nonintracranial bleeding. (Adapted from ref. *11*.)

half-dose reteplase, abciximab, and reduced-dose heparin *(12)*. This trial enrolled 16,588 patients who were within 6 h of evolving STEMI. At 30 d, the primary endpoint of all-cause mortality was not significantly different between the reteplase group and the combined reteplase and abciximab group. Although the combination regimen significantly reduced rates of reinfarction and emergent PCI within 7 d compared with fibrinolytic monotherapy, this did not result in improved 1-yr mortality *(12)*. No differences in rates of intracranial hemorrhage were seen overall, but non-ICH bleeding, transfusions, and thrombocytopenia were all increased in the combination therapy arm (Fig. 8).

ASSENT-3 was a multicenter, randomized study of 6095 patients with STEMI who were randomly assigned to one of three treatment regimens: full-dose tenecteplase and enoxaparin; half-dose tenecteplase, abciximab, and low-dose unfractionated heparin (UFH); or full-dose tenecteplase with UFH *(13)*. The tenexteplase-enoxaparin regimen will be discussed below. The findings in the combination arm (half-dose tenecteplase with abciximab) were virtually identical to those observed in GUSTO-V: nonfatal recurrent ischemic events were lower in the combination arm, but mortality was not reduced and bleeding complications were increased. Of particular importance, both GUSTO-V and ASSENT-3 showed that combination therapy was associated with increased rates of ICH in patients >75 yr old. In summary, despite great promise from phase II trials, appropriately powered endpoint trials have demonstrated that the combination of GP IIb/IIIa inhibitors with reduced doses of fibrinolytics are not superior to fibrinolytic monotherapy. These regimens cannot be recommended outside of an ongoing clinical trial, and are contraindicated in the elderly. Future studies will evaluate whether these regimens might have a role in facilitated PCI (*see* "Mechanical Perfusion" following).

Adjunctive Therapy With Unfractionated Heparin and Low-Molecular-Weight Heparin

In acute ST-segment elevation MI, unfractionated heparin (UFH) is also an important adjunctive agent to decrease reocclusion following administration of t-PA. Although no difference in infarct-related artery patency is seen at 90 min, patency is higher between 18 h and 5 d in patients randomized to receive intravenous heparin, suggesting that the benefit of heparin is a result of decreased reocclusion rather than enhanced fibrinolysis. Furthermore, long-term patency rates are highest in patients who are effectively anticoagulated at a target APTT range of 50–70 s.

Recently, it has become appreciated that the dose of intravenous heparin is also an important risk factor for the development of ICH. Therefore, the ACC/AHA guidelines recommend a reduced dose of UFH to be given with tPA, rPA, or TNK: a bolus of 60 U/kg (maximum 4000 U) and an infusion of 12 U/kg/h (maximum 1000 U/h).

Following streptokinase or anistreplase (APSAC), the role of heparin is less clear. Patients treated with streptokinase and intravenous or subcutaneous heparin in the GUSTO-I trial had similar infarct-related artery patency at 90 min and 24 h, but those receiving intravenous heparin had significantly higher patency at 5 to 7 d (84% vs 72%, $p = 0.04$). Nonetheless, overall mortality and the rate of clinical reinfarction were the same between these two groups. Therefore intravenous heparin may be considered optional in streptokinase-treated patients. Subcutaneous heparin has been shown to be of no benefit in preventing reinfarction or death.

Low-molecular-weight heparins (LMWHs) are created by depolymerization of standard, unfractionated heparin and selection of those fragments with lower molecular weight. As compared with unfractionated heparin, which has nearly equal anti-IIa and anti-Xa activity, LMWHs have increased ratios of anti-Xa to anti-IIa activity: either 2:1 (dalteparin) or 3:1 (enoxaparin or nadroparin). Greater factor Xa inhibition is thought to be responsible for the greater anticoagulant potency of LMWH over UFH. The high bioavailability and reproducible anticoagulant response of LMWH allows for subcutaneous administration without monitoring of the coagulation system. While this is an advantage in patients with non-ST elevation ACS, the long half-life of LMWH could be a disadvantage early in STEMI when patients are being considered for fibrinolytic therapy or primary PCI.

The ASSENT-3 trial evaluated the potential role of low-molecular-weight heparin used in combination with fibrinolytic therapy. As described above, ASSENT-3 randomized 6095 patients with STEMI to either full-dose tenectaplase and enoxaparin, the combination of reduced-dose tenecteplase, abciximab, and UFH, or full-dose tenecteplase with UFH *(13)*. Patients receiving enoxaparin were treated until hospital discharge, whereas those receiving UFH were treated for only 48 h, a design feature of the trial that has led to considerable criticism. Patients treated with full-dose tenecteplase plus enoxaparin had a significantly lower composite occurrence of mortality, in-hospital reinfarction, or refractory ischemia to 30 d compared with patients treated with tenecteplase plus UFH (11.4% vs 15.4%; $p = 0.0002$) *(13)*. The rate of ICH was comparable between the two treatment arms. The primary benefit of enoxaparin was a reduction in nonfatal recurrent MI, which is somewhat difficult to interpret because the duration of enoxaparin therapy was longer than UFH therapy. Similar results to ASSENT-3 were observed in the Enoxaparin and TNK-tPA with or without GP IIb/IIIa Inhibitor as Reperfusion Strategy in ST-Elevation MI (ENTIRE-TIMI)-23 trial.

While the results of ENTIRE-TIMI-23 and ASSENT-3 suggested that enoxaparin might be a potential replacement for UFH in multiple pharmacologic reperfusion strategies for STEMI, caution was raised after the ASSENT-3 PLUS trial was reported. This extension of the ASSENT-3 trial evaluated the safety and feasibility of reperfusion therapy with tenecteplase and enoxaparin in the prehospital setting *(14)*. In this trial, 1639 patients with STEMI were randomly assigned to treatment with tenecteplase and either enoxaparin or UFH. The composite of 30-d mortality or in-hospital reinfarction tended to be lower in the enoxaparin group; however, there was an increased risk of stroke and ICH in this group compared with UFH. The increased risk of stroke and ICH occurred exclusively in the older population (>75 yr). In summary, insufficient data are available to recommend enoxaparin as an adjunct to reperfusion therapy in STEMI. More data are needed to determine the efficacy and safety of enoxaparin in combination with fibrinolytics in the elderly. In an ongoing phase III trial, Enoxaparin and Thrombolysis Reperfusion for Acute Myocardial Infarction Trial (EXTRACT), the enoxaparin dose has been reduced for those greater than 75 yr of age. This trial will enroll more than 21,000 patients and should definitively determine the role for enoxaparin as an adjunct to fibrinolysis.

DIRECT THROMBIN INHIBITORS

Direct thrombin inhibitors have also undergone extensive evaluation. One such agent is the anticoagulant hirudin, which binds in a 1:1 relationship to thrombin, the last step in the coagulation cascade. In the TIMI 9B trial, although hirudin reduced the rate of recurrent MI following thrombolytic therapy, there was no difference in the primary endpoint, death, MI or severe CHF/shock at 30 d. Hirudin was compared with unfractionated heparin in more than 12,000 patients across the full spectrum of acute coronary syndromes in the GUSTO IIb trial. There was a reduction in reinfarction (5.4%

Table 3
Contraindications to Thrombolytic Therapy

Absolute contraindications	Relative contraindications
Active internal bleeding	Blood pressure consistently >180/110
History of CNS hemorrhage	History of stroke or AVM
Stroke of any kind within the last year	Known bleeding diathesis
Recent head trauma or CNS neoplasm	Active peptic ulcer
Suspected aortic dissection	Proliferative diabetic retinopathy?
	Prolonged CPR
	Prior exposure to SK or APSAC (5 d to 2 yr) or prior allergic reaction
	Pregnancy
	Major surgery or trauma within 2 wk
	Anticoagulation use
	Puncture of a noncompressible vessel

CNS, central nervous system; SK, streptokinase; APSAC, anisolylated plasminogen streptokinase activator complex (anistreplase).

vs 6.3%, $p = 0.04$) but only a trend toward reduction in death or MI at 30 d (8.9% vs 9.8%, $p = 0.06$) *(15)*. Bivalirudin, a synthetic polypeptide that forms a temporary high-affinity stoichiometric complex with thrombin, was evaluated in HERO-2 *(16)*. This trial compared bivalirudin with unfractionated heparin in more than 17,000 patients receiving streptokinase. No difference was observed in the primary outcome of death at 30 d; however, there was a 30% reduction in the incidence of new myocardial infarction in the bivalirudin group at 96 h, a benefit that was maintained out to 30 d. There was a small but significant excess of moderate bleeding with bivalirduin compared with heparin and a similar trend for excess severe bleeding (0.7% vs 0.5%, $p = 0.07$). In summary, multiple trial data do not support direct thrombin inhibitors as a replacement for UFH in patients treated with fibrinolytic therapy.

CURRENT GUIDELINES FOR FIBRINOLYTIC THERAPY

Fibrinolytic therapy is indicated for patients presenting within 12 h of symptom onset if they have ST segment elevation (or new left bundle branch block) provided they have no contraindications to thrombolytic therapy (Table 3). Less clear indications include patients who are older than 75 yr of age, those who present with ongoing pain between 12 and 24 h after the onset of acute MI, and those who are hypertensive but present with high-risk MI. Patients should not be treated if the time to treatment is >24 h, or if they present only with ST segment depression.

LIMITATIONS OF FIBRINOLYTIC THERAPY

Current fibrinolytic regimens achieve patency (TIMI grade 2 or 3 flow) in approx 80% of patients, but complete reperfusion (TIMI grade 3 flow) in only 50 to 60% of cases (Fig. 6). As described above, incomplete reperfusion is associated with a poor prognosis. In addition, even after successful fibrinolysis, 10 to 30% of patients suffer reocclusion of the infarct related artery and experience reinfarction in the following 3 mo *(17)*. Reocclusion and reinfarction are associated with a two- to threefold increase in mortality. Despite widespread availability of fibrinolytic agents, most patients who present with STEMI do not receive such therapy. A disproportionate number of patients eligible for receiving thrombolytic therapy include women, the elderly, and those with a history of prior myocardial infarction, multivessel coronary disease, or depressed left ventricular systolic function.

Finally, bleeding is the most common complication of fibrinolytic therapy; major hemorrhage, as defined by the TIMI criteria, occurs in 5 to 15% of patients. Intracranial hemorrhage (ICH) is the most devastating of the bleeding complications, causing death in the majority of patients affected and almost universal disability in survivors. In major clinical trials ICH has occurred in 0.6 to 1.4%

Table 4
Summary of 23 Randomized Trials
of Primary Angioplasty Versus Thrombolytic Therapy

Study group	PTCA	Thrombolytic therapy	p value
Mortality			
Short-term	7%	9%	0.0002
Long-term	9.6%	12.8%	0.0019
Nonfatal MI			
Short-term	3%	7%	<0.0001
Long-term	4.8%	10%	<0.0001
Total stroke			
Short-term	1%	2%	0.0004
Long-term	*	*	
Death, nonfatal MI or stroke			
Short-term	8%	14%	<0.0001
Long-term	12%	19%	<0.0001

[a]Data not available.

of patients receiving thrombolytic therapy. Patients at particularly high risk for ICH include elderly persons (particularly elderly females) and patients with low body weight.

Mechanical Reperfusion

PRIMARY PCI

The emerging method of achieving coronary reperfusion is the use of immediate or "primary" PCI. Many randomized controlled trials have evaluated both pharmacologic and mechanical reperfusion during STEMI. A meta-analysis of the 23 randomized controlled trials evaluated the short- and long-term clinical events among the 3872 patients randomized to primary PCI with the 3867 patients randomized to thrombolytic therapy (18). Primary PCI was superior to thrombolytic therapy in reducing mortality, nonfatal reinfarction, stroke, and the combined endpoint of death, nonfatal reinfarction, and stroke (Table 4). The reductions in mortality and recurrent MI were particularly striking. PCI remained a better option than thrombolytic therapy during long-term follow-up as well. These results are consistent with prior meta-analyses that have compared fibrinolytic therapy with primary PCI.

Recent clinical studies in patients with STEMI have sought to evaluate the effect of primary PCI among particular patient subsets. The relative benefits of primary PCI are greatest in patients at highest risk, including those with cardiogenic shock, right ventricular infarction, large anterior MI, and increased age (due partly to increased ICH rate with thrombolytic therapy). Primary PCI has traditionally been performed only in hospitals with surgical backup because of the potential for complications that might require immediate bypass surgery. The incidence of emergency bypass surgery with primary PCI, however, is now reported to be less than 0.5%. Coronary artery dissection and closure can be managed effectively with intracoronary stents. The Atlantic Cardiovascular Patient Outcomes Research Team (C-PORT) trial examined whether primary PCI could be performed safely at community hospitals with primary PCI programs but without access to on-site cardiac surgery. After a formal primary PCI development program was completed at all sites, 451 patients with STEMI of less than 12 h duration and eligible for thrombolytic therapy were enrolled. The incidence of the composite endpoint of death, reinfarction, and stroke was reduced in the primary PCI group at both 6 wk and 6 mo after index MI (19). Though this trial was small and underpowered, it suggests that PCI can be performed safely, promptly, and effectively in community hospitals following an extensive development program, even if these centers do not have an elective PCI or cardiac surgery program.

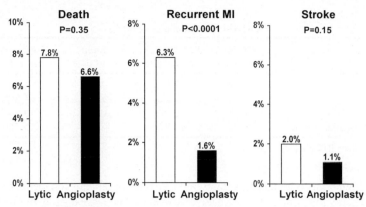

Fig. 9. Results of a randomized clinical trial comparing transfer for primary PCI with local fibrinolysis (DANAMI 2). (Adapted from Andersen HR, Nielsen TT, Rasmussen K for the DANAMI 2 Investigators. A comparison of coronary angioplasty with fibrinolytic therapy in acute myocardial infarction. N Engl J Med 2003;349:733–742.)

More recently, clinical trials have evaluated whether patients with STEMI should be transferred emergently to a site where PCI can be performed as compared with the administration of fibrinolytic therapy locally without transfer. A summary of DANAMI-2, PRAGUE-2, and Air PAMI trials reveals a benefit for catheter-based perfusion over on-site fibrinolytic therapy with respect to the combined endpoint of death, reinfarction, or stroke (Fig. 9). In all three transport trials, there is a similar rate of adverse events in the PCI group (8–8.5%) and in the fibrinolytic assigned patients (13.5–15%), demonstrating a 40 to 50% reduction of the combined endpoint. The aggregate data suggests that catheter-based reperfusion therapy reduces the composite outcome of death, reinfarction, and stroke. In addition the rate of ICH is virtually eliminated with primary PCI compared with thrombolysis.

Intracoronary Stenting

Intracoronary stents reduce the risk of early reocclusion and restenosis when used for elective PCI and have been investigated for the treatment of STEMI. In the first trial comparing stents to balloon angioplasty, 900 STEMI patients were randomly assigned to primary PTCA or implantation of a heparin-coated stent during primary PCI. Although there was no difference in death, reinfarction, or stroke, both reocclusion and restenosis occurred less frequently in the stent group at 6 mo. A recent trial showed a trend for decreased mortality rates at 6 mo for primary stenting versus primary balloon angioplasty with significant reductions in other major adverse events *(20)*.

More recently, stents coated with polymers that elute antiproliferative compounds have been introduced; these drug-eluting stents markedly lower rates of in-stent restenosis compared with traditional bare-metal stents in patients undergoing routine PCI. Although data on drug-eluting stents in the setting of primary PCI are limited, a recent observational study demonstrated an excellent safety profile and very low restenosis rates when these new stents were used in STEMI. It is highly likely that drug-eluting stents will become the standard of care when primary PCI is performed within a short time period.

GP IIb/IIIa Inhibitors as Adjuncts to Mechanical Reperfusion

GP IIb/IIIa inhibitors were originally shown to reduce the ischemic complications of urgent and elective PCI. As a result, these agents were evaluated in patients undergoing mechanical and pharmacologic reperfusion. The ADMIRAL trial recently demonstrated that abciximab therapy initiated before primary PCI with stenting improved outcomes in patients with STEMI *(21)*. In this 300-patient trial comparing primary PCI with and without abciximab pretreatment, the group receiving

Table 5
CADILLAC Outcomes at 6 Mo

	PTCA (n = 518)	PTCA + Abx (n = 528)	Stent (n = 512)	Stent + Abx (n = 524)	p value
Death	4.5%	2.5%	3.0%	4.2%	0.23
Recurrent MI	1.8%	2.7%	1.6%	2.2%	0.64
CVA	0.2%	0.2%	0.4%	0.4%	0.88
Target vessel revascularization	16.9%	14.8%	8.9%[a]	5.7%[a]	<0.001

[a]$p < 0.001$ vs either PTCA group.

abciximab had higher procedural success rates, reduced rates of reocclusion, better epicardial blood flow, and a markedly lower rate of clinical adverse events. The largest study of GP IIb/IIIa inhibitors during primary PCI was the CADILLAC study, which enrolled 2082 patients with STEMI. These patients were randomly assigned to primary percutaneous transluminal coronary angioplasty (PTCA) alone, primary PTCA plus abciximab, stenting alone, or stenting plus abciximab. Major adverse events occurred in 20% of patients in the primary PTCA group, 16.5% with primary PTCA plus abciximab, 11.5% with stenting alone, and 10.2% with stenting plus abciximab ($p < 0.001$) (20). As described previously, this study suggests primarily that stent implantation should be the preferred reperfusion strategy. In addition, the combination of abciximab and stenting leads to a modest but significant reduction in the need for repeat revascularization at 6 mo (Table 5). These studies support a consistent benefit when GP IIb/IIIa inhibitors are used for patients treated with mechanical reperfusion.

RESCUE PCI

Because failure of fibrinolytic therapy is associated with increased rates of morbidity and mortality, "rescue" PCI is frequently performed in such patients. Data to support rescue PCI in patients with persistent infarct artery occlusion are limited, but the totality of evidence supports rescue PCI in moderate or high-risk patients with an occluded IRA after fibrinolytic therapy. The relative benefits of rescue PCI have likely increased in recent years with the widespread utilization of intracoronary stenting and glycoprotein IIb/IIIa inhibitors.

Identifying candidates for rescue PCI remains a challenge, due to limitations of the noninvasive measures that determine either success or failure of reperfusion therapy. We recommend urgent catheterization and PCI for all patients with persistent ST elevation and ongoing chest pain 90 to 120 min after the administration of fibrinolytic therapy, unless they are at particularly low risk for complications. If chest pain has resolved but ST segments remain elevated, urgent catheterization should also be considered, particularly in high-risk patients such as those with older age, anterior infarction, or diabetes. Additional information may be obtained from evaluation of the early levels of cardiac markers, particularly myoglobin. A rapid rise in serum myoglobin (a ratio of myoglobin at 60 min/baseline >4.0) identifies patients who are highly likely to have a patent infarct artery. Urgent catheterization may not be needed in these patients even if persistent ST elevation is present.

ROUTINE IMMEDIATE PCI AFTER FIBRINOLYTIC THERAPY—"FACILITATED" PCI

While rescue PCI in patients with suspected failure of fibrinolysis is generally accepted, there has been considerable controversy as to the role of PCI after apparently successful fibrinolytic therapy. In the late 1980s, the ECSG, TAMI-1, and TIMI 2A investigators reported no benefit with respect to mortality, reinfarction, or vessel patency in patients randomized to an early invasive strategy (immediate catheterization and PTCA for suitable lesions) following administration of fibrinolytic therapy.

Since these trials were published, dramatic advances in interventional cardiology have taken place. Intracoronary stenting has significantly decreased the incidence of abrupt vessel closure after PTCA, the need for emergency coronary artery bypass surgery for failed PTCA, and the need

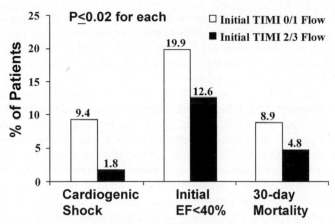

Fig. 10. Spontaneous reperfusion prior to primary PCI results in improved outcomes including less cardiogenic shock, better preservation of left ventricular function, and reduced mortality. (Adapted from Brodie BR, Stuckey TD, Hansen C, Muncy D. Benefit of coronary reperfusion before intervention on outcomes after primary angioplasty for acute myocardial infarction. Am J Cardiol 2000;85:13–18.)

for tar-get vessel reintervention due to restenosis. Glycoprotein IIb/IIIa inhibitors have further decreased complications following both elective and emergent procedures. In addition, the management of vascular access sites has changed in parallel. Today's sheaths are smaller and removed earlier after PCI; less heparin is used during procedures; and new percutaneous closure devices have been developed that can reduce local bleeding complications. These factors have combined to improve procedural efficacy and reduce complications, and have rekindled enthusiasm among interventional cardiologists to perform adjunctive PCI following fibrinolysis.

The term "facilitated" PCI has been coined to signify the administration of a pharmacologic reperfusion regimen en route to the cardiac catheterization laboratory for "primary" PCI. The rationale for facilitated PCI is as follows. First, it is well known that patients who arrive in the catheterization laboratory with a patent IRA prior to "primary" PCI, due either to spontaneous fibrinolysis or to pharmacologic reperfusion, have an extraordinarily low risk for mortality (Fig. 10). Second, it is clear that a range of agents, including fibrinolytics (in full or reduced dosages), GP IIb/IIIa inhibitors, or their combination, increase the probability of early reperfusion. Finally, it is known that after initial, successful fibrinolytic therapy, reocclusion and reinfarction are common, in contrast to primary PCI, which is associated with very low rates of reocclusion and reinfarction. Therefore, administration of a pharmacologic reperfusion regimen *prior* to primary PCI may increase the probability of reperfusion prior to PCI, minimizing myocardial necrosis and facilitating an excellent long-term result of PCI.

Results from the PACT trial support the safety of immediate PCI in the setting of fibrinolytic monotherapy *(22)*. In this study, patients were randomized to either reduced-dose tPA or to placebo and were then taken immediately to cardiac catheterization, where angioplasty was performed unless TIMI 3 flow was found. Patients receiving tPA prior to catheterization had higher initial rates of TIMI grade 3 flow than those receiving placebo (32.8% vs 14.8%); after PCI, TIMI flow grade was similar between the two groups, indicating that tPA administration did not adversely impact procedural outcomes. Most importantly, there were no significant differences in bleeding or recurrent ischemic complications, suggesting that angioplasty could be performed safely immediately after a reduced dose of tPA.

Other investigators have evaluated combination reperfusion regimens (reduced-dose lytics and GP IIb/IIIa inhibitors) prior to PCI. In a substudy of the TIMI 14 trial described above, early adjunctive PCI appeared to improve tissue perfusion (as reflected in greater resolution of ST elevation) after combination therapy, but not after fibrinolytic therapy alone, suggesting that abciximab may prevent distal embolization at the time of PCI in the platelet- and fibrin-rich milieu characteristic of AMI. The SPEED investigators have shown that this "facilitated" approach (combination reperfusion therapy followed by PCI 60–90 min later) was associated with very high TIMI 3 flow rates and improved clinical outcomes *(23)*. Patients treated with PCI after combination reperfusion therapy had significantly fewer episodes of recurrent MI and urgent revascularization without an increase in bleeding complications. It is important to acknowledge that the interventional strategy was not a randomized variable of the study. Selection bias, therefore, may explain part of the result.

A recent small randomized trial, the BRAVE study *(24)*, evaluated whether early administration of the combination of half-dose reteplase plus abciximab produced better results compared with abciximab alone in patients with acute MI referred for PCI. The primary outcome measure was assessment of the final infarct size according to a single-photon emission computed tomography perfusion imaging performed between 5 and 10 d after randomization in the 228 patients studied. As expected, patients who received combination therapy had higher coronary patency rates than those treated with abciximab alone (40% vs 18%, respectively) at the time of initial angiography. This angiographic advantage, however, did not translate into improved myocardial salvage as measured by nuclear scintigraphy. Moreover, bleeding rates were higher in the group receiving the combination of reteplase and abciximab prior to PCI. Other trials, including TIMI 14, GRAPE, TIGER PA, and RAPIER have shown have also suggested that GP IIb/IIIa inhibitors alone may be the best facilitation strategy prior to PCI. In each of these studies, administration of GP IIb/IIIa inhibitors in the emergency room resulted in significantly greater rates of TIMI grade 3 flow at the time of primary PCI.

Several large randomized trials are now under way evaluating a number of different strategies of facilitated PCI, including GP IIb/IIIa inhibitors alone, fibrinolytic monotherapy, and combination therapy with GP IIb/IIIa inhibitors and reduced-dose lytics. Until these trials have been completed, only GP IIb/IIIa inhibitors should be considered for facilitated PCI. GP IIb/IIIa inhibitors are safe (they do not increase ICH), they improve reperfusion rates prior to PCI, and they may prevent microvascular injury post-PCI. Moreover, data from the ADMIRAL study (discussed above), in which glycoprotein IIb/IIIa was started prior to PCI, support the role for this agent in facilitated PCI.

Long-Term Antithrombotic Therapy

ASPIRIN

In the setting of acute ST segment elevation MI, aspirin has been shown to decrease reocclusion after successful fibrinolysis by over 50%, reinfarction by nearly 50%, and mortality by 25% *(25)*. Aspirin should be given immediately on presentation (or preferably in the ambulance) in an oral dose of 160 to 325 mg daily. Following MI, aspirin also reduces subsequent cardiac events, a secondary prevention benefit that has now been observed to persist for up to 4 yr of follow-up. Low-dose aspirin, 75 to 81 mg, is now preferred as it is associated with lower rates of bleeding. Thus, aspirin has had a dramatic effect in reducing adverse clinical events and thus constitutes primary therapy for all acute coronary syndromes.

CLOPIDOGREL

Clopidogrel is a thienopyridine derivative that inhibits the binding of adenosine diphosphate (ADP) to its platelet receptor, blocking ADP-mediated platelet activation and aggregation. This agent has replaced its sister drug ticlopidine as an adjunctive agent following coronary stenting due to its more favorable safety and side effect profile. Recent studies have shown that a longer duration (1 yr) of treatment with clopidogrel following coronary stenting is associated with lower recurrent ischemic event rates than the standard one month regimen. Moreover, in patients with non-ST elevation acute coronary syndromes, the combination of clopidogrel and aspirin, administered for 3 to 12 mo, has been shown to reduce cardiac event rates vs therapy with aspirin alone *(26)*. Finally, among patients less than 75 yr of age who received fibrinolytic therapy and aspirin, the addition of clopidogrel prevents early reocclusion and reinfarction, as well as mortality, and should be considered as standard adjunctive therapy *(26a)*.

Table 6
Randomized Trial of β-Adrenergic Antagonists in AMI

Study	Agent	n	Duration	RR death (95% CI)	p value
During AMI					
ISIS-1	Atenolol	16,027	7 d	0.85 (0.73–0.99)	0.04
MIAMI	Metoprolol	5778	15 d	0.87 (0.67–1.08)	0.29
TIMI IIb	Metoprolol	1434	6 d	1.00	0.98
Therapy Started Post-AMI, LV Dysfunction					
Norwegian	Timolol	1884	33 mo	0.61 (0.46–0.80)	<0.001
BHAT	Propranolol	3837	25 mo	0.72 (0.64-0.80)	<0.005
CAPRICORN	Carvedilol	1959	1.3 yr	0.77 (0.60–0.98)	0.03

WARFARIN/ORAL ANTICOAGULATION

Results from a number of clinical trials suggest that warfarin monotherapy appears to be at least as effective as aspirin for secondary prevention post-MI. There are several circumstances in which the benefit or potential benefit with warfarin therapy exceeds that of aspirin. First, warfarin is superior to aspirin in preventing systemic emboli in patients with atrial fibrillation. In addition, warfarin has beneficial effects in reducing systemic emboli in patients post-MI with documented left ventricular dysfunction. Since there is a substantial risk of systemic embolization following a large anterior MI, even if thrombus is not visible on echocardiography, one should consider 3 to 6 mo of coumadin therapy in these patients if they are suitable candidates for anticoagulation. However, in patients who have undergone primary stenting and are maintained on aspirin and clopidogrel, we do not recommend the concomitant administration of warfarin unless thrombus is visualized on echocardiography.

Studies have also evaluated the combination of warfarin and aspirin post-MI. Neither fixed-dose warfarin nor low dose warfarin titrated to an international normalized ratio (INR) of ~1.5 appears to be superior to monotherapy with either agent alone, and the combination is associated with excess bleeding risk (27). More recently, several studies have shown benefit for the combination of low-dose aspirin and warfarin when the INR is maintained at a higher level consistently (28). However, these findings are of questionable significance in light of the results of the CURE trial, which has demonstrated similar benefits with a simpler regimen of aspirin and clopidogrel. Thus, warfarin plus low-dose aspirin may be a good choice in patients who have another indication for anticoagulation (such as atrial fibrillation or prosthetic valve) provided the bleeding risk is low and a warfarin clinic is available for very careful monitoring.

Antiischemic Therapy

β-BLOCKERS

β-Blockers exert their beneficial effect in acute MI by preventing catecholamine-mediated β_1 activation, leading to decreased contractility and heart rate, thereby improving the balance between oxygen supply and demand. These drugs also exert an antiarrhythmic effect, as evidenced by an increase in the threshold for ventricular fibrillation in animals and a reduction in complex ventricular arrhythmias in humans. β-Blockers may prevent plaque rupture by reducing the mechanical stresses imposed on the plaque. Finally, β-blockers appear to attenuate adverse remodeling post-MI and prevent the development of heart failure.

β-Blockers were among the first therapeutic interventions used to limit the size of an acute MI. Administration of a β-blocker very early following onset of acute MI decreases infarct size, recurrent MI, and mortality (Table 6). When β-blockers have been used in conjunction with thrombolytic therapy they provide incremental benefit, particularly if they can be administered early after the onset of infarct symptoms. Tabulation of the results from the available studies indicates a highly significant reduction of approx 30% in the incidence of sudden death and a nonsignificant reduction of only about 12% in the incidence of non-sudden death. The fact that β-blockers were particularly effective in reducing sudden death again suggests that they exert much of their early beneficial effect by reducing the frequency and severity of arrhythmias. In addition, β-blockers appear to significantly decrease the risk of cardiac rupture.

In addition to the early benefits of β-blockers, when given long-term, these agents significantly reduce the incidence of nonfatal reinfarction and also reduce long-term mortality (Table 6) *(29)*. The benefits from routine beta-blocker use seem to persist as long as the active agent is continued and appear to extend to most patient subgroups. The long-term mortality benefits of the β-blockers extend to most members of this class of agents. There does not seem to be a significant difference between agents with or without cardioselectivity. Considering the low cost of routine β-blocker use and its substantial benefit, such therapy has a very favorable cost-effectiveness ratio and represents one of the few "bargains" left in contemporary cardiology practice.

The Carvedilol Postinfarction Survival Control in Left Ventricular Dysfunction (CAPRICORN) trial examined the incremental effect of β-blockade (with carvedilol) in the post-MI setting over and above the effects of other established therapies, including ACE inhibitors. Over a 6-mo treatment period post-MI, the group treated with carvedilol had smaller LV volumes and improved LV ejection fraction and wall motion score index vs the placebo group. In addition, they also had a more favorable clinical course *(30)*. Thus, β-blockade appears to add favorable and independent effects on the post-MI remodeling process in the presence of ACE inhibition.

In summary, β-blockers remain a cornerstone of treatment for acute MI. Treatment should be initiated intravenously, especially if it can be administered within 12 h of symptom onset followed by continuous oral therapy. β-Blockers are consistently useful for secondary prevention following MI and should be maintained indefinitely.

NITRATES

The clinical effects of nitrates are mediated through several distinct mechanisms, including dilation of large coronary arteries and arterioles with redistribution of blood flow from epicardial to endocardial regions. Further, peripheral venodilation leads to an increase in venous capacitance and a substantial decrease in preload, thereby reducing myocardial oxygen demand. Finally, peripheral arterial dilation, typically of a modest degree, may decrease afterload. In addition, nitrates have been shown to relieve dynamic coronary constriction caused by vasospasm. Nitrates may also have an inhibitory effect on platelet aggregation, though the clinical significance of this finding is unclear.

More recent studies have investigated the use of nitrate therapy in the setting of routine use of thrombolytic therapy and aspirin. The GISSI-3 trial *(31)* randomly assigned 19,394 patients to a 24-h infusion of nitroglycerin (beginning within 24 h of onset of pain), followed by topical nitroglycerin (10 mg daily) for 6 wk (with patch removed at bedtime, allowing a 10-h nitrate-free interval to avoid tolerance), or placebo. There was a nonsignificant reduction in mortality at 6 wk in the group randomly assigned to nitrate therapy alone compared with the control group (6.5% vs 6.9%). The other large trial, ISIS-4 *(32)*, compared 28-d treatment of controlled-release oral isosorbide mononitrate with placebo control in 58,050 patients with suspected MI. Nitrate therapy was not associated with a reduction in 35-d mortality compared with the control group (7.34% vs 7.54%; $p =$ NS). In both GISSI-3 and ISIS-4, the power to detect potential beneficial effects of routine nitrate therapy was reduced by the extensive early use (greater than 50%) of off-protocol nitrates in patients in the control group.

A review of evidence from all pertinent randomized clinical trials does not support routine use of intermediate or long-term nitrate therapy in patients with uncomplicated acute MI. However, it is reasonable to use nitroglycerin for the first 24 to 48 h in patients with acute MI and recurrent ischemia, CHF, or hypertension. Intravenous administration is recommended in the early stage of acute MI because of its immediate onset of action, ease of titration, and the opportunity for prompt termination in the event of side effects.

CALCIUM-CHANNEL BLOCKERS

All of the currently available calcium-channel antagonists block the entry of calcium into cells via voltage-sensitive (L-type) calcium channels. In vascular smooth muscle cells, this causes coronary and peripheral vasodilation. In cardiac tissue, this blockade leads to depression of myocardial contractility, cardiac pacemaker function, and AV nodal conduction. The differences between the three classes of calcium-channel blockers relate to differences in their primary sites of actions.

Dihydropyridine calcium-channel antagonists can be viewed as almost pure vasodilators. They dilate resistance vessels in both the peripheral and coronary beds and improve coronary blood flow. However, this is countered by a reflex increase in heart rate, making the overall effect on oxygen demand unpredictable. This factor causes nifedipine to be potentially dangerous in the setting of acute MI. The addition of a β-blocker can block reflex tachycardia. Short-acting preparations of nifedipine appear to be responsible for most of the problems associated with this class of drugs, and short-acting nifedipine should not be used. Rapid hemodynamic fluctuations frequently occur, particularly in elderly patients with potentially serious adverse consequences. Sustained release preparations, on the other hand, appear to avoid these rapid hemodynamic changes and are safe when properly used. Amlodipine, a third-generation dihydropyridine agent, causes less reflex tachycardia than other dihydropyridines and usually has a neutral effect on heart rate. Dihydropyridines have been uniformly unsuccessful in reducing either mortality or the rate of reinfarction in multiple trials. Thus, while sustained-release dihydropyridine preparations remain useful for treating hypertension, they should be used in AMI only when other evidence-based medications such as β-blockers, ACE inhibitors, and angiotensin receptor blockers have been exhausted.

Verapamil and diltiazem can be considered together because their net pharmacologic effect is that of slowing the heart rate and, to some extent, reducing myocardial contractility and myocardial oxygen demand. Of the two agents, verapamil has greater negative inotropic and chronotropic effects. A recent pooled analysis indicated that verapamil and diltiazem had no effect on mortality following acute MI *(33)*. In patients with CHF or LV dysfunction, these agents have been associated with an *increase* in mortality. Although diltiazem and verapamil have been shown to reduce nonfatal MI, it must be noted that these studies compared diltiazem and verapamil with placebo and not with a β-blocker. Because β-blockers consistently reduce both mortality and reinfarction, they are recommended for all patients who can tolerate such medications. Verapamil or diltiazem may be a reasonable alternative for those patients who cannot tolerate a β-blocker provided they have no evidence of CHF and do not have severe LV dysfunction. It should be noted that many patients who cannot tolerate a β-blocker because of concern of excessive bradycardia or CHF may experience similar complications from diltiazem or verapamil.

ANTAGONISTS OF THE RENIN–ANGIOTENSIN–ALDOSTERONE SYSTEM

Inhibiting the renin–angiotensin–aldosterone system (RAAS) has proven to be one of the most fruitful therapeutic strategies in cardiovascular medicine. Many therapies that have proven beneficial in heart failure patients have also shown benefit in patients following MI. This is in part due to the fact that a large percentage of heart failure patients are survivors of MI and that many of the neurohormonal systems—including the RAAS—that are activated in heart failure are also activated following infarction. Additionally, the RAAS has been implicated in healing and remodeling following MI: angiotensin is directly involved in collagen synthesis and breakdown pathways and may mediate post-MI tissue repair.

ACE inhibitors have become a mainstay in the treatment of patients with acute MI because they prevent the deleterious left ventricular chamber remodeling and the progression of vascular pathology. LV remodeling is characterized by alterations in ventricular mass, chamber size, and shape, all of which result from myocardial injury, or pressure or volume overload. These processes, which occur in the noninfarcted myocardium, contribute to progressive LV remodeling and LV dysfunction. Substantial experimental and clinical data exist that support the pivotal role of the RAAS in contributing to these cellular processes.

Table 7
Randomized Trials of ACE Inhibitor Therapy Post-AMI

Study	Agent	n	Duration	RR death (95% CI)	p value
Therapy Started During Infarction					
ISIS-4	Captopril	58,050	35 d	0.93 (0.87–0.99)	0.02
GISSI-3	Lisinopril	19,394	42 d	0.88 (0.79–0.99)	0.03
CONSENSUS II	Enalaprilat	6090	41–180 d	1.11 (0.93–1.29)	0.26
Therapy Started Post-AMI, LV Dysfunction					
SAVE	Captopril	2231	42 mo	0.81 (0.68–0.97)	0.02
AIRE	Ramipril	2006	15 mo	0.73 (0.69–0.89)	0.002
TRACE	Trandolalapril	1749	24–50 mo	0.78 (0.70–0.86)	<0.001

An overview by the ACE Inhibitor Myocardial Infarction Collaborative Group, which included observations in almost 100,000 patients with acute MI treated within 36 h of the onset of chest pain, found a 7% reduction in 30-d mortality when ACE inhibitors were given to all patients with acute MI (Table 7). Most of the benefit was observed in the first week (34). The absolute benefit was particularly large in some high-risk groups such as those in Killip class II or III (23 lives saved per 1000 patients) and those with an anterior MI (11 lives saved per 1000 patients). ACE-inhibitor therapy also reduced the incidence of nonfatal CHF (14.6% vs 15.2%, $p = 0.01$), but was associated with an excess of persistent hypotension and renal dysfunction. In the overview >85% of the lives saved attributed to ACE inhibitor therapy occurred in the anterior MI subgroup, which represented 37% of the overall population.

Additional studies have suggested that ACE inhibitors may improve clinical outcomes by reducing LV remodeling and specifically LV enlargement. The effect of the ACE inhibitor on the remodeling process was initially examined in a subgroup of patients from the SAVE trial in whom serial quantitative evaluation of LV volumes demonstrated that treatment with captopril was associated with an attenuation of the process of LV enlargement. Subsequent analysis from the SAVE trial demonstrate that changes in LV area at 1 yr following MI were significantly related to long-term cardiovascular morbidity and mortality (Table 7). These data provide compelling evidence that the remodeling process itself, independent of drug effect, is associated with adverse natural history outcomes in patients with LV dysfunction. Those patients with more substantial post-MI LV dilation were at higher risk of death during follow-up.

Of note, ACE inhibitors may also protect against progression of atherosclerosis and the development of MI by their antiproliferative and antimigratory effects on smooth muscle cells, neutrophils, and mononuclear cells, by enhancing endogenous fibrinolysis, and by improving endothelial dysfunction. As seen initially in SAVE and now in HOPE and EUROPA, it is clear that patients with coronary disease who are treated with ACE inhibitors experience fewer MIs and episodes of unstable angina. As a result, ACE inhibitors are indicated to prevent recurrent ischemic events in patients with MI, an additional benefit to the antiremodeling effect described above. The benefits of ACE inhibition appear to be class specific, with little difference between agents (Table 7).

ACE inhibitors only partially block production of angiotensin II in the human heart because of the existence of ACE-independent pathways that convert angiontenins I to angiotensin II. This experimental finding led to the development of angiotensin-receptor antagonists that offer more complete protection against angiotensin II by directly blocking the angiotensin type I receptor. The Valsartan in Acute Myocardial Infarction (VALIANT) trial compared the effects of the angiotensin-receptor blocker valsartan, the ACE inhibitor captopril, and the combination of valsartan and captopril in 14,808 high-risk patients with clinical or radiologic evidence of heart failure, evidence of LV systolic dysfunction, or both after acute MI. During a median follow-up of 24.7 mo, mortality was 19.9% in the valsartan group, 19.5% in the captopril group, and 19.3% in the valsartan and captopril group *(35)*. The comparison of valsartan with captopril showed that these two agents were equivalent in terms of overall mortality and in terms of the rate of the composite end point of fatal and nonfatal cardiovascular events. The results of this study show that high-dose valsartan per day is as effective as a dose of captopril that has been shown to be superior to placebo in reducing morbidity and mortality among high-risk patients with acute myocardial infarction. On the other hand, more complete blockade of the renin-angiotensin system with the use of valsartan and captopril leads to an increase in the rate of adverse events without improving overall survival. Given the established benefits of ACE inhibitors post-MI and their low cost, we recommend that angiotensin receptor antagonists be reserved for those patients who are intolerant to ACE inhibitors.

The mineralocorticoid aldosterone is another component of the RAAS that may significantly contribute to the development of adverse ventricular remodeling in patients with LV systolic dysfunction. In addition, aldosterone may contribute to cardiac fibrosis post-MI. In the EPHESUS study, more than 6600 patients with AMI complicated by left ventricular dysfunction (left ventricular ejection fraction $\leq 40\%$) and signs of heart failure were randomized to the selective aldosterone inhibitor eplerenone or placebo in addition to standard therapy, which could include reperfusion, aspirin, statin, angiotensin-converting enzyme inhibitor (ACE-I)/angiotensin receptor blocker (ARB), and a β-blocker. Eplerenone, when administered at a dose of up to 50 mg daily between days 3 and 14 after infarction (mean 7.3 d), resulted in a 15% reduction in total mortality ($p = 0.008$) and a 17% reduction in cardiovascular mortality ($p = 0.005$), mainly due to a 21% reduction in sudden cardiac death ($p = 0.03$) *(36)*.

The results of EPHESUS suggest that aldosterone blockade will be an important addition to the current therapy of patients with acute myocardial infarction. Of the patients enrolled, 87% were already being treated with ACE inhibitors and 75% received β-blockers, indicating that the aldosterone inhibitor provided incremental benefit to optimal therapy. Further studies will be required to determine whether aldosterone blockade should be restricted to patients with early evidence of LV dysfunction or whether they should be used in a manner similar to ACE inhibitors and β-blockers in all patients with myocardial infarction, regardless of LVEF. Also, it remains to be determined whether a similar benefit would be expected with a less selective agent such as spironolactone.

IN-HOSPITAL MANAGEMENT FOLLOWING ACUTE MI

Risk Factor Modification

Correction of modifiable risk factors is essential for the treatment of patients following myocardial infarction. The benefits of aggressive risk factor modification are profound and are more dramatic than any of the expensive treatment strategies described in this chapter. Risk factor modification, including lipid-lowering therapy, is discussed in detail in Chapter 43.

Risk Stratification

Risk stratification in acute MI actually should begin the moment a patient arrives in the emergency room and should continue through hospital discharge and beyond. When the patient is first seen, historical, physical exam, ECG, and serum marker information are rapidly integrated both to arrive at a diagnosis and to estimate a patient's *a priori* risk for adverse outcome. For example, older age, female sex, presence of diabetes, and history of prior MI or CHF are all associated with increased risk. In addition, tachycardia or bradycardia, hypotension, and evidence of CHF are markers for increased risk that are easily obtained from a focused examination. The ECG provides incremental predictive power, in addition to distinguishing ST elevation from non-ST elevation MI. An anterior location of infarction (or an inferior infarction with RV extension or anterior ST depression), and greater ST deviation are associated with larger infarcts and increased risk. Finally, elevated serum markers at presentation, even in patients with known ST elevation, predict an increased risk for mortality. Scoring systems such as the TIMI Risk Score *(37)* for STEMI can be used to quantita-

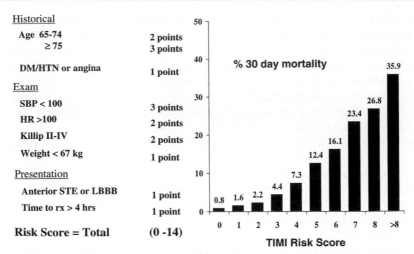

Historical

Age 65-74	2 points
≥ 75	3 points
DM/HTN or angina	1 point

Exam

SBP < 100	3 points
HR >100	2 points
Killip II-IV	2 points
Weight < 67 kg	1 point

Presentation

| Anterior STE or LBBB | 1 point |
| Time to rx > 4 hrs | 1 point |

Risk Score = Total   (0 -14)

Fig. 11. TIMI risk score and associated 30-d mortality for STEMI. (Adapted from Morrow DA, Antman EA, Charlesworth A, et al. TIMI risk score for ST-elevation myocardial infarction: a convenient, bedside, clinical score for risk assessment at presentation: An intravenous nPA for treatment of infarcting myocardium early II trial substudy. Circulation 2000;102:2031–2037.)

tively predict a patient's risk of adverse events following STEMI (Fig. 11). This scoring system has been validated in multiple different datasets.

After initial risk stratification is completed, subsequent risk-stratification steps should focus on identifying patients at risk for electrical, mechanical, and ischemic complications and to select those patients who will benefit most from particular therapies such as revascularization. It should be remembered that with many therapies, absolute risk reduction is highest in those patients at greatest risk; therefore, the higher the risk for an individual patient, the more aggressive the care should be.

Left Ventricular Function

Left ventricular function is the single most important determinant of long-term survival after myocardial infarction; for example, patients with significant left ventricular dysfunction (LVEF ≤40%) post-MI have a 5-yr mortality of >25%. In addition, patients with LV dysfunction and multivessel coronary artery disease derive significant benefit from surgical revascularization. Due to the importance of LV function to risk assessment, almost all patients should have an ejection fraction measurement following an acute MI. Since reversible LV dysfunction, termed myocardial stunning, may follow an ischemic insult, initial measurements may significantly underestimate true LV function. Therefore, unless clinically indicated because of congestive heart failure, suspected valvular heart disease, or pericardial effusion, measurement of ejection fraction can be deferred until approx 5 to 7 d post-MI. Although echocardiography, contrast ventriculography, and radionuclide angiography are all reliable methods for assessing LVEF, echocardiography has the advantage of providing structural information as well. Contrast ventriculography should be considered in patients in whom there is a strong suspicion for acute mitral regurgitation since transthoracic echocardiography may underestimate the amount of regurgitation.

Routine Coronary Angiography
and Revascularization Following Fibrinolytic Therapy

The potential role for immediate catheterization and PCI was discussed in the section on facilitated PCI above. The TIMI 2B trial evaluated a delayed invasive versus conservative (catheterization and PTCA for spontaneous or inducible ischemia only) strategy following t-PA administration. No differences in death or MI were seen between the two strategies through 3 yr of follow-up, despite the fact that revascularization rates were twice as high in the invasive arm. The current AHA/ACC guideline recommendation is to reserve cardiac catheterization after successful thrombolytic therapy to patients with spontaneous or inducible ischemia or those with significantly reduced left ventricular function (with "viable" myocardium). Of note, however, more recent observational studies have shown a lower rate of mortality in patients undergoing routine PCI after thrombolysis versus those managed conservatively *(17)*. Thus, it may be reasonable to perform catheterization in other high-risk patients who may benefit from revascularization, including those with prior MI and those with significant ventricular arrhythmias.

Conservative Management Strategies

As described above, a conservative diagnostic strategy is indicated for many patients after successful fibrinolysis for ST elevation MI. This strategy consists of noninvasive determination of left ventricular function and a modified exercise tolerance test (ETT) (with or without nuclear imaging) prior to discharge. Patients who complete a submaximum ETT without evidence of ischemia should subsequently have a symptom limited ETT 4 to 6 wk later before returning to full activity.

COMPLICATIONS OF ACUTE MI

Infarct Expansion and Remodeling

Following a large myocardial infarction, particularly if it involves the anterior wall and apex of the left ventricle, the infarct area may expand and cause thinning of the necrotic myocardium. Over weeks to months, the left ventricle may dilate and assume a more globular shape. This process, termed *left ventricular remodeling*, has been associated with an increased risk for the development of left ventricular dysfunction, heart failure, and death. Factors that have been found to affect remodeling favorably include ACE inhibitors, β-blockers (described above), and establishment of a patent infarct related artery. Indeed, one of the purported benefits of late reperfusion is improved tissue healing and the prevention of adverse left ventricular remodeling.

Recurrent Ischemia and Infarction

Following successful fibrinolysis, reocclusion of the infarct artery and subsequent reinfarction may occur in up to 10 to 15% of patients by hospital discharge and 30% of patients by 3 mo, a complication that is associated with a two- to threefold increase in mortality. As described above, fibrinolytic therapy itself may create a prothrombotic state that promotes reocclusion. Reocclusion rates after primary PCI are much lower, particularly if adjunctive stenting and GP IIb/IIIa inhibition are employed. Recurrent infarction may be difficult to diagnose, particularly if it occurs within the first 24 to 48 hr post-MI when cardiac enzymes remain elevated from the index event. Recurrent ST elevation, or a new "peak" in CKMB or myoglobin, is highly suggestive of MI. Recurrent ischemia without infarction is also a frequent complication post-MI. Since patients with postinfarction angina are at high risk for recurrent MI cardiac catheterization should be performed with a goal of target vessel revascularization.

Cardiogenic Shock

Cardiogenic shock is characterized by tissue hypoperfusion, hypotension, low cardiac output, and elevated filling pressures. When cardiogenic shock occurs post-MI, it is most commonly due to infarction of 40% or more of the left ventricle. In three large international series of patients with ST segment elevation myocardial infarction receiving thrombolytic therapy, the incidence of shock has ranged from 4.2 to 7.2% *(38)*. In the setting of an acute ischemic event, shock may occur in patients with either non-STEMI or STEMI, though it is about two times more common in the setting of transmural myocardial infarction.

Although shock typically results from a substantial amount of damage to the left ventricular myocardium, other etiologies must be considered. In the Should We Emergently Revascularize Occluded

Table 8
SHOCK Trial Results

	Revascularization	Medical therapy	p value
30-d mortality			
<75 yr	41%	57%	0.02
>75 yr	75%	53%	0.16
6-mo mortality			
<75 yr	45%	65%	0.002
>75 yr	79%	56%	0.09

Adapted from ref. *39*.

Coronaries for Cardiogenic Shock (SHOCK) registry *(39)*, predominant left ventricular failure was seen in 74.5% of patients. However, acute severe mitral regurgitation was seen in 8.3%, ventricular septal rupture in 4.6%, and right ventricular shock in 3.4%. Delineation of the specific etiology of shock has obvious importance for selecting an optimal treatment strategy.

Shock has been associated with a marked increase in mortality. Indeed, patients with shock account for the majority of all deaths related to acute infarction. As a result, intensive resources are both required and consumed in shock patients. Adjunctive therapy is important including vasopressor therapy, mechanical ventilatory support and intraaortic balloon pump counterpulsation (IABP). Though it is difficult to determine the independent effect of each of these interventions, IABP can stabilize some patients and may make revascularization safer. This approach, however, is underutilized in managing patients with shock. When an invasive approach with revascularization is considered, an IABP should usually be placed unless it is contraindicated such as in the presence of severe peripheral vascular disease or severe aortic regurgitation.

Revascularization for patients with cardiogenic shock has received considerable scrutiny. The SHOCK trial is the only completed randomized trial to evaluate an aggressive, invasive approach in managing patients with shock due to left ventricular failure. In this trial *(39)*, 152 patients were randomly assigned to emergency revascularization by either CABG or angioplasty and 150 patients were assigned to medical stabilization, which often included fibrinobolytic therapy. Intraaortic balloon counterpulsation was performed in 86% of the patients in both groups. The primary endpoint in this trial was 30-d mortality. The 30-d mortality rate in the invasive therapy arm was 46.7% compared with 56% in the conservative arm ($p = 0.11$). At 6 mo, however, mortality was significantly lower in the revascularization group: 50.3% compared with 63.1% in the medical therapy group ($p = 0.027$). Early revascularization benefits were seen only in patients younger than 75 yr (Table 8). The results of the SHOCK trial are relatively consistent with the other series in which revascularization is associated with improved outcome.

Despite successful revascularization, mortality in patients with cardiogenic shock remains very high. Therapies directed at improving hemodynamic parameters are under investigation in attempt to improve outcomes and make revascularization safer. Systemic hypothermia is being tested in the setting of acute MI without shock. Lowering core temperature to approx 33°C has been shown in experimental models to significantly improve myocardial salvage. In addition, therapy directed against inflammatory mediators such as inducible nitric oxide synthase (iNOS), which results in decreased production of nitric oxide, are under investigation. Experimental and preliminary clinical studies demonstrate improved survival when iNOS is absent or inhibited. SHOCK-2 (Should We Inhibit Nitric Oxide Synthase in Patients with Cardiogenic Shock?) is being designed to test an NO inhibitor, L-NMMA, among patients with persistent shock despite a patent IRA.

Right Ventricular MI

Right ventricular (RV) infarction is a frequent complication of inferior-wall MI (IMI) and is almost always caused by proximal occlusion of the right coronary artery. The diagnosis should

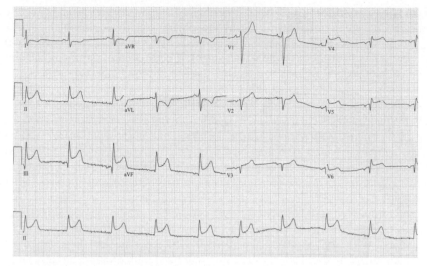

Fig. 12. ECG changes associated with right ventricular infarction. Note ST elevation in lead V4$_R$, a finding highly specific for RV infarction.

be suspected in patients with IMI and unsuspected hypotension, particularly when it occurs after small doses of nitrates. Patients will usually have jugular venous distention but will have clear lungs unless significant left ventricular infarction is present as well. A right-sided ECG should be standard in all patients with IMI because ST elevation of ≥0.1 mV in V$_4$R (Fig. 12) is sensitive and specific for the diagnosis of RV infarction. The hemodynamic profile is one of elevated right-sided filling pressures with reduced cardiac output, findings similar to those of pericardial tamponade. In patients without ECG evidence of RV infarction, therefore, echocardiography (or placement of a pulmonary artery [PA] catheter) is indicated to distinguish between the two diagnoses.

The hemodynamic derangements of RV infarction can be improved by expansion of intravascular volume with normal saline. Short-term morbidity and mortality are increased in patients with right ventricular MI compared with those with IMI alone. Several studies have suggested that primary PCI, rather than thrombolytic therapy, should be the preferred reperfusion method in these high-risk individuals. In patients who stabilize, the prognosis for full recovery of RV function is very good.

Free-Wall Rupture

Rupture of the free wall of the left ventricle is the most catastrophic mechanical complication of acute MI with a mortality rate in excess of 90%. The presentation is one of pericardial tamponade and hemodynamic collapse, often culminating in pulseless electrical activity. Survival is dependent on prompt recognition, emergent pericardiocentesis, and surgical repair.

The interaction of rupture and fibrinolytic therapy is complex. Although early fibrinolytic therapy lowers the risk for rupture, late fibrinolytic therapy, when given in the setting of a completed infarct with softened, necrotic tissue, may actually increase the incidence of rupture. In the fibrinolytic era, rupture appears to be occurring earlier after presentation. Although the most common time frame is 1 to 4 d post-MI, rupture may occur within the first 24 h. Rupture is associated with large transmural infarctions and is more common in the elderly, women, and patients *without* prior MI. Controversy exists about an association with glucocorticoids and nonsteroidal antiinflammatory drugs. The most common location of rupture is in the anterior and lateral distributions of the left anterior descending artery.

Incomplete free-wall rupture can lead to formation of a pseudoaneurysm. In this situation, the rupture site is sealed by hematoma and the pericardium itself. When the thrombus organizes, a pseudoaneurysm cavity is formed. The pseudoaneurysm is often quite large and typically remains filled with some degree of thrombus. In distinction to a true aneurysm, in which the wall is composed of myocardial tissue, a pseudoaneurysm communicates with the LV cavity via a narrow neck of myocardial tissue; the wall of the pseudoaneurysm is composed of thrombus and pericardium but no myocardial tissue. Early elective repair is indicated for all suitable patients.

Septal Rupture

Rupture of the intraventricular septum typically does not present in as catastrophic a manner as does free-wall rupture. Septal rupture causes an acute ventricular septal defect (VSD) with left-to-right flow across the lesion. The presentation is usually one of congestive heart failure that develops over hours to days (depending on the size of the defect) and is associated with a harsh holosystolic murmur, which may be difficult to distinguish from mitral regurgitation. Either Doppler echocardiography or insertion of a PA catheter can be used to confirm the diagnosis. A "step-up" in oxygen saturation seen at the level of the right ventricle is diagnostic of a VSD in this setting. Septal rupture is more common following anterior infarction where the apical regions of the septum are involved. With inferior infarction, the basal portions of the septum are involved, and the prognosis is somewhat worse. Patients should be stabilized with pressors, usually an IABP, and vasodilators (if tolerated) followed by surgical repair and revascularization.

Acute Mitral Regurgitation

Acute mitral regurgitation following AMI is caused by ischemic dysfunction or frank rupture of a papillary muscle. This complication is more common following inferior MI, since the postero-medial papillary muscle typically has a single blood supply from the right coronary artery, while the anterolateral papillary muscle has dual supply from the left anterior descending and circumflex arteries. As opposed to rupture, this complication may occur with relatively small but well localized, infarctions. As with septal rupture, a new holosystolic murmur is classically present in the setting of acute pulmonary edema, and even cardiogenic shock. As blood pressure falls, the murmur may disappear entirely. Doppler echocardiography is particularly helpful in distinguishing acute MR from septal rupture. Treatment for this complication requires initial stabilization, usually with an IABP, pressors, and vasodilators (if tolerated) followed by prompt surgical correction.

Ventricular Tachycardia and Ventricular Fibrillation
(see Chapters 16 and 17)

Ventricular tachycardia (VT) is common in patients during the first hours and days after myocardial infarction and does not appear to be associated with an increased risk for subsequent mortality if the arrhythmia is rapidly terminated. Ventricular tachycardia occurring after 24 to 48 h, however, is associated with a marked increase in mortality. *Monomorphic* VT is usually due to a reentrant focus around a scar, while *polymorphic* VT is more commonly a function of underlying ischemia, electrolyte abnormalities, or drug effects.

Ventricular fibrillation is felt to be the primary mechanism of arrhythmic sudden death. The incidence of primary ventricular fibrillation appears to have declined substantially in recent years. In patients with acute MI, the vast majority of the episodes of VF occur early (<4–12 h) after infarction. As with sustained VT, *late* VF occurs more frequently in patients with severe LV dysfunction or CHF, and is associated with a poor prognosis. Patients with VF or sustained VT associated with symptoms or hemodynamic compromise should be cardioverted emergently. Underlying metabolic and electrolyte abnormalities must be corrected, and ongoing ischemia should be addressed. Amiodarone is a particularly effective antiarrhythmic agent in the setting of acute MI and should be used to treat VF.

In patients with ventricular fibrillation or hemodynamically significant sustained ventricular tachycardia that takes place more than 48 h after STEMI, implantation of an implantable cardioverter defibrillator (ICD) is warranted when there appears to be no reversible cause of recurrent MI *(40)*.

Bradyarrhythmias (see *Chapters 16 and 17*)

Bradyarrhythmias are common in the setting of acute MI and may be due to either increased vagal tone or ischemia/infarction of conduction tissue. Sinus bradycardia is usually a result of stimulation of cardiac vagal receptors, which are located most prominently on the inferoposterior surface of the left ventricle. If the heart rate is extremely low (<40–50) or if hypotension is present, intravenous atropine should be given.

Mobitz Type I (Wenkebach) second-degree AV block is also very common in patients with inferior wall MI and may be a function of either ischemia or infarction of the AV node or increased vagal tone. The level of conduction block is usually within the AV node. As a result, the QRS complex is narrow and the risk for progression to complete heart block is minimal. Again, atropine can be used for patients with significant bradycardia, hypotension, or symptoms. Temporary pacing is rarely required unless there is hemodynamic or electrical instability. Mobitz Type II block is much less common than Mobitz Type I block in the setting of an inferior MI. As opposed to Mobitz Type I block, Mobitz type II block is more frequently associated with anterior MI, an infranodal lesion, and a wide QRS complex. Since Mobitz type II block can progress suddenly to complete heart block, a temporary pacemaker is indicated.

Although compete heart block may occur with either inferior or anterior MI, the implications differ considerably depending on the location of the infarct. With inferior MI, heart block often progresses from first-degree or Wenkebach to third-degree AV block. The level of block is usually within or above the level of the AV node, the escape rate is often stable, and the effect transient. Although temporary pacing is indicated for hemodynamic or electrical instability, a permanent pacemaker is rarely required. With anterior MI, complete heart block is usually a result of extensive infarction that involves the bundle branches. The escape rhythm is usually unstable and the AV block permanent. Mortality is extremely high, and permanent pacing is performed unless there are contraindications.

Supraventricular Arrhythmias (see *Chapters 16 and 17*)

Atrial fibrillation occurs in up to 15% of patients early after MI, with atrial flutter and paroxysmal supraventricular tachycardia occurring much less frequently. Ischemia itself is rarely a cause of atrial fibrillation except in rare cases of atrial infarction. Precipitants of atrial fibrillation post-MI include right or left ventricular failure and pericarditis. Although the arrhythmia itself is usually transient, it is a marker for increased morbidity and mortality. Management of supraventricular arrhythmias in the setting of acute MI is similar to management in other settings (*see* Chapter 16); however, in the setting of acute MI, the threshold for cardioversion should be lower and the urgency with which the ventricular response is controlled should be greater. Due to their beneficial effects in acute MI, β-blockers should be the first agents used to control rate. Diltiazem or verapamil are appropriate alternatives in patients without heart failure or significant LV dysfunction, and digoxin is indicated for patients with concomitant LV dysfunction. Of the antiarrhythmic agents available, amidarone is probably the safest in the peri-infarct setting.

Left Ventricular Aneurysm

A "true" left ventricular aneurysm is a discreet "outpouching" of a thinned, dyskinetic, myocardial segment. As opposed to a pseudoaneurysm, the wall of a true aneurysm contains cardiac and fibrous tissues, and the neck is broad-based. The most common site of aneurysm formation is the LV apex due to distal occlusion of a noncollateralized left anterior descending artery. As opposed to psuedoaneurysms, the risk of rupture is small. Aneurysms, however, are associated with increased morbidity and mortality. The dyskinetic aneurysmal segment may alter overall LV geometry and impair contractile performance. Additionally, thrombus frequently lines the thinned wall and may be a source for arterial embolus. Most importantly, the scarred aneurysmal tissue may be a source for malignant ventricular arrhythmias. Though rare, surgical aneurysmectomy is indicated to control malignant arrhythmias and to improve LV function. Anticoagulation with long-term warfarin therapy may be indicated to prevent the development of mural thrombus and embolization.

Left Ventricular Mural Thrombus

Left ventricular mural thrombus occurs in approx 40% of patients with transmural anterior MI. The incidence is lower in patients who receive thrombolytic and/or anticoagulant therapy. The risk for subsequent arterial embolization is ~10% and is higher in patients with mobile thrombus detected by echocardiography. Although echocardiography can detect mural thrombus in many cases, patients with large anterior MI remain at risk for systemic embolization even if no thrombus is seen. Heparin, followed by coumadin for 3 to 6 mo, is indicated as preventive therapy in patients who are candidates for long-term anticoagulation.

Pericarditis

Asymptomatic pericardial effusion occurs in as many as 25% of patients following transmural MI; these effusions are rarely associated with symptoms or hemodynamic compromise. Fibrinous pericarditis may also occur in the days to weeks following transmural infarction and may be confused with postinfarction angina or recurrent MI. The pain of pericarditis is usually pleuritic and positional and often radiates to the trapezius ridge. A pericardial friction rub may be present. Treatment should consist of aspirin, but nonsteroidal antiinflammatory agents should be avoided as they may inhibit healing of the infarct. If an effusion is seen on echocardiography in a patient with symptomatic pericarditis, anticoagulants should be held unless absolutely necessary. Dressler's syndrome is an immunologic phenomenon that is characterized by pericardial pain, generalized malaise, fever, elevated WBC, elevated erythrocyte sedimentation rate (ESR), and pericardial effusion. It occurs several weeks to several months post-MI and is felt to be immunologically mediated. Again, higher-dose aspirin should be used as primary therapy, avoiding steroids and nonsteroidal antiinflammatory drugs until the patient is at least 1 mo post-MI.

CONCLUSIONS

Dramatic advances have occurred in the management of ST elevation MI in recent years. The superiority of primary PCI over fibrinolytic therapy has been clearly demonstrated even in community hospitals. On the other hand, despite tremendous efforts, little progress has been made in the past 10 yr with pharmacologic reperfusion. Nevertheless, because most hospitals cannot offer high-quality primary PCI around the clock, pharmacologic reperfusion therapy remains the dominant mode of reperfusion therapy worldwide. Therefore, continued efforts are needed to improve reperfusion therapy for patients with STEMI. Advances have also occurred in medical therapy for patients with STEMI, including demonstration of the benefit of ACE inhibitors, beta-blockers, angiotensin receptor blockers, and aldosterone inhibitors.

REFERENCES

1. Diver DJ, Bier JD, Ferreira PE, et al. Clinical and arteriographic characterization of patients with unstable angina without critical coronary arterial narrowing (from the TIMI-IIIA Trial). Am J Cardiol 1994;74:531–537.
2. de Lemos JA, Morrow DA, Bentley JH, et al. The prognostic value of B-type natriuretic peptide in patients with acute coronary syndromes. N Engl J Med 2001;345:1014–1021.
3. Cannon CP, Braunwald E. GUSTO, TIMI and the case for rapid reperfusion. Acta Cardiol 1994;49:1–8.
4. de Lemos JA, Antman EM, Giugliano RP, et al. ST-segment resolution and infarct-related artery patency and flow after thrombolytic therapy. Thrombolysis in Myocardial Infarction (TIMI) 14 investigators. Am J Cardiol 2000;85: 299–304.
5. Ito H, Tomooka T, Sakai N, et al. Lack of myocardial perfusion immediately after successful thrombolysis. A predictor of poor recovery of left ventricular function in anterior myocardial infarction. Circulation 1992;85:1699–1705.
6. Indications for fibrinolytic therapy in suspected acute myocardial infarction: collaborative overview of early mortality and major morbidity results from all randomised trials of more than 1000 patients. Fibrinolytic Therapy Trialists' (FTT) Collaborative Group. Lancet 1994;343:311–322.
7. An international randomized trial comparing four thrombolytic strategies for acute myocardial infarction. The GUSTO investigators. N Engl J Med 1993;329:673–682.
8. A comparison of reteplase with alteplase for acute myocardial infarction. The Global Use of Strategies to Open Occluded Coronary Arteries (GUSTO III) Investigators. N Engl J Med 1997;337:1118–1123.

9. Single-bolus tenecteplase compared with front-loaded alteplase in acute myocardial infarction: the ASSENT-2 double-blind randomised trial. Assessment of the Safety and Efficacy of a New Thrombolytic Investigators. Lancet 1999;354:716–722.

10. Young JJ, Kereiakes DJ. Pharmacologic reperfusion strategies for the treatment of ST-segment elevation myocardial infarction. Rev Cardiovasc Med 2003;4:216–227.

11. Antman EM, Giugliano RP, Gibson CM, et al. Abciximab facilitates the rate and extent of thrombolysis: results of the thrombolysis in myocardial infarction (TIMI) 14 trial. The TIMI 14 Investigators. Circulation 1999;99:2720–2732.

12. Topol EJ. Reperfusion therapy for acute myocardial infarction with fibrinolytic therapy or combination reduced fibrinolytic therapy and platelet glycoprotein IIb/IIIa inhibition: the GUSTO V randomised trial. Lancet 2001;357:1905–1914.

13. Efficacy and safety of tenecteplase in combination with enoxaparin, abciximab, or unfractionated heparin: the ASSENT-3 randomised trial in acute myocardial infarction. Lancet 2001;358:605–613.

14. Wallentin L, Goldstein P, Armstrong PW, et al. Efficacy and safety of tenecteplase in combination with the low-molecular-weight heparin enoxaparin or unfractionated heparin in the prehospital setting: the Assessment of the Safety and Efficacy of a New Thrombolytic Regimen (ASSENT)-3 PLUS randomized trial in acute myocardial infarction. Circulation 2003;108:135–142.

15. A comparison of recombinant hirudin with heparin for the treatment of acute coronary syndromes. The Global Use of Strategies to Open Occluded Coronary Arteries (GUSTO) IIb investigators. N Engl J Med 1996;335:775–782.

16. White H. Thrombin-specific anticoagulation with bivalirudin versus heparin in patients receiving fibrinolytic therapy for acute myocardial infarction: the HERO-2 randomised trial. Lancet 2001;358:1855–1863.

17. Gibson CM, Karha J, Murphy SA, et al. Early and long-term clinical outcomes associated with reinfarction following fibrinolytic administration in the Thrombolysis in Myocardial Infarction trials. J Am Coll Cardiol 2003;42:7–16.

18. Keeley EC, Boura JA, Grines CL. Primary angioplasty versus intravenous thrombolytic therapy for acute myocardial infarction: a quantitative review of 23 randomised trials. Lancet 2003;361:13–20.

19. Aversano T, Aversano LT, Passamani E, et al. Thrombolytic therapy vs primary percutaneous coronary intervention for myocardial infarction in patients presenting to hospitals without on-site cardiac surgery: a randomized controlled trial. JAMA 2002;287:1943–1951.

20. Stone GW, Grines CL, Cox DA, et al. Comparison of angioplasty with stenting, with or without abciximab, in acute myocardial infarction. N Engl J Med 2002;346:957–966.

21. Montalescot G, Barragan P, Wittenberg O, et al. Platelet glycoprotein IIb/IIIa inhibition with coronary stenting for acute myocardial infarction. N Engl J Med 2001;344:1895–1903.

22. Ross AM, Coyne KS, Reiner JS, et al. A randomized trial comparing primary angioplasty with a strategy of short-acting thrombolysis and immediate planned rescue angioplasty in acute myocardial infarction: the PACT trial. PACT investigators. Plasminogen-activator Angioplasty Compatibility Trial. J Am Coll Cardiol 1999;34:1954–1962.

23. Herrmann HC, Moliterno DJ, Ohman EM, et al. Facilitation of early percutaneous coronary intervention after reteplase with or without abciximab in acute myocardial infarction: results from the SPEED (GUSTO-4 Pilot) Trial. J Am Coll Cardiol 2000;36:1489–1496.

24. Kastrati A, Mehilli J, Schlotterbeck K, et al. Early administration of reteplase plus abciximab vs abciximab alone in patients with acute myocardial infarction referred for percutaneous coronary intervention: a randomized controlled trial. JAMA 2004;291:947–954.

25. Roux S, Christeller S, Ludin E. Effects of aspirin on coronary reocclusion and recurrent ischemia after thrombolysis: a meta-analysis. J Am Coll Cardiol 1992;19:671–677.

26. Yusuf S, Zhao F, Mehta SR, et al. Effects of clopidogrel in addition to aspirin in patients with acute coronary syndromes without ST-segment elevation. N Engl J Med 2001;345:494–502.

26a. Sabatine MS, Cannon CP, Gibson CM, et al. Addition of clopidogrel to aspirin and fibrinolytic therapy for myocardial infarction with ST-segment elevation. N Engl J Med 2005;352:1179–1189.

27. Randomised double-blind trial of fixed low-dose warfarin with aspirin after myocardial infarction. Coumadin Aspirin Reinfarction Study (CARS) Investigators. Lancet 1997;350:389–396.

28. Hurlen M, Abdelnoor M, Smith P, et al. Warfarin, aspirin, or both after myocardial infarction. N Engl J Med 2002;347:969–974.

29. Borrello F, Beahan M, Klein L, Gheorghiade M. Reappraisal of beta-blocker therapy in the acute and chronic post-myocardial infarction period. Rev Cardiovasc Med 2003;4(Suppl 3):S13–S24.

30. Costalunga A, Gavazzi A. Effect of carvedilol on outcome after myocardial infarction in patients with left ventricular dysfunction: the CAPRICORN randomized trial. Ital Heart J 2001;2:1246–1247.

31. GISSI-3: effects of lisinopril and transdermal glyceryl trinitrate singly and together on 6-week mortality and ventricular function after acute myocardial infarction. Gruppo Italiano per lo Studio della Sopravvivenza nell'infarto Miocardico. Lancet 1994;343:1115–1122.

32. ISIS-4: a randomised factorial trial assessing early oral captopril, oral mononitrate, and intravenous magnesium sulphate in 58,050 patients with suspected acute myocardial infarction. ISIS-4 (Fourth International Study of Infarct Survival) Collaborative Group. Lancet 1995;345:669–685.

33. The effect of diltiazem on mortality and reinfarction after myocardial infarction. The Multicenter Diltiazem Postinfarction Trial Research Group. N Engl J Med 1988;319:385–392.

34. Indications for ACE inhibitors in the early treatment of acute myocardial infarction: systematic overview of individual data from 100,000 patients in randomized trials. ACE Inhibitor Myocardial Infarction Collaborative Group. Circulation 1998;97:2202–2212.

35. Pfeffer MA, McMurray JJ, Velazquez EJ, et al. Valsartan, captopril, or both in myocardial infarction complicated by heart failure, left ventricular dysfunction, or both. N Engl J Med 2003;349:1893–1906.

36. Pitt B, Remme W, Zannad F, et al. Eplerenone, a selective aldosterone blocker, in patients with left ventricular dysfunction after myocardial infarction. N Engl J Med 2003;348:1309–1321.

37. Morrow DA, Antman EM, Charlesworth A, et al. TIMI risk score for ST-elevation myocardial infarction: a convenient, bedside, clinical score for risk assessment at presentation: an intravenous nPA for treatment of infarcting myocardium early II trial substudy. Circulation 2000;102:2031–2037.

38. Holmes DR Jr. Cardiogenic shock: a lethal complication of acute myocardial infarction. Rev Cardiovasc Med 2003; 4:131–135.

39. Hochman JS, Sleeper LA, Webb JG, et al. Early revascularization in acute myocardial infarction complicated by cardiogenic shock. SHOCK Investigators. Should We Emergently Revascularize Occluded Coronaries for Cardiogenic Shock. N Engl J Med 1999;341:625–634.

40. Moss AJ, Zareba W, Hall WJ, et al. Prophylactic implantation of a defibrillator in patients with myocardial infarction and reduced ejection fraction. N Engl J Med 2002;346:877–883.

28   Cardiopulmonary Resuscitation

Joseph P. Ornato, MD

INTRODUCTION

Sudden cardiac death (SCD) due to unexpected cardiac arrest in adults claims the lives of an estimated 400,000 to 460,000 adult Americans each year *(1)*. Most episodes of unexpected SCD in adults occur in the home. The most common victim is a male who is 50 to 75 yr of age. The majority of SCD victims have underlying structural heart disease, usually in the form of coronary atherosclerosis and/or cardiomegaly. Although 75% of SCD victims have significant atherosclerotic narrowing (>75%) in one or more major coronary artery, fewer than half of all sudden deaths occur *during* an acute myocardial infarction (AMI).

SCD is usually caused by a chance arrhythmic event that is triggered by an interaction between structural heart abnormalities and transient, functional electrophysiological disturbances. In the majority of cases the initiating event is a ventricular tachyarrhythmia, either pulseless ventricular tachycardia (VT) that degenerates rapidly to ventricular fibrillation (VF) or "primary" VF *(2)*. The majority of neurologically intact survivors of sudden, unexpected cardiac arrest come from a subset of patients whose event is initiated by a ventricular tachyarrhythmia. In such cases, the single most important determinant of survival is the time interval from initiation of the cardiac arrest until defibrillation can be provided to terminate the ventricular tachyarrhythmia and restore a more normal rhythm accompanied by effective perfusion of vital organs.

PRINCIPLES OF RESUSCITATION

The American Heart Association (AHA) has introduced the "chain of survival" metaphor to represent the sequence of events that ideally should occur to maximize the odds of successful resuscitation from cardiac arrest in adults *(3)*. Fewer than 5% of all out-of-hospital cardiac arrest victims survive to leave the hospital with neurological functioning intact *(3)*. Survival from in-hospital cardiac arrest is not much better (averaging between 10 and 20%) *(4)*. There is substantial variability in the odds for survival among various geographic locations.

The outcome of resuscitation is influenced strongly by the patient's initial cardiac rhythm. The likelihood of survival is relatively high if the initial rhythm is VT or VF (particularly if the VF is "coarse," the arrest was witnessed, and prompt CPR and defibrillation are provided). The best outcomes from VT/VF in adults occur regularly in the electrophysiology laboratory, where prompt defibrillation (within 20–30 s) results in virtually 100% survival. The next best reported outcomes are in cardiac rehabilitation programs, where defibrillation occurs in 1 to 2 min, and survival is approx 85 to 90%. At Chicago's O'Hare and Midway airports, 61% of cardiac arrest patients whose initial rhythm was VF survived to hospital discharge *(5)*. Survival from out-of-hospital VT/VF treated by police officers equipped with automated external defibrillators (AEDs) in Rochester, MN has averaged 50% with a median time from collapse to defibrillation of about 5 min *(6)*. Outcomes in many locations with EMS systems that cannot provide defibrilation until 10 min or more

From: *Essential Cardiology: Principles and Practice, 2nd Ed.*
Edited by: C. Rosendorff © Humana Press Inc., Totowa, NJ

after patient collapse typically yield survival rates of <10%. Thus, survival from cardiac arrest due to ventricular tachyarrhythmias is highly dependent on the time interval from collapse to defibrillation. For every minute's delay from the patient's collapse to defibrillation the chance for survival diminishes by approx 7–10% *(3)*.

If the initial rhythm is not VT or VF, survival is typically <2–3% in most reported series. Asystolic patients whose cardiac arrest was unwitnessed rarely survive to hospital discharge neurologically intact, even when they are treated promptly with atropine, epinephrine, and/or an artificial pacemaker. The only common exceptions are witnessed cardiac arrest patients whose initial bradycardia or asystole (bradyasystole) is due to increased vagal tone or other relatively easily correctible factors (e.g., hypoxia of brief duration).

Pulseless electrical activity (PEA) is, by definition, the presence of an organized rhythm unaccompanied by a detectable pulse in an individual who is clinically in cardiac arrest. The latter part of the definition is important for exclusion of conditions in which the rescuer is unable to detect a pulse but there is unmistakable evidence that there is adequate blood pressure and cardiac output to maintain vital organ perfusion (e.g., a conscious patient with profound vasoconstriction due to hypothermia). The underlying physiological cause of PEA in most cases is a marked reduction in cardiac output that is due to either profound myocardial depression or mechanical factors that reduce venous return or otherwise impede the flow of blood through the cardiovascular system. Management of patients with PEA is directed at identifying and treating the underlying cause(s).

There are two fundamental goals in resuscitating an adult from cardiac arrest. First, a rhythm must be restored with a rate that is potentially capable of generating an adequate cardiac output and perfusion pressure. This may involve defibrillating a patient out of VF or speeding up a bradyasystolic rhythm with atropine or an artificial pacemaker. Once an acceptable rhythm has been restored, attention should be focused on optimizing cardiac output and perfusion pressure.

CPR

The technique and quality of CPR can affect critical organ perfusion pressure and blood flow dramatically. Maintenance of both the systolic and diastolic arterial pressure is even more vital for optimizing critical organ perfusion during CPR than in nonarrest conditions. Since flow to most vital organs (except the heart) occurs during the downstroke of closed chest compression (systole), a minimal systolic arterial pressure of 50 to 60 mmHg is usually required to resist arteriolar collapse. Diastolic pressure is particularly important during CPR because it is a critical determinant of the coronary perfusion pressure (CPP = aortic diastolic pressure – right atrial pressure). CPP is one of the best hemodynamic predictors of return of spontaneous circulation (ROSC) in both animal models and humans. A minimal threshold CPP gradient of approx 15 mmHg (usually corresponding to an aortic diastolic pressure of 30–40 mmHg) provides enough myocardial blood flow to meet minimum metabolic needs of the arrested myocardium and to achieve ROSC. Uninterrupted, or minimally interrupted, chest compressions appear to be helpful in maintaining an optimal CPP and improving ROSC in animal models and humans.

Understanding the mechanisms of blood flow during closed-chest CPR and real-time monitoring of hemodynamic parameters allows rescuers to modify chest compression techniques (the force of compression and the downstroke:upstroke ratio) when appropriate to optimize perfusion pressure and blood flow. It is now known that there are at least two major mechanisms of blood flow during closed-chest CPR: the "cardiac pump" and the "thoracic pump."

It was initially believed that blood flow during CPR was caused by direct compression of the heart between the sternum and the spine ("cardiac pump"). In the mid-1970s, the cardiac-pump theory began to be challenged by investigators who observed that increased intrathoracic pressure alone (without precordial compression) is capable of generating blood flow. A sudden increase in the intrathoracic pressure causes air trapping in the alveoli and small bronchioles during chest compression, creating a pressure gradient between the intrathoracic and extrathoracic cavities. In the thoracic-pump theory, the heart functions as a passive conduit. Pressurization of the thorax collapses veins at the thoracic inlet, preventing venous backflow. Forward flow occurs because the more muscular arteries remain open, particularly if epinephrine is administered.

Transesophageal echocardiography studies demonstrate that both mechanisms are operative during CPR *(7)*. Physiological studies in experimental models and humans suggest a strong, probably dominant, role for the thoracic pump during closed chest compression in adults. In addition, active decompression of the chest by application of negative pressure or suction to the sternum may further enhance cardiac output by improving venous inflow and/or by increasing the intrathoracic pressure difference between the upstroke and downstroke phase of chest compression (active compression-decompression CPR, also known as ACD-CPR). Unfortunately, ACD-CPR did not improve survival compared to standard CPR in a recent large, well-controlled, randomized clinical trial *(8)*. Other experimental techniques, such as interposing an abdominal compression between chest compressions (IAC-CPR) *(9)* or phased chest and abdominal compression *(10,11)* are designed to simulate the physiological effects of intraaortic balloon counterpulsation. Use of an inspiratory resistance valve in patients in cardiac arrest increases the efficiency of CPR and, when combined with other efficient forms of chest compression, can increase the diastolic arterial pressure to >50 mmHg *(12–15)*. It is not clear whether any of these techniques is clinically superior to well-performed standard CPR.

Chest compression delivers blood and oxygen to the myocardium, allowing a buildup of high-energy phosphates intracellularly. Interrupting chest compressions causes the coronary perfusion pressure and flow to fall precipitously, forcing cells to expend their high-energy phosphate reserves *(16)*. Even brief (i.e., 10–15 s) pauses or delays in performing chest compressions can decrease the probability of successful defibrillation and return of spontaneous circulation in animal models *(17)* and humans *(18)*.

CARDIOVASCULAR ASSESSMENT DURING RESUSCITATION

Echocardiography

Conventional transthoracic echocardiography is of value during CPR but is sometimes limited because it is difficult to image the heart when the chest wall is in motion. Transesophageal echocardiography provides high-resolution, real-time images during CPR and can be used to (1) better define the mechanism of blood flow during chest compression; (2) determine the presence of pericardial effusion, intracardiac tumor or clot, chamber enlargement or hypertrophy, severe volume depletion, pneumothorax, or thoracic aortic dissection; (3) better define the cause of PEA; (4) evaluate global and regional wall motion after ROSC; and (5) provide a visual guide for positioning intracardiac catheters and pacemaker wires.

Capnography

The percentage of carbon dioxide (CO_2) contained in the last few milliliters of gas exhaled from the lungs with each breath is termed the end-tidal carbon dioxide concentration ($P_{et}CO_2$). During normal respiration and circulation, the $P_{et}CO_2$ averages 4 to 5%. Two units of measure are popularly used in reporting the $P_{et}CO_2$: percentage and mmHg (1% is approx 7 mmHg). The $P_{et}CO_2$ can be used to confirm endotracheal (ET) tube airway placement, particularly in the noncardiac-arrest patient who has a pulse and an adequate blood pressure (where the sensitivity and specificity of the $P_{et}CO_2$ for detecting correct ET tube placement approach 100% and 90%, respectively) *(19)*. Ventilation through an ET tube that has been properly inserted in the trachea yields a $P_{et}CO_2$ of 4 to 5% in a patient with a normal cardiac output and no significant ventilation–perfusion gradient. Ventilation through an ET tube that has been inadvertently inserted into the esophagus results in a $P_{et}CO_2$ of <0.5%.

There is a logarithmic relationship between the $P_{et}CO_2$ and the cardiac output *(20)*. At normal or elevated levels of cardiac output, ventilation is the rate-limiting factor responsible for eliminating the large amount of CO_2 passing through the pulmonary circuit (e.g., hyperventilation lowers, and hypoventilation raises, the $P_{et}CO_2$). In this range, the $P_{et}CO_2$ closely approximates arterial CO_2 tension (P_aCO_2) and can be used as a "real-time" guide to the adequacy of ventilation. At low levels of cardiac output (below approx 50% of normal in animal models), ventilation has much less effect on the $P_{et}CO_2$. If ventilation is kept relatively constant in this range, an increase or a decrease in the cardiac output will usually be reflected by a rise or fall in the $P_{et}CO_2$, respectively. During CPR the $P_{et}CO_2$ is typically between one quarter and one third of normal, paralleling the low cardiac output and pulmonary blood flow (20,21). As CO_2 builds up in venous blood, hyperventilation cleanses the reduced quantity of venous blood traversing the lungs of CO_2, resulting in a low arterial (P_aCO_2) and a high central venous ($P_{cv}CO_2$) CO_2 concentration (a venoarterial CO_2 and pH gradient). Within seconds following ROSC, the improved cardiac output delivers large quantities of CO_2-rich venous blood to the lungs and the $P_{et}CO_2$ climbs suddenly to normal or above-normal levels (21–23). The dramatic change from a low to a high $P_{et}CO_2$ due to venous CO_2 washout is often the first clinical indicator that ROSC has occurred.

Monitoring the $P_{et}CO_2$ during CPR can be used as a guide to the patient's hemodynamic status. Inadequate chest compression is usually accompanied by a very low (i.e., <1%) $P_{et}CO_2$ that increases linearly with increasing sternal compression depth and force (24). Administration of sodium bicarbonate intravenously causes a transient rise in $P_{et}CO_2$ as the substance dissociates into water and CO_2. Disorders that cause significant ventilation–perfusion mismatch (e.g., pulmonary embolization), or decrease in production of CO_2 (e.g., hypothermia) are accompanied by a low $P_{et}CO_2$. The initial $P_{et}CO_2$ also has prognostic value. An end-tidal CO_2 level of ≤10 mmHg measured 20 min after the initiation of ACLS accurately predicts death in patients with cardiac arrest associated with electrical activity but no pulse. Cardiopulmonary resuscitation may be terminated in such patients (25).

ADVANCED AIRWAY MANAGEMENT

Endotracheal Intubation

One of the most important goals early in resuscitation is to establish a definitive airway that will allow delivery of oxygen in high concentrations, protect the airway from aspiration, and permit administration of aerosolized medications. Intubation of the trachea with an endotracheal (ET) tube serves all of these purposes and is generally considered to be the airway of choice during CPR. Medications that are commonly administered via the ET tube during resuscitation include epinephrine, lidocaine, atropine, and naloxone. Epinephrine should be given in higher dosages endotracheally (at least double the iv dosage).

Laryngeal Mask Airway and Combitube™ Airway

In the past several years, the laryngeal mask airway (LMA) has become a highly accepted alternative to endotracheal tube insertion for many elective operative procedures as well as for use during resuscitation. The device is easy to use, even in the hands of nurses and paramedics, and can generally be inserted much more quickly than an endotracheal tube. Insertion is performed blindly without the need for a laryngoscope. The Combitube airway is another suitable alternative that can permit minimally trained rescuers to ventilate adult cardiac arrest victims effectively.

Confirmation of Correct Airway Placement

The $P_{et}CO_2$ can be used to confirm whether an ET tube or LMA has been positioned in the trachea or the esophagus in the cardiac-arrest patient. If the $P_{et}CO_2$ during CPR is very low (below 0.5%) on at least the seventh breath following intubation, it is highly likely that inadvertent esophageal insertion of the ET tube has occurred. Conversely, a moderately low (above 0.5% but below 2.0%) $P_{et}CO_2$ does not necessarily indicate esophageal placement of the ET tube, as there are many other causes for this finding during CPR (Table 1). An alternative to the measurement of $P_{et}CO_2$ for confirmation of airway placement is the use of an aspiration syringe or bulb device. Such devices are attached to the ET tube immediately after it is inserted. Suction is applied to the

Table 1
Common Causes of Low (<2%) $P_{et}CO_2$ During CPR

Inadequate ventilation
    Unrecognized esophageal intubation
    Airway obstruction
Inadequate blood flow
    Inadequate chest compression
    Hypovolemia
    Tension pneumothorax
    Pericardial tamponade
Ventilation–perfusion mismatch
    Pulmonary embolism
Decreased metabolic production of carbon dioxide
    Hypothermia

ET tube using an aspiration syringe or bulb. If the tip of the ET tube is in the trachea, air is aspirated readily since the cartilage-containing trachea does not collapse. If the tip of the ET tube is in the esophagus, application of suction causes the esophagus to collapse. In such a case, there is resistance to the flow of air during aspiration.

USE OF VASOPRESSORS AND INOTROPIC AGENTS

Epinephrine

Epinephrine is the vasopressor of choice for use during CPR. It improves coronary and cerebral blood flow by increasing peripheral vasoconstriction. By enhancing coronary perfusion pressure, epinephrine facilitates the resynthesis of high-energy phosphates in myocardial mitochondria and enhances cellular viability and contractile force.

The optimal dose of epinephrine to augment aortic diastolic blood pressure in humans during CPR has been controversial. However, recent prospective, randomized clinical trials have not shown improved outcome with "high dose" (e.g., >1 mg in adults) compared to standard dose (0.5–1 mg) epinephrine *(26–29).* The AHA currently recommends an adult iv dose of 0.5 to 1.0 mg at intervals that do not exceed 3 to 5 min. The use of higher doses of epinephrine after the initial 1-mg dose during resuscitation is neither recommended nor discouraged. If the dose is given by peripheral injection, it should be followed by a 20-mL flush of iv fluid to ensure drug delivery into the central compartment.

During cardiac arrest epinephrine also may be administered by continuous iv infusion (add 30 mL of a 1:1000 solution to 250 mL of normal saline or D5W, infused at 100 mL/h and titrating to the desired hemodynamic endpoint). Continuous infusions of epinephrine should be administered centrally to reduce the risk of extravasation. Epinephrine should not be added to infusion bags or bottles that contain alkaline solutions.

Dopamine

Dopamine is less effective than epinephrine with respect to improving blood flow to vital organs during CPR. During resuscitation, treatment with dopamine is usually reserved for patients with hypotension and shock that occurs after return of spontaneous circulation. When used to treat shock, norepinephrine should be added if more than 20 µg/kg/min of dopamine is needed to maintain an adequate blood pressure.

Dobutamine

Dobutamine may be the ideal agent to use after ROSC, particularly if congestive heart failure rather than hypotension is present. In animal models, dobutamine that is initiated within 15 min of successful resuscitation can successfully overcome the global systolic and diastolic left ventricular dysfunction resulting from prolonged cardiac arrest and CPR *(30)*. At present, the AHA recommends giving 2.0 to 20 µg/kg/min of dobutamine (500 mg mixed in 250 mL of D5W or normal saline), using the smallest effective dose needed to improve hemodynamics. The maximum dose is 40 µg/kg/min.

Vasopressin

Vasopressin produces significantly higher coronary perfusion pressure and myocardial blood flow than epinephrine during closed-chest CPR in a pig model of ventricular fibrillation *(31)*. Both vasopressin and adrenocorticotropin concentrations are higher during CPR in patients in whom resuscitation is successful compared to those in whom it fails *(32)*. Because of these observations, there has been considerable interest in the use of vasopressin for supporting coronary perfusion pressure during CPR in humans.

In a small, blinded, randomized clinical study, 40 patients with out of hospital VF resistant to electrical defibrillation were treated with either epinephrine (1 mg iv; $n = 20$) or vasopressin (40 U iv; $n = 20$) during resuscitation *(33)*. Seven (35%) patients in the epinephrine group and 14 (70%) in the vasopressin group survived to hospital admission ($p = 0.06$). At 24 h, 4 (20%) epinephrine-treated patients and 12 (60%) vasopressin-treated patients were alive ($p = 0.02$). Three (15%) patients in the epinephrine group and eight (40%) in the vasopressin group survived to hospital discharge ($p = 0.16$). Neurological outcomes were similar in both groups.

Unfortunately, survival to hospital discharge did not differ for patients receiving either epinephrine or vasopressin during resuscitation in the emergency department, intensive care unit, or hospital inpatient units in a large, well-controlled, Canadian randomized clinical trial *(34)*. This finding has been explained by some to possibly represent the lack of difference between the two vasoconstrictors early in resuscitation. This leaves open the possibility that vasopressin might be superior to epinephrine later in resuscitation when adrenergic agents typically become less effective due to downregulation of receptors. Further study will be needed to determine whether vasopressin has advantages over epinephrine late in resuscitation. In addition, there is increasing evidence that the combination of vasopressin and epinephrine may be more effective than either alone *(35–37)*.

ACID-BASE MANAGEMENT

The marked fall in cardiac output during CPR reduces tissue oxygen delivery to critically low levels. Cells shift to anaerobic metabolism, causing a gradual building up of lactic acid. The PCO_2 level begins to increase inside cells, including heart muscle cells in which the concentration of CO_2 may reach very high levels (>400 mmHg), at which point PEA develops *(38)*.

There is a dynamic equilibrium between intracellular CO_2 and the blood traversing each capillary bed in the body. As CO_2 diffuses into capillary blood in exchange for oxygen, the CO_2 is transported to the heart and lungs in venous blood. Because of this, central (mixed) venous blood during closed chest compression is acidotic (pH approx 7.15) and hypercarbic (P_vCO_2 approx 74 mmHg). CO_2 is removed from the lungs during ventilation. During well-performed closed-chest compression, arterial blood pH is usually normal, slightly acidotic, or mildly alkalotic. Early in resuscitation, arterial blood can be slightly alkalotic while the venous blood is acidotic. Severe arterial acidosis early during closed chest compression is usually due to inadequate ventilation or other forms of acidosis (e.g., lactic acidosis). The best solution is usually to improve the technique of closed-chest compression and to increase ventilation, if possible. If severe acidosis is present despite confirmed proper endotracheal intubation, hyperventilation, and acceptably performed external chest compression, an alternate method for providing assisted circulation (e.g., open chest compressions or venoarterial bypass) should be considered.

In the past, administration of sodium bicarbonate was recommended for use early during closed-chest compression because of the belief that bicarbonate would buffer the H+ ion produced during anaerobic metabolism. However, sodium bicarbonate itself contains a large amount of CO_2 (260–280 mmHg). In plasma, the CO_2 is released and diffuses into cells more rapidly than HCO_3^-, causing a paradoxical rise in intracellular PCO_2 and a fall in intracellular pH. The increases in intracellular PCO_2 in heart muscle cells decrease cardiac contractility, cardiac output, and blood pressure. Sodium bicarbonate causes other potentially harmful effects, including paradoxical acidosis of cerebrospinal fluid, hyperosmolality, alkalemia, and sodium overload.

At present, there are no convincing data indicating that treatment with sodium bicarbonate is of benefit during closed-chest compression and it does not improve survival in experimental animals. The AHA no longer recommends routine administration of sodium bicarbonate during resuscitation because it provides minimal, if any, benefit and adds significant risk. If used at all, bicarbonate should not be given until proven interventions such as defibrillation, cardiac compression, support of ventilation including intubation, and pharmacological therapies such as epinephrine and antiarrhythmic agents have been employed. If used, the initial recommended dose of sodium bicarbonate is 1 mEq/kg. No more than half of the original dose should be given every 10 min thereafter. There are a small number of "special situations" in which sodium bicarbonate is indicated for use early and, in some cases, repeatedly during resuscitation. Such circumstances include severe hyperkalemia, known severe metabolic acidosis, and certain toxicological conditions (e.g., tricyclic antidepressant or barbiturate overdose). Alternate buffer agents do not appear to improve survival during cardiac resuscitation.

MANAGEMENT OF VENTRICULAR TACHYARRHYTHMIAS

Electrical countershock is the treatment of choice for VF and pulseless VT. If three initial countershocks at increasing energies (200, 200–300, and 360 J), intubation, epinephrine, and a fourth countershock (360 J) fail to terminate the arrhythmia (refractory VF or VT) or if, as in many cases, the arrhythmia rapidly recurs, antiarrhythmic drug therapy is usually recommended. Until recently, the agents most commonly used for this purpose included lidocaine, bretylium tosylate, procainamide, β-blockers, and magnesium sulfate. With one recent exception, there are no randomized, placebo-controlled clinical trials confirming whether these agents are any better than just repeating electrical countershocks, continuing CPR, and administering intermittent epinephrine.

Lidocaine Hydrochloride

For refractory VF and pulseless VT, the AHA guidelines suggest an initial lidocaine dosage of 1.5 mg/kg for all adult patients. After restoration of spontaneous circulation, lidocaine is continued as an iv infusion at a rate of 30 to 50 μg/kg/min (2–4 mg/min). The need for additional bolus doses of lidocaine is usually guided by clinical response and/or by plasma lidocaine concentrations. A recent European out-of-hospital cardiac arrest clinical trial showed no benefit from the use of lidocaine over placebo (which included repeated defibrillation attempts and epinephrine) for patients with recurrent and/or refractory VF (39).

Procainamide

Procainamide is a Type 1 antiarrhythmic agent with presynaptic ganglionic blocking, vasodilating, and modest negative inotropic properties. During resuscitation procainamide is usually given in a dosage of 1 gm administered at a rate of 20 to 30 mg/min, followed by a maintenance infusion of 1 to 4 mg/min. An alternative regimen that achieves therapeutic levels faster (in some patients in only 15 min) includes a loading dose of 17 mg/kg given over 1 h followed by a maintenance infusion of 2.8 mg/kg/h. In patients who might clear the agent slowly, the loading dose is reduced to 12 mg/kg and the infusion rate is reduced to 1.4 mg/kg/h. The rate of drug administration should be reduced or stopped temporarily if hypotension occurs or there is prolongation of the QT interval or QRS complex by 50% or more.

Other Antiarrhythmic Agents and Treatments

Other conventional antiarrhythmic agents that may be tried in patients with recurrent and/or refractory VT/VF include iv β-blockers or magnesium sulfate. Unfortunately, β-blockers have not been formally studied during cardiac arrest and recent randomized, placebo-controlled clinical trials have not shown benefit from IV magnesium sulfate *(40,41)*.

Recently there has been considerable interest in the use of iv amiodarone to treat patients with recurrent life-threatening ventricular arrhythmias. Studies on hospitalized patients have confirmed that this agent is active within minutes after iv administration. It is at least as effective as bretylium in terminating refractory and/or recurrent, life-threatening ventricular tachyarrhythmias but causes fewer side effects.

In a recent randomized, controlled clinical prehospital trial conducted on 504 cardiac arrest patients with recurrent and/or refractory ventricular tachyarrhythmias, the administration of a single 300-mg bolus of IV amiodarone at the time of the first IV epinephrine administration resulted in 26% greater survival to hospital admission compared to standard ACLS therapy *(42)*. The study was inadequately powered to answer the question of whether IV amiodarone increases survival to hospital discharge. Dorian et al. conducted a randomized, controlled, clinical trial in Toronto, Canada comparing IV amiodarone and lidocaine in 347 patients with out-of-hospital cardiac arrest. After treatment with amiodarone, 22.8% of 180 patients survived to hospital admission, as compared with 12.0% of 167 patients treated with lidocaine ($p = 0.009$; odds ratio, 2.17; 95% CI, 1.21–3.83).

Thus, as compared with lidocaine, amiodarone leads to substantially higher rates of survival to hospital admission in patients with shock-resistant out-of-hospital ventricular fibrillation. The principal side effects of iv amiodarone are hypotension and bradycardia, which usually respond readily to therapy (volume infusion and vasopressors; atropine and/or electrical pacing).

Other treatment strategies and troubleshooting checklists should be considered when the patient develops refractory or recurrent VT/VF. Underlying metabolic derangements, such as hypokalemia and/or hypomagnesemia, should be sought and corrected. Arterial hypoxemia and acidosis should be reversed or minimized by endotracheal intubation, ventilation with 100% oxygen, and proper CPR technique. Proarrhythmic drug effects, hypokalemia, and/or hypomagnesemia can induce ventricular arrhythmias such as torsade de pointes. Although magnesium sulfate can be tried, torsade de pointes is best managed with electrical pacing (or other forms of overdrive suppression such as with isoproterenol until pacing is available).

MANAGEMENT OF BRADYASYSTOLIC CARDIAC ARREST

Survival is poor regardless of therapy for cardiac arrest patients who present with bradyasystole. It is always important to exclude disconnection of a lead or monitor electrode prior to concluding that a "flat line" is the patient's rhythm, as some patients with such a tracing may have VF (a rhythm more amenable to treatment) masquerading as asystole. Whenever there is any doubt, the monitor lead should be switched quickly to another lead to confirm the diagnosis prior to treatment. Treatment with atropine sulfate may improve outcome in patients with bradyasystolic cardiac arrest that is due to excessive vagal stimulation, but atropine is less effective when asystole or pulseless idioventricular rhythms are the result of prolonged ischemia or mechanical injury in the myocardium.

For patients with bradyasystolic cardiac arrest, a 1-mg dose of atropine is administered iv and is repeated every 3 to 5 min if asystole persists. Three milligrams (0.04 mg/kg) given intravenously is a fully vagolytic dose in most adults patients. The administration of a total vagolytic dose of atropine should be reserved for patients with bradyasystolic cardiac arrest. Endotracheal atropine (1–2 mg diluted in 10 mL of sterile water or normal saline) produces a rapid onset of action similar to that observed with iv injection.

Pacing (transvenous, transthoracic, or transcutaneous) rarely influences survival in the unwitnessed cardiac arrest patient who is initially found with asystole or bradycardia without a pulse. However, pacing is extremely useful for bradycardic patients with a pulse and in selected patients in whom a pacemaker can be placed immediately after the development of the conduction disturbance. In such cases, a precordial thump can also stimulate ventricular complexes and a pulse ("fist pacing").

Endogenous adenosine released during myocardial hypoxia and ischemia relaxes vascular smooth muscle, decreases atrial and ventricular contractility, depresses pacemaker automaticity, and impairs AV conduction. The cellular electrophysiological effects of adenosine can be competitively antagonized by methylxanthines, but not by atropine. Aminophylline, a competitive nonspecific adenosine antagonist, has been shown to restore cardiac electrical activity within 30 s in 12 of 15 in-hospital, bradyasystolic cardiac arrest patients who were refractory to atropine and epinephrine *(43)*. Another small randomized clinical pilot study found that adenosine blockade may restore normal sinus rhythm in some bradyasystole patients who do not respond to conventional therapy *(44)*. Although further clinical research will be necessary to determine the potential value of adenosine blockade for bradyasystolic cardiac arrest, adenosine blockade should not be used when VF is present because use of this agent may make it more difficult to terminate this arrhythmia.

MANAGEMENT OF PULSELESS ELECTRICAL ACTIVITY

PEA is present when there is organized electrical activity on the electrocardiogram but no effective circulation, as manifest by a lack of a detectable pulse. There are many underlying potential causes, but the most common denominator may involve myocardial ischemia and dysfunction due to intramyocardial increases in CO_2. Prognosis is generally poor unless a discrete and treatable etiology for PEA can be discerned and corrected. Efforts should be directed toward detecting causes such as hypovolemia, hypoxemia, acidosis, tension pneumothorax, and pericardial tamponade.

REFERENCES

1. Centers for Disease Control and Prevention (CDC). State-specific mortality from sudden cardiac death—United States, 1999. MMWR 2002;51:123–126.
2. Bayes de Luna A, Coumel P, Leclercq JF. Ambulatory sudden cardiac death: mechanisms of production of fatal arrhythmia on the basis of data from 157 cases. Am Heart J 1989;117:151–159.
3. Cummins RO, Ornato JP, Thies WH, Pepe PE. Improving survival from sudden cardiac arrest: the "chain of survival" concept. A statement for health professionals from the Advanced Cardiac Life Support Subcommittee and the Emergency Cardiac Care Committee, American Heart Association. Circulation 1991;83:1832–1847.
4. Saklayen M, Liss H, Markert R. In-hospital cardiopulmonary resuscitation. Survival in 1 hospital and literature review. Medicine 1995;74:163–175.
5. Caffrey SL, Willoughby PJ, Pepe PE, Becker LB. Public use of automated external defibrillators. N Engl J Med 2002; 347:1242–1247.
6. White RD, Asplin BR, Bugliosi TF, Hankins DG. High discharge survival rate after out-of-hospital ventricular fibrillation with rapid defibrillation by police and paramedics. Ann Emerg Med 1996;28:480–485.
7. Porter TR, Ornato JP, Guard CS, et al. Transesophageal echocardiography to assess mitral valve function and flow during cardiopulmonary resuscitation. Am J Cardiol 1992;70:1056–1060.
8. Stiell IG, Hebert PC, Wells GA, et al. The Ontario trial of active compression-decompression cardiopulmonary resuscitation for in-hospital and prehospital cardiac arrest. JAMA 1996;275:1417–1423.
9. Sack JB, Kesselbrenner MB, Jarrad A. Interposed abdominal compression-cardiopulmonary resuscitation and resuscitation outcome during asystole and electromechanical dissociation Circulation 1992;86:1692–1700.
10. Halle AA, 3rd. Alternatives to conventional chest compression. New Horiz 1997;5:112–119.
11. Tang W, Weil MH, Schock RB, et al. Phased chest and abdominal compression-decompression. A new option for cardiopulmonary resuscitation. Circulation 1997;95:1335–1340.
12. Plaisance P, Lurie KG, Payen D. Inspiratory impedance during active compression-decompression cardiopulmonary resuscitation: a randomized evaluation in patients in cardiac arrest. Circulation 2000;101:989–994.
13. Voelckel WG, Lurie KG, Zielinski T, et al. The effects of positive end-expiratory pressure during active compression decompression cardiopulmonary resuscitation with the inspiratory threshold valve. Anesth Analg 2001;92: 967–974.
14. Lurie KG, Voelckel WG, Zielinski T, et al. Improving standard cardiopulmonary resuscitation with an inspiratory impedance threshold valve in a porcine model of cardiac arrest. Anesth Analg 2001;93:649–655.
15. Lurie K, Zielinski T, McKnite S, Sukhum P. Improving the efficiency of cardiopulmonary resuscitation with an inspiratory impedance threshold valve. Crit Care Med 2000;28(11 Suppl):N207–N209.
16. Kern KB, Hilwig RW, Berg RA, et al. Importance of continuous chest compressions during cardiopulmonary resuscitation: improved outcome during a simulated single lay-rescuer scenario. Circulation 2002;105:645–649.

17. Sato Y, Weil MH, Sun S, et al. Adverse effects of interrupting precordial compression during cardiopulmonary resuscitation. Crit Care Med 1997;25:733–736.
18. Eftestol T, Sunde K, Steen PA. Effects of interrupting precordial compressions on the calculated probability of defibrillation success during out-of-hospital cardiac arrest. Circulation 2002;105:2270–2273.
19. Ornato JP, Shipley JB, Racht EM, et al. Multicenter study of a portable, hand-size, colorimetric end-tidal carbon dioxide detection device. Ann Emerg Med 1992;21:518–523.
20. Ornato JP, Garnett AR, Glauser FL. Relationship between cardiac output and the end-tidal carbon dioxide tension. Ann Emerg Med 1990;19:1104–1106.
21. Garnett AR, Ornato JP, Gonzalez ER, Johnson EB. End-tidal carbon dioxide monitoring during cardiopulmonary resuscitation. JAMA1987;257:512–515.
22. Weil MH, Bisera J, Trevino RP, Rackow EC. Cardiac output and end-tidal carbon dioxide. Crit Care Med 1985;13: 907–909.
23. Falk JL, Rackow EC, Weil MH. End-tidal carbon dioxide concentration during cardiopulmonary resuscitation. N Engl J Med 1988;318:607–611.
24. Ornato JP, Levine RL, Young DS, et al. The effect of applied chest compression force on systemic arterial pressure and end-tidal carbon dioxide concentration during CPR in human beings. Ann Emerg Med 1989;18:732–737.
25. Levine RL, Wayne MA, Miller CC. End-tidal carbon dioxide and outcome of out-of-hospital cardiac arrest. N Engl J Med 1997;337:301–306.
26. Gueugniaud PY, Mols P, Goldstein P, et al. A comparison of repeated high doses and repeated standard doses of epinephrine for cardiac arrest outside the hospital. N Engl J Med 1998;339:1595–1601.
27. Callaham M, Madsen CD, Barton CW, et al. A randomized clinical trial of high-dose epinephrine and norepinephrine vs standard-dose epinephrine in prehospital cardiac arrest JAMA 1992;268:2667–2672.
28. Brown CG, Martin DR, Pepe PE, et al. A comparison of standard dose epinephrine and high dose epinephrine in cardiac arest outside the hospital. N Engl J Med 1992;327:1051–1055.
29. Stiell IG, Hebert PC, Weitzman BNea. A study of high-dose epinephrine in human CPR. N Engl J Med 1992;327: 1047–1050.
30. Kern KB, Hilwig RW, Berg RA, et al. Postresuscitation left ventricular systolic and diastolic dysfunction. Treatment with dobutamine. Circulation 1997;95:2610–2613.
31. Lindner KH, Prengel AW, Pfenninger EG, et al. Vasopressin improves vital organ blood flow during closed-chest cardiopulmonary resuscitation in pigs. Circulation 1995;91:215–221.
32. Lindner KH, Haak T, Keller A, et al. Release of endogenous vasopressors during and after cardiopulmonary resuscitation. Heart 1996;75:145–150.
33. Lindner KH, Dirks B, Strohmenger HU, et al. Randomised comparison of epinephrine and vasopressin in patients with out-of-hospital ventricular fibrillation. Lancet 1997;349:535–537.
34. Stiell IG, Hebert PC, Wells GA, et al. Vasopressin versus epinephrine for inhospital cardiac arrest: a randomised controlled trial. Lancet 2001;358:105–109.
35. Voelckel WG, Wenzel V, Lindner KH. Is one drug enough? Arginine vasopressin in pediatric cardiopulmonary resuscitation. Resuscitation 2002;52:157–158.
36. Voelckel WG, Lurie KG, McKnite S, et al. Effects of epinephrine and vasopressin in a piglet model of prolonged ventricular fibrillation and cardiopulmonary resuscitation. Crit Care Med 2002;30:957–962.
37. Lurie KG, Voelckel WG, Iskos DN, et al. Combination drug therapy with vasopressin, adrenaline (epinephrine) and nitroglycerin improves vital organ blood flow in a porcine model of ventricular fibrillation. Resuscitation 2002;54: 187–194.
38. Johnson BA, Weil MH, Tang W, et al. Mechanisms of myocardial hypercarbic acidosis during cardiac arrest. J Appl Physiol 1995;78:1579–1584.
39. Tunstall-Pedoe H, Woodward M, Chamberlain D. Lidocaine and bretylium in resistant ventricular fibrillation. Eur Heart J 2001;22:449.
40. Thel MC, Armstrong AL, McNulty SE, et al. Randomised trial of magnesium in in-hospital cardiac arrest. Duke Internal Medicine Housestaff. Lancet 1997;350:1272–1276.
41. Miller B, Craddock L, Hoffenberg S, et al. Pilot study of intravenous magnesium sulfate in refractory cardiac arrest: safety data and recommendations for future studies. Resuscitation 1995;30:3–14.
42. Kudenchuk PJ, Cobb LA, Copass MK, et al. Amiodarone for resuscitation after out-of-hospital cardiac arrest due to ventricular fibrillation. N Engl J Med 1999;341:871–878.
43. Viskin S, Belhassen B, Roth A, et al. Aminophylline for bradyasystolic cardiac arrest refractory to atropine and epinephrine. Ann Intern Med 1993;118:279–281.
44. Mader TJ, Gibson P. Adenosine receptor antagonism in refractory asystolic cardiac arrest: results of a human pilot study. Resuscitation 1997;35:3–7.

29 Rehabilitation After Acute MI

Fredric J. Pashkow, MD

INTRODUCTION

Cardiac rehabilitation as practiced today is a synthesis of exercise training, risk factor modification, psychosocial support, and education for the purpose of facilitating readaptation to normal life via improved functional performance and coronary heart disease risk factors.

Randomized studies performed mainly between 1975 and 1985 typically suggested a 20 to 30% reduction in cardiovascular mortality and sudden cardiac death, but generally failed to achieve individual statistical significance largely because of insufficient sample size (Table 1). Beyond traditional cardiac endpoints, improved quality of life and cost utility have also become important contemporary outcome goals.

Cardiac rehabilitation is rapidly changing with the dynamics of shortened length of hospital stays, a changing patient population, and the impact of large clinical trials of drugs that have an impact on the progression of the disease and that influence events. It is provided now via multiple models: institution- or center-based, community-based, or at-home. Studies suggest that patients stratified at low risk will benefit most by the modification of coronary risk factors and that patients previously thought to be poor candidates for rehabilitation (such as the elderly or those with significant left ventricular dysfunction and low work capacity) may experience substantial relative functional benefits.

Beyond exercise, the role of risk-factor modification in patients with known coronary artery disease (CAD) has become even more established. In addition to the reduction of future acute coronary events and the need for subsequent revascularization, newer data suggest the potential to arrest, and in some cases actually regress, coronary atherosclerosis.

CARDIAC REHABILITATION AS MODALITY OF THERAPY IN CURRENT TREATMENT OF CAD

Evolution of Cardiac Rehabilitation From Progressive Activity

Cardiac rehabilitation had its beginnings as a formalization of escalating physical activity after acute myocardial infarction (1). Up to the early 1950s, exercise following acute myocardial infarction was thought to be ill-advised and patients were prescribed extended periods of bed rest. Levine and others experimented with earlier activities such as chair sitting and progressive ambulating (2). By the late 1960s, 3 wk hospitalization after myocardial infarction was still routine in the United States. Research related to early mobilization burgeoned in the 1970s, particularly in the United Kingdom and in countries where the cost of hospitalization had already become a major social welfare issue. It evolved into structured exercise training before and/or after hospital discharge, but in the last decade it has matured into a multidisciplinary effort serving as a comprehensive preventive cardiac practice encompassing risk stratification, exercise training, secondary risk factor modification, and personal/vocational adjustment (3).

From: *Essential Cardiology: Principles and Practice, 2nd Ed.*
Edited by: C. Rosendorff © Humana Press Inc., Totowa, NJ

Table 1
Outcomes of Selected Prospective Cardiac Rehabilitation Trials

Study	Year	Subjects	Cardiovascular deaths				Nonfatal MIs		
			Follow-up (mo)	Treatment (%)	Control (%)	p	Treatment (%)	Control (%)	p
Kentala	1972	158	24	10.39	12.35	NS	7.79	4.94	NS
Wilhelmsen	1975	315	48	17.72	21.02	NS	15.82	17.83	NS
Palatsi	1976	380	29	4.20	5.80	NS	4.90	6.00	NS
Hakkila[a]	1977	350	23	10.40	12.30	NS			
Kallio[a]	1979	375	36	18.62	29.41	0.02	18.09	11.23	<.10
Shaw	1981	651	36	4.33	6.10	0.4	4.64	3.35	NS
Carson	1982	303	24	7.95	13.82	NS(1)	7.80	6.58	NS
Vermeulen	1983	98	60	4.26	9.80	NS	8.51	17.65	0.05
Rechnitzer	1983	733	48	3.96	3.67	NS	10.29	9.32	NS
Román	1983	193	108	13.98	24.00	NS(2)	9.68	8.00	NS(2)
WHO	1984	1360	36	11.91	13.44	NS	10.64	9.16	NS
Froelicher	1984	146	12	0.00	1.35	NS	1.39	2.70	NS
Marra	1985	167	55	5.95	4.82	NS	5.95	10.84	NS
Hedbäck[b]	1987	305	60	27.21	30.38	NS	17.30	33.30	0.02
Hämäläinen[a]	1989	375	120	35.10	47.10	0.02	25.60	19.30	NS
Hedbäck[b]	1993	305	120	36.70	48.10	<.001	28.60	39.90	<.001
Debusk	1994	585	12	3.80	3.10	NS			
Haskell	1994	300	48	1.38	1.94	NS	4.14	7.10	0.23

[a,b]Same study populations.
NS (1): significant for those with IWMI; $p < 0.01$.
NS (2): using life-table analysis; $p < 0.05$ using crude death rate.
Adapted from ref. 49.

The most recent trend is for cardiac rehabilitation programs to be combined or aligned with other programs, such as lipid clinics, that address management of risk factors or provide models of chronic disease management (4,5).

Physiology of Exercise Relevant to Conditioning in Patients With CAD

Peripheral adaptations, mainly consisting of more efficient oxygen extraction and utilization of oxygen by skeletal muscle, account for much of the improvement in functional capacity associated with exercise training. The reduction in activity-related symptoms experienced by many coronary disease patients who have received moderate-intensity exercise training is in large part a result of the diminished coronary blood supply required to meet the reduced myocardial oxygen demand required to perform a given amount of physical work. This is especially evident at submaximal workloads, below the anaerobic threshold. The anaerobic threshold is the highest oxygen uptake that can be maintained without an increase in lactate (6). It effectively delineates routine daily activities from athletic endeavors. Exercise results in a lowering of peripheral vascular resistance, heart rate, and intramyocardial wall tension during exercise, generally producing an improvement in exercise duration.

Exercise alone has not been studied in coronary angiographic regression trials. However, an intensive physical training program in association with a moderate diet intervention has been shown to favorably effect the progression of coronary atherosclerotic lesions and stress-induced myocardial ischemia in patients with stable angina pectoris (7). Furthermore, this same group has shown that the extent of improvement (progression, stabilization, regression) was associated with the weekly amount of physical exercise. Regression was seen only in patients exercising an average of 2200 kcal/wk, whereas angiographically determined slowing of coronary lesion progression was seen in patients averaging approx 1500 kcal/wk. The salutary effect of exercise training on peripheral vascular resistance, autonomic nervous system adaptations, blood coagulation, and platelet function will likely be linked to both the process of primary atherogenesis and to the role of plaque rupture leading to initiation of acute coronary events.

Consistent evidence that exercise stimulates development of coronary collateralization in humans has been lacking (8) but studies published in the mid- to late 1990s suggest that adaptations can occur that may improve coronary blood flow (9) and collateralization (10). Some studies suggest that regression is significantly related to a decrease in collateralization (11). Improvement in ventricular systolic function as a result of exercise training has been reported in elderly normals (12), but generally not in those with CAD (13).

Ejection fraction is a poor predictor of endurance functional capacity. This appears to be primarily related to the intrinsic capacity of the patient's heart rate to increase appropriately and, secondarily, the capability to improve stroke volume by changes in load or contractility. A patient with an extremely large heart and an adequate heart rate reserve (via a normal chronotropic response) may have adequate cardiac output to perform moderate endurance exercise despite a very low ejection fraction (14).

Components of Program Design

Cardiac rehabilitation programs have traditionally been designated by phases according to the temporal and functional status of the patient relative to an index coronary event. Although falling out of favor in some institutions, this designative system remains useful for classification purposes. Phase I rehabilitation is an inpatient therapy. The major goal for the physical activity portion of the Phase I program is to condition the patient for the exertional demands required after discharge. This has been a reasonably straightforward task since most activities of daily living in the home are below the 3 to 4 MET level (1 MET = **met**abolic oxygen requirement for resting conditions). However, shortening lengths of stay have reduced the time available for inpatient exercise training. The time available is not adequate to acquire the skills required for self-monitoring of exercise activity or for adequately achieving an understanding of the disease process. With patients often overwhelmed by the chaos of the acute coronary event, it is difficult to do more than begin the process of identifying risk factors and changing lifestyles. Thus, an appropriate trend in Phase I programs is to focus more on evaluation of risks and needs and motivate patients to participate in the appropriate outpatient (Phase II or III) rehabilitation program. Phase II programs are both ECG-monitored and supervised; Phase III programs are supervised only. Whether Phase II or III, current outpatient programs are generally center-based group experiences offering ECG monitoring, exercise supervision, education, and risk factor management. The exercise component occurs concurrently with education and psychosocial support for modification of coronary-prone behavior and for satisfactory return to a suitable and active lifestyle (15).

Using a multifactorial approach, all potential risk factors should be addressed (3). In patients of working age, there are usually vocational and job-specific issues as well (16). With an increasing emphasis on quality survival and economic valuation of the service (17), the major focus of many programs has gone well beyond the presumed impact of exercise training on mortality. Today, cardiac rehabilitation is being refashioned as a "soft technology" with great potential to influence outcomes including, but not limited to, long-term postinfarction survival. It is likely that in the future the emphasis will be on Phase III outpatient programs that can provide supervision and guidance to large numbers of patients in relatively low-cost, community-based (18) or at-home programs (19).

Risk Stratification

Cardiac rehabilitation has been the wellspring of several important concepts in contemporary cardiology, including progressive activity after MI, perceived exertion measurement, and risk stratification. The process of risk stratification has become an integral part of the management of patients during and after any acute myocardial event (20). Three factors determine the prognosis for any patient who has had a myocardial infarction: the amount of myocardium currently ischemic, the extent of LV dysfunction, and the patient's myocardial arrhythmic potential. The results of the risk

Table 2
Characteristics of Low-, Intermediate-, and High-Risk
Disease as Defined During Exercise Testing

Low-risk
 ≥8 METs 3 wk after cardiac event
 No symptoms
Intermediate-risk
 ≤8 METs 3 wk after cardiac event
 Angina with moderate or intense exercise
 History of congestive heart failure
High-risk
 ≤5 METs 3 wk after cardiac event
 Exercise-induced hypotension
 Ischemia induced at low levels of exercise
 Persistence of ischemia after exercise
 Sustained arrhythmia

METs, metabolic equivalents
Reprinted with permission from ref. 20.

stratification process thus serve as mileposts for patient management (Table 2). In addition, the results of risk stratification define the management of the patient throughout the rehabilitative process. The designations of low-, intermediate-, or high-risk are then applied for purposes of guidelines and standards used for program planning and operations, e.g., staffing and allocation of resources such as ECG telemetry and for reimbursement of program services (21,22).

IMPACT OF CARDIAC REHABILITATION ON SURVIVAL AND SUBSEQUENT MI

Trials of Exercise Alone or Exercise Plus Additional Interventions

Individual prospective studies performed mainly from the 1970s into the 1980s (Table 1) showed a trend toward reduced mortality in those participating after an acute myocardial infarction. Insufficient sample size, limited follow-up duration, and dropout rates as high as 50% resulted in insufficient statistical power for any single randomized trial of exercise training to prove its efficacy (23, 24). In 1988, Oldridge et al. published a meta-analysis of 10 randomized clinical trials that included 4347 patients that suggested a reduction in the incidence of overall and cardiovascular mortality of about 25% in those participating in exercise rehabilitation (23). Exercise training started between 8 and 36 wk postinfarction and duration varied between 6 and 48 mo. In these pooled data, there was a significant reduction in both all-cause and cardiovascular mortality with an odds ratio of 0.76 (95% confidence interval [CI] 0.63–0.92, $p = 0.004$). The reduction in mortality was more marked in those exercising for 52 wk or more and was only marginally significant among those exercising 12 to 52 wk. There was no statistically significant effect on mortality observed for those exercising 12 wk or less. This is especially noteworthy since most contemporary programs deliver (and are only maximally reimbursed for) 8 to 12 wk of program participation, with variable (and largely unknown) participation thereafter.

O'Connor et al. published a similar analysis the following year and came to a similar conclusion, namely, that cardiac rehabilitation reduced overall and cardiovascular mortality by 20%. They further noted that there was a 37% reduction in the incidence of sudden cardiac death (OR 0.63; 95% CI 0.41, 0.97) within the first year following exercise training. The odds ratios and 95% confidence intervals at 2 and 3 yr were 0.76 (0.54, 1.06) and 0.92 (0.69, 1.23), respectively, which suggest a benefit, but they are not statistically significant (24).

Other studies report that the incidence of sudden death is favorably influenced by exercise training. Exercise may contribute to improved electrical stability of the myocardium by virtue of a number of different mechanisms: decreased regional ischemia at submaximal exercise, decreased ambient catecholamines in myocardial substrate at rest and submaximal exercise, and increased ventricular fibrillation threshold due to reduction of cyclic AMP.

Other explanations for the impact on mortality have been postulated. An alteration of the balance between sympathetic and parasympathetic activity occurs in those undergoing endurance exercise training. This has been observed in the modification of heart rate variability observed by spectral analysis indicating an increase in vagal tone with physical training (25).

The increased surveillance present in the rehabilitation environment may in part explain the one-third reduction in the incidence of sudden death (18). The frequent regular contact with knowledgeable and experienced staff provides an opportunity for earlier discovery of potentially destabilizing factors such as decompensating ischemia or heart failure. The fact that patients do well when exercising under direct observation in the rehabilitation environment is further suggested by VanCamp and Peterson's 1986 survey that revealed only 3 deaths among 21 cardiac arrests occurring during more than 2 million patient-hours of exercise training (26). Thus cardiac rehabilitation may influence both the incidence of sudden death, as well as survival from sudden death.

Both the Oldrich and O'Connor meta-analyses failed to show any decrease in the prevention of nonfatal reinfarction following myocardial infarction with exercise-based cardiac rehabilitation programs. In addition to the possibility that this lack of effect is real, other factors may explain this observation, including inadequate attention to other risk factors, selection bias leading to lower participation in rehabilitation programs for patients with ongoing symptoms and risk of reinfarction, and finally, inadequate follow-up.

Modifications of Other Risk Factors for Coronary Artery Disease

Because of the manifold causes of coronary artery disease and the multidisciplinary interventions employed by contemporary cardiac rehabilitation programs, it is difficult to determine the benefits of individual interventions targeted to specific risk factors. Clearly, the trend toward a more aggressive secondary preventive approach has had an impact on both the design and, in all likelihood, the effects of cardiac rehabilitation programs. Several lines of evidence point to the benefits of the multifactorial approach. In addition to exercise, attention is appropriately directed to psychological factors; control of lipid abnormalities (Chapter 22), hypertension (Chapter 30), and diabetes, and smoking cessation (Chapters 22 and 41).

Advances in our understanding of the pathogenesis of acute coronary syndromes has led to an evolution of secondary preventive approaches that rationally combine multiple risk factor interventions targeted to an individual's unique combination of risk factors present. Understanding of patient-based lifestyle and behavioral factors relevant to modification of appropriate risk factors is ideally managed through the multidisciplinary individualized approach available in comprehensive postinfarct cardiac rehabilitation programs.

Psychological Stress and Depression, Their Impact on Cardiac Events and Survival, and Benefits of Exercise Training

The relationship between the heart and the brain has been the subject of speculation for ages, but an understanding of the details of this association and its impact on the prognosis and treatment of coronary artery disease is only relatively recent. A relationship between neural activity and ventricular fibrillation has been observed and the fact that psychological stress can predispose humans to sudden cardiac death has recently been documented (27).

The existence and association of certain specific personality characteristics with coronary artery disease has been controversial for many years since first being reported by Rosenman and Friedman (27a). The "Type A" personality profile includes such behavioral characteristics as aggressiveness/competitiveness, time urgency, and labile hostility. It has been linked to mortality from coronary artery disease as well as to the extent and progression of coronary atherosclerosis. However, studies over time have failed to consistently confirm this relationship and the current thought is that some element of the classical personality profile, such as anger/hostility, comprises the potentially destructive component *(28)*.

Depression is commonly present in the post-MI period *(29)*. Frasure-Smith et al. have shown that major depression following myocardial infarction has a significant *independent* impact on cardiac mortality over the first 6 mo following hospital discharge *(30)*. Depression was the most significant predictor of mortality (hazard ratio, 5.74; 95% CI, 4.61–6.87; $p = 0.0006$). The impact of depression remained significant even after control for left ventricular dysfunction and previous MI, which were also significant multivariate predictors of mortality (adjusted hazard ratio, 4.29; 95% CI, 3.14–5.44; $p = 0.013$).

Other manifestations of psychosocial dysfunction are important as well. These include social isolation and degree of life stress. Data also suggest that there is a lack of recognition and treatment of these serious comorbid psychosocial conditions.

Exercise has been popularly attributed to improve psychological well-being. Anecdotally, patients report significant subjective improvements in mood, anxiety, and self-confidence. The emphasis of studies relevant to this issue has generally been on specific alterations of psychological measures or personality such as positive self-concept and self-esteem. Neurophysiological improvements have also been observed. For example, in patients with ischemic heart disease, exercise training reduced plasma norepinephrine levels. The addition of psychosocial treatments to standard cardiac rehabilitation regimens reduces mortality and morbidity, psychological distress, and some biological risk factors *(31)*.

Thus, cardiac rehabilitation produces measurable worthwhile psychological effects in coronary heart disease patients and provides an alternative or adjunct for improving pathologic psychological conditions. Thus, it appears that affective and stress disorders are potentially important issues to be addressed in patients with coronary heart disease and the cardiac rehabilitation experience provides an excellent opportunity to address psychological issues.

OTHER GOALS AND ENDPOINTS
Quality of Life, an Alternative Endpoint

Quality of life has become an increasingly prominent issue in medicine and cardiology over the past decade *(32)*. Although interest has been focused on the impact of higher-cost modalities of therapy, such as coronary bypass surgery, on quality of life, many other approaches, regardless of their expense, will now increasingly be analyzed in the same way *(33)*. Cardiac rehabilitation is no exception, and as measures of quality of life become better understood and more standardized, these subjective outcomes will be more closely and appropriately scrutinized *(34)*.

Cardiac rehabilitation makes an important difference in perceived quality of life. Many participants enjoy and value their rehabilitation program, but measurable differences attributable to quality have been scarce *(35)*. In a study in which low-risk patients underwent a brief period of rehabilitation, little difference was observed between patients who participated in rehabilitation and those who received usual care *(36)*. Low-risk patients will likely recover normal performance of routine activities of daily living, regardless of whether they participate in an exercise rehabilitation program. Rehabilitation is less likely to affect their perception of quality of life.

However, the potential impact on quality of life is inherently greater the lower the functional capacity of the patient at the time of program entry. Assuming the absence of other major obstacles to exercise training, conditioning may result in sufficient capacity to perform most activities of daily living—for example, to maintain independence, assist an invalid spouse, or participate in most socially integrating activities (Fig. 1).

Reduction in Clinical Events as a Surrogate of Atherosclerotic Regression

During the past decade, there has been a heightened focus on secondary prevention of atherosclerotic coronary artery disease within the context of cardiac rehabilitation programs *(20)*. A number of clinically important studies using serial angiography have provided convincing evidence that

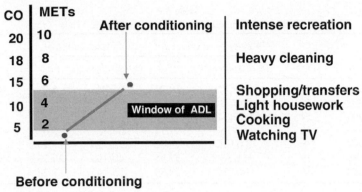

Fig. 1. The impact of exercise training on a hypothetical patient with restricted exercise tolerance at the time of entry. Note that the patient, who is essentially sedentary at the time of entry, can achieve a functional capacity that brackets the majority of activities of daily living by the completion of 8–12 wk of exercise training. CO, cardiac output; ADL, activities of daily living; METs, metabolic equivalents, where sitting at rest (1 MET) requires 3.5 mL O_2/kg/min.

a slowing of progression or actual regression of coronary atherosclerosis can occur with interventions *(37,38)*. Most studies have focused on strategies to improve serum lipids by the lowering of serum low-density lipoprotein cholesterol (LDL-C) and the raising of serum high-density lipoprotein cholesterol (HDL-C) through the use of drugs, diet, exercise, stress reduction, or in combination.

Ornish and colleagues published results from a prospective, randomized, controlled trial suggesting that comprehensive lifestyle changes can affect coronary atherosclerosis after only 1 yr *(38)*. Significant regression of atherosclerotic lesions following aggressive lipid-lowering treatment without lipid-lowering drugs has also been documented with angiographic studies by Schuler and associates *(7)*. They tested the appropriateness and effects of intensive physical exercise and low-fat diet on coronary morphology and myocardial perfusion in patients with coronary artery disease manifested as active angina. Following 12 mo of intensive physical exercise and low-fat, low-cholesterol diet (American Heart Association phase 3 diet), repeat coronary angiography showed relative and minimal diameter reductions using quantitative image processing. Stress-induced myocardial ischemia improved as well.

Haskell and associates found that intensive multiple risk factor reduction delivered via a nurse-managed, home-based model over an extended period (4 yr) can significantly reduce the rate of progression of atherosclerosis in the coronary arteries of men and women with coronary artery disease and decrease hospitalizations for clinical cardiac events *(39)*. In this study, a multifactorial risk reduction intervention analogous to a comprehensive long-term cardiac rehabilitation program plus cholesterol-lowering medication, when appropriate, resulted in highly significant improvements in several risk factors and a rate of narrowing of diseased coronary artery segments that was 47% less than that for subjects in the usual-care group. Perhaps more importantly, while an equal number of deaths (3) occurred in each group, there were 25 hospitalizations in the risk-reduction group compared with 44 in the usual-care group (rate ratio, 0.61; 95% CI, 0.4–0.9; p = .05).

While evidence of atherosclerotic regression by digital angiography has been the index piece of circumstantial evidence validating the concept of secondary risk factor reduction, the clinical benefit of the intervention (in terms of cardiac event reduction) tends to be of greater magnitude than expected from the angiographic improvement *(40)*. Perhaps this is due to a plaque-stabilizing effect of lipid-lowering therapy, with clinical events being prevented by interventions that, through a variety of potential mechanisms, render the atherosclerotic plaque less likely to become disrupted and, if destabilized, less likely to promote local thrombosis. Thus, multifactorial interventions that include cholesterol lowering with medication has resulted in a relative reduction of subsequent events of about 40 to 50% (Table 3).

Table 3
Outcomes of Selected Secondary Prevention Trials

Study	Year	Follow-up (mos)	CV events–experimental (# of subjects)	(%)	CV events–control (# of subjects)	(%)	Rate of change (%)	p
FATS	1990	30	10/52	19.23	05/94	5.32	−0.73	<0.05
STARS	1992	30	10/28	35.71	01/26	3.85	−0.80	<0.05
REGRESS	1992	24	93/434	21.43	59/450	13.11	−0.35	<0.002
PLAC	1993	36	13/76	17.11	05/75	6.67	−0.61	<0.04
MARS	1994	48	31/124	25.00	22/124	17.74	−0.32	N/S
MAAS	1994	48	51/88	57.95	40/193	20.73	−0.30	<0.05
SCRIP	1994	48	44/155	28.39	25/145	17.24	−0.40	<0.05

CHANGING DEMOGRAPHICS AND COMPLEXITY OF PATIENTS

Impact of Changing Patient Population

The patient population hospitalized for acute coronary syndromes is changing and, as a result, those referred for cardiac rehabilitation are changing as well. Patients are increasingly older, sicker, and more complex (1). These patients were formerly thought to pose increased risk and, because of compromise in their circulatory hemodynamics, to be poor candidates for the exercise portion of rehabilitation (41). Ironically, data suggest that formal exercise training may be of significant benefit to medically complex patients, including those with severe left ventricular dysfunction (42).

Exercise Training in Patients With Left Ventricular Dysfunction

Exercise intolerance in patients with significant LV dysfunction appears most consistently related to the early onset of anaerobic metabolism in peripheral muscle leading to the development of leg fatigue (41). This is thought to be due to both reduced muscle perfusion and reduced aerobic enzyme activity. In the majority of patients, it is not related to higher pulmonary capillary wedge pressures, or to increased pulmonary dead space and ventilation in relation to oxygen uptake. Despite the observation of inconsistent responses to exercise, there are theoretical as well as demonstrated benefits of exercise in heart failure patients. Patients with severe LV dysfunction can condition safely by gradually raising their heart rates above resting level. With time, they are able to extract more oxygen from the blood during exercise, thus widening the arterial–venous oxygen difference.

For a person who is severely limited, in distinction to the low-risk patient, even modest improvement is likely to have a noticeable impact on functional capacity (43). In a randomized, controlled, single-blind trial comparing 3 mo of supervised training, then 9 mo of home-based training with usual care, exercise training improved peak oxygen uptake and strength during the supervised training. Over the final 9 mo of the study, there was little further improvement, suggesting that some supervision is required for these patients (44). It is ironic that patients with severely reduced exercise tolerance were formerly excluded from exercise rehabilitation on the assumption that they would derive little tangible benefit. Similar reasoning applies to both the elderly and other subsets of patients who, with small increments in exercise capacity, have the capability of maintaining independence and provision of self-care. Four to five METs, a work capacity achievable by even some of the very elderly (45), is adequate to perform most activities of daily living, such as light housework, shopping, and other domestic functions (Fig. 1).

Gender Issues Relevant to Cardiac Rehabilitation

Women derive comparable benefits from cardiac rehabilitation, but unfortunately, in part because they are usually older and have other concomitant problems, they are not referred as often (46). There are also more obstacles for them to participate. Among these, physician referral appears to be the greatest obstacle. Compared to men, women appear to utilize cardiac rehabilitation programs less frequently than men, have higher dropout rates, and return to work less frequently and after a longer period of time. However, women completing cardiac rehabilitation can be expected to have similar improvement in risk factors and functional capacity compared with men *(47)*. While the risk factors for coronary disease, other than estrogen, are the same for women as for men, the frequency and relative impact of the risk factors differ *(48)*. These findings have very important implications for the design of rehabilitation programs.

SUMMARY

Cardiac rehabilitation has evolved from progressive ambulation after myocardial infarction into a multifactorial therapy of exercise training, psychosocial support, and education with the twin primary goals of returning patients to normalcy following heart attack, and reducing the chances of subsequent coronary events thereafter. This process especially appears to succeed in patients who are severely deconditioned at the time of program entry. Furthermore, survival itself is likely improved largely via a decrease in the incidence of sudden cardiac death, but the potential impact of this is hard to assess given the reduction in mortality associated with multiple other post-MI interventions. Improved quality of life and cost utility have also become important contemporary outcomes. Finally, the potential impact of risk factor modification on the fundamental pathologic process of coronary atherosclerosis, thereby reducing subsequent coronary events, may be the most exciting and important outcome of cardiac rehabilitation and the one with the most important potential.

REFERENCES

1. Pashkow FJ. Issues in contemporary cardiac rehabilitation: a historical perspective. J Am Coll Cardiol 1993;21: 822–834.
2. Levine S, Lown B. "Armchair" treatment of acute coronary thrombosis. JAMA 1952;148:1365–1369.
3. Wenger NK, Froelicher ES, Smith LK, et al. Cardiac Rehabilitation as Secondary Prevention. Department of Health and Human Services, Public Health Service, Agency for Health Care Policy and Research and National Heart, Lung, and Blood Institute, Publication No. 96-0672, October, 1995.
4. Williams MA, Fleg JL, Ades PA, et al. Secondary prevention of coronary heart disease in the elderly (with emphasis on patients > or = 75 years of age): an American Heart Association scientific statement from the Council on Clinical Cardiology Subcommittee on Exercise, Cardiac Rehabilitation, and Prevention. Circulation 2002;105:1735–1743.
5. Fonarow GC, Gawlinski A, Moughrabi S, Tillisch JH. Improved treatment of coronary heart disease by implementation of a Cardiac Hospitalization Atherosclerosis Management Program (CHAMP). Am J Cardiol 2001;87:819–822.
6. Wasserman K, Koike A. Is the anaerobic threshold truly anaerobic? Chest 1992;101:211S–218S.
7. Schuler G, Hambrecht R, Schlierf G, et al. Regular physical exercise and low-fat diet. Effects on progression of coronary artery disease. Circulation 1992;86:1–11.
8. Franklin BA. Exercise training and coronary collateral circulation. Med Sci Sports Exerc 1991;23:648–653.
9. McKirnan MD, Bloor CM. Clinical significance of coronary vascular adaptations to exercise training. Med Sci Sports Exerc 1994;26:1262–1268.
10. Senti S, Fleisch M, Billinger M, et al. Long-term physical exercise and quantitatively assessed human coronary collateral circulation. J Am Coll Cardiol 1998;32:49–56.
11. Niebauer J, Hambrecht R, Marburger C, et al. Impact of intensive physical exercise and low-fat diet on collateral vessel formation in stable angina pectoris and angiographically confirmed coronary artery disease. Am J Cardiol 1995;76:771–775.
12. Ehsani AA, Ogawa T, Miller TR, et al. Exercise training improves left ventricular systolic function in older men. Circulation 1991;83:96–103.
13. Jette M, Heller R, Landry F, Blumchen G. Randomized 4-week exercise program in patients with impaired left ventricular function [see comments]. Circulation 1991;84:1561–1567.
14. Litchfield RL, Kerber RE, Benge JW, et al. Normal exercise capacity in patients with severe left ventricular dysfunction: compensatory mechanisms. Circulation 1982;66:129–134.
15. Fletcher GF. Rehabilitative exercise for the cardiac patient. Early phase. Cardiol Clin 1993;11:267–275.
16. Dafoe W, Frabklin B, Cupper L. Vocational issues: maximizing the patient's potential for return to work. In: Pashkow F, Dafoe W, eds. Clinical Cardiac Rehabilitation: A Cardiologist's Guide, 2nd ed. Williams & Wilkins, Baltimore, 1999, pp. 304–323.
17. Oldridge N, Furlong W, Feeny D, et al. Economic evaluation of cardiac rehabilitation soon after acute myocardial infarction. Am J Cardiol 1993;72:154–161.

18. Pashkow FJ, Pashkow PS, Schafer MN. Successful Cardiac Rehabilitation: The Complete Guide for Building Cardiac Rehab Programs, 1st ed. The HeartWatchers Press, Loveland, CO, 1988.
19. Ades P, Pashkow F, Fletcher G, et al. A controlled trial of cardiac rehabilitation in the home setting: Improving accessibility. J Am Coll Cardiol 1996;27(Suppl A):150A.
20. Pashkow F, Dafoe W. Cardiac rehabilitation as a model of integrated cardiovascular care. In: Pashkow F, Dafoe W, eds. Clinical Cardiac Rehabilitation: A Cardiologist's Guide, 2nd ed. Williams & Wilkins, Baltimore, 1999, pp. 3–25.
21. American Association of Cardiovascular and Pulmonary Rehabilitation. Guidelines for Cardiac Rehabilitation Programs, 2nd ed. Human Kinetics Books, Champaign, IL, 1995.
22. Ryan TJ, Anderson JL, Antman EM, et al. ACC/AHA guidelines for the management of patients with acute myocardial infarction: executive summary. A report of the American College of Cardiology/American Heart Association Task Force on Practice Guidelines (Committee on Management of Acute Myocardial Infarction). Circulation 1996;94:2341–2350.
23. Oldridge NB, Guyatt GH, Fischer ME, Rimm AA. Cardiac rehabilitation after myocardial infarction. Combined experience of randomized clinical trials. JAMA 1988;260:945–950.
24. O'Connor GT, Buring JE, Yusuf S, et al. An overview of randomized trials of rehabilitation with exercise after myocardial infarction. Circulation 1989;80:234–244.
25. Seals DR, Chase PB. Influence of physical training on heart rate variability and baroreflex circulatory control. J Appl Physiol 1989;66:1886–1895.
26. VanCamp S, Peterson R. Cardiovascular complications of outpatient cardiac rehabilitation programs. JAMA 1986; 256:1160–1163.
27. Leor J, Poole WK, Kloner RA. Sudden cardiac death triggered by an earthquake. N Engl J Med 1996;334:413–419.
27a. Friedman M, Rosenman RH. Type A behavior pattern: its association with coronary heart disease. Ann Clin Res 1971;3:300–312.
28. Mittleman MA, Maclure M, Sherwood JB, et al. Triggering of acute myocardial infarction onset by episodes of anger. Determinants of Myocardial Infarction Onset Study Investigators. Circulation 1995;92:1720–1725.
29. Kavanagh T, Shephard RJ, Tuck JA. Depression after myocardial infarction. Can Med Assoc J 1975;113:23–27.
30. Frasure-Smith N, Lesperance F, Talajic M. Depression following myocardial infarction. Impact on 6-month survival [see comments]. JAMA 1993;270:1819–1825.
31. Linden W, Stossel C, Maurice J. Psychosocial interventions for patients with coronary artery disease: a meta-analysis. Arch Intern Med 1996;156:745–752.
32. Wenger N. Improvement of quality of life in the framework of cardiac rehabilitation. In: Pashkow F, Dafoe W, eds. Clinical Cardiac Rehabilitation: A Cardiologist's Guide, 2nd ed. Williams & Wilkins, Baltimore, 1999, pp. 43–51.
33. Ades PA, Pashkow FJ, Nestor JR. Cost-effectiveness of cardiac rehabilitation after myocardial infarction. J Cardiopulm Rehabil 1997;17:222–231.
34. Probstfield JL. How cost-effective are new preventive strategies for cardiovascular disease? Am J Cardiol 2003; 91:22G–27G.
35. Shephard RJ, Franklin B. Changes in the quality of life: a major goal of cardiac rehabilitation. J Cardiopulm Rehabil 2001;21:189–200.
36. Oldridge N, Guyatt G, Jones N, et al. Effects on quality of life with comprehensive rehabilitation after acute myocardial infarction. Am J Cardiol 1991;67:1084–1089.
37. Brown G, Albers JJ, Fisher LD, et al. Regression of coronary artery disease as a result of intensive lipid-lowering therapy in men with high levels of apolipoprotein B [see comments]. N Engl J Med 1990;323:1289–1298.
38. Ornish D, Brown SE, Scherwitz LW, et al. Can lifestyle changes reverse coronary heart disease? The Lifestyle Heart Trial. Lancet 1990;336:129–133.
39. Haskell WL, Alderman EL, Fair JM, et al. Effects of intensive multiple risk factor reduction on coronary atherosclerosis and clinical cardiac events in men and women with coronary artery disease. The Stanford Coronary Risk Intervention Project (SCRIP). Circulation 1994;89:975–990.
40. Brown BG, Zhao XQ, Sacco DE, Albers JJ. Arteriographic view of treatment to achieve regression of coronary atherosclerosis and to prevent plaque disruption and clinical cardiovascular events. Br Heart J 1993;69:S48–S53.
41. Sullivan MJ, Higginbotham MB, Cobb FR. Exercise training in patients with severe left ventricular dysfunction. Hemodynamic and metabolic effects. Circulation 1988;78:506–515.
42. Pashkow FJ. Rehabilitation strategies for the complex cardiac patient. Cleve Clin J Med 1991;58:70–75.
43. Sullivan MJ, Higginbotham MB, Cobb FR. Exercise training in patients with chronic heart failure delays ventilatory anaerobic threshold and improves submaximal exercise performance. Circulation 1989;79:324–329.
44. McKelvie RS, Teo KK, Roberts R, et al. Effects of exercise training in patients with heart failure: the Exercise Rehabilitation Trial (EXERT). Am Heart J 2002;144:23–30.
45. Lavie CJ, Milani RV, Littman AB. Benefits of cardiac rehabilitation and exercise training in secondary coronary prevention in the elderly. J Am Coll Cardiol 1993;22:678–683.
46. Limacher MC. Exercise and rehabilitation in women. Indications and outcomes. Cardiol Clin 1998;16:27–36.
47. Carhart RL Jr, Ades PA. Gender differences in cardiac rehabilitation. Cardiol Clin 1998;16:37–43.
48. Foody J, Pashkow F. Gender-specific issues related to coronary risk factors in women. In: Pashkow F, Dafoe W, eds. Clinical Cardiac Rehabilitation: A Cardiologist's Guide, 2nd ed. Williams & Wilkens, Baltimore, 1999, pp. 383–402.
49. Pashkow FJ, Pasternak R. Cardiac rehabilitation and risk factor modification. In: Fuster V, Ross R, Topol EJ, eds. Atherosclerosis and Coronary Artery Disease. Lippincott-Raven, Philadelphia/New York, 1996, pp. 1267–1282.

RECOMMENDED READING

Taylor RS, Brown A, Ebrahim S, et al. Exercise-based rehabilitation for patients with coronary heart disease: systematic review and meta-analysis of randomized controlled trials. Am J Med 2004;116:682–692.

Sanderson BK, Southard D, Oldridge N. Outcomes evaluation in cardiac rehabilitation/secondary prevention programs: improving patient care and program effectiveness. J Cardiopulm Rehabil 2004;24:68–79.

Dalal H, Evans PH, Campbell JL. Recent developments in secondary prevention and cardiac rehabilitation after acute myocardial infarction. BMJ 2004;328:693–697.

Newman S. Engaging patients in managing their cardiovascular health. Heart 2004;90(Suppl iv):9–13; discussion iv: 39–40.

Bittner V, Sanderson BK. Women in cardiac rehabilitation. J Am Med Womens Assoc 2003;58:227–235.

VIII VALVULAR HEART DISEASE

30

Rheumatic Fever and Valvular Heart Disease

Edmund A. W. Brice, MB ChB, PhD
and Patrick J. Commerford, MB ChB

INTRODUCTION

Rheumatic fever causes most cases of acquired heart disease in children and young adults worldwide. It is generally classified as a collagen vascular disease where the inflammatory insult is directed mainly against the tissues of the heart, joints, and the central nervous system. The inflammatory response, which is characterized by fibrinoid degeneration of collagen fibrils and connective tissue ground substance, is triggered by a throat infection with Group A β-hemolytic streptococci (GAS). The destructive effects on cardiac valve tissue accounts for most of the morbidity and mortality seen in the disease through the serious hemodynamic disturbances produced.

ACUTE RHEUMATIC FEVER

Epidemiology

During the 20th century, the two major influences in the reduction of rheumatic fever incidence in many parts of the world were the advent of penicillin and improvements in socioeconomic conditions. At the turn of the 20th century the reported incidence of rheumatic fever in the United States was 100 per 100,000 population; by 1960 this had fallen to 45 per 100,000. The most recent US figures show that some regions have rates as low as 2 per 100,000. In stark contrast to these figures are those in the developing world,where rates as high as 1500 to 2100 per 100,000 have been reported in various areas of Africa, Asia, and South America. In Soweto, South Africa, a prevalence of rheumatic carditis of 1900 per 100,000 was reported in the early 1970s *(1)*.

Pathogenesis

The role of GAS in the genesis of rheumatic fever has been supported by a variety of clinical, epidemiologic, and immunologic observational studies. Pharyngeal infection with this organism is the only known cause of rheumatic fever. In situations of overcrowding, such as in schools or in military facilities, epidemics of streptococcal throat infection have resulted in approx 3% of those affected developing rheumatic fever *(2)*.

Group A β-hemolytic streptococci have a variety of cell-wall antigens such as the M, T, and R proteins. It is the M-wall protein that is responsible for type-specific immunity and is widely regarded as determining streptococcal rheumatogenic potential. Patients with acute rheumatic fever are often found to have high titers of antibody to the M proteins.

The currently accepted mode of development of acute rheumatic fever is that GAS pharyngitis leads to a host response to the GAS antigens, with cross-reactivity of the GAS antibodies with antigens in human tissues such as heart and brain (molecular mimicry) *(3)*. This would explain the

From: *Essential Cardiology: Principles and Practice, 2nd Ed.*
Edited by: C. Rosendorff © Humana Press Inc., Totowa, NJ

Table 1
Modified Criteria for Diagnosis of Acute Rheumatic Fever (6)

Major	Minor
Carditis	Fever
Chorea	Arthralgia
Polyarthritis	Elevated ESR
Erythema marginatum	Elevated C-reactive protein
Subcutaneous nodules	Prolonged PR interval

frequent observation that, following pharyngeal infection, there is a 3-wk asymptomatic period and also the finding that rheumatic fever is rare in very young children. The peak incidence of rheumatic fever is between the ages of 5 and 18 yr.

Host factors such as HLA subtypes have also been cited as possible explanations in the varying susceptibility to disease. Approximately 60–70% of patients worldwide are positive for HLA-DR3, DR4, DR7, DRW53, or DQW2 (4).

Clinical Presentation

These is no test specific for the diagnosis of rheumatic fever; therefore, the diagnosis of a patient's first attack of rheumatic fever is usually made by fulfilling the clinical criteria first formulated by Jones (5) and subsequently modified (6). These are divided into major and minor criteria and, if preceded by a GAS infection, two major or one major and two minor criteria are found, a diagnosis of rheumatic fever can be made (Table 1).

Carditis is a pancarditis involving endo-, myo-, and pericardial tissues. Valvular involvement is frequent; if no evidence of this is found clinically despite myocarditis or pericarditis, rheumatic fever is unlikely. The mitral valve is most commonly involved, followed by the aortic valve, and gives rise to the frequent finding of regurgitant murmurs. A mitral systolic murmur, and occasionally even a mid-diastolic murmur (Carey-Coombs murmur: increased flow across the a mitral valve), detected during the course of an acute attack of rheumatic fever, do not necessarily indicate permanent valvular disease. An aortic early diastolic murmur rarely disappears and is evidence of established valve disease. Echocardiography is usually not required acutely and may give rise to overdiagnosis (7). As the progression to valvular stenosis through progressive scarring of the valve leaflets occurs gradually, early routine echocardiography seldom adds any information to that found clinically.

Arthritis is symmetrical, migratory, and involves the larger joints such as the wrists, elbows, knees, and ankles. If a patient presents with joint symptoms and evidence of recent GAS pharyngitis, but has insufficient criteria for a diagnosis of rheumatic fever, poststreptococcal reactive arthritis must be considered. This may give rise to delayed carditis and, therefore, patients should be followed closely.

Sydenham's chorea, characterized by purposeless involuntary movements, incoordination, and emotional lability, is seen in about 20% of patients with rheumatic fever. It often presents 3 mo after the onset of the preceding GAS pharyngitis. Even without treatment, symptoms often resolve within 2 wk.

Erythema marginatum, an erythematous macular rash of the trunk and proximal extremities, occurs in approx 5% of rheumatic fever cases. Lesions have pale centers with rounded or serpiginous pale-pink margins and are nonpruritic. They are transient and extremely difficult to detect, particularly in dark-skinned patients.

Subcutaneous nodules are found in 3% of rheumatic fever cases and are painless, mobile, 0.5- to 2-cm nodules on the extensor surfaces of joints, the occipital area of the scalp, and over spinous processes.

Peritoneal involvement is rare but may simulate an acute abdomen, mimicking acute appendicitis in children.

Often problematic is confirmation of the diagnosis of preceding GAS infection. Throat swab culture is positive in only approx 11% of patients at time of acute rheumatic fever diagnosis *(8)*. A rapid streptococcal antigen test has also been utilized to confirm recent GAS infection. Another confirmatory test is the finding of a rising titer of antistreptococcal antibodies, either antistreptolysin O (ASO) or antideoxyribonuclease B (anti-DNase B).

It is important to have a high level of suspicion of rheumatic fever in any patient presenting with a pyrexial illness, tachycardia, and a progressive symmetrical polyarthritis. While most patients are between the ages of 5 and 15 at first presentation, much older patients may occasionally develop acute rheumatic fever. Recurrence of rheumatic fever can occur at any age and must be distinguished from infective endocarditis.

Treatment

Once the diagnosis has been made, it is customary for patients to be prescribed bed rest. Although at the time of presentation for rheumatic fever throat swabs are frequently negative for GAS, a 10-d course of oral penicillin V or a single intramuscular injection of benzathine penicillin is empirically given to eradicate any GAS present.

In order to minimize inflammatory damage to the affected tissues, often joint and cardiac, high doses of oral salicylates (100 mg/kg/d in divided doses) is cost-effective therapy. For patients with severe carditis or for those whose valve lesions may require early surgical repair, prednisone (2 mg/kg/d) is often used instead of salicylates. The evidence for any real superiority of prednisone is weak but patients with carditis do appear to respond more rapidly to it *(9)*.

Duration of therapy is determined by clinical and laboratory evidence of resolution of inflammation. This is often achieved in milder cases after a month of salicylate therapy, although more severe cases may require 3 mo of steroid treatment and up to 5% of cases are still active at 6 mo.

Heart failure, due to severe valve regurgitation, is the usual cause of death and, when it is resistant to antifailure therapy, may necessitate urgent valve replacement surgery, even in the presence of active carditis *(10)*.

PRIMARY PREVENTION

Prompt recognition and effective treatment of GAS pharyngitis can prevent the development of rheumatic fever, reducing both morbidity and mortality.

Penicillin remains the most cost-effective agent in the treatment of GAS pharyngitis. Often a single intramuscular dose of benzathine penicillin (1.2 MU if ≥27 kg body weight) is effective. When compliance is not a concern an alternative oral regimen such as penicillin V (500 mg three times a day in adults) may be used. Erythromycin estolate (20–40 mg/kg/d in 2–4 daily doses) can be used in penicillin-allergic individuals.

True primary prevention of GAS pharyngitis can only be achieved through prevention of the conditions of squalor, overcrowding, and socioeconomic deprivation that promote frequent attacks of GAS pharyngitis in communities.

SECONDARY PREVENTION

Recurrent attacks of rheumatic fever are common and can be reduced through the use of prophylactic antibiotics. Duration of secondary prevention must be individualized for patients and extended for those in poor socioeconomic conditions. Generally patients should, following their first attack of rheumatic fever, receive antibiotics until 21 yr of age or for at least 5 yr. Those with persistent evidence of carditis should receive prolonged therapy, some authors recommending treatment until age 40 or at least 10 yr after the attack.

Antibiotic regimens whose efficacy is proven include 1.2 MU intramuscular benzathine penicillin every 3 wk *(11)*. Oral therapy is often used for patients on warfarin anticoagulation and 250 mg penicillin V twice daily is recommended. Penicillin-allergic individuals may use 250 mg erythromycin twice daily.

More recently, efforts have been made to develop vaccines incorporating recombinant M protein fragments in an effort to elicit a protective antibody response. Rabbits immunized with such

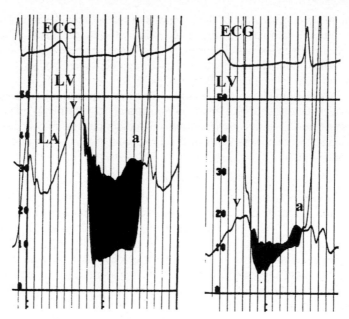

Fig. 1. Simultaneous recording of left atrial (LA) and left ventricular (LV) pressure in a patient with severe MS before (left) and immediately after (right) balloon valvuloplasty. Shaded area indicates the gradient.

a vaccine have been shown to be highly immunogenic and evoke protective antibodies *(12)*. Animal studies have thus shown the feasibility of this strategy and human studies are awaited.

MITRAL VALVE DISEASE

Mitral Stenosis

With the rare exception of congenital abnormalities, mitral stenosis (MS) due to abnormalities of the leaflets, commissures, and cusps of the valve is due to rheumatic fever *(13)*. Some 40% of patients with rheumatic heart disease have combined mitral stenosis and mitral regurgitation and a quarter have pure mitral stenosis. Mitral stenosis is more common in females. The reason for this female predominance is unclear.

Pathology

The rheumatic process affects the edges of the leaflets; resolution of the inflammatory process there is thickening, fibrosis, and fusion of the commissures. Involvement of the chordae tendineae results in thickening, fusion, and contraction with scarring extending down onto the papillary muscles. Dense fibrosis and calcification may reduce the normal delicate structure of the valve to a rigid, immobile, and funnel-shaped orifice.

Pathophysiology

The normal adult mitral valve orifice area is 4–6 cm^2. When MS reduces the orifice area to 2 cm^2 a higher-than-normal pressure is required to propel blood from the left atrium to the left ventricle. When stenosis is more severe (1–1.5 cm^2) a considerably elevated left atrial pressure is required to maintain a normal cardiac output even at rest, resulting in a pressure gradient across the valve (Fig. 1). The elevated left atrial pressure raises pulmonary capillary pressures, resulting in exertional dyspnea. Dyspnea usually first occurs with exercise, emotional stress, or infection that require an increased rate of flow across the mitral valve and hence a higher left atrial pressure. Patients with MS do not tolerate a tachycardia. An increase in heart rate shortens diastole proportionally more than systole and hence reduces the time available for blood flow across the mitral valve *(14)*; the development of atrial fibrillation (AF) with a rapid ventricular rate may precipitate pulmonary edema in previously asymptomatic patients with MS.

Pulmonary hypertension in patients with MS may result from passive backward transmission of the elevated left atrial pressure or organic obliterative changes in the pulmonary vasculature. Reactive pulmonary hypertension due to pulmonary arteriolar constriction triggered by left atrial and pulmonary venous hypertension may be important in some patients. Prolonged severe pulmonary hypertension results in dilation of the right ventricle and secondary tricuspid regurgitation.

Clinical Features

HISTORY

Subclinical or unrecognized attacks of acute rheumatic fever presumably account for the fact that fewer than half of all patients with MS clearly recollect the acute event.

Dyspnea, which may be accompanied by cough and wheezing, is the major symptom of mitral stenosis. This is initially only exertional but with progression orthopnea and paroxysmal nocturnal dyspnea develop. Patients with severe mitral stenosis may tolerate modest impairment of ordinary daily activities but are at risk of developing frank pulmonary edema, which may be precipitated by exercise, chest infections, fever, emotional stress, pregnancy, intercourse, or the advent of atrial fibrillation.

Classically several different kinds of hemoptysis are described as complicating mitral stenosis.

- Sudden profuse hemorrhage (pulmonary apoplexy) results from the rupture of thin-walled dilated bronchial veins *(15)*. It is more common early in the disease before bronchial veins thicken and are able to withstand the raised pressure. Often profuse and terrifying, it is rarely life-threatening.
- Pink frothy sputum of pulmonary edema.
- Blood-stained sputum associated with attacks of paroxysmal nocturnal dyspnea.
- Pulmonary infarction, which is a late complication of long-standing MS associated with heart failure.

Thromboembolism is an important and life-threatening complication of MS. Systemic emboli occur in approx 20% of patients at some time. Emboli are more common in older patients with a low cardiac output, a large left atrial appendage, and atrial fibrillation. Embolism may, however, occur in patients with mild MS and may occasionally be the presenting feature. Cerebral, renal, and coronary emboli may occur and occasionally a large embolus may block the aorta at its bifurcation (saddle embolus). Unexpected systemic or cerebral emboli in a young patient should prompt a careful search for MS.

Uncommon manifestations include *chest pain* indistinguishable from angina pectoris, which, in the absence of coronary disease, may be due to right ventricular or left atrial hypertension. Poorly explained, it resolves with successful treatment of the stenosis. *Hoarseness* caused by compression of the left recurrent laryngeal nerve by a dilated left atrium, lymph nodes, and dilated pulmonary artery occurs in isolated cases (Ortner's syndrome). Severe untreated MS with pulmonary hypertension and right heart failure produces symptoms due to systemic venous hypertension with hepatomegaly, edema, and ascites.

PHYSICAL EXAMINATION

The typical so-called *mitral facies* with pinkish-purple patches on the cheeks is rarely appreciated in dark-skinned patients in whom the disease is common. The *pulse* is normal in character but of small volume if the cardiac output is reduced. The *venous pressure* may be normal if pulmonary hypertension has not developed. When severe pulmonary hypertension is present a large "a" wave is found. Atrial fibrillation (AF) and tricuspid incompetence is associated with large "cv" waves and systolic hepatic pulsation. A typical feature on *palpation* is an easily palpable first heart sound (S_1). Pulmonary hypertension produces a right ventricular lift and a palpable pulmonic closure sound (P_2) in the left parasternal area.

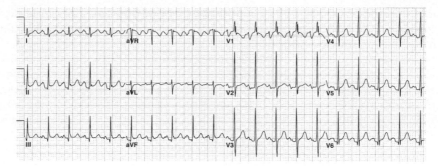

Fig. 2. Twelve-lead electrocardiogram in a patient with severe isolated mitral stenosis and pulmonary hypertension. It shows the combination of left atrial enlargement (P-wave broadened in lead II, biphasic in lead VI) and right ventricular hypertrophy (right axis deviation, dominant R in lead VI).

Auscultation is best performed with the patient turned into the left lateral position. The first heart sound is typically loud. This accentuation occurs when the anterior leaflet of the mitral valve remains pliable and is due to the abrupt crossover in pressure between left atrium and left ventricle at the onset of systole in mitral stenosis and the rapid acceleration of the closing leaflets *(16)*. Normally the leaflets drift closed toward the end of diastole. In MS they are held open by the transmitral pressure gradient. Marked calcification or fibrosis of the leaflets attenuates the accentuation. In patients with pulmonary hypertension, P_2 is accentuated. The mitral valve opening snap (OS) is heard only in patients with MS. Caused by sudden tensing of the anterior leaflet, it is best heard in the left parasternal area. The characteristic murmur is a low-pitched diastolic rumble best heard with the bell of the stethoscope and may be limited to the apex. Presystolic accentuation of the murmur occurs due to atrial contraction, which increases the gradient and flow across the mitral valve just prior to systole in patients in sinus rhythm. The auscultatory features of MS in obese and emphysematous patients are notoriously difficult. Simple bedside maneuvers (exercise) increase the heart rate and render the appreciation of the auscultatory features easier. Auscultation offers clues to *severity* of stenosis: The longer the murmur and the closer the OS is to the aortic component of the second sound (A2), the more severe the stenosis and *mobility* of the valve; a well-heard OS and loud, easily heard S_1 imply that the anterior leaflet is mobile.

The only important differential diagnosis to be considered is that of a *left atrial myxoma*, which may produce auscultatory features similar to those of MS. The characteristic inspiratory augmentation of the murmur of *tricuspid stenosis* should readily allow for its differentiation.

LABORATORY EXAMINATION

Electrocardiography is relatively insensitive but may reveal characteristic changes in patients with moderate or severe mitral stenosis (Fig. 2). The *chest radiograph* usually shows an enlarged atrial appendage and left atrial enlargement will be visible on the left lateral view. *Echocardiography* (Fig. 3) both confirms the diagnosis by demonstrating thickening, restricted motion and doming of the anterior leaflet and provides vital information on the mobility of the anterior leaflet, the presence and severity of calcification of the valve, and involvement of the subvalvular apparatus, which determine selection of treatment. Color-flow Doppler *echocardiography* demonstrates the high-velocity jet entering the left ventricle (Fig. 4; *see* Color Plate 7, following p. 268) and allows quantitation of severity.

Clinical evaluation and detailed echocardiographic examination including a Doppler study usually provides sufficient information to plan management without the need for *cardiac catheterization*, which can be reserved for patients in whom doubt remains about severity of associated mitral regurgitation, other valve lesions, or left ventricular function. *Coronary angiography* may be indicated in selected patients with chest pain syndromes or in those considered to be at risk of having coronary disease before elective valve replacement surgery.

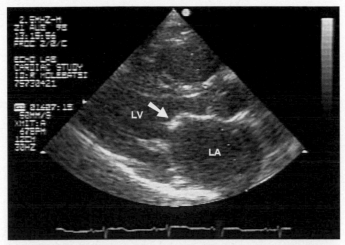

Fig. 3. Transthoracic echocardiographic images (parasternal long axis view) reveals left atrial (LA) enlargement and thickened domed anterior leaflet of the mitral valve (arrow).

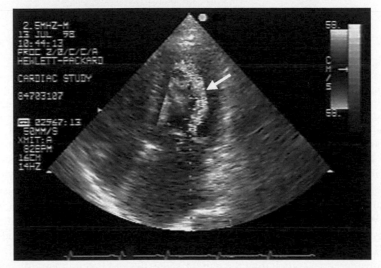

Fig. 4. Color-flow Doppler echocardiography demonstrates the high-velocity jet entering the left ventricle (arrow). (*See* Color Plate 7, following p. 268.)

TREATMENT

Medical treatment includes advice regarding lifestyle and pregnancy, long-term prophylaxis against recurrences of rheumatic fever if appropriate, antibiotic prophylaxis against infective endocarditis (although the risks are low), and prophylactic anticoagulation with warfarin if AF is present (sustained or paroxysmal). There is no clear evidence that warfarin anticoagulation is of benefit in patients in sinus rhythm who have not experienced an episode of systemic embolism. Diuretics and dietary sodium restriction reduce pulmonary congestion. β-Blockers increase exercise capacity by reducing heart rate *(17)*.

Surgical treatment: Mechanical relief of obstruction may be obtained by closed mitral valvotomy, open mitral valvotomy, percutaneous balloon mitral valvuloplasty (PBMV), or mitral valve replacement. Selection and timing of the procedure requires clinical judgment based on knowledge of the patient's symptoms, the severity of MS, and the risks of the procedure. PBMV has largely superseded surgical valvotomy in suitable patients with pliable leaflets and little or no significant calcification or mitral regurgitation (MR). A balloon catheter inserted via the femoral vein and a

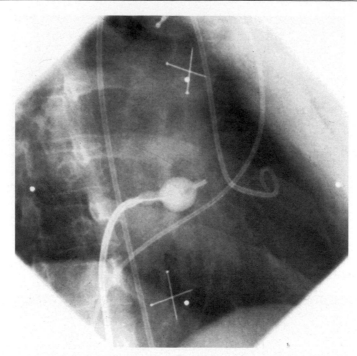

Fig. 5. An Inoue balloon catheter is positioned across the mitral valve. The indentation in the contrast-filled balloon as it ruptures the mitral valve commissures is evident.

transatrial puncture across the stenotic valve when dilated (Fig. 5) tears the fused commissures and partially relieves the obstruction. While palliative, PBMV preserves the patient's own valvular apparatus and defers mitral valve replacement with its attendant risks. Periprocedural risk is low (1–3%), it can be performed as an emergency or in pregnant patients, and it provides excellent relief of symptoms. Severe MR may follow rupture of one of the leaflets. PBMV is usually recommended in patients with significant MS (mitral valve area <1.5 cm^2) and symptoms NYHA Class II or greater. When the valve is badly deformed, heavily calcified, or there is associated significant MR, then mitral valve replacement surgery is the only option. This is usually recommended in patients with Class III or IV symptoms.

Clinical considerations—including the patient's age, desired level of activity, comorbid conditions, and, importantly in young women, desire for pregnancy—will influence decisions. Each patient with MS requires an individualized assessment recognizing that progression to severe stenosis is almost inevitable, medical treatment can offer only temporary relief, and valvotomy is palliative with restenosis inevitable, although the time to restenosis is unpredictable. Many patients who underwent successful closed mitral valvotomy when the procedure was introduced in the 1950s have had repeat procedures and lead successful and productive lives 40 yr later after inevitable mitral valve replacement.

Mitral Regurgitation

PATHOLOGY

A number of pathological processes may affect components of the mitral valve apparatus and cause it to become incompetent (Table 2). The rheumatic process leads to fibrosis with resultant scarring and contracture of the valve leaflets, and a similar process affecting the chordae with scarring of the papillary muscles results in mitral regurgitation. The severe mitral regurgitation seen in acute rheumatic fever in children or adolescents is usually secondary to prolapse of the anterior leaflet, elongation of the chordae, and dilation of the annulus *(18)*.

Table 2
Causes of Mitral Regurgitation

Chronic	Acute
Rheumatic heart disease	Infective endocarditis
Mitral valve prolapse	Chordal rupture
Mitral annular calcification	Trauma (surgery, PMBV)
Infective endocarditis	Ischemic papillary muscle dysfunction, rupture
Chordal rupture (spontaneous, infective, traumatic)	Prosthetic valve malfunction
Ischemic papillary muscle dysfunction	
Congenital clefts	
Systemic lupus erythematosus	

PATHOPHYSIOLOGY

Isolated or pure MR is uncommon in chronic rheumatic heart disease, and there is almost always a degree of associated stenosis. In chronic MR, the mitral orifice functions in parallel with the aortic valve and considerable regurgitation into the low-pressure left atrium may occur before the aortic valve opens. This systolic unloading of the ventricle may permit the patient with chronic MR many years of relatively symptom-free survival at the risk of developing progressive left ventricular dysfunction. The loading conditions in chronic MR are favorable, the lesion favors left ventricular emptying, and if myocardial function is normal the ejection fraction should be supernormal. An understanding of the complex hemodynamic adaptations that occur in chronic MR are important in planning patient management *(19)*.

When left ventricular function is impaired end-diastolic pressure rises, as does left atrial pressure, and pulmonary venous hypertension may increase the pulmonary artery pressure. Severe pulmonary hypertension is less frequent than in patients with isolated mitral stenosis.

When MR develops abruptly, the unprepared noncompliant left atrium is unable to accommodate the regurgitant load and acute heart failure is common.

CLINICAL FEATURES

History. *Dyspnea* is the usual presenting symptom. Most patients tolerate chronic mitral regurgitation very well unless there is a dramatic increase in the degree of MR. The great danger is that by the time that symptoms secondary to reduced cardiac output or pulmonary congestion become apparent, severe and irreversible left ventricular dysfunction may develop. *Hemoptysis* and *thromboemolism* are less common than in patients with MS. Untreated, severe chronic MR may result in pulmonary hypertension with secondary tricuspid regurgitation, hepatomegaly, and ascites with symptoms attributable to these.

Physical Examination. The *pulse* is usually normal in volume with a brisk upstroke. In the absence of pulmonary hypertension and associated tricuspid valve abnormalities, venous pressure may be normal. On precordial *palpation* the apex beat is volume-loaded and displaced to the left. A systolic lift in the left parasternal area, due to systolic expansion of the enlarged left atrium, may be difficult to differentiate from right ventricular enlargement secondary to pulmonary hypertension.

Auscultation: The first heart sound is usually soft and P_2 may be accentuated if pulmonary hypertension has developed. An apical pansystolic murmur commencing immediately after S_1 and continuing up to the second sound is characteristic of chronic severe mitral regurgitation. Best heard at the apex, it radiates to the axilla and back. In occasional patients in whom the regurgitant jet is directed medially, it may be heard maximally parasternally and even in the pulmonary area. The murmur, unlike that of aortic stenosis, varies little in intensity with alterations in cardiac cycle length. Severity of regurgitation does not correlate with loudness of the murmur. Failure of the murmur to accentuate with inspiration differentiates it from that of tricuspid regurgitation. An apical third heart sound frequently precedes a short mid-diastolic murmur, the result of the increased forward flow produced by the regurgitant volume and some degree of commissural fusion that is often present in rheumatic MR.

Laboratory Examination. *Electrocardiography* may be normal or show left atrial enlargement. A pattern of severe left ventricular hypertrophy with repolarization abnormalities is unusual and, when present, is an indication that the diagnosis may be incorrect and that the mitral regurgitation is secondary to left ventricular dilation (dilated cardiomyopathy) or that the differential diagnosis of the systolic murmur should be wider (aortic stenosis, hypertrophic cardiomyopathy). The *chest radiograph* usually reveals cardiomegaly and left atrial enlargement. *Echocardiography* confirms the diagnosis of mitral regurgitation, revealing a high-velocity jet in the left atrium during systole. In addition to its diagnostic role, echocardiography provides vital information on left ventricular function and mitral valve morphology, which together determine management and prognosis.

Treatment. *Medical treatment* in the asymptomatic patient must include advice regarding prophylaxis against recurrences of acute rheumatic fever, prophylaxis against infective endocarditis, and lifestyle, pregnancy, and the need for long-term medical supervision. Careful serial evaluation with noninvasive monitoring of left ventricular function is essential. Diuretics relieve symptoms of pulmonary congestion and digitalis is indicated in patients with severe MR and evidence of heart failure, particularly if atrial fibrillation is present. Chronic afterload reduction with angiotensin-converting enzyme inhibitors is logical but unproven therapy.

Surgical treatment: Mitral valve replacement results in symptomatic improvement, but long-term results are far from ideal. Mitral valve annuloplasty or repair is the preferred procedure. The timing of surgery in patients with MR is difficult. Patients with severe symptoms (NYHA Class III and IV) should be offered surgery. Asymptomatic patients or those with mild symptoms (NYHA Class II) can be observed or treated medically provided that left ventricular function is monitored meticulously; they are considered for surgery if the ejection fraction falls toward 60% or end-systolic dimension approaches 45 mm *(19)*. Mitral valve repair is, for technical reasons, often not possible in patients with rheumatic MR and when attempted, results are often unsatisfactory *(20)*.

Mixed Mitral Stenosis and Regurgitation

Rheumatic disease of the mitral valve results in a wide spectrum of clinical presentations that range from predominant MS to predominant MR. Common and particularly difficult management problems are patients in whom the disease process results in severe deformity of the valve, which is stenotic during diastole and leaks during systole.

Clinical and laboratory features depend on which pathology is dominant; no brief description can encompass the variety of clinical signs that may be detected. *Medical treatment* in both asymptomatic and symptomatic patients is the same as that for those with pure MS and pure MR. *Surgical treatment* by means of valve replacement provides symptomatic relief, but the risks of the procedure need to be weighed against the risks of the underlying disease. It is usually recommended to patients with NYHA Class III or IV disability.

AORTIC VALVE DISEASE
Aortic Stenosis

PATHOLOGY

Congenitally abnormal valves that may be bicuspid may be only mildly obstructive in childhood but the abnormal flow dynamics they cause damage the leaflets leading to fibrosis, rigidity, and increasing stenosis later in life. Ultimately the appearances of the congenitally abnormal valve resemble that of degenerative aortic stenosis. *Degenerative* or senile calcific disease is the most common cause of AS in older patients. Mechanical stress over many years on a valve originally normal ultimately results in deposits of calcium along the base of the cusps, rendering them immobile and obstructive.

The valvulitis of an attack of acute rheumatic fever results in adhesions along the edges of the cusps with fusion of the commissures. Fibrosis and scarring, which may be associated with calcification, result in thickening and contraction of the cusps so that the normal trileaflet structure becomes fused with a small central orifice. Varying degrees of regurgitation are common. Concentric left ventricular hypertrophy occurs and evidence of rheumatic mitral valve involvement is common.

PATHOPHYSIOLOGY

Minor degrees of commissural fusion produce murmurs due to turbulent blood flow but significant hemodynamic obstruction occurs only when the cross-sectional area of the valve is reduced to about one fourth of the normal size of 2.5 to 3.5 cm^2. The ventricle adapts to the gradually progressive obstruction by developing concentric left ventricular hypertrophy. Hypertrophy allows for maintenance of cardiac output in the face of a large gradient across the valve for many years without left ventricular dilation or the development of symptoms. The hypertrophied left ventricle is less distensible than normal, resulting in elevation of the left ventricular end-diastolic pressure.

CLINICAL FEATURES

Isolated severe aortic stenosis (AS) without clinically evident aortic regurgitation or concomitant mitral valve involvement is usually idiopathic and degenerative rather than rheumatic in origin *(21)*.

History. Characteristically, there is a long asymptomatic period. *Angina*, which is typical and indistinguishable from that due to atherosclerotic coronary disease, is common even though the coronary arteries are normal. It is caused by increased myocardial oxygen demand as a result of hypertrophy and reduced coronary flow reserve. *Syncope* is usually exertional and is attributed to failure of an increase in cardiac output to adapt to exercise-associated vasodilation because of the fixed obstruction at the valve. Alternatively, a vasodepressor mechanism in response to marked elevation of left ventricular systolic pressure is invoked. Premonitory symptoms, exertional dizziness, and "gray-outs" may predominate and bear the same significance as syncopal episodes. *Dyspnea* on exertion early in the clinical course is due to the elevated left ventricular end-diastolic pressure. Severe manifestations such as orthopnea or paroxysmal nocturnal dyspnea are manifest late in the natural history and, if prominent, suggest that there might be associated mitral valve disease.

Physical Examination. The *pulse* in mild AS is normal. In advanced AS it is of small volume and sustained (pulsus parvus et tardus). The distinctive character is best appreciated by palpating a larger vessel such as the carotid, where the radiation of the basal *systolic thrill* may also be detected. Recognition of the classical features of the pulse is difficult and they may not be present in older patients with an inelastic arterial bed or if there is associated aortic regurgitation. The *jugular venous pressure* may be normal unless there is heart failure or associated mitral valve disease. Prominent "a" waves occur due to reduced right ventricular compliance secondary to marked septal hypertrophy. Precordial *palpation* reveals a forceful sustained apical impulse that may not be greatly displaced in the early stage of the disease.

Auscultation typically reveals a normal or soft first heart sound. If accentuated, associated MS should be considered. In severe AS the second sound may be single due, in part, to immobility of the aortic leaflets and inaudibility of A$_2$. A presystolic gallop, due to a prominent fourth heart sound reflecting vigorous atrial contraction, may be heard. An aortic ejection systolic murmur is characteristic. Best heard to the right and left of the sternum and the base of the heart, it radiates to the neck and apex. Usually described as harsh and rasping in character, its intensity varies markedly. Severity of stenosis usually correlates with the duration of the murmur (long murmur, severe aortic stenosis) and the timing of the peak intensity (late peak, severe stenosis). Accentuation of the murmur after a postectopic pause is helpful in differentiating it from that of mitral regurgitation when it is well-heard at the apex. An early diastolic murmur of associated aortic regurgitation is often detected. Valvar aortic stenosis must be distinguished from other causes of left ventricular outflow obstruction (Table 3).

Clinical evaluation of the severity of aortic stenosis is notoriously difficult. Even experienced clinicians may fail to evaluate the pulse correctly. When left ventricular failure occurs and cardiac output falls, the murmur may soften or disappear completely. Operative intervention, even at this

Table 3
Differential Diagnosis of Aortic Stenosis

Type of stenosis	Maximum murmur and thrill	Aortic ejection sound	Aortic component of second sound	Regurgitant diastolic murmur	Arterial pulse
Acquired	Second right sternal border to neck; may be at apex in the aged	Uncommon	Decreased or absent	Common	Delayed upstroke; anacrotic notch; ± small amplitude
Hypertrophic subaortic	Fourth left sternal border to apex (± regurgitant systolic murmur at apex)	Rare	Normal or decreased	Very rare	Brisk upstroke, sometimes bisferiens
Congenital valvular	Second right sternal border to neck (along left sternal border in some infants)	Very common in children, disappearing with age	Normal or increased in childhood; decreased with decrease in valve mobility with age	Uncommon in in child; not not uncommon in adult	Delayed upstroke; anacrotic notch; ± small amplitude
Congenital subvalvular	Discrete: like valvular; tunnel: left sternal border	Rare	Not helpful (normal, increased, decreased or absent)	Almost all	Delayed upstroke; anacrotic notch; ± small amplitude
Congenital supravalvular	First right sternal border to neck and sometimes to medial aspect of right arm; occasionally greater in neck than in chest	Rare	Normal or decreased	Uncommon	Rapid upstroke in right carotid, delayed in left carotid; right arm pulse pressure greater than left

From ref. 27. Copyright 1987 Lippincott Williams & Wilkins.

556

Table 4
Causes of Aortic Regurgitation

Chronic	Acute
Rheumatic	Infective endocarditis
Degenerative	Dissecting aortic aneurysm
Chronic severe hypertension	Prosthetic valve malfunction
Syphilis	Trauma
Marfan's syndrome	
Infective endocarditis	
Discrete subaortic stenosis	
Ventricular septal defect with prolapse	
Rheumatoid arthritis	
Ankylosing spondylitis	
Congenital	

late stage, is often successful and clinical evaluation should be supplemented by echocardiography in any patient with unexplained heart failure. Associated MS may mask manifestations of AS *(22)*.

Laboratory Examination. Left ventricular hypertrophy with repolarization changes is manifested *electrocardiographically* in the majority of patients with severe AS. In rheumatic heart disease the pattern may be modified by the effects of concomitant mitral valve disease and pulmonary hypertension. The cardiac silhouette on *chest radiography* may be almost normal in pure AS, with some poststenotic dilation of the ascending aorta or calcification of the aortic valve the only clue to the diagnosis. This is unusual in rheumatic AS where associated AR or mitral valve disease often result in left ventricular or left atrial enlargement. *Echocardiography* demonstrates the thickened, poorly mobile leaflets, quantitates severity utilising the Bernoulli equation, and evaluates left ventricular size and function. Complete "hemodynamic" evaluation of most young patients can now be performed using this technique. *Cardiac catheterization and angiography* are indicated only in symptomatic patients being evaluated for valve replacement surgery in whom there is concern about the presence of coronary disease (because of symptoms of angina, age, or risk factor profile) or in whom doubt remains about the severity of stenosis or the presence or severity of other valve disease after detailed clinical and echocardiographic evaluation.

Treatment. An understanding of the natural history of the condition aids management. Survival of patients with asymptomatic AS is almost normal until symptoms develop, at which time prognosis worsens dramatically *(23)*.

Medical treatment for all patients should include prophylaxis against infective endocarditis and recurrences of rheumatic fever. Asymptomatic patients with severe AS should be advised to avoid vigorous physical activity, particularly competitive contact sports. All patients require education about the natural history of the condition, its gradually progressive nature, the need for regular medical supervision, and the importance of promptly reporting the onset of symptoms.

Aortic valve replacement surgery is the only effective form of treatment in adults with acquired AS. Aortic valve replacement should be advised in patients with severe aortic stenosis (aortic valve area <0.8 cm^2) and symptoms considered to be due to this. Although operative mortality is higher in patients with advanced disease, frank heart failure and apparently impaired systolic function by conventional measures, valve replacement often results in dramatic improvement in clinical state and left ventricular function. Given the poor prognosis of medical treatment, surgery is usually recommended.

Aortic Regurgitation

PATHOLOGY

Diseases affecting the aortic valve leaflets, the wall of the aortic root, or both structures may result in incompetence, which develops acutely or progresses slowly over many years (Table 4). The

Table 5
Eponymous Physical Signs of Chronic Severe Aortic Regurgitation

Corrigan's pulse	Bounding carotid pulse
De Musset's sign	Nodding of head with each heartbeat
Traube's sign	Pistol-shot sound heard over the femoral artery
Quincke's pulse	Capillary pulsation visible in nailbed with transillumination
Duroziez's sign	Diastolic murmur over femoral when compressed distal to stethoscope (Systolic murmur if compressed proximally)
Hill's sign	Popliteal systolic pressure exceeds brachial by >60 mmHg

inflammatory process of acute rheumatic valvulitis heals by fibrosis causing cusp retraction preventing apposition during diastole, thus allowing reflux of blood from the aorta to the left ventricle. Some commissural fusion may produce a degree of stenosis.

PATHOPHYSIOLOGY

Adaptive processes usually account for a long latent period in chronic AR. Diastolic reflux from aorta to left ventricle results in diastolic volume overload, increased end-diastolic volume, and a large stroke volume. Increased wall stress leads to eccentric left ventricular hypertrophy, a restoration of the ratio of wall thickness to cavity dimension toward normal, and hence tends to normalize end-diastolic wall stress. Despite a very large end-diastolic volume, end-diastolic pressure remains normal or only modestly elevated because of increased diastolic compliance. Ultimately, compensatory mechanisms fail, left ventricular contractile function deteriorates, the ventricle dilates further, and interstitial fibrosis contributes to a decline in compliance. The end-diastolic pressure rises and symptoms and signs of heart failure develop.

CLINICAL FEATURES

History. There may be a long latent period in chronic AR (10–15 yr) before adaptive mechanisms fail; thus the disease may first manifest when the characteristic murmur is recognized at routine examination of an asymptomatic patient. *Dyspnea* on exertion, with orthopnea and nocturnal dyspnea if presentation is delayed, are the most common symptoms. *Angina* is unusual but does occur in young patients with severe AR and normal coronary arteries. Often nocturnal, it is attributed to a slow heart rate, low diastolic blood pressure, and elevated left ventricular end-diastolic pressure resulting in reduced coronary perfusion. Symptoms of apical discomfort, awareness of the heart's activity when lying on the left side, or an awareness of pulsation in the neck and precordium are manifestations of ventricular dilation and a large stroke volume and may be manifest long before there is evidence of left ventricular dysfunction.

In *acute AR*, however, the situation is very different. The unprepared left ventricle is unable to tolerate the abrupt hemodynamic load. Acute cardiovascular collapse with hypotension and intense dyspnea may occur. The physical signs of acute AR are very different from those of the chronic state. Peripheral arterial signs are absent, the apex beat may not be prominent, and the murmur may be short, soft, and difficult to detect.

Physical Examination. The *pulse* in chronic severe aortic regurgitation is of large volume with a brisk upstroke and rapid descent (collapsing or water-hammer pulse). Systolic arterial pressure is elevated and diastolic abnormally low, with Korotkoff sounds persisting until zero. A bisferiens pulse, with both percussion and tidal waves palpable during systole, may be detected in the brachial or carotid arteries. The large pulse volume gives rise to an array of eponymous physical signs (Table 5). The *apex beat* is usually markedly displaced and is diffuse and volume-overloaded. A systolic thrill at the base may be a manifestation of a large stroke volume in pure AR or be due to a minor degree of commissural fusion in rheumatic disease.

Auscultation in chronic severe AR reveals a normal or soft first heart sound and a third sound may be present. The murmur of AR is an early diastolic decrescendo that commences immediately after the aortic component of the second heart sound. It is best heard with the patient sitting up, leaning forward with breath held in expiration, and the diaphragm of the stethoscope firmly applied between the apex and base. In general, the longer the murmur, the more severe the AR. A rumbling mid-diastolic murmur (Austin-Flint) is common and is attributed to antegrade flow across a normal mitral valve closing early because of the rapidly rising left ventricular end-diastolic pressure. It may be impossible to distinguish this from the murmur of mitral stenosis. The detection of a loud first heart sound and OS suggests associated MS, but absence of these does not exclude MS.

Laboratory Examination. The *electrocardiogram* in the early stages shows increased voltage in the precordial leads; with progression of the condition, repolarization abnormalities develop. *The chest radiograph* usually reveals cardiomegaly. Duration and severity of AR determines the degree of cardiac enlargement. In early, mild AR heart size may be almost normal, while it is markedly increased in chronic severe AR with dilation of the ascending aorta. Doppler *echocardiography* and color flow imaging readily detect even minor degrees of AR and allow quantification of severity by measuring the rate of decline in velocity of the regurgitant jet. Two-dimensional imaging of left ventricular size and function provides information on ventricular adaptation to the regurgitant load. Serial echocardiographic evaluation provides essential information on ventricular response to the regurgitant load and is vital in formulating a management plan for the asymptomatic patient. *Cardiac catheterization and angiography* are rarely necessary in young patients with rheumatic AR unless doubt remains about the severity of associated mitral valve disease after careful echocardiographic evaluation. Coronary angiography is indicated before valve replacement surgery in patients with angina and those considered to be at risk of coronary disease because of age or associated risk factors.

Treatment. Chronic aortic regurgitation may be well-tolerated for years. Once symptoms develop they are usually progressive, with death occurring in 2 to 4 yr if aortic valve replacement, the only definitive form of therapy, is not offered. *Medical treatment* for all patients includes prophylaxis against IE and recurrent ARF. Patients with severe AR, even if symptomatic, are conventionally advised against strenuous physical exertion. All asymptomatic patients with severe chronic AR and normal LV function should be informed of the natural history of the disease and advised to have regular evaluation at 6-mo intervals with serial measurement of left ventricular size and function.

Vasodilator therapy can logically be expected to reduce the degree of regurgitation and enhance LV performance, delaying the need for valve replacement in *asymptomatic* patients with preserved LV function. While this has been demonstrated with nifedipine *(24)*, it has not been well tested in young patients with rheumatic AR. Digoxin, diuretics, and vasodilators may temporarily stabilize patients with decompensated AR and heart failure awaiting valve replacement surgery. The need to prescribe any such agent, either for symptoms or evidence of LV dysfunction, should prompt consideration of aortic valve replacement.

Surgical treatment by aortic valve replacement should be offered to all patients with severe chronic AR as soon as possible after symptoms attributable to the condition have developed. Asymptomatic patients with impaired LV function require individualized assessment and evaluation, which needs to take into account the natural history of the condition and the risk of aortic valve replacement and anticoagulation. Single measures of LV function may be unreliable and serial repeated observations may be necessary. If these reveal consistent reproducible changes and the left ventricular ejection fraction falls below 50 to 55%, the left ventricular end-systolic diameter exceeds 55 mm or the left ventricular end diastolic diameter exceeds 70 mm, surgery is recommended *(25)*.

Occasional patients present very late in the course of the disease with severe heart failure, markedly impaired left ventricular function, and severe AR. Aortic valve replacement in this situation carries an increased operative mortality but the long-term outlook for survivors is unpredictable.

Most will obtain at least temporary relief of symptoms and, in some, ventricular function improves markedly with removal of the abnormal loading conditions. Short duration of symptoms may be helpful in predicting those who will obtain maximum benefit.

TRICUSPID VALVE DISEASE

Rheumatic involvement of the tricuspid valve is reported in autopsy series far more frequently than it is detected clinically. This may be due to relatively minor degrees of involvement or because the physical signs are often evanescent and rapidly modified by bed rest and diuretic therapy. Severe organic tricuspid valve disease, almost always associated with significant mitral valve disease as part of a syndrome of multiple valve involvement, poses a formidable therapeutic challenge and has a grave impact on prognosis.

Tricuspid Regurgitation

PATHOLOGY

Rheumatic tricuspid regurgitation (TR) is a result of scarring and deformity of the leaflets with fibrosis of chordae impairing mobility and preventing leaflet apposition. A degree of tricuspid stenosis (TS) is common. Infective endocarditis, carcinoid syndrome, and trauma are other causes. *Functional* tricuspid regurgitation secondary to tricuspid annular dilation may occur as a consequence of right ventricular failure secondary to pulmonary hypertension of any cause.

CLINICAL FEATURES

History. Symptoms due to associated involvement of left heart valves usually predominate. Peripheral edema, ascites, and painful hepatomegaly produce prominent symptoms if TR is severe.

Physical Examination. *Cachexia*, jaundice, ascites, and edema are prominent in untreated patients with severe TR presenting late in the course of the disease. The arterial pulse form is determined by associated valve lesions and atrial fibrillation is common. The *venous pressure* is always elevated with prominent "cv" waves and marked "y" collapse. A degree of associated TS renders the "y" descent less prominent. *Palpation* in severe TR reveals an atrial systolic impulse at the right lower sternal edge due to right atrial expansion. *Auscultation* reveals accentuation of P_2 and a pansystolic murmur, best heard in the fourth left intercostal space, which typically increases on inspiration. When TR is very severe this inspiratory accentuation may be very difficult to appreciate particularly if AF is present. If there is marked right ventricular dilation the murmur may be widespread, be heard at the apex and be easily mistaken for that of mitral regurgitation. All the clinical features of severe TR, particularly if it is functional in origin, may abate dramatically after a brief period of intense diuresis.

Laboratory Examination. *Electrocardiography* is unhelpful, usually showing atrial fibrillation and reflecting changes of pulmonary hypertension and the left-sided lesions responsible for its development. *Echocardiography* reveals dilation of the right atrium and ventricle with paradoxical septal motion. Color Doppler imaging readily demonstrates the regurgitant jet and evaluation of peak velocity of regurgitant flow allows estimation of pulmonary artery systolic pressure. *Cardiac catheterization* and *angiography*, which may be indicated to assess other valves, left ventricular function, or coronary anatomy, seldom add any information of note to that obtained by careful clinical and echocardiographic evaluation.

Tricuspid Stenosis

PATHOLOGY

Fusion of the leaflets at their commissures consequent on rheumatic valvulitis results in a narrowed central orifice. Shortening and fibrosis of chordae limit leaflet motion. The valve is obstructive in diastole and almost invariably there is a degree of systolic regurgitation. Pathological evidence of TS may be found in 15% of all patients with rheumatic heart disease but is the rarest clinical manifestation, occurring in only 5%.

CLINICAL FEATURES

The details on history and general physical examination are very similar to those in patients with rheumatic TR. A dominant "a" wave, which is sharp and flicking in the *jugular venous pressure* if sinus rhythm is present, is characteristic and more easily recognized than the slow "y" descent. Presystolic hepatic pulsation may be palpable.

On *auscultation* a diastolic murmur, loudest at the lower left sternal border with presystolic accentuation (if sinus rhythm is present), is heard. The murmur is accentuated on inspiration. A tricuspid opening snap is frequently recorded but clinically very difficult to distinguish from the OS of associated MS. As MS frequently coexists, only careful attention to respiratory variation will allow for differentiation of the two murmurs. A loud early diastolic murmur of AR in patients with multiple valve involvement may further confound clinical detection of the *murmur* of TS.

Laboratory Examination. Marked right atrial enlargement on *electrocardiography* in the absence of significant right ventricular hypertrophy is suggestive. Cardiomegaly on chest radiography is common with right atrial enlargement causing prominence of the right heart border. *Echocardiography* reveals thickening and doming, restricted motion, and reduced separation of the leaflets. Doppler echocardiography demonstrates increased antegrade velocity.

Treatment. Intensive *medical treatment* with bed rest, salt restriction, and diuretic therapy improves the symptoms and physical signs of systemic venous congestion, improves hepatic function, and reduces the risk of valve replacement surgery. *Surgical treatment* of rheumatic tricuspid valve disease is difficult and generally unsatisfactory but requires careful consideration at the time of correction of mitral and aortic valve abnormalities. Failure to correct significant tricuspid regurgitation may result in considerable disability in the long term.

The final decision as to what procedure is possible or necessary can often only be made by the surgeon after open inspection. Minor degrees of TS and TR, which have not caused significant venous pressure elevation, are best left alone. Although open commissurotomy may relieve TS, it may also produce severe TR and tricuspid valve replacement with a bioprosthesis is usually necessary. Minor degrees of functional TR improve dramatically with resolution of pulmonary hypertension after mitral valve surgery. Patients with severe functional or organic TR require repair with a ring annuloplasty. If the immediate result at surgery is unsatisfactory, valve replacement is necessary. Whenever possible tricuspid valve replacement is avoided, as all prostheses are inherently stenotic in this position and, while the operation relieves symptoms, the additional procedure increases the operative morbidity and mortality of mitral and aortic valve replacement.

MULTIPLE VALVE DISEASE

It is conventional and convenient to describe the various clinical syndromes of valvular heart disease in isolation. Clinical reality, however, is that a wide variety of combined lesions may occur, particularly in patients with rheumatic heart disease. Only some 25% of all patients with rheumatic heart disease have isolated MS. Others have mixed valve disease or a combination of valve lesions that may produce a wide array of clinical syndromes. Correct identification and correction of all lesions is important. Failure to identify and correct an associated severe lesion may increase operative risk. Disregard of mild or moderate associated disease at the time of surgery for the major abnormality may allow progression, necessitating reoperation with its attendant risks and thus negating benefit of the primary procedure.

When multiple valves are involved, the clinical and hemodynamic manifestations depend on the relative severity of each lesion. Generally, when lesions are of approximately equal severity, clinical manifestations produced by the more proximal (upstream) lesions predominate *(26)*. Careful clinical evaluation supplemented by two-dimensional and Doppler echocardiography usually serves to estimate the relative contribution of each valve to the clinical syndrome. If doubt remains, catheterization or angiography, specifically directed to answer unresolved issues, may be necessary. The final decision as to severity of individual lesions, the need for repair, and the method of repair, may only be possible at the time of operation.

SPECIAL CONSIDERATIONS

Acute rheumatic fever is a disease of poverty and overcrowding, and the majority of patients who suffer the sequelae of chronic valvular heart disease live in conditions where medical care is far from ideal. Availability of services and patients' access to and compliance with monitoring of anticoagulation, among many other factors, will influence decisions on timing and type of valve replacement surgery. Considerations of this nature, and the hemorrhagic risks attendant on poor supervision of warfarin anticoagulation, may prompt deferral of valve replacement in mildly symptomatic patients, even though measures of ventricular function suggest that under ideal circumstances it should be performed. Alternatively, despite the known risks of premature degeneration in young patients, bioprostheses may be used in patients who wish to return to rural homes that are remote from medical supervision and where warfarin anticoagulation is impossible. Thromboembolic complications of mechanical prostheses are inevitable if warfarin anticoagulation is not possible.

Pregnancy poses particular problems to young women with valvular heart disease. It often precipitates symptoms in previously asymptomatic patients with mitral stenosis. If the valve is suitable, then prophylactic PBMV may be possible prior to pregnancy or, if necessary, it may be done during pregnancy. Asymptomatic or mildly symptomatic patients with other lesions should be advised to complete their families as soon as possible and then, ideally, an effective form of contraception instituted before valve replacement surgery becomes necessary, thus avoiding the risks of warfarin to both mother and fetus.

REFERENCES

1. McLaren MJ, Hawkins DM, Koornhof HJ, et al. Epidemiology of rheumatic heart disease in black schoolchildren of Soweto, Johannesburg. Br Med J 1975;3:474–478.
2. Siegel AC, Johnson EE, Stollerman GH. Controlled studies of streptococcal pharyngitis in a pediatric population. 1. Factors related to the attack rate of rheumatic fever. N Engl J Med 1961; 265:559–565.
3. Dale JB, Beachey EH. Sequence of myosin cross-reactive epitopes of streptococcal M protein. J Exp Med 1986;164:1785–1790.
4. Haffejee I. Rheumatic fever and rheumatic heart disease: the current state of its immunology, diagnostic criteria and prophylaxis. Q J Med 1992;84:641–658.
5. Jones TD. Diagnosis of rheumatic fever. JAMA 1944;126:481–484.
6. Dajani AS, Ayoub EM, Bierman FZ, et al. Guidelines for the diagnosis of rheumatic fever: Jones criteria, updated 1992. JAMA 1992;268:2069–2073.
7. Vasan RS, Shrivastava S, Vijayakumar M, et al. Echocardiographic evaluation of patients with acute rheumatic fever and rheumatic carditis. Circulation 1996;94:73–82.
8. Dajani AS. Current status of nonsuppurative complications of Group A streptococci. Pediatr Infect Dis J 1991;10:S25–S27.
9. Albert DA, Harel L, Karrison T. The treatment of rheumatic carditis: a review and meta-analysis. Medicine (Baltimore) 1995;74:1–12.
10. Lewis BS, Geft IL, Milo S, Gotsman MS. Echocardiography and valve replacement in the critically ill patient with acute rheumatic carditis. Ann Thorac Surg 1979;27:529–535.
11. Lue HC, Wu MH, Wang JK, et al. Long-term outcome of patients with rheumatic fever receiving benzathine penicillin G prophylaxis every three weeks versus every four weeks. J Pediatr 1994;125:812–816.
12. Hu MC, Walls MA, Stroop SD, et al. Immunogenicity of a 26-valent Group A Streptococcal vaccine. Infect Immun 2002;70:2171–2177.
13. Olson LJ, Subramanian R, Ackermann DM, et al. Surgical pathology of the mitral valve. A study of 712 cases spanning 21 years. Mayo Clin Proc 1987;62:22–34.
14. Leavitt JI, Coats MH, Falk RH. Effects of exercise on transmitral gradient and pulmonary artery pressure in patients with mitral stenosis or a prosthetic mitral valve. A Doppler echocardiographic study. J Am Coll Cardiol 1991;17:1520–1526.
15. Ohmichi M, Tagaki S, Nomura N, et al. Endobronchial changes in chronic pulmonary venous hypertension. Chest 1988;94:1127–1132.
16. Barrington W W, Boudoulas J, Bashore T, et al. Mitral stenosis: Mitral dome excursion at M1 and the mitral opening snap—the concept of reciprocal heart sounds. Am Heart J 1998;115:1280–1290.
17. Klein HO, Sareli P, Schamroth CL, et al. Effects of atenolol on exercise capacity in patients with mitral stenosis with sinus rhythm. Am J Cardiol 1985;56:598–601.
18. Marcus RH, Sareli P, Pocock WA, Barlow JB. The spectrum of severe rheumatic mitral valve disease in a developing country: correlations among clinical presentations, surgical pathologic finding and haemodynamic sequelae. Ann Intern Med 1994;120:177–183.

19. Carabello BA, Crawford FA. Valvular heart disease. N Engl J Med 1997;337:32–41.
20. Rahimtoola SH. Valvular heart disease: a perspective. J Am Coll Cardiol 1983;1:199–215.
21. Passik CS, Ackermann DM, Pluth JR, Edwards WP. Temporal changes in the causes of aortic stenosis: a surgical pathologic study of 646 cases. Mayo Clin Proc 1987;62:119–123.
22. Zitnik RS, Piemme TE, Messer RJ, et al. The masking of aortic stenosis by mitral stenosis. Am Heart J 1965;69: 22–30.
23. Ross J Jr, Braunwald E. Aortic stenosis. Circulation 1968;38(Suppl V):V-61–V-67.
24. Scognamiglio R, Rahimtoola SH, Fasoli G, et al. Nifedipine in asymptomatic patients with severe aortic regurgitation and normal left ventricular function. N Engl J Med 1994;331:689–694.
25. Rahimtoola SH. Indications for surgery in aortic valve disease. In: Yusuf S, Cairns JA, Camm AJ, eds. Evidence Based Cardiology. BMJ Books, London, 1998, pp. 811–832.
26. Braunwald E. Valvular heart disease. In: Braunwald EB, ed. Heart Disease: a Textbook of Cardiovascular Medicine, 5th ed. W. B. Saunders, Philadelphia, 1997, pp. 1007–1076.
27. Levinson GE. Aortic stenosis. In: Dalen JE, Alpert JS, eds. Valvular Heart Disease, 2nd ed. Little, Brown, Boston, 1987, pp. 202–203.

RECOMMENDED READING

Bonow RO, Carabello B, de Leon AC Jr, et al. ACC/AHA guidelines for the management of patients with valvular heart disease: a report of the American College of Cardiology/American Heart Association Task Force on Practice Guidelines (Committee on Management of Patients with Valvular Heart Disease). J Am Coll Cardiol 1998;32:1486–1588.
Carabello BA. Mitral valve disease: indications for surgery. In: Yusuf S, Cairns JA, Camm AJ, eds. Evidence Based Cardiology. BMJ Books, London, 2003, pp. 758–766.
Dajani A, Taubert K, Ferrieri P, et al. Treatment of acute streptococcal pharyngitis and prevention of rheumatic fever: a statement for health professionals. Paediatrics 1995;96:758–764.
Otto CM, Burwask IG, Legget ME, et al. Prospective study of asymptomatic valvular aortic stenosis. clinical, echocardiographic, and exercise predictors of outcome. Circulation 1997;95:2262–2270.
Turi ZG. Balloon valvuloplasty: mitral valve. In: Yusuf S, Cairns JA, Camm AJ, eds. Evidence Based Cardiology. BMJ Books, London, 2003, pp. 796–808.

31

Infective Endocarditis

Adolf W. Karchmer, MD

INTRODUCTION

Infective endocarditis (IE) results when microbial agents infect the endothelial surface of the heart. Heart valves are the most common site for this process; however, occasionally infection develops on the low-pressure side of a ventricular septal defect, on chordae tendinae, or on mural endocardium that has been damaged by an aberrant jet of blood or an intracardiac foreign device (transvenous pacing lead, pulmonary artery catheter). Very rarely a similar process, infective endarteritis, arises when arteriovenous shunts, arterioarterial shunts (patent ductus arteriosus), or a coarctation of the aorta is involved. The cardinal lesion developing at these sites is the vegetation, a mass of platelets and fibrin, engendered by the procoagulant activity of infecting organisms and injured local tissue, wherein are enmeshed the causative microorganism and scant inflammatory cells.

A relatively infrequent disease, the incidence of IE generally has ranged from 1.5 to 6.2 cases per 100,000 population in developed countries over the past four decades (1,2). From 1988 to 1990 in a metropolitan area in the northeastern United States, the incidence was 9.3 cases per 100,000 population; notably, almost half of the cases occurred among injecting drug users (4.3 cases per 100,000 population) (1,3). The incidence increases progressively with age, reaching rates of 15 to 30 cases per 100,000 among persons in the sixth and later decades. In developed countries, prosthetic valve endocarditis (PVE) accounts for 7 to 25% of cases not involving injecting drug users (2,3). Based on actuarial estimates, PVE develops in 1.4 to 3.1% of valve recipients within the first year after surgery and in 3.2 to 5.7% after 5 yr have elapsed (4).

CLINICAL MANIFESTATIONS

Symptomatic IE likely arises within several weeks of the initiating bacteremia, although in some patients with perioperative infection of new implanted prosthetic valves, overt symptoms may be delayed for more than 2 mo (4). The IE syndrome may be acute in onset with hectic fevers and chills, multiple extracardiac manifestations, and rapid development of intracardiac complications or a very indolent illness with modest fevers, night sweats, anorexia, weight loss, infrequent extracardiac complications, and little or no progressive intracardiac injury. In fact, the presentations of IE are a continuum between these two extremes, i.e., between acute and subacute endocarditis. The temporal evolution of IE is in large part a function of the causative microorganism. *Staphylococcus aureus* and β-hemolytic streptococci usually result in acute presentations. In contrast, viridans streptococci, enterococci, coagulase-negative staphylococci, and the fastidious Gram-negative coccobacilli, organisms often referred to by the acronym HACEK (*Haemophilus parainfluenzae, Haemophilus aphrophilus, Haemophilus paraprophilus, Actinobacillus actinomycetemcomitans, Cardiobacterium hominis, Eikenella corrodens,* and *Kingella kingae*) give rise to subacute endocarditis. *Bartonella* species and *Coxiella burnetii* (the rickettsia-like agent that causes Q fever), organisms associated with blood culture-negative IE, also cause indolent IE.

From: *Essential Cardiology: Principles and Practice, 2nd Ed.*
Edited by: C. Rosendorff © Humana Press Inc., Totowa, NJ

Table 1
Signs and Symptoms in Patients With Infective Endocarditis

Symptoms	Percent	Signs	Percent
Fever	80–85	Fever	80–90
Chills	40–75	Heart murmur	80–85
Sweats	25	Changing or new murmur	10–40
Anorexia	25–55	Systemic emboli	20–50
Weight loss	25–35	Splenomegaly	15–50
Malaise	25–40	Clubbing	10–20
Cough	25	Osler's nodes	7–10
Stroke	15–20	Splinter hemorrhage	5–15
Headache	15–40	Janeway's lesions	2–10
Myalgia/arthralgia	15–30	Retinal lesions (Roth spots)	2–10
Back pain	7–14	Petechiae	10–40
Confusion	10–20		

Adapted from refs. *84, 85.*

Nonspecific signs and symptoms are characteristic of IE (Table 1); nevertheless, in the appropriate context these clinical features should suggest the diagnosis. These settings include patients with cardiac conditions that are substrates for infection, patients with behavior patterns that predispose to endocarditis (injecting drug use), and bacteremia due to organisms that commonly cause IE. In addition, progressive cardiac valvular dysfunction or arterial emboli in the context of a nonspecific febrile illness should prompt consideration of IE.

Fever, the most common clinical feature of IE, may be absent or minimal in those who are severely debilitated or who have congestive heart failure or chronic renal failure. IE caused by coagulase-negative staphylococci or *Tropheryma whippelii* (the cause of Whipple disease) may present with little or no fever *(5).* The purported increased frequency of muted presentations of IE among the elderly has not been confirmed *(6,7).*

Heart murmurs in patients with IE involving native heart valves (NVE) commonly reflects the valve pathology that predisposed the patient to IE. With acute *S. aureus* NVE, a process often engrafted on previously normal heart valves, murmurs are detected in only 30 to 45% of patients on presentation but ultimately develop in 85%. Murmurs are often not heard in tricuspid valve endocarditis or in pacemaker-related IE. Murmurs reflecting new or progressive valve dysfunction rather than alterations in cardiac output are most commonly encountered in patients with acute IE or PVE and are less frequent in subacute NVE.

The classic noncardiac manifestations of IE—splenomegaly, petechiae, Osler's nodes, Janeway lesions, Roth spots, and splinter hemorrhages—are found less frequently today than several decades ago. Since many of these occur as a consequence of long-standing infection, this change likely represents the increasingly prompt diagnosis of endocarditis. None of these are pathognomonic for IE. Splinter hemorrhages, linear or flame-shaped lesions beneath the nails of the fingers or toes, associated with IE are found proximally in the nails. Those seen at the distal nail margin are most likely due to trauma.

Arthralgias, myalgias, true arthritis with nonspecific inflammatory synovial fluid, and localized back pain are common symptoms that remit rapidly with antimicrobial therapy. These focal skeletal symptoms must be distinguished from metastatic infection, which may require additional therapy, including drainage.

Arterial emboli, which are evident clinically in up to 50% of patients and are also frequently subclinical, discovered only at autopsy, are associated with significant morbidity and mortality in NVE and PVE *(6,8,9).* Systemic emboli are more common in patients with left-sided vegetations that exceed 10 mm in diameter (by echocardiogram) and that are located on the mitral valve, particularly on the anterior leaflet *(10–13).* Emboli are often a presenting symptom in patients with

IE. After initiation of appropriate therapy the frequency of emboli decreases rapidly from 13 per 1000 patient days during the initial treatment week to <1.2 per 1000 patient days during the third week of effective therapy *(14)*. Emboli that occur late during treatment are not in themselves evidence of failed antimicrobial therapy. Renal emboli may cause gross or microscopic hematuria but rarely result in clinically important renal dysfunction.

Neurologic symptoms and complications occur in as many as 40% of patients and are particularly prominent when infection is due to *S. aureus (6,15–17)*. Embolic stroke syndromes occur in 10 to 25% of patients and are the most common neurologic consequences of IE; less common complications include mycotic aneurysm, intracranial hemorrhage, meningitis (either aseptic or occasionally purulent), cerebritis with microabscess formation, seizures, and encephalopathy *(15–17)*. Intracranial hemorrhage, which occurs in 5% of cases, results from hemorrhagic infarction, rupture of an artery due to septic arteritis at a site of embolic occlusion, or rupture of a mycotic aneurysm. Surgically drainable brain abscesses are uncommon in IE, whereas microabscesses of brain and meninges occur in patients with IE due to *S. aureus*.

Disruptions or distortion of left heart valves or rupture of chordae tendinae with subsequent valvular insufficiency may result in congestive heart failure. Heart failure due to aortic valve insufficiency generally progresses more rapidly than that due to mitral valve regurgitation. Similar hemodynamic consequences are seen with mechanical and bioprosthetic PVE due to valve dehiscence with paravalvular leakage or to destruction or disruption of valve parts. Bulky vegetations may obstruct the orifice of a mitral prosthesis, resulting in functional stenosis *(4)*.

Renal dysfunction in patients with IE most commonly results from reduced cardiac output or antimicrobial toxicity. Glomerulonephritis due to deposition of circulating immune complexes on the glomerular basement membrane results in renal dysfunction, which may progress during initial therapy but then gradually improves with continued antimicrobial treatment.

DIAGNOSIS

To avoid overlooking the diagnosis of IE a high index of suspicion must be maintained. A sensitive and specific diagnostic schema, the Duke criteria, was developed using predispositions plus the clinical, laboratory, and echocardiographic features of IE *(18)*. Using these clinical criteria, 74 and 26% of more than 300 pathologically proven IE cases were classified as definite and possible IE, respectively, and none were rejected *(19)*. Similarly, among 1395 clinically diagnosed cases, 55 and 35% were classified by the Duke criteria as definite or possible, respectively; the 10% rejection rate often resulted from a suboptimal echocardiographic evaluation at the time of initial diagnosis *(7,19)*. Study of rejected cases suggested that the negative predictive value and specificity were high *(19)*. However, the Duke criteria accepted as possible IE some cases considered by the experts to not have IE, i.e., made a false positive diagnosis by comparison with experts. To address the somewhat reduced specificity that resulted from the limited capability to reject cases and the resulting expanded possible category, Li and colleagues suggested a modification of the Duke criteria that has been widely accepted *(20)*. The modified Duke criteria (Tables 2 and 3) included evidence of infection by *C. burnetii* as a major criterion. Additionally, the modified criteria require that one major plus one minor criterion or three minor criteria be present before cases are classified as possible IE and treated *(20)*.

The Duke diagnostic schema appropriately emphasizes the role of bacteremia (blood cultures) and echocardiography in the evaluation of patients with potential IE. Endocarditis is characterized by sustained low-density (<100 organisms/mL) bacteremia. Among patients with IE who have not had prior antimicrobial therapy and who ultimately will have positive blood cultures, at least 95% of all blood cultures will be positive and in 98% of cases one of the first two sets will yield the causative organism. The diagnostic criteria give weight to both the persistence of bacteremia as well as the specific organism isolated. Bacteremia with organisms rarely encountered in the absence of IE (viridans streptococci, HACEK group) are thus highly suggestive, whereas organisms associated with endocarditis as well as other infections (enterococci) must be encountered in the absence

Table 2
Criteria for Diagnosis of Infective Endocarditis

Definitive infective endocarditis
  Pathologic criteria
    Microorganisms: demonstrated by culture or histology in a vegetation, *or* in a vegetation that has
      embolized, *or* in an intracardiac abscess, *or*
    Pathologic lesions: vegetation or intracardiac abscess present, confirmed by histology showing active
      endocarditis
  Clinical criteria, using specific definitions listed in Table 3
    2 major criteria, *or*
    1 major and 3 minor criteria, *or*
    5 minor criteria
Possible infective endocarditis
  1 major criterion and 1 minor criterion, *or*
  3 minor criteria
Rejected
  Firm alternative diagnosis for manifestations of endocarditis, *or*
  Sustained resolution of manifestations of endocarditis, with antibiotic therapy for 4 d or less, *or*
  No pathologic evidence of infective endocarditis at surgery or autopsy, after antibiotic therapy for 4 d or less

Adapted from ref. *20*.

Table 3
Terminology Used in Criteria for the Diagnosis of Infective Endocarditis (Table 2)

Major criteria
  Positive blood culture
    Typical microorganism for infective endocarditis from two separate blood cultures
      Viridans streptococci, *Streptococcus bovis*, HACEK group, *Staphylococcus aureus, or*
      Community-acquired enterococci, in the absence of a primary focus, *or*
    Persistently positive blood culture, defined as recovery of a microorganism consistent with infective
      endocarditis from:
      a. Blood cultures drawn more than 12 h apart, *or*
      b. All of three or a majority of four or more separate blood cultures, with first and last drawn at least
        1 h apart
    Positive blood culture for *C. burnetii* or antiphase I IgG antibody titer >1:800
  Evidence of endocardial involvement
    Positive echocardiogram
      a. Oscillating intracardiac mass, on valve or supporting structures, *or* in the path of regurgitant jets,
        or on implanted material, in the absence of an alternative anatomic explanation, *or*
      b. Abscess, *or*
      c. New partial dehiscence of prosthetic valve, *or*
    New valvular regurgitation (increase or change in preexisting murmur not sufficient)
Minor criteria
  Predisposition: predisposing heart condition *or* intravenous drug use
  Fever ≥38.0°C (100.4°F)
  Vascular phenomena: major arterial emboli, septic pulmonary infarcts, mycotic aneurysm, intracranial
    hemorrhage, conjunctival hemorrhages, Janeway lesions
  Immunologic phenomena: glomerulonephritis, Osler's nodes, Roth spots, rheumatoid factor
  Microbiologic evidence: positive blood culture but not meeting major criterion as noted previously[a]
    or serologic evidence of active infection with organism consistent with infective endocarditis

[a]Excluding single positive cultures for coagulase-negative staphylococci and organisms that do not cause endocarditis.
  HACEK, *Haemophilus* species, *Actinobacillus actinomycetemcomitans, Cardiobacterium hominis, Eikenella* species,
Kingella kingae. (Adapted from ref. *20*.)

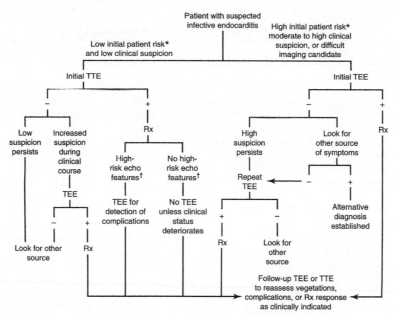

Fig. 1. An approach to the diagnostic use of echocardiography. *, *See* Table 9. †, High-risk echocardiographic features include large or mobile vegetation, valvular insufficiency, suggestion of perivalvular infection, prosthetic valve. (Adapted from ref. *19*.)

of another site of infection in order to rank as a major criterion. Organisms that commonly contaminate blood cultures, e.g., coagulase-negative staphylococci or diphtheroids, or that rarely cause IE, e.g., *Enterobacteriaceae*, must be isolated from blood repetitively or from multiple cultures as a single molecular clone (coagulase-negative staphylococci) and in the absence of an alternative infection in order to be used as a criterion *(18,19)*.

Incorporation of specifically defined echocardiographic findings characteristic of IE as a criterion markedly enhances the clinical utility of the schema and recognizes the high sensitivity and specificity of two-dimensional echocardiography *(21–25)*. Echocardiography is not recommended as a screening test for febrile or bacteremic patients when endocarditis is unlikely; however, all patients suspected of having IE should be studied by echocardiogram (Fig. 1) *(19)*.

DIAGNOSTIC TESTING

Blood Cultures

In patients with suspected endocarditis who have not received an antibiotic recently, three blood cultures, obtained from separate venipuncture sites and spaced over 24 h independent of temperature elevations, are sufficient to isolate the causative organism and to demonstrate the persistence of bacteremic characteristic of IE (Table 4, Fig. 2). If blood cultures remain negative after 48 to 72 h and fungi or fastidious organisms are suspected, additional cultures should be obtained, possibly using special techniques such as the lysis contrifugation system or a biphasic system *(19, 26)*. When initial routine blood cultures appear to be negative, the microbiology laboratory should be advised that IE is suspected so that it can prolong the incubation of the cultures and, where appropriate, to perform special subcultures to isolate unusual organisms *(1,19,26)*. From 5 to 15% of patients with IE diagnosed clinically have negative blood cultures *(27)*. Prior receipt of antimicrobials accounts for 35 to 50% of these blood culture-negative cases. The remainder are a consequence of infection with organisms that have fastidious growth requirements *(19,27)*. In hemodynamically stable patients with subacute presentations of suspected IE who have received antibiotics within the previous 2 wk, empiric antibiotic therapy should be delayed to allow time for additional

Table 4
Evaluation of Patients With Suspected Endocarditis[a]

Timing	Test or procedure	Comment
Admission (prior to admission if stable)	CBC[b], differential, 3 blood cultures[c], urine analysis, electrocardiogram, creatinine, bilirubin, AST[b], alkaline phosphatase, prothrombin time, chest roentgenogram	Tests, other than blood cultures, do not aid with diagnosis but establish baseline for assessing the complications of IE or treatment
After admission 24 to 48 h Blood culture positive	TTE	TEE is the initial study of choice with suspected prosthetic valve IE
48 to 72 h Blood cultures positive but TTE negative or blood cultures and TTE negative	TEE	See Fig. 2 and text regarding initiation of therapy
72 to 96 h Blood cultures negative	Two blood cultures daily for 2 days[c], ESR[b], rheumatoid factor, circulating immune complex titer	ESR, circulating immune complex titer, and rheumatoid factor add little value if blood cultures and echocardiogram are positive. May contribute to minor diagnostic criterion
Day 5 to 10 Blood cultures remain negative (no antibiotics given)	Serologic testing and special blood cultures for fastidious organisms Retrieve material embolic to a peripheral artery for culture histologic examination, molecular testing Repeat TEE if initially negative	See text: Diagnosis; Causative Microorganisms. Obtain infectious disease consultation and advice of microbiology laboratory director. Consider empiric therapy (Fig. 2, see text) Increases the yield for vegetations
Any time Focal central nervous system symptoms or finding suggesting localized event	Computerized tomography (with enhancement). If evidence of hemorrhage without mass effect, consider magnetic resonance angiogram or formal angiogram. If no mass effect, consider lumbar puncture	Consider mycotic aneurysm; with acute S. aureus IE or new focal symptoms without infarct, consider angiography
Left upper quadrant pain (with/without left shoulder pain)	Image spleen (and kidney) for abscess or infarct	
Intracardiac complication: hemodynamic deterioration, suspected paravalvular infection	Electrocardiogram, echocardiogram	Electrocardiographic conduction change insensitive indicator of paravalvular abscess. TEE optimal technique

[a]For patients who are hemodynamically stable and have a subacute presentation.
[b]CBC, complete blood count; AST, aspartate aminotransferase; ESR, erythrocyte sedimentation rate.
[c]Request that laboratory incubate blood cultures for 3 wk (indicate diagnosis of infective endocarditis). (Adapted from ref. 85.)

blood cultures to be obtained without the confounding effects of further antibiotic therapy *(19)*. This delay, while potentially enhancing culture yields, is unlikely to allow otherwise preventable complications. In contrast, among patients with acute presentations or with deteriorating hemodynamics, empiric therapy should be initiated immediately after the initial cultures have been obtained.

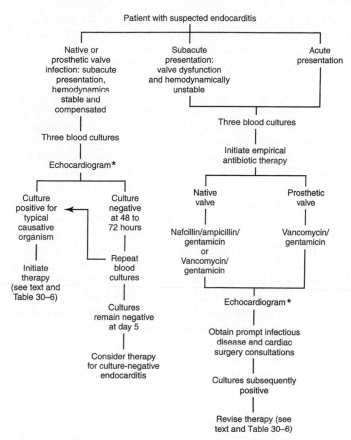

Fig. 2. An approach to the initiation of therapy in patients with suspected infective endocarditis. *Can initially evaluate by transthoracic approach; however, transesophageal views are required for maximal evaluation and are essential in patients with prosthetic valves.

If after 5 d initial blood cultures remain negative (not attributable to confounding antimicrobial therapy), serologic testing to identify infection caused by pathogens that are difficult or unlikely to be recovered from blood (*Brucella, Bartonella, Legionella, C. burnetii*, and some fungi) should be considered *(19,26)* (Table 4, Fig. 2). If valve tissue or embolized vegetations become available from these patients, not only should the material be cultured and examined by special microscopic techniques, but also the organism's identity should be sought by using the polymerase chain reaction to recover specific microbial DNA or 16S rRNA *(1,28)*.

Echocardiography

Echocardiographic evaluation with color flow and continuous as well as pulsed Doppler allows anatomic confirmation of IE, identifies intracardiac complications, and allows functional assessment of the heart. Transthoracic echocardiography (TTE), while noninvasive and 98% specific for vegetations, detects vegetations in about 65% of clinical or anatomically established IE *(10,23)*. TTE is limited by vegetation size (≤2 mm in diameter) and in 20% of adults by body habitus, chest wall configuration, or lung disease. Furthermore, TTE is not adequate for the assessment of prosthetic valves (especially in the mitral position), or the detection of perivalvular abscess, leaflet perforations, or intracardiac fistulae *(21,25,29–31)*. In contrast, transesophageal echocardiography (TEE), which while invasive is extremely safe in the hands of experienced operators, detects vegetations in more than 90% of patients with proven NVE and 82 to 94% of patients with clinically diagnosed IE *(10,23,24)*. In patients with PVE, the sensitivity for detecting vegetations by TEE ranged from 74 to 96% while the sensitivity with TTE was 13 to 36% *(30,31)*. TEE is clearly the optimal technique for the diagnosis of PVE and the identification of complications that affect management *(29–31)*. TEE is more sensitive than TTE (78 to 87% vs 28%) in detecting paravalvular abscesses, intracardiac fistulae, and subaortic invasive infection, without loss of specificity *(21, 32)*. Although the sensitivity of TEE for detecting abnormalities indicative of NVE and PVE is very high, false negative studies occur in 6 to 18% of patients *(23,24,31)*. The rate of false negative studies can be reduced (4 to 13%) by repeat TEE and multiplane examinations *(24,25)*.

Assuming that all patients with definite or possible IE by the modified Duke criteria require treatment for endocarditis, when clinical and laboratory findings are considered, the incremental information gained from a TEE beyond that from a TTE infrequently alters the decision to treat for endocarditis *(33,34)*. For example, among 114 patients with suspected endocarditis studied by both TTE and TEE, 22 classified as possible IE using the TTE data were reclassified as definite IE based on TEE findings. Only two patients for whom the diagnosis of IE had been rejected were reclassified as possible IE based on the TEE and required treatment. Of the 24 patients wherein the classification was changed, 12 had PVE, including both who would have been rejected *(34)*. In patients at low risk of NVE, a negative high-quality TTE is generally sufficient to rule out endocarditis (Fig. 1) *(19,35)*. In moderate-risk patients TEE may be required to exclude IE. For example, a TEE was required to establish the diagnosis of IE in 9 of 16 patients wherein endocarditis resulted from catheter-associated *S. aureus* bacteremia *(36)*. Furthermore, decision analysis studies suggest that a TEE as the initial imaging study in these patients is cost effective *(35,37)*. Still, in patients at high risk of IE, a negative TEE is not sufficient to override clinical evidence and exclude the diagnosis *(19,24)*. Cardiac catheterization, magnetic resonance imaging, and scintigraphy with various isotopes offer little beyond echocardiography in the anatomic assessment of IE.

Other Studies

Complete blood counts and differential, creatinine, selected liver function tests, prothrombin time, urine analysis, chest radiography, and electrocardiogram are often followed serially and may be important in patient management (Table 4). Erythrocyte sedimentation rate, C-reactive protein, quantitative circulating immune complexes, immunoglobulin or cryoglobulin measurements, and rheumatoid factor are commonly abnormal in subacute IE but do not yield significant value beyond clinical observations when monitoring response to therapy. They may be useful if incorporated into a minor criterion in the Duke schema.

CAUSATIVE MICROORGANISMS

Although almost any bacteria or fungal species can cause IE, in fact, a relatively small number of bacterial species cause the majority of cases of IE (Table 5). *S. aureus* is the major organism causing acute NVE, whereas streptococci, enterococci, coagulase-negative staphylococci, and the HACEK group are the major causes of subacute NVE. β-Hemolytic streptococci, *S. pneumoniae*, and *Staphylococcus lugdenensis*, a coagulase-negative staphylococcus species, are associated with valve destruction and an acute presentation. Nosocomial NVE occurs as a complication of bacteremia associated with intravascular devices and genitourinary tract manipulations and is caused primarily by staphylococci and enterococci. In recent series of *S. aureus* IE, 35 to 46% had nosocomial infection *(38,39)*.

Patients with PVE can be divided into three groups: those with infection developing from perioperative events and having onset within 60 d of surgery (early PVE), those with onset 1 yr or more after surgery and most likely resulting from community-acquired transient bacteremia (late PVE), and those developing PVE between 2 and 12 mo after valve surgery. The causes of early PVE are largely coagulase-negative staphylococci, *S. aureus*, Gram-negative bacilli, and fungi (primarily *Candida* species). The frequencies of organisms causing late-onset PVE are similar to those noted in community-acquired NVE, except that there is an increased frequency of coagulase-negative

Table 5
Microbiology of Infective Endocarditis in Specific Clinical Settings

| | Number of cases (%) | | | | | | | |
| | Native valve endocarditis | | Prosthetic valve endocarditis Time of onset after valve surgery | | | Endocarditis in drug addicts | | |
Organism	Community acquired n = 683	Nosocomial n = 82	<2 mo n = 144	2–12 mo n = 31	>12 mo n = 194	Right-sided n = 346	Left-sided n = 204	Total N = 675
Streptococci[a]	220 (32)	6 (7)	2 (1)	3 (9)	61 (31)	17 (5)	31 (15)	80 (12)
Pneumococci	8 (1)	—	—	—	—	—	—	—
Enterococci	57 (8)	13 (16)	12 (8)	4 (12)	22 (11)	7 (2)	49 (24)	59 (9)
Staphylococcus aureus	241 (35)	45 (55)	32 (22)	4 (12)	34 (18)	267 (77)	47 (23)	396 (57)
Coagulase-negative staphylococci	29 (4)	8 (10)	47 (33)	11 (32)	22 (11)	—	—	—
Fastidious Gram-negative coccobacilli (HACEK Group)[b]	22 (3)	—	—	—	11 (6)	—	—	—
Gram-negative bacilli	22 (3)	4 (5)	19 (13)	1 (3)	11 (6)	17 (5)	26 (13)	45 (7)
Fungi, Candida species	5 (1)	3 (4)	12 (8)	4 (12)	3 (1)	—	25 (12)	26 (4)
Polymicrobial/Miscellaneous	41 (6)	1 (1)	4 (3)	2 (6)	9 (5)	28 (8)	20 (10)	48 (7)
Diphtheroids	—	—	9 (6)	—	5 (3)	—	—	1 (0.1)
Culture negative	38 (5)	2 (2)	7 (5)	2 (6)	16 (8)	10 (3)	6 (3)	20 (3)

[a]Includes viridans streptococci, Streptococcus bovis, other nongroup A, groupable streptococci, Abiotrophic species (nutritionally variant streptococci).
[b]Includes Haemophilus species, Actinobacillus actinomycetemcomitans, Cardiobacterium hominis, Eikenella species, and Kingella kingae.
Adapted from ref. 85.

573

staphylococci. Coagulase-negative staphylococci causing PVE within 12 mo of valve surgery are predominantly *Staphylococcus epidermidis* and 85% are methicillin-resistant, whereas 50% of those causing PVE 1 yr or more after surgery are nonepidermidis species and only 30% are methicillin-resistant *(4)*.

Among injecting drug users, *S. aureus* causes more than 50% of all IE and 70% of tricuspid valve IE (Table 5). Streptococci and enterococci infect previously abnormal left heart valves in these patients. IE due to Gram-negative bacilli, particularly *Pseudomonas aeruginosa*, and fungi occur with increased frequency among drug users. Unusual organisms, e.g., *Corynebacterium, Lactobacillus, Bacillus cereus*, and polymicrobial infections, possibly related to injection of contaminated materials, are seen occasionally in drug users with IE. Infective endocarditis in patients with underlying human immunodeficiency virus (HIV) infection occurs primarily among injecting drug abusers; its microbiology is very similar to IE in drug abusers in general *(40)*.

Many unusual and fastidious organisms cause IE *(26)*. Some cause IE in unique epidemiologic settings, e.g., *C. burnetii* in Europe, *Brucella* in the Middle East and Mediterranean basin; others are associated with unique clinical situations, e.g., *Legionella* and *Mycobacterium chelonei*, and *Mycoplasma hominis* on prosthetic valves; and some appear to be sporadic events. *Bartonella* species have been implicated increasingly as a cause of IE, often with negative blood cultures, and may account for as many as 3% of cases of IE overall *(41)*. *T. whippelii* has been identified as a cause of very indolent, afebrile IE *(5)*.

ANTIMICROBIAL THERAPY

Antimicrobial therapy capable of killing (as opposed to only inhibiting growth of) the organism causing IE is required for optimal treatment. The recommended therapies are based on the precise susceptibility of the etiologic agent combined with prior clinical experience with that species, but must be adjusted in consideration of circumstances unique to the patient, i.e., allergies, end-organ dysfunction, interactions with other required medications or other perceived risks of adverse events. Accordingly, it is crucial to identify the causative organism (*see* Diagnostic Testing, Blood Cultures). The impact of beginning empiric antimicrobial therapy immediately after blood cultures have been obtained must be carefully considered (Fig. 2). In patients with acute endocarditis or with severely compromised hemodynamics who will require urgent valve surgery, rapid initiation of therapy may prevent further cardiac structural damage or reduce the risk of recrudescent infection after valve surgery. However, among hemodynamically stable patients with subacute IE, especially if antibiotics have been given during the prior 2 wk, therapy should be delayed for 2 to 5 d while awaiting blood culture results. If initial cultures remain negative, blood cultures should be repeated (Table 4, Fig. 2).

Organism-Specific Regimens

Expert committees have developed regimens for the treatment of IE caused by the more commonly encountered causative microorganisms (Table 6) *(1,42)*. Regimens for treatment of IE involving native and prosthetic valves are usually qualitatively similar (except for staphylococcal infection) but treatment for PVE is given for several weeks longer than that for NVE. In general, compromises in recommended dosing, duration, and route of administration should be avoided unless supported by medical literature and required by untoward events.

STREPTOCOCCAL IE

Most viridans streptococci and *Streptococcus bovis* that cause IE are susceptible to penicillin (minimum inhibitory concentration [MIC] ≤0.1 µg/mL). IE caused by these organisms can be treated with any of the recommended regimens (Table 6, 1A–E). IE caused by nutritionally deficient streptococci (now assigned to the genera *Abiotrophia*), PVE, or complicated streptococcal NVE should not be treated with the 2-wk regimen (Table 6, 1C). The ceftriaxone regimen (Table 6, 1D) can be used in patients with a history of an allergy to penicillin that does not result in urticaria or anaphylaxis-like symptoms (immediate-type allergy). In patients who have had an immediate-type

Table 6
Recommended Therapy for IE Caused by Specific Organisms

Infecting organism	Antibiotic	Dose and route[a]	Duration wk	Comments
1. Penicillin-susceptible viridans streptococci, *Streptococcus bovis*, and other streptococci, penicillin MIC ≤0.1 μg/mL	A. Penicillin G	12–18 million units iv daily in divided doses q4h	4	
	B. Penicillin G	12–18 million units iv daily in divided doses q4h	4	Avoid aminoglycoside-containing regimens when potential for nephrotoxicity or ototoxicity is increased
	plus gentamicin	1 mg/kg IM or iv q8h	2	
	C. Penicillin G plus gentamicin	Same doses as noted above	2	*See* text
	D. Ceftriaxone	2 g iv or IM daily as single dose	4	Can be used in patients with nonimmediate penicillin allergy; intramuscular ceftriaxone is painful
	E. Vancomycin[b]	30 mg/kg iv in divided doses q12h	4	Use for patients with immediate or severe penicillin or cephalosporin allergy. Infuse doses over 1 h to avoid histamine release reaction (red man syndrome)
2. Relatively penicillin-resistant streptococci Penicillin MIC 0.2 to 0.5 μg/mL	A. Penicillin G	18–24 million units iv daily in divided doses q4h	4	
	plus gentamicin	1 mg/kg im or iv q8h	2	
Penicillin MIC >0.5 μg/mL	B. Penicillin G plus gentamicin	*See* regimens recommended for enterococcal endocarditis	4	Preferred for nutritionally variant (pyridoxal- or cysteine-requiring) streptococci
3. Enterococci (in vitro evaluation for MIC to penicillin and vancomycin, β-lactamase production, and high-level resistance to gentamicin and streptomycin required)	A. Penicillin G	18–30 million units iv daily in divided doses q4h	4–6	*See* text for use of streptomycin instead of gentamicin in these regimens.
	plus gentamicin	1–1.5 mg/kg iv q8h		Four weeks of therapy recommended for patients with shorter history of illness (<3 mo) who respond promptly to treatment
	B. Ampicillin	12 g iv daily in divided doses q4h	4–6	
	plus gentamicin	Same dose as noted above	4–6	
	C. Vancomycin[b]	30 mg/kg iv daily in divided doses q12h	4–6	Use for patients with penicillin allergy; do not use cephalosporins
	plus gentamicin	Same dose as noted above	4–6	

(continued)

575

Table 6 (Continued)

Infecting organism	Antibiotic	Dose and route[a]	Duration wk	Comments
4. Staphylococci infecting native valves (assume penicillin resistance) Methicillin-susceptible	A. Nafcillin or oxacillin plus optimal addition of gentamicin	12 g iv daily in divided doses q4h	6	Penicillin 18–24 million units daily in divided doses q4h can be used instead of nafcillin, oxacillin, or cefazolin if strains do not produce β-lactamase.
		1 mg/kg iv q8h	3–5 d	
	B. Cefazolin plus optional addition of gentamicin	2 g iv q8h	6	Other first-generation cephalosporin in equivalent doses can be used
		Same dose as above	3–5 d	
	C. Vancomycin[b]	30 mg/kg iv in divided doses q12h	6	Use for patients with immediate penicillin allergy
5. Staphylococci infecting native valves, methicillin-resistant	A. Vancomycin[b]	30 mg/kg iv in divided doses q12h	6	
6. Staphylococci infecting prosthetic valves, methicillin-susceptible (assume penicillin-resistance)	A. Nafcillin or oxacillin plus gentamicin plus rifampin[c]	12 g iv daily in divided doses q4h	6	First-generation cephalosporin or vancomycin could be used in penicillin-allergic patients. Uses gentamicin during initial 2 wk. See text for alternatives for gentamicin. For patients with immediate penicillin allergy, use regimen 7.
		1 mg/kg iv or im q8h	2	
		300 mg po q8h	6	
7. Staphylococci infecting prosthetic valves, methicillin-resistant	A. Vancomycin[b]	30 mg/kg iv in divided doses q12h	6	Use gentamicin during the initial 2 wk of therapy. See text for alternatives to gentamicin. Do not substitute a cephalosporin or imipenem for vancomycin.
	plus gentamicin	1 mg/kg iv or im q8h	2	
	plus rifampin[c]	300 mg po q8h	6	
8. HACEK organisms[d]	A. Cefriaxone	2 g iv or im daily as a single dose	4	Cefotaxime or other third-generation cephalosporin in comparable doses may be used.
	B. Ampicillin	12 q iv daily in divided doses q4h	4	Test organism for β-lactamase production. Do not use this regimen if β-lactamase is produced.
	plus gentamicin	1 mg/kg iv or im q8h	4	

[a]Recommended doses are for adults with normal renal and hepatic function. Doses of gentamicin, streptomycin, and vancomycin must be adjusted in patients with renal dysfunction. Use ideal body weight to calculate doses (men = 50 kg + 2.3 kg per inch over 5 feet; women = 45.5 kg plus 2.3 kg per inch over 5 feet).

[b]Peak levels obtained 1 h after completion of the infusion should be 30 to 45 μg/mL.

[c]Rifampin increases the dose of warfarin or dicumarol required for effective anticoagulation.

[d]HACEK organisms are *Haemophilus parainfluenzae, Haemophilus aphrophilus, Actinobacillus actinomycetemcomitans, Cardiobacterium hominis, Eikenella corrodens, Kingella kingae.* (From ref. 86.)

MIC, minimum inhibitory concentration.

allergic reaction to penicillin or a cephalosporin, treatment with vancomycin is recommended (Table 6, 1E). In patients with normal renal function, uncomplicated NVE caused by penicillin-susceptible viridans streptococci has been effectively treated with a 2-wk regimen using 2 g ceftriaxone IV plus an aminoglycoside (netilmicin 4 mg/kg/d or gentamicin 3 mg/kg/d), each given as a single daily dose *(43,44)*. Because experience with short-course therapy using aminoglycosides in single daily doses is very limited, this approach has not been incorporated into recommendations. Combination therapy with penicillin or ceftriaxone for 6 wk plus gentamicin (1 mg/kg ideal body weight every 8 h) during the first 2 wk is advocated for treatment or PVE caused by penicillin-susceptible streptococci.

Endocarditis caused by streptococci that are relatively resistant to penicillin (MIC ≥0.2 µg/mL but <0.5 µg/mL) and IE caused by group B streptococci (*S. agalactiae*) is treated with combination therapy (Table 6, 2A). If these patients report an immediate-type β-lactam allergy, vancomycin therapy is recommended (Table 6, 1E), whereas for those with milder penicillin allergies ceftriaxone can be substituted for penicillin. IE caused by even more resistant streptococci (penicillin MIC >0.5 µg/mL) is treated with a regimen used for enterococcal IE (Table 6, 3A). IE caused by nutritionally deficient streptococci (*Abiotrophia* sp.) is treated with penicillin plus gentamicin or streptomycin (Table 6, 3A or B) or vancomycin alone for 6 wk.

ENTEROCOCCAL IE

Enterococci are inhibited but not killed by penicillin, ampicillin, or vancomycin and are resistant to cephalosporins and antistaphylococcal penicillinase-resistant penicillins, e.g., nafcillin, oxacillin, or cloxacillin. Optimal antimicrobial therapy for enterococcal IE requires a bactericidal synergistic interaction between a cell wall active antibiotic (penicillin, ampicillin, vancomycin, or teicoplanin [not available in the United States]) that at clinically achievable concentrations inhibits the organism and an aminoglycoside (gentamicin or streptomycin) for which the organism does not have high-level resistance *(45)*. If high concentrations of streptomycin (2000 µg/mL) or gentamicin (500 to 2000 µg/mL) fail to inhibit the growth of an enterococcus, i.e., there is high-level resistance, the aminoglycoside cannot exert a lethal effect or contribute to bactericidal synergism. High-level resistance to gentamicin predicts the inefficacy of kanamycin, amikacin, tobramycin, and netilmicin as well. Additionally, the ability of aminoglycosides other than streptomycin or gentamicin to contribute to synergy, even against organisms not highly resistant to gentamicin, is unpredictable; thus, they should not be used to treat enterococcal IE.

Each of the standard regimens recommended for the treatment of enterococcal IE combines a cell wall active agent and gentamicin and anticipates that a synergistic bactericidal effect will be achieved (Table 6, 3A–C). If the causative enterococcus does not exhibit high-level resistance to streptomycin, this aminoglycoside (9.5 mg/kg ideal body weight given intramuscularly or intravenously every 12 h to achieve peak serum concentrations of 20 µg/mL) can be used in lieu of gentamicin. When there is a history of an allergic reaction to a penicillin, the patient with enterococcal IE must be treated with vancomycin plus an aminoglycoside (Table 6, 3C) or undergo desensitization and subsequent treatment with a penicillin or ampicillin regimen (Table 6, 3A or B). Cephalosporins are ineffective. Aminoglycosides are not administered in single daily doses. A bacteriologic cure can be achieved in 85% of patients with enterococcal NVE or PVE who are treated with a synergistic combination regimen.

Enterococci have become increasingly resistant, and regimens that were previously predictably effective now require careful assessment. To structure an effective regimen, the enterococcus must be tested for its susceptibility to ampicillin and vancomycin, for β-lactamase production, and for high-level resistance to gentamicin and streptomycin. With this information, a synergistic bactericidal regimen can be designed, if possible, or alternative nonbactericidal single drug therapy can be considered (Table 7). Treatment with an aminoglycoside if synergy cannot be effected—e.g., high-level resistance is present to both streptomycin and gentamicin or treatment does not include a cell wall active antibiotic—is inappropriate; it offers no benefit and may result in significant toxicity.

Table 7
Strategy for Selecting Therapy for Enterococcal Endocarditis Caused by Strains Resistant to Components of the Standard Regimen

I.   Ideal therapy includes a cell-wall active agent plus an effective aminoglycoside (streptomycin or gentamicin) to achieve bactericidal synergy

II. Cell-wall active antimicrobial
   A. Determine MIC for ampicillin and vancomycin; test for β-lactamase production (nitrocefin test)
   B. If ampicillin- and vancomycin-susceptible, use ampicillin
   C. If ampicillin-resistant (MIC ≥16 μg/mL), use vancomycin
   D. If β-lactamase produced, use vancomycin or consider ampicillin-sulbactam
   E. If ampicillin-resistant and vancomycin-resistant (MIC ≥16 μg/mL), consider teicoplanin[a]
   F. If ampicillin-resistant and highly resistant to vancomycin and teicoplanin (MIC ≥256 μg/mL), *see* IV.

III. Aminoglycoside to be used with cell-wall active antimicrobial
   A. Test for high-level resistance to streptomycin (growth in media with 2000 μg/mL) and gentamicin (growth in media with 500–2000 μg/mL)
   B. If no high-level resistance, use gentamicin; if high-level resistance to gentamicin but no high-level resistance to streptomycin, use streptomycin
   C. If high-level resistance to gentamicin and streptomycin, omit aminoglycoside therapy; use prolonged therapy with cell-wall active antimicrobial (8–12 wk) (*see* II, B–E)

IV. Alternative regimens and approaches
   A. Treatment with chloramphenicol, tetracyclines, fluoroquinolones, rifampin, or trimethoprim-sulfamethoxazole of questionable efficacy
   B. Limited experience suggest possible efficacy of linezolid or daptomycin
   C. Consider quinupristin/dalfopristin therapy for IE due to susceptible *E. faecium*
   D. Consider surgery during suppressive therapy with cell-wall active antimicrobial (II) or an alternative regimen (IV B,C)

[a]Not approved by the Food and Drug Administration for use in the United States.

Prolonged administration of aminoglycosides, as recommended for treatment of enterococcal IE, is often associated with nephrotoxicity or otovestibular toxicity. If significant aminoglycoside toxicity arises, the aminoglycoside arm of the regimen often can be truncated without loss of efficacy. Among 93 patients with enterococcal IE, 75 (81%) were cured with combination regimens wherein the aminoglycoside component was administered a median of 15 d *(46)*. Of the 75 who were cured, 40 (who did undergo surgery) were cured with less than 22 d of aminoglycoside therapy.

STAPHYLOCOCCAL IE

More than 95% of *S. aureus* and coagulase-negative staphylococci produce a β-lactamase and thus are resistant to penicillin. Many *S. aureus,* those acquired both nosocomially and in the community, and many coagulase-negative staphylococci are resistant to methicillin also (which implies resistance to all available β-lactam antibiotics). These organisms remain largely susceptible to vancomycin. Although IE caused by a staphylococcus susceptible to penicillin could be effectively treated by that drug, such strains are so infrequent that the regimens recommended for the treatment of staphylococcal IE are organized around susceptibility or resistance to methicillin (the penicillinase-resistant penicillins) and the valve(s) involved, and infection of a prosthetic valve (Table 6, 4A–C, 5–7, Fig. 3). Whether strains are coagulase-positive (*S. aureus)* or negative does not affect antimicrobial selection beyond susceptibility data.

Methicillin-susceptible staphylococcal infection of a native aortic or mitral valve should be treated with a parenteral penicillinase-resistant penicillin, e.g., nafcillin or oxacillin, plus gentamicin during the initial 3 to 5 d of treatment (Table 6, 6A). The addition of gentamicin seeks to achieve more rapid control of infection through the synergistic interaction of combination therapy. Longer courses of gentamicin are not recommended because nephrotoxicity is increased. Combination therapy has reduced the duration of bacteremia in these patients but has not been shown to reduce the mortality rates. Patients with a history of penicillin allergy can be treated with cefazolin or vancomycin, based on the nature of the allergic reaction (Table 6, 6B–C). Infection caused by methicil-

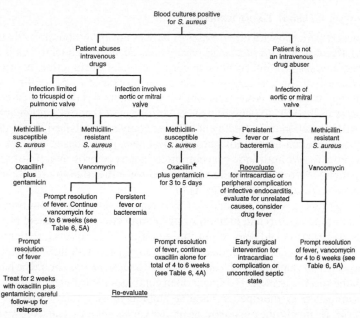

Fig. 3. Treatment of native valve endocarditis caused *by Staphylococcus aureus.* *, Can use nafcillin; for patient with penicillin allergy who is not anaphylactic/urticarial type, may use first-generation cephalosporin instead of oxacillin (Table 6, 4B). If patient has anaphylactic or immediate (urticarial) penicillin allergy, use vancomycin (Table 6, 4C) (Adapted from ref. *85*.)

lin-resistant staphylococci is treated with vancomycin (Table 6, 6C). In general, rifampin is not used to treat NVE due to staphylococci.

Isolated tricuspid valve endocarditis caused by methicillin-susceptible *S. aureus* that is not complicated by paravalvular extension or metastatic extracardiac focal infection can often be treated with a penicillinase-resistant penicillin plus gentamicin (1 mg/kg ideal body weight every 8 h) administered for only 2 wk *(47)*. A significant percentage of these patients may have prolonged fevers and require longer courses of treatment. Vancomycin does not appear to be a suitable alternative to the penicillinase-resistant penicillin in this short-course regimen, which effectively excludes highly penicillin-allergic patients and those infected with methicillin-resistant *S. aureus* from this short-course treatment.

A multiple drug regimen administered for 6 to 8 wk is recommended for the treatment of staphylococcal PVE (Table 6, 6A, 7A) *(4)*. Rifampin, because of its unique ability to kill staphylococci that are adherent to foreign materials or that are not replicating, is an essential component of optimal therapy. However, rifampin resistance emerges frequently in this setting even when rifampin is administered in combination with a β-lactam antibiotic or vancomycin. To prevent the emergence of rifampin resistance, a third antibiotic, preferably gentamicin if the staphylococcus is susceptible to achievable serum concentrations, is included in the initial 2 wk of treatment. If the staphylococcus is resistant to gentamicin, another aminoglycoside or a fluoroquinolone to which the organism is susceptible should be used *(4)*. Treatment for staphylococcal PVE should be initiated with a penicillinase-resistant penicillin or vancomycin plus gentamicin; rifampin should be added only after the susceptibility of the staphylococcus to gentamicin has been confirmed or an effective alternative to gentamicin has been initiated.

HACEK ENDOCARDITIS

β-lactamase production has been confirmed in some isolates resulting in resistance to ampicillin. Third-generation cephalosporins, to which HACEK organisms are exquisitely susceptible, are recommended for the treatment (Table 6, 8A).

OTHER ORGANISMS CAUSING ENDOCARDITIS

Limited clinical experience with other causes of IE does not allow consensus therapeutic recommendations *(26)*. IE caused by *Streptococcus pneumoniae* occurs infrequently but is highly destructive and often requires surgical intervention to correct valvular dysfunction. Mortality rates often exceed 35%. Because of the increasingly widespread resistance to penicillin among pneumococci, initial therapy with ceftriaxone plus vancomycin (Table 6, 1D and E) is recommended. If for the pneumococcus the MIC to penicillin or ceftriaxone is ≤1.0 μg/mL, either antimicrobial can be used; if the MIC is ≥2.0 μg/mL, treatment with vancomycin is advised. If pneumococcal IE is complicated by concomitant meningitis, therapy must be adjusted based on the susceptibility of the isolate to insure effective antibiotic concentrations in the cerebrospinal fluid *(48)*. Penicillin—or, in allergic patients, ceftriaxone—is recommended for initial therapy for the treatment of IE caused by *Streptococcus pyogenes* (Group A) *(42)*.

The preferred treatment for IE caused by *P. aeruginosa* combines an antipseudomonal penicillin (ticarcillin or piperacillin) and high doses of tobramycin (8 mg/kg ideal body weight daily in divided doses every 8 h to yield peak serum concentrations of 15 μg/mL). Patients with this form of endocarditis often experience intracardiac complications, persistent infection, and require valve replacement surgery. The treatment of IE caused by *Enterobacteriaceae* should be based on reported experience with the specific genera. Treatment often combines a third-generation cephalosporin or a carbapenem (imipenem or meropenem) and an aminoglycoside.

Corynebacterial IE involving prosthetic or native valves may be caused by various species, including *Corynebacterium jeikeium* and nontoxigenic *Corynebacterium diphtheriae*. Usually corynebacteria are susceptible to penicillin, aminoglycosides, and vancomycin. Aminoglycoside-susceptible strains are killed synergistically by these agents in combination with penicillin. Corynebacterial IE is generally treated with penicillin plus an aminoglycoside or with vancomycin *(49)*.

Optimum antibiotic therapy for *Bartonella* IE is not known. Aminoglycosides have bactericidal activity against *Bartonella*. Regimens that have included an aminoglycoside for two or more weeks, often administered in combination with a β-lactam antibiotic since therapy was initiated for apparently blood-culture-negative IE, have yielded higher cure rates than nonaminoglycoside-containing regimens *(50)*. Many of these patients have been undergoing valve replacement surgery. Some authors suggest several months of a fluoroquinolone as well. Outcomes have been inferior in patients treated with doxycycline without an aminoglycoside *(50)*.

Treatment of IE caused by *C. burnetii* with doxycycline plus a fluoroquinolone for periods ranging from 4 yr to indefinitely, with valve surgery as indicated, yields survival rates exceeding 90% *(51)*. Shorter courses (18 mo to 4 yr) of 100 mg doxycycline orally twice daily plus 200 mg hydroxychloroquine orally three times daily (adjusted subsequently to 150 to 800 mg daily to maintain a serum concentration of 0.8 to 1.2 μg/mL) were as effective as doxycycline plus a quinolone *(51)*. Photosensitivity, and potential phototoxicity, is a consequence of both regimens. Patients with acute Q fever who have valve abnormalities, especially with prosthetic valves, are at high risk of developing endocarditis. Endocarditis can be prevented by treating acute Q fever with doxycycline plus hydroxychloroquine for 1 to 15 mo *(52)*.

Amphotericin B, probably in a liposomal formulation and often combined with flucytosine, remains the antimicrobial of choice for treating fungal endocarditis, the majority of which is caused by *Candida* sp. and involves prosthetic valves *(53)*. Limited experience has suggested treatment of *Candida* IE should be followed by long-term, if not indefinite, suppression with fluconazole or an alternate trizole orally *(53)*.

CULTURE-NEGATIVE ENDOCARDITIS

In the absence of clinical or epidemiologic information that suggests a specific cause, culture-negative NVE is treated with ceftriaxone (or ampicillin) plus an aminoglycoside. Culture-negative PVE is treated with this regimen plus vancomycin. These recommendations are in part predicated on the unlikely possibility that, in the absence of confounding prior antimicrobial therapy, blood cultures would be negative if IE was caused by enterococci or *S. aureus* and that fastidious causes have been sought through serologic tests.

Monitoring Antimicrobial Therapy

Clinical and laboratory monitoring to assess the response to therapy and to allow prompt detection of complications of IE itself or of therapy is essential to allow timely revision of treatment and to insure an optimal outcome. Persistent fever beyond 7 to 10 d of presumably effective therapy can indicate treatment failure, paravalvular infection, or an extracardiac focal infection. Recrudescence of fever that had previously resolved suggests systemic emboli, processes unrelated or indirectly related to IE (catheter-related infection, deep vein thrombophlebitis, etc.) or drug fever, the latter particularly if fever recurs during the third or fourth week of β-lactam treatment *(54,55)*. The serum bactericidal titer, the highest dilution of a patient's serum that kills 99.9% of a standard inoculum of the infecting organism, is no longer recommended when patients are treated with a consensus recommendation. Vancomycin and aminoglycoside serum concentrations should be monitored to ensure appropriate dosing. Renal and hepatic function as well as complete blood counts should be monitored regularly when the treatment has the potential to adversely affect these areas. Repeat blood cultures should be obtained to assess persistent or recrudescent fever, to document cure 2 to 8 wk after completing therapy, and to assess relapse if fever recurs during the 2 to 3 mo after treatment. Electrocardiograms, echocardiograms, and special radiologic imaging studies should be obtained or repeated if intracardiac or focal extracardiac complications are suspected (Table 4).

Outpatient Antimicrobial Therapy

Patients who have responded to antimicrobial therapy and whose fever has resolved, who have no symptoms or signs suggesting threatening intracardiac or extracardiac complications, who are fully compliant, who have a stable, suitable home situation, and who can be followed carefully can be considered candidates for outpatient therapy. Most complications of IE arise during the initial 2 wk of therapy. Consequently, IE patients generally, and those at increased risk for complications (e.g., acute endocarditis, *S. aureus* endocarditis, PVE) in particular, should be treated in settings that allow daily physician monitoring (usually as inpatients) during this interval *(56)*. Thereafter they can be safely considered for outpatient therapy. Before beginning home therapy patients must be fully apprised of the potential complications of IE and instructed to immediately seek medical care if complications or unanticipated symptoms develop. Although outpatient therapy may reduce the cost of treatment, shifting therapy to the outpatient setting must not compromise antimicrobial therapy or the required clinical and laboratory monitoring.

SURGICAL TREATMENT

Although the mortality associated with IE can be attributed in part to the increased age of patients and comorbidities, intracardiac and central nervous system complications also contribute significantly. In a study of 513 patients with complicated left-sided IE and an overall mortality rate of 26%, 7 variables were, in a multivariate analysis, significantly associated with mortality at 6 mo. These were assigned a weighted point score based on the strength of the association: Charlson comorbidity score $\geq$2, 3 points; moderate to severe congestive heart failure, 3 points; altered mental status, 4 points; *S. aureus* infection, 6 points; nonstreptococcal infection other than *S. aureus*, 8 points; medical therapy only, 5 points. Surgical intervention was associated with reduced mortality (odds ratio 0.35, 95% confidence interval 0.23–0.54). Mortality could be predicted by the variable associated point score as follows: $\leq$6 points, 5 to 7%; 7 to 11 points, 15 to 19%; 12 to 16 points, 32%; >15 points, 59–69% *(57)*. As suggested by this study and published experience in general, some life-threatening intracardiac complications, as well as instances when antimicrobial therapy fails, can be effectively treated surgically and improve outcome. This clinical setting constitutes indications

Table 8
Clinical Circumstances Suggesting Cardiac Surgical Intervention in Patients With Endocarditis

Indications[a]
  Moderate to severe congestive heart failure due to valve dysfunction
  Rupture of perivalvular abscess into the pericardium
  Partially dehisced unstable prosthetic valve
  Rupture of a sinus of Valsalva aneurysm into the right heart
  Persistent bacteremia in the face of optimal antimicrobial therapy
  Absence of effective bactericidal therapy
  Fungal endocarditis, *Brucella* endocarditis, no effective antimicrobial therapy available
  S. aureus prosthetic valve endocarditis with an intracardiac complication
  Relapse of PVE after optimal antimicrobial therapy
  Persistent unexplained fever (≥10 d) in culture-negative PVE
Relative indications[b]
  Perivalvular extension of infection (myocardial, septal, or annulus abscess, intracardiac fistula)
  Poorly responsive *S. aureus* endocarditis involving the aortic or mitral valve
  Relapse of native valve IE after optimal antimicrobial therapy
  Large (>10 mm diameter) hypermobile vegetations
  Persistent unexplained fever (≥10 d) in culture-negative native valve endocarditis
  Endocarditis due to highly antibiotic-resistant enterococci or Gram-negative bacilli

[a]Cardiac surgery required for optimal outcome.
[b]Surgery, while not always required, must be carefully considered. (Adapted from ref. *85*.)

for cardiac surgery (Table 8). The clinical circumstances wherein surgical intervention is considered can be divided into relative and more absolute indications; however, even the latter circumstances are to some degree relative. The treatment of each patients requires that the risk-benefit ratio and the timing of surgery be carefully evaluated and the decisions individualized. Often it is a combination of findings, rather than a single observation, that indicate the need for surgery *(58,59)*.

Specific Indications

CONGESTIVE HEART FAILURE DUE TO VALVE DYSFUNCTION

Moderate to severe heart failure due to valve dysfunction portends a very poor prognosis; however, this can be improved by surgical intervention. Mortality rates of 60 to 90% are seen within 6 mo when IE complicated by new onset valve dysfunction and moderate to severe heart failure (New York Heart Association class III or IV) is treated medically. Among patients with comparable hemodynamic dysfunction who are treated surgically, mortality rates are reduced to 20 to 40% in NVE and 35 to 55% in PVE *(4,58,60)*. In a retrospective, but rigorously controlled analysis of patients with left-sided IE, after adjustments for clinical circumstances associated with mortality and indications for surgical intervention, mortality at 6 mo for those with moderate to severe heart failure treated surgically was 12% as was mortality for those with mild or no heart failure treated medically or surgically, whereas mortality for those with moderate to severe heart failure treated medically was significantly greater, 50% *(61)*. Functional stenosis due to vegetation that obstructs the valve orifice may also cause congestive heart failure and necessitate surgery. Repair of mitral valve fenestrations and ruptured chordae tendinae allows correction of valve dysfunction in the setting of either active or healed IE without the enduring burden of a prosthetic valve.

PERIVALVULAR INFECTION

In 10 to 15% of patients with NVE and 45 to 60% of those with PVE, perivalvular infection complicates endocarditis *(4,32,62–64)*. In NVE this complication occurs primarily with aortic valve infection. In patients with PVE or endocarditis involving native aortic valves clinical findings may suggest perivalvular infection: persistent unexplained fever after 10 d of appropriate antibiotic therapy, pericarditis, or new-onset persistent electrocardiographic conduction disturbance *(4,32,54,63)*. As an indicator of perivalvular abscess, new conduction disturbances have low sensitivity (28 to 53%) *(32,63,64)*. The most sensitive method for detection of perivalvular infection is multiplane TEE with color Doppler *(21,25,32)*. Among the clinical findings that suggest a need for cardiac surgery, partially dehisced unstable prosthetic valve, rupture of a periaortic abscess into the pericardial space, rupture of a sinus of Valsalva aneurysm into the right heart, and relapse of PVE after optimal therapy, are often manifestations of invasive infection *(58)*. Occasional patients with perivalvular infection will be cured with medical treatment alone; the majority, however, require surgical intervention *(58)*.

UNCONTROLLED INFECTION

The major manifestations of uncontrolled infection are continued positive blood cultures during therapy and persistent fever. Other causes of continued fever must be excluded before fever can be judged to be due to failure of antimicrobial therapy. Undrained perivalvular abscess may result in failure of antimicrobial therapy. For some organisms predictable effective bactericidal therapy is not available and surgical excision of infected valves is necessary to cure IE: fungi, *P. aeruginosa*, other highly resistant Gram-negative bacilli, enterococci for which synergistic killing cannot be effected, *Brucella* species, possibly *C. burnetii (58)*.

S. AUREUS IE

Mortality rates of 22 to 46% have been associated with *S. aureus* infection of native aortic or mitral valves and prosthetic valves *(38,39,65)*. Retrospective studies suggest that the survival of patients with *S. aureus* left-sided NVE who appear to have perivalvular infection, remain septic during the initial week of treatment (with or without bacteremia), or who have TTE-demonstrable vegetations may be improved by early aggressive surgical intervention *(38,66,67)*. Mortality in patients with *S. aureus* PVE is significantly increased among those with intracardiac complications and is significantly reduced by surgical intervention during active disease *(65)*. Endocarditis due to *S. aureus* that is restricted to the tricuspid valve can usually be cured without surgical intervention in spite of persistent fever and pulmonary emboli.

UNRESPONSIVE CULTURE-NEGATIVE IE

Patients with echocardiographically confirmed but blood culture-negative IE who fail to become afebrile during empiric antibiotic therapy should be considered for valve replacement. This clinical scenario suggests that either empiric therapy is not effective or there is invasive infection. Before proceeding with surgery, especially when valve function is intact, it is important to rule out other causes of persistent fever, including drug reaction, focal undrained metastatic infection, intercurrent complications, and noninfectious endocardial involvement (e.g., atrial myxoma, marantic endocarditis, antiphospholipid antibody syndrome, lupus erythematosus with valvular disease).

PREVENTION OF SYSTEMIC EMBOLI (VEGETATIONS >10 MM IN DIAMETER)

Vegetations on the aortic or mitral valve greater than 10 mm in diameter are associated with a higher frequency of systemic emboli than are smaller vegetations (37 vs 19%) *(13,68,69)*. Furthermore, systemic emboli occurring after initial echocardiography are significantly associated with larger vegetations (>10 mm diameter), and location on the mitral valve, particularly its anterior leaflet *(10,12)*. The risk of embolization, however, is markedly reduced after 2 wk of effective antimicrobial therapy *(58)*. Additionally, the mortality and residual morbidity associated with embolic events is largely confined to those emboli that lodge in the central nervous system or the coronary arteries. It is not possible to predict, based on echocardiographic findings, which patients would experience enhanced survival and reduced morbidity from surgical intervention, particularly when the hazards of surgery and the burden of a prosthetic valve are considered. Consequently, the role of surgery to prevent emboli remains controversial. Surgery is often considered after one or more embolic events during the initial 10 d of antibiotic therapy when there is a large residual vegetation *(58)*; however, even here the risk, including perioperative neurologic deterioration (*see* Timing of Cardiac Surgery section), and benefits must be weighed. Rarely is vegetation size alone an indication for surgery (perhaps only with exceptionally large hypermobile vegetations). Benefit from surgery in terms of reduced embolic events is most likely when surgery is undertaken early in therapy, the vegetation has characteristics associated with increased embolic risk, and other clinical features suggest that surgery may be beneficial, e.g., valve dysfunction with moderate congestive heart failure, an antibiotic-resistant organism, suspected paravalvular infection. Vegetectomy and repair of the mitral valve, particularly with younger patients, may reduce the risk of postoperative morbidity and thus enhance the net benefit of surgery in this circumstance *(58)*.

Timing of Cardiac Surgery

Surgery to correct valvular dysfunction that has resulted in congestive heart failure must be performed before intractable hemodynamic deterioration results. Delaying surgery under these circumstances risks additional hemodynamic deterioration and a consequent dramatic increase in perioperative mortality. Thus, the timing of surgical intervention to correct valvular dysfunction should be based on hemodynamic status and should be independent of the duration of prior antimicrobial therapy *(58,70)*. Similarly, surgery should not be delayed when the indication is uncontrolled infection *(58,70–72)*. Additional antibiotic therapy in this setting does not improve outcome. In fact, only 2 to 3.5% of patients develop recrudescent endocarditis when a prosthetic valve is inserted in patients with active NVE *(70)*. Although the presence of perivalvular infection increases the risk of surgical failure and recrudescent infection, approx 85 to 90% of patients survive after surgery for perivalvular abscess and relapse of IE is rare *(70,72,73)*. Even with surgical treatment of PVE where the new valve is typically inserted into an infected annulus that has been debrided and reconstructed, survival approaches 85% and only 15 to 25% of patients develop recurrent endocarditis or require additional cardiac surgery *(70,74–76)*. Among patients with valve dysfunction that will warrant surgery but who are hemodynamically stable and have controlled infection, surgery can often be safely delayed but other considerations may affect timing. For example, in this circumstance a large anterior mitral leaflet vegetation that threatened to embolize could justify early surgery.

Patients who have experienced a neurologic complication of IE and undergo cardiac surgery may experience further neurologic deterioration. Morbidity and mortality can be reduced by adjusting the interval between the neurologic complication and surgery or by treating the neurologic complication, e.g., clipping a ruptured mycotic aneurysm, before surgery. Among IE patients with an embolic cerebral infarction, the frequency of neurologic deterioration postoperatively decreases as the interval between the infarct and surgery increases: within 0 to 7 d, 45% deterioration, from 8 to 14 d, 15%; 15 to 28 d, 10%; greater than 29 d, 2%. Cardiac surgery performed 4 wk after intracerebral hemorrhage complicating IE is associated with neurologic deterioration in 20% of patients *(77)*. Depending on the urgency of cardiac surgery, among patients who have had an embolic stroke without hemorrhage surgery should be delayed for 2 to 3 wk; among those with a hemorrhagic embolic stroke (no aneurysm) an interval of 4 wk between the neurologic event and surgery is advised; and with hemorrhage due to rupture of a mycotic aneurysm, the aneurysm should be clipped and cerebral edema allowed to resolve (usually 2 to 3 wk after neurosurgery) before cardiac surgery *(77,78)*.

Antibiotic Therapy After Cardiac Surgery

The duration of antibiotic therapy after cardiac surgery is contingent on the ease with which the causative organism is eradicated, the duration of the preoperative therapy, whether recent blood cultures or intraoperative cultures yield the organism, and the pathology encountered at surgery. Patients with endocarditis caused by a highly susceptible, easily eradicated organism, with negative cultures at surgery, and where there is no perivalvular invasive infection should complete the remainder of the standard regimen for that organism. In contrast, patients with endocarditis caused by treatment-recalcitrant organisms, who are culture-positive perioperatively, or who have perivalvular invasive infection (especially if it looks active or is suboptimally debrided) should receive a full course of therapy postoperatively. Most patients with PVE and perivalvular infection receive a full course of therapy after surgery *(4,70)*. Although valve cultures are generally sterile, organisms remain visible on Gram stain of vegetations resected from patients who have received 75 to 100% of standard (per organism) antibiotic treatment in 50 to 65% of cases and from those who have successfully completed therapy from 1 to 6 mo earlier in 20 to 25% of cases *(79)*. Because of the delay in clearing nonviable organisms from vegetations, valve culture and histopathologic evidence of acute inflammation should be used to judge adequacy of prior therapy rather than Gram stain.

EXTRACARDIAC COMPLICATIONS

From 3 to 5% of patients with IE develop a splenic abscess. Although a splenic defect is easily identified with ultrasonography or computed tomography (CT), the distinction between abscess and infarct is difficult. Progressive enlargement of a lesion suggests an abscess, which can be confirmed by guided percutaneous needle aspiration. Successful therapy of splenic abscess requires percutaneous drainage or splenectomy.

Approximately 2 to 12% of patients with IE develop mycotic aneurysm and half of the aneurysms involve cerebral arteries. In 0.5 to 2% of patients with IE, cerebral mycotic aneurysms rupture *(16, 17)*. Focal neurologic symptoms and persistent headache may be premonitory symptoms. Based on serial angiograms, 50% of mycotic aneurysms resolve with effective antimicrobial treatment of IE *(80)*. The risk that an asymptomatic cerebral aneurysm will rupture after completion of effective antimicrobial therapy is estimated to be low *(81)*. Cerebral angiography is not recommended for all patients with IE and a neurologic deficit; however, head CT with enhancement is advised if there are neurologic symptoms. If intracerebral hemorrhage is detected, angiography is recommended. Ruptured cerebral mycotic aneurysms should be resected. Unruptured cerebral aneurysms should be followed by angiography and those that persist or enlarge during therapy should be resected if feasible. Extracranial mycotic aneurysms are managed in an analogous fashion; persistent aneurysms involving intraabdominal arteries should be resected.

PREVENTION OF ENDOCARDITIS

Although the benefit of periprocedure antibiotic use to prevent IE has not been proved and can be debated, an expert committee of the American Heart Association has identified patients who are at risk for IE, procedures that might increase the risk of IE among endocarditis-prone patients, and regimens that might be used prior to selected procedures to prevent endocarditis (Tables 9–13) *(82)*. Patients with cardiac abnormalities can be divided into groups with high, moderate, or low to negligible risk for developing IE (Table 9). Prophylaxis is not recommended for those at low to negligible risk. Patients with a secundum atrial septal defect (ASD) or those lacking other endocarditis-vulnerable defects who have undergo successful repair of an ASD, patent ductus arteriosus, or ventricular septal defect are at negligible risk for IE *(83)*. In spite of corrective surgery, patients with all other forms of congenital heart disease or coarctation of the aorta remain at high risk for IE; this is in large part the result of coincident unrepaired abnormalities, failed repairs, or placement of prosthetic valves during the repair *(83)*. Prophylaxis in patients with mitral valve prolapse (MVP) is controversial. The risk is increased relative to the general population but is still significantly less than that among patients with rheumatic heart disease. Prophylaxis is recommended for patients with MVP and a murmur of mitral regurgitation and for those over 45 yr of age who, on echocardiography, have MVP and thickened valve leaflets even in the absence of mitral regurgitation at rest.

Prophylaxis has been advised for those procedures likely to induce bacteremia with bacteria causally associated with IE (Tables 10 and 11). Maintenance of good dental health reduces the risk of IE. Similarly, patients should have dental disease treated before they undergo cardiac valve surgery.

Table 9
Risk of Infective Endocarditis Associated With Cardiac Abnormalities

High risk	Moderate risk	Low or negligible risk
Prosthetic heart valves	Congenital cardiac malformations (other than high-/low-risk lesions)	Isolated secundum atrial septic defect
Prior bacterial endocarditis	Acquired valvular dysfunction	Surgical repair of atrial or ventricular septic defect or patent ductus arteriosus
Complex cyanotic congenital heart disease	Hypertrophic cardiomyopathy	Prior coronary artery bypass surgery
Surgically constructed systemic-pulmonary shunts	Mitral valve prolapse with valvular regurgitation and/or thickened leaflets	Mitral valve prolapse without valvular regurgitation
		Physiologic, functional, or innocent heart murmurs
		Prior Kawasaki disease or rheumatic fever without valvular dysfunction
		Cardiac pacemakers and implanted defibrillators

Adapted from ref. 82.

Table 10
Dental Procedures for Which Endocarditis Prophylaxis is Considered

Prophylaxis recommended	Prophylaxis not recommended
Dental extractions	Restorative dentistry (operative and prosthodontic) with/without retraction cord
Periodontal procedures (surgery, scaling, root planing, probing)	Local anesthetic injection (not intraligamentary)
Dental implant placement, reimplantation of avulsed teeth	Intracanal endodontic treatment (post placement and buildup)
Endodontic instrumentation (root canal) or surgery beyond the apex	Placement of rubber dams
Subgingival placement of antibiotic fibers/strips	Suture removal
Initial placement of orthodontic bands (not brackets)	Placement of removable prosthodontic/orthodontic appliances
Intraligamentary local anesthetic injections	Taking oral impressions or radiographs
Prophylactic cleaning of teeth or implants where bleeding is anticipated	Orthodontic appliance adjustment
	Shedding primary teeth

Adapted from ref. 82.

Among endocarditis-prone patients with infection in the genitourinary tract, the infection should be eradicated before proceeding with genitourinary manipulation.

The regimens recommended for use in the prophylaxis of IE have been selected because they kill or inhibit the endocarditis-causing bacteria present at the site to be manipulated (Tables 12 and 13). Penicillin regimens used to prevent acute rheumatic fever are not suitable for IE prophylaxis; patients receiving them may have oral and gingival flora that are resistant to penicillins. Accordingly, clindamycin or clarithromycin should be used for prophylaxis in patients receiving penicillin repetitively. Surgical procedures on infected tissues and skin infections may be associated with

Table 11
Procedures for Which Endocarditis Prophylaxis is Considered

Prophylaxis recommended	Prophylaxis not recommended[c]
Respiratory tract	Respiratory tract
Surgical operation involving mucosa	Endotracheal intubation
Bronchoscopy with rigid bronchoscope	Bronchoscopy with flexible bronchoscope with or without biopsy[a]
	Tympanostomy tube insertion
Gastrointestinal tract[b]	Gastrointestinal tract[b]
Sclerotherapy for esophageal varices	Transesophageal echocardiography
Dilation of esophageal stricture	Endoscopy with or without biopsy[a]
Endoscopic retrograde cholangiography with biliary obstruction	
Biliary tract surgery	
Surgery involving intestinal mucosa	
Genitourinary tract	Genitourinary tract
Prostate surgery	Vaginal hysterectomy[a]
Cytoscopy	Vaginal delivery[a]
Urethral dilation	Cesarean section
	In the absence of infection:
	Uretural catheterization, cervical dilation and uterine curettage, therapeutic abortion, sterilization, insertion/removal of intrauterine device
	Cardiac catheterization, coronary angioplasty
	Implantation of pacemakers, defibrillators, coronary stents
	Clean surgery
	Circumcision

[a]Prophylaxis is optional for high-risk patients.
[b]Recommended for high-risk patients; optional for moderate-risk group.
[c]Prophylaxis may be recommended for a procedure itself, e.g., pacemaker implantation. (Adapted from ref. 82.)

Table 12
Regimens for Endocarditis Prophylaxis in Adults: Oral, Respiratory Tract, or Esophageal Procedures

Setting	Antibiotic	Regimen[a]
Standard	Amoxicillin	2.0 g po 1 h before procedure
Unable to take oral medication	Ampicillin	2.0 g im or iv within 30 min of procedure
Penicillin-allergic	Clindamycin	600 mg po 1 h before procedure or iv 30 min before procedure
	Cephalexin[b]	2.0 gm po 1 h before procedure
	Cefazolin[b]	1.0 gm iv or im 30 min before procedure
	Cefadroxil[b]	2.0 gm po 1 h before procedure
	Clarithromycin	500 mg po 1 h before procedure

[a]For patients in high-risk group, administer half the dose 6 h after the initial dose; dosing for children: amoxicillin, ampicillin, cephalexin or cefadroxil use 50 mg/kg po; cefazolin iv 25 mg/kg; clindamycin 20 mg/kg po, 25 mg/kg iv; clarithromycin 15 mg/kg po.
[b]Do not use cephalosporins in patients with immediate hypersensitivity (urticaria, angioedema, anaphylaxis) to penicillin. (Adapted from ref. 82.)

bacteremia and an increased risk for IE. Antibiotic prophylaxis for IE is recommended for selected surgical procedures. Similarly, skin and wound infections caused by *S. aureus* should be treated vigorously when they occur in IE-prone patients.

Table 13
Regimens for Endocarditis Prophylaxis in Adults: Genitourinary and Gastrointestinal^a Tract Procedures

Setting	Antibiotic	Regimen^b
High-risk patients	Ampicillin plus gentamicin	Ampicillin 2.0 g iv/im plus gentamicin 1.5 mg/kg within 30 min of procedure; repeat ampicillin 1.0 g iv/im or amoxicillin 1.0 g po 6 h later
High-risk, penicillin-allergic patients	Vancomycin plus gentamicin	Vancomycin 1.0 g iv over 1–2 h plus gentamicin 1.5 mg/kg im/iv infused or injected 30 min before procedure. No second dose recommended
Moderate-risk patients	Amoxicillin or ampicillin	Amoxicillin 2.0 g po 1 h before procedure or ampicillin 2.0 g im/iv 30 min before procedure
Moderate-risk, penicillin-allergic patients	Vancomycin	Vancomycin 1.0 g iv infused over 1–2 h and completed within 30 min of procedure

^{a}Excludes esophageal procedures (*see* Table 10).

^{b}Dosing for children: ampicillin 50 mg/kg iv/im, vancomycin 20 mg/kg iv, gentamicin 1.5 mg/kg iv/im (children's doses should not exceed adult doses). (Adapted from ref. 82.)

REFERENCES

1. Mylonakis E, Calderwood SB. Infective endocarditis in adults. N Engl J Med 2001;345:1318–1330.
2. Hoen B, Alla F, Selton-Suty C, et al. Changing profile of infective endocarditis: results of a 1-year survey in France. JAMA 2002;288:75–81.
3. Berlin JA, Abrutyn E, Strom BL, et al. Incidence of infective endocarditis in the Delaware Valley, 1988–1990. Am J Cardiol 1995;76:933–936.
4. Karchmer AW, Longworth DL. Infections of intracardiac devices. Infect Dis Clin N Am 2002;16:477–505.
5. Fenollar F, Lepidi H, Raoult D. Whipple's endocarditis: review of the literature and comparisons with Q fever, *Bartonella* infection, and blood culture-positive endocarditis. Clin Infect Dis 2001;33:1309–1316.
6. Gagliardi JP, Nettles RE, McCarty DE, et al. Native valve infective endocarditis in elderly and younger adult patients: comparison of clinical features and outcomes with use of the Duke criteria and the Duke endocarditis data base. Clin Infect Dis 1998;26:1165–1168.
7. Werner GS, Schulz R, Fuchs JB, et al. Infective endocarditis in the elderly in the era of transesophageal echocardiography: clinical features and prognosis compared with younger patients. Am J Med 1996;100:90–97.
8. Tornos MP, Permanyer-Miralda G, Olona M, et al. Long-term complications of native valve infective endocarditis in non-addicts: a 15-year follow-up study. Ann Int Med 1992;117:567–572.
9. Tornos P, Almirante B, Olona M, et al. Clinical outcome and long-term prognosis of late prosthetic valve endocarditis: a 20-year experience. Clin Infect Dis 1997;24:381–386.
10. Mugge A, Daniel WC, Frank G, Lichtlen PR. Echocardiography in infective endocarditis: reassessment of prognostic implications of vegetation size determined by the transthoracic and transesophageal approach. J Am Coll Cardiol 1989;14:631–638.
11. Rohman S, Erbel R, Darius H. Prediction of rapid versus prolonged healing of infective endocarditis by monitoring vegetation size. J Amer Soc Echocardiogr 1991;4:465–474.
12. Rohman S, Erbel R, George G, et al. Clinical relevance of vegetation localization by transesophageal echocardiography in infective endocarditis. Eur Heart J 1992;13:446–452.
13. Aragam JR, Weyman AE. Echocardiographic findings in infective endocarditis. In: Weyman AE, ed. Principles and Practice of Echocardiography. 2nd ed. Lea & Febiger, Philadelphia, 1994, pp. 1178–1197.
14. Steckelberg JM, Murphy JG, Ballard D, et al. Emboli in infective endocarditis: the prognostic value of echocardiography. Ann Int Med 1991;114:635–640.
15. Pruitt AA, Rubin RH, Karchmer AW, Duncan GW. Neurologic complications of bacterial endocarditis. Medicine 1978;57:329–343.
16. Salgado AV, Furlan AJ, Keys TF, et al. Neurologic complications of endocarditis: a 12-year experience. Neurology 1989;39:173–178.
17. Kanter MC, Hart RG. Neurologic complications of infective endocarditis. Neurology 1991;41:1015–1020.
18. Durack DT, Lukes AS, Bright DK. New criteria for diagnosis of infective endocarditis: utilization of specific echocardiographic findings. Am J Med 1994;96:200–209.

19. Bayer AS, Bolger AF, Taubert KA, et al. Diagnosis and management of infective endocarditis and its complications. Circulation 1998;98:2936–2948.
20. Li JS, Sexton DJ, Mick N, et al. Proposed modifications to the Duke criteria for the diagnosis of infective endocarditis. Clin Infect Dis 2000;30:633–638.
21. Daniel WG, Mugge A, Martin RP, et al. Improvement in the diagnosis of abscesses associated with endocarditis by transesophageal echocardiography. N Engl J Med 1991;324:795–800.
22. Mugge A. Echocardiographic detection of cardiac valve vegetations and prognostic implications. Infect Dis Clin N Am 1993;7:877–898.
23. Shively BK, Gurule FT, Roldan CA, et al. Diagnostic value of transesophageal compared with transthoracic echocardiography in infective endocarditis. J Am Coll Cardiol 1991;18:391–397.
24. Sochowski RA, Chan KL. Implication of negative results on a monoplane transesophageal echocardiographic study in patients with suspected infective endocarditis. J Am Coll Cardiol 1993;21:216–221.
25. Job FP, Franke S, Lethen H, et al. Incremental value of biplane and multiplane transesophageal echocardiography for the assessment of active infective endocarditis. Am J Cardiol 1995;75:1033–1037.
26. Brouqui P, Raoult D. Endocarditis due to rare and fastidious bacteria. Clin Micro Rev 2001;14:177–207.
27. Hoen B, Selton-Suty C, Lacassin F, et al. Infective endocarditis in patients with negative blood cultures: analysis of 88 cases from a one-year nationwide survey in France. Clin Infect Dis 1995;20:501–506.
28. Goldenberger D, Kunzli A, Vogt P, et al. Molecular diagnosis of bacterial endocarditis by broad-range PCR amplification and direct sequencing. J Clin Micro 1992;35:2733–2739.
29. Khandheria BK. Transesophageal echocardiography in the evaluation of prosthetic valves. Am J Cardiac Imag 1995;9:106–114.
30. Daniel WG, Mugge A, Grote J, et al. Comparison of transthoracic and transesophageal echocardiography for detection of abnormalities of prosthetic and bioprosthetic valves in the mitral and aortic positions. Am J Cardiol 1993;71:210–215.
31. Morguet AJ, Werner GS, Andreas S, Kreuzer H. Diagnostic value of transesophageal compared with transthoracic echocardiography in suspected prosthetic valve endocarditis. Herz 1995;20:390–398.
32. Blumberg EA, Karalis DA, Chandrasekaran K, et al. Endocarditis-associated paravalvular abscess. Do clinical parameters predict the presence of abscess? Chest 1995;107:898–903.
33. Lindner JR, Case A, Dent JM, et al. Diagnostic value of echocardiography in suspected endocarditis: an evaluation based on the pretest probability of disease. Circulation 1996;93:730–736.
34. Roe MT, Abramson MA, Li J, et al. Clinical information determines the impact of transesophageal echocardiography on the diagnosis of infective endocarditis by the Duke criteria. Am Heart J 2000;139:945–951.
35. Heidenreich PA, Masoudi FA, Maini B, et al. Echocardiography in patients with suspected endocarditis: a cost-effectiveness analysis. Am J Med 1999;107:198–208.
36. Fowler VG Jr, Li J, Corey GR, et al. Role of echocardiography in evaluation of patients with *Staphylococcus aureus* bacteremia: experience in 103 patients. J Am Coll Cardiol 1997;30:1072–1078.
37. Rosen AB, Fowler VG Jr, Corey GR, et al. Cost-effectiveness of transesophageal echocardiography to determine the duration of therapy for intravascular catheter-associated *Staphylococcus aureus* bacteremia. Ann Int Med 1999;130:810–820.
38. Fowler VG Jr, Sanders LL, Kong LK, et al. Infective endocarditis due to *Staphylococcus aureus*: 59 prospectively identified cases with follow-up. Clin Infect Dis 1999;28:106–114.
39. Roder BL, Wandall DA, Frimodt-Moller N, et al. Clinical features of *Staphylococcus aureus* endocarditis: a 10-year experience in Denmark. Arch Intern Med 1999;159:462–469.
40. Ribera E, Miro JM, Cortes E, et al. Influence of human immunodeficiency virus 1 infection and degree of immunosuppression in the clinical characteristics and outcome of infective endocarditis in intravenous drug users. Arch Intern Med 1998;158:2043–2050.
41. Raoult D, Fournier PE, Drancourt M, et al. Diagnosis of 22 new cases of *Bartonella* endocarditis. Ann Int Med 1996;125:646–652.
42. Wilson WR, Karchmer AW, Bisno AL, et al. Antibiotic treatment of adults with infective endocarditis due to viridans streptococci, enterococci, other streptococci, staphylococci, and HACEK microorganisms. JAMA 1995;274:1706–1713.
43. Francioli P, Ruch W, Stamboulian D, The International Infective Endocarditis Study Group. Treatment of streptococcal endocarditis with a single daily dose of ceftriaxone and netilmicin for 14 days: a prospective multicenter study. Clin Infect Dis 1995;21:1406–1410.
44. Sexton DJ, Tenenbaum MJ, Wilson WR, et al. Ceftriaxone once daily for four weeks compared with ceftriaxone plus gentamicin once daily for two weeks for treatment of endocarditis due to penicillin-susceptible streptococci. Clin Infect Dis 1998;27:1470–1474.
45. Eliopoulos GM. Aminoglycoside resistant enterococcal endocarditis. Infect Dis Clin N Am 1993;7:117–133.
46. Olaison L, Schadewitz K, The Swedish Society for Infectious Diseases Quality Assurance Study Group for Endocarditis. Enterococcal endocarditis in Sweden, 1995–1999: can shorter therapy with aminoglycosides be used? Clin Infect Dis 2002;34:159–166.
47. Torres-Tortosa M, de Cueto M, Vergara A, et al. Prospective evaluation of a two-week course of intravenous antibiotics in intravenous drug addicts with infective endocarditis. Eur J Clin Microbiol Infect Dis 1994;13:559–564.
48. Martinez E, Miro JM, Almirante B, et al. Effect of penicillin resistance of *Streptococcus pneumoniae* on the presentation, prognosis, and treatment of pneumococcal endocarditis in adults. Clin Infect Dis 2002;35:130–139.

49. Petit AIC, Bok JW, Thompson J, et al. Native-valve endocarditis due to CDC coryneform group ANF-3: report of a case and review of corynebacterial endocarditis. Clin Infect Dis 1994;19:897–901.
50. Raoult D, Fournier PE, Vandenesch F, et al. Outcome and treatment of *Bartonella* endocarditis. Arch Intern Med 2003;163:226–230.
51. Raoult D, Houpikian P, Tissot Dupont H, et al. Treatment of Q fever endocarditis: comparison of 2 regimens containing doxycycline and ofloxacin or hydroxychloroquine. Arch Intern Med 1999;159:167–173.
52. Fenollar F, Fournier PE, Carrieri MP, et al. Risk factors and prevention of Q fever endocarditis. Clin Infect Dis 2001;33:312–316.
53. Ellis ME, Al-Abdely H, Sandridge A, et al. Fungal endocarditis: evidence in the world literature, 1965–1995. Clin Infect Dis 2001;32:50–62.
54. Douglas A, Moore-Gillon J, Eykyn S. Fever during treatment of infective endocarditis. Lancet 1986;i:1341–1343.
55. Olaison L, Hogevik H, Alestig K. Fever, C-reactive protein, and other acute-phase reactants during treatment of infective endocarditis. Arch Intern Med 1997;157:885–892.
56. Andrews MM, von Reyn CF. Patient selection criteria and management guidelines for outpatient parenteral antibiotic therapy for native valve infective endocarditis. Clin Infect Dis 2001;33:203–209.
57. Hasbun R, Vikram HR, Barakat LA, et al. Complicated left-sided native valve endocarditis in adults: risk classification for mortality. JAMA 2003;289:1933–1940.
58. Olaison L, Pettersson G. Current best practices and guidelines: indications for surgical intervention in infective endocarditis. Infect Dis Clin N Am 2002;16:453–475.
59. Alsip SG, Blackstone EH, Kirklin JW, Cobbs CG. Indications for cardiac surgery in patients with active infective endocarditis. Am J Med 1985;78(Suppl 6B):138–148.
60. Croft CH, Woodward W, Elliott A, et al. Analysis of surgical versus medical therapy in active complicated native valve infective endocarditis. Am J Cardiol 1983;51:1650–1655.
61. Vikram HR, Buenconsejo J, Hasbun R, Quagliarello VJ. Impact of valve surgery on 6-month mortality in adults with complicated, left-sided native valve endocarditis: a propensity analysis. JAMA 2003;290:3207–3214.
62. Sandre RM, Shafran SD. Infective endocarditis: review of 135 cases over 9 years. Clin Infect Dis 1996;22:276–286.
63. DiNubile MJ, Calderwood SB, Steinhaus DM, Karchmer AW. Cardiac conduction abnormalities complicating native valve active infective endocarditis. Am J Cardiol 1986;58:1213–1217.
64. Meine TJ, Nettles RE, Anderson DJ, et al. Cardiac conduction abnormalities in endocarditis defined by the Duke criteria. Am Heart J 2001;142:280–285.
65. John MVD, Hibberd PL, Karchmer AW, et al. *Staphylococcus aureus* prosthetic valve endocarditis: optimal management and risk factors for death. Clin Infect Dis 1998;26:1302–1309.
66. Richardson JV, Karp RB, Kirklin JW, Dismukes WE. Treatment of infective endocarditis: a 10-year comparative analysis. Circulation 1978;58:589–597.
67. Bishara J, Leibovici L, Gartman-Israel D, et al. Long-term outcome of infective endocarditis: the impact of early surgical intervention. Clin Infect Dis 2001;33:1636–1643.
68. Tischler MD, Vaitkus PT. The ability of vegetation size on echocardiography to predict clinical complications: a meta-analysis. J Am Soc Echocardiograph 1997;10:562–568.
69. Mangoni ED, Adinolfi LE, Tripodi MF, et al. Risk factors for "major" embolic events in hospitalized patients with infective endocarditis. Am Heart J 2003;146:311–316.
70. Alexiou C, Langley SM, Stafford H, et al. Surgery for active culture-positive endocarditis: determinants of early and late outcome. Ann Thorac Surg 2000;69:1448–1454.
71. Baumgartner WA, Miller DC, Reitz BA, et al. Surgical treatment of prosthetic valve endocarditis. Ann Thorac Surg 1983;35:87–102.
72. Baumgartner FJ, Omari BO, Robertson JM, et al. Annular abscesses in surgical endocarditis: anatomic, clinical and operative features. Ann Thorac Surg 2000;70:442–447.
73. d'Udekem Y, David TE, Feindel CM, et al. Long-term results of operation for paravalvular abscess. Ann Thorac Surg 1996;62:48–53.
74. Jault F, Gandjbakheh I, Chastre JC, et al. Prosthetic valve endocarditis with ring abscesses: surgical management and long-term results. J Thorac Cardiovasc Surg 1993;105:1106–1113.
75. Lytle BW, Priest BP, Taylor PC, et al. Surgery for acquired heart disease: surgical treatment of prosthetic valve endocarditis. J Thorac Cardiovasc Surg 1996;111:198–210.
76. Pansini S, di Summa M, Patane F, et al. Risk of recurrence after reoperation for prosthetic valve endocarditis. J Heart Valve Dis 1997;6:84–87.
77. Eishi K, Kawazoe K, Kuriyama Y, et al. Surgical management of infective endocarditis associated with cerebral complications: multicenter retrospective study in Japan. J Thorac Cardiovasc Surg 1995;110:1745–1755.
78. Gillinov AM, Shah RV, Curtis WE, et al. Valve replacement in patients with endocarditis and acute neurologic deficit. Ann Thorac Surg 1996;61:1125–1130.
79. Morris AJ, Drinkovic D, Pottumarthy S, et al. Gram stain, culture, and histopathological examination findings for heart valves removed because of infective endocarditis. Clin Infect Dis 2003;36:697–704.
80. Brust JCM, Dickinson PCT, Hughes JEO, Holtzman RNN. The diagnosis and treatment of cerebral mycotic aneurysms. Ann Neurol 1990;27:238–246.
81. Salgado AV, Furlan AJ, Keys TF. Mycotic aneurysm, subarachnoid hemorrhage, and indications for cerebral angiography in infective endocarditis. Stroke 1987;18:1057–1060.

82. Dajani AS, Taubert KA, Wilson W, et al. Prevention of bacterial endocarditis: recommendations by the American Heart Association, from the Committee on Rheumatic Fever, Endocarditis, and Kawasaki Disease, Council on Cardiovascular Diseases in the Young. JAMA 1997;277:1794–1801.
83. Morris CD, Reller MD, Menashe VD. Thirty-year incidence of infective endocarditis after surgery for congenital heart defect. JAMA 1998;279:599–603.
84. Karchmer AW. Infective endocarditis. In: Braunwald E, ed. Heart Disease: A Textbook of Cardiovascular Medicine, 5th ed. W. B. Saunders, Philadelphia, 1996, pp. 1084.
85. Karchmer AW. Approach to the patient with infective endocarditis. In: Goldman L, Braunwald E, eds. Primary Cardiology. W. B. Saunders, Philadelphia, 1998, p. 202.
86. Karchmer AW. Prevention and treatment of infective endocarditis. In: Antman EM, ed. Cardiovascular Therapeutics, 2nd ed. W. B. Saunders, Philadelphia, pp. 1082–1099.

RECOMMENDED READING

Baddour LM, Bettmann MA, Bolger AF, et al. Nonvalvular cardiovascular device-related infections. Circulation 2003; 108:2015–2031.
Bayer AS, Bolger AF, Taubert KA, et al. Diagnosis and management of infective endocarditis and its complications. Circulation 1998;98:2936–2948.
Brouqui P, Raoult D. Endocarditis due to rare and fastidious bacteria. Clin Micro Rev 2001;14:177–207.
Durack DT (guest ed.). Infective endocarditis. Infect Dis Clin N Am 2002;16:255–533.
Durack DT. Prevention of infective endocarditis. N Engl J Med 1995;332:38–44.
Karchmer AW, Longworth DL. Infections of intracardiac devices. Infect Dis Clin N Am 2002;16:477–505.
Mylonakis E, Calderwood SB. Infective endocarditis in adults. N Engl J Med 2001;345:1318–1330.
Wilson WR, Karchmer AW, Bisno AL, et al. Antibiotic treatment of adults with infective endocarditis due to viridans streptococci, enterococci, other streptococci, staphylococci, and HACEK microorganisms. JAMA 1995;274:1706–1713.

IX   HYPERTENSION

32 Hypertension

Mechanisms and Diagnosis

Clive Rosendorff, MD, PhD

INTRODUCTION

Cardiovascular disease is by far the leading cause of death, in males and females, in industrialized nations. In the United States this year. about a million deaths will be due to diseases of the heart and circulation, more than twice the number for the next most frequent cause of death, cancer. The most common fatal cardiovascular diseases are coronary artery disease, congestive heart failure, and stroke; these, together with renovascular disease, all have hypertension as a major risk factor. High blood pressure is therefore a highly lethal disease.

The relationship between blood pressure and the relative risks of stroke and coronary heart disease is direct, continuous, and independent, and no evidence has been put forward of any "threshold" level of blood pressure below which humans are entirely safe *(1)*. In general, men are at greater risk for hypertension-related death than women, black persons than white, and older ones than younger ones. With increasing age, the prevalence of isolated systolic hypertension with a normal diastolic pressure increases considerably, and it is now generally accepted that in adults systolic blood pressure may be a more accurate predictor of cardiovascular risk than diastolic pressure.

An enormous amount of data—experimental, epidemiologic, and clinical—now indicates that reducing elevated blood pressure is beneficial. The first definitive proof of this came from the Veterans Administration (VA) Cooperative Study begun in 1963, and it has been confirmed in a host of studies since, most of which utilized diuretics or β-blockers as antihypertensive agents. Since then, there have been numerous clinical trials of many different classes of antihypertensive drugs, which have shown huge reductions in cardiovascular morbidity and mortality.

In spite of the demonstrated benefits of blood pressure reduction, physicians and other health care professionals who are responsible for identifying and treating patients with hypertension are not doing a great job. From 1976 to 1980 and 1988 to 1989, the percentages of Americans who were aware that they had high blood pressure increased from 51% to 73%, but since 1991 that figure has dropped back to 68%. The proportion who were treated at all increased from 31% from 1976 to 1980 to 55% from 1988 to 1991, but it declined to 54% in 1991 to 1994. Most depressing of all were the data for patients whose blood pressure was controlled to normal values: 10% in 1976 to 1980, up to 29% in 1988 to 1991, but back to 27% since then. So, of every 100 patients with hypertension, 68 are aware of the fact, 54 are receiving treatment, and only 27 are "controlled" *(2)*. This may explain why the dramatic reductions in age-adjusted stroke and coronary heart disease mortality since the 1970s seem to be faltering; the stroke rate has risen slightly since 1993, and the slope of the decline in coronary heart disease appears to be leveling off *(3)*. Furthermore, rates have increased for end-stage renal disease, for which high blood pressure is the second most common antecedent, and for heart failure, which in a large majority of patients is associated with hypertension *(4,5)*.

From: *Essential Cardiology: Principles and Practice, 2nd Ed.*
Edited by: C. Rosendorff © Humana Press Inc., Totowa, NJ

DEFINITION AND CLASSIFICATION

Blood pressure is a continuous variable in any population, with a distribution along a bell-shaped curve. The difference between "normotensive" and "hypertensive" blood pressure values is, therefore, somewhat arbitrary, but since cardiovascular risk increases with blood pressure, various operational definitions of hypertension have been developed.

The Seventh Joint National Committee on Detection, Evaluation, and Treatment of High Blood Pressure (JNC VII) *(2)* defined hypertension as a systolic blood pressure (SBP) of 140 mmHg or greater, or diastolic blood pressure (DBP) of 90 mmHg or greater. JNC VII subdivided "hypertension" into two categories: stage 1 with a blood pressure range of 140 to 159 mmHg (SBP) or 90 to 99 mmHg (DBP), and stage 2 with blood pressure ≥160 mmHg (SBP) or ≥100 mmHg (DBP). The utility of such a classification is, first, to provide an appropriate basis for comparing patients in epidemiologic and clinical studies, and, second, as an indicator of the urgency of starting therapy. For example, a patient with a blood pressure of 142/92 mmHg (stage 1) need not be treated with antihypertensive therapy right away; repeat visits to the office or clinic should be arranged to confirm the hypertension, and possibly to establish the antihypertensive efficacy of nonpharmacologic interventions (*see* Chapter 33). On the other hand, a patient with a blood pressure of 220/118 mmHg (Stage 2) usually requires antihypertensive therapy without delay.

JNC VII also labeled as "prehypertensive" individuals with blood pressures in the 120–139 mmHg (SBP) or 80–89 mmHg (DBP) range. This will clearly cause much unnecessary anxiety in an essentially healthy population.

MEASUREMENT OF BLOOD PRESSURE

Blood pressure is usually measured *(6,7)* with a mercury sphygmomanometer, an aneroid manometer, or an electronic manometer, with a 12-by-26-cm cuff. The bladder of the cuff should encircle at least 80% of the arm, so for patients with arms of greater than 30 cm circumference, pressure should be measured with a large cuff (13-by-36 cm). If an aneroid or electronic manometer is used, it should be calibrated against a mercury manometer at regular intervals. Blood pressures should be measured with subjects both lying and standing, or sitting and standing, and repeated 5 min later when possible. The cuff should be placed over the brachial artery and the bell of the stethoscope over the artery distal to the cuff; the environment should be quiet and the patient relaxed. Serial measurements should be taken at the same time of day, preferably in the morning, before the patient has taken any antihypertensive medication (i.e., at the trough of the plasma concentration).

The cuff is pumped up to about 20 mmHg above the systolic level, which point is signaled by the disappearance of the radial pulse, and then the pressure lowered by about 2 mmHg per second. The systolic blood pressure is the pressure at which the first faint, consistent, tapping sounds are heard (Korotkoff sounds, phase I). The diastolic pressure is the level at which the last regular blood pressure sound is heard and after which all sound disappears (Korotkoff sound, phase V). Below Korotkoff phase I there is sometimes a period of silence referred to as the *auscultatory gap*; otherwise there is a continuum of sound, including swishing beats (Korotkoff II), crisper and louder sounds (Korotkoff III), and muffling of the sound (Korotkoff IV). If the sounds continue down to zero, Korotkoff IV is recorded as the diastolic pressure.

Since blood pressure can vary by as much as 10 mmHg between arms (and more in conditions such as coarctation of the aorta), it should be measured in both arms, at least at the initial visit. The higher pressure is recorded. All blood pressures should be read to the nearest 2 mmHg, not rounded off to the nearest 5 or 10 mmHg, as is done so often.

There are many sources of variability of blood pressure. These include poor technique, faulty equipment, a stressful setting or an anxious patient, and a patient who has been smoking or has had caffeine or alcohol. A common error is the failure to remove patients' garments with tight sleeves. The considerable interobserver variability in blood pressure measurements can be minimized by meticulous attention to correct technique.

Among the biologic variations are short-term ones driven by changes in the autonomic nervous system and a slower, circadian, variability. Blood pressure usually falls about 15% at night, during sleep, to rise to daytime levels an hour or two before awakening. Pressure usually peaks in the late afternoon and evening. Some patients (so-called *non-dippers*) have a smaller fall of BP during sleep, sometimes none; these patients seem to be at greater risk for cardiovascular disease, a more rapid progression of hypertensive renal disease, and even cognitive dysfunction. The converse, namely an excessive fall of nocturnal blood pressure, also carries risk, especially for stroke and myocardial ischemia. The early-morning surge of pressure, after arising from sleep, is also associated with more cardiovascular catastrophes, compared with the remainder of the 24-h period.

The *white-coat effect* refers to the higher pressures seen in the clinic or the doctor's office as compared with those measured at home, whether by the patient or by 24-h ambulatory monitoring, and it is quite usual. *White-coat hypertension* is an entity in which clinic or office blood pressure is in the hypertensive range but at home is normal. The best current evidence indicates that white-coat hypertension is a low-risk, but not entirely harmless, clinical entity, and these patients should be monitored closely for the appearance of (1) features that would require antihypertensive therapy, especially daytime ambulatory blood pressure or home self-measured pressure greater than 130/85 mmHg, or (2) target organ damage.

INITIAL WORKUP OF THE HYPERTENSIVE PATIENT

The initial evaluation of patients with hypertension has three objectives: (1) to find clues to secondary causes of hypertension; (2) to assess target organ damage; and (3) to determine whether there are other risk factors for cardiovascular disease. This requires careful history taking, a complete physical examination, some basic laboratory tests, and electrocardiography (ECG).

The first step is to establish the diagnosis of sustained hypertension. Blood pressure should be measured on at least two occasions. If the hypertension is stage 1, measurements should be made within 1 mo of each other; if stage 2, within a week; and, if severe, immediate action is necessary to complete the workup and treat the hypertension.

Secondary Hypertension

Table 1 lists the common causes of secondary hypertension. If none of these causes is present, the hypertension is primary. The term *primary hypertension* is preferred to *essential hypertension,* because the latter refers to an obsolete and incorrect concept—that the hypertension is "essential" to achieve perfusion of organs through arteries narrowed by arteriosclerotic disease.

Of the secondary causes of hypertension, some are often fairly easy to recognize. For example, by the time Cushing syndrome is severe enough to cause hypertension, the clinical features are usually obvious on physical examination. The same is true of acromegaly. Many cases of coarctation of the aorta are detected in infancy or childhood. However, most of the causes of secondary hypertension need to be carefully excluded in the history, the physical examination, and the laboratory workup. Tables 2 and 3 propose a simple and general approach to this process. Some of the commonest causes of secondary hypertension are described in more detail later in this chapter.

Target Organ Damage

VASCULAR HYPERTROPHY

Hypertrophy (8,9) refers to growth brought about by an increase in cell *size* rather than *number.* (An increase in cell number is hyperplasia.) In adults, the vascular smooth muscle cells (VSMC) are relatively quiescent, having an extremely low (<5%) mitotic index. In persons with hypertension and atherosclerosis, however, VSMC undergo phenotypic modulation with hypertrophy and/or hyperplasia, altered receptor expression, altered lipid handling, and migration from the vascular media to the subintimal portion of the vessel, and the vessel shows enhanced extracellular matrix deposition. All these result in an increase in stiffness (lower compliance) of the arteries of hypertensive

Table 1
Causes of Secondary Hypertension

Renal parenchymal hypertension
Renovascular disease
Coarctation of the aorta
Adrenal disorders
  Adrenocortical hypertension:
    Mineralocorticoid hypertension (e.g., Conn's syndrome)
    Glucocorticoid hypertension (e.g., Cushing's syndrome)
Other hormonal disorders
  Hypothyroidism
  Hyperthyroidism
  Hyperparathyroidism
  Acromegaly
Neurologic disorders: increased intracranial pressure
Drugs, especially oral contraceptives, exogenous steroids, erythropoietin, cyclosporine, licorice,
  sympathomimetic drugs, cocaine, tricyclic antidepressants, prostaglandin synthesis inhibitors
  (e.g., nonsteroidal antiinflammatory drugs interfere with the effects of many antihypertensive drugs),
  anabolic steroids

Table 2
Hypertension Workup: History and Physical Examination

Symptoms and signs	Diagnosis
Secondary Hypertension	
Abdominal or flank masses	Polycystic kidneys
Abdominal bruit	Renovascular hypertension
Delayed/absent femoral pulses, blood pressure gradient between arm and leg	Aortic coarctation
Truncal obesity, moonface, purple striae, buffalo hump	Cushing's syndrome
Tachycardia, tremor, pallor, sweating	Pheochromocytoma
Flank pain, frequency dysuria, hematuria, prostatism, edema	Renal parenchymal disease
Target Organ Damage	
Vision, fundoscopy	Retinopathy
Dyspnea, fatigue, signs of left ventricular failure	Left ventricular failure
Angina, previous myocardial infarction	Coronary artery disease
Focal neurologic symptoms and signs	Cerebrovascular disease
Symptoms and signs of renal failure	Hypertensive renal disease
Risk Factor Profiling	
Hypertension, age, gender, body mass index, family history, smoking, coronary artery, cerebrovascular, or peripheral vascular disease, left ventricular hypertrophy	

patients. This diffuse arteriosclerosis of hypertension increases with age. Superimposed on this may be accelerated development of atherosclerotic lesions.

Factors that stimulate vascular smooth muscle hypertrophy or hyperplasia in hypertension include endothelin, which activates the ETA subtype of the endothelin receptor to activate an intracellular transduction pathway involving phospholipase C (PLC), inositol 1,4,5-trisphosphate ($1P_3$), and 1,2-diacylglycerol (DAG); release of cytosolic calcium from the endoplasmic reticulum; and, possibly, the mitogen-activated protein (MAP) kinase system. Angiotensin II, acting via the AT_1 receptor subtype, has a similar intracellular transduction pathway. Other hormones or autocrine or paracrine factors that affect VSMC growth are vasopressin, catecholamines, insulin-like growth factor 1 (IGF-1), platelet-derived growth factor (PDGF), fibroblast growth factor (FGF), and transforming growth factor (TGF)-β, which all stimulate growth, and nitric oxide, atrial natriuretic

Table 3
Hypertension Workup: Screening Laboratory Tests

Test	Rationale
Blood chemistry	
Blood urea nitrogen	Impaired renal function
Creatinine	Impaired renal function
Potassium	Primary aldosteronism
	Cushing's syndrome
	Renal failure
Calcium/phosphate	Hyperparathyroidism
Cholesterol (total, HDL and LDL), triglycerides, glucose, C-reactive protein, uric acid	Risk factors for cardiovascular disease
Thyroid-stimulating hormone assay	Hyperthyroidism
	Hypothyroidism
Urinalysis	Renal disease
Electrocardiography	LVH
Complete blood count	All new patients should have one

peptide, estrogens, and prostacyclin, which are inhibitory. This inhibition is thought to be due to an increase in apoptosis, reversing VSMC proliferation. Many studies have shown improvement in VSMC hypertrophy and hyperplasia in hypertensive patients who take drugs that inhibit the action of angiotensin II (ACE inhibitors or AT_1 receptor blockers) or calcium (calcium-channel blockers), and it could be predicted that the same effects would occur with agents that enhance inhibitory factors, such as those neutral endopeptidase inhibitors that reduce the breakdown of atrial natriuretic peptide.

LEFT VENTRICULAR HYPERTROPHY

Left ventricular hypertrophy (LVH) *(10)* is a consequence of mechanical forces such as chronic increased systolic afterloading of the cardiac myofibrils in hypertension. As they do to VSMC hypertrophy, important neurohormonal stimuli contribute to LVH, particularly the renin–angiotensin system (angiotensin II), the sympathetic nervous system, and the other growth factors listed earlier for VSMC. The clinical significance of the prohypertrophic actions of angiotensin II, for instance, is that ACE inhibitors or AT_1 receptor blockers could be expected to prevent, or even reverse, LVH more than antihypertensive drugs that reduce blood pressure by the same amount but have no direct action on myocardial cells *(11)*. This is important, because of the very adverse effect of LVH on the prognosis for patients with hypertension.

Patients with LVH (and many hypertensive patients without LVH) usually have diastolic dysfunction: their left ventricle is stiffer (i.e., less compliant) and thus requires greater distending pressure during diastole. These patients may have dyspnea (secondary to raised pulmonary venous filling pressure), left atrial hypertrophy, a fourth heart sound, and late diastolic flow across the mitral valve (A wave) that is larger than early diastolic flow (E wave). LVH may progress toward the syndrome of systolic dysfunction and dilated cardiomyopathy with congestive heart failure.

HEART ATTACK AND BRAIN ATTACK *(12,13)*

Hypertension is a significant risk factor for both acute myocardial infarction and stroke. Both situations are marked by hypertension-induced vascular hypertrophy and/or hyperplasia, endothelial dysfunction, and accelerated atherosclerosis, caused by migration of VSMC into the subintima, subendothelial infiltration of monocytes, cholesterol deposition and oxidation, and calcification. Additional elements in acute myocardial infarction are plaque disruption, platelet adhesion and aggregation, and thrombosis. Patients with hypertension are at much greater risk of coronary events, because of the malignant combination of decreased oxygen supply and the increased oxygen demand.

The limitation of oxygen supply is due to either decreased coronary flow, or more commonly a decreased capacity of the arteriosclerotic coronary arteries to vasodilate (impaired coronary flow reserve) in response to the increased oxygen demand of LVH and the increased output impedance of the left ventricle.

Strokes, however, are more varied in their pathogenesis. Hypertension is the major cause of stroke. In hypertension, about 80% of strokes are ischemic, and about 15% are hemorrhagic. Reduction of cerebral blood flow due to arterial stenosis or thrombosis may produce any degree of tissue injury from asymptomatic and isolated neuronal dropout to huge infarction and cavitary necrosis. The extent of the ischemic injury depends on the duration and the intensity of the ischemia, and these, in turn, depend on the efficiency of the collateral circulation and the cardiac output. Hemorrhagic stroke in hypertension is probably due to rupture of microaneurysms of the small intracerebral arteries. Hypertension can also cause focal damage to small intracerebral arteries (lipohyalinosis) marked by occlusion of the vessels and the production of small ischemic cavities in the brain known as *lacunar infarcts,* frequently seen in the MRIs of patients with vascular dementia. Last, hypertension is a risk factor for berry aneurysms and subarachnoid hemorrhage.

HYPERTENSIVE ENCEPHALOPATHY

Hypertensive encephalopathy *(14)* is an acute syndrome of severe hypertension, cerebrovascular dysfunction, and neurologic impairment that resolves rapidly with treatment. The pathophysiologic mechanism is segmental dilation along the cerebral arterioles (sausage-string appearance); when, in severe hypertension, the autoregulatory capacity of vessels is exceeded, segments of the vessel are stretched and dilated. There is then leakage of fluid into the perivascular tissue causing edema and the syndrome of hypertensive encephalopathy. Clinical features are those of encephalopathy (headache, nausea, projectile vomiting, visual blurring, drowsiness, confusion, seizures, coma) in association with severe hypertension. Papilledema, usually with retinal hemorrhages and exudates, may be present, and the sausage-string arteries may be seen in the retina. The differential diagnosis includes cerebral infarction, intracerebral hemorrhage, subarachnoid hemorrhage, subdural hematoma, brain tumor, encephalitis, and epilepsy. These lesions are usually identified by their distinctive clinical features and by computed tomography (CT). Drugs, such as intravenous amphetamines and cocaine, and ingestion of tyramine by patients taking monoamine oxidase inhibitors can produce a similar clinical picture, as can lupus vasculitis, polyarteritis, or uremic encephalopathy.

HYPERTENSION-RELATED RENAL DAMAGE

Hypertension is both a cause and a consequence of glomerulosclerosis, the hallmark lesion of progressive renal disease (*see* Chapter 40) *(15,16)*. It is a cause of end-stage renal disease, second only to diabetes, particularly in African-American patients. About 15% of patients with primary hypertension have microalbuminuria, and this finding in any patient is predictive of increased cardiovascular risk, but whether hypertensive nephropathy will develop in these patients is not known. The pathologic processes of hypertensive renal injury consist of vascular intimal thickening and fibrosis and hyalinization of arterioles (arteriosclerosis). There may be focal glomerulosderosis with atrophic tubules. Mechanisms of the hypertensive renal injury include ischemia and increased glomerular capillary pressure. Other mechanisms whose roles are not clearly understood involve free oxygen radicals, glomerular capillary endothelial cell dysfunction, and proteinuria induced by the increased glomerular capillary pressure. However some authorities who have questioned the causal relationship between hypertension and renal disease, suggest that the focal glomerulo-sclerosis is always primary.

HYPERTENSIVE RETINOPATHY

Table 4 summarizes the features of hypertensive retinopathy *(17)*, using the Keith and Wagener classification first proposed in 1939. The optic fundi should be examined in every new hypertensive patient; with some practice this can often be done without having to dilate the pupils. The

Table 4
Keith-Wagener Classification of Hypertensive Retinopathy

Degree	A-V Ratio	Hemorrhages	Exudates	Papilledema	Other findings
Normal	3:4	0	0	0	
Grade I	1:2	0	0	0	
Grade II	1:3	0	0	0	"Copper wire" arterioles,
Grade III	1:4	+	+	0	arteriovenous nipping
Grade IV	1:4	+	+	+	"Silver wire" arterioles

0, none; +, at least one.

presence of hemorrhages, exudates, or optic disk swelling should prompt earlier and more aggressive therapy. In addition to retinopathy, hypertensive choroidopathy occurs, but rarely. In addition to the lesions listed in Table 4, hypertension is associated with an increased incidence of central retinal vein occlusion, cotton-wool spots or cytoid bodies (areas of infarction in the retina), capillary microaneurysms (more common in diabetes), arteriolar macroaneurysms, and large, flame-shaped hemorrhages. Because of the frequent association of hypertension and diabetes, diabetic retinopathy is common.

HYPERTENSIVE EMERGENCIES AND URGENCIES

Hypertensive emergencies are situations in which severe hypertension is associated with acute or rapidly progressive target organ damage. This condition is sometimes referred to as *malignant hypertension* or *accelerated malignant hypertension,* and a frequent, but not universal feature is papilledema (grade IV retinopathy). The mechanism of the often extremely high blood pressure with rapid deterioration of target organ function is not known; hypotheses include vascular endothelial damage with myointimal proliferation, and pressure natriuresis producing hypovolemia with activation of vasoconstrictor hormones such as catecholamines, endothelin, and the renin–angiotensin system. Plasma renin activity is usually very high. Usually, but not always, the diastolic blood pressure is over 120 mmHg and at least one of the features of rapid target organ damage is evident, such as cerebrovasular (hypertensive encephalopathy, stroke) or cardiac (acute left ventricular failure, myocardial infarction, aortic dissection) lesions or acute renal failure. Obviously, these patients require urgent therapy with parenteral antihypertensive agents (*see* Chapter 33), although care should be taken not to drop mean arterial pressure too suddenly or below the lower limit of cerebrovascular autoregulation, which could induce an ischemic stroke. *Hypertensive urgencies* describe situations of very high blood pressure (>180 mmHg SBP or >110 mmHg DBP) not related to severe symptoms or acute progressive target organ damage. For this condition the blood pressure should be reduced by oral agents without delay.

Risk Factor Profiling

The third objective of the initial evaluation of a patient with hypertension is to get a full picture of the cardiovascular risk factors for that patient; what risk factors, other than hypertension, are present? There is a cluster of atherogenic risk factors that often accompanies hypertension, referred to as "metabolic syndrome." This consists of hypertension, abdominal obesity (waist circumference: men >40 in [>102 cm], women >35 in [>88 cm]), dyslipidemia (triglycerides >150 mg/dL, HDL-cholesterol <40 mg/dL [men] and <50 mg/dL [women], insulin resistance or glucose intolerance (fasting blood glucose >110 mg/dL), a proinflammatory state (elevated C-reactive protein), and a prothrombotic state (elevated plasma plasminogen activator inhibitor (PAI)-1) *(18)*. Other potent risk factors include age, gender, smoking, LDL-cholesterol, a positive history of premature cardiovacular events in first-degree relatives, left ventricular hypertrophy and hyperuricemia. More recently homocysteine, fibrinogen, factor VII, t-PA, and lipoprotein(a) have been shown to predict cardiovascular morbidity and mortality. These are discussed more fully in Chapter 1.

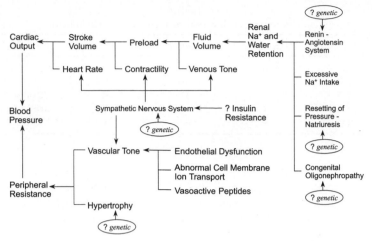

Fig. 1. Hemodynamic and renal control of blood pressure.

PATHOGENESIS OF PRIMARY HYPERTENSION

Most of the causes of secondary hypertension (*see* "Common Causes of Secondary Hypertension" section) have been well-characterized, and their pathophysiologic mechanisms are reasonably well-understood. These causes, however, account for only 5 to 10% of all hypertension cases seen by physicians, and the remaining 90 to 95% of patients with primary hypertension have a disease that is as poorly understood as it is common. Consequently, enormous research efforts have been mobilized to study the pathogenesis of primary hypertension, using animal models, human patients, and, more recently, the powerful tools of cell and molecular biology. The result has been a plethora of mechanisms and theories, not all mutually exclusive, that support the concept devised by Irvine Page of a "mosaic" of mechanisms, each operating in different organs and at different levels of organization. A brief and selective survey of this topic follows.

Genetic Predisposition

Monogenic syndromes are covered in the section on secondary hypertension. Primary hypertension also tends to cluster in families, but a specific genotype has not been identified. A number of associations have been suggested, but none has been confirmed. These include mutations in the genes for angiotensinogen, renin, 11β-hydroxylase, aldosterone synthase, and the α_1-adreno receptors; a negative association with transforming growth factor β_1 (TGF-β_1) and the adducin protein which affects the assembly of the actin-based cytoskeleton; and polymorphisms in about 25 genes, including those for angiotensinogen, angiotensin-converting enzyme (ACE), and the angiotensin II type 1 receptor.

Increased Cardiac Output

Blood pressure is proportional to cardiac output (CO) and total peripheral resistance (TPR). Some young "borderline hypertensives" have a hyperkinetic circulation with increased heart rate and CO (Fig. 1). This, in turn, may be due to increased preload associated with increased blood volume or to increased myocardial contractility. Also, LVH has been described in the still normotensive children of hypertensive parents, an observation that suggests that the LVH is not only a consequence of increased arterial pressure but that it may itself reflect some mechanism, such as hyperactivity of the sympathetic nervous system or the renin–angiotensin system, that causes both LVH and hypertension. In mature primary hypertension the CO is normal and the TPR elevated. The switch from elevated CO to elevated TPR may be due to autoregulatory vasoconstriction in response to organ hyperperfusion; thereafter the hypertension becomes self-sustaining due to the

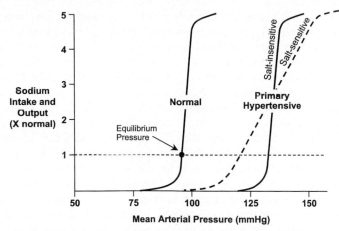

Fig. 2. Steady-state relations between blood pressure and sodium intake and output in normotensive subjects and in patients with salt-sensitive or salt-insensitive hypertension. Normally, an increase in sodium intake will result in a small increase in mean arterial pressure that is sufficient to increase sodium output by pressure natriuresis, so that the "equilibrium pressure" is restored. In salt-insensitive hypertension, the steep curve is retained but is shifted to the right (i.e., reset at a higher mean arterial pressure). In salt-sensitive hypertension, there is a shift to the right and flattening of the curve so that sodium loading increases blood pressure by a greater amount. (Modified from ref. *33.*)

accelerated arteriosclerosis. Plasma volume is usually normal or slightly lower than normal in established primary hypertension; however, some investigators have suggested that the volumes are still higher than they should be, given the elevated blood pressure, which should produce substantial pressure natriuresis and diuresis.

Excessive Dietary Sodium

We ingest many times more sodium than we need; there is much epidemiologic and experimental evidence to show an association between salt intake and hypertension. Sodium excess activates some pressor mechanisms (such as increases of intracellular calcium and plasma catecholamines, and an upregulation of angiotensin II type 1 receptors), and it increases insulin resistance. About half of hypertensive patients are particularly salt-sensitive (as defined by the blood pressure rise induced by sodium loading), as compared with about a quarter of normotensive controls. Sodium sensitivity becomes greater with age and has a strong genetic component. The mechanism of sodium sensitivity may be renal sodium retention (*see* later). More than 100 trials have shown an average reduction of blood pressure of 5/2 mmHg in hypertensive patients who lower their sodium intake to approx 100 mmol/d.

Renal Sodium Retention

Four mechanisms have been advanced to explain renal sodium retention in hypertension; resetting of the renal pressure-natriuresis curve, an endogenous sodium pump inhibitor, inappropriately high renin levels, and reduced nephron number.

Abnormal renal sodium handling may be due to a rightward shift of the pressure-natriuresis curve of the kidney (Fig. 2) *(19)*. When the arterial pressure is raised, the normal kidney excretes more salt and water; balance normally occurs at a mean perfusion pressure of around 100 mmHg, producing sodium excretion of about 150 mEq/d. Increased salt intake transiently raises blood pressure, and the pressure-natriuresis effectively restores total body sodium to normal. In patients with primary hypertension, this pressure-natriuresis curve is reset to a higher blood pressure, preventing return of the blood pressure to normal. There is some evidence in certain animal models and in humans that the rightward shift in the pressure-natriuresis curve is inherited.

A variation on this theme is a hormonal mediator of salt sensitivity, a sodium pump inhibitor, endogenous ouabain, which is secreted by the adrenal cortex and is natriuretic in sodium-loaded animals *(20)*. Renal sodium retention stimulates ouabain release, which, by its inhibition of the sodium pump, increases intracellular sodium. In turn, sodium-calcium exchange is inhibited, and the rise in intracellular calcium causes increased vascular tone and vascular hypertrophy. This is discussed further in the "Abnormal Cell Membrane Ion Transport," section.

Some investigators believe that a more important role for the kidney is the generation of more renin from nephrons that are ischemic, owing to afferent arteriolar vasoconstriction or structural narrowing of the lumen *(21)*. Some patients with primary hypertension have elevated plasma renin activity, but, even in those with normal levels, it may be inappropriately high, as we would expect the hypertension to suppress renin *(22)*. Others have developed the idea that hypertension may arise from a congenital reduction in the number of nephrons or in the filtration surface area per glomerulus that limits the ability of the kidney to excrete sodium, raising blood pressure, which destroys more glomeruli, thus setting up a vicious cycle of hypertension and renal glomerular dysfunction. This idea has support from the observation that low-birth-weight babies are more likely to become hypertensive later in life.

Increased Activity of the Renin–Angiotensin System

The components of the renin–angiotensin system, the biosynthesis and actions of angiotensin II, and angiotensin II signal transduction in VSMC are all described in Chapter 44. Plasma renin activity is nearly always low in association with primary aldosteronism, high with renovascular or accelerated-malignant hypertension, and low, normal, or high with primary hypertension. Primary hypertension with sodium retention would be expected to depress plasma renin levels; under these circumstances "normal" values are inappropriately high. Three explanations for this have been developed. The first, cited earlier, is that a population of ischemic nephrons contributes excess renin. The second is that the sympathetic hyperactivity associated with primary hypertension stimulates β-adrenergic receptors in the juxtaglomerular apparatus of the nephron to activate renin release. The third proposes that many of the patients with inappropriately normal or even high renin levels have defective regulation of the relationship of sodium and the renin–angiotensin system—that they are "nonmodulators." This results in abnormal adrenal and renal responses to salt loads; in particular, salt loading does not reduce angiotensin II *(23)*. In low-renin hypertension, the hypertension is primarily due to volume overload, but may in rarer cases be explained by hyperaldosteronism *(see* below), or excess 18-hydroxylated steroids, or with high levels of cortisone from inhibition of 11β-hydroxysteroid dehydrogenase. High- or normal-renin hypertensives have a higher rate of cardiovascular complications than those with low renin. Also it has been suggested that, since high- and normal-renin hypertensives are vasoconstricted, the drug of first choice in their treatment should be one that antagonizes the renin–angiotensin system, and because low-renin hypertensives are volume-overloaded, they should be treated in the first instance with a diuretic.

Increased Sympathetic Activity

There is much evidence of sympathetic hyperactivity in patients with primary hypertension. Heart rate and stroke volume are increased, at least in the early, labile phase of blood pressure elevation, and at least part of the increased vascular resistance of the established phase of hypertension may be due to the increased sympathetic tone. It is not surprising that psychogenic stress seems to predispose to high blood pressure, tension causing hypertension. Baroreceptor sensitivity is reduced in some patients with hypertension, presumably because of the arteriosclerotic stiffness of the vessels that house baroreceptors, so that a given increase in blood pressure decreases heart rate less than it normally would. In other patients there is resetting of the baroreceptor reflex, with baroreceptor reflexes operating normally, but around a higher setpoint of arterial pressure.

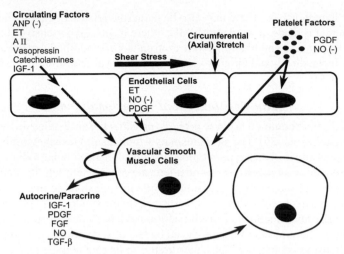

Fig. 3. Stimuli to vascular smooth muscle growth. ANP, atrial natriuretic peptide; El, endothelin; AII, angiotensin II; PDGF, platelet-derived growth factor; NO, nitric oxide; IGF-l, insulin-like growth factor-1; FGF, fibroblast growth factor; TGF-β, transforming growth factor β; (–), inhibitory to hypertrophy/hyperplasia.

Increased Peripheral Resistance

Small arteries and arterioles are responsible for most of the peripheral resistance, but the microvasculature is difficult to study in humans. It is much easier to study larger arteries, especially by noninvasive methods such as ultrasonography. We can make measurements of morphology such as wall thickness and wall:lumen ratio, and of physiologic processes, such as compliance or distensibility (lumen cross-sectional diameter or area change per unit pressure change). Patients with hypertension very frequently have large arteries (e.g., brachial, carotid, femoral) that are thick (owing to hypertrophy, increased wall:lumen ratio) and stiff (owing to decreased compliance). These effects are due to vascular smooth muscle cell hypertrophy in the media. Smaller arteries probably undergo cither hyperplasia or remodeling, which is a rearrangement of existing cells around a smaller lumen. The growth factors responsible for these changes are summarized in Fig. 3 and are discussed in more detail in Chapter 4.

Abnormal Cell Membrane Ion Transport

Because it is so easy to measure red cell cation concentrations, and therefore the kinetics of transmembrane cation flux, the literature on abnormalities of these in primary hypertension is voluminous. There seems to be general agreement that there is decreased activity of the Na^+-K^+-ATPase pump (which pumps Na^+ *out* of the cell), possibly the result of an excess of the endogenous inhibitor ouabain (*see* earlier in the section on renal sodium retention). There may also be increased activity of the Na^+-H^+ exchange antiporter (which pumps Na^+ *into* the cell). Both mechanisms increase intracellular sodium. This high intracellular sodium concentration (and low intracellular pH) inhibits Na^+-Ca^{2+} exchange (normally Na^+ *in* and Ca^{2+} *out*) to increase intracellular Ca^{2+}, which increases vascular tone and stimulates hypertrophy. Hyperactivity of the Na^+-H^+ exchanger in renal proximal tubule cells may also cause increased sodium reabsorption and intravascular volume expansion *(24)*.

Endothelial Dysfunction

Impaired biosynthesis or release of nitric oxide, the vascular endothelium-derived relaxing factor, has been described in animal models of hypertension and in human hypertension *(9)*. Endothelin, a 21-amino-acid vasoconstrictor made by endothelial cells, is present in increased amounts in the plasma of hypertensives. There may also be paracrine release of endothelin from the endo-thelial cells, where it is made, toward the VSMC, where it acts. Hypertensives have an increased vasoconstrictor response to endothelin, as well as an enhanced endothelial expression of the endo-thelin gene. Prostaglandin H_2 and thromboxane A_2 are other vasoconstrictors made by endothelial cells (*see* Chapter 4).

Insulin Resistance and Hyperinsulinemia

Hypertension is more common in obese persons, possibly because of insulin resistance and the resulting hyperinsulinemia *(25)*. The mechanism by which insulin resistance or hyperinsulinemia increases blood pressure is obscure; possibilities include enhanced renal sodium and water reab-sorption, increased renin–angiotensin or sympathetic nervous system activity, and vascular hyper-trophy, all firmly established actions of insulin. While the physiologic role of insulin resistance and hyperinsulinemia has been studied most intensively in the syndrome of obesity, hypertension, and diabetes, similar abnormalities of insulin action have been described in lean hypertensives who are not diabetic. Leptin, a hormone produced by fat cells, stimulates the sympathetic nervous and renin–angiotensin systems, but is also natriuretic, so its role in hypertension is not yet clear.

Other Possible Mechanisms

The many other possible mechanisms that have been investigated are supported by more or less solid evidence. Notable ones are abnormal patterns of biosynthesis or secretion of adrenocortical hormones in response to various stimuli; adrenomedullin (an adrenomedullary vasodilator pep-tide); the kallikrein-kinin system, including bradykinin; other vasoactive peptides (natriuretic pep-tide, calcitonin gene-related peptide, neuropeptide Y, opioid peptides, vasopressin); dopamine; serotonin; prostaglandins; and medullipin (a renomedullary vasodepressor lipid). In addition to all the postulated mechanisms for primary hypertension, many other factors may contribute to high blood pressure in susceptible persons. Examples are increased urinary calcium with a low plasma calcium concentration, potassium and magnesium deficiency, smoking, excessive consumption of caffeine or alcohol, physical inactivity, and hyperuricemia.

COMMON CAUSES OF SECONDARY HYPERTENSION

"Common" is an overstatement. As a rough estimate, only about 5% of all patients who present with hypertension have a demonstrable cause that therefore may qualify the condition as *secondary*. It is, however, critically important to recognize these conditions when they occur, as many are curable—by surgery or some other means.

Renovascular Hypertension

Renal hypoperfusion as a result of renovascular disease accounts for about 1% of all cases of hypertension, but it is much more likely to be the cause when hypertension is rapidly progressive, accelerated, or malignant, or is associated with coronary, carotid, or peripheral vascular disease *(26–28)*. The mechanism of renovascular hypertension has been firmly established in animal models (based on those developed by Harry Goldblatt in the 1930s). When both renal arteries in the dog are partially occluded by clamps, or when one artery is clamped and the other kidney removed, sustained hypertension develops. The two-clip–two-kidney model resembles bilateral renovascular hypertension, and the one-clip–one-kidney animal is a model for renovascular hyper-tension plus chronic renal parenchymal disease. A more useful model for the common form of reno-vascular hypertension, unilateral renal artery stenosis, is the one-clip–two-kidney model.

MECHANISMS

Bilateral renovascular hypertension and *renovascular hypertension (unilateral or bilateral) with chronic renal parenchymal disease* have similar mechanisms. The decreased intrarenal vascular pressure results in increased secretion of renin from the juxtaglomerular apparatus, and, consequently, increased activity of angiotensin II and aldosterone. The systemic vasoconstriction produced by angiotensin II raises the blood pressure (renin-dependent hypertension). With time, however, the renin–angiotensin dependency of the systemic hypertension wanes because of progressive retention of sodium and water, which leads to increases in extracellular fluid volume, blood volume, and blood pressure. Sodium and water retention are consequences of a reduction in the functional renal mass subjected to reduced perfusion pressure, with the associated rightward shift of the pressure-natriuresis curve (*see* Fig. 2), and are secondary to the effects of angiotensin II, namely intrarenal vasoconstriction, increased net tubular sodium reabsorption, and increased aldosterone levels. At this stage, the hypertension is mainly volume-dependent. With progressive diminution in renin release and in circulating angiotensin II levels, salt and water balance is restored, but at the expense of high arterial blood pressure.

This dual mechanism has important therapeutic implications. Therapy with vasodilators reduces the renal perfusion pressure even further and exacerbates volume retention. Diuretics reduce the extracellular fluid volume and enhance the activity of the renin–angiotensin system. Vasodilator drugs in combination with volume depletion can decrease the glomerular filtration rate and can even cause acute renal failure. ACE inhibitors or angiotensin II receptor blockers may also be dangerous because they remove the selective vasoconstrictor action of angiotensin II on efferent arterioles to maintain glomerular filtration pressure.

Unilateral renovascular hypertension is much more common than bilateral stenosis in humans. Here, the stenotic kidney releases renin, elevating circulating levels of angiotensin II to increase blood pressure. This hypertension should increase sodium excretion in the nonstenotic kidney to restore blood pressure to normal; however, this pressure-natriuresis effect (*see* Fig. 2) is blunted by the increased angiotensin II levels, because of angiotensin II and aldosterone-mediated sodium reabsorption, and because of angiotensin II renal vasoconstriction with reduction in renal plasma flow and glomerular filtration rate (GFR). Since the pressure distal to the stenosis is never completely restored to normal, even with high systemic blood pressure, the levels of renin and angiotensin II remain high and the hypertension is "renin-dependent."

Treatment of unilateral renovascular hypertension with ACE inhibitors or angiotensin II receptor blockers reduces glomerular filtration pressure and GFR in the stenotic kidney but increases renal blood flow and GFR in the nonstenotic kidney. In some patients, the sustained hypertension of unilateral renovascular disease can cause hypertensive glomerular injury in the nonstenotic kidney, which further compromises renal function and exacerbates the hypertension. In these patients, ACE inhibitors and angiotensin II receptor blockers may further impair renal function, for the reasons described earlier.

Pathology

The most common cause of renovascular hypertension is atherosclerotic stenosis of a main renal artery. Affected patients are relatively older and usually have vascular disease elsewhere. The second condition is fibromuscular dysplasia, which can be subdivided into intimal fibroplasia, medial fibromuscular dysplasia, and periadventitial fibrosis. Of these, the most common is medial fibromuscular dysplasia (or medial fibroplasia), usually a condition of young women. Other, rare, causes are renal artery aneurysms, emboli, and Takayasu's arteritis and other vasculitides.

Clinical Features

The only unique clinical finding, an abdominal bruit, is heard in about half of those who have renal artery stenosis. In general, renal artery stenosis should be suspected in severe hypertension associated with any one of the following: progressive renal insufficiency, refractoriness to aggressive treatment, other evidence of occlusive vascular disease, in young women, or in patients whose serum creatinine value rises quickly after they start taking an ACE inhibitor. Laboratory findings often include proteinuria, elevated renin and aldosterone levels, and a low serum potassium value.

DIAGNOSIS

The most cost-effective screening test is color Doppler ultrasonography. A more traditional modality of screening is the captopril renal scan. Reduced renal uptake of technetium 99m diethylenetriamine pentaacetic acid (^{99m}Tc-DTPA) or reduced renal excretion of iodine 121 (^{121}I) hippurate or ^{99m}Tc-mercaptoacetyltriglycine (^{99m}Tc-MAG$_3$) are measures of renal function in stenotic kidneys. Renal function can be reduced further after a single dose of the ACE inhibitor captopril. If the ultrasonogram or the captopril scan is positive, then gadolinium-enhanced magnetic resonance angiography (MRA) or spiral CT angiography should be done. Other useful imaging tests include digital subtraction intravenous angiography and renal arteriography. Various tests detect hypersecretion of renin from the hypoperfused kidney: these are peripherial blood plasma renin activity (PRA), captopril-augmented peripheral blood PRA, and the renal vein renin ratio (ratio of PRA between the two renal veins; a ratio >1.5:1 is diagnostic).

THERAPY

For most patients, renal angioplasty (with or without stenting) or surgery is the treatment of choice. If, however, the hypertension is very well-controlled and renal function does not decline under close monitoring, antihypertensive drug therapy may be appropriate. ACE inhibitors or angiotensin II receptor antagonists should not be used.

Renal Parenchymal Hypertension (29)

Renal parenchymal hypertension is discussed in more detail in Chapter 40. Renal disease is the most common cause of secondary hypertension, which is present in about 80% of patients with chronic renal failure (CRF). Primary hypertension also damages the kidneys; in the United States, hypertension ranks just below diabetes among causes of end-stage renal disease. Hypertension is, therefore, both a cause and a consequence of renal disease, and often there is a vicious circle: hypertension causes renal damage, which exacerbates hypertension.

PATHOPHYSIOLOGIC MECHANISMS

The following mechanisms have been identified.

Glomerular Hypertension. A high systemic blood pressure may be transmitted to the glomerular capillaries, particularly if the autoregulatory vasoconstrictor response of the afferent arterioles is defective. This causes an increased filtration pressure, and an increased filtration rate of individual glomeruli, increased pressure within Bowman's capsule, and damage to glomerular epithelial cells. This results in a protein leak through the glomerular membrane, and the protein may then damage tubule cells. The renal damage will eventually result in a decrease of whole-kidney glomerular filtration rate, sodium and water retention, and worsening of the hypertension.

Sodium and Volume Status. A severely reduced GFR (<50 mL/min) causes sodium retention and volume expansion and, therefore, increased cardiac output. The disorder of sodium homeostasis may also be due to increased amounts of an endogenous ouabain-like natriuretic factor that inhibits the Na$^+$-K$^+$-ATPase pump.

Renin–Angiotensin–Aldosterone System. The renin–angiotensin–aldosterone system is activated in CRF because of diffuse intrarenal ischemia. The aldosterone contributes to sodium retention. Eventually, however, the expanded fluid volume inhibits renin release, and plasma renin activity may become normal. Even "normal" plasma concentrations of renin are, however, inappropriately high in relation to the state of sodium and water balance, and the hypertension remains partly due to an angiotensin-dependent increase in peripheral vascular resistance.

Autonomic Nervous System. CRF activates renal baroreceptors, which effect increases sympathetic nervous system activity and elevates plasma norepinephrine levels (as does reduced catecholamine clearance).

Other Mechanisms. In uremic patients increased plasma levels of an endogenous compound, asymmetrical dimethylarginine (ADMA), a nitric oxide synthase inhibitor, contribute to the hypertension. Recombinant human erythropoietin (rHu-EPO), used extensively to treat the anemia of CRF, exacerbates hypertension, though how it does so is not known. The secondary hyperparathyroidism of CRF makes the hypertension worse. The mechanism, as yet undefined, is somehow related to the increase in intracellular calcium concentration.

MANAGEMENT

The problem in treating hypertension in patients with CRF is that diuretics and other antihypertensive agents often produce a transient drop in renal blood flow and GFR and an increase in serum creatinine; thus, management is often a delicate balancing act between achieving blood pressure control and maintaining whatever renal function is left. In general, diuretics and ACE inhibitors or angiotensin receptor blockers are the antihypertensive drugs of choice (see Chapter 33).

Pheochromocytoma

About 0.5% of hypertensives have pheochromocytomas as the cause of the high blood pressure *(30)*. Pheochromocytomas can occur at any age, and they arise from neuroectodermal chromaffin cells, mostly in the adrenal medulla (85%) but sometimes elsewhere, usually in the abdomen or pelvis (15%). About 10% of adrenal and about 30 to 40% of extraadrenal tumors are malignant. Ten percent are familial and autosomal-dominant. The familial form seems to be due to mutations of the RET protooncogene on chromosome 10 and may be intercurrent with other tumors as a syndrome of multiple endocrine neoplasia (MEN). In MEN 2A, pheochromocytoma is associated with medullary thyroid carcinoma (MTC) and hyperparathyroidism, whereas in MEN 2B there is no parathyroid disease but there is a characteristic phenotype (marfanoid appearance, neuromas of the lips and tongue, thickened corneal nerves, intestinal ganglioneuromatosis). Other familial syndromes with pheochromocytoma include von-Hippel-Lindau syndrome and von Recklinghausen's disease.

Pheochromocytomas secrete mainly norepinephrine (NE) and less epinephrine, plus a variety of peptide hormones, adrenocorticotropin (ACTH), erythropoietin, parathyroid hormone, calcitonin gene-related protein, atrial natriuretic peptide, vasoactive intestinal peptide, and others. Most patients have hypertension; in about half it is sustained, with or without paroxysms, and in the other half blood pressure is normal between paroxysms. Paroxysms of hypertension may be signaled by severe headaches, sweating, palpitations with tachycardia, pallor, anxiety, and tremor. Also described are orthostatic hypotension, nausea and vomiting, and weight loss. Any patient with this symptom complex should be screened for pheochromocytoma with measurement of the plasma or urinary concentrations of the catecholamine metabolites, metanephrine and normetanephrine. There are, however, some problems with these tests. Results can be normal in patients with paroxysmal hypertension if the test is done during a normotensive interval. Plasma or urinary metabolites of an antihypertensive drug, labetalol, may cause a false-positive result. Other medications, particularly tricyclic antidepressants, may also give false-positive results.

If plasma catecholamines are only moderately elevated (600 to 2000 pg/mL), the differential diagnosis includes neurogenic hypertension and hypertension associated with increased sympathetic activity. Here, the clonidine suppression test is useful; clonidine decreases plasma catecholamine levels to normal in neurogenic hypertension, but not in pheochromocytoma. If blood or urine test findings are positive, the next step is to localize the tumor using CT or MRI. In patients with elevated metanephrines but a negative CT or MRI, scintigraphy using ^{131}I-metaiodobenzylguanidine (^{131}I-MIBG) should be done. Definitive treatment is surgery, but great care must be taken to prevent severe hypertension or hypotension during the operation or in the immediate postoperative period, utilizing α- and β-adrenergic blocking drugs and careful management of fluid balance.

Mineralocorticoid Hypertension

Aldosterone, the most abundant mineralocorticoid hormone, is synthesized by aldosterone synthase in the outer zone of the adrenal cortex (zona glomerulosa). Its synthesis and release are controlled by adrenocorticotropic hormone (ACTH) and blood levels peak in the early morning, but angiotensin II and the serum concentration of potassium also affect it. Aldosterone increases distal tubular reabsorption of sodium and chloride and secretion of potassium and hydrogen ions. Another mineralocorticoid hormone, deoxycorticosterone, produced by the inner zone of the adrenal cortex (zona fasciculata), is a much weaker mineralocorticoid than aldosterone, but it can cause hypertension when produced in large quantities.

The hypertension produced by mineralocorticoid excess is due to the increase in total exchangeable sodium, but many patients with chronic mineralocorticoid excess have normal plasma volume, because the initial increase in extracellular fluid volume is restored to normal by an increased natriuresis and diuresis due to decreased sodium reabsorption in segments of the nephron other than the distal tubule (mineralocorticoid escape). The hypertension is sustained by increased vascular resistance (possibly due to augmented vascular sensitivity to catecholamines) or by central nervous system mineralocorticoid receptors, which activate the sympathetic nervous system.

Primary hyperaldosteronism (Conn's syndrome) *(31)* is due either to a benign aldosterone-producing adenoma (APA) or, more rarely, to bilateral hyperplasia (BH). The classic clinical features of primary hyperaldosteronism are hypertension, excessive urinary potassium excretion, hypokalemia, hypernatremia, and metabolic alkalosis. The 24-h urinary potassium excretion exceeds 30 mEq/d, and the plasma aldosterone will be high and the renin low. The normal plasma aldosterone concentration is 5 to 20 ng/dL and the normal plasma renin activity is 1 to 3 ng/mL/h. This give a plasma aldosterone:renin ratio of approx 10, whereas in patients with primary aldosteronism the ratio is well above 20 (or above 900 using SI units). A hypertensive patient who is treated with diuretics or who has diarrhea may also have a low serum potassium concentration. In this situation, the serum potassium value returns to normal after recovery from the diarrhea or a few weeks after the diuretic is discontinued. Diuretics raise both PRA and aldosterone levels. Another test sometimes done to confirm the diagnosis is based on the failure of volume expansion to suppress aldosterone (plasma aldosterone is >10 ng/dL after 2 L normal saline iv over 4 h). CT or MRI of the adrenal glands completes the workup. If the imaging shows normal adrenals or bilateral nodularity or an adrenal mass of less than 1 cm, then serum 18-hydroxycorticosterone, the precursor of aldosterone, should be measured; serum 18-hydroxycorticosterone levels are higher than 65 ng/dL with APA and lower than 65 ng/dL with BH. Bilateral adrenal venous sampling is a highly specialized procedure that may reveal a unilateral source of excess aldosterone.

Glucocorticoid Hypertension (32)

The principal glucocorticoid in humans, cortisol, is synthesized in the zona fasciculata under the control of ACTH. While cortisol has only a weak mineralocorticoid effect, the circulating levels of the hormone in Cushing's syndrome are usually hundreds of times the normal value. Since most patients with Cushing's syndrome, however, do not have other findings of hypermineralocorticoidism, particularly hypokalemia, and since spironolactone, a mineralocorticoid antagonist, does not blunt the hypertensive effect of cortisol, other mechanisms must be operating. Possibilities include the glucocorticoids activating gene transcription of angiotensinogen in the liver, or increasing vascular reactivity to vasoconstrictor amines, or inhibition of the extraneuronal uptake and degradation of norepinephrine, or inhibition of vasodilators such as endothelial nitric oxide, kinins, and some prostaglandins, or a shift of sodium from cells to the extracellular compartment with an increase in plasma volume and, thus, in cardiac output. Also, in Cushing's syndrome, the ACTH excess may stimulate production and release of endogenous mineralocorticoids, especially 11-deoxycorticosterone (Fig. 4).

Other Clinical Syndromes of Adrenocortical Hypertension

GLUCOCORTICOID-REMEDIABLE HYPERALDOSTERONISM (GRA)

GRA is an autosomal-dominant disorder in which the classic features of primary hyperaldosteronism are completely relieved by glucocorticoids such as dexamethasone. Because dexamethasone

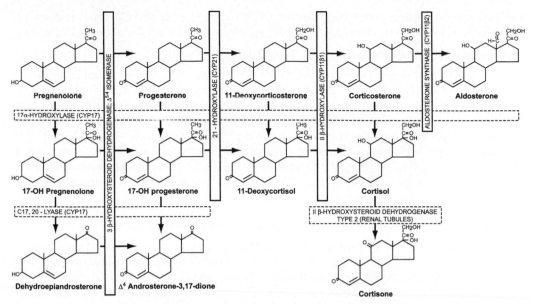

Fig. 4. Pathways of steroid biosynthesis in the adrenal cortex.

suppresses ACTH, the concept was developed of increased adrenal sensitivity to the aldosterone-stimulating effects of ACTH. Recently it has been shown that this syndrome is due to a chimeric gene produced by unequal crossing over of the 5' regulatory region of 11β-hydroxylase (CYP11β1) and the 3' coding sequence of aldosterone synthase (CYP11β2) (Fig. 4). As a result, aldosterone synthase, normally found in the zona glomerulosa, is expressed in the zona fasciculata under the control of the ACTH-sensitive 11β-hydroxylase regulatory sequence, which accounts for the aldosterone elevation and the excess formation of products of 11β-hydroxylase activity, such as cortisol. This is the first description of a gene mutation as a cause of hypertension in humans.

PSEUDOHYPERALDOSTERONISM (LIDDLE'S SYNDROME)

In 1963, Liddle described members of a family with hypertension and hypokalemic alkalosis who had low levels of aldosterone and no elevations of other mineralocorticoids. Treatment with the mineralocorticoid antagonist spironolactone or with other inhibitors of mineralocorticoid biosynthesis had no effect, but amiloride and triamterene, both inhibitors of distal nephron sodium reabsorption, improved hypertension and hypokalemia. Affected patients have a mutation of the β- or γ-subunits of the renal epithelial sodium channel that increases sodium reabsorption in the distal nephron.

Enzyme Deficiencies

11β-HYDROXYLASE (CYP11β1) DEFICIENCY

11β-Hydroxylase converts 11-deoxycorticosterone to corticosterone and 11-deoxycortisol to cortisol (Fig. 4). Deficiency of this enzyme leads to reduced cortisol levels, increased ACTH secretion, and increased production of 11-deoxycorticosterone in the zona fasciculata. The 11-deoxycorticosterone induces volume expansion and hypertension. The adrenal steroid pathway is also redirected toward androgen production, so that these patients also have virilization, usually recognized in infancy.

17α-HYDROXYLASE (CYP17) DEFICIENCY

17α-hydroxylase converts pregnenolone to 17-hydroxypregnenolone, progesterone to 17-hydroxyprogesterone, 11-deoxycorticosterone to 11-deoxycortisol, and corticosterone to cortisol (Fig. 4).

Deficiency of 17α-hydroxylase reduces cortisol levels, causing increased ACTH and increased 11-deoxycorticosterone, corticosterone and aldosterone levels. There is an absence of sex hormones.

11β-HYDROXYSTEROID DEHYDROGENASE TYPE 2 DEFICIENCY

The normal renal mineralocorticoid receptor binds glucocorticoids with a similar affinity to mineralocorticoids. The 11β-hydroxysteroid dehydrogenase type 2 isoform enzyme in the renal tubules normally converts the large amounts of fully active cortisol to the inactive cortisone (Fig. 4), thereby leaving the renal mineralocorticoid receptors open to the effects of aldosterone. A deficiency of this enzyme in the kidney allows for high renal levels of cortisol, producing all of the features of the hypermineralocorticoid state but with low mineralocorticoid levels (the syndrome of *apparent mineralocorticoid excess*). An acquired form of this syndrome develops in adults who eat large quantities of licorice. The active alkaloid in licorice, glycyrrhetinic acid, is an inhibitor of 11β-hydroxysteroid dehydrogenase.

Miscellaneous Causes of Secondary Hypertension

Other causes of secondary hypertension include coarctation of the aorta, hypo- and hyperthyroidism, hyperparathyroidism, sleep apnea, brain tumors and increased intracranial pressure, erythropoietin, polycythemia, inappropriate antidiuretic hormone, and a host of drugs and other chemical agents, notably exogenous steroids, cyclosporine, tacrolimus, pseudoephedrine (in nasal decongestants), monoamine oxidase inhibitors, tricyclic antidepressants, nonsteroidal antiinflammatory drugs, herbal remedies containing ephedrine, yohimbine, or licorice, and street drugs such as amphetamines and cocaine.

REFERENCES

1. MacMahon S, Peto R, Cutler J, et al. Blood pressure, stroke, and coronary heart disease. Part I. Prolonged differences in blood pressure: prospective observational studies corrected for the regression dilution bias. Lancet 1990; 335:765–773.
2. Chobanian AV, Bakris GL, Black HR, et al. Seventh Report of the Joint National Committee on Prevention, Detection, Evaluation, and Treatment of High Blood Pressure. Hypertension 2003;42:1206–1252.
3. National Institutes of Health; National Heart, Lung and Blood Institute. Fact Book, Fiscal Year 1996. National Institutes of Health, Bethesda, MD, 1997.
4. National Institute of Diabetes and Digestive and Kidney Disease. U.S. Renal Data System Annual Report. US Department of Health and Human Services, Bethesda, MD, 1997.
5. Levy D, Larson MG, Vasan RS, et al. The progression from hypertension to congestive heart failure. JAMA 1996; 275:1557–1562.
6. American Society of Hypertension. Recommendations for routine blood pressure measurement by indirect cuff sphygmomanometry. Am J Hypertens 1992;5:207–209.
7. Peloff D, Grim C, Flack J, et al. Human blood pressure determination by sphygmomanometry. Circulation 1993;88: 2460–2470.
8. Rosendorff C. The renin-angiotensin system and vascular hypertrophy. J Am Coll Cardiol 1996;28:803–812.
9. Rosendorff C. Endothelin, vascular hypertrophy and hypertension. Cardiovasc Drugs Ther 1996;10:795–802.
10. Lorell BH, Carabello BA. Left ventricular hypertrophy. Circulation 2000;102:470–479.
11. Schmieder RE, Martus P, Klingbeil A. Reversal of left ventricular hypertrophy in essential hypertension: a meta-analysis of randomized double-blind studies. JAMA 1996;275:1507–1513.
12. Rosendorff C. Treatment of hypertension patients with ischemic heart disease. In: Izzo JL Jr, Black HR, eds. Hypertension Primer: The Essentials of Blood Pressure, 3rd ed. American Heart Association, Council for High Blood Pressure Research, Dallas, TX, 2003, pp. 456–459.
13. Rosendorff C. Stroke in the elderly—risk factors and some projections. Cardiovasc Rev Reports 1999;20:244–248.
14. Healton EB, Brust JC, Feinfeld DA, Thomson GE. Hypertensive encephalopathy and the neurological manifestations of malignant hypertension. Neurology 1982;32:127–132.
15. Mountokalalds TD. The renal consequences of arterial hypertension. Kidney Int 1997;51:1639–1653.
16. Rennke HG, Anderson S, Brenner BM. Structural and functional correlations in the progression of renal disease. In: Tisher CC, Brenner PM, eds. Renal Pathology, 2nd ed. Lippincott, Philadelphia, 1994, pp. 116–142.
17. Frank RN. The eye in hypertension. In: Izzo JL Jr, Black HR, eds. Hypertension Primer: The Essentials of High Blood Pressure, 3rd ed. Council for High Blood Pressure Research, American Heart Association, Dallas, TX, 2003, pp. 209–211.
18. Third Report of the National Cholesterol Education Program (NCEP) expert panel on detection, evaluation, and treatment of high blood cholesterol in adults (Adult Treatment Panel III). Final report. Circulation 2002;106: 3143–3421.

19. Guyton AC. Kidneys and fluids in pressure regulation. Small volume but large pressure changes. Hypertension 1992; 19(Suppl 1):2–8.
20. de Wardener HE. Sodium transport inhibitors and hypertension. J Hypertens 1996;14(Suppl 5):S9–518.
21. Laragh JH. Renin-angiotensin-aldosterone system for blood pressure and electrolyte homeostasis and its involvement in hypertension, in congestive heart failure and in associated cardiovascular damage (myocardial infarction and stroke). J Hum Hypertens 1995;9:385–390.
22. Brenner BM, Chertow GM. Congenital oligonephropathy and the etiology of adult hypertension and progressive renal injury. Am J Kidney Dis 1994;23:171–175.
23. Williams GH, Hollenberg NK. Non-modulating hypertension. A subset of sodium-sensitive hypertension. Hypertension 1991;17(Suppl 1):181–185.
24. Swales JD. Functional disturbance of ions in hypertension. Cardiovasc Drug Ther 1990;4:367–372.
25. Reaven GM, Lithell H, Landsberg L. Hypertension and associated abnormalities—the role of insulin resistance and the sympathoadrenal system. N Engl J Med 1996;334:374–381.
26. Martinez-Maldonado M. Pathophysiology of renovascular hypertension. Hypertension 1991;17:707–719.
27. Ploth DW. Renovascular hypertension. In: Jacobson HR, Striker GE, Klahr S, eds. The Principles and Practice of Nephrology, 2nd ed. Mosby—Year Book, St. Louis, 1995, pp. 379–386.
28. Pohi MA. Renal artery stenosis, renal vascular hypertension and ischemic nephropathy. In: Schrier RW, Gottschalk CW, eds. Diseases of the Kidney, 6th ed. Little, Brown, Boston, 1997, pp. 1367–1423.
29. Working Group: 1995 Update of the Working Group Reports on Chronic Renal Failure and Renovascular Hypertension. NIH Publication No. 95-3791. National Heart, Lung and Blood Institute, Washington, DC, 1995.
30. Manger WM, Gifford RW Jr. Pheochromocytoma: diagnosis and treatment. J Clin Hypert 2002;4:62–72.
31. Ganguly A. Primary aldosteronism. N Engl J Med 1998;339:1828–1834.
32. Stern N, Tuck M. Pathophysiology of adrenal cortical hypertension. In: Izzo JL Jr, Black HR, eds. Hypertension Primer; The Essentials of High Blood Pressure, 3rd ed. American Heart Association Council for High Blood Pressure Research, Dallas, TX, 2003, pp. 144–148.
33. Hall JE, Brands MW, Shek EW. Central role of the kidney and abnormal fluid volume control in hypertension. J Hum Hypertens 1996;10:633–639.

RECOMMENDED READING

Izzo JL Jr, Black HR, eds. Hypertension Primer. The Essentials of High Blood Pressure, 3rd ed. Council on High Blood Pressure Research, American Heart Association, Dallas, TX, 2003.
Kaplan NK. Kaplan's Clinical Hypertension, 8th ed. Lippincott Williams & Wilkins, Philadelphia, 2002.
The Seventh Report of the Joint National Committee on Prevention, Detection, Evaluation, and Treatment of High Blood Pressure. No. 98-4080. National Institutes of Health, Bethesda, MD, 1997.

33 Hypertension Therapy

Norman M. Kaplan, MD

INTRODUCTION

Hypertension is almost always easy to treat but often exceedingly difficult to keep under control. As documented in the latest survey of a representative sample of the US population, more than half of hypertensives are being treated but only 34% have their blood pressure controlled, defined as below 140/90 mmHg on three measurements at two different times *(1)*. Although hypertension remains the most common reason for nonpregnant adults to visit a physician in the US *(2)*, these disappointing rates of control point to a number of problems: Many hypertensive patients have not been diagnosed or started on treatment, and many physicians have not provided adequate amounts of medications. But the most likely problem is inherent to the nature of hypertension: a lifelong condition that is usually asymptomatic for many years but that requires daily therapy that may in itself induce symptoms.

As described in the previous chapter, most hypertension is of unknown cause and therefore cannot be prevented with certainty. Nonetheless, in view of the inherent difficulty of treating the condition after it has developed, attention will first be given to the lifestyle modifications that may help delay, if not stop, the onset of the condition. All these are also of value in treating those with established hypertension; if offered to the prehypertensive, they may provide prevention as well *(3)*.

LIFESTYLE MODIFICATIONS

As described in all recent expert guidelines *(1,4,5)*, lifestyle modifications are often the only therapy indicated for patients with relatively mild hypertension and little overall cardiovascular risk, and they are always indicated along with drug therapy for the remainder.

The tendency for most physicians is to immediately proceed to drug therapy for any degree of hypertension. Drugs are a known quantity that are easy to prescribe and likely to be effective. Instructing, motivating, and following patients in the use of lifestyle modifications is costly in time and energy, costs that are not compensated by the insurance payers.

But the effort is worthwhile. Even if the degrees of weight loss and sodium restriction are relatively small, marked benefits have been shown as among the elderly hypertensives enrolled in the Nonpharmacologic Interventions in the Elderly (TONE) study *(6)* and the prediabetics in the Diabetes Prevention Program *(7)*. Moreover, other cardiovascular risk factors—dyslipidemia, glucose intolerance and diabetes, physical inactivity, cigarette smoking—may thereby be relieved, multiplying the benefits far beyond the reduction in blood pressure. The lifestyle modifications recommended in the Seventh Report of the Joint National Committee on Prevention, Detection, Evaluation and Treatment of High Blood Pressure (JNC-VII) for treatment are also applicable to prevention (Table 1).

Prevention of Intrauterine Growth Retardation

Though not included in the list of lifestyle modifications, another effective preventive measure is the prevention of intrauterine growth retardation and rapid postnatal "catch-up" weight gain *(8)*.

From: *Essential Cardiology: Principles and Practice, 2nd Ed.*
Edited by: C. Rosendorff © Humana Press Inc., Totowa, NJ

Table 1
Lifestyle Modifications to Manage Hypertension[a]

Modification	Recommendation	Approximate systolic BP reduction, range
Weight reduction	Maintain normal body weight (BMI, 18.5–24.9)	5–20 mmHg/10-kg weight loss
Adopt DASH eating plan	Consume a diet rich in fruits, vegetables, and low-fat dairy products with a reduced content of saturated and total fat	8–14 mmHg
Dietary sodium reduction	Reduce dietary sodium intake to no more than 100 mEq/L (2.4 g sodium or 6 g sodium chloride)	2–8 mmHg
Physical activity	Engage in regular aerobic physical activity such as brisk walking (at least 30 min per day, most days of the week)	4–9 mmHg
Moderation of alcohol consumption	Limit consumption to no more than 2 drinks per day (1 oz or 30 mL ethanol [e.g., 24 oz beer, 10 oz wine, or 3 oz 80-proof whiskey]) in most men or no more than 1 drink per day in women and lighter-weight persons	2–4 mmHg

BMI, body mass index (calculated as weight in kilograms divided by the square of height in meters); BP, blood pressure; DASH, Dietary Approaches to Stop Hypertension.

[a]For overall cardiovascular risk reduction, stop smoking. The effects of implementing these modifications are dose and time dependent and could be higher for some individuals. (From ref. *1*.)

A number of epidemiological surveys have documented an increased prevalence of hypertension in adults whose birth weight was low for their gestational age *(9)*.

The mechanism for this is uncertain, with the most attractive hypothesis being congenital oligonephropathy—a reduced number of nephrons at birth that leads to both systemic and glomerular hypertension *(10)*. Regardless of how low birth weight predisposes to hypertension (as well as diabetes and coronary heart disease), the prevention of low birth weight may very well be an effective and achievable way to prevent these adult diseases.

Low birth weight is more likely in disadvantaged populations, in particular among African-Americans (who have a much higher prevalence of both hypertension and renal insufficiency). Associations with low-birth-weight babies have been noted with teenage pregnancy, shorter intervals between pregnancies, inadequate nutrition, familial aggregation, and other unknown factors linked to the African-American population. The opportunity for overcoming most of these contributing factors is obvious. However, recent cutbacks in support for teenage contraception, maternal nutrition, and prenatal care in the United States suggest that we will continue to pay billions for the eventual care of hypertension-related end-stage renal disease, strokes, and heart attacks instead of millions for preventive care of the disadvantaged.

Prevention of Obesity

As difficult as it may be to overcome low birth weight, it likely will be even harder to correct the three major environmental contributors to the pathogenesis of hypertension: obesity, excess sodium, and stress. Of these three, obesity is growing most rapidly, with 65% of all adult Americans now overweight, defined as a body mass index (BMI) above 25, and 30% obese, defined as a BMI above 30. The association of weight gain and hypertension was shown clearly among the 82,500 female nurses 30 to 55 yr of age followed every 2 yr from 1976 to 1992 *(11)*. As seen in Fig. 1, a weight gain of only 5 kg (12 lb) from age 18 was responsible for almost a doubling of the incidence of hypertension; a 10-kg gain tripled the incidence.

When obesity is predominantly upper-body or visceral in distribution, the dangers for hypertension, diabetes, and dyslipidemia are even greater, with a marked increase in coronary disease

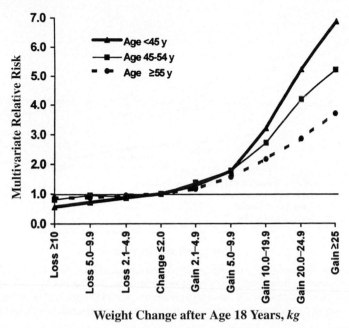

Weight Change after Age 18 Years, *kg*

Fig. 1. Multivariate relative risk for hypertension according to weight change after age 18 yr within strata of age. Adjusted for age, body mass index at age 18 yr, height, family history of myocardial infarction, parity, oral contraceptive use, menopausal status, postmenopausal use of hormones, and smoking status. (Adapted from ref. *11*.)

as a consequence of metabolic syndrome *(12)*. Moreover, upper-body obesity is associated with obstructive sleep apnea, which is increasingly being recognized as a cause of hypertension *(13)*.

The problem is obvious, the solution perhaps unattainable. As children and their parents become couch potatoes, rising only begrudgingly to change the TV channel or computer game, and eat increasingly "empty calorie" fast and junk food, the future looks even worse in regard to obesity. Nonetheless, even small amounts of weight loss can protect against a rise in blood pressure *(6)*. In the TONE trial, almost 1000 elderly patients with hypertension that was well controlled on one or two drugs voluntarily discontinued their drug therapy and were randomly assigned to one of four regimes: weight loss by caloric restriction and physical activity; sodium restriction; both weight loss and sodium restriction; or nothing (usual care). After 30 mo, those who lost an average of 4.7 kg (10 lb) on the weight-loss regimen had a 50% greater likelihood of staying normotensive and free of cardiovascular complications than did those with no weight loss (Fig. 2).

This study was done in elderly hypertensives but equally small amounts of weight loss have been shown to decrease the incidence of hypertension and diabetes in young subjects as well *(7)*. Therefore, the effort is worthwhile, best directed at young people to prevent them from becoming obese but also in adults to help them lose even more weight.

The DASH Diet

The Dietary Approaches to Stop Hypertension (DASH) diet has been shown to lower blood pressure in prehypertensives *(14)*. The DASH diet uses eight to nine daily portions of fruits and vegetables and more low-fat dairy products, providing more potassium, calcium, fiber, and protein and less saturated fat. However, the addition of the DASH diet to a regimen of weight loss, increased physical activity, moderate sodium reduction, and moderation of alcohol intake provided little additional antihypertensive effect *(15)*. Regardless, the DASH diet may be cardioprotective in ways beyond its blood pressure effect.

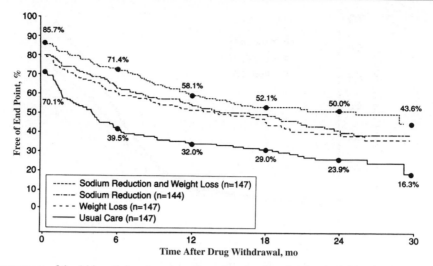

Fig. 2. Percentages of the 144 participants assigned to reduced sodium intake, the 147 assigned to weight loss, the 147 assigned to reduced sodium intake and weight loss combined, and the 147 assigned to usual care (i.e., no lifestyle intervention) who remained free of cardiovascular events and high blood pressure and did not have an antihypertensive agent prescribed during follow-up. CI, confidence interval. (Adapted from ref. *6*.)

Reduction of Sodium Intake

This goal could most easily be accomplished by a lowering of the amount of sodium added to processed foods, the source of 80% of overall sodium intake, since it is difficult to get individuals to reduce their intake by more than 30 mmol/d (*16*). As amply documented in many controlled trials, a reduction of 40 to 50 mmol/d, about one fourth to one third of the usual intake, will provide a 4 to 6 mmHg fall in systolic blood pressure among hypertensives and a 1 to 2 mmHg fall in blood pressure among normotensives (*17*). The TONE trial provides further evidence: Those who reduced daily sodium intake an average of 40 mmol/d had a 50% greater chance of remaining normotensive and free of cardiovascular events than did those on no sodium restriction (*6*) (Fig. 2).

The few-mmHg fall in blood pressure that would occur in normotensives by such moderate sodium restriction could have a very considerable impact on the incidence of hypertension and the development of cardiovascular disease. As noted by Rose (*18*), "All the life-saving benefits achieved by current antihypertensive treatment may be equaled by a downward shift of the whole blood pressure distributed by a mere 2–3 mmHg. The benefits from a mass approach in which everybody received a small benefit may be unexpectedly large."

DOUBTS ABOUT UNIVERSAL SODIUM RESTRICTION

A few hypertension experts question both the role of sodium excess in the pathogenesis of hypertension and the wisdom of advocating a populationwide strategy of moderate sodium restriction. The evidence, although only circumstantial, for a causal role for the high sodium content only recently introduced into the food supply of industrialized societies is so extensive that most are convinced that excess sodium intake is necessary, though not sufficient, for the pathogenesis of hypertension. Absolute proof for the role of high sodium may never be obtained since it is not possible to monitor the sodium intake of thousands of people almost from birth through midlife and observe the effects, particularly as there is considerable variability in the pressor sensitivity of people to sodium intake. Convincing evidence for direct and specific hypertensive effect of amounts of sodium typically consumed by humans has been obtained in chimpanzees, the species closest to man.

Those who object to the recommendations for universal sodium restriction point to evidence from short-term, profound reductions in sodium intake wherein hormonal and lipid perturbations are induced. Such perturbations do not occur with moderate sodium restriction as advocated by most experts and practiced by most patients. Therefore, a populationwide modest reduction in sodium will almost certainly be beneficial. It can be easily achieved while we wait for food processors to reduce the amount of salt they add by simply reading the labels and avoiding those with more than 300 mg of sodium per portion.

Potassium Deficiency

Rather than placing the blame on an excessive sodium intake, some evidence points to an imbalance between too much sodium and too little potassium in the diet. For example, surveys have noted a lower-than-recommended intake of potassium but no greater intake of sodium in poor African-Americans, particularly in the southern United States, who have a greater prevalence of hypertension. The lesser intake of potassium presumably reflects lesser consumption of meats, fresh fruits, and vegetables by the poor.

Potassium supplements will lower blood pressure in those who are on a low-potassium diet and the salutary effects of a diet rich in fruits and vegetables on blood pressure may have been provided by the increased potassium intake *(14)*. Potassium supplements cannot be recommended for prevention but more fresh fruits and vegetables will likely be beneficial.

Relief From Stress

Although the evidence is not sufficient to include this lifestyle modification in Table 1, data support a role for stress in the pathogenesis of hypertension, likely interacting with multiple other factors to increase vascular resistance. Nonetheless, it has not been possible to show that relief of stress as provided by various relaxation methods will prevent hypertension, much less provide more than a placebo effect in lowering the pressure in those with established hypertension, with rare exceptions *(19)*.

Increased Physical Activity

One way to help overcome stress may be physical activity. Whether or not that is the way physical activity lowers blood pressure, most well-controlled studies do show that regular aerobic exercise will lower blood pressure in hypertensive people and numerous surveys show a lesser incidence of hypertension in those who are physically fit. This protection likely involves a dampening of sympathetic nervous activity and the inflammatory response *(20)*.

Moderation of Alcohol

Excessive alcohol consumption certainly serves as a pressor mechanism, responsible for 5 to 10% of the hypertension found among men. About half of all published data show the pressor effect only when average daily consumption is greater than two drinks, the equivalent of one ounce of ethanol. Some even show a lower pressure among women who consume no more than one drink per day compared with those who drink nothing *(21)*. Whether or not such small amounts of alcohol lower blood pressure, there is clearly a reduced risk of heart attack and stroke *(22)* and perhaps dementia *(23)* with such moderate consumption.

Cessation of Smoking

Although only a footnote in Table 1, cessation of smoking should be the first item addressed if the patient smokes. Cessation of smoking will reduce overall cardiovascular risk beyond any other maneuver, including normalization of blood pressure. Moreover, each cigarette raises blood pressure acutely and 20 or more cigarettes a day keeps the blood pressure higher throughout the time the patient is awake. Unfortunately, the pressor effect of smoking is usually not recognized. Since smoking is not allowed in clinics and physicians' offices, the pressor effect of the last cigarette will almost certainly be gone by the time the blood pressure is measured. Therefore, it is essential that the smoker take his or her own blood pressure while smoking and the physician should use that blood pressure as the criterion for therapy. Hopefully, the recognition of this additional insult

Table 2
Trials of Lifestyle Modifications and Their Effects on the Incidence of Hypertension

Table 2
Trials of Lifestyle Modifications and Their Effects on the Incidence of Hypertension

Trial (Reference)	Number	Duration (yr)	Reduction of incidence (%)
Primary Prevention (Stamler et al., 1989)	201	5	54
Hypertension Prevention (HPTR, 1990)	252	3	23
Trials of Hypertension Prevention			
I (TOHP, 1992)	564	1.5	51
II (TOHP, 1997)	495	4	21

will help motivate the smoker to quit. If not, the physician should consider use of the available pharmacological aids to smoking cessation. Those that include small amounts of nicotine rarely raise the blood pressure.

Reduction of Dietary Saturated Fat and Cholesterol

Correction of dyslipidemia provides a small but significant lowering of elevated blood pressure, likely by a virtually immediate improvement in endothelial function that promotes vasodilation. Even without a further lowering of blood pressure, statin therapy provides a significant cardiovascular protection to hypertensive patients (24).

Maintenance of Adequate Intake of Calcium and Magnesium

Although calcium and magnesium supplements continue to be advocated by a few enthusiasts, multiple controlled trials have shown little if any lowering of blood pressure with them. An adequate intake of both can be provided by a balanced diet that includes low-fat dairy products.

Caffeine

Although the first cup of coffee will transiently raise the blood pressure by 5 to 20 mmHg, tolerance to this pressor effect usually develops and most surveys do not demonstrate a relationship between hypertension and caffeine intake.

A host of other lifestyle modifications, mostly dietary, have been advocated both to prevent and to control hypertension. None of these have been documented to be effective in large-scale, randomized controlled trials so we are left with the maneuvers previously described. Although the evidence that they will prevent hypertension is not conclusive, in those controlled trials combining sodium restriction, weight loss, exercise, and moderation of alcohol in subjects with "high-normal" blood pressure, a uniform decrease in the incidence of overt hypertension has been seen (Table 2).

ANTIHYPERTENSIVE DRUG THERAPY

Drug therapy should begin if blood pressure remains above the goal of therapy after assiduous application of lifestyle modifications or if the patient starts with a blood pressure so high or cardiovascular risk so great as to mandate immediate institution of treatment with antihypertensive drugs as shown in Fig. 3.

Goal of Therapy

It is critically important to recognize a goal for therapy at the very onset and to define that goal for the patient. Otherwise simply taking a medication may be incorrectly construed as fulfilling the need for treatment. In the JNC-VII treatment algorithm (Fig. 3), the goal of therapy is given as 140/90 mmHg except for patients known to require further reductions, including patients with diabetes

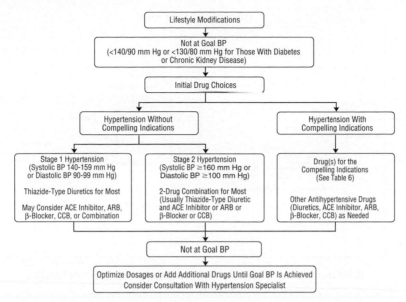

Fig. 3. Joint National Committee. The seventh report of the Joint Committee on Prevention, Detection, Evaluation, and Treatment of High Blood Pressure (JNC-7 Express). (Adapted from ref. *1*.)

or renal insufficiency. Until recently, that goal has been based on conjecture. Fortunately, the level of blood pressure that provides the best protection against cardiovascular morbidity and mortality has been ascertained in a properly designed prospective trial involving more than 19,000 patients with diastolic blood pressure between 100 and 115 mmHg, the Hypertension Optimal Treatment (HOT) trial *(25)*, in which patients were randomly allocated to achieve three levels of diastolic blood pressure—80, 85, and 90 mmHg. In this trial, the lowest rate of major cardiovascular events and mortality overall was at a blood pressure of 139/84 mmHg. Therefore, the appropriate goal for most, relatively uncomplicated hypertension likely should be 140/85, rather than 140/90 as given in the JNC-VII and the European guidelines *(1,4)*. Diastolic pressures below 80 mmHg were more protective in the 1500 diabetics enrolled in the HOT trial, in keeping with the JNC-VII and European recommendations for lower goals in diabetics and other high-risk patients.

THE J-CURVE

Most patients, even when enrolled in clinical trials wherein adherence to therapy should be maximized, are not adequately controlled *(26)*. The diastolic goal of less than either 90 or 85 mmHg is usually reached but the systolic goal of less than 140 mmHg is rarely achieved. This largely reflects the increasing role of atherosclerotic stiffness of capacitance vessels in the elderly with isolated systolic hypertension (ISH), an issue that will be addressed subsequently. Such structural stiffness may be much more difficult to overcome than the functional constriction present in younger hypertensives.

Nonetheless, concerns have been raised as to dangers from lowering blood pressure too much, to a level below which it is possible to maintain adequate perfusion of vital organs. A plot of the relationship between the degree of systolic blood pressure reduction (beyond that achieved by placebo) in 27 randomized controlled trials and cardiovascular mortality shows a continuous decrease to as low as a level as achieved in the trials *(27)* (Fig. 4). However, a J-curve seems present for cardiovascular morbidity (events) with greater reductions in systolic pressure.

More evidence for a J-curve has been seen with reductions in diastolic pressure, including the results of the HOT trial *(28)*. The myocardium may be uniquely susceptible to reduced perfusion from lower diastolic levels for multiple reasons: all coronary flow is during diastole; the myocardium usually hypertrophies and needs more blood flow, whereas the brain and kidney often shrink

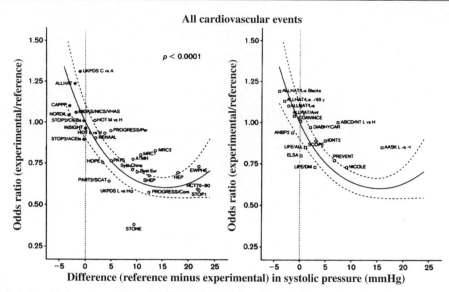

Fig. 4. Relationship between odds ratios for cardiovascular events and corresponding differences in systolic blood pressure (left panel). Odds ratios were calculated for experimental versus reference treatment. Blood pressure differences were obtained by subtracting achieved levels in experimental groups from those in reference groups. Negative values indicate tighter blood pressure on control than on reference treatment. The regression lines were plotted with 95% confidence interval and were weighted for the inverse of the variance of the individual odds ratios. Results of recent trials were plotted superimposed on the meta-regression line (right panel). (Adapted from ref. *27*.)

in size; unlike the brain and kidneys, with increased demands the heart cannot extract any more oxygen than under basal conditions; and the atherosclerotic coronary vessels may not be able to vasodilate to increase blood flow when perfusion pressure falls, i.e., poor autoregulation. Therefore, caution remains advisable in reducing diastolic blood pressure much below 85 mmHg in those who start with elevated diastolic levels with known CHD or in whom unrecognized CHD is very likely.

In the elderly with isolated systolic hypertension and "naturally" occurring low diastolic pressures, an increase in stroke has been noted in two populations when diastolic pressures were further reduced to below 65 mmHg with antihypertensive therapy *(28)*, so caution seems appropriate in these patients as well.

Initial Choice of Therapy

A great deal of attention has been directed toward the "best" choice for initial therapy. As noted in the Antihypertensive and Lipid-Lowering Treatment to Prevent Heart Attack Trial (ALLHAT), most patients—even those with initial levels of blood pressure only of 155/90, as in ALLHAT—require two or more drugs to reach the goal of 140/90 or lower *(29)*. Therefore, JNC-VII acknowledges the need for starting therapy with two drugs in those with initial blood pressure above 160/100 (*see* Fig. 3).

For the rest, a low-dose thiazide diuretic is recommended for the initial choice, as such therapy was equal or superior to the other three choices in ALLHAT—an ACE inhibitor (ACEI), an α-blocker, or a calcium-channel blocker (CCB). The rationale for starting with a diuretic and continuing with that diuretic, even if another agent needs to be added, has been confirmed in many trials in addition to ALLHAT (Fig. 5) *(30)*. When compared against all other classes, low-dose diuretics are as good or, in most ways, better at protecting against various outcomes.

The European guidelines *(3)* continue to include all major classes—diuretics, β-blockers, CCBs, ACEIs, and angiotensin-receptor blockers (ARBs)—as appropriate choices for initial therapy, stating, "The main benefits of antihypertensive therapy are due to lowering of blood pressure per se."

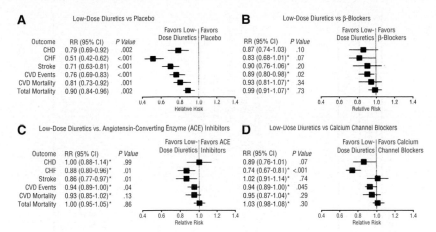

Fig. 5. Meta-analysis of outcomes with various first-line treatments in randomized controlled trials of hypertension. (Modified from ref. *30*.)

In fact, all guidelines recognize the need for agents other than diuretics for patients with certain "compelling" indications (Table 3). This list from the European guidelines *(4)* is broader than that given in JNC-VII, since it only "favors the use" of various agents rather than specifying only "compelling" indications. For me, a low-dose diuretic for most patients seems appropriate, in part because, without one, control is often negated by reactive sodium retention and, with one, the effectiveness of all other classes is enhanced.

A word of caution is needed as to the meaning of "low-dose" diuretic. In the ALLHAT trial, the rarely prescribed chlorthalidone was chosen over the commonly prescribed hydrochlorothiazide (HCTZ). If HCTZ is chosen, 12.5 mg/d is recommended as the starting dose and 25 mg/d the maximum for most patients. Chlorthalidone is more potent than HCTZ so that 25 mg would be equivalent to about 40 mg of HCTZ, a level that likely will cause more metabolic mischief then 25 mg of HCTZ. Even though only a minimal fall in serum potassium should be seen with a dose of 12.5 mg, the combination of HCTZ with a potassium-sparing agent will blunt the fall in potassium at little extra cost. The most popular potassium-sparing agent has been triamterene. The aldosterone blocker, spironolactone, will do as well in sparing potassium and at the same time reduce cardiac, renal, and vascular fibrosis. A more specific aldosterone blocker, eplerenone, has been approved, which does not cause the side effects of androgen or progesterone blockade seen with spironolactone *(31)*. Eplerenone may become the potassium-sparer of choice.

Low doses of the other long-acting diuretic, indapamide, do as well as HCTZ, possibly with fewer biochemical changes and additional antihypertensive effects. For the uncomplicated hypertensive, loop diuretics are not needed and, if given as one daily dose of furosemide, almost totally ineffective. In those with renal insufficiency, loop diuretics are needed but either metolazone or torsemide will provide efficacy with one dose a day, whereas two to three doses of short-acting furosemide will be needed.

The antihypertensive effect of low doses of diuretic may be overcome by very high dietary intake of sodium and blunted by nephrosclerosis that has not yet induced renal insufficiency. For most uncomplicated hypertensives, a single morning dose of HCTZ works well.

SAFETY OF CALCIUM-CHANNEL BLOCKERS

As seen in Table 3, long-acting dihydropyridine (DHP) calcium antagonists are favored for the elderly with isolated systolic hypertension and non-DHPs are recommended for other comorbid conditions. The various indications for members of this family are partly responsible for their current position as the most commonly prescribed drugs for the treatment of hypertension in the US with one of them, amlodipine, now being the most popular antihypertensive worldwide.

Table 3

Indications and Contraindications for Major Classes of Antihypertensive Drugs

Class	Conditions favoring the use	Contraindications	
		Compelling	Possible
Diuretics (thiazides)	Congestive heart failure; elderly hypertensives; isolated systolic hypertension; hypertensives of African origin	Gout	Pregnancy
Diuretics (loop)	Renal insufficiency; congestive heart failure		
Diuretics (anti-aldosterone)	Congestive heart failure; postmyocardial infarction	Renal failure; hyperkalemia	
β-Blockers	Angina pectoris; postmyocardial infarction; congestive heart failure (up-titration); pregnancy; tachyarrhythmias	Asthma; chronic obstructive pulmonary disease; A-V block (grade 2 or 3)	Peripheral vascular disease; glucose intolerance; athletes and physically active patients
Calcium antagonists (dihydropyridines)	Elderly patients; isolated systolic hypertension; angina pectoris; peripheral vascular disease; carotid atherosclerosis; pregnancy		Tachyarrhythmias; congestive heart failure
Calcium antagonists (verapamil, diltiazem)	Angina pectoris; carotid atherosclerosis; supraventricular tachycardia	A-V block (grade 2 or 3); congestive heart failure	
Angiotensin-converting enzyme (ACE) inhibitors	Congestive heart failure; LV dysfunction; post-myocardial infarction; nondiabetic nephropathy; type 1 diabetic nephropathy; proteinuria	Pregnancy; hyperkalemia; bilateral renal artery stenosis	
Angiotensin II receptor antagonists (AT_1-blockers)	Type 2 diabetic nephropathy; diabetic micro-albuminuria; proteinuria; left ventricular hypertrophy; ACE-inhibitor cough	Pregnancy; hyperkalemia; bilateral renal artery stenosis	
α-Blockers	Prostatic hyperplasia (BPH); hyperlipidaemia	Orthostatic hypotension	Congestive heart failure

A-V, atrioventricular; LV, left ventricular.
From ref. 4.

In addition, effective marketing has almost certainly played a major role in the popularity of these drugs. However, marketing would not translate into usage if these drugs were not both effective and well tolerated. Nonetheless, a series of reports have appeared over the past few years incriminating various calcium-channel blockers as being responsible for an increased incidence of coronary disease, cancer, gastrointestinal bleeding, and suicide.

The majority of these reports were uncontrolled retrospective case-control studies comparing the frequency of the use of various CCBs against other drugs in patients found to have coronary disease, cancer, GI bleeding, and attempted suicide. Almost all of these reports involved short-acting formulations of verapamil, diltiazem, or nifedipine, but the long-acting formulations were also faulted in the manner of guilt by association. Whereas large doses of such short-acting agents may aggravate coronary disease by the sympathetic activation induced by abrupt falls in blood pressure, long-acting agents do not induce such reactions and they clearly should not have been incriminated.

The results of the multiple prospective controlled trials have negated these highly publicized incriminations. In particular, in the largest trial, ALLHAT, in which more than 9000 patients on amlodipine were closely observed, "the mortality from non-cardiovascular causes was significantly lower in the CCB group" *(29)*.

Perhaps the only other positive outcome of this misguided campaign is the recognition that sublingual nifedipine was being greatly overused for the treatment of hypertensive "pseudocrises." In truth, the dangers of sublingual nifedipine may be no greater than seen with other drugs that rapidly lower blood pressure and the larger number of reports of adverse effects may simply reflect its much wider use. Nonetheless, sublingual nifedipine should be used only when life-threatening hypertension cannot be properly managed with a parenteral agent, as will be described later in this chapter. Other than in this situation, there is no reason to use short-acting nifedipine in hypertension. For the majority of patients with nonthreatening but severe hypertension that needs to be lowered in a matter of hours, one or more of a variety of rapidly acting oral agents should be used.

General Recommendations

With whatever drug is chosen for initial therapy, three additional general recommendations are appropriate: Start with a low dose and gradually titrate upward; use a once-a-day, long-acting formulation; and, if appropriate to the needs of the patient, use combinations as recommended in JNC-VII for those with blood pressure of 160/100 or higher.

Low Starting Doses

Many patients and most physicians are in a hurry to bring hypertension under control. The motives are usually good: Reduce the time and money needed to control the disease, thereby more quickly protecting the patient from the dangers of untreated hypertension. (Limitations imposed by managed care may further the push toward "quick and easy" control.)

Unfortunately, the consequences are often bad: Fast and marked falls in blood pressure often provoke symptoms of tiredness, fatigue, and dizziness, likely a consequence of reduced perfusion to the brain when systemic pressure is lowered even to levels that are not "hypotensive" and that are well tolerated by normotensive people (Fig. 6). As shown, autoregulation maintains normal cerebral blood flow over a range of arterial blood pressure from as low as 90/50 mmHg to 180/120 mmHg in normotensives. In hypertensives, the autoregulatory curve is shifted to the right as thickened vessels are able to maintain perfusion despite pressures that could not be tolerated in normotensives. On the other hand, if blood pressure is lowered in hypertensives below a mean pressure of 100 to 110 mmHg, i.e., 140/90 mmHg, cerebral blood flow falls. Fortunately, over time, treated patients shift their curve toward the left so that lower pressures can be tolerated.

Other organs may also be underperfused if blood pressure is abruptly lowered. These include the heart, kidneys, and perhaps most bothersome to many men, the penis. Penile blood flow must increase almost 10-fold to achieve and maintain an erection. Particularly when blood flow to the genitals is already compromised by atherosclerotic narrowing, an abrupt fall in systemic pressure may induce impotence, whereas a slower and less marked fall in pressure may be tolerated.

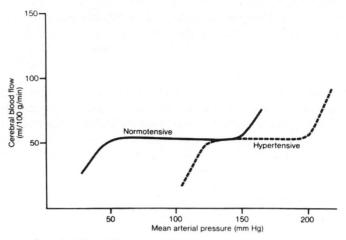

Fig. 6. Idealized curves of cerebral blood flow at varying levels of systemic blood pressure in normotensive and hypertensive subjects. Rightward shift is shown in autoregulation with chronic hypertension. (Adapted from ref. *47*.)

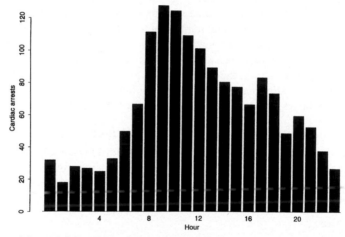

Fig. 7. Distribution of time of dispatch for 1558 unwitnessed, untreated cardiac-etiology episodes of cardiac arrests. (Adapted from ref. *48*.)

By "starting low and going slow," good control should be achieved within a few months, with fewer if any symptoms related to tissue hypoperfusion. If patients monitor their own blood pressure with home devices, manipulations of therapy can easily be made without the need for office visits. For most patients in no distress, upward titrations should be made only after 4 to 6 wk to enable the full effectiveness of the previous dose to be expressed.

ONCE-A-DAY DOSING

Long-acting formulations of drugs that provide 24-h efficacy are preferred over short-acting agents for many reasons: (1) adherence is better with once-daily dosing; (2) for some agents, fewer tablets incur lower cost; (3) control of hypertension is persistent and smooth rather than intermittent; and (4) protection is provided against the risk for sudden death, heart attack, and stroke that is due to the abrupt increase of blood pressure after arising from overnight sleep. Agents with a duration of action beyond 24 h, such as amlodipine and trandolapril, are attractive because many patients inadvertently miss at least one dose of medication each week.

The first three reasons are obvious. The fourth deserves additional comment, as all cardiovascular catastrophes occur at a greater frequency in the first few hours after arising from sleep (Fig. 7).

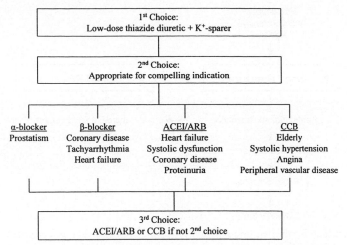

Fig. 8. An algorithm for treatment of hypertension in the absence of renal insufficiency.

If drugs with less than full 24-h efficacy are taken only once a day in the morning, the patient's blood pressure will be poorly controlled in the hours just before and after arising from sleep when the need for control is most critical. Therefore drugs with full 24-h effectiveness should be chosen, hopefully to thereby provide full protection from early morning catastrophes.

A special formulation of the calcium antagonist verapamil, i.e., CoVera HS®, has been marketed that does not release the drug for 4 to 6 h. It is to be taken at bedtime, thereby ensuring early morning efficacy. Although this "choronobiologic approach" is rational, equal efficacy was seen with therapy beginning with either a β-blocker or a diuretic *(32)*. If, as is true of many formulations, the maximal effect occurs within 2 to 6 h, bedtime dosing could induce nocturnal tissue hypoperfusion as blood pressure usually falls spontaneously during sleep. The author's preference is to give all antihypertensive drugs with 24-h efficacy as early in the morning as possible. If the patient awakes because of nocturia, some 2 to 3 h before arising for the day, the medications can be taken at that time.

COMBINATION THERAPY

As noted, two types of combinations have been widely used—a thiazide diuretic with a potassium-sparing diuretic and a thiazide diuretic with a β-blocker, angiotensin-converting enzyme inhibitor, or angiotensin-receptor blocker. According to JNC-VII, more of the second type of combination should be used as initial therapy and, in those started only with a diuretic but in need of another drug, they are logical second choices.

In addition, combinations of an ACEI with a CCB are available. Not only may they be indicated for those who require three or more drugs but they also will decrease the incidence of the most common side effect of CCBs—pedal edema *(33)*.

Second Step in Therapy

As noted previously, as many as 70% of patients who take their medication faithfully will not reach the goal of therapy with the first drug alone. As shown in Fig. 8, the second choice should be appropriate to the individual's specific needs. The list of compelling indications in Fig. 8 is similar to that shown in Table 3 but is predicated upon the first choice being a diuretic.

The need for some diuretic is based on the principles of pressure-natriuresis that were clearly elucidated by the late Arthur Guyton, describing the usual relationship between systemic blood pressure and renal sodium excretion that must be reset in order for hypertension to develop and persist. If not, the higher pressure would effect a natriuresis and the shrinkage in fluid volume would

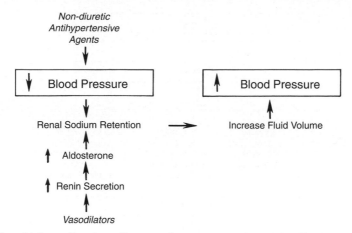

Fig. 9. Manner by which nondiuretic antihypertensive agents may lose their effectiveness by reactive renal sodium retention. (Adapted from ref. *49*.)

return the pressure to normal. Only by a rightward shift of the relation should hypertension persist. As a corollary to this rightward shift, when blood pressure is lowered by a nondiuretic agent, the kidney perceives the pressure to be so low as to interfere with its normal functions and intrinsically retains extra sodium and water. Consequently, circulating fluid volume is expanded and the blood pressure rises (Fig. 9). The problem is even worse with direct vasodilators such as minoxidil, which stimulate renin secretion.

Such reactive fluid retention was recognized soon after the introduction of nondiuretic antihypertensive agents that were found to lose their effectiveness over time when used alone, only to regain full efficacy after addition of a diuretic. The problem may be less with newer agents such as calcium antagonists, which have some intrinsic natriuretic action, or with ACEIs and ARBs, which blunt the renin–angiotensin–aldosterone mechanism. Nonetheless, such reactive sodium retention may still preclude the full expression of the efficacy of those agents and their efficacy is clearly increased by the addition of a diuretic.

Third Step in Therapy

If the goal has still not been reached, agents from other classes should sequentially be added, even if four or five are needed. Fortunately only about 5% of patients will not respond to moderate doses of three drugs, with a diuretic being one. As will be described in the next section, resistance to therapy is usually defined as blood pressure above 140/90 despite the use of three drugs.

If resistance persists and cannot be overcome by the steps described in the next section, referral to a hypertension specialist should be considered. If the practitioner is not aware of such specialists, they are listed by the American Society of Hypertension (www.ash-us.org), which certifies those with particular expertise in dealing with complicated hypertensives.

MANAGEMENT OF RESISTANT HYPERTENSION

If office blood pressure readings are persistently elevated despite increasing therapy, the possibility of pseudoresistance from the white-coat effect should be considered. As shown in Fig. 10, if significant target organ damage is occurring, the assumption must be that true resistance is present and additional therapy is needed. But, in the absence of progressing target organ damage, home blood pressure readings and, if available, ambulatory monitoring should be obtained before proceeding with more therapy.

Of all the causes for true resistance to therapy shown in Table 4, the most common is likely nonadherence to therapy. If the patient is taking the prescribed medications, search should be made

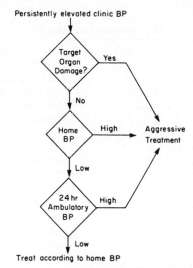

Fig. 10. Proposed schema of blood pressure measurement for patients with apparently resistant hypertension. (Adapted from ref. *50.*)

Table 4
Causes for Inadequate Responsiveness to Therapy

Pseudoresistance	Associated conditions
White-coat or office elevations	Smoking
Pseudohypertension in the elderly	Increasing obesity
Nonadherence to therapy	Sleep apnea
Side effects or costs of medication	Insulin resistance or hyperinsulinemia
Lack of consistent and continuous primary care	Ethanol intake more than 1 oz a day
Inconvenient and chaotic dosing schedules	Anxiety-induced hyperventilation or panic attacks
Instructions not understood	Chronic pain
Organic brain syndrome (e.g., memory deficit)	Intense vasoconstriction (Raynaud's phenomenon, arthritis)
Drug-related causes	Identifiable causes of hypertension
Doses too low	Renal parenchymal disease
Inappropriate combinations	Renovascular disease
Rapid inactivation (e.g. hydralazine)	Primary aldosteronism
Drug actions and interactions	Pheochromocytoma, etc.
NSAIDS	Volume overload
Sympathomimetics	Excess sodium intake
Nasal decongestants	Progressive renal damage (nephrosclerosis)
Appetite suppressants	Fluid retention from reduction of blood pressure
Cocaine and other street drugs	Inadequate diuretic therapy
Caffeine	
Oral contraceptives	
Adrenal steroids	
Licorice (as may be found in chewing tobacco)	
Cyclosporine, tacrolimus	
Erythropoietin	

Modified from ref. *51.*

for drug interactions, one or another associated conditions, or identifiable (secondary) forms of hypertension.

In a number of studies of such groups of patients, the most common cause for resistance has turned out to be volume overload from multiple causes, most likely inadequate diuretic therapy.

Table 5
Hypertension Emergencies

Accelerated-malignant hypertension with papilledema	Excess circulating catecholamines
Cerebrovascular	Pheochromocytoma crisis
Hypertensive encephalopathy	Food or drug interactions with monamine
Atherothrombotic brain infarction with severe	oxidase inhibitors
hypertension	Sympathomimetic drug use (cocaine)
Intracerebral hemorrhage	Rebound hypertension after sudden cessation
Subarachnoid hemorrhage	of antihypertensive drugs
Head trauma	Automatic hyperreflexia after spinal cord injury
	Eclampsia
Cardiac	Surgical
Acute aortic dissection	Severe hypertension in patients requiring
Acute left ventricular failure	immediate surgery
Acute or impending myocardial infarction	Postoperative hypertension
After coronary bypass surgery	Postoperative bleeding from vascular suture lines
Renal	Severe body burns
Acute glomerulonephritis	Severe epistaxis
Renovascular hypertension	Thrombotic thrombocytopenic purpura
Renal crises from collagen vascular diseases	
Severe hypertension after kidney transplantation	

Adapted from ref. 52.

In turn, this is often due to the use of a single dose a day of the short-acting loop diuretic, furosemide. When used once a day, the short duration of action provides only a transient natriuresis and contraction of effective blood volume. When lunch or dinner are eaten, all of the sodium initially excreted is retained so, at the end of the day, the patient is no different than before, other than for the discomfort of having to empty a full bladder for the first 2 or 3 h after taking the diuretic.

For patients with intact renal function, a single morning dose of a thiazide will usually provide the continued shrinkage of fluid volume that is needed to lower blood pressure. In those with markedly high blood pressure who are taking one or more other drugs, the tendency for reactive sodium retention shown in Fig. 9 may require the use of larger doses than needed for most patients.

For those with renal insufficiency, two or three doses of a short-acting loop diuretic may work, but better control will likely be achieved with one dose a day of such long-acting and potent agents as metolazone or torsemide. In addition, caution is needed when nonsteroidal antiinflammatory drugs are taken. They may counteract the efficacy of most antihypertensive drugs (34) and precipitate acute renal failure in some with preexisting renal insufficiency.

THERAPY OF HYPERTENSIVE EMERGENCIES

The small number of patients who present with a hypertensive emergency (Table 5) almost always should receive parenteral therapy (Table 6) in an intensive care facility where careful monitoring is feasible. The choice of drug will usually be based on the experience of the caregiver but, as noted in Table 6, certain types of emergencies are best treated with specific parenteral agents.

Many patients with markedly elevated blood pressure but no advancing target organ damage or other features of a true hypertensive emergency have been considered to have a hypertensive "urgency," i.e., to be in need of immediate reduction of blood pressure but not requiring parenteral therapy. By far the most common therapy for such patients had been sublingual nifedipine, but the use of this agent has diminished since ischemic events were described with its use (35). Such hypertensive sequelae are neither unexpected nor unique to sublingual nifedipine. They have been observed with almost every fast-acting antihypertensive agent given to patients with markedly high blood pressure. It is almost certain that the apparently larger number of adverse effects reported with sublingual nifedipine reflects a much larger number of patients given this agent.

Table 6

Parenteral Drugs for Treatment of Hypertensive Emergency

Drug[a]	Dose	Onset of action	Duration of action	Adverse effects[b]	Special indications
Diuretics					
Furosemide	20–40 mg in 1–2 min, repeated and higher doses with renal insufficiency	5–15 min	2–3 h	Volume depletion, hypokalemia	Usually needed to maintain efficacy of other drugs
Vasodilators					
Nitroprusside (Nipride, Nitropress)	0.25–10 µg/kg/min as iv infusion	Immediate	1–2 min	Nausea, vomiting, muscle twitching, sweating, thiocyanate and cyanide intoxication	Most hypertensive emergencies; caution with high intracranial pressure or azotemia
Nitroglycerin (Nitro-bid IV)	5–100 µg/min as iv infusion	2–5 min	5–10 min	Headache, vomiting, methemoglobinemia, tolerance with prolonged use	Coronary ischemia
Fenoldopam (Corlopam)	0.1–0.6 µg/kg/min as iv infusion	4–5 min	10–15 min	Reflex tachycardia, increase intraocular pressure, headache	Renal insufficiency, postoperative
Nicardipine[c] (Cardene IV)	5–15 mg iv	5–10 min	1–4 h	Headache, nausea, flushing, tachycardia, local phlebitis	Most hypertensive emergencies; caution with acute heart failure
Hydralazine (Apresoline)	10–20 mg iv 10–10 mg im	10–20 min 20–30 min	3–8 h	Tachycardia, flushing, headache, vomiting, aggravation of angina	Eclampsia; caution with high intracranial pressure
Enalaprilat (Vasotec IV)	1.25–5 mg every 6 h	15 min	6 h	Precipitous fall in pressure in high-renin states; response variable	Acute left ventricular failure
Adrenergic inhibitors					
Phentolamine	5–15 mg iv	1–2 min	3–10 min	Tachycardia, flushing, headache	Catecholamine excess
Esmolol (Brevibloc)	200–500 µg/kg/min for 4 min, then 50–300 µg/kg/min iv	1–2 min	10–20 min	Hypotension, nausea	Aortic dissection, postoperative
Labetalol (Normodyne, Trandate)	20–80 mg iv bolus every 10 min 2 mg/min iv infusion	5–10 min	3–6 h	Vomiting, scalp tingling, burning in throat, dizziness, nausea, heart block, orthostatic hypotension	Most hypertensive emergencies except acute heart failure

[a]In order of rapidity of action.

[b]Hypotension may occur with any.

[c]Intravenous formulations of other calcium-channel blockers are also available. (Modified from ref. 52.)

631

Table 7
Relative Risk Reduction of Fatal Events and Combined Fatal and Nonfatal Events
in Patients on Active Antihypertensive Treatment vs Placebo or No Treatment

	Systolic-diastolic hypertension		Isolated systolic hypertension	
	Risk reduction	p	Risk reduction	p
Mortality				
All cause	−14%	<0.01	−13%	0.02
Cardiovascular	−21%	<0.001	−18%	0.01
Noncardiovascular	− 1%	NS		NS
Fatal and Nonfatal Events				
Stroke	−42%	<0.001	−30%	<0.001
Coronary	−14%	<0.01	−23%	<0.001

Adapted from ref. *4.*

It is likely that the relative danger of sublingual nifedipine has been exaggerated since many millions of hypertensive patients swallowed nifedipine capsules for decades, before long-acting calcium antagonists became available, without inciting acute ischemic events. Nonetheless, Grossman et al. *(35)* are certainly correct in describing gross overuse of this agent in patients with a "pseudoemergency," i.e., high blood pressure but no other indications for rapid reduction of the pressure.

There are, however, a sizable number of patients who need fairly fast treatment, including most hypertensives who are found to have a sustained blood pressure above 210/120 mmHg. The prudent physician will treat such patients immediately until their blood pressure is at a safer level, likely below 180/110 mmHg. Several oral agents are available that begin working within 30 to 60 min and bring the blood pressure down in 2 to 6 h, not so fast as to induce ischemia but fast enough to allow the patient to be sent home on a regimen of long-acting medications with close follow-up to ensure that control is achieved and necessary evaluation is performed. These agents include oral furosemide, propranolol, captopril, nicardipine, felodipine, or nifedipine among the fast-acting agents.

TREATMENT OF SPECIAL POPULATIONS

Limitations of space preclude coverage of all the special populations that clinicians may encounter—from neonates to children to pregnant women, and patients with a variety of comorbid conditions. Additional attention will be given to three groups of hypertensives because they are both common and in need of special considerations: the elderly, those with diabetes, and those with coexisting cardiac diseases.

Pregnant women with preexisting hypertension can be safely continued on drugs used before pregnancy with the exception of ACEIs and ARBs, which must be stopped as soon as the pregnancy is recognized. Since few trials have documented the safety of newer drugs for the fetus as has been shown with methyldopa, this drug is still chosen by most US obstetricians, along with parenteral hydralazine if needed.

The Elderly Hypertensive

The largest and most rapidly expanding portion of the hypertensive population are those over age 65. More than half are hypertensive, and almost two thirds have isolated systolic hypertension. ISH is a serious risk factor for all cardiovascular complications, particularly stroke but including myocardial infarction. Fortunately, treatment of the elderly with either ISH or combined systolic and diastolic hypertension provides excellent protection against all these morbidities (Table 7) *(4)*. Over the relatively short duration of most randomized clinical trials in the elderly, even greater protection against coronary events was noted among elderly patients than younger, likely because the elderly start at so much greater immediate risk. In most trials of the elderly, therapy began with

Table 8
Possible Contributors to Increased Risk From Drug Treatment of Hypertension in Elderly Persons

Factor	Potential complications
Diminished baroreceptor activity	Orthostatic hypotension
Impaired cerebral autoregulation	Cerebral ischemia with small falls in systemic pressure
Decreased intravascular volume	Orthostatic hypotension; volume depletion; hyponatremia
Sensitivity to hypokalemia	Arrhythmia; muscle weakness
Decreased renal and hepatic function	Drug accumulation
Polypharmacy	Drug interaction
Central nervous system changes	Depression, confusion

a low dose of diuretic or a long-acting dihydropyridine calcium antagonist, and these drugs are given preference in the European guidelines for treatment of the elderly with ISH. However, ACEI-based therapy was more protective than diuretic-based therapy among the male subjects in the recent large Australian study of patients whose mean age was 72 and mean blood pressure was 167/91 mmHg *(36)*. Moreover, the combination of an ACEI and diuretic reduced recurrent stroke and cognitive decline in elderly patients who had survived a stroke *(37)*.

Since other drugs work well in the elderly, if comorbid conditions require such agents, they may logically be used alone or, preferably, with a low dose of diuretic. This is particularly true of β-blockers: In the two RCTs involving elderly hypertensives, β-blockers given alone did not reduce coronary or overall mortality *(38)*. Therefore, if an elderly hypertensive is deemed in need of a β-blocker, as after an acute myocardial infarction, it should be given with a low dose of diuretic.

Avoid Risks of Therapy

The elderly are more susceptible to a variety of potential risks from antihypertensive drug therapy (Table 8). In particular, they frequently have postural and postprandial hypotension *(39)*, which may be converted from an occasional but tolerable nuisance to a frequent intolerable danger by the addition of antihypertensive therapy. Often, their supine and seated hypertension can be treated only after their postural and postprandial hypotension is managed by a variety of helpful maneuvers including slow rising, elevation of the head of the bed, isometric exercises, support hose, and small meals. A few will require additional drugs, including the α-antagonist midodrine or octreotide.

Since the only medical condition more frequent than hypertension in the elderly is osteoarthritis, many use nonsteroidal antiinflammatory drugs (NSAIDs). As noted, all NSAIDs may interfere with the antihypertensive efficacy of all antihypertensives, with the probable exception of CCBs. Therefore, whenever possible, other analgesics including acetaminophen should be used instead of NSAIDs.

Since the elderly are susceptible to both over- and undertreatment, home blood pressure self-monitoring is particularly useful for them. Thereby, the white-coat effect, which is quantitatively greater in the elderly, can be recognized and assurance provided that therapy is enough but not excessive.

Diabetic Hypertensives

Diabetics are more likely to have hypertension than nondiabetics, and more hypertensives than normotensives have diabetes. The combination is deadly: All diabetic micro- and macrovascular complications are accelerated by the presence of hypertension. As diabetics survive longer, they are prone to develop cardiomyopathy and nephropathy, both worsened by hypertension and now the leading causes of their premature mortality. Antihypertensive therapy should be started at lower levels of blood pressure in diabetics, at a level above 130/80 and the goal of therapy is even lower *(1,4)*. Since most diabetics are obese, weight reduction must be vigorously pursued by caloric restriction and physical activity. If drugs are needed, ACEIs or, particularly in type 2 diabetics with nephropathy, ARBs should be the first drug, with an appropriate dose of diuretic as second. ACEIs and ARBs may protect the kidneys of diabetic hypertensives better than do CCBs or other drugs *(40)*. However, the overriding need is to lower the systemic blood pressure to below 130/80 mmHg if possible.

Hypertensives With Cardiac Diseases

Since these various diseases are extensively covered elsewhere in this book, only a few specific issues relative to the coexistence of hypertension will be highlighted.

LEFT VENTRICULAR HYPERTROPHY

Left ventricular hypertrophy (LVH) is recognizable by electrocardiography in perhaps 25% of hypertensives and by echocardiography in more than half. As an independent risk factor for coronary mortality in hypertensives, LVH is being more diligently looked for and its regression is being used as a surrogate endpoint for effective therapy. Data still do not document that knowledge of either the presence or the regression of LVH add enough useful information to make routine echocardiography worthwhile.

Nonetheless, numerous studies have examined the relative ability of various antihypertensive drugs to regress LVH with the assumption that regression in itself is beneficial beyond the value of simply lowering the blood pressure. All lifestyle modifications and antihypertensive drugs except direct vasodilators will regress LVH, with ACEIs and ARBs perhaps somewhat better than other classes of drugs that provide equal antihypertensive efficacy *(41)*.

HEART FAILURE

LVH is often the progenitor of heart failure. In the Framingham study population, hypertension was a factor in more than 90% of patients with heart failure. The role of hypertension may not be recognized because as cardiac output falls, systemic blood pressure may fall despite the activation of vasoconstrictor neurohormonal mechanisms.

Therapy will usually include a diuretic, an ACEI, or an ARB in those who cough, the α-β blocker, carvedilol, and an aldosterone blocker. If needed to treat angina or hypertension in patients with heart failure, the long-acting dihydropyridine calcium antagonists amlodipine and felodipine have been found to be safe.

CORONARY HEART DISEASE

Beyond the particular ability of β-blockers and long-acting CCBs to treat both angina and hypertension, β-blockers, ACEIs, and aldosterone blockers have been shown to be protective in patients with systolic dysfunction after an acute myocardial infarction.

Two caveats are needed in hypertensives with coronary heart disease (CHD). First, the diastolic blood pressure, if initially above 90 mmHg, should not be lowered below 80 mmHg because of the likely presence of a J-curve. Second, short-acting calcium antagonists should be avoided since they may abruptly lower blood pressure and thereby stir up the sympathetic nervous system, further stressing the already compromised myocardium.

THE NEED TO IMPROVE ADHERENCE TO THERAPY

As noted at the beginning of this chapter, most hypertensives in the US and elsewhere are not being treated adequately. A good deal of the blame can be laid on physicians who are noncompliant with the need to push therapy to the goal. Even more is due to patient nonadherence to therapy.

Only a few interventions have been proven to be effective in improving patient adherence to therapy *(42)*. These include more convenient care, special pill containers that monitor removal of the contents, home self-monitoring of blood pressure, and special staff who provide reminders, support, feedback, and reinforcement. These maneuvers may cost a bit more and require greater involvement of physician and staff, but the benefits outweigh the costs.

Easier-to-use medications should help. The quality of life has been shown to be improved by once-a-day, effective drug therapy as well as by weight loss and increased physical activity *(43)*. On the other hand, male sexual potency may be diminished by the use of the type of drug that is most frequently recommended—low doses of diuretic *(44)*. Obviously, care should be taken to recognize any sexual dysfunction related to the treatment of hypertension. Fortunately, the most widely used treatment for impotence, sildenafil, does not react adversely with any oral antihypertensive drug, but should be used with caution in patients with coronary artery disease and not at all if the patient is on nitrates.

THE PAST AND THE FUTURE

The treatment of hypertension has improved greatly over the past 30 yr. Despite the evidence that only 59% of current US hypertensives are being treated and only 34% are well controlled *(1)*, recognition should be given to the fact that these figures are much improved over those from 1980. These improvements have clearly played a significant role in the marked decreases in mortality from CHD and stroke in the US population.

Just as clearly, more needs to be done. Even among presumably well-treated hypertensives, long-term rates of cardiovascular disease remain higher than among normotensives *(45)*. In particular, hypertensives with high levels of overall cardiovascular risk from other known risk factors have not been well protected from morbidity and mortality despite successful antihypertensive therapy *(46)*.

More intensive antihypertensive therapy always pushed to the appropriate goal of therapy is one likely solution to the problem. New, and hopefully better, antihypertensive drugs are being developed so that it may be easier to accomplish good blood pressure control. Beyond that, greater attention to other cardiovascular risk factors must be given so that the full benefits of health care can be provided to all hypertensive patients.

REFERENCES

1. Joint National Committee. The seventh report of the Joint Committee on Prevention, Detection, Evaluation, and Treatment of High Blood Pressure. JAMA 2003; 289:2560–2571.
2. Cherry DK, Woodwell DA. National ambulatory medical care survey: 2000 summary. Advance Data (CDC) 2002; 328.
3. Whelton PK, He J, Appel LJ, et al. Primary prevention of hypertension: clinical and public health advisory from the National High Blood Pressure Education Program. JAMA 2002;288:1882–1888.
4. Guidelines Committee. 2003 European Society of Hypertension-European Society of Cardiology guidelines for the management of arterial hypertension. J Hypertens 2003;21:1011–1053.
5. International Society of Hypertension Writing Group. International Society of Hypertension (ISH): statement on blood pressure lowering and stroke prevention. J Hypertens 2003;21:651–663.
6. Whelton PK, Appel, LJ, Espeland MA, et al. Sodium, reduction, and weight loss in the treatment of hypertension in older persons. JAMA 1998;279:839–846.
7. Diabetes Prevention Program Research Group. Reduction in the incidence of type 2 diabetes with lifestyle intervention or metformin. N Engl J Med 2002;346:393–403.
8. Law CM, Shiell AW, Newsome CS, et al. Fetal, infant, and childhood growth and adult blood pressure: a longitudinal study from birth to 22 years of age. Circulation 2002;105:1088–1092.
9. Huxley R, Neil A, Collins R. Unravelling the fetal origins hypothesis: is there really an inverse association between birthweight and subsequent blood pressure? Lancet 2002;360:659–665.
10. Kaplan NM. Primary hypertension: pathogenesis. In: Kaplan's Clinical Hypertension, 8th ed. Lippincott Williams & Wilkins, Philadelphia, 2003, pp. 77–80.
11. Huang Z, Willett WC, Manson JE, et al. Body weight, weight change and risk for hypertension in women. Ann Intern Med 1998;128:81–88.
12. Park Y-W, Zhu S, Palaniappan L, et al. The metabolic syndrome: prevalence and associated risk factor findings in the US population from the Third National Health and Nutrition Examination Survey, 1988–1994. Ann Intern Med 2003;163:427–436.
13. Tishler PV, Larkin EK, Schluchter MD, Redline S. Incidence of sleep-disordered breathing in an urban adult population: the relative importance of risk factors in the development of sleep-disordered breathing. JAMA 2003;289:2230–2237.
14. Sacks FM, Svetkey LP, Vollmer WM, et al. Effects of blood pressure on reduced dietary sodium and the Dietary Approaches to Stop Hypertension (DASH) diet. N Engl J Med 2001;344:3–10.

15. PREMIER Collaborative Research Group. Effects of comprehensive lifestyle modification on blood pressure control: main results of the PREMIER clinical trial. JAMA 2003;289:2083–2093.
16. Hooper L, Bartlett C, Davey Smith G, Ebrahim S. Systematic review of long term effects of advice to reduce dietary salt in adults. Br Med J 2002;325:628.
17. He FJ, MacGregor GA. Effect of modest salt reduction on blood pressure: a meta-analysis of randomized trials. Implications for public health. J Human Hypertens 2002;16:761–770.
18. Rose G. Strategy of prevention. Br Med J 1981;282:1847–1849.
19. Linden W, Lenz JW, Con AH. Individualized stress management for primary hypertension: a randomized trial. Arch Intern Med 2001;161:1071–1080.
20. Rothenbacher D, Hoffmeister A, Brenner J, Koenig W. Physical activity, coronary heart disease, and inflammatory response. Arch Intern Med 2003;163:1200–1205.
21. Thadhani R, Camargo CA JR, Stampfer MJ, et al. Prospective study of moderate alcohol consumption and risk of hypertension in young women. Arch Intern Med 2002;162:569–574.
22. Di Castelnuovo A, Rotondo S, Iacoviello L, et al. Meta-analysis of wine and beer consumption in relation to vascular risk. Circulation 2002;105:2836–2844.
23. Mukamal KJ, Kuller LH, Fitzpatrick AL, et al. Prospective study of alcohol consumption and risk of dementia in older adults. JAMA 2003;289:1405–1413.
24. Sever PS, Dahlöf B, Poulter NR, et al. Prevention of coronary and stroke events with atorvastatin in hypertensive patients who have average or lower-than-average cholesterol concentrations, in the Anglo-Scandinavian Cardiac Outcomes Trial—Lipid Lowering Arm (ASCOT-LLA): a multicentre randomised controlled trial. Lancet 2003;361: 1149–1158.
25. Zanchetti A, Hansson L, Clement D, et al. Benefits and risks of more intensive blood pressure lowering in hypertensive patients of the HOT study with different risk profiles: does a J-shaped curve exist in smokers? J Hypertens 2003; 21:797–804.
26. Mancia G, Grassi G. Systolic and diastolic blood pressure control in antihypertensive drug trials. J Hypertens 2002; 20:1461–1464.
27. Staessen JA, Wang J-G, Thijs L. Cardiovascular prevention and blood pressure reduction: a quantitative overview updated until 1 March 2003. J Hypertens 2003;21:1055–1076.
28. Kaplan NM. What is goal blood pressure for the treatment of hypertension? Arch Intern Med 2001;161:1480–1482.
29. ALLHAT Officers. Major outcomes in high-risk hypertensive patients randomized to angiotensin-converting enzyme inhibitor or calcium channel blocker vs diuretic. JAMA 2002;288:2981–2997.
30. Psaty BM, Lumley T, Furber CD, et al. Health outcomes associated with various antihypertensive therapies used as first-line agents: a network meta-analysis. JAMA 2003;289:2534–2544.
31. Brown NJ. Eplerenone: cardiovascular protection. Circulation 2003;107:2512–2518.
32. Black HR, Elliott WJ, Grandits G, et al. Principal results of the Controlled Onset Verapamil Investigation of Cardiovascular End Points (CONVINCE) trial. JAMA 2003;289:2073–2082.
33. Gogari R, Malamani GD, Zoppi A, et al. Effect of benazepril addition to amlodipine on ankle oedema and subcutaneous tissue pressure in hypertensive patients. J Human Hypertens 2003;17:207–212.
34. Whelton A, White WB, Bello AE, et al. Effects of celecoxib and rofecoxib on blood pressure and edema in patients ≥65 years of age with systemic hypertension and osteoarthritis. Am J Cardiol 2002;90:959–963.
35. Grossman E, Messerli FH, Grodzicki T, Kowey P. Should a moratorium be placed on sublingual nifedipine capsules given for hypertensive emergencies and pseudoemergencies? JAMA 1996;276:1328–1331.
36. Wing LMH, Reid CM, Ryan P, et al. A comparison of outcomes with angiotensin-converting-enzyme inhibitors and diuretics for hypertension in the elderly. N Engl J Med 2003;348:583–592.
37. PROGRESS Collaborative Group. Effects of blood pressure lowering with perindopril and indapamide therapy on dementia and cognitive decline in patients with cerebrovascular disease. Arch Intern Med 2003;163:1069–1075.
38. Messerli FH, Grossman E, Goldbout U. Are β-blockers efficacious as first-line therapy for hypertension in the elderly? JAMA 1998;279:1903–1908.
39. Weiss A, Grossman E, Beloosesky Y, Grinblat J. Orthostatic hypotension in acute geriatric ward: is it a consistent finding? Arch Intern Med 2002;162:2369–2374.
40. Snow V, Weiss KB, Mottur-Pilson C. The evidence base for tight blood pressure control in the management of type 2 diabetes mellitus. Ann Intern Med 2003;138:587–592.
41. Kjeldsen SE, Dahlöf B, Devereux RB, et al. Effects of losartan on cardiovascular morbidity and mortality in patients with isolated systolic hypertension and left ventricular hypertrophy: a Losartan Intervention for Endpoint Reduction (LIFE) substudy. JAMA 2002;288:1491–1498.
42. Haynes RB, McDonald HP, Garg AX. Helping patients follow prescribed treatment: clinical applications. JAMA 2002;288:2880–2883.
43. Grimm RH Jr, Grandits GA, Cutler JA, et al. Relationships of quality-of-life measures to long-term lifestyle and drug treatment in the Treatment of Mild Hypertension Study. Arch Intern Med 1997;157:638–648.
44. Grimm RH Jr, Grandits GA, Prineas RJ, et al. Long-term effects on sexual function of five antihypertensive drugs and nutritional hygienic treatment in hypertensive men and women. Hypertension 1997;29:8–14.
45. Anderson OK, Almgren T, Persson B, et al. Survival in treated hypertension: follow up study after two decades. Br Med J 1998;317:167–171.
46. Alderman MH, Cohen H, Madhavan S. Distribution and determinants of cardiovascular events during 20 years of successful antihypertensive treatment. J Hypertens 1998;16:761–769.

47. Strangdaard S, Olesen J, Skinhoj E, Lassen NA. Autoregulation of brain circulation in severe arterial hypertension. Br Med J 1973;1:507–510.
48. Peckova M, Fahrenbruch CE, Cobb LA, Hallstrom AP. Circadian variations in the occurrence of cardiac arrests. Circulation 1998;98:31–39.
49. Kaplan NM. Treatment of hypertension: drug therapy. In: Kaplan's Clinical Hypertension, 8th ed. Lippincott Williams & Wilkins, Philadelphia, 2002, pp. 237–338.
50. Pickering TG. Blood pressure monitoring outside the office for the evaluation of patients with resistant hypertension. Hypertension 1998;11(Suppl 2):II96–II100.
51. Joint National Committee. The sixth report of the Joint National Committee on Detection, Evaluation, and Treatment of High Blood Pressure (JNC-VI). Arch Intern Med 1997;157:2413–2446.
52. Kaplan's Clinical Hypertension, 8th ed. Lippincott Williams & Wilkins, Baltimore, 2002, p. 340.

RECOMMENDED READING

Chobanian AV, Bakris GL, Black HR, et al. Joint National Committee. The seventh report of the Joint Committee on Prevention, Detection, Evaluation, and Treatment of High Blood Pressure. JAMA 2003;289:2560–2571.
Chobanian AV, Bakris GL, Black HR, et al. Seventh report of the Joint National Committee on Prevention, Detection, Evaluation, and Treatment of High Blood Pressure. Hypertension 2003;42:1206–1252.
Kaplan NM. Kaplan's Clinical Hypertension, 8th ed. Lippincott Williams & Wilkins, Philadelphia, 2002.

X   OTHER CONDITIONS AFFECTING THE HEART

34   Cardiomyopathies and Myocarditis

Edward K. Kasper, MD

INTRODUCTION

Cardiomyopathies are diseases of the heart muscle associated with cardiac dysfunction. The World Health Organization/International Society and Federation of Cardiology task force on the definition and classification of cardiomyopathies has defined five subtypes of cardiomyopathy *(1)*: dilated, hypertrophic, restrictive, arrhythmogenic right ventricular dysplasia, and unclassified cardiomyopathies. The term *specific cardiomyopathy* is used in reference to cardiomypathies associated with specific, usually systemic, disorders. Table 1 lists echocardiographic characteristics of the major types of cardiomyopathy.

DILATED CARDIOMYOPATHY

Left ventricular enlargement and decreased contractility are the defining elements of dilated cardiomyopathy. The right ventricle is often involved as well. Dilated cardiomyopathy is the most common form of cardiomyopathy, accounting for more than 90% of all cardiomyopathies. The most common presentation is with signs and symptoms of heart failure, although perhaps as many as 50% of the cases are asymptomatic or undiagnosed.

Causes of Dilated Cardiomyopathy

A variety of insults can cause dilated cardiomyopathy. We have had a long-standing interest in the causes of cardiomyopathy. Table 2 reviews the causes of initially unexplained cardiomyopathy in our tertiary care referral center experience *(2,3)*. All patients underwent a complete evaluation for the etiology of the cardiomyopathy, including endomyocardial biopsy, laboratory studies, and cardiac catheterization if appropriate. In population-based studies, coronary disease and hypertension are the major causes of cardiomyopathy. In our referral cohort of 1278 patients, no cause could be found in 51% of the cases. Myocarditis occurred in about 9% of the cases, a finding similar to that seen in the Myocarditis Treatment Trial *(4)*.

Familial cardiomyopathy may be a more common finding than reported in our series, as we did not evaluate first-degree relatives of patients with idiopathic dilated cardiomyopathy with echocardiography. When this was done by Michels and colleagues, 20% of patients with idiopathic dilated cardiomyopathy had first-degree relatives with the disease *(5)*. Indeed, studies of families with dilated cardiomyopathy have demonstrated autosomal dominant, autosomal recessive, X-linked, and mitochondrial modes of inheritance *(6)*. There are several distinct phenotypes, including dilated cardiomyopathy, dilated cardiomyopathy with conduction system disease, dilated cardiomyopathy with skeletal myopathy, and dilated cardiomyopathy with hearing loss. The first disease gene to be located was actin. Furthermore, mutations in a number of sarcomeric genes first associated with hypertrophic cardiomyopathy have also been shown to cause dilated cardiomyopathy including B-myosin heavy chain and cardiac troponin T. A more complete list of the causes of dilated cardiomyopathy can be found in Table 3.

From: *Essential Cardiology: Principles and Practice, 2nd Ed.*
Edited by: C. Rosendorff © Humana Press Inc., Totowa, NJ

Table 1
Echocardiographic Findings in Cardiomyopathy

	Dilated	Hypertrophic	Restrictive
Ventricular volume	Increased	Decreased	Decreased or normal
LV contractility	Decreased	Increased	Usually normal
Atrial size	Increased	Usually normal	Markedly increased
Other findings	Often MR	LVOT gradient	Diastolic dysfunction

Natural History of Clinical Course

Prognosis is tied to the underlying cause of unexplained cardiomyopathy *(2)*. As compared to patients with idiopathic cardiomyopathy, patients with peripartum cardiomyopathy had better survival. Patients with infiltrative cardiomyopathies, HIV infection, or a cardiomyopathy caused by doxorubicin had significantly worse survival when compared with idiopathic cardiomyopathy (Fig. 1). In addition, not all infiltrative cardiomyopathies are associated with equally poor survival. Patients with a cardiomyopathy due to sarcoidosis have better survival than do patients with either hemochromatosis or amyloidosis and a cardiomyopathy (Fig. 2). With the exception of peripartum cardiomyopathy, the natural history of dilated cardiomyopathy is one of progressive heart failure, arrhythmia, and eventual death or heart transplantation. Current therapies for heart failure, including angiotensin-converting enzyme (ACE) inhibitors, β-blockers, and aldosterone antagonists have improved this prognosis *(7)*.

Evaluation of Dilated Cardiomyopathy

The ACC/AHA Guidelines for the Evaluation and Management of Chronic Heart Failure in the Adult suggest that physicians should focus their evaluation of the etiology of dilated cardiomyopathy on those diagnoses with the potential for improvement *(7)*. A complete history and physical examination, including a family history of cardiomyopathy, heart failure, and early sudden death, is the foundation. The history should focus on possible causes such as hypertension, coronary disease, diabetes, valvular disease, rheumatic fever, chest irradiation, cardiotoxic agents, illicit drugs, alcohol, systemic disorders, and possible infectious etiologies. Screening for thyroid disease with a TSH is suggested, while laboratory screening for specific cardiomyopathies rests on clinical suspicion. ECG should be done to look for evidence of prior infarct and the presence of rhythm and conduction disturbances. Echocardiography is the most cost-efficient means to understand the anatomy of the heart, including not only left ventricular function but also valvular and pericardial function. Coronary arteriography may be important if revascularization proves to be an effective treatment for left ventricular dysfunction. Endomyocardial biopsy has a limited role in the diagnosis of infiltrative diseases when clinically suspected, but should not be done routinely.

Treatment of Dilated Cardiomyopathy

Treatment rests on the diagnosis of a specific disorder: for example, replacement of thyroid hormone in hypothyroidism. In general, the treatment for dilated cardiomyopathy is outlined in the chapter on heart failure.

HYPERTROPHIC CARDIOMYOPATHY

The findings in hypertrophic cardiomyopathy include left or right ventricular hypertrophy, often asymmetric and involving the ventricular septum. A maximal left ventricular wall thickness greater than or equal to 15 mm is the usual diagnostic finding, but abnormal genotypes are associated with almost any degree of LV wall thickness. Mildly increased LV wall thickness (13 to 14 mm) can also be seen in highly trained athletes and must be differentiated from hypertrophic cardiomyopathy. Obstructive and nonobstructive forms of hypertrophic cardiomyopathy exist, with the nonobstruc-

Table 2
Final Diagnoses in 1230 Patients
With Initially Unexplained Cardiomyopathy

Diagnosis	Number (%)
Idiopathic cardiomyopathy	616 (50)
Myocarditis	111 (9)
Ischemic heart disease	91 (7)
Infiltrative disease	59 (5)
Amyloid	36
Sarcoidosis	14
Hemochromatosis	9
Peripartum cardiomyopathy	51 (4)
Hypertension	49 (4)
HIV	45 (4)
Connective-tissue disease	39 (3)
Scleroderma	12
Systemic lupus erythematosus	9
Marfan's syndrome	3
Polyarteritis nodosa	3
Dermatomyositis or polymyositis	3
Nonspecific connective-tissue disease	3
Ankylosing spondylitis	2
Rheumatoid arthritis	1
Relapsing polychondritis	1
Wegener's granulomatosis	1
Mixed connective-tissue disease	1
Substance abuse	37 (3)
Alcohol	28
Cocaine	9
Doxorubicin therapy	15 (1)
Other causes	117 (10)
Restrictive cardiomyopathy	28
Familial	25
Valvular heart disease	19
Endocrine dysfunction	
Thyroid disease	7
Carcinoid	2
Pheochromocytoma	1
Acromegaly	1
Neuromuscular disease	7
Neoplastic heart disease	6
Congenital heart disease	4
Complication of coronary bypass surgery	4
Radiation	3
Critical illness	3
Endomyocardial fibroelastosis	1
Thrombotic thrombocytopenic purpura	1
Rheumatic carditis	1
Drug therapy (not including doxorubicin)	
Leukotrienes	2
Lithium	1
Prednisone	1
Total	1230 (100)

Adapted from ref. 2.

Table 3
Causes of Cardiomyopathy

Dilated cardiomyopathy	Connective-tissue disease
Idiopathic	Systemic lupus erythematosus
Familial/genetic	Polyarteritis nodosa
Myocarditis/immune (*see* Table 4)	Scleroderma
Drug toxicity	Rheumatoid arthritis
Alcohol	Dermatomyositis/polymyositis
Antidepressants	Muscular dystrophies and neuromuscular disorder
Catecholamines	Tachycardia
Cobalt	Hypertension
Cocaine	Radiation
Doxorubicin	Sepsis/critical illness
Interferon	Hypertrophic cardiomyopathy
Lithium	Familial/genetic
Prednisone	Aortic stenosis
Metabolic	Renal failure
Thyroid disease	Hypertension
Diabetes mellitus	Fabry disease
Carcinoid	Restrictive cardiomyopathy
Pheochromocytoma	Idiopathic
Acromegaly	Familial/genetic
Hypocalcemia	Metastatic tumors
Infiltrative disease	Infiltrative
Amyloid	Amyloid
Sarcoidosis	Sarcoidosis
Hemochromatosis	Storage diseases
Storage diseases	Endocardial
Nutritional	Endomyocardial fibrosis
Beriberi	Hypereosinophilic syndrome
Carnitine	Radiation
Pellagra	Carcinoid heart disease
Selenium	Arrhythmogenic right ventricular dysplasia
	Noncompacted myocardium

This is a relatively complete list.

tive form being more common. For this reason, the term *hypertrophic cardiomyopathy* is now preferred over previous terms, such as hypertrophic subaortic stenosis, that tended to emphasize the obstructive component.

Hypertrophic cardiomyopathy is one of the more common inherited cardiac disorders, with a prevalence in young adults of about 1 in 500. It is the second most common subtype of cardiomyopathy after dilated cardiomyopathy. It is a frequent cause of sudden death in competitive athletes *(8)*.

Left Ventricular Outflow Tract Obstruction

Outflow tract obstruction is caused by hypertrophy of the basal portion of the septum in association with an elongated mitral valve leaflet and systolic anterior motion of the mitral valve. This leads to a narrowed outflow tract, an outflow tract gradient, and often mitral regurgitation as the mitral valve leaflets fail to coapt. The pressure gradient is responsible for the murmur usually described as harsh, located along the lower left sternal border, and made worse by release of Valsalva strain or standing from a squat position. In perhaps 5% of the cases, the obstruction is midventricular rather than subaortic. The pressure gradient is often dynamic, made worse by increased contractility and decreased ventricular volume. Therefore, the gradient, usually defined as 30 mmHg or more, may be present in the resting state, provocable, or absent entirely.

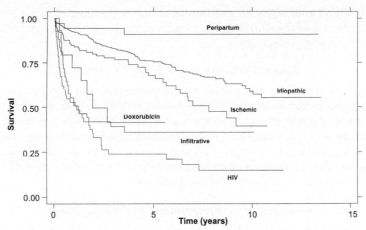

Fig. 1. Kaplan-Meier estimates of survival according to underlying cause of cardiomyopathy. (From ref. 2. Copyright 2000 Massachusetts Medical Society. All rights reserved.)

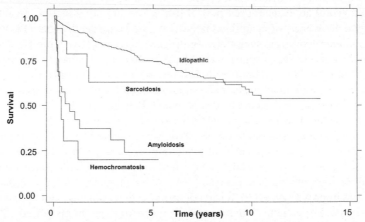

Fig. 2. Kaplan-Meier estimates of survival among patients with infiltrative cardiomyopathy. (From ref. 2. Copyright 2000 Massachusetts Medical Society. All rights reserved.)

Causes of Hypertrophic Cardiomyopathy

Hypertrophic cardiomyopathy is inherited as an autosomal dominant trait. It is caused by at least 12 different disease genes, with more being reported every day *(6,8)*. Most of these genes encode protein components of the cardiac sarcomere, such as β myosin heavy chain, cardiac troponin T, cardiac troponin C, cardiac myosin binding protein C, and so on. Several genes encode nonsarcomeric proteins. Adding to this complexity is that for each disease gene, a variety of different mutations have been reported. These mutations account for perhaps 50 to 70% of all cases of hypertrophic cardiomyopathy and thus new mutations will certainly be described. The extent of left ventricular hypertrophy varies between different genes. Hypertrophy confined to the apex (apical hypertrophic cardiomyopathy) has been associated with cardiac troponin I mutations. Prognosis varies with the mutation, with β myosin heavy chain mutations presenting early in life and cardiac myosin binding protein C mutations presenting in the elderly. Finally, not all individuals with an abnormal genotype will express the phenotype of hypertrophic cardiomyopathy.

An important management point is the importance of family screening of new cases of hypertrophic cardiomyopathy. It is recommended that screening consist of a history and physical examination, 12-lead ECG, and two-dimensional echocardiography at annual evaluation during the adolescent years *(8)*. Adults with normal screening evaluations should be reevaluated every 5 yr, as hypertrophic cardiomyoapthy may present in later life. Genetic screening remains a research tool but may some day allow more directed screening.

Natural History and Clinical Course

The prognosis and clinical course of patients with hypertrophic cardiomyopathy is likewise variable. Patients may remain stable over long periods and reach normal longevity, while others present with sudden death. In general, patients who are symptomatic follow one or more of several pathways: (1) sudden death; (2) progressive dyspnea, chest pain, and presyncope/syncope in the face of normal or even supranormal LV function; (3) progression to LV systolic dysfunction and a dilated cardiomyopathy; or (4) atrial fibrillation with associated clinical deterioration or stroke *(8)*. Management is directed at each of these possible clinical pathways.

Treatment of Hypertrophic Cardiomyopathy

Treatment is directed at symptom alleviation and prevention of sudden death. In asymptomatic patients, it may not be necessary to do anything other than explain the importance of avoiding competitive athletics and reporting symptoms of presyncope/syncope immediately. Pharmacological therapy is usually initiated with the onset of disabling symptoms. β-Blockers such as propranolol, atenolol, or metoprolol are usually used first. If β-blockers are not effective, a trial of verapamil may be warranted. However, verapamil has been associated with death in patients with resting LV outflow tract gradients and severe symptoms. Both agents have negative inotropic actions and slow heart rate. The response to such drugs is variable; few clinical trials have examined treatment in hypertropic cardiomyopathy, so therapy remains somewhat of a "trial and error" event. If a patient develops a dilated cardiomyopathy, he or she should be treated with agents shown to be effective for that disorder, and verapamil should be discontinued. Patients with LV outflow tract obstruction or intrinsic mitral valve disease deserve infective endocarditis prophylaxis.

For patients with severe drug refractory symptoms and marked LV outflow tract gradients (50 mmHg at rest or on stress testing), surgical myectomy or catheter-based alcohol septal ablation is often performed. Both of these procedures work best in patients with LV outflow tract obstruction rather than mid-cavitary obstruction. Both surgery and alcohol septal ablation reduce LV outflow tract gradients and improve symptoms. It is recommended that both procedures be confined to centers with experience. For patients with severe drug refractory symptoms but no LV outflow tract gradient, heart transplantation may be necessary.

Those who survive sudden cardiac death are treated with an implanted cardioverter-defibrillator. The difficult issue is risk stratification to prevent sudden death. The highest risk has been associated with prior cardiac arrest, sustained ventricular tachycardia, family history of sudden cardiac death, nonsustained ventricular tachycardia on Holter monitoring, abnormal blood pressure response on stress testing, extreme LV hypertrophy (wall thickness 30 mm or more), and the presence of a high-risk genotype. Annual evaluation for patients with hypertrophic cardiomyopathy at risk for sudden death should include a history directed toward presyncope and syncope, an echocardiogram, a stress test, and possibly a Holter monitor for 24 h *(8)*.

Atrial fibrillation is usually poorly tolerated and because of this justifies aggressive attempts at maintenance of sinus rhythm. Warfarin is indicated for those with both paroxysmal and chronic atrial fibrillation.

RESTRICTIVE CARDIOMYOPATHY

This heart muscle disease is characterized by impaired ventricular filling and reduced diastolic ventricular volumes associated with normal or near-normal left ventricular function, normal wall thickness, and biatrial enlargement *(9)*. It is a rare cause of cardiomyopathy, but more common in parts of the tropics. The key component is decreased ventricular compliance, without increased wall thickness in most cases, leading to decreased ventricular filling and hence biatrial enlargement.

Causes of Restrictive Cardiomyopathy

Outside the tropics, amyloidosis is probably the most frequent cause of restrictive cardiomyopathy. Other infiltrative causes include hemochromatosis, sarcoidosis, Fabry's disease, and a variety of other uncommon disorders. In the tropics, endomyocardial fibrosis with and without eosinophilia is more common. Radiation, metastatic tumors, and familial inheritance may also cause restrictive cardiomyopathy. Finally, cases may be idiopathic.

Natural History and Clinical Course

Prognosis varies with the cause of the restrictive cardiomyopathy. Amyloidosis is again associated with a poor prognosis. Others causes of restrictive cardiomyopathy arc associated with a prolonged course, often of right heart failure with pronounced venous congestion. Dyspnea is often present as well, due to left atrial hypertension.

Treatment of Restrictive Cardiomyopathy

Treatment is often frustrating and is directed at the relief of congestion, as well as the underlying cause. Digoxin should be avoided in patients with amyloidosis. Otherwise, diuretics remain the mainstay of therapy. Constrictive pericarditis needs to be excluded, as this treatable disorder is easily confused with restrictive cardiomyopathy.

ARRYTHMOGENIC RIGHT VENTRICULAR DYSPLASIA

Arrythmogenic right ventricular dysplasia (ARVD) is characterized by an enlarged right ventricle due to fibrofatty infiltration of the right ventricular free wall *(10)*. Patients present with ventricular tachycardia of left bundle branch morphology or sudden death. The disease is frequently familial, and mutations in at least three genes have been associated with ARVD. It should be suspected in young patients resuscitated from sudden death without overt left ventricular dysfunction or underlying congenital heart disease.

Evaluation and Treatment of ARVD

The evaluation includes echocardiography, magnetic resonance imaging, and sometimes endomyocardial biopsy. In general, an enlarged, hypocontractile right ventricle is seen with evidence of fat infiltration on magnetic resonance imaging. Cardiac sarcoid may at times also present in a similar manner. Treatment includes the screening of family members and the placement of an automatic implantable cardioverter-defibrillator. Given the rarity of ARVD, referral to a center with expertise in this disorder is warranted.

MYOCARDITIS

Myocarditis is an inflammatory disease of the myocardium, which can lead to a dilated cardiomyopathy. It has been associated with a variety of infectious organisms, including bacteria, parasites, and fungi, as well as hypersensitivity drug reactions and autoimmune diseases (*see* Table 4). The key concept is that some form of myocardial injury, usually viral, leads to an autoimmune reaction. This, in turn, causes a dilated cardiomyopathy. This section will concentrate on primary myocarditis, which most believe is a postviral autoimmune disease.

Causes of Myocarditis

As early as the 1800s, it was recognized that cardiac symptoms could be associated with mumps. Sometime about 1929, cardiac inflammation was found in association with influenza. Enteroviruses, particularly the poliomyelitis virus, were associated with myocarditis in the late 1920s. Since then, a number of viruses have been identified in association with myocarditis including both DNA and RNA core viruses (Table 4), but cardiotropic strains of Coxsackie viruses were felt to be the most common cause of myocarditis. By polymerase chain reaction (PCR), viral genome was recently

Table 4
Causes of Myocarditis

Infections
  Viral: Coxsackie virus, echovirus, poliovirus, influenza, vaccinia, cytomegalovirus, adenovirus,
    parvovirus, herpes simplex, respiratory syncytial virus, Epstein-Barr virus, hepatitis, varicella
    zoster, human immunodeficiency virus
  Bacterial: *Streptococcus pyogenes, Staphylococcus aureus, Salmonella, Leptospira, Borellia burgdorferi,*
    Mycoplasma pneumoniae, Chlamydia, Rickettsia
  Fungi: *Aspergillus, Candida*
  Parasites: *Trypanosoma cruzii, Toxoplasma*
Smallpox vaccination
Peripartum
Giant cell
Eosinophilic
Chemical or drug hypersensitivity
Multiple antibiotics, diuretics, anticonvulsants, interferon
Radiation

found in 38% of 624 patients with myocarditis and only 1.4% of control samples *(11)*. The myocardial samples came from endomyocardial biopsy, autopsy, and explanted hearts. The most common virus genome identified in both children and adults with myocarditis was adenovirus followed
by enterovirus, cytomegalovirus, parvovirus, influenza A, herpes simplex virus, Epstein-Barr virus,
and respiratory syncitial virus. There were 26 patients with infection with two different viruses.

That adenoviruses and enteroviruses, such as Coxsackie, cause myocarditis should not be too
surprising as both use common cellular receptors for entry into myocardial cells, and differences
in affinity for the receptor may account for differences in susceptibility and pathogenesis. Other
viruses that have been described as causes of myocarditis include human immunodeficiency virus
and hepatitis C. In addition, myocarditis has recently been confirmed following smallpox vaccination in US military personnel *(12,13)*.

Natural History and Clinical Course

The natural history is variable. The majority of patients probably have subclinical cardiac inflammation that clears spontaneously *(14)*. A much smaller percentage present with overt disease.
Four clinicopathologic forms of myocarditis have been described (Table 5). Patients with *fulminant myocarditis* are usually young and have a distinct onset with a recent, recognizable viral illness.
They present abruptly with poor left ventricular function and near-normal-sized left ventricles. Ventricular walls are often thick due to a combination of lymphocytic infiltration and edema. Patients
either spontaneously recover completely or die of cardiogenic shock or ventricular arrhythmias
(15,16). We do not believe that immunosuppression has a role in the management of these patients.
Patients with *acute myocarditis* have an indistinct onset of symptoms, moderate to severe left ventricular dysfunction, and active or borderline myocarditis on endomyocardial biopsy. Such patients
may respond to immunosuppression. *Chronic active myocarditis* has an indistinct onset and progressive left ventricular dysfunction, resulting in a restrictive picture. Endomyocardial biopsy shows
inflammation and severe fibrosis, which does not respond to immunosuppression. Patients with
chronic persistent myocarditis present with atypical chest pain or ventricular arrhythmias. Left
ventricular dysfunction is not present. Endomyocardial biopsy shows inflammation.

Giant-cell myocarditis has a particularly poor prognosis, with a median survival of 5.5 mo after
the development of symptoms as documented in the largest registry of such patients *(17)*. The course
is characterized by progressive heart failure with refractory ventricular arrhythmias. Patients tend
to present in their 40s, and many have had a previous autoimmune disease. It is known to recur in
transplanted hearts, but heart transplantation is the only therapy likely to offer a significant survival

Table 5
Clinicopathologic Forms of Myocarditis

	Fulminant	Acute	Chronic active	Chronic persistent
Onset	Distinct	Indistinct	Indistinct	Indistinct
LV function	Severe dysfunction	Moderate dysfunction	Moderate dysfunction	Normal
Biopsy	Multiple foci active	Active or borderline	Active or borderline	Active or borderline
Clinical prognosis	Complete recovery or death	Dilated cardiomyopathy	Restrictive cardiomyopathy	Normal
Histologic prognosis	Resolution	Resolution	Ongoing inflammation and fibrosis	Ongoing myocarditis

advantage. Endomyocardial biopsy shows a diffuse, aggressive lymphocytic infiltrate with myocyte necrosis and the presence of giant cells without well-formed granuloma. Giant-cell myocarditis is different from cardiac sarcoidosis. The pathology is different, with cardiac sarcoidosis presenting with a patchy infiltrate and well-formed granuloma. The prognosis of cardiac sarcoid is better and patients with sarcoid are more likely to present with heart block and a long duration of symptoms *(18)*.

Evaluation of Myocarditis

Diagnosis is based on endomyocardial biopsy. In general, the Dallas criteria remain the benchmark for histologic diagnosis *(19)*. Myocarditis is characterized by myocyte necrosis associated with an adjacent inflammatory infiltrate. Borderline myocarditis is diagnosed if there is no evident myocyte damage. Myocarditis can be suspected in patients who present with a nondilated, hypocontractile heart and an antecedent viral syndrome. Troponins may be elevated and sometimes pericarditis symptoms predominate.

Treatment of Myocarditis

Treatment remains controversial. The largest trial of immunosuppressive therapy for myocarditis did not support the use of such agents. There was no significant difference in survival *(4)*. Since then, a number of reports have suggested that patients with cardiac inflammation may respond if the correct patients are chosen. In a trial of 22 patients with PCR-proven enteroviral or adenoviral genomes and persistent left ventricular dysfunction, treatment with interferon-β for 6 mo resulted in the elimination of viral genomes in all patients and improvement in left ventricular function in 15 of 22 patients *(20)*. In another study of 112 patients with a histologic diagnosis of myocarditis, patients with circulating cardiac autoantibodies and no viral genome were most likely to respond to immunosuppression *(21)*. Wojnicz et al. showed no difference in survival in 84 patients with dilated cardiomyopathy and increased myocyte HLA expression randomized to 3 mo of immunosuppression versus placebo *(22)*. Approximately 27% of patients in this trial had myocarditis as diagnosed by the Dallas Criteria. Intravenous immunoglobulin did not augment left ventricular function when compared to placebo in adult patients with recent-onset dilated cardiomyopathy *(23)*. However, left ventricular function did improve to a similar degree, about 16 EF units, in both groups. Only about 16% of patients in this trial had myocarditis as defined by the Dallas Criteria.

Currently, the treatment of myocarditis is in evolution. Patients with a fulminant presentation usually will not need immunosuppression. In patients with chronic active myocarditis and chronic persistent myocarditis, immunosuppression is either ineffective or unwarranted. Patients with giant-cell myocarditis are treated with immunosuppression, but this is rarely effective. In the future we should be able to predict which patients with acute myocarditis will respond to immunosuppression, and likely tailor therapy to the stage of the disease.

Peripartum Cardiomyopathy

Peripartum cardiomyopathy is included here because in our experience 62% of patients had myocarditis on endomyocardial biopsy *(24)*. In the United States, this occurs in 1 of every 1300 to 4000 deliveries. It is defined as left ventricular systolic dysfunction developing in the final month of pregnancy or within 5 mo after delivery in the absence of preexisting heart disease. In our experience, recovery of left ventricular function occurs in the majority of patients and the 5-yr survival is excellent. Subsequent pregnancies have been associated with a reoccurrence of left ventricular dysfunction *(25)*. In 28 women whose left ventricular function had returned to normal, there was no mortality but 21% of patients developed symptoms of heart failure. In 16 women whose heart function had failed to normalize, the mortality was 19% and 44% of the women developed heart failure. These data are helpful in counseling women regarding future pregnancies.

CONCLUSION

Diseases of the myocardium, cardiomyopathies, leading to heart failure represent fertile ground for further research. I expect molecular techniques to substantially affect our ability to diagnose and care for patients with cardiomyopathy. The next decade will likely see the advent of biologically based therapies to both prevent the phenotypic development of cardiomyopathy and to manage the disease once present.

REFERENCES

1. Report of the 1995 World Health Organization/International Society and Federation of Cardiology Task Force on the Definition and Classification of Cardiomyopathies. Circulation 1996;93:841–842.
2. Felker GM, Thompson RE, Hare JM, et al. Underlying causes and long-term survival in patients with initially unexplained cardiomyopathy. N Engl J Med 2000;342:1077–1084.
3. Felker GM, Hu W, Hare JM, et al. The spectrum of dilated cardiomyopathy. The Johns Hopkins experience with 1,278 patients. Medicine (Baltimore) 1999;78:270–283.
4. Mason JW, O'Connell JB, Herskowitz A, et al. A clinical trial of immunosuppressive therapy for myocarditis. The Myocarditis Treatment Trial Investigators. N Engl J Med 1995;333:269–275.
5. Michels VV, Moll PP, Miller FA, et al. The frequency of familial dilated cardiomyopathy in a series of patients with idiopathic dilated cardiomyopathy. N Engl J Med 1992;326:77–82.
6. Fatkin D, Graham RM. Molecular mechanisms of inherited cardiomyopathies. Physiol Rev 2002;82:945–980.
7. Hunt SA, Baker DW, Chin MH, et al. ACC/AHA Guidelines for the Evaluation and Management of Chronic Heart Failure in the Adult: Executive Summary A Report of the American College of Cardiology/American Heart Association Task Force on Practice Guidelines (Committee to Revise the 1995 Guidelines for the Evaluation and Management of Heart Failure): Developed in Collaboration with the International Society for Heart and Lung Transplantation; Endorsed by the Heart Failure Society of America. Circulation 2001;104:2996–3007.
8. Maron BJ, McKenna WJ, Danielson GK, et al. ACC/ESC clinical expert consensus document on hypertrophic cardiomyopathy: a report of the American Colege of Cardiology Task Force on Clinical Expert Consensus Documents and the European Society of Cardiology Committee for Practice Guidelines. J Am Coll Cardiol 2003;42:1687–1713.
9. Kushwaha SS, Fallon JT, Fuster V. Restrictive cardiomyopathy. N Engl J Med 1997;336:267–276.
10. Marcus F, Towbin JA, Zareba W, et al. Arrhythmogenic right ventricular dysplasia/cardiomyopathy (ARVD/C): a multidisciplinary study: design and protocol. Circulation 2003;107:2975–2978.
11. Bowles NE, Ni J, Kearney DL, et al. Detection of viruses in myocardial tissues by polymerase chain reaction. evidence of adenovirus as a common cause of myocarditis in children and adults. J Am Coll Cardiol 2003;42:466–472.
12. Halsell JS, Riddle JR, Atwood JE, et al. Myopericarditis following smallpox vaccination among vaccinia-naive US military personnel. JAMA 2003;289:3283–3289.
13. Murphy JG, Wright RS, Bruce GK, et al. Eosinophilic-lymphocytic myocarditis after smallpox vaccination. Lancet 2003;362:1378–1380.
14. Lieberman EB, Herskowitz A, Rose NR, Baughman KL. A clinicopathologic description of myocarditis. Clin Immunol Immunopathol 1993;68:191–196.
15. McCarthy RE, Boehmer JP, Hruban RH, et al. Long-term outcome of fulminant myocarditis as compared with acute (nonfulminant) myocarditis. N Engl J Med 2000;342:690–695.
16. Felker GM, Boehmer JP, Hruban RH, et al. Echocardiographic findings in fulminant and acute myocarditis. J Am Coll Cardiol 2000;36:227–232.
17. Cooper LT Jr, Berry GJ, Shabetai R. Idiopathic giant-cell myocarditis—natural history and treatment. Multicenter Giant Cell Myocarditis Study Group Investigators. N Engl J Med 1997;336:1860–1866.
18. Okura Y, Dec GW, Hare JM, et al. A clinical and histopathologic comparison of cardiac sarcoidosis and idiopathic giant cell myocarditis. J Am Coll Cardiol 2003;41:322–329.

19. Aretz HT. Myocarditis: the Dallas criteria. Hum Pathol 1987;18:619–624.
20. Kuhl U, Pauschinger M, Schwimmbeck PL, et al. Interferon-beta treatment eliminates cardiotropic viruses and improves left ventricular function in patients with myocardial persistence of viral genomes and left ventricular dysfunction. Circulation 2003;107:2793–2798.
21. Frustaci A, Chimenti C, Calabrese F, et al. Immunosuppressive therapy for active lymphocytic myocarditis: virological and immunologic profile of responders versus nonresponders. Circulation 2003;107:857–863.
22. Wojnicz R, Nowalany-Kozielska E, Wojciechowska C, et al. Randomized, placebo-controlled study for immunosuppressive treatment of inflammatory dilated cardiomyopathy: two-year follow up results. Circulation 2001;104: 39–45.
23. McNamara DM, Holubkov R, Starling RC, et al. Controlled trial of intravenous immune globulin in recent-onset dilated cardiomyopathy. Circulation 2001;103:2254–2259.
24. Felker GM, Jaeger CJ, Klodas E, et al. Myocarditis and long-term survival in peripartum cardiomyopathy. Am Heart J 2000;140:785–791.
25. Elkayam U, Tummala PP, Rao K, et al. Maternal and fetal outcomes of subsequent pregnancies in women with peripartum cardiomyopathy. N Engl J Med 2001;344:1567–1571.

RECOMMENDED READING

Report of the 1995 World Health Organization/International Society and Federation of Cardiology Task Force on the Definition and Classification of Cardiomyopathies. Circulation 1996;93:841–842.
Felker GM, Thompson RE, Hare JM, et al. Underlying causes and long-term survival in patients with initially unexplained cardiomyopathy. N Engl J Med 2000;342:1077–1084.
Hunt SA, Baker DW, Chin MH, et al. ACC/AHA Guidelines for the Evaluation and Management of Chronic Heart Failure in the Adult: Executive Summary A Report of the American College of Cardiology/American Heart Association Task Force on Practice Guidelines (Committee to Revise the 1995 Guidelines for the Evaluation and Management of Heart Failure): Developed in Collaboration With the International Society for Heart and Lung Transplantation; Endorsed by the Heart Failure Society of America. Circulation 2001;104:2996–3007.
Maron BJ, McKenna WJ, Danielson GK, et al. ACC/ESC clinical expert consensus document on hypertrophic cardiomyopathy: a report of the American Colege of Cardiology Task Force on Clinical Expert Consensus Documents and the European Society of Cardiology Committee for Practice Guidelines. J Am Coll Cardiol 2003;42:1687–1713.
Kushwaha SS, Fallon JT, Fuster V. Restrictive cardiomyopathy. N Engl J Med 1997;336:267–276.

35

Pericardial Disease

David H. Spodick, MD, DSc

INTRODUCTION

The pericardium is a complex, mesothelium-lined serous sac surrounding the heart and clasped externally by a fibrous sac so that the layer on the heart (visceral pericardium) is mesothelium, while the external portion (parietal pericardium) is composed of mesothelium internally and fibrosa externally. Normally, 15 to 35 mL of serous fluid surrounds the heart. The normal microphysiology of the visceral and parietal pericardia is complex and is discussed in detail elsewhere (1). The pericardium is involved in every known kind of disease, and abnormal fluid accumulation in it frequently seriously compromises cardiac function (tamponade) and raises important questions in differential diagnosis and treatment.

Table 1 lists the nine major categories of pericardial disease, each of which must be considered in any new case. A vast array of individual conditions under each of these categories is described in detail elsewhere (2).

CONGENITAL PERICARDIAL DEFECTS AND CYSTS

Gaps in the pericardium, although usually left-sided, may occur anywhere and have the potential to compress herniating cardiac structures, including parts of chambers and coronary vessels. Predictable syndromes, however, may be difficult to identify, although imaging is usually successful, especially magnetic resonance imaging (MRI). Congenital cysts, the majority occurring in the right cardiophrenic angle, usually require imaging to distinguish them from solid tumors or cardiac aneurysms.

PERICARDIAL INFLAMMATIONS: ACUTE PERICARDITIS

Acute pericarditis is the most common—and therefore the most important—of all pericardial disorders, although subclinical cases may be missed. Every category of inflammatory, including infectious, agent has been identified. Most patients, particularly younger ones, present with "idiopathic pericarditis syndrome." There is no proved cause, but it is most likely viral. This syndrome is typically the epitome of acute pericarditis, because it includes any and all the classic manifestations: pain, pericardial rubs, and electrocardiographic (ECG) changes (3). Coxsackie virus and other enteroviruses are the most common agents in the United States. Effusion is frequent, usually without tamponade. Adhesions are undetectable except by imaging, but constrictive scarring occurs occasionally. The differential diagnosis includes systemic diseases such as lupus erythematosus and other vasculitides that frequently involve the pericardium.

CLINICALLY DRY ACUTE PERICARDITIS

Clinically dry indicates either that the condition is without effusion or that any effusion has no clinical significance; it is the most common presentation of acute pericarditis. Onset may be gradual or sudden with central chest pain, usually pleuritic, that is exacerbated by body movements and by

From: *Essential Cardiology: Principles and Practice, 2nd Ed.*
Edited by: C. Rosendorff © Humana Press Inc., Totowa, NJ

Table 1
Causes and Pathogenesis of Acquired Diseases of the Pericardium[a]

I	Idiopathic pericarditis (syndromes)
II	Living agents: infections, parasitoses
III	Vasculitis, connective tissue disease
IV	Immunopathies/hypersensitivity states
V	Diseases of contiguous structures
VI	Disorders of metabolism
VII	Trauma, direct or indirect
VIII	Neoplasms: primary, metastatic
IX	Of uncertain pathogenesis or in association with many syndromes

[a]Considerable overlap (e.g., categories III and IV; V and VII). (Modified from ref. 2.)

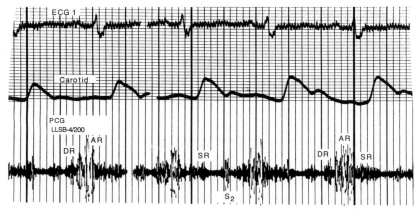

Fig. 1. Electrocardiogram (ECG 1), carotid displacement pulse (carotid), and phonocardiogram (PCG) show a quasidiagnostic, three-part pericardial rub. DR, late diastolic component; AR, atrial component; SR, ventricular systolic component. In this example, the AR is the most intense. (From ref. 2, with permission.)

breathing. Occasionally it mimics ischemic forms of chest pain, including substernal pressure sensations. The pain is simultaneously (or occasionally only) perceived in one or both trapezius ridges, a finding *virtually pathognomonic for acute pericarditis*. Frequently, the onset follows an upper respiratory tract infection. Fever varies according to the cause but is usually between 37° and 38.8°C. A pericardial friction sound (rub) is usual *(4)*: it has a high frequency, is often loud, is nearly always strongest at the left lower to middle sternal edge, and has a peculiar shuffling, grating, scratching, or, rarely, creaking quality. Usually, three components are distinguishable by careful auscultation: presystolic (atrial), systolic, and early diastolic (Fig. 1). Biphasic—and even monophasic—rubs are relatively common. When all three components are distinguishable, this rules out similar-sounding murmurs. Rubs are supposedly due to friction between pericardial surfaces, yet inflammatory effusions, including large effusions, often occur with rubs. Moderate leukocytosis is common, but the infective agent or any systemic disorder causing the pericarditis dictates the variation in cell count, sedimentation rate, and other acute-phase reactants. Cardiac enzyme studies vary widely, from normal to small increases depending directly on the extent of any accompanying myocarditis. Indeed, some degree of myocarditis is entirely responsible for electrocardiographic (ECG) PR segment and ST-T changes. When typical, ECG changes are quasidiagnostic, particularly Stage 1 (Fig. 2) of four sequential stages. J-point (ST) elevations with normal-looking T waves in all leads except a VR and occasionally V_1 and V_2 characterize stage 1 *(5)*. Atypical ECG variants are described in detail elsewhere *(6)*. In Stage 2, all J points return to the baseline together with little change in the T waves until later, when T waves progressively flatten and invert. In Stage 3, T waves are com-

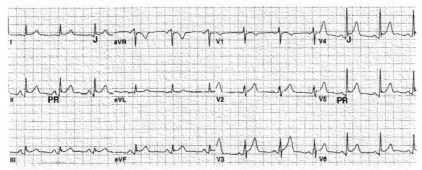

Fig. 2. A 12-lead ECG shows typical, quasidiagnostic stage 1 changes of acute pericarditis. The J points (ST segments) are elevated in most leads. (AVR is always an exception, and V_1 nearly always; aVL is almost algebraically zero.) PR segments are oppositely deviated, reflecting the atrial T waves due to atrial pericarditis. (From ref. *2*, with permission.)

pletely inverted. Stage 4 is a recovery stage. A typical transition from Stage 1 to 2 to 3 is diagnostic; however, in modern times, many patients stop at Stage 2, because of antiinflammatory treatment. Equally characteristic are PR segment deviations, mostly depression, occurring in most leads. These tend to appear earlier than ST elevations and may be the only ECG abnormality. Heart rate is quite variable and is proportional to the systemic reaction. Usually, it is relatively rapid (>90 beats/min), but it can be slow, especially in uremic patients. Rhythm abnormalities are due not to pericarditis but to an accompanying heart disorder, such as severe myocarditis or prior valve or myocardial disease.

A similar ECG pattern, "early repolarization," must be distinguished, occurring mainly in males younger than 40 yr. Here, PR segment deviations are uncommon and never generalized, while the J-point elevation, unlike in pericarditis, is usually less than 25% of the T-wave height in lead V_6. T voltages tend to be high, and RV_4 tends to be the tallest R.

PERICARDIAL EFFUSION

Inflammation of the pericardium or a fluid-retaining state (e.g., congestive heart failure) can cause pericardial effusion if fluid is produced too fast to be reabsorbed. There may be one of four general consequences: clinically insignificant amounts; a larger effusion without apparent physiologic effects; a relatively large effusion compressing the heart but checked at least temporarily by compensatory mechanisms; and frank cardiac tamponade: cardiac compression limiting cardiac input and therefore output with life-threatening consequences. Heart sounds may be distant, especially with tamponade. Large effusions may be asymptomatic but can compress adjacent organs, causing dyspnea, cough, hoarseness, abdominal fullness, hiccups, and nausea.

Ordinary chest X-rays show cardiomegaly often with a "water flask" outline and clear lung fields in the absence of independent pulmonary disease. Echocardiography (Fig. 3) is the standard for identifying and following the course of pericardial effusion. Other imaging modalities may be required. Pleural effusions, especially on the left, are common. Larger effusions, particularly with tamponade, permit "swinging" of the heart, producing electric alternation on the ECG.

ACUTE CARDIAC TAMPONADE

Tamponade is the decompensated phase of cardiac compression resulting from an unchecked increase in pericardial fluid pressure. Tamponade may be slow to develop, owing to slow effusion, or sudden, usually due to hemorrhage. In either case, compression of the heart must be relieved by drainage. Clinically, patients have signs of low-output state, including air hunger, which often resembles congestive heart failure, but without pulmonary edema. There is equalization of diastolic pressures throughout the heart. Pulsus paradoxus, a drop in systolic blood pressure greater than

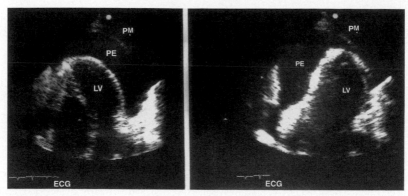

Fig. 3. Large circumcardiac pericardial effusion is compressing the heart. Apical 4-chamber echocardiogram. (From ref. 2, with permission.)

10 mmHg during normal inspiration, is usual. Imaging, particularly Doppler echocardiography, usually shows right ventricular and/or atrial diastolic collapse, and occasionally left atrial collapse and a swinging heart. In volume-expanded patients, however, chamber collapses may not be present, whereas hypovolemia can produce collapses without tamponade.

PERICARDIAL CONSTRICTION

Pericardial inflammation may heal with tight or thick scar tissue, compressing the heart much as tamponade does, but more slowly. Some degree of pericardial bleeding has been necessary to produce experimental constrictive scarring. Constrictive pericarditis was formerly regarded as a chronic disease, but earlier diagnosis by better trained and equipped modern physicians, and a shift in its major causes, now make most cases subacute or even relatively acute. Any pericardial inflammation (except rheumatic) can cause constriction. Tuberculosis was the major detectable cause but it is no longer so in developed countries, where often relatively rapid constriction after cardiac surgery is an increasingly important factor. The acute pericardial inflammation may have been manifest, but if totally silent some patients present with constrictive pericarditis *de novo*.

The pathophysiology of constrictive pericarditis is distinct from that of tamponade. Catheterization traces usually show a diastolic "dip" and plateau (square-root sign). As a rule, atrial *x* and *y* descents are deep. Chest films are of no use unless there is pericardial calcification, which is best seen in lateral views. Doppler echocardiography, CT and MRI, and other imaging modalities usually give the diagnosis. It is sometimes difficult to distinguish constriction from its mimic, restrictive cardiomyopathy.

Pedal edema is common, especially in chronic constriction. Ascites, with or without edema, is most common with chronic constriction. Symptoms correspond to those of congestive heart failure without pulmonary edema. There is frequently a loud early third heart sound, which is sometimes palpable and may have a "knocking" quality. ECG changes are nonspecific, although they may resemble Stage 3 of the acute pericarditis ECG, with frequent interatrial block (usually notched, wide P waves).

In *effusive-constrictive pericarditis*, concomitant pericardial effusion produces acute and subacute clinical pictures. The clinical and physiologic signs depend on whether tamponade or constriction predominates. Drainage of the effusion without significant effect on the abnormal hemodynamics often reveals this lesion. The treatment for all forms of constriction is pericardiectomy, except in the relatively uncommon, undiscovered *transient constriction*.

IDIOPATHIC PERICARDITIS

Cases in which the cause cannot be established can be considered "idiopathic," although in this case most patients have a viral pericardial syndrome and the designation of "idiopathic" persists because it is usually not productive to search for a particular virus. As in acute viral pericarditis, tamponade and constriction occur occasionally and recurrences are common (15–25%).

INFECTIOUS ACUTE PERICARDITIS

Viruses are perhaps the most common cause of infectious acute pericarditis in the United States, especially coxsackieviruses and other enteroviruses. Other viral etiologies include the agents for hepatitis, mumps, and other childhood diseases. Elements of myopericarditis or perimyocarditis are common, especially in children. Although the pericardial syndrome dominates, patients may have dyspnea, cough, and pulmonary infiltrates. Viral pericarditis is much more common in men, usually young, healthy male patients. Patients less likely to have a viral infection always raise questions of acute myocardial infarction, tuberculosis, and vasculitis. Patients may have recurrent attacks within the first few months, but others have attacks for years owing to a persistent immunopathy in the absence of living organisms.

BACTERIAL PERICARDITIS

Bacterial infection is the most serious of the common infectious forms of pericarditis. The control of bacteria, except in compromised hosts, has reduced its incidence; but serious tamponade and constriction are much more likely with aggressive bacterial infections, which are more destructive of tissues than most viral infections. These appear to be increasingly evident in hospitalized patients and may be dramatic, with septic manifestations, though in many elderly patients with severe systemic diseases they are silent. Tachycardia is the rule, and about half the patients have a very high fever. Leukocytosis with a marked leftward shift is characteristic. Blood culture may help, but pericardial fluid culture is more specific. Pericardial drainage with resection for any signs of constriction of the pericardium or loculation is virtually mandatory.

Tuberculosis—although its prevalence is decreasing, except in AIDS patients—is still a significant cause, particularly in immunocompromised hosts, who may also have atypical organisms. There is a broad spectrum of tuberculous pericarditis from painful acute pericarditis with minimal to large effusions to tamponade. Others may lack acute symptoms, except fever. Some patients have chronic pericardial effusions and pericardial calcifications with or without hemodynamic impairment. Tuberculin testing is of little help for the diagnosis. Treatment is drainage for tamponade and surgical resection for any suggestion of pericardial constriction, under multiple antituberculous drug therapy.

FUNGAL PERICARDITIS

Fungal pericarditis is seen increasingly in immunocompromised patients. Organisms include fungi such as *Histoplasma* and *Coccidioides*, each with a geographic distribution that makes consideration of these diagnoses important in endemic areas. Many other fungi also attack the pericardium. Treatment is with an agent specific for a particular fungus, except histoplasmosis, as well as amphotericin, as indicated.

PARASITIC PERICARDIAL DISEASE

Parasitic infestations are mainly geographically endemic, particularly echinococcosis, amebiasis, and toxoplasmosis. Indeed, any parasite may attack the pericardium. Patients returning from endemic areas should always raise the question of parasitosis.

PERICARDITIS IN DISEASES OF CONTIGUOUS STRUCTURES

Pericarditis is common in anatomically *transmural myocardial infarction* and usually has no clinical importance. Occasionally, rubs and pleuritic pain are associated. Most cases are self-limited. Fluid retention may cause hydropericardium. Tamponade is usually due to hemorrhagic effusion

Table 2
Acute Pericarditis vs Acute Myocardial Ischemia[a]

	Acute pericarditis	Acute myocardial ischemia
ECG		
J-ST	Diffuse elevation usually concave, without reciprocal depressions	Localized deviation usually convex (with reciprocals in infarct)
PR segment depression	Frequent	Almost never
Abnormal Q waves	None unless with infarction	Common with infarction (Q wave infarcts)
T waves	Inverted after J points return to baseline	Inverted while ST segment still elevated (infarct)
Arrhythmia	None (in absence of heart disease)	Frequent
Conduction Abnormalties	None (in absence of heart disease)	Frequent
Pain		
Onset	More often sudden	Usually gradual, crescendo
Main location	Substernal or left precordial	Same or confined to zones of radiation
Radiation	May be the same as ischemic, also trapezius ridge(s)	Shoulders, arms, neck, jaw, back; not trapezius ridge(s)
Quality	Usually sharp, stabbing; "background" ache or dull and oppressive	Usually "heavy" (pressure sensation) or burning
Inspiration	Worse	No effect unless with infarction pericarditis
Duration	Persistent; may wax and wane	Usually intermittent; <30 min each recurrence, longer for unstable angina
Body movements	Increased	Usually no effect
Posture	Worse on recumbency; improved on sitting, leaning forward	No effect or improvement on sitting
Nitroglycerin	No effect	Usually relief

From ref. 2.

but is rare unless there is antithrombotic therapy or cardiac rupture. The ECG does not show diagnostic changes unless there is a postinfarction (Dressler) syndrome, which can occur weeks after (and sometimes with) the acute infarct and may cause tamponade or constriction. Table 2 summarizes the clinical differential diagnosis between acute pericarditis and acute ischemia.

Type 1 aortic dissections commonly rupture into the pericardium with rapid hemopericardium and tamponade. Although the pericardium may be irritated if blood leaks beneath the epicardium producing signs and symptoms of acute pericarditis, a compressed coronary vessel may rarely cause infarction. Emergency surgical management is virtually mandatory.

Pulmonary diseases, including pneumonia and pulmonary embolism, can involve the pericardium. *Esophageal disorders*, including inflammation, ulcers, and malignancies, can extend to the pericardium, usually with tamponade and a stormy clinical picture, although, rarely, they are relatively silent.

Postmyocardial and *pericardial injury syndromes* are considered to be immunopathic with common features, including response to corticosteroids, latent period, recurrences, fever with pulmonary infiltrates and pleuritis, and sterile blood and pericardial fluid cultures. Immunopathies also include postmyocardial infarction and related syndromes.

Traumatic pericarditis due to penetrating wounds or nonpenetrating chest injuries (including radiation) produces the signs typical of acute pericarditis or pericardial effusion, with or without tamponade or constriction.

VASCULITIS-CONNECTIVE TISSUE DISEASE GROUP

Every member of this group, notably *rheumatoid arthritis*, produces pericardial lesions of every description, except acute rheumatic fever, which scars the pericardium but does not provoke constriction. The differential diagnosis includes idiopathic (presumably viral) pericarditis, which in itself can present with arthropathy. *Systemic lupus erythematosus* is particularly important in this group and must be ruled out in women with "idiopathic" or viral pericardial syndrome, since the latter are so common in men and lupus so frequent in women. Antiinflammatory agents suppress most attacks unless there are complications.

DISORDERS OF METABOLISM

In *renal failure*, especially when chronic, pericarditis is quite common, though it occasionally accompanies uncomplicated acute renal failure. Bacterial or viral infection can occur, although bacteria are much less common in the antibiotic era. ECG usually is not helpful. A stubborn form in patients on dialysis, *dialysis pericarditis*, is difficult to treat and sometimes causes huge effusions with variable symptoms. Resection of the pericardium is often necessary.

Myxedema, increasingly rare, produces large pericardial effusions that are often asymptomatic and often with small eletrocardiographic voltage. Tamponade is rare.

NEOPLASTIC PERICARDIAL DISEASES

Primary malignant tumors are rare, and benign tumors (like fibromas and lipomas) are relatively uncommon. Mesothelioma is the most dangerous malignancy, masquerading as acute pericarditis pericardial effusion or constriction.

RECURRENT AND INCESSANT PERICARDITIS

Patients with acute pericarditis, particularly those receiving corticosteroid therapy, may have frequently recurring pericarditis requiring new therapy. The term "incessant pericarditis" applies to patients who are asymptomatic only when taking medication. This difficult problem is discussed in detail elsewhere *(7)*.

REFERENCES

1. Spodick DH. Macro- and microphysiology and anatomy of the pericardium. Am Heart J 1992;124:1046–1051.
2. Spodick DH. The Pericardium: A Comprehensive Textbook. Marcel Dekker, New York, 1997, pp. 98–100.
3. Permanyer-Miralda G, Sagrista-Sauleda J, Soler-Soler J. Primary acute pericardial disease: a prospective series of 231 consecutive patients. Am J Cardiol 1985;56:623–630.
4. Spodick DH. The pericardial rub: a prospective, multiple observer investigation of pericardial friction in 100 patients. Am J Cardiol 1975;35:357–362.
5. Spodick DH. Diagnostic eletrocardiographic sequences in acute pericarditis: significance of PR segment and PR vector changes. Circulation 1973;48:575–580.
6. Bruce MA, Spodick DH. Atypical electrocardiogram in acute pericarditis: characteristics and prevalence. J Electrocardiol 1980;13:61–66.
7. Spodick DH. Recurrent and incessant pericarditis. In: Spodick DH. The Pericardium: A Comprehensive Textbook. Marcel Dekker, New York, 1997, pp. 422–431.

RECOMMENDED READING

Fowler NO. The Pericardium in Health and Disease. Futura, Mt. Kisco, NY, 1985.
Reddy PS, Leon DF, Shaver JA, eds. Pericardial Disease. Raven, New York, 1982.
Shabetai R. The Pericardium. Grune & Stratton, New York, 1981.
Spodick DH. The Pericardium: A Comprehensive Textbook. Marcel Dekker, New York, 1997.

36   Pulmonary Vascular Disease

Dermot O'Callaghan, MD
and Sean P. Gaine, MD, PhD

INTRODUCTION

Disorders of the pulmonary circulation constitute a diverse group of conditions that arise primarily either from within the lung (e.g., idiopathic pulmonary arterial hypertension [IPAH]), or as a consequence of diseases that originate outside the lungs (e.g., pulmonary embolism [PE]). This chapter will outline the major causes of pulmonary vascular disease and describe the chief complications of these disorders—pulmonary hypertension and cor pulmonale.

PULMONARY HYPERTENSION

Classification of Disorders of Pulmonary Circulation

In 1998, the World Symposium on Primary Pulmonary Hypertension was held in Evian, France *(1)*. One of the more significant outcomes of the Evian symposium was a new, more clinically useful, classification system for pulmonary hypertension, dividing the causes into categories based on their anticipated response to treatment. Primary pulmonary hypertension (PPH) was now classified in a new category, pulmonary arterial hypertension (PAH), that included diseases that produce similar pathologic abnormalities in the wall of small pulmonary arteries despite the heterogeneous nature of the underlying conditions. This category also includes various collagen vascular diseases associated with the development of pulmonary hypertension, including scleroderma, lupus erythematosus, and rheumatoid arthritis, as well as pulmonary hypertension occurring in the setting of congenital heart defects, including the so-called Eisenmenger's syndrome. Four other categories were described: pulmonary venous hypertension, pulmonary hypertension secondary to chronic thrombotic disease and/or embolic disease, disorders directly affecting the pulmonary vasculature, and disorders of the respiratory system and/or hypoxemia. The classification system was updated and refined at the subsequent conference in Venice in 2003 (Table 1). At the Venice conference, PPH was replaced with the term idiopathic pulmonary arterial hypertension.

Clinical Presentation

SIGNS AND SYMPTOMS

The earliest symptom of pulmonary hypertension is exertional shortness of breath, the gradual onset of which can result in a considerable delay in diagnosis. Other common symptoms include chest pain (related to right ventricular ischemia), easy fatiguability, peripheral edema, and lightheadedness or frank syncope. The degree of symptomatic involvement can be assessed by using the modified New York Heart Association classification system grading symptoms I through IV (Table 2).

Physical examination may suggest the presence of a systemic disease associated with pulmonary hypertension. Scleroderma may be identified by cutaneous telangiectasias and sclerodactyly, while

From: *Essential Cardiology: Principles and Practice, 2nd Ed.*
Edited by: C. Rosendorff © Humana Press Inc., Totowa, NJ

Table 1
Venice Classification of Causes of Pulmonary Hypertension

1. Pulmonary arterial hypertension
   1.1. Idiopathic pulmonary atrial hypertension (formerly primary pulmonary hypertension or PPH)
     a. Sporadic
     b. Familial
     c. Pulmonary venoocclusive disease (formerly classified in category 2)
   1.2. Related to:
     a. Collagen vascular disease
     b. Congenital systemic to pulmonary shunts
     c. Portal hypertension
     d. HIV infection
     e. Drugs/toxins
       i. Anorexigens
       ii. Other
     f. Persistent pulmonary hypertension of the newborn
     g. Other
2. Pulmonary hypertension with left heart disease (formerly pulmonary venous hypertension)
   2.1. Left-sided atrial or ventricular heart disease
   2.2. Left-sided valvular heart disease
3. Pulmonary hypertension associated with disorders of the respiratory system and/or hypoxemia
   3.1. Chronic obstructive pulmonary disease
   3.2. Interstitial lung disease
   3.3. Sleep disordered breathing
   3.4. Alveolar hypoventilation disorders
   3.5. Chronic exposure to high altitude
   3.6. Neonatal lung disease
   3.7. Alveolar-capillary dysplasia
   3.8. Other
4. Pulmonary hypertension due to chronic thrombotic disease and/or embolic disease
   4.1. Thromboembolic obstruction of proximal pulmonary arteries
   4.2. Obstruction of distal pulmonary arteries
     a. Pulmonary embolism (thrombus, tumor, ova and/or parasites, foreign material)
     b. *In situ* thrombosis
     c. Sickle cell disease
5. Pulmonary hypertension due to disorders directly affecting the pulmonary vasculature
   5.1. Inflammatory
     a. Schistosomiasis
     b. Sarcoidosis
     c. Other
   5.2. Pulmonary capillary hemaniogmatosis
   5.2. Extrinsic compression of central pulmonary veins
     a. Fibrosing mediastinitis
     b. Adenopathy/tumors

Adapted from ref. 62.

the presence of significant systemic hypertension may suggest underlying obstructive sleep apnea or left ventricular diastolic dysfunction. Clubbing is not seen in IPAH; therefore, its presence suggests alternative diagnoses such as congenital heart disease or lung or liver disease.

    The findings on physical examination in pulmonary hypertension depend on the severity of disease. The most common findings are an accentuated second heart sound in the pulmonic region and a right ventricular S_4. These may be difficult to appreciate in patients with hyperinflation secondary to emphysema. Patients with severe right ventricular hypertrophy may have a heave palpable along the left sternal border or in the epigastrium. Examination of the neck veins may manifest a prominent "a" wave, indicating a noncompliant right ventricle and as the right ventricle enlarges,

Table 2
World Health Organization Functional Class in Pulmonary Arterial Hypertension

Class I	Patients in with pulmonary hypertension, but without resulting limitation of physical activity. Ordinary physical activity does not cause undue dyspnea or fatigue, chest pain, or near-syncope.
Class II	Patients with pulmonary hypertension resulting in slight limitation of physical activity. Patients are comfortable at rest, but ordinary physical activity causes undue dyspnea or fatigue, chest pain, or near-syncope.
Class III	Patients with pulmonary hypertension resulting in marked limitation of physical activity. Patients are comfortable at rest, but less than ordinary physical activity cause undue dyspnea or fatigue, chest pain, or near-syncope.
Class IV	Patients with pulmonary hypertension resulting in inability to perform any physical activity without symptoms. Patients manifest signs of right heart failure. Dyspnea and/or fatigue may be present at rest, and discomfort is increased by any physical activity.

Adapted from ref. *62*.

"v" waves indicative of tricuspid regurgitation may be seen. When right ventricular decompensation and right heart failure finally develop, the jugular venous pressure increases. Dilation of the pulmonic valve annulus or right ventricular outflow tract can produce a soft-blowing diastolic murmur along the upper left sternal border: the Graham Steell murmur of pulmonary regurgitation. The presence of a right ventricular S_3 gallop signifies more advanced right heart dysfunction.

Diagnostic Testing

An extensive battery of diagnostic tests is required in the evaluation of the patient with pulmonary hypertension to define the etiology of the condition. If all tests are negative, then a diagnosis of IPAH or PPH can be made (Fig. 1). Screening blood tests should include an evaluation of liver function, antibodies to human immunodeficiency virus (HIV), and serologic studies to exclude occult collagen vascular disease. The antinuclear antibody (ANA) may be positive in primary pulmonary hypertension, usually in a low titer and without other evidence of connective tissue disease *(2)*.

The chest X-ray demonstrates prominence of the central pulmonary arteries and clear lung fields in individuals with intrinsic pulmonary vascular disease but will reveal evidence of interstitial pulmonary fibrosis (IPF) or emphysema in pulmonary hypertension secondary to parenchymal lung disease. The presence of kerley B lines and pulmonary edema will suggest left heart or postcapillary causes for the pulmonary hypertension. The electrocardiogram will usually demonstrate right axis deviation, right ventricular hypertrophy, and T wave changes suggesting strain. Echocardiography is helpful in excluding congenital heart disease or postcapillary causes of pulmonary hypertension, such as mitral valve disease or left ventricular dysfunction, and may be useful in monitoring the response to therapy *(3)*. The echocardiographic findings of pulmonary hypertension include right heart chamber dilation, right ventricular hypertrophy, and paradoxical movement of the septum. Left ventricular filling may be impaired, with severe dilation of the right heart chambers. Doppler studies can estimate the pulmonary artery systolic pressure by measuring either systolic flow velocity across the pulmonic valve or the regurgitant flow across the tricuspid valve. Transesophageal echocardiography is more sensitive than transthoracic studies in evaluating intracardiac defects such as a patent foramen ovale.

Pulmonary function tests are essential to detect the presence of significant parenchymal or airway disease. Arterial blood gases frequently show a chronic respiratory alkalosis, perhaps due to increased activity of intrapulmonary stretch receptors or intravascular baroreceptors. An increased PCO_2 may be seen in individuals with underlying obstructive lung disease or obesity hypoventilation. Mild hypoxemia, when present in PAH, is frequently secondary to ventilation-perfusion mismatching; however, more severe hypoxia, when present, may be due to parenchymal lung disease, a decreased cardiac output, or intracardiac shunting through a patent foramen ovale. Formal cardiopulmonary exercise testing may be used to quantify disease severity and response to treat-

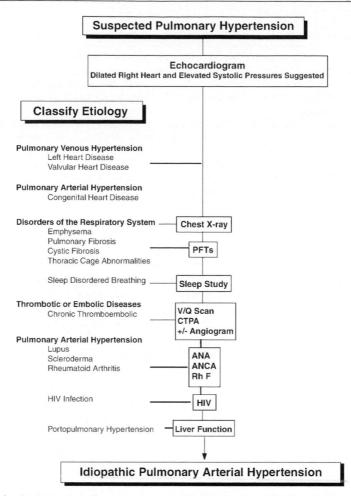

Fig. 1. Algorithm for the evaluation of suspected pulmonary hypertension. V/Q, ventilation perfusion; CTPA, CT pulmonary angiogram; ANA, antinuclear antibody; ANCA, antineutrophilic cytoplasmic antibody; RhF, rheumatoid factor; PFTs, pulmonary function tests.

ment. However, the 6-min walk test, a simpler and safer measure of exercise tolerance, has been demonstrated to correlate with both resting hemodynamics and survival in patients with PPH and is currently the most widely accepted noninvasive endpoint in pulmonary hypertension therapeutic trials *(4)*. Measurement of plasma B-type natriuretic peptide (BNP) has been demonstrated to correlate with disease severity and is gaining in popularity as a noninvasive method of following response to treatment *(5)*.

The ventilation-perfusion lung scan is essential to exclude chronic thromboembolic disease with pulmonary angiography indicated only when segmental or subsegmental perfusion defects are persistently present and suggestive of large-vessel, unresolved chronic thromboembolic disease *(6)*. CT pulmonary angiography is effective in ruling out acute pulmonary emboli but cannot replace the ventilation and perfusion (VQ) in ruling out chronic thromboembolic disease. The potential benefits of cardiac MRI are becoming apparent, especially in congenital heart disease, where measurements of both structure and function are possible noninvasively. Cardiac MRI will very likely become a standard part of the diagnostic algorithm within a few years. Polysomnography is recommended in patients with daytime hypersomnolence, as sleep apnea is associated with the development of pulmonary hypertension *(7,8)*. Lung biopsy is rarely necessary to make the diagnosis of pulmonary hypertension and is reserved for cases in which the clinical diagnosis is unclear.

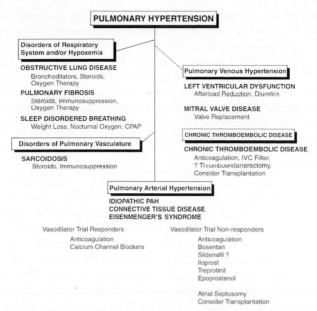

Fig. 2. Algorithm for the treatment of pulmonary hypertension.

Management

GENERAL APPROACH

The first step in the management of pulmonary hypertension is to identify and treat the underlying cause. Therefore, in pulmonary hypertension secondary to disorders of the respiratory system, improving gas exchange with bronchodilators and reversing hypoxia with oxygen therapy may significantly improve pulmonary hypertension. Similarly, patients with IPF may experience improvement in their pulmonary hypertension in response to oxygen, high-dose steroids, and immunosuppression. Individuals with disorders of ventilation, such as obstructive sleep apnea, may benefit from nocturnal chronic positive airway pressure (CPAP) (Fig. 2) *(8)*. Surgical intervention may be warranted in selected patients with chronic thromboembolic disease *(6)*.

In all patients with significant pulmonary hypertension general measures recommended include limiting physical activity to tolerance and avoidance of concomitant medications that can aggravate pulmonary hypertension, such as vasoactive decongestants, cardiodepressant antihypertensives such as β-adrenergic blockers, and agents that interfere with warfarin or potentiate the degree of anticoagulation. Environments with reduced oxygen levels, such unpressurized aircraft or high altitude, can worsen the condition, and individuals with borderline oxygenation may need supplemental oxygen. The hemodynamic stresses of pregnancy are poorly tolerated. Female patients with pulmonary hypertension should be counseled on effective contraception. Hormone replacement therapy appears to be without significant adverse effects in the postmenopausal population.

AN APPROACH TO VASODILATOR THERAPY

Smooth-muscle hypertrophy and vasoconstriction are present to varying degrees in pulmonary hypertension. However, while vasodilators may be beneficial in many types of intrinsic pulmonary vascular disease such as IPAH, they do not have a role in pulmonary hypertension secondary to parenchymal lung disease or disorders of left heart filling. Treatment with vasodilators in pulmonary hypertension can be unpredictable and hazardous, and great care must be exercised to decrease the risk of serious adverse events.

Patients with PAH should undergo a right heart catheterization and vasodilator trial before initiating empirical vasodilator therapy. Hemodynamic assessment at catheterization will determine the degree of pulmonary hypertension, exclude left heart filling problems, and allow prediction of survival. The completion of a vasodilator trial using short-acting agents such as inhaled nitric oxide, epoprostenol, or adenosine at the time of catheterization will also provide a guide to therapy. A decrease in mean pulmonary artery pressure of at least 10 mmHg and an increase or no change in cardiac output identifies patients with PAH who tend to have sustained hemodynamic improvement and prolonged survival or oral vasodilators (9). While approx 10% of patients with IPAH demonstrate an acute response to vasodilators, the number is even smaller in other causes of PAH such as scleroderma. Oral vasodilators are contraindicated in patients who have an adverse hemodynamic response such as drop in systemic pressure or drop in oxygen saturation with a decrease in cardiac output during the vasodilator trial (Fig. 3).

CALCIUM-CHANNEL BLOCKERS

Patients with PAH who have a favorable response to an acute vasodilator trial during right-heart catheterization demonstrate improved survival and regression of right ventricular hypertrophy with calcium-channel blockers. Indiscriminate use of calcium-channel blockers without first determining an individual's response during a vasodilator trial, however, may result in worsening gas exchange, depressed systolic function, and right heart failure, hypotension, or death. While calcium-channel blockers are initiated cautiously at low dose, the final dose attained in order to achieve benefit is generally higher than that used to treat systemic hypertension. The most commonly used agents are amblodipine (2.5–20 mg/d), nifedipine (30–240 mg/d), and diltiazem (120–900 mg/d). Abrupt discontinuation can lead to fatal rebound pulmonary hypertension. It is important that the response to calcium-channel blocker therapy is confirmed with a follow-up catheterization and alternative therapeutic options explored if the initial response has waned.

ENDOTHELIN ANTAGONISTS

The vasoconstrictor peptide, endothelin, is elevated in patients with pulmonary hypertension and the level correlates with patient outcome (10). Bosentan, an endothelin A and B receptor antagonist, was the first oral therapy approved for PAH and has been demonstrated to improve dyspnea, exercise tolerance, functional class, hemodynamics, and survival (11,12). Bosentan is contraindicated in pregnancy. There is a dose-related risk of hepatic injury, and monthly monitoring of liver function tests is recommended. Two new endothelin antagonists specific for endothelin-A receptors—sitaxsenstan and ambrisentan—are currently in development. Bosentan should be considered first-line therapy in patients with PAH who have Class III symptoms of PAH.

EPOPROSTENOL (PROSTACYCLIN, PGI$_2$, FLOLAN®)

Epoprostenol is a potent vasodilator that is delivered through a permanent indwelling catheter by a continuous infusion pump because of its short half-life (3–5 min). Individuals with severe PAH who do not demonstrate a favorable response to bosentan are considered for continuous intravenous epoprostenol. In a randomized trial, epoprostenol improved hemodynamics, exercise tolerance, and prolonged survival in severe IPAH (NYHA III–IV) (13). Epoprostenol has also been shown to have benefits in scleroderma and systemic lupus erythematosus (14,15). Furthermore, epoprostenol may be a bridge to transplant in patients with IPAH or it may also function to defer or avoid lung transplantation (16,17).

Minor side effects of epoprostenol include jaw pain, headache, rash, diarrhea, and joint pain. More serious side effects are related predominantly to the drug delivery system and include life-threatening line sepsis or discontinuation of drug delivery (18). Dose increments are frequently required during the first year of therapy. Epoprostenol should be avoided in postcapillary pulmonary hypertension because of the risk of acute pulmonary edema.

PROSTACYCLIN ANALOGS

Prostacyclin analogs can be given by alternative routes and thus eliminate catheter-related complications. Inhaled therapy with iloprost is widely available in Europe, but not yet studied in the United States. Iloprost is administered via an ultrasonic nebulizer every 3 h with demonstrated

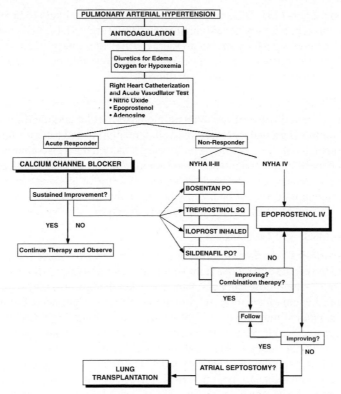

Fig. 3. Algorithm for the management of pulmonary arterial hypertension (PAH). NYHA, New York Heart Association.

benefits in symptoms and exercise tolerence *(19)*. Treprostinil, which is biologically active when delivered subcutaneously, is approved for patients with NYHA Class II–IV symptoms with PAH. Treprostinil, a more stable prostacyclin analog with a half-life of 3 to 4 h, also improves exercise capacity, dyspnea indices, and pulmonary hemodynamics in patients with IPAH, PAH associated with connective tissue disease, and congenital heart disease *(20)*. However, in addition to the side effects typical of all prostacyclin-based treatments (jaw pain, flushing, diarrhea), patients on treprostinil may have significant pain at the infusion site, which can limit its usefulness. Delivery of treprostinil via the inhaled route is currently under investigation.

SILDENAFIL

Sildenafil, a phosphodiesterase (type 5) inhibitor, may be an effective treatment for pulmonary hypertension. Numerous reports have demonstrated that sildenafil may improve pulmonary hemodynamics and 6-min walk distances in patients with IPAH and in patients with inoperable chronic thromboembolic disease *(21,22)*. Side effects of sildenafil include headache, visual disturbances, flushing, dyspepsia, and rhinitis. The results of a large multinational clinical trial of sildenafil in PAH are awaited.

CHRONIC OXYGEN THERAPY

Chronic oxygen therapy is indicated in patients with pulmonary hypertension who have documented hypoxemia, either at rest or with exercise. Patients with intrinsic vascular disease such as primary pulmonary hypertension usually do not have significant hypoxemia; when it is present it is usually as a result of right-to-left intracardiac shunting or reduced cardiac output. However, hypoxemia is frequently observed in parenchymal lung disease such as chronic obstructive pulmonary disease (COPD) and IPF. In these patients survival is improved when hypoxemia is corrected by chronic oxygen therapy *(23)*. The benefits of oxygen therapy are likely to be multifactorial, as the effects of oxygen on pulmonary hemodymamics in COPD are variable and improvements slow to develop *(24)*. Continuous positive airway pressure (CPAP) or biphasic positive airway pressure (BiPAP) are used to treat obstructive sleep apnea or chronic alveolar hypoventilation and the hypercarbia that can exacerbate the pulmonary hypertension.

ANTICOAGULATION

Local thrombus formation on dysfunctional pulmonary vascular endothelium and the development of venous thrombosis secondary to right heart failure, diminished cardiac output and impaired mobility are all potential risks in all forms of pulmonary hypertension. Two nonrandomized studies have suggested a benefit of anticoagulation in prolonging life in PPH *(9,25)*. Recommendations for anticoagulation have been extrapolated to include all forms of moderate to severe pulmonary hypertension. Particular care should be taken when initiating warfarin in patients with a history of hemoptysis or with right heart failure and liver dysfunction.

DIURETICS, INOTROPES, AND GLYCOSIDES

Diuretic therapy, with a loop diuretic alone or in combination with spironolactone, is frequently required to control the edema and reduce right ventricular end-diastolic volume in advancing right heart failure. Patients on high-dose calcium-channel blocker therapy also may require diuretic therapy for drug-induced edema formation. In patients with severe right heart failure, chronic low-dose ambulatory dopamine may improve right ventricular contractility and enhance diuresis. In parenchymal lung disease ankle edema may occur as a result of salt retention secondary to hypoxia or steroid use and may not indicate deterioration in right heart function.

Digoxin has been shown to be of benefit in patients with hypoxemic pulmonary hypertension when there is concomitant left heart dysfunction *(26)*. However, the role of digoxin in other forms of pulmonary hypertension is controversial. Digoxin may also have a role in counteracting the negative inotropic effect of calcium-channel blockers and in antagonizing the neurohumoral activation of right heart failure *(27,28)*.

SURGICAL THERAPY

The right ventricular dysfunction in pulmonary hypertension is reversible upon restoration of normal pulmonary artery pressures; therefore, double lung transplantation has become the treatment of choice for patients with pulmonary hypertension failing medical therapy, reserving heart-lung transplantation for patients with left heart disease or congenital structural abnormalities. Approximately 10% of lung transplants are performed for pulmonary hypertension *(29)*. Single-lung transplantation has also been successfully used as an alternative for patients with pulmonary hypertension. Patients with functional class IV disease or starting prostacyclin therapy should be considered for listing for transplantation given the prolonged waiting time for organs. Survival after transplantation is 40 to 45% at 3 yr *(17,29)*. Atrial septostomy, the controlled opening of a right-to-left shunt at the atrial level during right heart catheterization, is reserved for patients with severe right-sided heart failure or recurrent syncope. The procedure, by decompressing the right ventricle and improving cardiac output, may provide palliation and improved survival *(30)*. It is hoped that the impact of oxygen desaturation that results will be offset by the overall increase in cardiac output and systemic oxygen delivery.

Summary

Disorders of the pulmonary circulation that develop abruptly may result in acute right ventricular failure, while more chronically progressive disorders allow the right ventricle to adapt while pulmonary hypertension develops. However, inevitably if the afterload is not reduced—either with chronic oxygen therapy, pharmacologically with oral or intravenous vasodilators, or by surgical intervention with a thromboendarterectomy or lung transplantation—the right ventricle becomes increasingly dysfunctional, resulting in cor pulmonale and inevitably death from right heart failure.

While a significant number of the disorders affecting the pulmonary circulation are idiopathic, the majority can be prevented by either effective prophylaxis against venous thromboembolism or rigorous attention to smoking cessation. While the treatment modalities remain few, significant progress has occurred over the past decade and further advances can be expected over the next few years.

VENOUS THROMBOEMBOLISM

Venous thromboembolism (VTE) represents an extremely common syndrome that encompasses a spectrum from asymptomatic deep-vein thrombosis (DVT) to life-threatening pulmonary embolism (PE). The thromboembolic process may be seen as a continuum; in up to 50% of cases of proximal DVT there is evidence of radiological evidence of PE (even if the patient is asymptomatic) *(31)*. Similarly, 95% of pulmonary emboli originate in leg veins, though only in a minority of cases are there symptoms related to DVT *(32)*.

Though the exact incidence of VTE is uncertain, it is estimated that PE may account for up to 200,000 *(33,34)* deaths annually in the United States. Half of all cases occur in hospitalized patients or nursing home residents in whom the 3-mo mortality rate following a PE approaches 20%. When a fatal PE occurs, the majority of patients die within 1 h of presentation, predominantly as a consequence of underdiagnosis *(35,36)*. Conversely, survival approaches 90% when PE is identified early and adequate therapy instituted. Without treatment, the mortality rate rises to approximately 30%, mostly a result of recurrent embolism *(34)*.

Deep Venous Thrombosis

RISK FACTORS

Venous thrombosis develops in the setting of abnormal blood flow, vessel wall integrity, or blood constituents (Virchow's triad). A number of major and minor risk factors for the development of venous thrombosis have been identified (Table 3). It is estimated that "idiopathic" thromboembolism, or thrombosis in the absence of an identifiable risk factor, is associated with an underlying malignancy in more than 10% of patients with the majority of cases (75%) being diagnosed within 1 yr of presentation of the VTE *(37)*.

Advances in molecular biology have allowed an ever-increasing number of inherited and acquired abnormalities of clotting predisposing to thrombus formation to be identified (Table 4). At least one of these clinical entities may be identified in up to 25% of cases of venous thromboembolism; however, there is usually an additional predisposing factor present. The prevalence of the factor V Leiden mutation, which represents an inherited form of resistance to activated protein C, is estimated at 5% of Caucasians. The combination of this mutation and certain oral contraceptive therapies confers a 40-fold increased risk of thrombosis in some series *(38)*.

PREVENTION

Given the considerable morbidity and mortality associated with venous thromboembolism, every effort should be made to prevent its occurrence in at-risk patients. The widespread practice of *pharmaceutical prophylaxis* with low-molecular-weight (LMW) heparin among medical *(39)* and surgical *(40)* patients has led to a significant reduction in the incidence of both DVT and PE. However, it is now established that most cases of postoperative thromboembolism occur after discharge from the hospital, and several studies have demonstrated a benefit to extended prophylaxis (administered in the community setting) following major orthopedic surgery *(41)*.

Use of *mechanical methods* of prophylaxis such as graded compression stockings or pneumatic compression devices is also highly effective in lowering thrombosis risk, and combining one of these with a LMW heparin confers additional benefit. Where anticoagulation is contraindicated or ineffective, an inferior vena cava filter may be inserted to prevent propagation of lower extremity thrombus (Fig. 4). Filter placement may also be considered in cases of recurrent embolism despite adequate anticoagulation and chronic thromboembolic pulmonary hypertension. Unfortunately, these devices themselves predispose to thrombosis and are associated with higher readmission rates.

Table 3
Risk Factors Associated
With Venous Thromboembolism

Major risk factors
    Surgery (within previous 3 mo)
    Major trauma
    Malignancy
    Previous VTE
    Immobilization/stroke
    Pregnancy and puerperium
    Varicose veins
Minor risk factors
    Hormonal replacement
    Thrombophilia
    Long-haul travel
    Obesity
    Cigarette smoking
    Hypertension
    Age

Table 4
Inherited and Acquired
Thrombophilias

Factor V Leiden deficiency
Prothrombin gene variant 20210A
Antiphospholipid antibody
Hyperhomocysteimaemia
Protein C deficiency
Protein S deficiency
Antithrombin deficiency
Elevated Factor VIII, XI
Dysfibrinogenemia

In cases of temporarily increased risk of VTE, there are emerging data on the use of removable filters *(42)*.

DIAGNOSIS

Clinical assessment of suspected deep-vein thrombosis is notoriously unreliable; however, incorporation of assessment of clinical probability helps improve the diagnostic power of imaging techniques. *Compression ultrasonography* has become the investigation of choice for a first suspected DVT, as it is accurate and noninvasive. The presence of DVT is inferred by demonstration of a noncompressible segment of the common femoral vein, popliteal vein, or at the calf vein trifurcation; scanning of the calf veins is generally considered unnecessary. In equivocal cases, serial noninvasive evaluations may improve diagnostic yield, though *contrast venography* remains the gold standard (Fig. 5). There is emerging evidence on the role of novel scanning methods, including computed tomographic (CT) angiography of the leg veins (usually performed in the context of CT pulmonary angiography) and MRI venography. Used alone, MRI has an overall sensitivity of 95% and is particularly useful for the diagnosis of isolated calf, pelvic, and recurrent DVT *(43)*.

When venous thromboembolism occurs, activation of endogenous thrombolytic pathways results in production and release into the systemic circulation of degradation products of cross-linked fibrin, known as *D-dimers*. Virtually all cases of VTE are associated with a rise in D-dimers, though similar increases may occur in a variety of settings including cancer, trauma, surgery, inflammatory conditions, and advancing age. Hence, D-dimer measurement is of negative predictive value only. Some

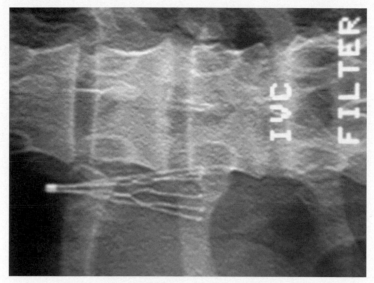

Fig. 4. IVC filter (image on side).

of the several commercially available assays have sensitivities approaching 100%, though there is considerable intertest variability. Furthermore, testing should not be considered a stand-alone screening device, but should be reserved for assessment of outpatients and performed only in those without strong clinical suspicion of thromboembolism. Conversely, where clinical likelihood is low and D-dimers are negative, further investigations are not required.

Pulmonary Embolism

CLINICAL FEATURES

The presenting features of PE vary depending on its extent and the degree of cardiorespiratory embarrassment caused (Table 5). Isolated subsegmental embolism may be asymptomatic, while larger proximal emboli may result in syncope secondary to circulatory compromise. While clinical assessment does not allow the diagnosis of PE to be made or eliminated confidently, it serves to identify patients in whom further investigation is required (Table 6). Dyspnea and pleuritic chest pain are the most frequently identified symptoms. Hemoptysis usually occurs in the context of pulmonary infarction. Tachypnea is almost universally present in PE, though tachycardia is present only 40% of the time and rarely exceeds 120 beats/min. A low-grade fever is not uncommon, and is frequently associated with pulmonary infarction. The finding of rales is present in over half of patients. Systemic arterial pressure may be misleading and can be normal even in the presence of massive PE; the presence of hypotension commonly portends a poor outcome. Identification of features of RV dysfunction is crucial in determining which patients are at high risk of adverse outcome. Evidence of elevated jugular venous pulse, prominence of the pulmonic component of the second heart sound and right ventricular added heart sounds, or the presence of a tricuspid regurgitant murmur are useful clinical markers of increased right heart pressure and strain.

PATHOPHYSIOLOGY

Respiratory Consequences. The degree of cardiopulmonary compromise following an acute pulmonary embolism correlates with the extent of occlusion and the degree of underlying cardiopulmonary disease. Almost every variety of abnormal gas exchange has been described in pulmonary embolism. Hypoxemia and hypocarbia occur most commonly mainly as a result of ventilation–perfusion mismatching. Portions of the lung remain ventilated though they no longer receive vascular supply and as a result other lung units experience perfusion out of proportion to the degree

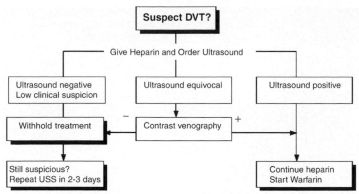

Fig. 5. Clinical investigation of DVT.

Table 5
Symptoms and Signs Associated With Pulmonary Embolism

Symptoms		Signs	
Symptom	Frequency (%)	Clinical finding	Frequency (%)
Dyspnea	73	Tachypnea	70
Pleuritic pain	66	Rales	51
Cough	37	Tachycardia	30
Leg wwelling	28	Fourth heart sound	24
Leg pain	26	Prominent P_2	23
Hemoptysis	13	Deep vein thrombosis	11
Palpitations	10	Diaphoresis	11
Wheezing	9	Fever	7
Angina-like pain	4	Wheeze	5

Adapted from ref. *63*.

of ventilation. Furthermore, areas distal to embolic obstruction develop atelectasis due to loss of surfactant as well as due to localized bronchoconstriction.

Impairment of right ventricular function may reduce cardiac output, promoting increased tissue oxygen extraction resulting in a decrease in mixed venous oxygen saturation and therefore worsening arterial hypoxemia. Furthermore, acute elevation of right-sided heart pressures may open a patent foramen ovale (PFO), leading to a right-to-left shunt. Inflammatory mediators such as serotonin are recognized as having a central role in changing vascular permeability and promoting shunting and atelectasis. Lung infarction occurs in approx 10%, most commonly in the relatively underperfused periphery of the lung.

Hemodynamic Consequences. The degree of obstruction that arises once a clot has become lodged in pulmonary artery branches largely determines the degree of hemodynamic compromise. Massive PE causing complete obstruction of the outflow to the right ventricle will cause acute right heart failure and death. Unless there is preexisting cardiorespiratory disease, the maximum mean pulmonary artery pressure capable of being generated by the nonadapted right heart is in the region of 40 mmHg. In general, only after more than 50% of the pulmonary vascular bed is occluded will pulmonary hypertension develop. The acutely dilated right heart may impede left ventricular filling due to septal flattening, resulting in a fall in cardiac output resulting in underperfusion of the right ventricle; systemic hypotension is thus a late and ominous sign in pulmonary embolism. Moreover, as the wall tension of the right ventricle increases, coronary perfusion pressure decreases, leading to RV ischemia and a further decrease in function.

Table 6
Scoring System for Clinical Assessment of Pulmonary Embolism

Clinical symptoms of DVT	3
Other diagnosis less likely than PE	3
Heart rate >100 bpm	1.5
Immobilization/surgery in previous 4 wk	1.5
Previous DVT or PE	1.5
Hemoptysis	1
Malignancy	1
Clinical Probability	Score
High	>6
Intermediate	2–6
Low	<2

Adapted from ref. *64.*

INVESTIGATIONS

The standard laboratory tests enhance the clinician's suspicion that an acute pulmonary embolism has indeed occurred. The predominant usefulness of electrocardiography (ECG) and chest radiography lies in identifying alternative diagnoses to PE, such as pneumonia, pneumothorax or acute myocardial infarction (AMI).

The *ECG* is abnormal in 90% of cases of PE, with tachycardia and nonspecific ST/T-wave changes the most common findings. Features of right ventricular strain may be seen, such as P-pulmonale, rightward axis deviation, and partial or complete right bundle branch block. The classic S_1, Q_3, T_3 pattern is distinctly uncommon.

With a reported sensitivity of 50%, *echocardiography* is usually unhelpful as a diagnostic modality although occasionally a clot may be identified in the main pulmonary artery or right ventricle. It also allows distinction of PE from other diagnostic considerations such as pericardial tamponade, aortic dissection, and myocardial infarction. Where echocardiography appears of most use is in allowing accurate and rapid risk assessment, defining the extent of cardiac dysfunction and by inference the extent of the clot and thus determining the appropriate level of therapeutic intervention. Findings of moderate or severe right ventricular compromise, pulmonary hypertension, or a patent foramen ovale predict those at risk of death or recurrent embolism and thereby prompt further intervention.

The *chest radiograph* may similarly be normal in acute PE. Cardiac enlargement is the most common abnormality identified *(44)*, while other nonspecific findings include focal atelectasis, pleural effusions, or localized infiltrates. The finding of decreased peripheral pulmonary vascularity due to central obstruction is termed *Westermark sign.*

Arterial blood gas analysis will typically demonstrate hypoxemia, often associated with a respiratory alkalosis due to hyperventilation. Unfortunately, it does not improve diagnostic accuracy in suspected PE as otherwise healthy young patients may maintain normoxia, while massive embolism may cause hypercarbia. Similarly, although a widened alveolar-arterial oxygen gradient is suggestive of the diagnosis, its absence cannot be used to exclude PE.

Data are accumulating on the sensitivities of several *D-dimer assays* for the diagnosis of PE. In patients with moderate clinical suspicion for PE presenting to the emergency department, negative values allow the diagnosis to be confidently excluded without the need for further studies. However, the negative predictive value of D-dimer falls as clinical suspicion for VTE increases, thereby limiting its usefulness as a screening tool.

Recently, novel *biomarkers* have been identified that reflect right ventricular strain and help stratify patients according to risk of adverse outcome. When significant PE occurs, B-type natriuretic peptide (BNP) is released from cardiac myocytes as a consequence of increase in right heart afterload; moreover, right ventricular microinfarction produces a rise in serum troponin. Although of limited diagnostic value, measurements of BNP and troponin provide useful prognostic information, and may in the future help influence treatment strategies.

The Prospective Investigation of Pulmonary Embolism Diagnosis (PIOPED) investigators (an international collaborative group that examined the role of lung scintigraphy in suspected PE) reported that only in a minority of cases does isotope *ventilation/perfusion lung scanning* allow a diagnosis of PE to be confidently made or excluded *(45)*. However, nuclear medicine still has an important role in the assessment of suspected PE provided the chest radiograph is normal and there is an absence of coexisting cardiorespiratory disease. A normal scan effectively rules out the diagnosis, while the presence of two or more filling defects, associated with a normal ventilation scan, represent a high probability of emboli. Scans should be reported according to standard criteria, and results interpreted only in the light of pretest clinical probability.

Increasingly however, helical *computed tomographic pulmonary angiography* (CTPA) is becoming the initial investigation of choice (Fig. 6A–C). It is quick, reliable, and may detect alternate or additional diagnoses to PE. Newer, thin-column multidetector row scanners have even greater than the 90% sensitivity and specificity rates associated with standard helical CT *(17,46)*. The main disadvantage of CTPA is its relative insensitivity in identifying clots in segmental or subsegmental pulmonary artery branches, which comprise some 20% of cases of PE. Even though a "negative" CTPA does not completely exclude the diagnosis, the clinical relevance of subsegmental PE is uncertain *(47)*.

Several studies have also reported excellent sensitivity and specificity rates for *magnetic resonance imaging* (MRI), which has the advantage over CTPA of less ionizing radiation. Use of real-time MR imaging further improves diagnostic accuracy, though the precise role of this imaging modality with regard to subsegmental pulmonary embolism remains to be clarified. Where doubt remains, pulmonary angiography remains the gold standard tool in identifying PE (Fig. 7).

INTEGRATION OF DIAGNOSTIC STRATEGIES

Rarely are physical assessment, laboratory data, or radiological techniques by themselves sufficiently sensitive to confirm or rule out the presence of thromboembolic disease. Consequently, algorithms incorporating multimodality testing have become standard. However, to reduce the necessity for invasive procedures, it is essential to incorporate the *clinical likelihood* of PE into diagnostic strategies. The likelihood is estimated on the basis of consistent symptoms, the identification of known risk factors for thromboembolism, and consideration of an alternative diagnosis. This allows patients to be stratified as high, intermediate, or low probability, prior to interpreting the findings of any investigations performed (Table 6). Alternatively, clinical prediction models may be employed to provide scores that estimate the pretest probability of VTE. The importance of this approach is underscored by the finding of the PIOPED group of investigators that where lung scintigraphy is reported as low likelihood for PE, a high clinical probability is nevertheless associated with angiographic evidence of embolism in 40% of cases.

In considering venous thromboembolism as a continuum, use of *lower-limb studies* to detect DVT where lung scintigraphy is equivocal or at odds with the clinical picture allows a further reduction in the numbers requiring formal angiography. Indeed, where a high clinical suspicion of PE exists and a diagnosis of DVT is made, further testing to pursue the diagnosis of PE are unnecessary (Fig. 8). Likewise, several management studies have demonstrated that anticoagulation may be safely withheld if (1) pulmonary angiogram or perfusion lung scanning is normal; (2) serial venous doppler examinations are negative where perfusion scanning is nondiagnostic or CTPA is nondiagnostic or negative; and (3) D-dimer levels are normal in combination with a low clinical probability for PE in the outpatient setting.

TREATMENT

The initial management of suspected PE is supportive, with supplementary oxygen, fluid hydration, or plasma expanders to preserve adequate right ventricular preload and analgesia where appropriate. Opiates such as morphine should be used with caution, given their propensity to cause

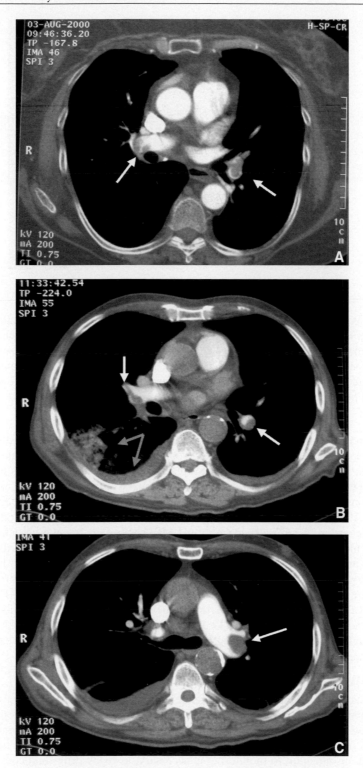

Fig. 6. (A) CT pulmonary angiogram with bilateral clot. **(B)** CT pulmonary angiogram with clot. Right base pleural effusion and wedge-shaped infiltrate (gray arrows). **(C)** CT pulmonary angiogram within left main pulmonary artery clot. Pleural effusion right base.

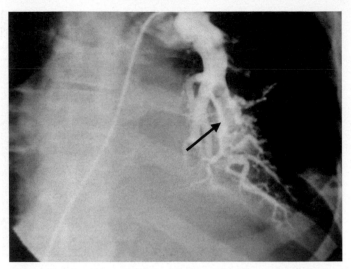

Fig. 7. Pulmonary angiogram with clot visible in left lower lobe.

hypotension. When inotropic support is required to maintain adequate systemic arterial blood pressure, norepinephrine appears to be the most effective agent. Since extensive occlusion of the pulmonary arterial tree may result in diminished blood flow, pulmonary arterial pressure may remain deceptively normal even when massive embolism has occurred. Hence, estimation of central venous pressure (CVP) or right atrial pressure (as a surrogate of right ventricular function) provides a more useful hemodynamic index to follow.

HEPARIN

If acute venous thromboembolism is suspected, treatment with heparin is begun while investigations proceed. Because of their safety, ease of administration, and predictable dose-response characteristics, LMW heparins have all but replaced unfractionated heparin as the mainstay of treatment in acute VTE. Administered subcutaneously once or twice daily, they exhibit predictable dose-response characteristics so that routine monitoring of activity is not required. This facilitates the initial treatment of selected stable patients with both DVT and PE in the outpatient setting at considerable cost saving (48,49). In addition, LMW heparin treatment is associated with fewer episodes of hemorrhage or recurrence of thromboembolism in comparison to intravenous heparin in some meta-analyses (50,51); the principal advantage of the latter is its short half-life, which allows rapid reversal of its effects if necessary. When standard heparin therapy is required, dosing adjustments are made according to the activated partial thromboplastin time (APTT). Measurement of anti-Xa levels allows precise determination of LMW heparin activity; this may be necessary in pregnancy and in the very obese. Usual practice is to continue heparin or LMW heparin for 5 to 7 d, although in instances of massive PE or extensive iliofemoral DVT, some experts advocate a more prolonged duration of initial therapy.

ORAL ANTICOAGULANTS

In most instances, oral anticoagulation can be started together with heparin or LMW heparin. Warfarin, which acts by inhibition of vitamin K-dependent clotting factors, is the mainstay of chronic therapy in VTE; the risk of recurrence is reduced by approx 90%. The dosing of warfarin is titrated to a therapeutic International Normalized Ratio, with a target of 2.5 and a range of 2.0 to 3.0. Meticulous attention to monitoring is necessary, as many drugs and coexisting medical conditions influence warfarin metabolism. Warfarin has teratogenic side effects and is therefore contraindicated in pregnancy. The optimal duration of oral anticoagulation therapy remains a matter of debate. Where a transient risk factor is identified (e.g., surgery), 3 mo of therapy is generally

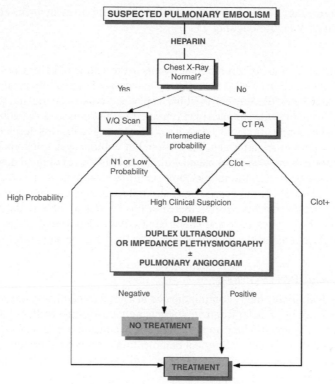

Fig. 8. Investigations for suspected pulmonary embolism.

recommended although there is evidence to support stopping therapy after 6 wk, given the extremely low recurrence rate in this cohort *(52)*. Conversely, several studies have demonstrated that discontinuation of warfarin after 6 mo for idiopathic VTE is associated with an absolute recurrence risk of 5 to 10% in the subsequent 12 mo *(53)*. The emerging consensus is that indefinite anticoagulation is probably appropriate for this group of patients and in patients with proven recurrent thromboembolism, although this strategy is hampered by an increase in serious bleeding episodes. Conversely, it is probably safe to withhold anticoagulation in those with isolated calf DVT, provided that repeated scanning does not demonstrate proximal clot extension. Nonetheless, this approach remains somewhat contentious, as repeated scanning is cumbersome and labor-intensive, and accordingly many programs will automatically treat for at least 6 wk empirically.

NOVEL ANTICOAGULANTS

There are emerging data on the use of novel anticoagulant therapies directed toward specific points on the coagulation cascade. Fondaparinux, a pentasaccharide with specific action against factor Xa, represents the first of a novel class of drug. Its extended half-life allows once-daily subcutaneous dosing, and this agent is less likely than either unfractionated or LMW heparin to be associated with thrombocytopenia. Fondaparinux has been granted FDA approval for DVT prophylaxis in patients undergoing hip or knee surgery, with superior efficacy to LMW heparin *(54)*. Studies have confirmed it to be at least as effective and safe as standard heparin for initial treatment of DVT and hemodynamically stable PE *(55)*.

The efficacy and safety of ximelagatran, a direct thrombin inhibitor, have been confirmed in phase III studies for prevention of thromboembolism in the context of orthopedic surgery *(32)*. Ximelagatran is orally active as a fixed twice-daily dose and represents an attractive alternative to warfarin, as routine monitoring is not required. Larger studies to evaluate its efficacy in prevention and treatment of VTE are ongoing.

THROMBOLYSIS

Although the criteria for use of thrombolytic agents in the setting of PE are less well studied than in acute myocardial infarction (AMI), their efficacy in massive PE resulting in hemodynamic instability has been established *(56)*. A recently published placebo-controlled trial has reported improved outcomes in the setting of acute submassive PE treated with alteplase (a recombinant tissue plasminogen activator) in conjunction with heparin *(57)*. Submassive PE was defined as right ventricular dysfunction or pulmonary arterial hypertension, but without systemic hypotension or shock. In this study, alteplase therapy was associated with fewer episodes of clinical deterioration requiring emergency intervention (e.g., thrombolectomy, inotrope requirement), albeit evidence for a survival advantage was lacking. Thrombolytics may also reduce incidence of postthrombotic syndrome in massive iliofemoral thrombosis. Overall there is a 1 to 3% risk of intracranial hemorrhage associated with thrombolysis. Urokinase and streptokinase have also been evaluated as treatment of VTE, though alteplase remains the only drug approved by the Food and Drug Administration for this indication.

NONPHARMACOLOGIC INTERVENTIONS

When thrombolysis is absolutely contraindicated in a hemodynamically unstable patient, physical disruption of a clot by catheter fragmentation using jets of saline and/or clot aspiration under fluoroscopy may be attempted. These approaches require considerable expertise, have substantial mortality, and are seldom available. Surgical embolectomy offers an alternative approach in centers with sufficient expertise. With careful patient selection this can be a life-saving procedure with excellent survival rates.

REFERENCES

1. Rich S. Executive summary of the World Symposium on PPH. Available at www.who.int/ncd/cvd/pph.html. Accessed Dec. 2003.
2. Rich S, et al. Antinuclear antibodies in primary pulmonary hypertension. J Am Coll Cardiol 1986;8:1307–1311.
3. Hinderliter AL, et al. Effects of long-term infusion of prostacyclin (epoprostenol) on echocardiographic measures of right ventricular structure and function in primary pulmonary hypertension. Primary Pulmonary Hypertension Study Group. Circulation 1997;95:1479–1486.
4. Miyamoto S, et al. Clinical correlates and prognostic significance of six-minute walk test in patients with primary pulmonary hypertension comparison with cardiopulmonary exercise testing. Am J Respir Crit Care Med 2000;161: 487–492.
5. Nagaya N, et al. Plasma brain natriuretic peptide as a prognostic indicator in patients with primary pulmonary hypertension. Circulation 2000;102:865–870.
6. Fedullo P, et al. Chronic thromboembolic pulmonary hypertension. N Engl J Med 2001;345:1465–1472.
7. Weitzenblum E, et al. Daytime pulmonary hypertension in patients with obstructive sleep apnea syndrome. Am Rev Respir Dis 1988;138:345–349.
8. Kessler R, et al. Pulmonary hypertension in the obstructive sleep apnea syndrome: prevalence, causes and therapeutic consequences. Eur Respir J 1996;9:787–794.
9. Rich S, Kaufmann E, Levy PS. The effect of high doses of calcium-channel blockers on survival in primary pulmonary hypertension. N Engl J Med 1992;327:76–81.
10. Rubens C, et al. Big endothelin-1 and endothelin-1 plasma levels are correlated with the severity of primary pulmonary hypertension. Chest 2001;120:1562–1569.
11. Channick R, et al. Effects of the dual endothelin receptor antagonist bosentan in patients with pulmonary hypertension: a placebo-controlled study. J Heart Lung Transplant 2001;20:262–263.
12. Rubin L, et al. Bosentan therapy for pulmonary arterial hypertension. N Engl J Med 2002;346:896–903.
13. Barst RJ, et al. A comparison of continuous intravenous epoprostenol (prostacyclin) with conventional therapy for primary pulmonary hypertension. The Primary Pulmonary Hypertension Study Group. N Engl J Med 1996;334: 296–302.
14. Badesch D, et al. A comparison of continuous intravenous epoprostenol with conventional therapy for pulmonary hypertension secondary to the scleroderma spectrum of diseases. Ann Intern Med 2000;132:425–434.
15. Robbins I, et al. Epoprostenol for treatment of pulmonary hypertension in patients with systemic lupus erythematosus. Chest 2000;117:14–18.

16. McLaughlin V, Shillington A, Rich S. Survival in primary pulmonary hypertension: the impact of epoprostenol therapy. Circulation 2002;106:1477–1482.
17. Conte JV, et al. Continuous intravenous prostacyclin as a bridge to lung transplantation. J Heart Lung Transplant 1998;17:679–685.
18. Gaine S. Pulmonary hypertension. JAMA 2000;284:3160–3168.
19. Olschewski H, et al. Aerosolized prostacyclin and iloprost in severe pulmonary hypertension. Ann Intern Med 1996; 124:820–824.
20. Simonneau G, et al. Continuous subcutaneous infusion of treprostinil, a prostacyclin analogue, in patients with pulmonary arterial hypertension: a double-blind, randomized, placebo-controlled trial. Am J Respir Crit Care Med 2002;165:800–804.
21. Ghofrani H, et al. Sildenafil for long-term treatment of nonoperable chronic thromboembolic pulmonary hypertension. Am J Respir Crit Care Med 2003;167:1139–1141.
22. Stiebellehner L, et al. Long-term treatment with oral sildenafil in addition to continuous IV epoprostenol in patients with pulmonary arterial hypertension. Chest 2003;123:1293–1295.
23. Nocturnal Oxygen Therapy Group. Continuous or nocturnal oxygen therapy in hypoxemic chronic obstructive lung disease. Ann Intern Med 1980;93:391–398.
24. Timms R, Khaja F, Williams GEA. Hemodynamic response to oxygen therapy in chronic obstructive pulmonary disease. Ann Intern Med 1985;102:29–36.
25. Fuster V, et al. Primary pulmonary hypertension: natural history and the importance of thrombosis. Circulation 1984; 70:580–587.
26. Mathur P, et al. Effect of digoxin on right ventricular function in severe chronic airflow obstruction. Ann Intern Med 1981;95:283–288.
27. Nootens M, et al. Neurohumoral activation in patients with right ventricular failure from pulmonary hypertension: relation to hemodynamics and endothelin levels. J Am Coll Cardiol 1995;26:1581–1585.
28. Rich S, et al. The short-term effects of digoxin in patients with right ventricular dysfunction from pulmonary hypertension. Chest 1998;114:787–792.
29. Charman S, et al. Assessment of survival benefit after lung transplantation by patient diagnosis. J Heart Lung Transplant 2002;21:226–232.
30. Sandoval J, et al. Graded balloon dilation atrial septostomy in severe primary pulmonary hypertension. A therapeutic alternative for patients nonresponsive to vasodilator treatment. J Am Coll Cardiol 1998;32:297–304.
31. Huisman M, et al. Unexpected high prevalence of silent pulmonary embolism in patients with deep venous thrombosis. Chest 1989;95:498–502.
32. Francis C, Berkowitz SD, Comp PC, et al. Comparison of ximelagatran with warfarin for the prevention of venous thromboembolism after total knee replacement. N Engl J Med 2003;349:1703–1712.
33. Horlander K, Mannino D, Leeper K. Pulmonary embolism mortality in the United States, 1979–1998: an analysis using multiple-cause mortality data. Arch Intern Med 2003;163:1711–1717.
34. Dalen J, Alpert J. Natural history of pulmonary embolism. Prog Cardiovasc Dis 1975;17:259–270.
35. Stein P, Henry J. Prevalence of acute pulmonary embolism among patients in a general hospital and at autopsy. Chest 1995;108:978–981.
36. Wood K. Major pulmonary embolism: review of a pathophysiologic approach to the golden hour of hemodynamically significant pulmonary embolism. Chest 2002;121:877–905.
37. Lee A, Levine M. Venous thromboembolism and cancer: risks and outcomes. Circulation 2003;107:Suppl 1:I17–I21.
38. Bloemenkamp K, et al. Enhancement by factor V Leiden mutation of risk of deep-vein thrombosis associated with oral contraceptives containing a third-generation progestagen. Lancet 1995;346:1593–1596.
39. Samama M, et al. A comparison of enoxaparin with placebo for the prevention of venous thromboembolism in acutely ill medical patients: Prophylaxis In Medical Patients with Enoxaparin Study Group. N Engl J Med 1999; 341:793–800.
40. Imperiale T, Speroff T. A meta-analysis of methods to prevent VTE following total hip replacement. JAMA 1994; 271:1780–1785.
41. Eikelboom J, Quinlan D, Douketis J. Extended-duration prophylaxis against venous thromboembolism after total hip or knee replacement: a meta-analysis of the randomised trials. Lancet 2001;358:9–15.
42. Offner P, et al. The role of temporary inferior vena cava filters in critically ill surgical patients. Arch Surg 2003;138: 591–594.
43. Fraser D, et al. Diagnosis of lower-limb deep venous thrombosis: a prospective blinded study of magnetic resonance direct thrombus imaging. Ann Intern Med 2002;136:89–98.
44. Elliott C, et al. Chest radiographs in acute pulmonary embolism results from the international cooperative pulmonary embolism registry. Chest 2000;118:33–38.
45. PIOPED. Prospective Investigation of Pulmonary Embolism Diagnosis. Value of the ventilation/perfusion scan in acute pulmonary embolism: results of the Prospective Investigation of Pulmonary Embolism Diagnosis (PIOPED). JAMA 1990;263:2753–2759.
46. Rathbun S, Raskob G, Whitsett T. Sensitivity and specificity of helical computed tomography in the diagnosis of pulmonary embolism: a systematic review. Ann Intern Med 2000;132:227–232.
47. Musset D, et al. Diagnostic strategy for patients with suspected pulmonary embolism: a prospective multicentre outcome study. Lancet 2002;360:1914–1920.

48. Segal J, et al. Outpatient therapy with low molecular weight heparin for the treatment of venous thromboembolism: a review of efficacy, safety, and costs. Am J Med Sci 2003;115:298–308.

49. Spyropoulos A, et al. Management of acute proximal deep vein thrombosis: pharmacoeconomic evaluation of outpatient treatment with enoxaparin vs inpatient treatment with unfractionated heparin. Chest 2002;122:108–114.

50. Gould M, et al. Low-molecular-weight heparins compared with unfractionated heparin for treatment of acute deep venous thrombosis. A meta-analysis of randomized, controlled trials. Ann Intern Med 1999;130:800–809.

51. Mismetti P, et al. Prevention of venous thromboembolism in internal medicine with unfractionated or low-molecular-weight heparins: a meta-analysis of randomised clinical trials. Thromb Haemost 2000;83:14–19.

52. Schulman S, et al. A comparison of six weeks with six months of oral anticoagulant therapy after a first episode of venous thromboembolism. Duration of Anticoagulation Trial Study Group. N Engl J Med 1995;332:1661–1665.

53. van Dongen C, et al. The incidence of recurrent venous thromboembolism after treatment with vitamin K antagonists in relation to time since first event: a meta-analysis. Arch Intern Med 2003;163:1285–1293.

54. Bauer K, Eriksson BI, Lassen MR, et al. Fondaparinux compared with enoxaparin for the prevention of venous thromboembolism after elective major knee surgery. N Engl J Med 2001;345;1305–1310.

55. Buller H, et al. Subcutaneous fondaparinux versus intravenous unfractionated heparin in the initial treatment of pulmonary embolism. N Engl J Med 2003;349:1695–1702.

56. Dalen J, Alpert J. Thrombolytic therapy for pulmonary embolism: is it effective? is it safe? when is it indicated? Arch Intern Med 1997;157:2550–2556.

57. Konstantinides S, et al. Heparin plus alteplase compared with heparin alone in patients with submassive pulmonary. N Engl J Med 2002;347:1143–1150.

58. D'Alonzo G, Bower J. The mechanism of abnormal gas exchange in acute massive pulmonary embolism. Am Rev Respir Dis 1983;128:170–172.

59. D'Alonzo G, et al. Survival in patients with primary pulmonary hypertension. Results from a national prospective registry. Ann Intern Med 1991;115:343–349.

60. Gaine S, Rubin L. Primary pulmonary hypertension. Lancet 1998;352:9124.

61. Hyers T. Venous thromboembolism: state of the art. Am J Respir Crit Care Med 1999;159:1–14.

62. Simonneau G, Galie N, Rubin LJ, et al. Clinical classification of pulmonary hypertension. J Am Coll Cardiol 2004; 43(12 Suppl S):5S–12S.

63. Stein PD, Terrin ML, Hales CA, et al. Clinical, laboratory, roentgenographic, and electrocardiographic findings in patients with acute pulmonary embolism and no pre-existing cardiac or pulmonary disease. Chest 1991;100: 598–603.

64. Wells PS, Anderson DR, Bormanis J, et al. Value of assessment of pretest probability of deep-vein thrombosis in clinical management. Lancet 1997;350:1795–1798.

RECOMMENDED READING

Rubin LJ, Rich S, eds. Primary Pulmonary Hypertension. Lung Biology in Health and Disease vol 99. Marcel Dekker, New York, 1997.

D'Alonzo G, Bower J, et al. The mechanism of abnormal gas exchange in acute massive pulmonary embolism. Am Rev Respir Dis 1983;128:170–172.

Dalen J, Alpert J. Natural history of pulmonary embolism. Prog Cardiovasc Dis 1975;17:259–270.

Fedullo P, et al. Chronic thromboembolic pulmonary hypertension. N Engl J Med 2001;345:1465–1472.

37 Diseases of the Aorta

Eric M. Isselbacher, MD

INTRODUCTION

The largest artery in the body, the aorta receives blood pumps from the left ventricle and distributes it distally to the branch arteries. While it is one continuous vessel, its segments have been distinguished anatomically. The aorta begins in the anterior mediastinum above the aortic valve as the ascending aorta, the most proximal portion of which is also called the aortic root. This is followed in the superior mediastinum by the aortic arch, which gives rise to the brachiocephalic arteries. The descending thoracic aorta then courses in the posterior mediastinum to the level of the diaphragm, after which it becomes the abdominal aorta that then bifurcates distally into the common iliac arteries.

AORTIC ANEURYSMS

Aortic aneurysms, defined as pathologic dilatation of the aorta, are one of the most commonly encountered aortic diseases. Aneurysms may involve any part of the aorta, but occur much more commonly in the abdominal than in the thoracic aorta. Abdominal aortic aneurysms have a prevalence of at least 3% in a population greater than 50 yr old *(1)*—although the exact prevalence varies with the age and risk of the population studied—and are five to 10 times more common in men than in women. The infrarenal aorta is the segment most often involved. Among thoracic aortic aneurysms, aneurysms of the ascending aorta are most common. When aneurysms involve the descending thoracic aortic aorta, they often extend distally and involve the abdominal aorta as well, producing a *thoracoabdominal* aortic aneurysm.

Etiology

Atherosclerosis has long been recognized as a major underlying cause of abdominal aortic aneurysms. While the mechanism by which atherosclerosis promotes the growth of aneurysms is uncertain, it appears that the atherosclerotic thickening of the aortic intima reduces diffusion of oxygen and nutrients from the aortic lumen to the media, in turn causing degeneration of the elastic elements of the media and a weakening of the aortic wall *(2)*. More recent research suggests that inflammation within the aortic wall may lead to degradation of the extracellular matrix, and thus also contribute to the development of abdominal aortic aneurysms *(3)*. Once the aorta begins to dilate, tension on the wall increases, thereby promoting further expansion of the aneurysm. There also appears to be a genetic predisposition to the development of abdominal aortic aneurysms, as 13 to 32% of first-degree relatives of those with abdominal aneurysms may be affected, compared with the 2 to 5% risk in the general population.

Atherosclerosis is also a common cause of aneurysms of the descending thoracic aorta. However, the most important etiology of ascending thoracic aortic aneurysms is a process known as *cystic medial necrosis* or *degeneration*, which appears histologically as smooth muscle cell necrosis and degeneration of elastic layers within the media. Cystic medial necrosis is found in almost all patients with Marfan's syndrome, placing this group at very high risk for aortic aneurysm formation at a

From: *Essential Cardiology: Principles and Practice, 2nd Ed.*
Edited by: C. Rosendorff © Humana Press Inc., Totowa, NJ

relatively young age. Among patients without overt evidence of connective tissue disease, ascending thoracic aortic aneurysms occur commonly among those with an underlying bicuspid aortic valve, and also among those with a family history of similar aneurysms (i.e., familial thoracic aortic aneurysm syndrome). In addition, a history of long-standing hypertension is a common risk factor. Syphilis was once a common cause of thoracic aortic aneurysms, but is now a rarity. Less common causes of thoracic aortic aneurysms include great-vessel arteritis (aortitis), aortic trauma, and aortic dissection. Often thoracic aortic aneurysms are idiopathic.

Clinical Manifestations

The large majority of patients with abdominal and thoracic aortic aneurysms are asymptomatic and the aneurysms are discovered incidentally on a routine physical exam or imaging study. When patients with abdominal aortic aneurysms do experience symptoms, the most frequent complaint is of pain in the hypogastrium or lower back. The pain typically has a steady gnawing quality and may last for hours or days. New or worsening pain may herald aneurysm expansion or impending rupture. Rupture of an abdominal aneurysm is often accompanied by the triad of pain, hypotension, and the presence of a pulsatile abdominal mass. Those with thoracic aortic aneurysms may experience chest or back pain from aneurysm expansion or compression of adjacent structures. Aneurysms of the ascending aorta often will produce aortic insufficiency (due to dilatation of the aortic root), so patients may present with congestive heart failure or a diastolic murmur.

Diagnosis

Abdominal aortic aneurysms may be palpable on physical examination, although even large aneurysms are sometimes obscured by body habitus (4). Typically abdominal aortic aneurysms are hard to size accurately by physical examination alone, as adjacent structures often make an aneurysm feel larger than it actually is. Thoracic aortic aneurysms, on the other hand, cannot be palpated at all on physical examination.

The definitive diagnosis of an aortic aneurysm is made by radiologic examination. Abdominal aortic aneurysms can be detected and sized by either abdominal ultrasonography or computed tomography (CT). Ultrasound is extremely sensitive and is the most practical method to use in screening for abdominal aortic aneurysms. While mass screening of the population has not yet become widely accepted, screening with ultrasound is generally recommended for patients considered to be at risk for aortic aneurysms (5). CT is even more accurate and can size aneurysms to within a diameter of ± 2 mm, and is therefore the preferred modality for following aneurysm growth over time (Fig. 1).

Thoracic aortic aneurysms are frequently recognized on chest radiographs, often producing widening of the mediastinal silhouette, enlargement of the aortic knob, or displacement of the trachea from midline. CT is an excellent modality for detecting and sizing thoracic aneurysms and for following growth over time. Transthoracic echocardiography, which generally visualizes the aortic root and ascending aorta well, is useful for screening patients with Marfan's syndrome because they are at particular risk for aneurysms in this location.

Prognosis

Most aneurysms expand over time, and the rate of growth tends to increase with increasing aneurysm size. The major risk associated with an aortic aneurysm in any location is that of rupture. The risk of rupture rises with increasing aneurysm size because—in accordance with Laplace's law (which states that wall tension is proportional to the product of pressure and radius)—as the diameter of the aorta increases its wall tension rises. Abdominal aortic aneurysms of less than 4.0 cm in size have only a 0.3% annual risk of rupture, those 4.0 to 4.9 cm have a 1.5% annual risk of rupture, and those 5.0 to 5.9 cm have a 6.5% annual risk of rupture (6). For aneurysms 6.0 cm or greater the risk of rupture rises sharply, although an exact risk cannot be estimated. The overall mortality from rupture of an abdominal aortic aneurysm is 80%, with a mortality of 50% even for those who

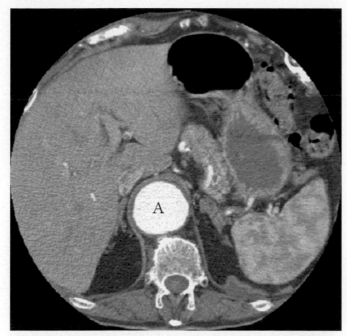

Fig. 1. A contrast-enhanced CT scan of the abdomen showing a 5.1 × 5.6 cm suprarenal abdominal aortic aneurysm (A).

reach the hospital. Thoracic aneurysms of less than 5.0 cm in size typically expand slowly and rarely rupture, but the rate of growth and risk of rupture increase significantly when the aneurysms are 6.0 cm or larger. Rupture of thoracic aneurysms carries an early mortality of 76% at 24 h *(7)*.

Treatment

Patients whose aneurysms are not at significant risk of rupture should be managed medically. The goal of medical therapy is to reduce the rate of aneurysm expansion and risk of future rupture. The use of β-blockers is the mainstay of this approach, but additional antihypertensive agents are often required. Both thoracic and abdominal aortic aneurysms should be followed closely with serial imaging studies (such as CT) to detect progressive enlargement over time that may indicate the need for surgical repair.

Size is the major indicator for repair of aortic aneurysms. Abdominal aortic aneurysms larger than 5.0 to 5.5 cm should be repaired in good operative candidates, and aneurysms greater than 4.0 cm is size should be monitored every 6 to 12 mo. Patients with ascending thoracic aortic aneurysms of greater than 5.5 cm in size should undergo surgical repair, while those with Marfan's syndrome should have repair when the aneurysm is ≥5.0 cm in size. Aneurysms of the descending thoracic aorta should be repaired when they are ≥6.0 cm in size.

Surgical repair consists of resection of the aneurysmal portion of the aorta and insertion of a synthetic prosthetic tube graft. When aneurysms involve aortic segments with branch arteries, such branches may need to be reimplanted into the graft. Similarly, when a dilated aortic root must be replaced in the repair of an ascending thoracic aortic aneurysm, the coronary arteries must be reimplanted.

A less-invasive alternative approach for repair of many abdominal and some descending thoracic aortic aneurysms is the placement of an expandable endovascular stent-graft inside the aneurysm via a percutaneous catheter-based approach. The device consists of a collapsible prosthetic tube graft that is inserted remotely (e.g., via the femoral artery), advanced transluminally across

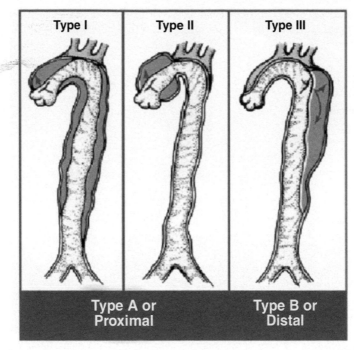

Fig. 2. Classification systems for aortic dissection. (From ref. *18*. Copyright 1998; with permission from Elsevier.)

the aneurysm under fluoroscopic guidance, and then secured at both its proximal and distal ends with an expandable stent attachment system. Once deployed the stent-graft serves to bridge the region of the aneurysm, thereby excluding it from the circulation while allowing aortic blood flow to continue distally through the prosthetic stent-graft lumen. However, only 30 to 60% of patients with abdominal aortic aneurysms—and fewer with descending thoracic aortic aneurysms—have aneurysm anatomy suitable for endovascular repair. The success rate of stent-graft implantation has been high, but in some instances patients are left with *endoleaks,* which means there is some residual blood flow into the aneurysm sac because of failure to completely exclude the aneurysm from the aortic circulation. Moreover, the long-term outcomes of endovascular repair versus conventional surgical repair are not yet known. Therefore, at present the use of stent-grafts for endovascular repair of abdominal aortic aneurysms has generally been limited to a subset of patients, typically older patients or those at high operative risk.

AORTIC DISSECTION

While far less common than aortic aneurysms, aortic dissection is a life-threatening condition with an early mortality as high as 1 to 2% per hour. However, with prompt early diagnosis and treatment, survival can be dramatically improved. The process of aortic dissection begins with a tear in the aortic intima that exposes a diseased medial layer to the systemic pressure of blood within the aortic lumen. The systolic force of aortic blood flow may cleave the media longitudinally into two layers, producing a blood-filled false lumen within the aortic wall that propagates distally (or sometimes retrograde) for a variable distance. The result is the presence of both a true and a false lumen separated by an intimal flap.

Aortic dissections are classified according to location, based on one of several systems as depicted in Fig. 2. Two thirds of aortic dissections are type A and the remainder are type B. The classification schemes are intended to distinguish those dissections that involve the ascending aorta from those that do not. Involvement of the ascending aorta carries a high risk of early aortic rupture and death from cardiac tamponade, while those not involving the ascending aorta carry a much lower risk. Therefore prognosis and management differ according to the extent of aortic involvement.

Etiology

Disease of the aortic media, with degeneration of the medial collagen and elastin, is the most common predisposing factor for aortic dissection. Patients with Marfan's syndrome have classic cystic medial degeneration and are at particularly high risk of aortic dissection at a relatively young age. The peak incidence of aortic dissection in patients without Marfan's syndrome is in the sixth and seventh decades of life, with men affected twice as often as women *(8)*. A history of hypertension is present in the large majority of cases. A bicuspid aortic valve is a less common risk factor. Iatrogenic trauma from catheterization procedures or cardiac surgery may also cause aortic dissection.

Clinical Manifestations

The most common presenting symptom of aortic dissection is severe pain, occurring in 80% of cases *(8)*. The pain is typically retrosternal or interscapular, but it may also appear in the neck or throat, in the lower back, in the abdomen, or in the lower extremities, depending on the location of the aortic dissection. In fact, the pain may migrate as the dissection propagates distally. The pain is often of abrupt onset and at its most severe at the start. It is most often described as "sharp" or "stabbing," or alternatively as "tearing" or "ripping," in quality *(8)*. On the other hand, the description of the pain is sometimes relatively nonspecific. Less typical presentations include congestive heart failure (due to acute aortic insufficiency), syncope, stroke, or mesenteric ischemia.

Hypertension on presentation is a common finding, especially among most of those with type B aortic dissection. Hypotension may also occur, particularly among those with type A dissections, and suggests the presence of rupture into the pericardium (causing cardiac tamponade) or the presence of severe aortic insufficiency. It is essential to recognize the presence of *pseudohypotension*, which represents a falsely low measure of blood pressure due to involvement of the affected extremity's subclavian artery by the dissection. Pulse deficits are a common finding on physical examination when there is involvement of any of the subclavian, carotid, or femoral arteries. Acute aortic insufficiency may occur in up to one-half of those with type A dissection. While the presence of congestive heart failure or a widened pulse pressure should raise one's suspicion of acute aortic insufficiency, the diastolic murmur is often difficult to appreciate.

Involvement of branch arteries by the aortic dissection may produce a variety of vascular complications. Compromise of the ostium of a coronary artery—the right is most often involved—may cause myocardial ischemia or acute infarction. Involvement of the brachiocephalic or left common carotid artery may produce a stroke or coma. When a dissection extends into the abdominal aorta it may compromise flow to one or both renal arteries, producing acute renal failure with an exacerbation of hypertension. Another consequence may be mesenteric ischemia presenting as abdominal pain. Finally, an extensive dissection may compromise one of the common iliac arteries, causing femoral pulse deficits or lower-extremity ischemia.

The findings on chest roentgenography are typically nonspecific and rarely diagnostic. An enlarged mediastinal silhouette is present in 62% of cases *(8)*, and is often the factor that first prompts suspicion of aortic dissection among patients with chest pain. A small left pleural effusion (an exudate produced by the inflamed aortic wall) is commonly seen when there is involvement of the descending thoracic aorta. It should be emphasized that under no circumstances does a normal chest roentgenogram exclude the diagnosis of aortic dissection, as the chest roentgenogram is indeed normal in 12% of cases *(8)*.

Diagnosis

When the possibility of aortic dissection is being considered it is essential that one promptly confirms or excludes the diagnosis with an appropriate imaging study. Computed tomography,

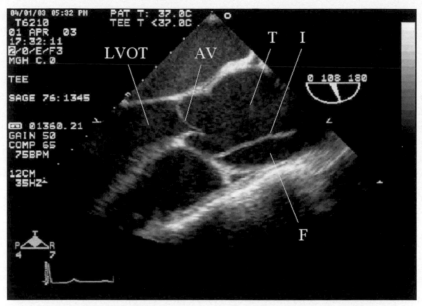

Fig. 3. A transesophageal echocardiogram of the ascending aorta in long-axis in a patient with a type A aortic dissection. The left ventricular outflow tract (LVOT) and aortic valve (AV) are on the left and the ascending aorta extends to the right. Within the aorta is an intimal flap (I) that originates at the level of the sinotubular junction. The true (T) and the false (F) lumens are separated by the intimal flap.

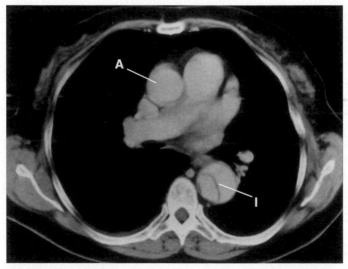

Fig. 4. A contrast-enhanced CT scan of the chest showing an intimal flap (I) separating the two lumens of the descending thoracic aorta in a type B aortic dissection. Note that there is no evidence of a dissection flap in the ascending aorta (A).

magnetic resonance imaging (MRI), transesophageal echocardiography (TEE), and aortography can accurately diagnose the presence of aortic dissection. In a tertiary care center when suspicion of aortic dissection is high, a transesophageal echocardiogram (Fig. 3) is often the study of choice as this examination provides sufficient detail to enable the surgeon to take the patient directly to the operating room for aortic repair if necessary *(1)*. When one's clinical suspicion is lower and the goal is to "rule out" aortic dissection, contrast-enhanced CT scanning (Fig. 4) is generally preferred since it is entirely noninvasive. In community hospitals where TEE is not readily available contrast-enhanced CT scanning should be performed in all cases; if positive the patient can then be transferred promptly to a tertiary center for definitive treatment. When clinically significant branch artery involvement is suspected, aortography may be necessary to adequately define the arterial anatomy *(1)*. However, a good CT angiogram may be sufficient to provide the same anatomical detail.

TREATMENT

The goal of medical therapy is to halt any further progression of the aortic dissection and to reduce the risk of rupture. Whenever there is a suspicion of aortic dissection medical therapy should be instituted immediately while imaging studies are ordered, rather than waiting for the diagnosis to be confirmed. The primary goal of therapy is to reduce the systolic force of blood ejected from the heart into the aortic lumen by reducing *dP/dt*. The secondary goal is to reduce systolic blood pressure to 100 to 120 mmHg, or to the lowest level that maintains cerebral, cardiac, and renal perfusion. β-blockers are the first-line therapy to achieve these goals, and intravenous agents such as propranolol, metoprolol, or esmolol (ultra-short-acting) should be administered. Intravenous labetalol, which acts as both an α- and a β-blocker, may be particularly useful in aortic dissection for reducing both *dP/dt* and hypertension. Finally, after β-blockers have been initiated intravenous nitroprusside may be added to control hypertension more precisely on a minute-by-minute basis.

When a patient first presents with aortic dissection one must always document which arm has the higher blood pressure and then use only that arm for subsequent hemodynamic monitoring. Moreover, when patients present with significant hypotension, *pseudohypotension* should be carefully excluded. When true hypotension occurs due to hemopericardium and cardiac tamponade, patients should be treated with volume expansion and taken to surgery without delay, as early mortality in this setting is extremely high. Pericardiocentesis should be performed only as a last resort in this setting as it may precipitate hemodynamic collapse and death *(9)*.

After the diagnosis of aortic dissection has been confirmed, one must choose between medical and surgical therapy. Whenever an acute dissection involves the ascending aorta, surgical repair is indicated in order to minimize the risk of life-threatening complications such as rupture, cardiac tamponade, or severe aortic insufficiency. Conversely, if the dissection is confined to the descending aorta patients have been found to fare as well with medical therapy as with surgical repair *(10)*. However, when a type B dissection is associated with a serious complication, such as end-organ ischemia, surgery is indicated. Over the past decade there have been advances in endovascular techniques that can be used, in some cases, for nonsurgical management of acute vascular complications of aortic dissection.

Prognosis

Whether treated medically or surgically, patients with acute aortic dissection who survive the initial hospitalization generally do well thereafter. However, potential late complications include aneurysm formation (and possible rupture), recurrent dissection, and aortic insufficiency. Medications to reduce *dP/dt* and control hypertension can dramatically reduce the incidence of such late complications and should therefore be continued indefinitely *(11)*. β-blockers are the drug of choice in this setting, but typically additional medications will be needed to achieve the goal of a systolic blood pressure below 130 mmHg. Patients are at highest risk of complications during the first 2 yr after aortic dissection. Progressive aneurysm expansion typically occurs without symptoms, so patients must be followed closely with serial aortic imaging. This can be done using CT, MRI, or TEE, although most prefer CT. All patients should have a baseline imaging study prior to hospital discharge, with follow-up examinations performed at 6-mo intervals initially and then annually thereafter, provided that the anatomy is stable.

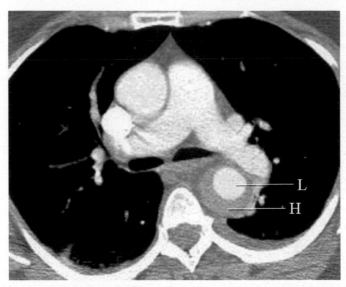

Fig. 5. Intramural hematoma of the aorta. A contrast-enhanced CT scan of the chest demonstrates crescentic thickening of the aortic wall consistent with an intramural hematoma (H). Note that there is no intimal flap within the lumen (L), nor does any contrast enter the hematoma. A small left pleural effusion is also present.

Intramural Hematoma of the Aorta

Intramural hematoma of the aorta is best defined as an atypical form of classic aortic dissection. Its etiology is not entirely certain, but it likely occurs when there is rupture of the vasa vasorum within the aortic media, resulting in a contained hemorrhage within the aortic wall. This hematoma may then propagate longitudinally along a variable length of the aorta, but since the intimal layer remains intact the hematoma does not communicate with the aortic lumen. While intramural hematoma of the aorta is clinically indistinguishable from aortic dissection, on cross-sectional imaging it appears as a crescentic thickening around the aortic wall (Fig. 5) rather than as true and false lumens separated by an intimal flap. It is important to note that the presence of an intramural hematoma may go undetected on aortography. The prognosis and management of intramural hematoma is essentially the same as that of classic aortic dissection *(12)*.

TAKAYASU'S ARTERITIS

Takayasu's arteritis is a chronic inflammatory disease of unknown etiology that involves the aorta and its branches. It typically affects young women, with a mean age of onset of 29 and women affected eight times as often as men *(13)*. It occurs more often in Asia and Africa than in Europe or North America. It typically has two stages. The first is an early stage in which there is active inflammation involving the aorta and its branches. This then progresses at a variable rate to a later sclerotic stage in which there is intimal hyperplasia, medial degeneration, and obliterative changes of the aorta and affected arteries. The majority of the resulting arterial lesions are stenotic, but aneurysms may occur as well. The aortic arch and brachiocephalic vessels are most often affected, but the abdominal aorta is also commonly involved. The pulmonary artery is occasionally involved. The disease may be diffuse or patchy, with affected areas separated by lengths of normal aorta.

Clinical Manifestations

Most patients present initially with symptoms of a systemic inflammatory process, such as fever, night sweats, arthralgia, and weight loss. However, there is often a delay of months to years between the onset of symptoms and the time the diagnosis is made. Indeed, at the time of diagnosis 90% of patients have already entered the sclerotic phase and suffer symptoms of vascular insufficiency, typically with pain in the upper (or less often lower) extremities *(14)*. There will often be absent pulses and diminished blood pressures in the upper extremities, and there may be bruits over affected arteries. Significant hypertension due to renal artery involvement occurs in more than half of patients, but its presence may be difficult to recognize due to the diminished pulses. Aortic insufficiency may result from proximal aortic involvement. Congestive heart failure may result from either the hypertension or aortic insufficiency. Involvement of the coronary artery ostia may cause angina or myocardial infarction, and carotid artery involvement may cause cerebral ischemia or stroke. Abdominal angina may result from mesenteric artery compromise. The overall 15-yr survival for those diagnosed with Takayasu's arteritis is 83%, with the majority of deaths due to stroke, myocardial infarction, or congestive heart failure *(15)*. The survival rate for those with major complications of the disease is as low as 66%, while it may be as high as 96% for those without a major complication.

Diagnosis

During the acute phase, laboratory abnormalities include an elevated erythrocyte sedimentation rate, mild leukocytosis, anemia, and elevated immunoglobulin levels. The diagnosis is most accurately made, however, by the angiographic findings of stenosis of the aorta and stenosis or occlusion of its branch vessels, often with poststenotic dilation or associated aneurysms. Specific clinical criteria have been proposed for making a definitive diagnosis of Takayasu's arteritis *(16)*.

Treatment

The primary therapy for those in the acute inflammatory stage of Takayasu's arteritis is corticosteroids, which may be effective in improving the constitutional symptoms, lowering the erythrocyte sedimentation rate, and slowing disease progression *(17)*. When steroid therapy is ineffective cyclophosphamide or methotrexate may be added. Nevertheless, it remains unknown whether medical therapy actually reduces the risk of major complications or prolongs life. Surgery may be necessary to bypass or reconstruct segments of the aorta or branch arteries. Most commonly surgery is performed to bypass the coronary, carotid, or renal arteries, or to treat aortic insufficiency. More recently, as an alternative to surgery, balloon angioplasty has been used to successfully dilate stenotic lesions of either the aorta or renal arteries.

REFERENCES

1. Bengtsson H, Bergquist D, Sternby NH. Increasing prevalence of abdominal aortic aneurysms: a necropsy study. Eur J Surg 1992;158:19–23.
2. Holmes DR, Liao S, Parks WC, Thompson RW. Medial neovascularization in abdominal aortic aneurysms: a histopathologic marker of aneurysm degeneration with pathophysiologic implications. J Vasc Surg 1995;21:761–771.
3. Lindholt JS, Juul S, Ashton HA, Scott RAP. Indicators of infection *Chlamydia pneumoniae* are associated with expansion of abdominal aortic aneurysm. J Vasc Surg 2001;34:212–215.
4. Lederle FA, Simel DL. Does this patient have abdominal aortic aneurysm? J Am Med Assoc 1999;281:77–82.
5. Cole CW. Prospects for screening for abdominal aortic aneurysms. Lancet 1997;349:1490–1491.
6. Brown LC, Powell JT. Risk factors for aneurysm rupture in patients kept under ultrasound surveillance. UK Small Aneurysm Trial Participants. Ann Surg 1999;230:289–296.
7. Johansson G, Markström U, Swedenborg J. Ruptured thoracic aortic aneurysms: a study of incidence and mortality rates. J Vasc Surg 1995;21:985–988.
8. Hagan PG, Nienaber CA, Isselbacher EM, et al. The International Registry of Acute Aortic Dissection (IRAD)— New insights into an old disease. JAMA 2000;283:897–903.
9. Isselbacher EM, Cigarroa JE, Eagle KA. Cardiac tamponade complicating proximal aortic dissection: is pericardiocentesis harmful? Circulation 1994;90:2375–2378.
10. Glower DD, Fann JI, Speier RH, et al. Comparison of medical and surgical therapy for uncomplicated descending aortic dissection. Circulation 1990;82(Suppl IV):IV-39–46.
11. Neya K, Omoto R, Kyo S, et al. Outcome of Stanford type B acute aortic dissection. Circulation 1992;86(Suppl II): II-1–7.
12. Nienaber CA, von Kodolitsch Y, Petersen B, et al. Intramural hemorrhage of the thoracic aorta. Circulation 1995;92: 1465–1472.

13. Procter CD, Hollier LH. Takayasu's arteritis and temporal arteritis. Ann Vasc Surg 1992;6:195–198.
14. Lupi-Herrera E, Sanchez-Torres G, Marcushamer J, et al. Takayasu's arteritis. Clinical study of 107 cases. Am Heart J 1977;93:94–103.
15. Ishikawa K, Maetani S. Long term outcome for 120 Japanese patients with Takayasu's disease. Circulation 1994;90: 1855–1860.
16. Ishikawa K. Diagnostic approach and proposed criteria for the clinical diagnosis of Takayasu's arteriopathy. J Am Coll Cardiol 1988;12:964–972.
17. Shelhamer JH, Volkman DJ, Parrillo JE, et al. Takayasu's arteritis and its therapy. Ann Int Med 1985;103:121–126.
18. Isselbacher EM, Eagle KA, DeSanctis RW. Diseases of the aorta. In: Braunwald E, ed. Heart Disease: A Textbook of Cardiovascular Medicine, 5th ed. W. B. Saunders, Philadelphia, 1997, pp. 1555.

RECOMMENDED READING

Hagan PG, Nienaber CA, Isselbacher EM, et al. The International Registry of Acute Aortic Dissection (IRAD)—New insights into an old disease. JAMA 2000;283:897–903.

Isselbacher EM. Diseases of the aorta. In: Braunwald E, Zipes DP, Libby P, Bonow RO, eds. Braunwald's Heart Disease: A Textbook of Cardiovascular Medicine, 7th ed. W. B. Saunders, Philadelphia, 2004.

Lederle FA, Wilson ES, Johnson GR, et al. Immediate repair compared with surveillance of small abdominal aortic aneurysms. N Engl J Med 2002;346:1437–1444.

Moore AG, Eagle KA, Bruckman D, et al. Choice of computed tomography, transesophageal echocardiography, magnetic resonance imaging, and aortography in acute aortic dissection: International Registry of Acute Aortic Dissection (IRAD). Am J Cardiol 2002;89:1235–1238.

Nienaber CA, von Kodolitsch Y, Petersen B, et al. Intramural hemorrhage of the thoracic aorta. Circulation 1995;92: 1465–1472.

XI ADDITIONAL TOPICS

38   Pregnancy and
Cardiovascular Disease

Samuel C. B. Siu, MD, SM
and Jack M. Colman, MD

INTRODUCTION

During pregnancy, hormonally mediated changes in blood volume, red cell mass, and heart rate result in a 50% increase in intravascular volume and cardiac output, peaking during the second trimester and remaining constant through the remainder of the pregnancy *(1)*. Gestational hormones, circulating prostaglandins, and the low-resistance vascular bed in the placenta result in concomitant decreases in peripheral vascular resistance and blood pressure. During labor and delivery, pain and uterine contractions result in additional increases in cardiac output and blood pressure. Immediately following delivery, relief of caval compression and autotransfusion from the emptied and contracted uterus produce a further increase in cardiac output. The hemodynamic changes of pregnancy persist for at least several days postpartum and may not fully resolve until the sixth postpartum month.

As a result of physiologic changes, many pregnant women without cardiac disease may have symptoms mimicking those associated with cardiac pathology. Common symptoms experienced by pregnant women without heart disease include fatigue, dyspnea, and lightheadedness. A displaced apical impulse, prominent jugular venous pulsations, widely split first and second heart sounds, and soft ejection systolic murmur are frequent findings during normal pregnancy. Sinus tachycardia, premature atrial or ventricular ectopic beats, right or left axis deviation, ST segment depression, and T-wave changes have been observed on 12-lead electrocardiograms obtained in normal pregnant women. There may be straightening of the left upper heart border and increased lung markings on the chest roentgenogram. In the postpartum period, small pleural effusions can be present. Echocardiographic studies of normal pregnant women have described a mild increase in left ventricular diastolic dimension with preservation of contractility and ejection fraction. Functional tricuspid and mitral regurgitation and small pericardial effusion are normal findings.

OUTCOMES ASSOCIATED WITH SPECIFIC CARDIAC LESIONS

In the presence of maternal heart disease, the physiologic changes of pregnancy can lead to maternal and fetal deterioration. With the exception of patients with Eisenmenger's syndrome, pulmonary vascular obstructive disease, and Marfan's syndrome with aortopathy, maternal death during pregnancy in women with heart disease is rare *(2–7)*.

However, pregnant women with heart disease remain at risk for other complications including heart failure, arrhythmia, and stroke *(2–6)*. They are also at increased risk for neonatal complications *(2,3,8)*. With advances in the pediatric treatment of congenital heart disease, women with congenital heart disease now comprise the majority of pregnant women with heart disease seen at referral centers in developed countries *(6)*, whereas in developing countries, rheumatic heart disease

From: *Essential Cardiology: Principles and Practice, 2nd Ed.*
Edited by: C. Rosendorff © Humana Press Inc., Totowa, NJ

remains the most common lesion encountered *(7)*. Hypertension, whether preexisting or gestational, is commonly encountered. Peripartum cardiomyopathy is infrequent but is mentioned in view of its unique relationship to pregnancy. Isolated mitral valve prolapse is surely the most prevalent cardiac lesion to be encountered in the pregnant woman. However, patients with this condition may not be referred to a cardiovascular specialist in view of their excellent outcomes during pregnancy *(9)*.

Congenital Heart Lesions

LEFT-TO-RIGHT CARDIAC SHUNTS

The main lesions in this group are atrial septal defect (ASD), ventricular septal defect (VSD), and patent ductus arteriosus (PDA). The effect of increase in cardiac output of pregnancy on the volume-loaded right ventricle in ASD, or left ventricle in VSD and PDA, may be counterbalanced by the decrease in peripheral vascular resistance such that the increase in left-to-right shunt is attenuated. In the absence of pulmonary hypertension, pregnancy, labor, and delivery are well tolerated *(3,5,6,10)*. However, arrhythmias, ventricular dysfunction, and progression of pulmonary hypertension may occur, especially when the shunt is large, or when there is preexisting elevation of pulmonary artery pressure. Infrequently, particularly in ASDs, paradoxical embolization may be encountered when systemic vasodilation and/or elevation of pulmonary resistance promote transient right-to-left shunting.

BICUSPID AORTIC VALVE; LEFT VENTRICULAR OUTFLOW TRACT OBSTRUCTION

Bicuspid aortic valve (BAV) is often functionally normal. Its presence is an indication for endocarditis prophylaxis and a reminder to exclude associated aortic coarctation or ascending aortopathy. When aortic stenosis (AS) complicates pregnancy it is usually due to congenital BAV; other causes of left ventricular (LV) outflow tract obstruction at, below, and above the valve have similar hemodynamic consequences. Women with symptomatic AS should delay pregnancy until after surgical correction. However, the absence of symptoms antepartum is not sufficient assurance that pregnancy will be well-tolerated; patients with suspected AS should be assessed by transthoracic echocardiography to define the level and severity of the obstruction and the degree of LV dysfunction. In a pregnant woman with severe AS, limited ability to augment cardiac output may result in abnormal elevation of LV systolic and filling pressures, which in turn may lead to heart failure or ischemia. In addition the noncompliant, hypertrophied ventricle is sensitive to falls in preload such as those that may occur due to inferior vena cava compression in late pregnancy, vasodilator effects of anaesthetic agents, peripartum blood loss, or bearing down maneuvers. The consequent exaggerated drop in cardiac output may lead to hypotension. In a 1993 compilation of many small published series, 65 patients were followed through 106 pregnancies with a maternal mortality of 11% and a perinatal mortality of 4% *(11)*. In a series of 49 pregnancies (39 women) with congenital aortic stenosis managed between 1986 and 2000 (severe AS in 59%), there was no mortality *(12)*. Adverse maternal cardiac events occurred in 6% and adverse fetal events in 10% of the pregnancies. In follow-up, 41% of the women required surgical intervention a mean of 2.6 ± 2 yr after pregnancy *(12)*. Intrapartum palliation by balloon valvuloplasty may be helpful in selected cases. Aortic dissection has also been reported in association with pregnancy in some patients with BAV and ascending aortopathy *(13)*. Although the risk of dissection is less in this group relative to the risk in Marfan's syndrome with aortopathy, perhaps a similar management strategy should be employed.

COARCTATION OF THE AORTA

Coarctation of the aorta will often have been corrected prior to pregnancy. It is commonly associated with a bicuspid aortic valve; other associations include aneurysm of the circle of Willis, VSD, and Turner's syndrome. Maternal mortality with uncorrected coarctation has been reported as 3 to 4%, higher in the presence of associated cardiac defects, aortopathy, or long-standing hypertension. Aortic rupture is a risk in the third trimester as well as during labor. However, recent studies of corrected and uncorrected patients have been encouraging, with only one maternal death reported in 182 pregnancies *(14)*. The death occurred in a woman who had previously undergone coarctation repair, emphasizing that while prior repair reduces maternal risk, it does not eliminate it *(5,6,14)*. Pregnant women with repaired coarctation are at increased risk for pregnancy-induced hypertension *(5,6,14)*, likely as a result of residual abnormalities in aortic compliance. Satisfactory control of upper-body hypertension during pregnancy may lead to excessive hypotension below the coarctation site, compromising the fetus. In unrepaired coarctation, the incidence of intrauterine growth restriction and premature labor is increased.

PULMONARY STENOSIS

Echocardiographic estimation of the pressure gradient allows classification into mild (<49 mmHg), moderate (50–79 mmHg), and severe (≥80 mmHg) pulmonic stenosis (PS). However gradients increase with cardiac output during pregnancy, so the severity of the stenosis may be overestimated if no antenatal study is available. Mild PS or PS that has been alleviated by valvuloplasty or surgery is well tolerated during pregnancy *(5,6)*. Fetal outcome in pregnancy complicated by PS is favorable. Even though a woman with severe pulmonic stenosis may be asymptomatic, the increased hemodynamic load of pregnancy may precipitate right heart failure or atrial arrhythmias. Such a patient should be considered for correction prior to pregnancy. Even during pregnancy, balloon valvuloplasty may be feasible if symptoms of pulmonary stenosis progress.

CYANOTIC HEART DISEASE: UNREPAIRED AND REPAIRED

Tetralogy of Fallot is the most common form of cyanotic congenital heart disease. Its essential features are right ventricular outflow tract obstruction and a large nonrestrictive ventricular septal defect. In uncorrected or palliated pregnant patients with tetralogy, the usual pregnancy-associated fall in systemic vascular resistance and rise in cardiac output exacerbate right-to-left shunting, leading to increased maternal hypoxemia and cyanosis. Fetal loss may be as high as 30% and maternal mortality is reported as 4 to 15%, with risk increasing proportional to hematocrit. In a study of 96 pregnancies in 44 women with a variety of cyanotic congenital heart defects, there was a high rate of maternal cardiac events (32% including 1 death), prematurity (37%) and a low live birth rate (43%) *(15)*. The lowest live birth rate (12%) was observed in mothers with arterial oxygen saturation ≤85%.

Pregnancy risk is low in women who have had successful correction of tetralogy *(3,5,6)*. However, residua and sequelae such as residual shunt, right ventricular outflow tract obstruction, arrhythmias, pulmonary regurgitation, right ventricular systolic dysfunction, pulmonary hypertension (due to the effects of a previous palliative shunt), or LV dysfunction (due to previous volume overload) increase the likelihood of pregnancy complications and require independent consideration.

Women who have had an atrial repair for complete transposition of the great arteries (i.e., Mustard or Senning procedure) are subject to late adult complications such as sinus node dysfunction, atrial arrhythmias, and dysfunction of the systemic right ventricle. In 43 pregnancies in 31 women described in recent reports, there was one late maternal death *(16,17)*. There was a 14% incidence of maternal heart failure, arrhythmias, or cardiac deterioration. No studies of pregnancy outcome in women who received the current repair of choice for complete transposition, the arterial switch procedure, have yet been reported. However, in the absence of ventricular dysfunction, coronary obstruction, or severe valve dysfunction, a good outcome is expected.

The Fontan operation for patients with univentricular circulation involves diversion of systemic venous return to the pulmonary artery without a functional subpulmonary ventricle. Cyanosis and volume overload of the functioning systemic ventricle are both eliminated but patients have a limited ability to increase cardiac output. In a review of 33 pregnancies in 21 women who were doing well after the Fontan operation, there were 15 (45%) term pregnancies with no maternal mortality although two women (14%) had cardiac complications and the incidence of first-trimester abortion was high (39%) *(18)*.

MARFAN'S SYNDROME

Marfan's syndrome is a heritable autosomal dominant connective tissue disorder. Life-threatening aortic complications are due to medial aortopathy resulting in dilation, dissection, and valvular regurgitation. Risk is increased in pregnancy due to hemodynamic stress and perhaps to hormonal effects. Although older case reports suggested a very high mortality risk in the range of 30%, more recent data suggested an overall maternal mortality of 1% and fetal mortality of 22%. A prospective evaluation of 45 pregnancies in 21 patients reported no increase in obstetrical complications or significant change in aortic root size in most patients. Importantly, in the 8 patients with a dilated aortic root (>40 mm) or prior aortic root surgery, 3 of their 9 pregnancies were complicated by either aortic dissection (2 patients) or rapid aortic dilation (1 patient) *(19)*. Thus patients with aortic root involvement should receive preconception counseling emphasizing their risk and if seen in early pregnancy should be offered termination. In contrast, women with little cardiovascular involvement and with aortic root diameter by echocardiography less than 40 mm may tolerate pregnancy well, though serial echocardiography should be used to identify progressive aortic root dilation, prophylactic β-blockers should be administered, and the possibility of dissection even with a normal aortic root should be acknowledged *(20)*. The aortopathy in Marfan's syndrome is a generalized process. Patients who already demonstrate root dilation likely have more severe aortic pathology than those whose ascending aortic dimension is still normal; hence prophylactic root replacement prior to pregnancy may not fully eliminate the risk of dissection of the residual native aorta.

EISENMENGER'S SYNDROME AND PULMONARY VASCULAR OBSTRUCTIVE DISEASE

Eisenmenger's syndrome consists of pulmonary vascular obstructive disease that develops as a consequence of a preexisting left-to-right shunt such that pulmonary pressures approach systemic levels and the direction of shunt flow becomes bidirectional or right-to-left. Maternal mortality approximates 30% in each pregnancy *(21)*. The preponderance of complications occurs at term and during the first postpartum week. Preconception counseling should stress the extreme pregnancy-associated risks. Termination of pregnancy should always be offered to such patients, as should sterilization. Fetal outcome is also poor. Spontaneous abortion is common, intrauterine growth restriction is seen in 50% of pregnancies, and preterm labor is frequent. Perinatal mortality is due mainly to prematurity and is seen in as many as 28% of pregnancies. A 1998 review of 52 pregnancies in patients with primary and secondary pulmonary hypertension reported maternal mortality to be 36 and 30% in the primary pulmonary and secondary pulmonary hypertension groups respectively. The overall neonatal mortality was 12% *(22)*.

Rheumatic Heart Disease

Mitral stenosis is the most common rheumatic valvular lesion encountered during pregnancy. The hypervolemia and tachycardia associated with pregnancy exacerbate the impact of mitral valve obstruction. The resultant elevation in left atrial pressure increases the likelihood of atrial fibrillation. Thus, even patients with only mild to moderate mitral stenosis who are asymptomatic prior to pregnancy may develop atrial fibrillation and heart failure during the ante- and peripartum periods. Atrial fibrillation is a precipitant of heart failure in pregnant patients with mitral stenosis primarily due to uncontrolled ventricular rate, and equivalent tachycardia of any cause may produce the same detrimental effect. Earlier studies examining a pregnant population comprised predominantly of women with rheumatic mitral disease showed that mortality rate varied directly with worsening antenatal maternal functional class *(4)*. More recent studies found no mortality but described substantial morbidity from heart failure and arrhythmia *(5,6,23,24)*. The risk for complications was higher in women with a history of prior cardiac events (arrhythmias, stroke, or pulmonary edema) and/or with moderate/severe mitral stenosis *(5,6,23,24)*. The risk of adverse fetal or neonatal outcomes also increased with increasing severity of mitral stenosis *(24)*. Percutaneous mitral valvuloplasty should be considered in patients with functional class III or IV symptoms despite optimal medical therapy and hospitalization.

Pregnant women whose dominant lesion is rheumatic aortic stenosis have a similar outcome to those with congenital aortic stenosis. Severe aortic or mitral regurgitation is generally well tolerated during pregnancy, although deterioration in maternal functional class has been observed.

Hypertensive Disorders in Pregnancy

Hypertensive disorders of pregnancy are the second most common cause of maternal mortality, accounting for 15% of all obstetrical deaths *(25)*. They also predispose to other complications such as placental abruption, stroke, disseminated intravascular coagulation, renal and/or hepatic failure, and congestive heart failure *(26)*. The fetus is at increased risk for intrauterine growth restriction, preterm birth, or perinatal death.

There have been recent attempts to standardize definitions and criteria for diagnosis *(26–29)*. The recommendations of the Canadian Hypertension Society and the Society of Obstetricians and Gynaecologists of Canada define hypertension in pregnancy as *preexisting hypertension* (chronic hypertension, renal hypertension, underlying hypertension, essential hypertension, or secondary hypertension), *gestational hypertension without proteinuria and other adverse conditions* (pregnancy-induced hypertension, transient hypertension of pregnancy) or *gestational hypertension with proteinuria or other adverse conditions* (preeclampsia, eclampsia, HELLP [hemolysis, elevated liver enzymes, low platelets] syndrome, gestational proteinuric hypertension) *(26–29)*.

Hypertension in pregnancy is defined as seated systolic blood pressure (BP) ≥140 and/or diastolic blood pressure ≥90 mmHg (using Korotkoff phase V [disappearance of sound] to determine diastolic pressure) *(25)*. The BP elevation should be noted on repeated measurements. Proteinuria in pregnancy is significant when there is >0.3 g protein in a 24-h urine collection. Severe hypertension is defined as a systolic blood pressure ≥160 and/or a diastolic blood pressure ≥110 mmHg and severe proteinuria as a 24-h urine protein excretion >2 g. Gestational hypertension may be *superimposed* on preexisting hypertension. In the absence of proteinuria and other adverse conditions, gestational hypertension that resolves postpartum is called *transient hypertension of pregnancy* or *benign gestational hypertension*, whereas if it persists postpartum it is understood as pregnancy-induced unmasking of preexisting (or chronic) hypertension.

The pathophysiology of gestational hypertension differs from other forms of hypertension. As a result of placental dysfunction, the normal cardiovascular adaptations to pregnancy (increased plasma volume and decreased peripheral resistance) fail to occur. There is reduced perfusion to placenta, liver, kidneys, and brain. It is thought that endothelial activation and dysfunction, perhaps a result of oxidative stress and increased sensitivity to endogenous vasoactive substances, are responsible for most manifestations of gestational hypertension *(30)*. Thus, hypertension is but one effect, not a cause, of the clinical syndrome.

Certain adverse conditions are associated with worse outcomes. Frontal headache, severe nausea and vomiting, visual disturbances, chest pain and shortness of breath, and right upper quadrant pain are significant symptoms. The components of HELLP syndrome may be found individually or combined. Other adverse maternal manifestations are severe hypertension, severe proteinuria, hypo-albuminemia (<18 g/L) oliguria, pulmonary edema, and convulsions. Fetal compromise may be revealed by oligohydramnios, absent or reversed umbilical artery end-diastolic flow, and abnormalities in fetal biophysical profile. Intrauterine growth restriction, prematurity, and placental abruption are the serious adverse feto-placental consequences. Chronic hypertension does increase the risk of growth-restricted infants, but otherwise its main acute effect is the increased risk of superimposed preeclampsia.

Peripartum Cardiomyopathy

Peripartum cardiomyopathy is a form of idiopathic dilated cardiomyopathy diagnosed by otherwise unexplained LV systolic dysfunction, confirmed echocardiographically, presenting during the last antepartum month or in the first 5 postpartum months *(31)*. It usually manifests as heart failure, although arrhythmias and embolic events also occur. Many affected women will show improvement in functional status and ventricular function postpartum, but others may have persistent or progressive dysfunction. The relapse rate during subsequent pregnancies is substantial in women with evidence of persisting cardiac enlargement or LV dysfunction. However, pregnancy may not be risk-free even in those with recovery of systolic function, as subclinical abnormalities may persist *(32)*. A multicenter survey examining the outcomes of 60 pregnancies in women with peripartum cardiomyopathy diagnosed during a prior pregnancy reported that 44% of women with LV ejection fraction <0.50 developed symptoms of congestive heart failure during subsequent pregnancies, with an associated mortality rate of 19%, whereas symptoms of congestive heart failure developed in 21% of women with LV ejection fraction ≥0.50 and none of this group died *(33)*. A smaller single-center prospective study of 26 pregnancies confirmed the higher risk in patients with persistent LV dysfunction compared with pregnancies in women whose LV function had normalized *(34)*.

MANAGEMENT

Risk Stratification and Counseling

Risk stratification and counseling of women with heart disease is best accomplished prior to conception. The data required for risk stratification can be readily acquired from a thorough cardiovascular history and examination, 12-lead electrocardiogram, and transthoracic echocardiogram. In patients with cyanosis, arterial oxygen saturation should be assessed by percutaneous oximetry. In counseling, the following six areas should be considered: the underlying cardiac lesion, maternal functional status, the possibility of further palliative or corrective surgery, additional associated risk factors, maternal life expectancy and ability to care for a child, and the risk of congenital heart disease in offspring.

Defining the *underlying cardiac lesion* is an important part of stratifying risk and determining management. The nature of residua and sequelae should be clarified, especially ventricular function, pulmonary pressure, severity of obstructive lesions, persistence of shunts, and presence of hypoxemia. Low-risk patients include those with small left-to-right shunts, repaired lesions without residual cardiac dysfunction, isolated mitral valve prolapse without significant regurgitation, bicuspid aortic valve without stenosis, mild to moderate pulmonic stenosis, or valvular regurgitation with normal ventricular systolic function. Intermediate risk lesions include unrepaired or palliated cyanotic congenital heart disease, large left-to-right shunt, uncorrected coarctation of the aorta, mitral stenosis, moderate aortic stenosis, prosthetic valves, severe pulmonic stenosis, or moderate to severe systemic ventricular dysfunction. Those at high risk include patients with New York Heart Association (NYHA) class III or IV symptoms, significant pulmonary hypertension, Marfan's syndrome with aortic root or major valvular involvement, or severe aortic stenosis.

Maternal functional status is an important predictor of outcome, and most often defined by NYHA functional class. In a landmark 1982 study of 482 pregnancies in women with congenital heart disease, cardiovascular morbidity was less (8% vs 30%) and live birth rate higher (80% vs 68%) in mothers with NYHA functional class I compared with the others *(2)*. In recent studies, we found NYHA class >2 to be an independent predictor of adverse maternal cardiac events during pregnancy *(5,6)*.

Both maternal and fetal outcomes are improved by *further palliative or corrective surgery* to correct cyanosis, which should be undertaken prior to conception when possible *(3)*. Similarly, patients with symptomatic obstructive lesions should undergo intervention prior to pregnancy *(35)*. During pregnancy, the result of cardiovascular surgery is less favorable, with maternal and fetal mortality of 6% and 30% respectively *(36)*. The lack of ideal choices once severe valve disease is present argues for completing families earlier, before age-dependent progression necessitates valve-replacement surgery and raises the difficult issues of anticoagulation required by mechanical valves, or predictable need for earlier reoperation if a tissue valve is used.

Additional associated risk factors that may complicate pregnancy include a history of arrhythmia or heart failure, prosthetic valves and conduits, anticoagulant therapy, and the use of teratogenic drugs such as warfarin or angiotensin-converting enzyme inhibitors.

Maternal life expectancy and ability to care for her child: A patient with limited physical capacity or with a condition that may result in premature maternal death should be advised of her potential inability to look after her child. Women whose condition imparts a high likelihood of fetal complications, such as those with cyanosis or on anticoagulants, must be apprised of these added risks.

The *risk of recurrence of congenital heart disease in offspring* should be addressed in the context of a 0.4 to 0.6% risk in the general population. If a first-degree relative is affected, the risk increases about 10-fold. Left heart obstructive lesions have a higher recurrence rate. Certain conditions such as Marfan's syndrome and the 22q11 deletion syndromes are autosomal-dominant, conferring a 50% risk of recurrence in an offspring. Patients with congenital heart disease who reach reproductive age should be offered genetic assessment and counseling so that they are fully informed of the mode of inheritance and recurrence risk as well as the prenatal diagnosis options available to them. Preventive strategies to decrease the incidence of congenital defects such as preconception use of multivitamins can be discussed at the time of prepregnancy counseling *(37)*.

Systematic stratification of risk–risk index: Canadian investigators analyzed maternal and fetal outcomes in 851 completed pregnancies, 252 in a retrospective study and subsequently 599 in a prospective multicenter study *(5,6)*. In the prospective study, poor functional status (NYHA > class II) or cyanosis, left ventricular systolic dysfunction, left heart obstruction, and history of cardiac events prior to pregnancy (arrhythmia, stroke, or pulmonary edema) were independent predictors of adverse maternal cardiac events in pregnancy *(6)*. A risk index was developed incorporating these maternal risk factors, which are definable prior to or early in pregnancy. The risk of a cardiac event (cardiac death, stroke, pulmonary edema, or arrhythmia) during pregnancy increased with the number of predictors present during the antepartum evaluation. In a woman with heart disease and a risk index of 0, the likelihood of a cardiac event during pregnancy is about 5%, whereas with a risk index of 1 it rises to 25%, and with a risk index >1, the likelihood is 75% *(6)*. This index should be used in conjunction with lesion-specific risk estimates where available, since certain populations with known lesion-specific risks are not defined by the global risk index. This is at least partially because patients with previously established high risk (e.g., Marfan's with dilated root, Eisenmenger's), were underrepresented in the contemporary population of pregnant women with heart disease from which the global risk index was derived (Table 1).

Women with heart disease have an increased risk of neonatal adverse events *(2–6,8)*. In a prospective study incorporating a control group of pregnant women without heart disease, we showed that the risk of neonatal complications (premature birth, small-for-gestational-age birth weight, respiratory distress syndrome, intraventricular hemorrhage, fetal or neonatal death) is higher in women with heart disease, especially in the presence of poor maternal functional class, cyanosis, or left heart obstruction, and further amplified if there are concomitant maternal noncardiac (obstetrical and other) risk factors for neonatal complications (Table 1) *(8)*.

Women with a high risk score (≥1) for cardiac complications, those with lesion-specific risks, and those at risk for neonatal complications should benefit from enhanced multidisciplinary surveillance in a high-risk obstetrics unit, whereas those with no such risk factors may do well with normal obstetrical and cardiac care in the community *(5,6)*.

Antepartum Management

Pregnant women with heart disease may be at particular risk for congestive heart failure, arrhythmias, thrombosis, emboli, and adverse effects of anticoagulants.

When ventricular dysfunction is a concern, activity limitation is helpful and in severely affected women with class III or IV symptoms, hospital admission by mid-second trimester may be advisable. Pregnancy-induced hypertension, hyperthyroidism, infection, and anemia should be identified early and treated vigorously. For patients with functionally significant mitral stenosis, β-adrenergic blockers rather than digoxin should be used to control heart rate. We also offer empiric therapy with β-adrenergic blockers to patients with coarctation, to Marfan's patients, and to other patients with ascending aortopathy (e.g., BAV).

Table 1
Risk Factors for Maternal Cardiac and Neonatal Adverse Events
in Pregnancy in Women With Heart Disease

Nature of risk	Risk factor
Maternal cardiac adverse event (pulmonary edema, arrhythmia, stroke, death)	Poor functional class (NYHA class > II) or cyanosis[a]
	Systemic ventricular systolic dysfunction (EF <0.40)[a]
	Left heart obstruction (mitral valve area <2.0 cm^2, aortic valve area <1.5 cm^2, or peak LVOT gradient >30 mmHg)[a]
	Cardiac event (arrhythmia, stroke, TIA, pulmonary edema) prior to pregnancy[a]
	Known lesion-specific risk
Neonatal adverse event (premature birth, small-for-gestational age birth weight, respiratory distress syndrome, intraventricular hemorrhage, fetal or neonatal death)	Presence of maternal heart disease (increased risk amplified by the additional presence of risk factors listed below)
	Poor maternal functional class (NYHA class > II) or cyanosis
	Maternal left heart obstruction
	Maternal age <20 or >35 yr old
	Obstetric risk factors for adverse neonatal events[b]
	Multiple gestation
	Smoking during pregnancy
	Anticoagulant therapy

[a]These risk factors may be used to constitute a risk index: the risk of a maternal cardiac adverse event with 0 risk factors present is <5%, with 1 risk factor present is 25%, and with more than one risk factor present is 75% (from ref. 6).

[b]History of premature delivery or rupture of membranes, incompetent cervix, or Caesarean section; or intrauterine growth retardation, antepartum bleeding after 12 wk gestation, febrile illness or uterine/placental abnormalities during present pregnancy. From: Colman JM, Siu SC. Pregnancy in adult patients with congenital heart disease. Prog Paed Cardiol vol. 17. 53–60, copyright 2003, with permission from Elsevier.

Arrhythmias in the form of premature atrial or ventricular beats are common in normal pregnancy, although sustained tachyarrhythmias have also been reported. In those with preexisting arrhythmias, pregnancy may exacerbate the frequency or hemodynamic severity of arrhythmic episodes. Pharmacologic treatment of arrhythmias is usually reserved for patients with severe symptoms or when sustained episodes are poorly tolerated in the presence of ventricular hypertrophy, ventricular dysfunction, or valvular obstruction. Sustained tachyarrhythmias such as atrial flutter or atrial fibrillation should be treated promptly, avoiding teratogenic antiarrhythmic drugs. Digoxin, β-adrenergic blockers (possibly excluding atenolol), and adenosine are antiarrhythmic drugs of choice in view of their established safety profiles *(38)*. Quinidine, sotalol, lidocaine, flecanide, and propafenone may be considered but published data on their use during pregnancy are more limited *(39)*. There are case reports describing successful use of amiodarone, although it is classified as contraindicated in pregnancy in standard texts. It is not teratogenic, but may impair neonatal thyroid function *(40,41)*. All antiarrhythmic drugs should be avoided during the first trimester if possible. Electrical cardioversion is safe in pregnancy. A report of 44 pregnancies in women with implantable cardioverter-defibrillators reported favorable maternal and fetal outcomes *(42)*.

There is no perfect anticoagulation strategy during pregnancy, and controversy about the optimal strategy will not be resolved without clinical trials. Oral anticoagulation with warfarin is effective and logistically easier. Warfarin embryopathy may be produced during organogenesis, though there is some evidence that a daily warfarin dose of ≤5 mg may not be teratogenic *(43)*. Fetal intracranial bleeding can occur throughout pregnancy when the mother takes warfarin, and is a particular risk during vaginal delivery unless warfarin has been stopped at least 2 wk prior to labor. Adjusted-dose subcutaneous heparin has no teratogenic effects, as the drug does not cross the placenta, but heparin may cause maternal thrombocytopenia and osteoporosis, and is less effective in preventing thromboses in patients with prosthetic valves. In a systematic overview of studies examining the relationship of anticoagulation regimen and pregnancy outcomes in women with prosthetic heart valves, the overall pooled maternal mortality was 2.9% *(44)*. The use of oral anticoagulant through-out pregnancy was associated with the lowest rate of valve thrombosis/systemic embolism (4%). The use of unfractionated heparin between 6 wk and 12 wk gestational age only was associated with an increased risk of valve thrombosis (9%). Recent practice guidelines have favored use of either warfarin plus low-dose aspirin during the entire pregnancy or warfarin substituted by heparin only during the peak teratogenic period (6th to 12th week gestation) *(35)*. The warfarin/aspirin only strategy may be most appropriate if therapeutic anticoagulation can be achieved with a warfarin dose ≤5 mg/d *(43)*. Low-molecular-weight heparin is easier to administer and has been suggested as an alternative to adjusted-dose unfractionated heparin *(45)*. Adjunctive use of low-dose ASA with heparin should also be considered. ASA in low dose is safe for the fetus, even at term *(46)*, although high maternal doses may promote premature duct closure.

If a woman with Eisenmenger's syndrome does not accept counseling to terminate, or presents late in pregnancy, meticulous antepartum management is necessary, including early hospitalization, supplemental oxygen, and possibly empiric anticoagulation.

Multidisciplinary Approach and High-Risk Pregnancy Units

Women with heart disease who are at intermediate or high risk for complications should be managed in a high-risk pregnancy unit by a multidisciplinary team from obstetrics, cardiology, anesthesia, and pediatrics. When dealing with a complex problem the team should meet early in the pregnancy. At this time the nature of the cardiac lesion, anticipated effects of pregnancy, and potential problems are explored. Since it is often not possible for every member of the team to be at the patient's bedside at a moment of crisis, it is helpful to develop a written management plan for most contingencies. Women with heart disease in "low risk" groups can be managed in a community hospital setting, but if there is doubt about the mother's status or the risk, a consultation at a regional referral center should be arranged.

Labor and Delivery

Vaginal delivery is recommended with very few exceptions. The only cardiac indications for Cesarean section are aortic dissection, patients with Marfan's syndrome with dilated aortic root, and a woman on anticoagulants who has not stopped warfarin at least 2 wk prior to labor. Preterm induction is uncommon, but once fetal lung maturity is assured, a planned induction and delivery in high-risk situations will ensure availability of appropriate staff and equipment. Although there is no consensus on the use of invasive hemodynamic monitoring during labor and delivery, we commonly utilize intraarterial monitoring, and may use central venous pressure monitoring as well in cases where there are concerns about the interpretation and deleterious effects of a sudden drop in systemic blood pressure (e.g., patients with severe aortic stenosis, pulmonary hypertension, severe systemic ventricular systolic dysfunction, or preload-dependent physiology such as Fontan). The clinical utility of an indwelling pulmonary artery catheter has not been studied in pregnancy. A PA catheter is utilized, rarely, in situations where the information sought is not available otherwise and warrants the risk of the procedure, considering also that the risk of its insertion may be increased because of complex anatomy such as atrial baffles, or in the setting of pulmonary hypertension because of possible pulmonary infarction or rupture.

Heparin anticoagulation is discontinued at least 12 h prior to induction, or reversed with protamine if spontaneous labor develops, and can usually be resumed 6 to 12 h postpartum.

Many centers with extensive experience in caring for pregnant women with heart disease utilize endocarditis prophylaxis routinely but there is no evidence to support this common practice, which, according to current American Heart Association guidelines, is not recommended for Cesarean section delivery or for uncomplicated vaginal delivery in absence of infection. If unanticipated bacteremia is suspected during vaginal delivery, intravenous antibiotics can be administered at the time.

Epidural anesthesia with adequate volume preloading is the technique of choice. Epidural fentanyl is particularly advantageous in cyanotic patients with shunt lesions or those with significant aortic stenosis, as it does not lower peripheral vascular resistance. In the presence of a shunt, air and particulate filters should be placed in all intravenous lines.

Labor is conducted in the left lateral decubitus position to attenuate hemodynamic fluctuations associated with contractions in the supine position. The latter part of the second stage of labor is shortened and delivery is assisted by forceps or vacuum extraction. As hemodynamics do not return to baseline for many days after delivery, patients at intermediate or high risk may require monitoring for a minimum of 72 h postpartum. Patients with Eisenmenger's syndrome require longer close postpartum observation, since mortality risk persists for up to 7 d.

Management of Hypertensive Disorders in Pregnancy

Mild preexisting hypertension may not require pharmacotherapy in pregnancy, as fetal outcomes are unaffected, maternal blood pressure falls lower than baseline during the first 20 wk of gestation, and excessive lowering of maternal blood pressure may compromise placental perfusion with no proven maternal benefit *(25)*. Therapy should be initiated or reinstituted if moderate-severe hypertension develops (systolic BP ≥150–160; diastolic BP ≥100–110; or both), or there is target organ damage. It is not clear whether treatment of mild-moderate preexisting (chronic) hypertension reduces the risk of developing superimposed gestational hypertension with proteinuria (preeclampsia). If treatment is indicated, drug therapy established as safe includes methyldopa, labetalol and some other β-blockers *(47)*, and nifedipine *(48)*. Caution has been advocated in use of atenolol in particular, due to intrauterine growth restriction, though the data are limited, the effect may be explained by the fall in blood pressure itself and not be specific to the drug used, and the long-term implications of the finding are not yet clear *(49)*. A meta-analysis has raised doubt about hydralazine as first-line therapy *(47)*. Diuretics are indicated for the management of volume overload in renal failure or heart failure, may be used as adjuncts in the management of preexisting (chronic) hypertension, but should be avoided in gestational hypertension (preeclampsia), which is a volume-contracted state *(25,50)*. Treatment, once instituted during pregnancy, should be continued for several weeks postpartum as the hypertensive effects of preeclampsia may persist that long. Angiotensin-converting enzyme inhibitors and angiotensin receptor-blocking agents are contraindicated after the first trimester of pregnancy, and so should be stopped either before conception or in first trimester as soon as pregnancy is diagnosed *(51,52)*.

ACKNOWLEDGMENT

This work is supported in part by an operating grant from the Canadian Institutes for Health Research.

REFERENCES

1. Elkayam U, Gleicher N. Hemodynamics and cardiac function during normal pregnancy and the puerperium. In: Elkayam U, Gleicher N, eds. Cardiac Problems in Pregnancy: Diagnosis and Management of Maternal and Fetal Disease, 3rd ed. Wiley-Liss, New York, 1998, pp. 3–19.
2. Whittemore R, Hobbins J, Engle M. Pregnancy and its outcome in women with and without surgical treatment of congenital heart disease. Am J Cardiol 1982;50:641–651.
3. Shime J, Mocarski E, Hastings D, et al. Congenital heart disease in pregnancy: short- and long-term implications. Am J Obstet Gynecol 1987;156:313–322.
4. McFaul P, Dornan J, Lamki H, Boyle D. Pregnancy complicated by maternal heart disease. A review of 519 women. Br J Obstet Gynaecol 1988;95:861–867.
5. Siu SC, Sermer M, Harrison DA, et al. Risk and predictors for pregnancy-related complications in women with heart disease. Circulation 1997;96:2789–2794.
6. Siu SC, Sermer M, Colman JM, et al. Prospective multicenter study of pregnancy outcomes in women with heart disease. Circulation 2001;104:515–521.
7. Avila WS, Rossi EG, Ramires JA, et al. Pregnancy in patients with heart disease: experience with 1,000 cases. Clin Cardiol 2003;26:135–142.
8. Siu SC, Colman JM, Sorensen S, et al. Adverse neonatal and cardiac outcomes are more common in pregnant women with heart disease. Circulation 2002;105:2179–2184.
9. Rayburn W. Mitral valve prolapse and pregnancy. In: Elkayam U, Gleicher N, eds. Cardiac Problems in Pregnancy: Diagnosis and Management of Maternal and Fetal Heart Disease, 3rd ed. Wiley-Liss, New York, 1998, pp. 175–182.

10. Zuber M, Gautschi N, Oechslin E, et al. Outcome of pregnancy in women with congenital shunt lesions. Heart 1999; 81:271–275.
11. Lao T, Sermer M, MaGee L, et al. Congenital aortic stenosis and pregnancy—a reappraisal. Am J Obstet Gynecol 1993;169:540–545.
12. Silversides CK, Colman JM, Sermer M, et al. Early and intermediate-term outcomes of pregnancy with congenital aortic stenosis. Am J Cardiol 2003;91:1386–1389.
13. Immer FF, Bansi AG, Immer-Bansi AS, et al. Aortic dissection in pregnancy: analysis of risk factors and outcome. Ann Thorac Surg 2003;76:309–314.
14. Beauchesne LM, Connolly HM, Ammash NM, Warnes CA. Coarctation of the aorta: outcome of pregnancy. J Am Coll Cardiol 2001;38:1728–1733.
15. Presbitero P, Somerville J, Stone S, et al. Pregnancy in cyanotic congenital heart disease. Outcome of mother and fetus. Circulation 1994;89:2673–2676.
16. Clarkson P, Wilson N, Neutze J, et al. Outcome of pregnancy after the Mustard operation for transposition of the great arteries with intact ventricular septum. J Am Coll Cardiol 1994;24:190–193.
17. Genoni M, Jenni R, Hoerstrup SP, et al. Pregnancy after atrial repair for transposition of the great arteries. Heart 1999; 81:276–277.
18. Canobbio M, Mair D, van der Velde M, Koos B. Pregnancy outcomes after the Fontan repair. J Am Coll Cardiol 1996; 28:763–767.
19. Rossiter J, Repke J, Morales A, et al. A prospective longitudinal evaluation of pregnancy in the Marfan syndrome. Am J Obstet Gynecol 1995;173:1599–1606.
20. Shores J, Berger K, Murphy E, Pyeritz R. Progression of aortic dilatation and the benefit of long-term B-adrenergic blockade in Marfan's syndrome. N Engl J Med 1994;330:1335–1341.
21. Gleicher N, Midwall J, Hochberger D, Jaffin H. Eisenmenger's syndrome and pregnancy. Obstet Gynecol Surv 1979; 34:721–741.
22. Weiss B, Zemp L, Seifert B, Hess O. Outcome of pulmonary vascular disease in pregnancy: a systematic overview from 1978 through 1996. J Am Coll Cardiol 1998;31:1650–1657.
23. Hameed A, Karaalp IS, Tummala PP, et al. The effect of valvular heart disease on maternal and fetal outcome of pregnancy. J Am Coll Cardiol 2001;37:893–899.
24. Silversides CK, Colman JM, Sermer M, Siu SC. Cardiac risk in pregnant women with rheumatic mitral stenosis. Am J Cardiol 2003;91:1382–1385.
25. Report of the National High Blood Pressure Education Program Working Group on High Blood Pressure in Pregnancy. Am J Obstet Gynecol 2000;183:S1–S22.
26. Helewa M, Burrows R, Smith J, et al. Report of the Canadian Hypertension Society Consensus Conference: 1. Definitions, evaluation and classification of hypertensive disorders in pregnancy. CMAJ 1997;157:715–725.
27. Brown MA, Hague WM, Higgins J, et al. The detection, investigation and management of hypertension in pregnancy: full consensus statement. Aust NZ J Obstet Gynaecol 2000;40:139–155.
28. Moutquin J, Garner P, Burrows R, et al. Report of the Canadian Hypertension Society Consensus Conference: 2. Nonpharmacologic management and prevention of hypertensive disorders in pregnancy. CMAJ 1997;157:907–919.
29. Rey E, LeLorier J, Burgess E, et al. Report of the Canadian Hypertension Society Consensus Conference: 3. Pharmacologic treatment of hypertensive disorders in pregnancy. CMAJ 1997;157:1245–1254.
30. Roberts JM, Pearson G, Cutler J, Lindheimer M. Summary of the NHLBI Working Group on Research on Hypertension During Pregnancy. Hypertension 2003;41:437–445.
31. Pearson GD, Veille JC, Rahimtoola S, et al. Peripartum cardiomyopathy: National Heart, Lung, and Blood Institute and Office of Rare Diseases (National Institutes of Health) workshop recommendations and review. JAMA 2000; 283:1183–1188.
32. Lampert MB, Weinert L, Hibbard J, et al. Contractile reserve in patients with peripartum cardiomyopathy and recovered left ventricular function. Am J Obstet Gynecol 1997;176:189–195.
33. Elkayam U, Tummala PP, Rao K, et al. Maternal and fetal outcomes of subsequent pregnancies in women with peripartum cardiomyopathy. N Engl J Med 2001;344:1567–1571.
34. Avila WS, de Carvalho ME, Tschaen CK, et al. Pregnancy and peripartum cardiomyopathy. A comparative and prospective study. Arq Bras Cardiol 2002;79:484–493.
35. Bonow RO, Carabello B, de Leon AC Jr, et al. ACC/AHA Guidelines for the management of patients with valvular heart disease: a report of the American College of Cardiology/American Heart Association Task Force on Practice Guidelines (Committee on Management of Patients with Valvular Heart Disease). J Am Coll Cardiol 1998;32:1486–1588.
36. Weiss BM, von Segesser LK, Alon E, et al. Outcome of cardiovascular surgery and pregnancy: a systematic review of the period 1984–1996. Am J Obstet Gynecol 1998;179:1643–1653.
37. Czeizel A. Reduction of urinary tract and cardiovascular defects by periconceptional multivitamin supplementation. Am J Med Genet 1996;62:179–183.
38. Chow T, Galvin J, McGovern B. Antiarrhythmic drug therapy in pregnancy and lactation. Am J Cardiol 1998;82: 58I–62I.
39. Blomstrom-Lundqvist C, Scheinman MM, Aliot EM, et al. ACC/AHA/ESC guidelines for the management of patients with supraventricular arrhythmias—executive summary. A report of the American College of Cardiology/ American Heart Association task force on practice guidelines and the European Society of Cardiology committee

for practice guidelines (writing committee to develop guidelines for the management of patients with supraventricular arrhythmias) developed in collaboration with NASPE-Heart Rhythm Society. J Am Coll Cardiol 2003;42: 1493–1531.

40. Magee LA, Downar E, Sermer M, et al. Pregnancy outcome after gestational exposure to amiodarone in Canada. Am J Obstet Gynecol 1995;172:1307–1311.
41. Bartalena L, Bogazzi F, Braverman LE, Martino E. Effects of amiodarone administration during pregnancy on neonatal thyroid function and subsequent neurodevelopment. J Endocrinol Invest 2001;24:116–130.
42. Natale A, Davidson T, Geiger M, Newby K. Implantable cardioverter-defibrillators and pregnancy: a safe combination? Circulation 1997;96:2808–2812.
43. Cotrufo M, De Feo M, De Santo LS, et al. Risk of warfarin during pregnancy with mechanical valve prostheses. Obstet Gynecol 2002;99:35–40.
44. Chan WS, Anand S, Ginsberg JS. Anticoagulation of pregnant women with mechanical heart valves: a systematic review of the literature. Arch Intern Med 2000;160:191–196.
45. Ginsberg JS, Greer I, Hirsh J. Use of antithrombotic agents during pregnancy. Chest 2001;119:122S–131S.
46. CLASP: a randomised trial of low-dose aspirin for the prevention and treatment of pre-eclampsia among 9364 pregnant women. CLASP (Collaborative Low-dose Aspirin Study in Pregnancy) Collaborative Group. Lancet 1994;343: 619–629.
47. Magee LA, Ornstein MP, von Dadelszen P. Fortnightly review: management of hypertension in pregnancy. BMJ 1999;318:1332–1336.
48. Magee LA, Schick B, Donnenfeld AE, et al. The safety of calcium channel blockers in human pregnancy: a prospective, multicenter cohort study. Am J Obstet Gynecol 1996;174:823–828.
49. Magee LA, Duley L. Oral beta-blockers for mild to moderate hypertension during pregnancy. Cochrane Database Syst Rev 2003:CD002863.
50. Collins R, Yusuf S, Peto R. Overview of randomised trials of diuretics in pregnancy. Br Med J (Clin Res Ed) 1985; 290:17–23.
51. Hanssens M, Keirse MJ, Vankelecom F, Van Assche FA. Fetal and neonatal effects of treatment with angiotensin-converting enzyme inhibitors in pregnancy. Obstet Gynecol 1991;78:128–135.
52. Piper JM, Ray WA, Rosa FW. Pregnancy outcome following exposure to angiotensin-converting enzyme inhibitors. Obstet Gynecol 1992;80:429–432.

RECOMMENDED READING

Bonow RO, Carabello B, de Leon AC Jr, et al. ACC/AHA Guidelines for the management of patients with valvular heart disease: a report of the American College of Cardiology/American Heart Association Task Force on Practice Guidelines (Committee on Management of Patients with Valvular Heart Disease). J Am Coll Cardiol 1998;32:1486–1588.
Ginsberg JS, Greer I, Hirsh J. Use of antithrombotic agents during pregnancy. Chest 2001;119:122S–131S.
Helewa M, Burrows R, Smith J, et al. Report of the Canadian Hypertension Society Consensus Conference: 1. Definitions, evaluation and classification of hypertensive disorders in pregnancy. CMAJ 1997;157:715–725.
Pearson GD, Veille JC, Rahimtoola S, et al. Peripartum cardiomyopathy: National Heart, Lung, and Blood Institute and Office of Rare Diseases (National Institutes of Health) workshop recommendations and review. JAMA 2000;283: 1183–1188.
Presbitero P, Somerville J, Stone S, et al. Pregnancy in cyanotic congenital heart disease. Outcome of mother and fetus. Circulation 1994;89:2673–2676.
Roberts JM, Pearson G, Cutler J, Lindheimer M. Summary of the NHLBI Working Group on Research on Hypertension During Pregnancy. Hypertension 2003;41:437–445.
Siu SC, Colman JM, Sorensen S, et al. Adverse neonatal and cardiac outcomes are more common in pregnant women with heart disease. Circulation 2002;105:2179–2184.
Siu SC, Sermer M, Colman JM, et al. Prospective multicenter study of pregnancy outcomes in women with heart disease. Circulation 2001;104:515–521.
Weiss B, Zemp L, Seifert B, Hess O. Outcome of pulmonary vascular disease in pregnancy: a systematic overview from 1978 through 1996. J Am Coll Cardiol 1998;31:1650–1657.

39 Heart Disease in the Elderly

Michael W. Rich, MD

INTRODUCTION

The 20th century has seen a dramatic shift in the demographics of the US population, as average life expectancy at birth has increased from approx 49 yr in 1900 to almost 80 yr today. As a result, both the absolute number and the relative proportion of older individuals in the population has increased exponentially, and these trends are expected to continue well into the current century. Of particular note is that the "oldest old," defined as individuals aged 85 yr or older, is the most rapidly growing segment of the US population.

Cardiovascular disease is the leading cause of death and major disability in the US, and a disproportionate number of individuals with cardiovascular disease are over 65 yr of age. Indeed, it is estimated that 70% of individuals over age 70 have clinically manifest cardiovascular disease (including hypertension). In addition, 84% of all deaths attributable to cardiovascular disease occur in patients over age 65, and 64% are in patients over the age of 75. The elderly also account for 65% of all cardiovascular hospitalizations, as well as an increasing proportion of all cardiovascular procedures (Table 1).

For these reasons, it is important for the practitioner to have an understanding of the effects of aging on the cardiovascular system, a working knowledge of cardiovascular therapeutics in the elderly, and an appreciation of the limitations of currently available data relevant to the treatment of older cardiac patients.

EFFECTS OF AGING ON THE CARDIOVASCULAR SYSTEM

Aging is associated with diffuse changes in cardiovascular structure and function (Table 2) *(1)*. From the clinical perspective, the principal effects of aging are as follows:

- Increased vascular stiffness, resulting in increased impedance to left ventricular ejection
- Impaired ventricular filling, due to altered relaxation and decreased ventricular compliance
- Diminished responsiveness to β-adrenergic stimulation
- Reduced capacity to augment adenosine triphosphate (ATP) production in response to increased demands
- Impaired endothelial function
- Progressive decline in sinus node function

These changes affect disease expression, clinical manifestations, and response to therapy in older patients. Thus, increased vascular stiffness contributes to the progressive rise in systolic blood pressure with advancing age. In turn, systolic hypertension is a key risk factor for coronary heart disease, heart failure, and stroke in the elderly.

Impaired diastolic filling, a hallmark of cardiovascular aging, is caused by increased interstitial collagen deposition, compensatory myocyte hypertrophy, and altered calcium flux leading to impaired relaxation during early diastole. These changes result in decreased filling during early and

From: *Essential Cardiology: Principles and Practice, 2nd Ed.*
Edited by: C. Rosendorff © Humana Press Inc., Totowa, NJ

Table 1
Major Cardiovascular Procedures by Age: 2000

	<45		Age, yr 45–64		≥65	
	No.[a]	%	No.[a]	%	No.[a]	%
Cardiac catheterization	122	(9.3)	550	(41.7)	646	(49.0)
Percutaneous coronary revascularization	62	(6.1)	437	(42.7)	524	(51.2)
Coronary bypass surgery	17	(3.3)	216	(41.6)	286	(55.1)
Permanent pacemaker	—	(NA)	20	(13.4)	129	(86.6)
Implanted cardioverter-defibrillator	—	(NA)	10	(31.2)	22	(68.8)
Carotid endarterectomy	—	(NA)	32	(26.0)	91	(74.0)

[a]In thousands. (Adapted from ref. *111*.)

Table 2
Effects of Aging on the Cardiovascular System

Gross anatomy
    Increased left ventricular wall thickness
    Decreased left ventricular cavity size
    Endocardial thickening and sclerosis
    Increased left atrial size
    Valvular fibrosis and sclerosis
    Increased epicardial fat
Histology
    Increased lipid and amyloid deposition
    Increased collagen degeneration and fibrosis
    Calcification of fibrous skeleton, valve rings, and coronary arteries
    Shrinkage of myocardial fibers with focal hypertrophy
    Decreased mitochondria, altered mitochondrial membranes
    Decreased nucleus:myofibril size ratio
Biochemical changes
    Decreased protein elasticity
    Numerous changes in enzyme content and activity affecting most metabolic pathways, but no change
        in myosin ATPase activity
    Decreased catechol synthesis, esp. norepinephrine
    Decreased acetylcholine synthesis
Conduction system
    Degeneration of sinus node pacemaker and transition cells
    Decreased number of conducting cells in the AV-node and HIS–Purkinje system
    Increased connective tissue, fat, and amyloid
    Increased calcification around conduction system
Vasculature
    Decreased distensibility of large and medium-sized arteries
    Aorta and muscular arteries become dilated, elongated, and tortuous
    Increased wall thickness
    Increased connective tissue and calcification
Autonomic nervous system
    Decreased responsiveness to β-adrenergic stimulation
    Increased circulating catecholamines, decreased tissue catecholamines
    Decreased α-adrenergic receptors in left ventricle
    Decreased cholinergic responsiveness
    Diminished response to Valsalva and baroreceptor stimulation
    Decreased heart rate variability

Table 3
Effects of Aging on Other Organ Systems

Kidneys
    Gradual decline in glomerular filtration rate, ~8 cc/min/decade
    Impaired fluid and electrolyte homeostasis
Lungs
    Reduced ventilatory capacity
    Increased ventilation/perfusion mismatching
Neurohumoral system
    Reduced cerebral perfusion autoregulatory capacity
    Diminished reflex responsiveness
    Impaired thirst mechanism
Hemostatic system
    Increased levels of coagulation factors
    Increased platelet activity and aggregability
    Increased inflammatory cytokines and C-reactive protein
    Increased inhibitors of fibrinolysis and angiogenesis

mid-diastole, and are accompanied by increased reliance on atrial contraction to optimize left ventricular end-diastolic volume. Clinical implications of these alterations include a progressive rise in the prevalence of atrial fibrillation and in the syndrome of heart failure with normal left ventricular systolic function, and a diminished capacity to augment stroke volume via the Frank-Starling mechanism *(2)*.

The effects of reduced responsiveness to β-adrenergic stimulation include a linear decline of approx 10 beats per decade in the maximum attainable heart rate, reduced ability to augment contractility, and impaired β_2-mediated vasodilation. Taken together, these effects greatly reduce the capacity of the older heart to increase cardiac output in response to increased demands, and this capacity is further diminished by the inability of cardiac mitochondria to maximally upregulate ATP production in response to increased energy requirements.

Impaired endothelial function contributes to the development of atherosclerosis and limits coronary artery vasodilation, thereby reducing maximum coronary blood flow. These changes predispose older adults to the development of coronary heart disease and also lower the coronary ischemic threshold.

Finally, degenerative changes in the sinus node and atrial conducting tissues result in a rising prevalence of "sick sinus syndrome" with advancing age, and predispose older individuals to the development of supraventricular tachyarrhythmias, especially atrial fibrillation. As shown in Table 1, more than 80% of permanent pacemakers are implanted in individuals over 65 yr of age, and sinus node dysfunction is by far the most common indication for pacemaker insertion.

In addition to age-related changes in the cardiovascular system, there are also important changes in renal, pulmonary, neurohumoral, and hemostatic function that have important implications for older patients with cardiovascular disease (Table 3). Older patients are also subject to numerous medical, behavioral, psychosocial, and financial influences that may have an impact on symptomatology, adherence to prescribed therapy, and overall prognosis. Finally, aging is associated with significant changes in the absorption, distribution, metabolism, and elimination of virtually all medications.

CARDIOVASCULAR RISK FACTORS

In general, the major risk factors for cardiovascular disease are similar in older and younger patients, but the relative importance of some risk factors (e.g., smoking, total cholesterol) declines with age. However, since the prevalence of cardiovascular disease increases with age, the clinical significance of these risk factors is maintained or even increases with age.

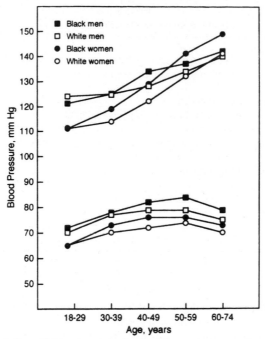

Fig. 1. Average systolic and diastolic blood pressure in the US population as a function of age, sex, and race: NHANES III. (From ref. *112*, reproduced with permission. Copyright 1995 Lippincott Williams & Wilkins.)

Relative vs Attributable Risk

Relative risk refers to the likelihood that an individual with a given risk factor will develop a specific disease, as compared to an individual without that risk factor. *Attributable risk* refers to the actual number of cases of a disease that can be attributed to the presence of a specific risk factor. As such, the attributable risk reflects both relative risk and disease prevalence, and it provides a more accurate estimate of the potential impact of risk factor modification (i.e., the number of cases prevented by the eradication of a given risk factor). Stated another way, since older individuals are at higher risk for developing cardiovascular disease, the potential benefit of treating a specific risk factor is often greater in older than in younger patients, even though the relative risk may be lower in the elderly.

Hypertension

As shown in Fig. 1, systolic blood pressure increases with age in both men and women, whereas diastolic blood pressure tends to peak and plateau in middle age, then declines slightly at older age. Although systolic and diastolic blood pressure are each independent risk factors for cardiovascular disease in the elderly, systolic hypertension is more common, and it is also a more powerful risk factor.

To date there have been at least 10 prospective, randomized, placebo-controlled clinical trials evaluating the effects of antihypertensive therapy in the elderly (Table 4) *(3–13)*. Six of these studies focused on diastolic hypertension *(3–9)*, three enrolled patients with isolated systolic hypertension *(10–12)*, and one included subjects with either systolic or diastolic hypertension *(13)*. These studies provide compelling evidence that treatment of systolic and diastolic hypertension substantially reduces the incidence of stroke, coronary heart disease, and cardiac failure in older adults. Moreover, the benefits of treating diastolic hypertension persist at least up to the age of 80, while the benefits of treating systolic hypertension are apparent at least up to the age of 90.

Table 4
Trials of Antihypertensive Treatment in the Elderly

Trial (ref.)	n	Age	Risk reduction (%)			
			CVA	CAD	CHF	All CVD
Australian (3)	582	60–69	33%	18%	NR	31%
EWPHE (4)	840	>60	36%	20%	22%	29%
Coope (5)	884	60–79	42%	−3%	32%	24%
STOP-HTN (6)	1627	70–84	47%	13%	51%	40%
MRC (7)	4396	65–74	25%	19%	NR	17%
HDFP (8,9)	2374	60–69	44%	15%	NR	16%
SHEP (10)	4736	≥60	33%	27%	55%	32%
Syst-Eur (11)	4695	≥60	42%	26%	36%	31%
STONE (13)	1632	60–79	57%	6%	68%	60%
Syst-China (12)	2394	≥60	38%	33%	38%	37%

CAD, coronary artery disease; CHF, congestive heart failure; CVA, cerebrovascular accident; CVD, cardiovascular disease; EWPHE, European Working Party on High Blood Pressure in the Elderly; HDFP, Hypertension Detection and Follow-up Program; MRC, Medical Research Council; NR, not reported; SHEP, Systolic Hypertension in the Elderly Program; STONE, Shanghai Trial of Nifedipine in the Elderly; STOP-HTN, Swedish Trial in Old Patients with Hypertension; Syst-China, Systolic Hypertension in China; Syst-Eur, Systolic Hypertension in Europe.

Treatment of hypertension is similar in older and younger patients (14). However, older patients are more susceptible to adverse drug reactions, so therapy should generally be initiated with lower drug dosages, and close follow-up is essential to assess efficacy and tolerability.

Hyperlipidemia

In men, total cholesterol levels tend to peak in late middle age, then decline modestly at older age (15). In the absence of estrogen replacement, cholesterol levels rise rapidly after menopause in women, surpassing those in men after the age of 60. In the Framingham Heart Study, the importance of total cholesterol as a risk factor for coronary heart disease declined with age, but the ratio of total cholesterol to high-density lipoprotein cholesterol (HDL-C) remained a strong independent risk factor in both men and women at older age (16). Similar findings from other studies confirm the importance of hyperlipidemia as a cardiovascular risk factor in the elderly.

In the Heart Protection Study, 40 mg simvastatin daily was associated with significant reductions in death, myocardial infarction, and stroke in patients 40 to 80 yr of age with vascular disease or diabetes, and the benefits were similar in older and younger patients (17). More recently, the PROSPER study (**PRO**spective **S**tudy of **P**ravastatin in the **E**lderly at **R**isk) showed that 40 mg/d pravastatin reduced the risk of myocardial infarction, stroke, or coronary heart disease death by 15% in patients 70 to 82 yr of age with established vascular disease, diabetes, hypertension, or current smoking (18). Age-specific subgroup analyses from several earlier trials also provide strong evidence that treatment with an HMG-CoA reductase inhibitor ("statin") reduces mortality and nonfatal coronary events in patients up to the age of 75 (Table 5) (19–22). Based on these trials, an HMG-CoA reductase inhibitor, in conjunction with an appropriate low-fat diet, is recommended for older individuals with manifest coronary heart disease, peripheral arterial disease, or prevalent risk factors in the absence of other major life-limiting illnesses.

Diabetes

The prevalence of diabetes increases with age, approaching 20% in persons over age 65. Diabetes is somewhat more common in older men than in older women, and it is significantly more common in African-Americans and Hispanics than in Caucasians. Diabetes remains a potent independent

Table 5
Impact of HMG-CoA Reductase Inhibitors on Coronary Events

		Risk reduction (%)	
	n	Coronary events	Death
4S (19)			
<65 yr	3423	34%	28%
65–70 yr	1021	34%	34%
CARE (20)			
<65 yr	2876	19%	−11%
65–75 yr	1283	32%	45%
LIPID (21)			
<65 yr	5500	23%	NR
65–75 yr	3514	21%	NR
AFCAPS/TexCAPS (22)			
≤median age[a]	3425	46%	NR
>median age	3180	30%	NR

[a]57 Years in men, 62 yr in women.
4S, Scandinavian Simvastatin Survival Study; CARE, Cholesterol and Recurrent Events; LIPID, Long-Term Intervention with Pravastatin in Ischemic Disease; AFCAPS/TexCAPS, Air Force/Texas Coronary Atherosclerosis Prevention Study; NR, not reported.

risk factor for coronary heart disease and other cardiovascular diseases at older age. In the Framingham Heart Study, the relative risk for coronary heart disease in diabetic men over age 65 was 1.4, while in women diabetes conferred a relative risk of 2.1. In both men and women, the excess risk for coronary heart disease in diabetics is greater in persons over 65 yr of age than in younger individuals.

Management of diabetes is similar in younger and older patients. In addition to maintaining effective glucose control, hypertension should be treated to a target blood pressure of <130/80 mmHg (14), the LDL-cholesterol fraction should be reduced to <100 mg/dL (23), weight should be maintained in a desirable range (body mass index <25 kg/m^2), regular exercise should be encouraged, and tobacco use should be strongly discouraged. As noted above, the Heart Protection Study provides strong evidence that statin therapy reduces mortality and nonfatal vascular events in older diabetics (17,24). In addition, data from the Heart Outcomes Prevention Evaluation (HOPE) indicate that an angiotensin-converting enzyme inhibitor is effective in reducing cardiovascular morbidity and mortality in diabetic patients over age 55 (25,26).

Smoking

Smoking prevalence declines with age due to smoking-related mortality and successful smoking cessation. Nonetheless, continued smoking remains an important risk factor for myocardial infarction and stroke in older individuals. Moreover, there is strong evidence that smoking cessation is beneficial at all ages. In the Coronary Artery Surgery Study (CASS) Registry, for example, coronary patients over 70 yr of age who continued to smoke had a 3.3-fold higher risk of death and a 2.9-fold higher risk of death or myocardial infarction during a 6-yr follow-up period compared with those who stopped smoking (27).

The efficacy of smoking cessation programs, nicotine replacement therapy, and other medications (e.g., bupropion) in elderly smokers is unknown, but older smokers tend to be more receptive to counseling interventions than younger individuals. In addition, the motivation to quit smoking often peaks following an index cardiovascular event, and the importance of smoking cessation should be strongly emphasized in individuals of all ages who suffer such an event.

Other Risk Factors

Left ventricular hypertrophy, physical inactivity, obesity, and elevated levels of C-reactive protein, fibrinogen, and homocysteine are all associated with increased risk for cardiovascular disease in older men and women. In addition, data from the Cardiovascular Health Study indicate that increased carotid artery intima-medial thickness and an ankle-arm blood pressure index less than 0.9 are predictive of an increased risk for incident cardiovascular events in older adults *(28)*. The impact of treating these risk factors in elderly patients is presently unknown.

CORONARY ARTERY DISEASE

Acute Myocardial Infarction

The incidence of acute myocardial infarction (MI) increases with age in both men and women. In 1999, 61.4% of patients hospitalized with acute MI in the US were over 65 yr of age, and 36.8% were over the age of 75. Case fatality rates increase with age, and 84% of deaths due to acute MI occur in patients over age 65, while 60% occur in patients over age 75. In addition, women comprise nearly half of all patients with acute MI over age 65, and MI is the leading cause of death in both men and women in this age group.

CLINICAL MANIFESTATIONS

After age 75, patients with acute MI are less likely to present with typical ischemic chest discomfort, and shortness of breath is the most common initial symptom in patients over the age of 80 *(29)*. Diaphoresis occurs less frequently at older age, whereas nonspecific neurological symptoms, such as lightheadedness, confusion, or syncope, are more common in the elderly, and may be the presenting manifestation in up to 20% of MI patients over the age of 85.

Older MI patients often present with nondiagnostic electrocardiograms (ECGs), due to the presence of preexisting ECG abnormalities (e.g., paced rhythm, left bundle branch block, or left ventricular hypertrophy) and a high prevalence of non-ST elevation MI (NSTEMI). The combination of atypical symptomatology and a nondiagnostic ECG may obfuscate the diagnosis unless a high index of suspicion is maintained. Lack of diagnostic certainty is also an important factor contributing to reduced utilization of reperfusion therapy and other interventions in older patients.

In addition to increased mortality, older patients with acute MI are more likely to develop heart failure, hypotension, atrial fibrillation, conduction abnormalities, myocardial rupture, and cardiogenic shock. Although ventricular arrhythmias are also more common in the elderly, older patients are less likely to develop primary ventricular fibrillation.

REPERFUSION THERAPY

A series of prospective randomized placebo-controlled trials completed in the 1980s established the efficacy of fibrinolytic therapy for reducing mortality in patients up to 75 yr of age with acute MI, but the value of fibrinolysis in patients over age 75 has been somewhat controversial *(30,31)*. However, a recent reanalysis of data from the large Fibrinolytic Therapy Trialists' overview confirmed that fibrinolytic treatment is associated with lower mortality in patients over age 75 with ST elevation or left bundle branch block MI who present within 12 h of symptom onset (Table 6) *(32)*. Note that the absolute mortality benefit, as defined by the number of lives saved per 1000 patients treated, was twofold greater in patients over age 75 than in patients under age 55, and similar to that seen in patients 55 to 74 yr of age *(32)*.

Intracranial hemorrhage occurs in 0.3 to 0.5% of patients receiving fibrinolytic therapy for acute MI, but the risk increases with advancing age. Other major bleeding complications occur slightly more frequently in patients receiving fibrinolysis, but the risk is not age-dependent *(33)*.

The choice of fibrinolytic agent in patients over the age of 75 remains controversial. In the Global Utilization of Streptokinase and rt-PA for Occluded Arteries (GUSTO-I) trial, recombinant tissue plasminogen activator (rt-PA) was associated with a somewhat lower mortality rate than streptokinase in patients over age 75 (19.3% vs 20.6%), but the difference was not statistically

Table 6
Effect of Fibrinolytic Treatment on 35-d Mortality in Patients With ST-Elevation
or Left Bundle Branch Block Myocardial Infarction Presenting Within 12 h
of Symptom Onset: Reanalysis of Data From the Fibrinolytic Therapy Trialists' Overview

Age (yr)	n	Mortality, control	Mortality, fibrinolysis	Relative risk reduction	Lives saved/ 1000 patients
<55	10,047	5.4%	3.8%	29.6%	16
55–64	12,252	10.7%	8.1%	24.3%	26
65–74	10,053	19.0%	15.0%	21.1%	40
≥75	3322	29.4%	26.0%	11.6%	34

significant *(34)*. In addition, rt-PA was associated with more intracranial hemorrhages in this age group (2.1% vs 1.2% with streptokinase, *p* < .05).

Percutaneous transluminal coronary angioplasty (PTCA) is an effective alternative to thrombolytic therapy in patients with acute MI, and it is associated with improved patency rates and fewer intracranial hemorrhages than thrombolysis. Among 300 patients over age 70 enrolled in the GUSTO-IIb trial, which compared PTCA with rt-PA in patients with acute MI, the composite endpoint of death, reinfarction, or disabling stroke tended to occur less frequently in patients randomized to PTCA *(35)*. More recently, de Boer and colleagues found that PTCA was associated with improved outcomes relative to streptokinase in a small randomized trial involving 87 patients 75 yr of age or older with acute MI *(36)*. These findings suggest that primary PTCA may be the preferred reperfusion strategy in appropriately selected elderly patients. However, to date very few patients over the age of 80 have been studied, and the value of PTCA in this age group remains undefined.

ASPIRIN

Among 3411 patients over 70 yr of age enrolled in the ISIS-2 trial, the administration of 162.5 mg aspirin daily to patients with acute myocardial infarction was associated with a 21% mortality reduction at 35 d *(37)*. Moreover, the *absolute* benefit of aspirin increased with advancing age, from 1.0% in patients under age 60 to 4.7% in those age 70 or older. Long-term aspirin use following MI also reduces the incidence of death, reinfarction, or stroke by approx 25% in patients of all ages.

CLOPIDOGREL

The addition of clopidogrel to aspirin reduces the risk of cardiovascular death, MI, or stroke by about 20% compared to aspirin alone during the 12-mo period following hospitalization for unstable angina or NSTEMI, with similar absolute benefits in patients younger or older than age 65 *(38)*. The value of clopidogrel in patients over age 75 and in those with STEMI is unknown, and the cost-effectiveness of routine clopidogrel therapy is uncertain *(39)*.

HEPARIN

Although older patients with acute MI often receive intravenous heparin, the value of this treatment is unproven. In a study involving 6935 Medicare patients hospitalized with acute MI, heparin use was associated with more bleeding complications and an increased length of hospital stay, but there was no evidence of a beneficial effect on mortality or reinfarction *(40)*.

Low-molecular-weight heparins (LMWHs) such as enoxaparin and dalteparin offer several advantages over conventional unfractionated heparin (UFH), and recent studies indicate that these agents are associated with improved clinical outcomes in patients with unstable coronary syndromes, including the elderly *(41–43)*. Based on these findings, subcutaneous LMWH is now preferred over intravenous UFH in the management of patients with acute MI or unstable angina.

GLYCOPROTEIN IIB/IIIA INHIBITORS

Glycoprotein IIb/IIIa inhibitors improve clinical outcomes in selected patients up to the age of 75 *(44–48)*, but the value of these agents in older patients is less clear. For example, in a trial involv-

Table 7
Mortality in 3 Large Trials of Intravenous β-Blockers:
Pooled Results by Age (Total *N* = 23,200)

	Younger (n = 14,687)	Older (n = 8513)
Mortality		
Control group	2.6%	8.9%
β-blocker group	2.5%	6.9%
Mortality reduction	5.0%	23.2%
Lives saved/100 patients	0.1	2.1
p-value	NS	0.0005

NS, not significant.

ing more than 10,000 patients, eptifibatide reduced the risk of death or nonfatal MI in patients up to the age of 80, but there was an increase in event rates among patients over 80 yr of age receiving eptifibatide *(48)*. In another study involving 1915 patients, tirofiban was associated with improved outcomes in patients younger or older than age 65, but outcomes for patients over age 75 were not reported *(47)*. Based on currently available evidence, the addition of a glycoprotein IIb/IIIa inhibitor to aspirin and heparin is recommended for patients with acute MI who are likely to undergo percutaneous coronary intervention. Treatment with either eptifibatide or tirofiban is also recommended for high-risk patients, including those over age 75, who are not expected to undergo early cardiac catheterization. It should be noted, however, that the risk of bleeding complications increases with age, and this may attenuate the benefit of glycoprotein IIb/IIIa inhibitors in the very elderly.

WARFARIN

Long-term warfarin following acute MI reduces the risk of death, reinfarction, and stroke in elderly patients *(49)*, and two recent studies found that the combination of aspirin and full-dose warfarin was superior to aspirin alone in reducing recurrent events after MI *(50,51)*. However, combination therapy was associated with an increased risk of bleeding, and very few patients over age 75 were included in these trials. For these reasons, warfarin use in the very elderly is generally restricted to patients who are intolerant of aspirin, and to those who have clear indications for long-term anticoagulation (e.g., chronic atrial fibrillation).

β-BLOCKERS

Table 7 summarizes data from three large randomized trials evaluating the use of intravenous β-blockers in patients with acute MI *(52)*. Intravenous β-blockade reduced mortality by 23% in older patients, but there was no significant effect in younger patients. In these trials, β-blockers also reduced the incidence of both supraventricular and ventricular arrhythmias, as well as recurrent ischemic events. Although these studies were conducted prior to the advent of reperfusion therapy, the results of these trials remain applicable today, since the majority of older patients with acute MI do not receive thrombolytic therapy or undergo primary PTCA.

Long-term β-blocker therapy is also associated with greater benefits in older than in younger patients (6.0 vs 2.1 lives saved per 100 treated patients) *(52)*. In addition, since event rates are higher in the elderly, β-blockade is more cost-effective in older than in younger individuals.

NITRATES

Nitrates can be administered safely to most elderly patients with acute MI, and data from the GISSI-3 trial indicate that early treatment with transdermal nitroglycerin is associated with favorable trends in mortality and in the combined endpoint of death, heart failure, or severe left ventricular dysfunction in patients over 70 yr of age *(53)*. The value of long-term nitroglycerin therapy following MI is unknown.

ANGIOTENSIN-CONVERTING ENZYME (ACE) INHIBITORS

In the GISSI-3 trial, treatment with lisinopril within 24 h of symptom onset reduced the combined endpoint of death, heart failure, or severe left ventricular dysfunction by 17% in patients over 70 yr of age (53). Similarly, in patients with anterior MI not receiving a thrombolytic agent, early treatment with zofenopril reduced the incidence of death or severe heart failure by 34%, and the absolute benefit was threefold greater in patients over 65 yr of age than in younger patients (54).

In patients with acute MI complicated by heart failure or left ventricular dysfunction (ejection fraction ≤40%), long-term ACE inhibitor therapy reduces mortality, hospitalizations, and heart failure progression, and the benefits of treatment are at least as great in older as in younger patients (55,56). Indeed, in the Acute Infarction Ramipril Efficacy (AIRE) trial, the mortality benefit of ramipril was limited to older patients (56). Since older patients are at greater risk for drug-induced hypotension and renal dysfunction, the use of these agents must be carefully monitored.

ANGIOTENSIN-RECEPTOR BLOCKERS

In the recently completed OPTIMAAL study (Optimal Trial in Myocardial Infarction with Angiotensin II Antagonist Losartan), which included 5477 patients 50 yr of age or older with acute MI complicated by heart failure or left ventricular dysfunction, mortality was higher (without reaching statistical significance) with the angiotensin-receptor blocker losartan than with the ACE inhibitor captopril, and these findings were consistent across age groups (57). Therefore, ACE inhibitors remain the preferred agents in post-MI patients. However, losartan was better tolerated than captopril, and angiotensin-receptor blockers are an acceptable alternative in patients who are unable to take an ACE inhibitor.

ALDOSTERONE ANTAGONISTS

Eplerenone is a selective aldosterone antagonist that has been shown to reduce mortality and cardiovascular hospitalizations following acute MI in patients with left ventricular dysfunction and heart failure (58). Although the efficacy of eplerenone was similar in younger and older patients, the role of this agent and other aldosterone antagonists in the routine management of older post-MI patients remains to be established.

ANTIARRHYTHMIC AGENTS

Antiarrhythmic agents have not been shown to reduce mortality or improve clinical outcomes in elderly MI patients, and the routine use of these agents is not recommended.

Non-ST Elevation MI

Non-ST elevation MI (NSTEMI) increases in frequency with advancing age, and accounts for more than 50% of all MIs in patients over the age of 70. Although the short-term prognosis following NSTEMI is more favorable than that following ST elevation MI, NSTEMI patients are at increased risk for reinfarction and death during follow-up.

In general, the treatment of NSTEMI is similar in younger and older patients (see Chapter 26), and recent studies indicate that early coronary angiography followed by percutaneous or surgical revascularization is associated with improved outcomes relative to conservative management in high-risk patients, including the elderly (59–61).

Chronic Coronary Artery Disease

Coronary artery disease (CAD) is highly prevalent in the elderly, and older patients account for more than half of hospital admissions for angina pectoris. Older CAD patients usually have more diffuse disease than younger patients, and they are more likely to have multivessel and left main coronary disease. Because older patients tend to be more sedentary than their younger counterparts, they are more likely to be asymptomatic or minimally symptomatic despite having more severe CAD. Older patients also have a higher prevalence of silent ischemia and infarction than younger patients.

The treatment of chronic CAD is similar in older and younger patients (*see* Chapter 25) and will not be reviewed here. However, a brief discussion of revascularization procedures is in order.

PERCUTANEOUS TRANSLUMINAL CORONARY ANGIOPLASTY

As shown in Table 1, more than 50% of PTCAs in the US are performed in patients over 65 yr of age. Compared with younger patients, older patients referred for PTCA are more likely to be female and have more severe symptoms, more comorbidity, and more complex "target" lesions *(62)*. These factors, in conjunction with age-related reductions in cardiovascular reserve, result in increased procedure-related morbidity and mortality in older patients, particularly those over the age of 80, and hospital mortality following elective PTCA in octogenarians ranges from 1 to 7% *(62)*. In addition, although late survival following successful PTCA in older patients is good, there is a higher incidence of recurrent angina than in younger patients, primarily due to incomplete revascularization.

CORONARY BYPASS SURGERY

Over 50% of all coronary artery bypass graft (CABG) operations in the US are performed in patients over age 65. As with PTCA, older patients referred for CABG are more likely to be female, have more advanced coronary disease, are more symptomatic, and have more comorbidity than younger patients. Perioperative mortality rates range from 5 to 10% in patients over age 75 undergoing isolated CABG, as compared to 1 to 2% in patients under age 65 *(63)*. Older patients also have a higher incidence of perioperative complications, including atrial fibrillation, heart failure, stroke, bleeding, cognitive dysfunction, respiratory disorders, and renal insufficiency. As a result, postoperative length of stay is substantially longer in older patients. Despite these difficulties, the long-term results following CABG in older patients are excellent, with up to 90% of patients experiencing sustained symptomatic improvement, and the majority reporting improved functional capacity and quality of life. In addition, a recent randomized trial comparing CABG to medical therapy in elderly patients with symptomatic angina found that CABG had a more favorable effect on symptoms and quality of life than medical therapy *(64)*.

VALVULAR HEART DISEASE

Aortic Valve

Aortic stenosis severe enough to warrant surgical consideration occurs in 2 to 3% of individuals over the age of 75, and aortic valve replacement is the second most common major cardiac operation in this age group (after CABG) *(65,66)*. Age-related degenerative changes occurring on a normal trileaflet aortic valve account for the majority of cases. Other causes include a congenitally bicuspid valve and rheumatic disease.

Aortic stenosis in the elderly is often occult because sedentary older individuals may experience few symptoms, or they may attribute their symptoms to "old age." Similarly, the physician may ascribe the symptoms of aortic stenosis to other causes. In addition, the murmur of aortic stenosis in older patients may be less prominent due to changes in chest wall geometry (increased anteroposterior diameter) and reduced stroke volume. An S_4 gallop is a nonspecific finding in older individuals, but the *absence* of an S_4 during sinus rhythm makes the diagnosis of severe aortic stenosis unlikely. The A_2 component of the second heart sound is frequently diminished in older patients with severe aortic stenosis, but this may be difficult to appreciate on routine examination. As a result of decreased vascular compliance, the carotid upstrokes may be well-preserved in older patients with severe aortic stenosis. In addition, although the electrocardiogram usually shows left ventricular hypertrophy with ST-segment and T-wave changes, these findings may be attributed to long-standing hypertension or other causes. For these reasons, echocardiography should be performed in all elderly patients with unexplained symptoms that could potentially be due to aortic stenosis. Cardiac catheterization should also be performed in patients with severe aortic stenosis who are suitable candidates for valve replacement.

Aortic valve replacement is the treatment of choice for severe aortic stenosis in adults of all ages. However, some elderly patients, such as those with dementia, advanced frailty, or major comorbidity, may not be suitable candidates for the procedure. The results of aortic valve replacement in the elderly are excellent, even in octogenarians, with several series reporting perioperative mortality rates of 4 to 7% for isolated valve replacement *(66)*. Mortality rates are somewhat higher when valve replacement is combined with CABG. The majority of patients experience marked improvement in symptoms and functional capacity following the procedure *(67,68)*, and long-term survival is comparable to the general population at similar age.

The prevalence of aortic regurgitation increases with age, but most cases are of insufficient severity to require surgery. Causes of acute aortic regurgitation in the elderly include type A aortic dissection, infective endocarditis, prosthetic valve dysfunction, and sinus of Valsalva rupture. Causes of chronic aortic regurgitation include rheumatic or calcific aortic valve disease, healed endocarditis, and aneurysms of the aortic root due to atherosclerosis, syphilis, or other disorders. Treatment of aortic regurgitation is similar in older and younger adults.

Mitral Valve

Mitral stenosis in the elderly is usually rheumatic in origin, but severe mitral valve annulus calcification can occasionally cause mitral stenosis in patients with small left ventricular cavities *(65)*. As in younger patients, the symptoms of mitral stenosis are often insidious, and it is not unusual for the diagnosis to be clinically unsuspected until echocardiography is performed. In most elderly patients with mitral stenosis, the valve apparatus is heavily calcified or there is significant mitral regurgitation, thus precluding percutaneous valvuloplasty or open commissurotomy. However, in elderly patients who are suitable candidates for valvuloplasty, the procedure can be performed safely, and it produces significant hemodynamic and clinical improvement in the majority of cases. In other patients with severe symptoms, mitral valve replacement offers the only viable therapeutic option *(66)*. As with aortic valve replacement, mitral valve surgery in elderly patients is associated with increased morbidity and mortality. The perioperative mortality rate for elective mitral valve surgery in elderly patients is 10 to 20%, although some centers are now reporting mortality rates of less than 10%.

Mitral regurgitation is the most common valvular lesion in elderly patients, but in most cases it is not severe enough to require surgical intervention. Common causes of mitral regurgitation in the elderly include ischemic mitral valve dysfunction, ischemic or nonischemic dilated cardiomyopathy, mitral valve prolapse, rheumatic heart disease, and mitral valve annulus calcification *(65)*. Less commonly, mitral regurgitation may be due to infective or noninfective endocarditis, prosthetic valve dysfunction, or hypertrophic cardiomyopathy. In patients with mild to moderate mitral regurgitation, medical management with afterload reduction (e.g., ACE inhibitors, hydralazine) is appropriate. In patients with severe symptomatic mitral regurgitation and satisfactory left ventricular function, surgical treatment should be considered. As in younger patients, mitral valve repair, when feasible, is associated with more favorable outcomes. Long-term results following successful mitral valve repair or replacement in elderly patients are generally favorable, with significant symptomatic improvement occurring in the majority of cases.

Infective Endocarditis

The incidence of infective endocarditis increases progressively with age, reflecting age-related changes in valve structure, the increasing prevalence of specific valvular pathologies in the elderly, and the increased prevalence of potential sources of bacteremia (e.g., poor dentition, respiratory and urinary tract infections, and procedures such as cystoscopy) *(69)*. The diagnosis of endocarditis in the elderly is often difficult, as the clinical manifestations are usually nonspecific and protean. The classical peripheral manifestations of endocarditis, such as Roth spots, Osler nodes, and Janeway lesions, are also uncommon in elderly patients.

In general, the causative organisms of endocarditis are similar in older and younger patients, with streptococci, staphylococci, and enterococci being the most common agents, followed by Gram-

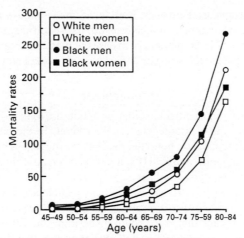

Fig. 2. Mortality rates for heart failure per 100,000 persons in the US by age, sex, and race: 1990. BF, black female; BM, black male; WF, white female; WM, white male. (Adapted from ref. *113*. Copyright 1993 with permission from Elsevier.)

negative bacilli and other less common pathogens. In addition, up to 10% of cases may be culture-negative, usually due to the initiation of antibiotic therapy prior to obtaining an adequate number of blood cultures. As in younger patients, vegetations are visualized with transthoracic echocardiography in less than 50% of cases, but the yield is substantially higher with the transesophageal approach. The treatment and complications of endocarditis are similar in older and younger patients, although mortality is higher in the elderly.

HEART FAILURE

The effects of aging on the cardiovascular system serve to markedly reduce cardiovascular reserve and predispose the older patient to the development of heart failure (HF). The prevalence of cardiovascular disease, particularly hypertension and CAD, also increases with age, and these factors combine to produce an exponential rise in HF with increasing age *(70)*. Indeed, HF is relatively uncommon in younger adults, but the prevalence doubles with each decade after age 45, and HF affects 1 in 10 individuals over the age of 80. As a result, HF is the most common indication for hospitalization in persons over age 65, and it is the most costly diagnosis-related group (DRG) by a factor of almost 2. HF is also a major cause of chronic disability in the elderly, and mortality rates from HF increase progressively with age (Fig. 2).

Hypertension is the most common antecedent illness in elderly patients with HF, and 70 to 80% of cases can be attributed to either hypertension or CAD. Valvular disease is the third most common cause of HF in the elderly, followed by nonischemic cardiomyopathy. Importantly, the prevalence of HF with preserved systolic function (so-called "diastolic HF") increases with age, and accounts for over 50% of cases after the age of 80.

HF in the elderly is both overdiagnosed and underdiagnosed. The cardinal symptoms of HF—shortness of breath, edema, fatigue, and exercise intolerance—are common in the elderly, and these symptoms are often attributed to HF even when caused by other disorders. Conversely, sedentary elderly individuals may not report exertional symptoms, and neurological symptoms, such as altered sensorium or irritability, or gastrointestinal disturbances, such as anorexia or bloating, may be the only overt manifestations of HF. Similarly, the physical findings are often nonspecific, and the chest radiograph may be difficult to interpret in patients with mild HF.

Recently, plasma B-type natriuretic peptide (BNP) levels have been shown to be a valuable aid in distinguishing dyspnea due to HF from that related to other causes, such as pulmonary disorders *(71)*. BNP levels tend to be elevated in both systolic and diastolic HF, and they also correlate with response to therapy and prognosis. However, BNP levels also increase with age in healthy individuals without HF, particularly women, and, as a result, the specificity and predictive accuracy of BNP levels decline with age *(72)*. Nonetheless, in cases of diagnostic uncertainty, a low or normal BNP level effectively excludes HF, whereas a markedly elevated level provides strong evidence in support of the diagnosis.

Management

The principal goals of HF management in elderly patients are to maximize quality of life, reduce medical resource utilization, and extend functional survival. In the past 25 yr, there have been major advances in the treatment of HF, but older patients are much less likely to receive aggressive therapy. In addition, management of older HF patients is often confounded by a variety of behavioral and psychosocial factors, particularly noncompliance, which contribute to the high rate of repetitive hospitalizations *(73)*. For these reasons, many centers are now utilizing a multidisciplinary disease management strategy for optimizing medication prescribing practices, enhancing compliance with medications and diet, and providing appropriate followup for older HF patients. Several studies have documented the efficacy of this approach in reducing hospitalizations and cost of care, while improving quality of life and overall compliance *(74,75)*.

Medical Therapy

In general, the pharmacologic treatment of patients with systolic HF is similar in older and younger patients (*see* Chapter 20). Considerations specific to the elderly are discussed briefly in the following paragraphs.

ACE INHIBITORS

Although none of the ACE inhibitor trials have specifically targeted older patients, the average age of patients in CONSENSUS (Cooperative North Scandinavian Enalapril Survival Study) was 71 yr *(76)*, and the beneficial effects of enalapril were also similar in older and younger patients enrolled in the SOLVD (Studies of Left Ventricular Dysfunction) trials *(77,78)*. Moreover, in the post-MI ACE inhibitor trials, the benefits of ACE inhibitors were, if anything, greater in older patients *(55,56)*, and meta-analyses of all the ACE inhibitor studies have concluded that there is substantial benefit in all age groups, including the elderly *(79,80)*. Thus, ACE inhibitors are indicated in all elderly individuals with significant left ventricular systolic dysfunction (ejection fraction <40–45%), whether or not overt HF symptoms are present. As in younger patients, the ACE inhibitor dosage should be gradually titrated to achieve a target daily dose of 150 mg captopril, 20 mg enalapril, or the equivalent. ACE inhibitors are usually well-tolerated in older patients, but hyperkalemia and renal dysfunction occur more frequently than in younger patients.

ANGIOTENSIN-RECEPTOR BLOCKERS

Angiotensin II receptor blockers (ARBs) have a more favorable side-effect profile than ACE inhibitors, and both valsartan and candesartan have been shown to improve clinical outcomes in patients with symptomatic HF and reduced left ventricular systolic function who are intolerant to ACE inhibitors *(81,82)*. Similarly, these agents have been shown to reduce mortality and hospitalizations when added to an ACE inhibitor *(83,84)*. In all these studies, the beneficial effects were similar in older and younger patients *(83,85)*. On the other hand, the effect of ARBs on mortality has not been shown to be equivalent to that of ACE inhibitors *(57,86)*, so that ACE inhibitors remain the preferred agents for patients with HF and impaired left ventricular systolic function.

OTHER VASODILATORS

The combination of hydralazine and isosorbide dinitrate increased survival relative to placebo in V-HeFT-I (**V**eterans **A**dministration **H**eart **F**ailure **T**rial) *(87)*, but was less effective than enalapril in V-HeFT-II *(88)*. Although few elderly patients were enrolled in these trials, this combination is an acceptable alternative to ACE inhibitors or ARBs in appropriately selected patients.

β-Blockers

Data from four large trials indicate that β-blockers improve ventricular function and reduce mortality and hospitalizations in patients with symptomatic systolic HF, including those with New York Heart Association class IV symptoms and persons up to 80 yr of age *(89–92)*. Use of β-blockers in older patients may be limited by a higher prevalence of bradyarrhythmias and severe chronic lung disease, and older patients may also be more susceptible to the development of fatigue and impaired exercise tolerance during long-term β-blocker administration. Nonetheless, β-blockers should be considered standard therapy in older patients with stable HF and no contraindications, especially those with underlying coronary heart disease or an elevated resting heart rate.

Digoxin

Digoxin improves symptoms and reduces hospitalizations in patients with symptomatic systolic HF treated with ACE inhibitors and diuretics, but has no effect on total or cardiovascular mortality *(93)*. Although these effects are similar in younger and older patients, including octogenarians *(94)*, a recent retrospective analysis has questioned the value of digoxin in women *(95)*.

The volume of distribution and renal clearance of digoxin decline with age. In addition, recent data indicate that the optimal therapeutic concentration for digoxin is 0.5 to 0.8 ng/mL *(96)*. For most older patients with preserved renal function (est. creatinine clearance ≥50 cc/min), 0.125 mg digoxin daily provides a therapeutic effect. Lower dosages should be used in patients with renal insufficiency. Although older patients are often thought to be at increased risk for digitalis toxicity, this was not confirmed in an analysis from the Digitalis Investigation Group (DIG) *(94)*.

Diuretics

Although conventional diuretics such as furosemide may not improve long-term outcomes in HF patients, diuretics remain a cornerstone of therapy due to their efficacy in relieving congestive symptoms and edema. Older patients are more susceptible to dehydration and to diuretic-induced electrolyte disturbances, so older patients receiving chronic diuretic therapy should be monitored closely with daily weights and periodic electrolyte assessments.

Aldosterone Antagonists

Spironolactone 12.5–50 mg daily added to standard therapy has been shown to reduce mortality by 30% in patients with class III–IV systolic HF, with similar benefits in older and younger patients *(97)*. Eplerenone, a selective aldosterone antagonist, has also been shown to reduce mortality and sudden cardiac death in patients with left ventricular dysfunction following acute myocardial infarction *(58)*. Spironolactone is contraindicated in patients with severe renal insufficiency or hyperkalemia, and up to 10% of patients develop painful gynecomastia. In addition, older patients receiving spironolactone in combination with an ACE inhibitor may be at increased risk for hyperkalemia, particularly in the presence of preexisting renal insufficiency or diabetes, and at doses in excess of 25 mg/d *(98)*.

Diastolic Heart Failure

As noted previously, up to 50% of older HF patients have preserved left ventricular systolic function; this represents a major clinical problem because few large-scale clinical trials have focused on treatment of this disorder.

Diuretics are effective in relieving congestion and edema, but they must be used cautiously because patients with diastolic dysfunction are dependent on a sufficient preload to maintain adequate stroke volume. Such patients are often "volume sensitive," and are prone to developing pulmonary edema with modest volume overload, while volume contraction and prerenal azotemia may occur in response to overdiuresis.

The only major trial reported to date that was specifically designed to address the treatment of patients with HF and preserved left ventricular systolic function is CHARM-Preserved (Candesartan

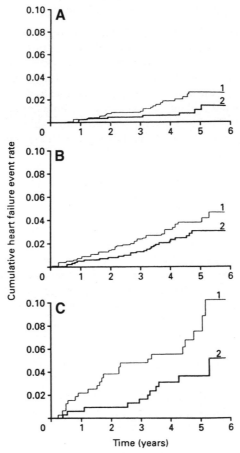

Fig. 3. Effect of antihypertensive drug therapy on the incidence of heart failure in the Systolic Hypertension in the Elderly Program (SHEP). (**A**) 60–69 yr; (**B**) 70–79 yr; (**C**) 80 yr and older. In each panel, line 1 represents placebo and line 2 represents active treatment. (From ref. *100*, reproduced with permission. Copyright 1997 American Medical Association.)

in **H**eart **F**ailure **A**ssessment of **R**eduction in **M**ortality and Morbidity) *(99)*. In this study, candesartan reduced HF hospitalizations but had no effect on mortality in patients with class II–IV HF and an ejection fraction >40%. Pending results from several ongoing studies, candesartan should be considered first-line therapy for the treatment of older patients with HF and preserved left ventricular systolic function. Additionally, data from the DIG ancillary study indicate that digoxin may reduce HF hospitalizations in patients with class II–III HF and an ejection fraction of 45% or greater *(93,94)*. Thus, digoxin may play a role in the management of patients with diastolic HF unresponsive to other agents.

Prevention

Given the high rates of morbidity and mortality in older patients with established HF, prevention of this disorder is clearly desirable. At the present time, the best preventive measures include aggressive treatment of hypertension and other known coronary risk factors. Indeed, based on data from the Systolic Hypertension in the Elderly Program (SHEP), treatment of hypertension may reduce the risk of incident HF by as much as 50% during a 5-yr followup period, and the benefit is most pronounced in patients 80 yr of age or older (Fig. 3) *(100)*.

ARRHYTHMIAS AND CONDUCTION DISORDERS

Supraventricular, ventricular, and bradyarrhythmias all increase in frequency with advancing age, as do supranodal, nodal, and infranodal conduction abnormalities. Each of these disorders is discussed briefly in the following paragraphs.

Supraventricular Arrhythmias

Atrial fibrillation is the most common and clinically important sustained supraventricular arrhythmia in older adults. The prevalence of atrial fibrillation increases from less than 1% in individuals under age 40 to more than 10% in those over the age of 80, and the median age of patients with atrial fibrillation is 75 yr. Atrial fibrillation is more common in men than in women at all ages, but the proportion of women increases with age.

Atrial fibrillation in the elderly is almost always associated with significant underlying cardiac disease, with hypertension, CAD, valvular heart disease, and sick-sinus syndrome being the most common precursors. Hyperthyroidism, alcoholism, nonischemic cardiomyopathies, chronic lung disease, and electrolyte disturbances (especially hypokalemia) are also important causes of atrial fibrillation in the elderly. In addition, atrial fibrillation frequently complicates major cardiac and noncardiac surgery in older patients.

The symptomatology of atrial fibrillation in the elderly is highly variable. Many patients are asymptomatic or experience only mild palpitations. Other patients describe fatigue, shortness of breath, or poor exercise tolerance, while still others present with acute pulmonary edema or stroke. In the Framingham Heart Study, the proportion of strokes attributable to atrial fibrillation increased from 1.5% in patients 50 to 59 yr of age to 23.5% in patients over the age of 80 *(101)*, thus demonstrating the importance of atrial fibrillation as a cause of stroke at older age.

Although it is clear that the risk of stroke in patients with atrial fibrillation increases with age, particularly after age 75, the management of atrial fibrillation in the very elderly remains somewhat controversial. The greatest effect of warfarin in reducing the absolute risk of thromboembolic stroke occurs in patients over age 75, but the risk of major bleeding complications, including intracranial hemorrhage, is also highest in this age group. However, despite concerns about bleeding risk, most experts recommend that patients over age 75 with chronic atrial fibrillation and no major contraindications be treated with warfarin to maintain an international normalized ratio (INR) in the range of 2.0 to 3.0. Aspirin is a less-effective alternative in patients who are ineligible for warfarin.

In patients with recent-onset atrial fibrillation, i.e., within 6 to 12 mo, many clinicians attempt cardioversion at least once, and prescribe antiarrhythmic drug therapy to maintain sinus rhythm following successful cardioversion. However, data from the AFFIRM (**A**trial **F**ibrillation **F**ollow-up **I**nvestigation of **R**hythm **M**anagement) trial and other studies indicate that a strategy of anticoagulation and rate control is associated with superior outcomes in patients with atrial fibrillation who are minimally symptomatic *(102,103)*.

The treatment of other supraventricular arrhythmias, including atrial flutter, is generally similar in older and younger patients, but the risk of antiarrhythmic drug toxicity is greater in the elderly.

Ventricular Arrhythmias

The prevalence and complexity of ventricular ectopic activity increase with age, with men being affected more often than women *(104)*. As in younger patients, the prognostic significance of ventricular arrhythmias is primarily related to the underlying cardiac disease. Therefore, therapy should be directed at the primary disorder (e.g., CAD, hypertension), and the arrhythmias should be treated only if they are highly symptomatic or life-threatening. When indicated, treatment is similar in older and younger patients. In particular, age is not a contraindication to an implanted cardioverter-defibrillator (ICD). Indeed, the majority of ICD recipients are over age 65 (Table 1), and long-term survival is similar in older and younger patients.

Bradyarrhythmias and Conduction Disturbances

Aging is associated with degenerative changes throughout the conduction system, and the prevalence of virtually all bradyarrhythmias and conduction abnormalities increases with age. From the clinical perspective, "sick sinus syndrome" is the most important disorder of the conduction system in older adults (105). Increasing age is associated with a decline in the number of functioning pacemaker cells in the sinus node, and by age 75 only about 10% of the cells remain capable of initiating an impulse. In addition, conduction of the impulse from the sinus node to the atrial tissues may be impaired (sinus exit block), and conduction within the atria and through the AV node may also be delayed. Sick sinus syndrome thus represents a generalized disorder of sinoatrial function that is often manifested by both bradyarrhythmias and supraventricular tachyarrhythmias (tachy-brady syndrome). Importantly, most medications used to treat the tachyarrhythmias, including β-blockers, diltiazem, verapamil, and antiarrhythmic agents, may exacerbate the bradyarrhythmias.

Bradyarrhythmias commonly associated with sick sinus syndrome include marked sinus bradycardia, sinus pauses and sinus arrest, sinus exit block, advanced AV-nodal block, and atrial fibrillation with slow ventricular response. These arrhythmias can produce a spectrum of symptoms ranging from fatigue, shortness of breath, angina, or reduced exercise tolerance to dizziness, impaired cognition, or syncope. In patients with major symptoms directly attributable to bradycardia, permanent pacemaker implantation is indicated. In the US, more than 80% of all pacemakers are inserted in older individuals (Table 1), and sick sinus syndrome is the most common underlying disorder. For patients in sinus rhythm, dual-chamber pacing is associated with a lower risk for developing atrial fibrillation, fewer hospitalizations for HF, and an improved quality of life compared to single-chamber ventricular pacing (106).

Cardiopulmonary Resuscitation

The value of cardiopulmonary resuscitation (CPR) in elderly patients remains a matter of debate. Fewer than 10% of older patients who suffer cardiac arrest and receive CPR survive beyond 30 d with favorable neurological outcomes (107). In addition, there is little difference in outcome whether the arrest occurs in a hospital, nursing home, or community setting. Despite these grim statistics, a subgroup of older patients with substantially better outcomes can be identified. For example, previously healthy individuals who receive prompt CPR for a witnessed cardiac arrest and who are subsequently found to be in ventricular fibrillation have a 25 to 40% likelihood of surviving with a good neurological outcome. Thus, although the decision to initiate CPR must be based on both clinical and psychosocial considerations, the results of CPR can be quite gratifying in selected patients, even at an elderly age.

EXERCISE AND CARDIAC REHABILITATION

As in younger patients, physical inactivity is a risk factor for cardiovascular events in older adults, and regular physical exercise is associated with improved health status and sense of well-being in the elderly. In addition, the benefits of cardiac rehabilitation following myocardial infarction or cardiac surgery are comparable in older and younger patients (108,109). Despite these considerations, physicians are less likely to recommend regular exercise or cardiac rehabilitation for older patients with or without cardiovascular disease. Nonetheless, the dictum "use it or lose it" is most applicable in the elderly, and maintaining a physically, intellectually, and emotionally active lifestyle is perhaps the best approach for preserving independence and ensuring a high quality of life in older individuals.

ETHICAL ISSUES AND END-OF-LIFE CARE

As discussed throughout this chapter, older patients with cardiovascular disease are at increased risk for a multitude of complications, including death. Elderly individuals maintain widely divergent views about the use of life-sustaining interventions and other invasive medical procedures, as well as what constitutes an acceptable quality of life in the face of chronic or terminal illness *(110)*. Moreover, studies have shown that patient surrogates, including spouses and physicians, are unable to reliably predict a patient's wishes in specific end-of-life scenarios. In order to ensure that a patient's wishes are honored if and when the patient is no longer capable of communicating his or her preferences, the physician should make an effort to address these issues at a time when the patient is still competent and lucid. The patient should also be encouraged to develop a living will and appoint a durable power of attorney. In addition, in patients with a progressive illness such as HF, it is helpful to discuss where the patient wishes to spend his or her final days. Potentially suitable environments include the home, a chronic-care facility, or a hospital. Palliative care through a reputable hospice should also be considered in older patients with terminal cardiovascular disease.

SUMMARY AND CONCLUSIONS

Aging is associated with extensive changes in cardiovascular structure and physiology, many of which have a direct impact on the clinical manifestations, response to treatment, and prognosis of cardiovascular disease in older adults. As a general principle, older patients are at increased risk for adverse outcomes, and the potential benefits to be derived from specific therapeutic interventions are therefore greater in older than in younger patients. Although additional research is needed to define the precise role of many therapies in older patients, the available evidence strongly suggests that age alone is not a sufficient justification for withholding treatment. Similarly, it is evident that more effective preventive strategies are needed to reduce the tremendous physical, emotional, and financial burden imposed on our society by cardiovascular disease in our ever-expanding elderly population.

REFERENCES

1. Lakatta EG. Age-associated cardiovascular changes in health: impact on cardiovascular disease in older persons. Heart Failure Reviews 2002;7:29–49.
2. Kitzman DW, Higginbotham MB, Cobb FR, et al. Exercise intolerance in patients with heart failure and preserved left ventricular systolic function: failure of the Frank-Starling mechanism. J Am Coll Cardiol 1991;17:1065–1072.
3. Management Committee. Treatment of mild hypertension in the elderly. Med J Aust 1981;II:398–402.
4. Amery A, Birkenhager W, Brixko P, et al. Mortality and morbidity results from the European Working Party on High Blood Pressure in the Elderly Trial. Lancet 1985;I:1349–1354.
5. Coope J, Warrender TS. Randomised trial of treatment of hypertension in elderly patients in primary care. BMJ 1986;293:1145–1151.
6. Dahlof B, Lindholm LH, Hannson L, et al. Morbidity and mortality in the Swedish Trial in Old Patients with Hypertension (STOP-Hypertension). Lancet 1991;338:1281–1285.
7. MRC Working Party. Medical Research Council Trial of Treatment of Hypertension in Older Adults: principal results. BMJ 1992;304:405–412.
8. Hypertension Detection and Follow-up Program Cooperative Group. Five-year findings of the Hypertension Detection and Follow-up Program. I. Reduction in mortality of persons with high blood pressure, including mild hypertension. JAMA 1979;242:2562–2571.
9. Hypertension Detection and Follow-up Program Cooperative Group. Five-year findings of the Hypertension Detection and Follow-up Program. II. Mortality by race, sex and age. JAMA 1979;242:2572–2577.
10. The Systolic Hypertension in the Elderly Program (SHEP) Cooperative Research Group. Prevention of stroke by antihypertensive drug treatment in older persons with isolated systolic hypertension: final results of SHEP. JAMA 1991;265:3255–3264.
11. Staessen JA, Fagard R, Thijs L, et al. Randomised double-blind comparison of placebo and active treatment for older patients with isolated systolic hypertension. The Systolic Hypertension in Europe (Syst-Eur) Trial Investigators. Lancet 1997;350:757–764.
12. Liu L, Wang JG, Gong L, et al. Comparison of active treatment and placebo in older Chinese patients with isolated systolic hypertension. Systolic Hypertension in China (Syst-China) Collaborative Group. J Hypertens 1998;16:1823–1829.
13. Gong L, Zhang W, Zhu Y, et al. Shanghai Trial of Nifedipine in the Elderly (STONE). J Hypertens 1996;14:1237–1245.
14. Chobanian AV, Bakris GL, Black HR, et al. The Seventh Report of the Joint National Committee on Prevention, Detection, Evaluation, and Treatment of High Blood Pressure: the JNC 7 report. JAMA 2003;289:2560–2572.

15. Johnson CL, Rifkind BM, Sempos CT, et al. Declining serum total cholesterol levels among U.S. adults. The National Health and Nutrition Examination Surveys. JAMA 1993;269:3002–3008.

16. Kannel WB, Wilson PWF. An update on coronary risk factors. Med Clin North Am 1995;79:951–971.

17. Heart Protection Study Collaborative Group. MRC/BHF Heart Protection Study of cholesterol lowering with simvastatin in 20,536 high-risk individuals: a randomised placebo-controlled trial. Lancet 2002;360:7–22.

18. Shepherd J, Blauw GJ, Murphy MB, et al. Pravastatin in elderly individuals at risk of vascular disease (PROSPER): a randomised controlled trial. Lancet 2002;360:1623–1630.

19. Miettinen TA, Pyorala K, Olsson AG, et al. Cholesterol-lowering therapy in women and elderly patients with myocardial infarction or angina pectoris. Findings from the Scandinavian Simvastatin Survival Study (4S). Circulation 1997;96:4211–4218.

20. Lewis SJ, Moye LA, Sacks FM, et al. Effect of pravastatin on cardiovascular events in older patients with myocardial infarction and cholesterol levels in the average range. Results of the Cholesterol and Recurrent Events (CARE) Trial. Ann Intern Med 1998;129:681–689.

21. The Long-Term Intervention with Pravastatin in Ischaemic Disease (LIPID) Study Group. Prevention of cardiovascular events and death with pravastatin in patients with coronary heart disease and a broad range of initial cholesterol levels. N Engl J Med 1998;339:1349–1357.

22. Downs JR, Clearfield M, Weis S, et al. Primary prevention of acute coronary events with lovastatin in men and women with average cholesterol levels: results of AFCAPS/TexCAPS. Air Force/Texas Coronary Atherosclerosis Prevention Study. JAMA 1998;279:1615–1622.

23. National Cholesterol Education Program (NCEP) Expert Panel on Detection, Evaluation, and Treatment of High Blood Cholesterol in Adults (Adult Treatment Panel III). Third Report of the National Cholesterol Education Program (NCEP) Expert Panel on Detection, Evaluation, and Treatment of High Blood Cholesterol in Adults (Adult Treatment Panel III) final report. Circulation 2002;106:3143–3421.

24. Collins R, Armitage J, Parish S, et al. MRC/BHF Heart Protection Study of cholesterol-lowering with simvastatin in 5963 people with diabetes: a randomised placebo-controlled trial. Lancet 2003;361:2005–2016.

25. Yusuf S, Sleight P, Pogue J, et al. Effects of an angiotensin-converting-enzyme inhibitor, ramipril, on cardiovascular events in high-risk patients. The Heart Outcomes Prevention Evaluation Study Investigators. N Engl J Med 2000;342:145–153.

26. Heart Outcomes Prevention Evaluation Study Investigators. Effects of ramipril on cardiovascular and microvascular outcomes in people with diabetes mellitus: results of the HOPE study and MICRO-HOPE substudy. Lancet 2000;355:253–259.

27. Hermanson B, Omenn GS, Kronmal RA, Gersh BJ, and participants in the Coronary Artery Surgery Study. Beneficial six-year outcome of smoking cessation in older men and women with coronary artery disease. N Engl J Med 1988;319:1365–1369.

28. Psaty BM, Furberg CD, Kuller LH, et al. Traditional risk factors and subclinical disease measures as predictors of first myocardial infarction in older adults: the Cardiovascular Health Study. Arch Intern Med 1999;159:1339–1347.

29. Tresch DD. Management of the older patient with acute myocardial infarction: difference in clinical presentations between older and younger patients. J Am Geriatr Soc 1998;46:1157–1162.

30. Thiemann DR, Coresh J, Schulman SP, et al. Lack of benefit for intravenous thrombolysis in patients with myocardial infarction who are older than 75 years. Circulation 2000;101:2239–2246.

31. Berger AK, Radford MJ, Wang Y, Krumholz HM. Thrombolytic therapy in older patients. J Am Coll Cardiol 2000;36:366–374.

32. White HD. Thrombolytic therapy in the elderly. Lancet 2000;356:2028–2030.

33. Fibrinolytic Therapy Trialists' (FTT) Collaborative Group. Indications for fibrinolytic therapy in suspected acute myocardial infarction: collaborative overview of early mortality and major morbidity results from all randomised trials of more than 1000 patients. Lancet 1994;343:311–322.

34. The GUSTO Investigators. An international randomized trial comparing four thrombolytic strategies for acute myocardial infarction. N Engl J Med 1993;329:673–682.

35. The Global Use of Strategies to Open Occluded Coronary Arteries in Acute Coronary Syndromes (GUSTO IIb) Angioplasty Substudy Investigators. A clinical trial comparing primary coronary angioplasty with tissue plasminogen activator for acute myocardial infarction. N Engl J Med 1997;336:1621–1628.

36. de Boer MJ, Ottervanger JP, van't Hof AW, et al. Reperfusion therapy in elderly patients with acute myocardial infarction: a randomized comparison of primary angioplasty and thrombolytic therapy. J Am Coll Cardiol 2002; 39:1723–1728.

37. ISIS-2 (Second International Study of Infarct Survival) Collaborative Group. Randomised trial of intravenous streptokinase, oral aspirin, both, or neither among 17187 cases of suspected acute myocardial infarction: ISIS-2. Lancet 1988;II:349–360.

38. The Clopidogrel in Unstable Angina to Prevent Recurrent Events Trial Investigators. Effects of clopidogrel in addition to aspirin in patients with acute coronary syndromes without ST-segment elevation. N Engl J Med 2001; 345:494–502.

39. Gaspoz JM, Coxson PG, Goldman PA, et al. Cost effectiveness of aspirin, clopidogrel, or both for secondary prevention of coronary heart disease. N Engl J Med 2002;346:1800–1806.

40. Krumholz HM, Hennen J, Ridker PM, et al. Use and effectiveness of intravenous heparin therapy for treatment of acute myocardial infarction in the elderly. J Am Coll Cardiol 1998;31:973–979.

41. Cohen M, Demers C, Gurfinkel EP, et al. A comparison of low molecular weight heparin with unfractionated heparin for unstable coronary artery disease. Efficacy and Safety of Subcutaneous Enoxaparin in Non-Q-Wave Coronary Events Study Group. N Engl J Med 1997;337:447–452.

42. Antman EM, McCabe CH, Gurfinkel EP, et al. Enoxaparin prevents death and cardiac ischemic events in unstable angina/non-Q-wave myocardial infarction. Results of the thrombolysis in myocardial infarction (TIMI) IIB trial. Circulation 1999;100:1593–1601.

43. Fragmin and Fast Revascularization during InStability in Coronary artery disease Investigators. Long-term low-molecular-mass heparin in unstable coronary-artery disease: FRISC II prospective randomised multicentre study. Lancet 1999;354:701–707.

44. The EPIC Investigators. Use of a monoclonal antibody directed against the platelet glycoprotein IIb/IIIa receptor in high-risk coronary angioplasty. N Engl J Med 1994;330:956–961.

45. The EPILOG Investigators. Platelet glycoprotein IIb/IIIa receptor blockade and low-dose heparin during percutaneous coronary revascularization. N Engl J Med 1997;336:1689–1696.

46. Platelet Receptor Inhibition in Ischemic Syndrome Management (PRISM) Study Investigators. A comparison of aspirin plus tirofiban with aspirin plus heparin for unstable angina. N Engl J Med 1998;338:1498–1505.

47. Platelet Receptor Inhibition in Ischemic Syndrome Management in Patients Limited by Unstable Signs and Symptoms (PRISM-PLUS) Study Investigators. Inhibition of the platelet glycoprotein IIb/IIIa receptor with tirofiban in unstable angina and non-Q-wave myocardial infarction. N Engl J Med 1998;338:1488–1497.

48. The PURSUIT Investigators. Inhibition of platelet glycoprotein IIb/IIIa with eptifibatide in patients with acute coronary syndromes. N Engl J Med 1998;339:436–443.

49. Aronow WS. Management of older persons after myocardial infarction. J Am Geriatr Soc 1998;46:1459–1468.

50. Hurlen M, Abdelnoor M, Smith P, et al. Warfarin, aspirin, or both after myocardial infarction. N Engl J Med 2002; 347:969–974.

51. van Es RF, Jonker JJC, Verheugt FWA, et al. Aspirin and coumadin after acute coronary syndromes (the ASPECT-2 study): a randomised controlled trial. Lancet 2002;360:109–113.

52. Rich MW. Therapy for acute myocardial infarction in older persons. J Am Geriatr Soc 1998;46:1302–1307.

53. Gruppo Italiano per lo Studio della Sopravvivenza nell'Infarto Miocardico. GISSI-3: effects of lisinopril and transdermal glyceryl trinitrate singly and together on 6-week mortality and ventricular function after acute myocardial infarction. Lancet 1994;343:1115–1122.

54. Ambrosioni E, Borghi C, Magnani B, for the Survival of Myocardial Infarction Long-Term Evaluation (SMILE) Study Investigators. The effect of the angiotensin-converting-enzyme inhibitor zofenopril on mortality and morbidity after anterior myocardial infarction. N Engl J Med 1995;332:80–85.

55. Pfeffer MA, Braunwald E, Moye LA, et al. Effect of captopril on mortality and morbidity in patients with left ventricular dysfunction after myocardial infarction. Results of the Survival and Ventricular Enlargement Trial. N Engl J Med 1992;327:669–677.

56. The Acute Infarction Ramipril Efficacy (AIRE) Study Investigators. Effect of ramipril on mortality and morbidity of survivors of acute myocardial infarction with clinical evidence of heart failure. Lancet 1993;342:821–828.

57. Dickstein K, Kjekshus J. Effects of losartan and captopril on mortality and morbidity in high-risk patients after acute myocardial infarction: the OPTIMAAL randomised trial. Lancet 2002;360:752–760.

58. Pitt B, Remme W, Zannad F, et al. Eplerenone, a selective aldosterone blocker, in patients with left ventricular dysfunction after myocardial infarction. N Engl J Med 2003;348:1309–1321.

59. Fragmin and Fast Revascularization during InStability in Coronary artery disease Investigators. Invasive compared with non-invasive treatment in unstable coronary-artery disease: FRISC II prospective randomised multicentre study. Lancet 1999;354:708–715.

60. Wallentin L, Lagerqvist B, Husted S, Kontny F, Stahle E, Swahn E. Outcome at 1 year after an invasive compared with a non-invasive strategy in unstable coronary-artery disease: the FRISC II invasive randomised trial. Lancet 2000;356:9–16.

61. Cannon CP, Weintraub WS, Demopoulos LA, et al. Comparison of early invasive and conservative strategies in patients with unstable coronary syndromes treated with the glycoprotein IIb/IIIa inhibitor tirofiban. N Engl J Med 2001;344:1879–1887.

62. Batchelor WB, Anstrom KJ, Muhlbaier LH, et al. Contemporary outcome trends in the elderly undergoing percutaneous coronary interventions: results in 7,472 octogenarians. National Cardiovascular Network Collaboration. J Am Coll Cardiol 2000;36:723–730.

63. Alexander KP, Anstrom KJ, Muhlbaier LH, et al. Outcomes of cardiac surgery in patients ≥80 years: results from the National Cardiovascular Network. J Am Coll Cardiol 2000;35:731–738.

64. The TIME Investigators. Trial of invasive versus medical therapy in elderly patients with chronic symptomatic coronary artery disease (TIME): a randomised trial. Lancet 2001;358:951–957.

65. Cheitlin MD. Valve disease in the octogenarian. In: Wenger NK, ed. Cardiovascular Disease in the Octogenarian and Beyond. Martin Dunitz Publishers, London, 1999, pp. 255–266.

66. Aranki SF, Nathan M, Cohn LH. Surgery for valvular heart disease in the octogenarian. In: Wenger NK, ed. Cardiovascular Disease in the Octogenarian and Beyond. Martin Dunitz Publishers London, 1999, pp. 267–277.

67. Sundt TM, Bailey MS, Moon MR, et al. Quality of life after aortic valve replacement at the age of > 80 years. Circulation 2000;102(Suppl 3):III70–III74.

68. Sedrakyan A, Vaccarino V, Paltiel AD, et al. Age does not limit quality of life improvement in cardiac valve surgery. J Am Coll Cardiol 2003;42:1208–1214.

69. Erbelding EJ, Gerding DN, Chesler E. Infective endocarditis. In: Chesler, ed. Clinical Cardiology in the Elderly. Futura Publishing Co., Inc. Armonk, NY, 1994, pp. 427–445.

70. Rich MW. Epidemiology, pathophysiology, and etiology of congestive heart failure in older adults. J Am Geriatr Soc 1997;45:968–974.

71. Maisel AS, Krishnaswamy P, Nowak RM, et al. Rapid measurement of B-type natriuretic peptide in the emergency diagnosis of heart failure. N Engl J Med 2002;347:161–167.

72. Redfield MM, Rodeheffer RJ, Jacobsen SJ, et al. Plasma brain natriuretic peptide concentration: impact of age and gender. J Am Coll Cardiol 2002;40:976–982.

73. Krumholz HM, Parent EM, Tu N, et al. Readmission after hospitalization for congestive heart failure among Medicare beneficiaries. Arch Intern Med 1997;157:99–104.

74. Rich MW. Heart failure disease management: a critical review. J Cardiac Failure 1999;5:64–75.

75. McAlister FA, Lawson FM, Teo KK, Armstrong PW. A systematic review of randomized trials of disease management programs in heart failure. Am J Med 2001;110:378–384.

76. The CONSENSUS Trial Study Group. Effects of enalapril on mortality in severe congestive heart failure. Results of the Cooperative North Scandinavian Enalapril Survival Study. N Engl J Med 1987;316:1429–1435.

77. The SOLVD Investigators. Effect of enalapril on mortality and the development of heart failure in asymptomatic patients with reduced left ventricular ejection fractions. N Engl J Med 1992;327:685–691.

78. The SOLVD Investigators. Effect of enalapril on survival in patients with reduced left ventricular ejection fractions and congestive heart failure. N Engl J Med 1991;325:293–302.

79. Garg R, Yusuf S, for the Collaborative Group on ACE Inhibitor Trials. Overview of randomized trials of angiotensin-converting enzyme inhibitors on mortality and morbidity in patients with heart failure. JAMA 1995;273: 1450–1456.

80. Flather MD, Yusuf S, Køber L, et al. Long-term ACE-inhibitor therapy in patients with heart failure or left-ventricular dysfunction: a systematic overview of data from individual patients. Lancet 2000;355:1575–1581.

81. Maggioni AP, Anand I, Gottlieb SO, et al. Effects of valsartan on morbidity and mortality in patients with heart failure not receiving angiotensin-converting enzyme inhibitors. J Am Coll Cardiol 2002;40:1414–1421.

82. Granger CB, McMurray JJV, Yusuf S, et al. Effects of candesartan in patients with chronic heart failure and reduced left-ventricular systolic function intolerant to angiotensin-converting-enzyme inhibitors: the CHARM-Alternative trial. Lancet 2003;362:772–776.

83. Cohn JN, Tognoni G, and the Valsartan Heart Failure Trial Investigators. A randomized trial of the angiotensin-receptor blocker valsartan in chronic heart failure. N Engl J Med 2001;345:1667–1675.

84. McMurray JJV, Ostergren J, Swedberg K, et al. Effects of candesartan in patients with chronic heart failure and reduced left-ventricular systolic function taking angiotensin-converting-enzyme inhibitors: the CHARM-Added trial. Lancet 2003;362:767–771.

85. Pfeffer MA, Swedberg K, Granger CB, et al. Effects of candesartan on mortality and morbidity in patients with chronic heart failure: the CHARM-Overall programme. Lancet 2003;362:759–766.

86. Pitt B, Poole-Wilson PA, Segal R, et al. Effect of losartan compared with captopril on mortality in patients with symptomatic heart failure: randomized trial—the Losartan Heart Failure Survival Study ELITE II. Lancet 2000; 355:1582–1587.

87. Cohn JN, Archibald DG, Ziesche S, et al. Effect of vasodilator therapy on mortality in chronic congestive heart failure. Results of a Veterans Administration Cooperative Study N Engl J Med 1986;314:1547–1552.

88. Cohn JN, Johnson G, Ziesche S, et al. A comparison of enalapril with hydralazine-isosorbide dinitrate in the treatment of chronic congestive heart failure. N Engl J Med 1991;325:303–310.

89. Packer M, Bristow MR, Cohn JN, et al. The effect of carvedilol on morbidity and mortality in patients with chronic heart failure. N Engl J Med 1996;334:1349–1355.

90. CIBIS-II Investigators and Committees. The Cardiac Insufficiency Bisoprolol Study II (CIBIS II): a randomized trial. Lancet 1999;353:9–13.

91. Merit-HF Study Group. Effect of metoprolol CR/XL in chronic heart failure: Metoprolol CR/XL Randomised Intervention Trial in Congestive Heart Failure (MERIT-HF). Lancet 1999;353:2001–2007.

92. Packer M, Coats AJS, Fowler MB, et al. Effect of carvedilol on survival in severe chronic heart failure. N Engl J Med 2001;344:1651–1658.

93. The Digitalis Investigation Group. The effect of digoxin on mortality and morbidity in patients with heart failure. N Engl J Med 1997;336:525–533.

94. Rich MW, McSherry F, Williford WO, Yusuf S, for the Digitalis Investigation Group. Effect of age on mortality, hospitalizations, and response to digoxin in patients with heart failure: the DIG Study. J Am Coll Cardiol 2001;38: 806–813.

95. Rathore SS, Wang Y, Krumholz HM. Sex-based differences in the effect of digoxin for the treatment of heart failure. N Engl J Med 2002;347:1403–1411.

96. Rathore SS, Curtis JP, Wang Y, et al. Association of serum digoxin concentration and outcomes in patients with heart failure. JAMA 2003;289:871–878.

97. Pitt B, Zannad F, Remme WJ, et al. The effect of spironolactone on morbidity and mortality in patients with severe heart failure. Randomized Aldactone Evaluation Study Investigators. N Engl J Med 1999;341:709–717.

98. Wrenger E, Muller R, Moesenthin M, et al. Interaction of spironolactone with ACE inhibitors or angiotensin receptor blockers: analysis of 44 cases. BMJ 2003;327:147–149.

99. Yusuf S, Pfeffer MA, Swedberg K, et al. Effects of candesartan in patients with chronic heart failure and preserved left-ventricular ejection fraction: the CHARM-Preserved trial. Lancet 2003;362:777–781.
100. Kostis JB, Davis BR, Cutler J, et al. Prevention of heart failure by antihypertensive drug treatment in older persons with isolated systolic hypertension. JAMA 1997;278:212–216.
101. Wolf PA, Abbott RD, Kannel WB. Atrial fibrillation as an independent risk factor for stroke: the Framingham Study. Stroke 1991;22:983–988.
102. Wyse DG, Waldo AL, DiMarco JP, et al. A comparison of rate control and rhythm control in patients with atrial fibrillation. N Engl J Med 2002;347:1825–1833.
103. Van Gelder IC, Hagens VE, Bosker HA, et al. A comparison of rate control and rhythm control in patients with recurrent persistent atrial fibrillation. N Engl J Med 2002;347:1834–1840.
104. Fleg JL. Arrhythmias and conduction disturbances in the octogenarian: epidemiology and progression. In: Wenger NK, ed. Cardiovascular Disease in the Octogenarian and Beyond. Martin Dunitz Publishers, London, 1999, pp. 279–290.
105. Adan V, Crown LA. Diagnosis and treatment of sick sinus syndrome. Am Fam Phys 2003;67:1725–1732.
106. Lamas GA, Lee KL, Silverman R, et al. Ventricular pacing or dual-chamber pacing for sinus-node dysfunction. N Engl J Med 2002;346:1854–1862.
107. Tresch DD, Amirani H. Cardiopulmonary resuscitation in the elderly: beneficial or an exercise in futility? In: Wenger NK, ed. Cardiovascular Disease in the Octogenarian and Beyond. Martin Dunitz Publishers, London, 1999, pp. 291–304.
108. Lavie CJ, Milani RV. Effects of cardiac rehabilitation programs on exercise capacity, coronary risk factors, behavioral characteristics, and quality of life in a large elderly cohort. Am J Cardiol 1995;76:177–179.
109. Lavie CJ, Milani RV. Effects of cardiac rehabilitation and exercise training programs in patients ≥75 years of age. Am J Cardiol 1996;78:675–677.
110. Hofmann JC, Wenger NS, Davis RB, et al. Patient preferences for communication with physicians about end-of-life decisions. SUPPORT Investigators. Study to Understand Prognoses and Preference for Outcomes and Risks of Treatment. Ann Intern Med 1997;127:1–12.
111. American Heart Association. Heart Disease and Stroke Statistics—2003 Update. American Heart Association, Dallas, TX, 2002.
112. Burt VL, Whelton P, Roccella EJ, et al. Prevalence of hypertension in the US adult population. Results from the Third National Health and Nutrition Examination Survey, 1988–1991. Hypertension 1995;25:305–313.
113. Gillum RF. Epidemiology of heart failure in the United States. Am Heart J 1993;126:1042–1047.

RECOMMENDED READING

Aronow WS, Fleg JL, eds. Cardiovascular Disease in the Elderly Patient, 3rd ed. Marcel Dekker, New York, 2004.
Gerstenblith G, ed. Cardiovascular Disease in the Elderly. Humana Press, Totowa, NJ, 2004.
Wenger NK, ed. Cardiovascular Disease in the Octogenarian and Beyond. Martin Dunitz Publishers, London, 1999.

40

Cardiovascular Complications in Patients With Renal Disease

Richard A. Preston, MD, MBA,
Simon Chakko, MD, *and Murray Epstein,* MD

INTRODUCTION

The heart and kidney are invariably intertwined. Heart failure is associated with the important alterations in renal hemodynamics and function that constitute a major problem of clinical management. Conversely, in chronic renal disease, rarely does the heart escape consequences. Cardiovascular complications comprise the major cause of death in the end-stage renal disease (ESRD) population. The effects of chronic renal failure on the heart are diverse and involve numerous anatomical and functional aspects of the cardiovascular system.

Given the broad scope of this subject, we have elected to focus our review primarily on the more common cardiovascular alterations that complicate the course of progressive renal disease: pericarditis, renal parenchymal hypertension, coronary arteriosclerosis, and left ventricular dysfunction. Finally, we have included a discussion of ischemic renal disease, a common but underdiagnosed disorder that is an important complication of systemic arteriosclerosis.

PERICARDITIS

Pericarditis *(1–11)* is a common and often severe complication of advanced chronic renal failure. Before emergency dialysis was available the appearance of a pericardial friction rub in a patient with ESRD was a harbinger of death within the ensuing 2 wk. Many authorities group pericarditis associated with ESRD into two main categories *(1–3)*. *Early* or *uremic pericarditis* occurs in the ESRD patient prior to the initiation of chronic dialysis therapy and is probably secondary to the biochemical perturbations of uremia per se. Early or uremic pericarditis generally responds rapidly to renal replacement therapy in the majority of patients. *Late* or *dialysis-associated pericarditis* occurs in patients who are already receiving renal replacement therapy. In general, dialysis-associated pericarditis tends to be more severe, has a higher rate of complications, responds less readily to dialysis, and is more likely to result in pericardial tamponade *(1–4)*.

Incidence

In 1968, a 41% incidence of uremic pericarditis was reported in patients beginning dialysis *(5)*. The incidence of uremic pericarditis has fallen in recent years, probably because of the greater availability and earlier initiation of renal replacement therapy. More recent reports indicate a much lower incidence, less than 10% *(6)*. Pericarditis has been found to occur in approx 10 to 20% of patients receiving regular dialysis therapy. The 10 to 20% incidence of dialysis-associated pericarditis has not changed appreciably over the past decade.

From: *Essential Cardiology: Principles and Practice, 2nd Ed.*
Edited by: C. Rosendorff © Humana Press Inc., Totowa, NJ

Table 1
Clinical Features of Pericarditis Associated With ESRD

Pericardial rub	95%
Chest pain	60–70%
Hypotension	13–56%
Fever	63–76%
Leukocytosis	35–71%
ECG (classical changes)	2–5%
Arrhythmias	20–28%
Pericardial effusion (echocardiogram)	89%

Pathology

The basic pathologic process of pericarditis associated with ESRD is an aseptic inflammatory reaction with fibrin formation. The process is similar in both uremic pericarditis and dialysis-associated pericarditis. Both parietal and visceral pericardia are covered with a fibrinous exudate. Fibrinous bands are usually present and form adhesions and areas of loculation between the two layers. The effusion is usually serosanguinous, but is uniformly hemorrhagic in cases of tamponade. The white blood cell count in the effusion is variable but usually in the $500–700/mm^3$ range with a variable proportion of polymorphonuclear and mononuclear leukocytes. Cultures are routinely negative.

Pathogenesis

Pericarditis in ESRD patients who have not yet begun dialysis is most likely related to the biochemical milieu of untreated uremia, as evidenced by the rapid response to the initiation of dialysis and the clinical correlation with biochemical control of uremia in the majority of patients (1–4, 6,8). Dialysis-associated pericarditis, on the other hand, is less well understood. It is not clear why a substantial percentage of patients receiving regular renal replacement should develop pericarditis. Dialysis-associated pericarditis may be related to underdialysis in some patients, but this is not always the case. The etiology of dialysis-associated pericarditis is probably multifactorial, and is not well understood (1–4,6).

A number of potential pathogenic factors have been proposed to explain dialysis-associate pericarditis, including inadequate dialysis therapy, hypercatabolic states, poorly controlled hyperparathyroidism, heparin received during dialysis, and an abnormal immunologic response. Underdialysis has been noted in a significant percent of patients developing dialysis-associated pericarditis, often as a result of vascular access failure or missing dialysis. In addition, pericarditis has been observed to occur during periods of hypercatabolism such as following major surgery or during sepsis (1–4).

Clinical Features

The presentation of pericarditis in a patient with ESRD (1–11) may be dramatic, marked by a fulminant course resulting in acute tamponade. On the other hand, a patient may present with only vague chest pain or mild constitutional symptoms. Dialysis-associated pericarditis may occasionally present as recurrent hypotension during hemodialysis. Clinical and laboratory features of the pericarditis of ESRD are summarized in Table 1 (5,8–11). Pericardial friction rub and chest pain are important in the diagnosis of pericarditis but are not always present. Dialysis-associated pericarditis is often associated with a more severe clinical illness, more systemic manifestations, a higher likelihood of tamponade, and a less favorable response to dialysis (1–4).

Chest pain occurs in the majority of patients and may be variable in character and severity. The pain may be located anywhere in the precordium and may precede the development of a friction rub. There is often a pleuritic component to the pain, and the pain may be aggravated by lying supine and partially relieved by sitting forward. A pericardial friction rub may be detected in more than 90%

of patients. The rub is typically evanescent in nature and may change in quality with time. Therefore, the absence of a rub on any given physical examination does not rule out pericarditis.

Hemodynamic compromise, including hypotension during hemodialysis, may occur as a presenting clinical feature *(1–3,7,8)*. Dialysis-associated pericarditis should be suspected and sought in any patient suffering from repeated episodes of hypotension during dialysis or in patients with ESRD presenting with hypotension despite signs of fluid overload.

Fever and leukocytosis may be present more commonly in dialysis-associated pericarditis, and, if severe, may predict a less favorable response to an intensification of the dialysis regimen *(7)*. The ECG is of very limited usefulness in the diagnosis of pericarditis in ESRD. ECG abnormalities are common but lack specificity. The classic ST segment elevations described in several types of acute pericarditis are uncommon in this form of pericarditis; the most common findings are nonspecific ST and T-wave abnormalities. Atrial arrhythmias, including atrial flutter and fibrillation, have been observed in a significant number of cases.

Echocardiography is the easiest and most accurate method for diagnosing pericardial effusion, provides useful information regarding the size of a pericardial effusion, and can detect early or impending tamponade. This information concerning quantity of effusion and hemodynamic significance is important when reaching a decision regarding early management of uremic pericarditis. A large effusion or one that causes hemodynamic embarrassment will generally not respond to conservative management with dialysis alone, but will often require surgical drainage.

Acute cardiac tamponade is the most serious and potentially lethal complication of pericarditis associated with ESRD, and is more common in dialysis-associated pericarditis than in uremic pericarditis. Tamponade may occur during or shortly following a dialysis session. It may be difficult to distinguish acute tamponade from hypovolemia-induced hypotension. In cases of unexplained hypotension during or shortly following dialysis, the echocardiogram may be very useful in making this important differential diagnosis. It is important to maintain a high index of suspicion for pericarditis-related tamponade in patients with hypotension during hemodialysis because it is potentially reversible.

Management

When uremic pericarditis presents in a patient with renal disease reaching ESRD, then the initiation of renal replacement therapy is indicated. Cardiac tamponade is unusual in this form of pericarditis and most patients will respond well to dialysis therapy with resolution of the signs and symptoms of pericarditis.

Management of dialysis-associated pericarditis has been less satisfactory. The initial treatment is determined by the hemodynamic stability of the patient. In the stable patient who does not have evidence of tamponade or impending tamponade, the first line of treatment is generally intensification of dialysis therapy, monitored by repeat echocardiographic evaluation of effusion size. This approach has yielded a response rate of approx 60 to 70%. In the majority of cases, the response is seen within the first 10 to 14 d of initiating intensive dialysis therapy. If hemodynamic compromise develops or the effusion fails to reduce in size or becomes larger over a course of 10 to 14 d, then a drainage procedure should be undertaken.

A positive effect from the use of nonsteroidal antiinflammatory agents in the treatment of pericarditis has been difficult to prove and is associated with gastrointestinal toxicity and bleeding complications. Similarly, systemic corticosteroids have been reported to improve the clinical course of pericarditis but are associated with side effects and do not seem to prevent the development of constrictive pericarditis. Nonsteroidal antiinflammatory agents and steroids in pericarditis associated with ESRD are controversial.

There are several clinical features that predict the failure of intensive dialytic intervention and hence the need for early surgical drainage in the treatment of pericarditis. A report by De Pace et al. *(7)* suggests that in the presence of a large pericardial effusion, temperature greater than 102°F, and rales, peritoneal dialysis is required because the patient is too hemodynamically unstable to permit hemodialysis. Systolic blood pressure under 100 mmHg, jugular venous distention, white blood cell count over 15,000/mm^3, and white blood cell count left shift all correlate with poor out-come of dialysis treatment alone. The simultaneous presence of several of these features describes a patient at risk of failing to respond favorably to intensive dialysis therapy. Thus, the febrile, toxic patient with a large effusion and evidence of hemodynamic compromise is at high risk of failing to respond to dialysis treatment alone, and the need for a drainage procedure should be anticipated.

Pericardiocentesis is associated with a high rate of severe complications including laceration of atrial or ventricular wall or coronary arteries. Most series report a high morbidity and mortality rate with pericardiocentesis. In addition, pericardiocentesis has a high rate of reaccumulation of pericardial fluid and thus does not represent a definitive procedure. Because purulent pericarditis is rare in patients with ESRD, there is little need for a diagnostic pericardiocentesis. Therefore, pericardiocentesis is generally recommended only for extreme emergency situations as a last-resort measure.

Subxiphoid pericardiotomy is considered a relatively safe and effective procedure to achieve pericardial drainage. It is generally well tolerated in the uremic patient who is ill and often with hemodynamic compromise in comparison with the more extensive (albeit more definitive) pericardiectomy. Subxiphoid pericardiotomy is associated with a 6% failure rate, but a low rate of complications.

Pericardiectomy is a definitive surgical procedure with essentially a nonexistent rate of fluid reaccumulation and the prevention of the late complication of constrictive pericarditis. It is, however, an extensive major surgical intervention requiring general anesthesia and either a median sternotomy or anterior thoracotomy. Pericardiectomy remains the treatment of choice for constrictive pericarditis.

RENAL PARENCHYMAL HYPERTENSION

Any consideration of cardiovascular complications in renal disease must a priori consider the generation of renal parenchymal hypertension and its effects on cardiac structure and function. Renal parenchymal hypertension *(12–22)* is hypertension that is caused by kidney disease and is the most common cause of secondary hypertension. Chronic renal disease and systemic hypertension may coexist in three very different clinical settings. First, primary hypertension is an important cause of chronic renal disease. Poorly controlled, severe, sustained hypertension over an extended period results in hypertensive nephrosclerosis. In the second situation, renal parenchymal disease is a well established and important cause of secondary hypertension. Therefore, hypertension is both a cause and a consequence of renal disease. Renal parenchymal hypertension is the most common secondary form of hypertension and accounts for 3.0 to 5.0% of all cases of systemic hypertension. The secondary hypertension produced by the diseased kidneys may accelerate the decline in renal function if inadequately controlled. Sometimes it may be difficult to distinguish clinically between primary hypertension causing nephrosclerosis and renal disease causing hypertension. The third clinical setting in which chronic renal disease and hypertension may coexist is ischemic renal disease, which will be discussed briefly later in this chapter.

Renal parenchymal hypertension may be caused by almost any disease of the renal parenchyma (Table 2). A patient who appears to have primary hypertension may have an underlying renal disease causing the hypertension. The initial evaluation of all hypertensive patients should include a screen for renal disease. Determination of blood urea nitrogen and serum creatinine values, and careful urinalysis with examination of the urinary sediment, often, but not invariably, will exclude significant underlying renal disease. Urinary findings that suggest that a renal disease is causing the hypertension are cellular and granular casts, significant hematuria, pyuria, and urine protein excretion >150 mg/24 h.

Pathogenesis

Renal parenchymal hypertension most probably represents the combined interactions of many independent mechanisms: potential factors include sodium retention leading to volume expansion, increases in endogenous pressor activity, and decreases in endogenous vasodepressor compounds. The precise mechanisms that lead to hypertension in chronic renal failure have not been completely

Table 2
Common Etiologies of Renal Parenchymal Hypertension

Glomerular diseases
    Postinfectious glomerulonephritis
    Focal segmental sclerosis
    Membranous glomerulonephritis
    Renal vasculitis
    Diabetic nephropathy
    Crescentic glomerulonephritis
    Systemic lupus erythematosis nephritis
Interstitial diseases
    Polycystic kidney disease
    Chronic interstitial nephritis

defined, but recent investigations have provided exciting new insights. The traditional focus has been on volume-mediated mechanisms, the renin-angiotensin system, and renal prostaglandins; recently, increasing attention has been given to other pressor and vasodilator systems, including endogenous digitalis-like factor, endothelin and endothelium-derived relaxing factor, and nitric oxide (NO). The sodium intake and the volume-mediated mechanisms of renal parenchymal hypertension are of central importance to management and will be discussed in more detail.

Sodium Intake

Impaired renal sodium excretion leads to positive sodium balance and contributes to the development of renal parenchymal hypertension. Abnormal renal sodium excretion is the most important mechanism of renal parenchymal hypertension from a clinical standpoint. Patients with renal failure have increased total extracellular fluid volume (ECFV) sodium compared with normal controls or patients with primary hypertension. This increase in ECFV sodium correlates directly with an increased ECFV and with hypertension. Changes in sodium intake directly influence blood pressure in patients with chronic renal failure, and this relationship seems stronger at lower levels of renal function. Increasing sodium intake in patients with chronic renal failure increases ECFV and blood pressure. The increment in blood pressure for a given increase in ECFV tends to be greater in the patients with further advanced renal failure. Reduction of dietary sodium will lower ECFV and blood pressure in many patients with chronic renal insufficiency. This sodium sensitivity of the hypertension caused by renal disease is key to appropriate antihypertensive therapy.

Despite the importance of impaired sodium excretion and ECFV expansion in the genesis of renal parenchymal hypertension, the most consistently observed hemodynamic alteration in established cases is an elevation of peripheral vascular resistance rather than an increase in cardiac output. The mechanism(s) for this elevation in peripheral vascular resistance is not known exactly: The relationship of ECFV expansion to pressure elevation appears to be complex and may involve alterations in autonomic function, in neurohumoral control of blood pressure, and possibly in local vascular factors such as increased cytosolic calcium concentration in vascular smooth muscle. There is a complex connection between volume expansion and peripheral vascular resistance in patients with the sodium-sensitive hypertension of chronic renal disease.

Treatment of Renal Parenchymal Hypertension: Focus on Sodium Balance

Regardless of the mechanisms leading from ECFV expansion to hypertension, sodium retention with associated ECFV expansion plays a central role in the pathogenesis of renal parenchymal hypertension. Consequently, therapeutic modalities that reduce total body sodium are frequently very effective in lowering blood pressure in patients with renal parenchymal hypertension. Even small net gains in total body sodium can produce significant increases in blood pressure. The first step in managing renal parenchymal hypertension is reduction of ECFV sodium.

Table 3
Dietary Sodium Restriction in Chronic Renal Failure

1. Initiate Na restriction with 2 g/d (88 mEq/d)
2. Serial measurements of weight and blood pressure
3. Serial measurements of blood urea nitrogen and creatinine
4. If $NaHCO_3$ replacement is required, monitor Na intake
5. Avoid potassium-containing salt substitutes

The management of patients with hypertension secondary to chronic renal insufficiency is a common and often perplexing problem confronting the general internist. Elevated systemic arterial blood pressure indicates a poor prognosis in a number of renal disorders, and there is extensive evidence that hypertension of any cause accelerates the deterioration of renal function. Therefore, preservation of renal function is a compelling reason for early identification and vigorous treatment of hypertension: Regardless of the mechanism(s) involved, treatment of hypertension has been shown to retard the rate of progression of renal impairment in several disease states. Because both the prevalence and the severity of hypertension increase as the glomerular filtration rate (GFR) declines, it is important to continue close follow-up and frequent reassessment of therapy.

Sodium Restriction

As discussed, renal sodium retention with associated ECFV expansion plays a central role in the genesis of renal parenchymal hypertension and therapeutic measures that will reduce extracellular fluid sodium are frequently very effective in lowering blood pressure. Sodium restriction and diuretics constitute critical components of effective antihypertensive therapy in patients with renal disease. Control of blood pressure in patients with chronic renal disease is difficult, if not impossible, without dietary sodium restriction.

Reasonable guidelines for dietary sodium restriction are summarized in Table 3. Realistically, 2 g sodium/d (i.e., 88 mEq sodium) is the minimum sodium intake attainable on an outpatient basis. To maintain this modestly low level of sodium intake requires intensive dietary education and patient cooperation. For example, processed foods, such as canned vegetables and soups, prepared meat products, and most so-called "fast foods," are extremely high in sodium content, as are most seasonings. The preparation of many processed foods adds a great deal of sodium. A variety of educational material listing the sodium contents of different foods for sodium-restricted diets is readily available, and we find repeated counseling and education by clinical dietitians along with diligent follow up to be quite useful. Patients should be cautioned about the use of salt substitutes: Many contain potassium and should be avoided altogether in patients with renal impairment and diminished potassium excretory capacity.

Because the chronically diseased kidney may adapt poorly to rapid changes in sodium intake, sodium restriction should be initiated under close observation. When confronted with an abrupt decrease of dietary sodium, some patients may not be able to reduce urinary sodium excretion quickly and a period of negative sodium balance may ensue. This sodium-wasting tendency is generally reversible after several weeks but early negative sodium balance may decrease ECFV and lead to prerenal azotemia.

Sodium intake must be individualized and carefully monitored. Every renal patient should be followed carefully for signs of ECFV depletion (orthostatic blood pressure change or rapid decline in body weight) or worsening azotemia. Serial measurements of body weight and blood chemistries are often useful to identify an "ideal" weight (ECFV) for optimal blood pressure control.

Diuretic Therapy

Because attempts to lower blood pressure by rigid dietary salt restriction are often not tolerated by patients, particularly in view of the concomitant dietary restrictions often needed to manage renal failure (i.e., protein restriction), in most cases the next step to control sodium balance is a trial of diuretic therapy. If a trial of sodium restriction is not tolerated or does not produce an adequate reduction of total body sodium, then a diuretic should be added to the antihypertensive regimen.

THIAZIDE DIURETICS

Thiazides alone are not usually effective natriuretics in a patient with a serum creatinine above 2.0 mg/dL or a creatinine clearance below 30 mL/min, probably due to diminished delivery of the sodium load to the distal nephron and of the drug to its site of action. Therefore, the use of thiazide diuretics alone is not recommended at low levels of renal function.

LOOP DIURETICS

The loop-acting diuretics (furosemide, ethacrynic acid, bumetanide, torasemide) are the agents of choice for the management of extracellular fluid volume and hypertension when the GFR falls below 30 mL/min. Unlike the thiazides, the loop agents are effective natriuretics at GFRs well below 30 mL/min, even when used alone, although very high doses may be required as renal failure progresses. The loop diuretics act by inhibiting chloride (and sodium) reabsorption at the medullary thick ascending limb of the loop of Henle, which reabsorbs approx 25 to 30% of the filtered sodium load. Because so much filtered sodium is reabsorbed in this nephron segment, it is understandable why these agents are such potent natriuretics.

Because these agents act from the luminal side, they must enter the tubular lumen, both by glomerular filtration and by tubular secretion, before they can act. The dose-response curve of the loop diuretics is sigmoidal, because the natriuretic response depends on a threshold concentration of drug being delivered to its site of action. One approach to obtaining the optimal diuretic dose is to increase the dosage of diuretic carefully until the desired natriuresis occurs. This dosage would correspond to some point on the "steep" part of the curve, where a small increase in diuretic delivery results in a large increase in natriuresis.

A common pitfall in the practical use of loop diuretics is increasing dose frequency rather than dose size: A dosage is tried that produces an insufficient natriuresis, but rather than increasing the dose, the clinician repeatedly administers the *same* dose, mistakenly expecting an additive response. The single dose should be increased until a satisfactory natriuresis is achieved. If still more natriuresis is desired, either the dose size or the dose frequency can be increased. Note that the dose-response curve flattens above a certain dose. Beyond this point there is no advantage to increasing the single dose. If further sodium excretion is required than is produced with the maximum single effective dose, then additional *effective* doses of the diuretic may be prescribed. In general, furosemide requires twice daily dosing whereas bumetanide is usually given once daily. If the response is insufficient, single doses can be increased to a maximum of about 480 mg. Larger single doses are unlikely to be more effective, and increase the risk of ototoxicity.

Continued dietary sodium restriction is important during diuretic therapy because sodium retention may occur between doses of diuretic. This sodium retention may be sufficient to completely neutralize the natriuretic effects of the loop diuretics if sodium restriction is not imposed.

In our clinical practice, we have found daily weight to be the most useful indicator of changes in extracellular sodium. When done at the same time of day and on the same scale, daily weight is quite helpful in determining net changes in sodium balance. An "ideal" weight can often be established, at which the blood pressure becomes easier to manage. Measurements of 24-h urinary excretion of sodium are somewhat time-consuming and cumbersome, but may be useful for the evaluation of patient compliance with sodium restriction or suspected sodium wasting.

Patients with nephrotic syndrome may demonstrate diuretic resistance even with a preserved GFR, possibly due to intraluminal binding of the diuretic by albumin, which inactivates the diuretic before it reaches its site of action at the loop of Henle. Conclusive human data have been difficult to obtain, but diuretic resistance in nephrotic patients is a serious clinical problem.

The initial dose of furosemide in patients with a 50% or greater reduction in GFR is about 40 mg iv or 80 mg po. The corresponding dosage of bumetanide is about 1 mg iv or po. Furosemide may be titrated as high as 120 to 160 mg iv or 240 to 320 mg po and bumetanide may be titrated as high as 4 to 6 mg iv or po.

Hypokalemia and glucose intolerance may complicate therapy with the loop diuretics. The risk of their ototoxicity is increased by renal insufficiency and by concomitant administration of aminoglycosides. In addition, care must be exercised to avoid overdiuresis, with consequent intravascular volume depletion and prerenal azotemia.

Blockade of Renin-Angiotensin System

There is a body of evidence suggesting that blockade of the renin-angiotensin system affords renal protection in the patient with hypertension and renal parenchymal disease beyond its effects on blood pressure (16–22). There have been several clinical trials demonstrating the benefit of ACE inhibitors in type I diabetic nephropathy, nondiabetic renal disease, and hypertensive nephrosclerosis (17–19). More recently several trials have emerged that suggest a preferential benefit of angiotensin AT1 receptor blockers in type 2 diabetes mellitus with nephropathy (20–22). In the IDNT trial (21), a total of 1715 hypertensive patients with type 2 diabetes and nephropathy were allocated to treatment with 300 mg irbesartan daily, 10 mg amlodipine daily, or placebo. The mean duration of follow-up was 2.6 yr, and the goal blood pressure was 135/85 mmHg. Treatment with irbesartan was associated with a risk of the primary composite endpoint of a doubling of the baseline serum creatinine concentration, the development of end-stage renal disease, or death from any cause that was 20% lower than that in the placebo group ($p = 0.02$) and 23% lower than that in the amlodipine group ($p = 0.006$). These differences were not explained by differences in the blood pressures that were achieved. In the IDNT trial, although irbesartan had more favorable effects on ESRD than did amlodipine, there were no significant differences between the two treatment groups in the rates of death from any cause, or in the cardiovascular composite endpoint.

The RENAAL study (20) compared 50 to 100 mg losartan once daily with placebo in patients with type 2 diabetes with nephropathy for a mean of 3.4 yr. The primary outcome was the composite of a doubling of the baseline serum creatinine concentration, end-stage renal disease, or death. A total of 327 patients in the losartan group reached the primary endpoint, as compared with 359 in the placebo group (risk reduction, 16%; $p = 0.02$). The benefit exceeded that attributable to changes in blood pressure. The level of proteinuria declined by 35% with losartan ($p < 0.001$ for the comparison with placebo).

These studies suggest that blockade of the renin-angiotensin system is perhaps a logical initial choice of antihypertensive agent along with control of the extracellular fluid volume.

Calcium-Channel Antagonists and Renal Parenchymal Hypertension

Two randomized trials in patients with chronic kidney disease have delineated the role of calcium-channel antagonists in the antihypertensive armamentarium to retard the progression of renal disease. In the IDNT trial patients treated with amlodipine or with placebo had greater probability of progression of renal disease than patients treated with irbesartan (21). The AASK trial was designed to compare the effects of three different treatments on progression of renal disease in African-Americans with a clinical diagnosis of hypertensive nephrosclerosis (17). One group received amlodipine, one received an ACE inhibitor and one a β-blocker as initial therapy. Additional drugs were used to achieve two levels of mean arterial pressure, 92 or 107 mmHg. The amlodipine arm was stopped prematurely because of a more rapid decline in GFR in patients treated with amlodipine than in those treated with the ACE inhibitor. The difference, however, was significant only in patients with proteinuria greater than 220 mg/g creatinine, whereas no difference was apparent in the majority of patients with less proteinuria.

Whereas a body of evidence indicates that CCBs, when used as first-line therapy, may be less protective against progression of kidney diseases than ACE inhibitors or angiotensin AT1 receptor blockers even when similar blood pressure control is achieved, in clinical practice it is unlikely that monotherapy with an ACE inhibitor or angiotensin AT1 receptor blocker alone will suffice

(17,20,21). On average, patients with significant renal parenchymal disease and renal functional impairment will require at least three to four antihypertensives to reach goal BP *(20,21)*. Indeed, an efficacious antihypertensive regimen includes multiple agents, in which diuretics and calcium antagonists constitute integral parts. For example, in a given patient with renal parenchymal hypertension, one might begin with a diuretic combined with an ACE inhibitor or angiotensin AT1 receptor blocker with a CCB added to reach the recommended goal blood pressure of 130/80.

In conclusion, the body of evidence seems to indicate that, when used as first-line therapy, ACE-inhibitors and AT1 antagonists appear to provide greater renal protection in patients with nephropathy and significant proteinuria than other classes of antihypertensive drugs, including CCBs. In contrast, in patients without significant proteinuria, there is no conclusive evidence that one class of drugs offers benefits over the other. Because the majority of hypertensive patients with renal disease require multiple antihypertensive agents to achieve adequate control, it appears that administration of CCBs in addition to ACE inhibitors or ARBs is effective and safe. Further, there is no substantial clinical evidence to suggest that dihydropyridine CCBs are inferior to non-dihydropyridine in the management of hypertension in patients with chronic kidney disease with or without diabetes mellitus, particularly when these agents are used in combination with ACE inhibitors or ARBs.

Importance of End-Stage Renal Disease to the Cardiologist

Because many patients with cardiovascular disease also have concomitant renal disease, and because this often progresses to end-stage renal disease, it is extremely important for the cardiologist to consider the importance of treating to an appropriate goal pressure in this population *(23–25)*. Among patients with end-stage renal disease, the annual mortality rate is nearly 25%. Cardiovascular diseases are the leading cause of death in patients receiving maintenance hemodialysis, especially in the first year of treatment. A history of long-lasting arterial hypertension is associated with an increase in cardiovascular deaths in these patients. Controlled studies are not available on the beneficial effect of antihypertensive therapy on patients in hemodialysis. However, there is unanimity that maintaining a controlled blood pressure is of great importance for long-term survival. Hypertension is the single most important predictor of coronary artery disease in uremic patients, even more so than cigarette smoking and hypertriglyceridemia. There is a paucity of studies comparing different antihypertensive regimens in this patient population and in clinical practice most nephrologists need to extrapolate results obtained from patients with relatively normal kidney function to patients with advanced kidney disease.

A recent study supports the safety of calcium antagonists in hemodialysis patients. Tepel et al. *(25)* have retrospectively studied the association of calcium-channel blockers and mortality in 188 hemodialysis patients. After a follow up of 30 mo, 51 patients (27%) had died, and 72% of those died of cardiovascular causes. In the deceased group, age was significantly higher, smoking was more frequent, and body mass index was lower compared with the group that survived. The percentage of patients taking CCBs was significantly higher in the survival group than in the group of patients that died. Among patients assigned to CCB therapy, there was a significant reduction in mortality of 67% ($p < 0.001$). Because of the retrospective nature of this study, a cause-effect relationship between CCB use and mortality cannot be established with certainty; however, at the very least, the study suggests that use of CCBs in hemodialysis patients may be considered safe.

CORONARY ATHEROSCLEROSIS

Ischemic heart disease is common in patients with ESRD. In the United States Renal Data System, ischemic heart disease was already present in 40.8% of 3399 patients starting chronic hemodialysis *(26)*. The incidence of ischemic heart disease is even higher among patients receiving dialysis therapy. In the Canadian Hemodialysis Morbidity Study, the annual incidence of myocardial infarction or angina requiring hospitalization was 10% per year *(24)*. Patients with chronic pyelonephritis or interstitial renal disease develop coronary artery disease more frequently than those with other forms of renal failure *(27)*.

The development and progression of coronary atherosclerosis is accelerated in the presence of renal failure. In general, risk factors for coronary artery disease in the general population applies to patients with ESRD. Advancing age is associated with increased risk for arteriographic coronary disease inpatients with ESRD. Hypertension and diabetes mellitus are common among these patients. Glucose intolerance and insulin resistance have been demonstrated in the absence of overt diabetes. Decreased fibrinolytic activity, platelet dysfunction, and vascular calcification may increase the risk for cardiac events. Lipid abnormalities have been reported in ESRD. Total cholesterol level may be normal. Elevated triglyceride levels and decreased HDL levels are seen in hemodialysis patients and also in peritoneal dialysis patients who may also have high LDL levels (28). Hypertriglyceridemia is caused by impaired degradation of very low-density lipoprotein. Lp(a) levels are increased in hemodialysis patients; in these patients, Lp(a) is an independent risk factor for cardiovascular disease. Caucasian men with ESRD have lower levels of HDL when compared to African-Americans (27). In nephrotic syndrome, elevated total cholesterol and LDL and low HDL are present. Elevated homocysteine, a risk factor for atherosclerosis, is also common in ESRD patients.

Clinical presentation of ischemic heart disease in patients with ESRD may be atypical. Myocardial ischemia may be silent due to autonomic neuropathy induced by diabetes mellitus or other diseases. Symptomatic myocardial ischemia may occur in the absence of significant obstructive disease of epicardial coronary arteries. Small-vessel coronary disease has been reported in hypertension, left ventricular hypertrophy, and diabetes, which are common among patients with ESRD. Increase in myocardial oxygen demand may result from left ventricular hypertrophy, volume and pressure overload, and high output state from anemia and AV fistula. Anemia worsens myocardial oxygen delivery. Electrocardiographic findings such as ST segment and T-wave abnormalities, which suggest ischemia, are common in many ESRD patients without coronary disease. The specificity of stress test with thallium imaging to diagnose coronary disease is poor in these patients (29). Dobutamine stress echocardiography may be a better diagnostic test (30). Coronary angiography may be necessary for definitive diagnosis.

Management of ischemic heart disease is similar to that used in patients without kidney disease. Dosages of drugs that are excreted by the kidney need to be lowered. Maintaining the hematocrit above 30 using erythropoietin improves exercise capacity (31,32). Patients on long-term dialysis have a poor prognosis following acute myocardial infarction. Mortality from cardiac causes was 41% at 1 yr, 52% at 2 yr and 70% at 5 yr following acute myocardial infarction (33). Thus an aggressive approach toward the prevention and treatment of acute myocardial infarction is justified. If coronary angiography is performed nonionic contrast media is preferred. Pre- and postprocedural hydration, and ultrafiltration, and possibly N-acetyl cysteine, may reduce the risk (34). Coronary angioplasty provides good results initially but restenosis rate is high. Coronary bypass surgery is a good option for selected patients but the mortality rate is increased to about 10% and the perioperative morbidity rate is also higher (35).

LEFT VENTRICULAR FUNCTION

Among chronic renal failure patients, alterations in cardiac structure and function have been demonstrated using hemodynamic and echocardiographic studies (37). The etiology of these alterations is multifactorial (Table 4). They can be divided into four major categories: (1) loading conditions that affect the myocardial function; (2) conditions that impair systolic function directly by their negative inotropic effect or indirectly by causing myocardial damage; (3) impaired diastolic filling of the heart; and (4) alterations in neural control of circulation.

Loading Conditions

Low cardiac output stimulates the sympathetic nervous system, renin-angiotensin-aldosterone axis, and arginine-vasopressin, which results in salt and water retention. In accordance with the Frank-Starling mechanism, the increase in preload (left ventricular end-diastolic volume or pressure) leads to an increase in stroke volume. However, an increase in preload beyond an optimal

Table 4
Factors Affecting Myocardial
Function in Chronic Renal Failure

Loading conditions
  Anemia
  Hypertension
  Fluid retention
  A-V fistula
  Thiamine deficiency
Systolic dysfunction
  Myocardial ischemia, infarction
  Hyperkalemia
  Hypocalcemia
  Metabolic acidosis
  Uremic toxins (?)
  Myocardial fibrosis
  Valvular disease
Diastolic filling
  Pericardial disease
  Left ventricular hypertrophy
  Myocardial fibrosis
Neural control
  Autonomic neuropathy

level causes pulmonary venous congestion. Usually pulmonary capillary wedge pressure >20 mmHg leads to pulmonary congestion and >30 mmHg leads to pulmonary edema. However, if the pulmonary capillary permeability is increased or plasma oncotic pressure is low, pulmonary congestion and edema may result at lower pressures. Retention of water and sodium may cause pulmonary edema in patients with acute renal failure or in chronic renal failure when fluid intake is excessive. In addition, an increase in pulmonary capillary permeability leading to pulmonary edema, even in the absence of elevated pulmonary capillary wedge pressure, has been reported in end-stage renal failure (36). The ease with which these patients develop pleural and pericardial effusions supports this possible mechanism. Diluting effect of volume overload on plasma protein concentration, which may already be reduced if significant proteinuria is a feature of the underlying nephropathy, accentuates the tendency for fluid transudation and edema formation.

While increases in afterload have little effect on the stroke volume of the normal ventricle, it can lead to a marked decrease in stroke volume when myocardial dysfunction is present. Most patients with chronic renal failure are hypertensive. In end-stage renal failure and in the dialysis population, severe hypertension is usually secondary to sodium and water retention. Such hypertension is usually present even in anephric patients and is exquisitely dependent on blood volume. In some patients, the hypertension is secondary to elevation of peripheral resistance due to increased plasma renin activity; it is not controlled by lowering the blood volume but responds to bilateral nephrectomy. Thus retention of water and sodium leads to increases in both preload and afterload in chronic renal failure and may precipitate congestive heart failure. Chronic renal failure causes reduced compliance of the aorta and large arteries, thus increasing the afterload. Pressure and volume overload leads to concentric and eccentric left ventricular hypertrophy, respectively. Regression of left ventricular hypertrophy may follow renal transplantation.

Heart failure exists when the cardiac output is insufficient to meet the demands of the metabolizing tissue. In anemia and arteriovenous fistula, a high cardiac output state is present; cardiac output and mean arterial pressure are elevated but the systemic vascular resistance is normal. Using hypertrophy and dilation as compensatory mechanisms, the normal heart can maintain tissue oxygenation for prolonged periods. But when myocardial function is impaired, these compensatory mechanisms are insufficient and the high cardiac output state will lead to clinical manifestations of heart failure. An increase in cardiac output occurs when the hematocrit falls below 25%; lowered blood viscosity is the major cause of increased cardiac output. In patients with congestive heart failure who are receiving hemodialysis, use of erythropoietin raised the hematocrit and provided symptom relief but did not improve survival *(31,32)*. Many end-stage renal failure patients treated with erythropoietin experience an increase in arterial pressure due to an increase in peripheral vascular resistance. Tissue hypoxia resulting from anemia can lead to an autonomic reflex response resulting in reduced arteriolar resistance.

High-output heart failure resulting from the arteriovenous shunts, surgically constructed for vascular access for hemodialysis, is not uncommon *(38)*. Mean flow rate through these shunts is 1.5 L/min. However, cardiac outputs as high as 11 L/min/m^2, which decrease substantially during the occlusion of the shunt, have been reported. Although anemia may play role in such high cardiac output states, the added hemodynamic burden of the shunt may explain heart failure. Banding or revising the fistula to an appropriate size may relieve heart failure symptoms. Water soluble vitamins are dialyzable, and it has been suggested that loss of thiamine may rarely lead to high-output heart failure due to beriberi.

Systolic Dysfunction

Although the presence of a cardiomyopathy caused by "uremic toxins" has been suspected for five decades, its existence as a separate entity has not been clearly demonstrated. Since uremic patients often have other conditions that may alter myocardial function—e.g., anemia, arteriovenous fistula, hypertension, and coronary artery disease—it is difficult to establish the independent contribution of uremia per se to ventricular dysfunction. In an echocardiographic study, uremic patients had left ventricular dilation, hypertrophy, and a higher ratio of left ventricular radius to wall thickness, indicating inadequate hypertrophy. Myocardial dysfunction associated with uremia is often multifactorial, but is reversible. Left ventricular systolic function may improve after peritoneal and hemodialysis. However, such improvement may be secondary to reductions in preload and afterload. Following renal transplantation, four patients with dilated cardiomyopathy, normal coronary angiograms, and severe left ventricular dysfunction were reported to have resolution of heart failure symptoms and return of left ventricular ejection fraction to normal *(39)*. Thus, although the existence of uremic cardiomyopathy is controversial, it is important to remember that the idiopathic cardiomyopathy seen in uremia may be reversible.

Calcium is fundamental to the process of myocardial contraction since its influx through sarcolemmal channels regulates the force of contraction. However, chronic hypocalcemia usually does not cause heart failure. Severe hypocalcemia (<6 mg/dL) in association with congestive heart failure has been described in dialysis patients after parathyroidectomy, with prompt improvement in cardiac function and resolution of heart failure following intravenous calcium replacement. Parathyroid hormone may be a myocardial depressant since cardiac function reportedly improves after parathyroidectomy but the negative inotropic effect of parathyroid hormone has not been established. Hyperkalemia has a negative inotropic effect but the principal detrimental effect is in its electrical effect on the heart. Severe metabolic acidosis impairs calcium release from the sarcoplasmic reticulum and myocardial contractility is impaired at a systemic pH below 7.2. Dystrophic calcification of the myocardial fibers occurs in secondary hyperparathyroidism of chronic renal failure. An increased incidence of calcific aortic stenosis and mitral annular calcification is noted in chronic renal failure. When valvular lesions are severe, myocardial dysfunction may result.

Diastolic Filling

Recently it has become apparent that diastolic dysfunction may lead to heart failure even in the presence of normal systolic function, especially in patients with left ventricular hypertrophy and in the older population. Doppler echocardiography is now used to evaluate the diastolic function of the ventricles; numerous studies have shown that diastolic filling is abnormal in the majority of patients with ventricular hypertrophy. Echocardiographic left ventricular hypertrophy is common among patients with chronic renal failure. Left ventricular hypertrophy often develops and progresses with time on dialysis. Asymmetric septal hypertrophy has also been reported, but this is an unusual manifestation of the hypertrophy resulting from hemodynamic stress and is not associated with left ventricular outflow obstruction.

Development of hypotension during dialysis that cannot be explained by changes in intravascular volume is a clue to impaired diastolic filling. Effect of hemodialysis on diastolic filling has been evaluated using Doppler echocardiography. Fluid removal during hemodialysis reduces the left ventricular preload to the extent that early diastolic filling becomes impaired without a compensatory increase in the atrial phase of filling. Hemodialysis without fluid removal does not alter the left ventricular diastolic filling pattern *(40)*.

Management of heart failure in ESRD patients includes correction of reversible conditions (e.g., coronary revascularization), improving exacerbating conditions (e.g., correction of severe anemia, hypocalcemia) and optimizing the volume status and blood pressure. Angiotensin-converting enzyme inhibitors, vasodilators, β-adrenergic blockers, and low dose digoxin therapy are all useful.

ISCHEMIC RENAL DISEASE

To this point, our review has been confined to a discussion of cardiac problems that arise in patients with renal disease. Ischemic renal disease (IRD), however, is a renal disease that occurs in cardiac patients. We include a discussion of this entity because IRD is very common in patients with arteriosclerotic cardiovascular disease, and consequently, the cardiologist may encounter the patient with IRD well in advance of the nephrologist. IRD is now recognized as an important and *potentially reversible* cause of end-stage renal disease that is often unrecognized by physicians caring for patients with arteriosclerotic complications. In addition, the prevalence of IRD is increasing. For these reasons, we feel that a working knowledge of when to suspect IRD, how to recognize its chief clinical manifestations, and an understanding of the potential benefits of intervention before ESRD supervenes can be of great utility to the practicing cardiologist.

Ischemic renal disease is defined as a clinically significant reduction in glomerular filtration rate and/or loss of renal parenchyma caused by hemodynamically significant arteriosclerotic renal artery stenosis *(41–54)*. IRD is an important cause of progressive renal disease, and the prevalence of IRD is increasing, especially in older patients *(41–54)*. Ischemic renal disease is an important and common consequence of arteriosclerotic renal artery stenosis that is separate and distinct from the problem of renovascular hypertension. In the past, the focus of treatment of patients with renal artery stenosis has primarily been on the goal of lowering blood pressure, but it has been recognized that renal artery stenosis secondary to atherosclerosis may produce progressive loss of renal function due to renal ischemia. Renal ischemia is now understood to be an important and potentially reversible cause of end-stage renal disease (ESRD). With increasing awareness of ischemic nephropathy as a common and important clinical entity there is greater potential for favorably impacting the course of this disease. Consequently, recent interest in renovascular disease has been directed at *preservation of renal function* in addition to correction of hypertension.

Prevalence of IRD

Unsuspected renal artery stenosis is commonly found in patients with coronary artery disease. Patients screened for renal artery disease with abdominal aortography while undergoing elective cardiac catheterization have been found to have a high prevalence of renal artery disease. A study of 1302 of 1651 consecutive cardiac catheterizations revealed significant unilateral renal artery stenosis in 11% of the patients and bilateral renal artery stenosis in 4% *(47)*. Other large studies estimate that 18 to 30% of patients undergoing cardiac catheterization had significant renal artery stenosis.

Natural History of IRD

Stenosis of the renal arteries, when high-grade, has a high likelihood of progressing over a 2-yr period, and progression is associated with loss of renal mass and function. Progressive arterial obstruction occurs in 42 to 53% of patients with renal artery stenosis, with progression to complete

Table 5
Clinical Presentations Suggesting Ischemic Renal Disease

1. Acute renal failure (ARF) caused by the treatment of hypertension, especially with angiotensin-converting enzyme (ACE) inhibitors
2. Progressive azotemia in a patient with known renovascular hypertension
3. Acute pulmonary edema superimposed on poorly controlled hypertension and renal failure
4. Progressive azotemia in an elderly patient with refractory or severe hypertension
5. Progressive azotemia in an elderly patient with evidence of atherosclerotic disease
6. Unexplained progressive azotemia in an elderly patient

renal artery occlusion ranging from 9 to 16%. Complete occlusion is more likely to occur in patients with high-grade stenosis on initial examination (41–46).

The prevalence of IRD as the etiology of ESRD may be between 11 and 14% (65–70,73). Moreover, patients with IRD as the cause of their ESRD have a high mortality rate following the initiation of renal replacement therapy, possibly because of the severity of the underlying atherosclerotic disease (50). IRD patients have a median survival of 27 mo and 5- and 10-yr survival rates of 18% and 5%, respectively. Patients with renal insufficiency secondary to IRD are often considered to be poor candidates for intervention, but the poor survival of these patients once they reach ESRD makes intervention with PTRA or surgical revascularization a reasonable alternative to "conservative" medical therapy.

Pathophysiology of IRD

Reduction in glomerular filtration rate sufficient to cause an elevation of the serum creatinine concentration requires injury to *both* kidneys. Therefore, IRD may arise from one of two principal clinical situations. The first situation is bilateral hemodynamically significant renal artery stenosis leading to bilateral renal ischemia. The second situation is hemodynamically significant renal artery stenosis in a solitary functioning kidney, or in a kidney that is providing the majority of a patient's glomerular filtration. In the second situation, the stenotic kidney suffers from chronic ischemia, while the contralateral kidney has been damaged from other causes. Possible causes of impaired function of the contralateral kidney are damage from severe renovascular hypertension induced by the stenotic kidney and from renal diseases that are typically unilateral, such as pyelonephritis and trauma.

Chronic reduction of blood low to the kidney results in decreased renal size: the well-known clinical hallmark of chronic renal ischemia from atherosclerotic renovascular disease is a unilateral small kidney.

Diagnosis of IRD

Clinical features that suggest renovascular hypertension point to IRD as the cause of renal insufficiency in a patient with coexisting renal failure and hypertension. The lengths of the two kidneys normally differ by less than 1 to 1.5 cm. Asymmetry of renal size in a hypertensive patient strongly suggests IRD. Hypertension is often abrupt in onset, severe, drug-resistant, and may present first after age 50. An abdominal bruit that is localized over the kidneys, prolonged into diastole, or heard in the flank suggests renovascular disease. In addition, there are six major clinical settings in which the clinician could suspect IRD (51,52) (Table 5).

A typical clinical presentation of a patient likely to have IRD is that of an older (>50 yr) patient with generalized atherosclerosis and refractory hypertension demonstrating progressive azotemia in conjunction with antihypertensive drug therapy (41–45). Patients with unsuspected arteriosclerotic IRD may present with acute renal failure caused by treatment of hypertension, particularly with angiotensin-converting enzyme (ACE) inhibitors. A reversible worsening of azotemia during ACE inhibitor therapy should raise the suspicion of IRD. ACE inhibitors may acutely alter intrarenal hemodynamics. The stenotic kidney depends on angiotensin II to maintain GFR. All causes vasoconstriction of both afferent and efferent arterioles, but with preferential effects on the efferent arterioles. This differential vasoconstriction increases the glomerular capillary pressure and therefore maintains or increases the single-nephron glomerular filtration rate (SNGFR). When the vasoconstrictor effect of angiotensin II on the efferent arteriole is blocked by an ACE inhibitor, efferent arteriolar constriction relaxes and glomerular capillary filtration pressures and glomerular filtration rate decrease. Although ACE inhibitor-induced acute renal failure (ARF) is an important clinical marker for IRD, the absence of ARF does not rule out the possibility of significant IRD because only 6–38% of patients with significant renal vascular disease will develop ARF when treated with these agents (53). The ARF associated with the use of antihypertensive agents in patients with IRD is generally reversible and indicates further clinical evaluation.

Recurrent acute pulmonary edema in patients with poorly controlled hypertension and renal insufficiency has also been reported to be a marker of severe bilateral atherosclerotic renal artery disease (51,52). Volume-dependent renovascular hypertension caused by bilateral renal artery stenoses appears to be the dominant factor in producing the pulmonary edema. Patients with pulmonary edema, uncontrolled hypertension, and azotemia have not been prospectively evaluated to establish what percent of patients with this scenario have IRD, but this clinical picture should alert the clinician to the possibility of IRD. The episodes of pulmonary edema may cease following renal revascularization.

A common presentation of IRD is unexplained progressive azotemia in an elderly patient with evidence of atherosclerotic disease. As discussed previously, angiographic studies have indicated a high prevalence of renal artery stenosis among patients with atherosclerotic disease in other vessels. Therefore, a history or physical findings of generalized are strongly suggestive of ischemic nephropathy.

POST-ACE INHIBITOR RENOGRAPHY

ACE inhibitor renography is the most accurate noninvasive functional test for diagnosing *renovascular hypertension*, but its accuracy is diminished in the setting of renal failure. ACE inhibitor renography generally has difficulty differentiating ischemic renal disease from intrinsic renal disease.

DUPLEX DOPPLER SONOGRAPHY

Duplex Doppler sonography (DDS) is useful for diagnosing IRD. DDS combines ultrasound and Doppler techniques to locate the renal artery and assess renal artery blood flow velocity. DDS has several major advantages: it is useful in the presence of azotemia; it is not necessary to discontinue antihypertensive agents as in ACE inhibitor renography; there is no risk of contrast nephropathy or cholesterol embolization; and bilateral renal artery stenosis can be assessed. Even total obstruction of a renal artery can be diagnosed by scanning over the kidney. The main limitation of DDS is inadequate studies because of patient obesity, the presence of bowel gas, and previous abdominal surgery.

Magnetic resonance angiography and spiral computed tomography (spiral CT) angiography are recently developed techniques that have been used to detect renal vascular disease with a high sensitivity and specificity, but 100 to 150 mL of contrast medium must be given in the latter procedure.

Treatment of IRD

SELECTION OF PATIENTS FOR INTERVENTION

The prognosis of medically treated IRD is poor, with many patients showing a deterioration of renal function during follow-up. Patients with high-grade (>75%) arterial stenosis bilaterally or involving a solitary functioning kidney are at risk of complete renal arterial occlusion. Intervention is indicated to restore renal arterial blood flow to preserve renal function. Total occlusion of the renal artery does not always indicate irreversible ischemic parenchymal damage because the viability of the kidney can be maintained through development of collateral arterial supply. This situation occurs when the arterial occlusion is gradual. Several clinical clues suggest that reestablishment of renal arterial flow can lead to recovery of renal function: (1) kidney size more than 9 cm; (2) evidence of acceptable function of the involved kidney on isotope renography; (3) angiographic filling of the distal renal arterial tree by collateral circulation in patients with total renal arterial occlusion proximally; (4) renal biopsy demonstrating well-preserved glomeruli with minimal arteriolar sclerosis; (5) preoperative serum creatinine levels of less than 3.0 mg/dL; and (6) presentation with acute deterioration of renal function after initiation of medical antihypertensive therapy, especially with an ACE inhibitor *(41–45)*.

The rate of decline in renal function is also an important determinant of the outcome after intervention in atherosclerotic ischemic renal disease. Rapid deterioration of renal function in a patient with renal artery stenosis (especially in association with ACE inhibitor therapy), suggests a strong possibility of retrieval of function by intervention to restore renal arterial flow. Patients with chronic severe azotemia (serum creatinine >4 mg/dL) are likely to have severe renal parenchymal disease, and improvement in renal function following revascularization or angioplasty is less likely. Exceptions to this observation are cases of total main renal artery occlusion, wherein kidney viability is maintained via collateral circulation.

PERCUTANEOUS TRANSLUMINAL RENAL ANGIOPLASTY

Percutaneous transluminal renal angioplasty (PTRA) does not require general anesthesia and can be repeated if needed. In patients with nonostial renal artery disease, the success rate of PTRA has been excellent. PTRA is less effective treatment for ostial lesions. Restenosis is the predominant cause of failure in patients with ostial lesions, due either to elastic recoil of the dilated artery, neointimal hyperplasia, or recurrent atheromatous disease. Technical difficulties and complications of angiographic investigation and PTRA in these patients include contrast media-induced acute renal failure and atheroembolic renal disease.

Endovascular stents are a newer treatment option for patients with ostial lesions or who are considered poor risks for surgical revascularization *(53)*. Early recurrent arterial stenosis is a problem. This technique requires further experience and evaluation, but offers promise to patients with ostial lesions who are not candidates for surgery.

SURGICAL REVASCULARIZATION

The surgical treatment of renovascular disease has been recently reviewed by Novick *(78)*. Surgical revascularization to preserve renal function in patients with high-grade atherosclerotic arterial occlusive disease affecting both kidneys or a solitary kidney may result in improvement or stabilization of renal function postoperatively in 75–89% of patients. For example, the Cleveland Clinic performed surgical revascularization for preservation of renal function in 161 patients with critical stenosis bilaterally or in a solitary kidney and achieved postoperative improvement in renal function in 93 patients (58%), stabilization in 50 patients (31%), and deterioration in only 18 patients (11%).

Surgical renal vascular reconstruction can be performed with operative mortality rates in the range of 2.1–6.1% and a high technical success rate. An increased risk of operative mortality has been observed with bilateral simultaneous renal revascularization, or when renal revascularization is performed in conjunction with another major vascular operation such as aortic replacement. Most studies have indicated a high technical success rate for surgical vascular reconstruction with postoperative thrombosis or stenosis rates of less than 10%.

SUMMARY

It is readily apparent that progressive renal disease is complicated by several common cardiovascular alterations including pericarditis, renal parenchymal hypertension, primary arteriosclerosis, and left ventricular dysfunction. We have reviewed the pathogenesis, clinical features, and management of the cardiovascular disorders. In addition, we have included a reviewed of ischemic renal disease (IRD), a common, albeit underdiagnosed, disorder that cardiologists may frequently encounter well in advance of the nephrologist. Increasing recognition that IRD is a *potentially reversible* cause of end-stage renal disease underscores the importance of its inclusion in our review. We are hopeful that the management approaches proposed in this chapter will facilitate the optimal care of these difficult patients.

REFERENCES

1. Rostand SG, Rutsky EA. Cardiac disease in dialysis patients. In: Nissenson AR, Fine RN, Gentile DE, eds. Clinical Dialysis, 3rd ed. Appleton and Lange, Norwalk, CT, 1995, pp. 652–698.
2. Lundin AP. Cardiovascular system in uremia. Part 1. Pericarditis. In: Massry SG, Glassock RJ, eds. Textbook of Nephrology, 3rd ed. Williams and Wilkins, Baltimore, 1995, pp. 1339–1363.
3. Preston RA, Chakko S, Materson BJ. End-stage renal disease. In: Rapaport E, ed. Cardiology and Co-existing Disease. Churchill Livingstone, NY, 1994, pp. 175–196.
4. Lazarus MJ, Denker BM, Owen WF Jr. Hemodialysis. In: Brenner BM, ed. Brenner and Rector's The Kidney, 5th ed. W. B. Saunders, Philadelphia, 1996, pp. 2424–2506.
5. Bailey GL, Hampers CL, Hager EB, Merrill JP. Uremic pericarditis. Clinical features and management. Circulation 1968;38:582–591.
6. Rutsky EA, Rostand SG. Pericarditis in end-stage renal disease: clinical characteristics and management. Semin Dial 1989;2:25–30.
7. De Pace NL, Nestico PF, Schwartz AB, et al. Predicting success of intensive dialysis in the treatment of uremic pericarditis. Am J Med 1984;76:38–46.
8. Rutsky EA, Rostand SG. Treatment of uremic pericarditis and pericardial effusion. Am J Kidney Dis 1987;10:2–8.
9. Silverberg S, Oreopoulos DG, Wise DJ, et al. Pericarditis in patients undergoing long-term hemodialysis and peritoneal dialysis. Incidence, complications and management. Am J Med 1977;63:874–880.
10. Comty CM, Cohen SL, Shapiro FL. Pericarditis in chronic uremia and its sequels. Ann Intern Med 1971;75:173–183.
11. Ribot S, Frankel HJ, Gielchinsky I, et al. Treatment of uremic pericarditis. Clin Nephrol 1974;2:127–130.
12. Preston RA, Epstein M. Hypertension and renal parenchymal disease. Seminars in Nephrology 1995;15:138–151.
13. Preston RA, Singer I, Epstein M. Renal parenchymal hypertension: current concepts of pathogenesis and management. Arch Intern Med 1996;154:637–642.
14. Campese VM. Salt sensitivity in hypertension. Renal and cardiovascular implications. Hypertension 1994;23: 531–550.
15. Brater DC. Diuretic therapy. N Engl J Med 1998;339:387–395.
16. Lewis EJ, Hunsicker LG, Bain RP, Rohde RD. The effect of angiotensin-converting-enzyme inhibition on diabetic nephropathy. N Engl J Med 1993;329:1456–1462.
17. Agodoa LY, Appel L, Bakris GL, et al. African American Study of Kidney Disease and Hypertension (AASK) Study Group. Effect of ramipril vs amlodipine on renal outcomes in hypertensive nephrosclerosis: a randomized controlled trial. JAMA 2001;285:2719–2728.
18. Maschio G, Alberti D, Janin G, et al. Effect of the angiotensin-converting enzyme inhibitor benazepril on the progression of chronic renal insufficiency. N Engl J Med 1996;334:939–945.
19. The GISEN Group. Randomized placebo controlled trial of effect of ramipril on decline in glomerular filtration rate and risk of terminal renal failure in proteinuric, non-diabetic nephropathy. Lancet 1997;349:1857–1863.
20. Brenner BM, Cooper ME, de Zeeuw D, et al. RENAAL Study Investigators. Effects of losartan on renal and cardiovascular outcomes in patients with type 2 diabetes and nephropathy. N Engl J Med 2001;345:861–869.
21. Lewis EJ, Hunsicker LG, Clarke WR, et al. Collaborative Study Group. Renoprotective effect of the angiotensin-receptor antagonist irbesartan in patients with nephropathy due to type 2 diabetes. N Engl J Med 2001;345:851–860.
22. Parving HH, Lehnert H, Brochner-Mortensen J, et al. Irbesartan in Patients with Type 2 Diabetes and Microalbuminuria Study Group. The effect of irbesartan on the development of diabetic nephropathy in patients with type 2 diabetes. N Engl J Med 2001;345:870–878.
23. Foley RN, Harnett JD, Parfrey PS. Cardiovascular complications of end-stage renal disease. In: Schrier RW, Gottschalk CW, eds. Diseases of the Kidney. Little, Brown, Boston, 1997, pp. 2647–2660.
24. Churchill DN, Taylor DW, Cook RJ. Canadian Hemodialysis Morbidity Study. Am J Kidney Dis 1992;19:214–234.
25. Tepel M, van der Giet M, Park A, Zidek W. Association of calcium channel blockers and mortality in hemodialysis patients. Clin Sci 2002;103:511–515.
26. United States Renal Data System. Am J Kidney Dis 2003;42(6 Suppl 5):1–230.
27. Boudoulas H, leier CV. Renal disorders and cardiovascular disease. In: Braunwald E, ed. Heart Disease. W. B. Saunders, Philadelphia, 2001, pp. 1856–1874.
28. Toto R, Lena Vega GL, Grundy SM. Mechanisms and treatment of dyslipidemia of renal diseases. Curr Opin Nephrol Hypertens 1993;2:784–790.
29. Holley J, Fenton RA, Arthur RS. Thallium stress testing does not predict cardiovascular disease in diabetic patients with end-stage renal disease undergoing cadaveric renal transplantation. Am J Med 1990;90:563–570.
30. Reis G, Marcovitz PA, Leichtman AB, et al. Usefulness of dobutamine stress echocardiography in detecting coronary artery disease in end-stage renal disease. Am J Cardiol 1995;75:707–710.
31. Besarab A, Bolton WK, Browne JK, et al. The effects of normal as compared with low hematocrit values in patients with cardiac disease who are receiving hemodialysis and epoetin. N Engl J Med 1998;339:584–590.

32. The US Recombinant Human Erythropoietin Predialysis Study Group. Double-blind, placebo-controlled study of the therapeutic use of recombinant human erythropoietin for anemia associated with chronic renal failure in pre-dialysis patients. Am J Kidney Dis 1991;18:50–59.

33. Herzog CA, Ma JZ, Collins AJ. Poor long-term survival after acute myocardial infarction among patients on long-term dialysis. N Engl J Med 1998;339:799–805.

34. Marenzi G, Marana I, Lauri G, et al. The prevention and mangement of radiocontrast agent induced nephropathy by hemofiltration. N Engl J Med 2003;349:1333–1340.

35. Rao V, Weisel RD, Buth KJ, et al. Coronary artery bypass grafting in non-dialysis dependent renal insufficiency. Circulation 1996;Supplement II:38.

36. Crosbie WA, Snowden S, Parsons V. Changes in pulmonary capillary permeability in renal failure. Br Med J 1972;4: 388–390.

37. Kleiger RE, deMello VR, Malone D, et al. Left ventricular function in end-stage renal disease. Echocardiographic classification. South Med J 1981;74:819–824.

38. Anderson CB, Codd JR, Graff RA, et al. Cardiac failure as a complication of upper extremity arteriovenous dialysis fistulas. Arch Intern Med 1976;136:292–297.

39. Burt RK, Burt SG, Suki WN, et al. Reversal of left ventricular dysfunction after renal transplantation. Ann Intern Med 1989;111:635–640.

40. Chakko S, Girgis I, Contreras G, et al. Effects of hemodialysis on left ventricular diastolic filling. Am J Cardiol 1997; 79:106–108.

41. Preston RA, Epstein M. Ischemic renal disease: an emerging cause of chronic renal failure and end-stage renal disease. J Hypertens 1997;15:1365–1377.

42. Preston RA, Epstein M. Ischemic renal disease. Am J Therapeutics 1998;5:203–210.

43. Greco BA, Breyer JA. The natural history of renal artery stenosis: who should be evaluated for ischemic nephropa-thy? Sem Nephrol 1996;16:2–11.

44. Greco BA, Breyer JA. Atherosclerotic ischemic renal disease. Am J Kidney Dis 1997;29:167–187.

45. Pohl MA. Renal artery stenosis, renal vascular hypertension, and ischemic nephropathy. In: Schrier RW, Gottschalk CW, eds. Diseases of the Kidney. Little, Brown, Boston, 1997, pp. 1367–1423.

46. Alcazar JM, Caramelo CA, Alegre ER, Abad J. Ischaemic renal injury. Curr Opin Nephrol Hypertens 1997;6:157–165.

47. Harding MB, Smith LR, Himmestein SI, et al. Renal artery stenosis: prevalence and associated risk factors in patients undergoing routine cardiac catheterization. J Am Soc Nephrol 1992;2:1608–1616.

48. Zierler RE, Bergelin RO, Isaacson AJ, Strandness DE Jr. Natural history of renal artery stenosis: a prospective study with duplex ultrasound. J Vasc Surg 1994;19:250–258.

49. Mailloux LU, Napolitano B, Bellucci AG, et al. Renal vascular disease causing end-stage renal disease, incidence, clinical correlates, and outcomes: a 20-year clinical experience. Am J Kidney Dis 1994;24:622–629.

50. Mallioux LU, Bellucci AG, Mossey RT. Predictors of survival in patients undergoing dialysis. Am J Med 1988;84: 855–862.

51. Pickering TG, Herman L, Devereux RB, et al. Recurrent pulmonary oedema in hypertension due to bilateral renal artery stenosis: treatment by angioplasty or surgical revascularization. Lancet 1988;2:551–552.

52. Messina LM, Zelenock GB, Yao KA, Stanley JC. Renal revascularization for recurrent pulmonary edema in patients with poorly controlled hypertension and renal insufficiency: a distinct subgroup of patients with arteriosclerotic renal artery occlusive disease. J Vasc Surg 1992;15:73–82.

53. Dorros G, Jaff M, Jain A, Dufek C, Mathiak L. Follow-up of primary Palmaz-Shatz stent placement for atheroscle-rotic renal artery stenosis. Am J Cardiol 1995;75:1051–1055.

54. Textor SC. Ischemic nephropathy: where are we now? J Am Soc Nephrol 2004;15:1974–1982.

RECOMMENDED READING

Bakris GL, Williams M, Dworkin L, et al. Preserving renal function in adults with hypertension and diabetes: a consensus approach. National Kidney Foundation Hypertension and Diabetes Executive Committees Working Group. Am J Kidney Dis 2000;36:646–661.

Epstein M, Campese VM. Evolving role of calcium antagonists in the management of hypertension. Med Clin North Am 2004;88:149–165.

Foley RN, Wright JR, Parfrey PS. Cardiac function and cardiac disease in renal failure. In: Greenberg A, ed. Primer on Kidney Diseases. National Kidney Foundation.Academic Press, San Diego, CA, 2001, pp. 434–438.

Gunukula SR, Spodick DH. Pericardial disease in renal patients. Sem Nephrol 2001;21:52–56.

Sowers JR, Epstein M, Frohlich ED. Diabetes, hypertension and cardiovascular disease: an update. Hypertension 2001; 37:1053–1059.

41 Assessment of Patients With Heart Disease for Fitness for Noncardiac Surgery

Joseph Savino, MD and Lee A. Fleisher, MD

INTRODUCTION

The tendency in medicine over the past decade is to decrease preoperative testing, as the evidence for improved outcomes for these often expensive procedures is lacking. Population-based management decisions are often steered by clinical trials, cost-effectiveness analysis, and resource allocation. However, few doctors take care of populations. Most of us care for individuals. Evidence-based paradigms based on "population medicine" define the most effective management scheme for the vast majority of patients, but not for every patient. Individual patient decisions by attending physicians are not consistently based on evidence but are often made in the context of "what would I do if it was my mother?" with the premise that more information is better. Should every patient undergoing repair of an abdominal aortic aneurysm undergo dipyridamole or dobutamine stress testing? The evidence supports not. Nonetheless, the practice in many centers is to obtain a dipyridamole or adenosine thallium stress test even if the patient is asymptomatic. Despite the reassurances provided by large clinical trials, practitioners do not consistently adhere to their recommendations and often rely on tradition, anecdote, and impression in their decision-making. If physicians are to remain the dispensers of medical care and resources, then we need to be cognizant of the effects of our decisions on all patients, not just the one sitting in the examination room. Exorbitant sums spent on unnecessary testing exhausts valuable resources that could be diverted to the more needy. Unfortunately, the risk of uncertainty and medicolegal liability results in more testing than is often indicated.

The evaluation of the patient scheduled for anesthesia for noncardiac surgery remains a diagnostic dilemma because of competing issues of economics, expediency, and the desire to have a complete knowledge base regarding the extent of cardiovascular disease. Multiple medical specialties are involved in the evaluation of the high-risk patient, each of which may have complementary or redundant contributions. In many institutions, anesthesiologists have established preoperative evaluation clinics and the surgeon will defer to the anesthesiologist's judgment regarding the need for extensive cardiovascular consultation *(1)*. However, these same "preoperative clinics" are at a significant cost to the hospital or the physician practices as their activity is not independently reimbursable by payers, and their cost-effectiveness has never been determined. Not uncommonly, the surgeon may initiate a cardiology consultation. The most effective paradigm to accomplish the preoperative assessment of cardiovascular fitness may be institution dependent, based on allocation of resources and expertise of staff. A preoperative evaluation clinic and a preoperative medical clearance by the primary physician for all patients seems redundant and unnecessary. Whatever the model, the goal of all individuals involved in the care of the surgical patient with heart disease

From: *Essential Cardiology: Principles and Practice, 2nd Ed.*
Edited by: C. Rosendorff © Humana Press Inc., Totowa, NJ

is to ensure that critical information is attained and communicated to the appropriate personnel so that optimal care can be provided.

CONCEPTS FOR PREOPERATIVE CARDIAC EVALUATION

The underlying premise for the need for preoperative evaluation is that the information will be used to modify perioperative care and improve outcome. The preoperative evaluation will also be used to provide the patient and physicians with information to assess risk and to determine if the benefits of the planned procedure outweigh these risks. The benefits of some elective surgeries may be small or may not accrue for several years. Alternatives to complex surgery, such as external beam or seed radiation implants for the treatment of prostate cancer, may be preferable for the patient at high risk of perioperative cardiac morbidity. Endovascular stents for the treatment of aortic aneurysm have revolutionized the discipline of vascular surgery (2). Initially considered an alternative for the aortic aneurysm patient who was considered at high risk for surgery and aortic clamping, stenting has rapidly become the treatment of choice for many patients, even in the absence of comorbidity.

The most important role is the evaluation of patients with unstable symptoms, as these patients have been shown to be at prohibitive risk (3). Management of unstable cardiovascular symptoms is achieved prior to elective surgery because the risk of tachycardia, hypercoagulability, and plaque rupture may be greater during the perioperative period. Coronary revascularization should be considered for patients with unstable angina, although the culprit lesion for a postoperative myocardial infarction is not reliably the coronary artery with the angiographically most significant stenosis (4). Alternative treatment strategies need to be considered if the procedure is emergent. The use of invasive monitoring during anesthesia and surgery is not without cost and risks. The use of a pulmonary artery catheter is unlikely to change outcome (5). The preoperative evaluation should be used to identify those individuals for whom postoperative intensive care is warranted.

ROLE OF THE CONSULTANT

As outlined in the recent American Heart Association/American College of Cardiology Guidelines on Perioperative Cardiovascular Evaluation for Noncardiac Surgery, the role of the consultant is to define the extent and stability of a patient's cardiac disease and determine if the patient is in optimum medical condition (6). Unfortunately, there is no assurance that optimization of preoperative disease leads to improved outcome, although it appears that postoperative myocardial infarction and death are more likely to occur in patients with preexisting left main or three-vessel coronary artery disease (4). If these patients can be identified in advance of their surgery, treatment or alternatives to surgery can be sought. There is a small but growing body of data that suggests that risk modification may actually improve outcome in the operative setting. The treatment of active coronary artery disease is efficacious before surgery. The perceived benefit of treatment of heart failure before surgery is based on the increased morbidity associated with NYHA class III and IV heart failure. Systolic or diastolic dysfunction leading to heart failure may produce the greatest cardiovascular risk, especially if the etiology is ischemic heart disease (7). The incidence of diastolic dysfunction and abnormal ventricular filling is often ignored during preoperative assessment, despite its marked prevalence in the aged (8). Although studies in surgical patients are lacking, diastolic dysfunction has been associated with significant increases in "all-cause" mortality during long term follow-up after adjustment for age, gender, and ventricular ejection fraction (9). An asymptomatic systolic murmur warrants an echocardiogram to assess aortic and mitral valve function. Occult aortic stenosis can lead to a catastrophic response to the vasodilatory effects of anesthetic induction or neuroaxial blockade and sympathectomy. Mitral regurgitation is typically better tolerated, as the vasodilation during anesthesia typically decreases regurgitant fraction and improves forward flow. Rheumatic mitral stenosis is much less common, but may become symptomatic during the perioperative period, especially during pregnancy. Severe pulmonary hypertension with mitral disease may lead to right heart failure and circulatory instability. Patients with prosthetic valves need meticulous attention to bacterial prophylaxis, depending on the nature of the operation. A growing population in the United States is adults with corrected congenital heart disease who often present with complex reconstruction of the great vessels of the mediastinum, residual shunts, pulmonary hypertension, and increased risk of endocarditis. Pathophysiology can vary significantly among cohorts of patients who carry the same diagnosis. Their response to intraoperative derangements may differ substantially, not allowing them to be considered under the same rubric (10). Preoperative assessment often includes echocardiography, electrocardiogram, and chest radiograph. Age-related cardiovascular disorders, as well as postoperative cardiac residua, need to be considered in their preparation for noncardiac surgery. Aggressive control of blood glucose levels during and after surgery leads to a decrease in wound infection, renal insufficiency, other major comorbidities, and mortality in surgical patients in the intensive care unit (11). It is appropriate to suggest that aggressive perioperative glucose control in diabetics begins with the preoperative period and the preoperative assessment. The benefits of preoperative "optimization" of hypertension, hypercholesterolemia, and smoking cessation are less clear. From the anesthesiologist's perspective, the necessary critical factors that modify intraoperative technique and monitoring are preexisting disease and the complexity of the operative procedure. The guidelines state that the specific choice of anesthetic technique and agents are best determined by the anesthesia providers (6). Inhalation anesthetics pose a potential advantage (preconditioning) and disadvantage (steal effect) in patients with coronary artery disease (12–14). The choice of anesthetic technique and agents does not influence cardiovascular outcome. There appears to be no evidence to support the use of regional (epidural and spinal) anesthesia over general anesthesia. Hence, the preoperative evaluation should target not the type of anesthetic, but rather the patient's condition in the context of the planned operation.

PATHOPHYSIOLOGY OF PERIOPERATIVE CARDIAC EVENTS

The pathophysiology underlying perioperative cardiac events is multifactorial, which influences the potential value of preoperative cardiac testing. There has been a great deal of attention focused on the association of perioperative myocardial ischemia and cardiac morbidity. In several large-scale studies, the presence of postoperative ischemia had the strongest association with myocardial infarction and cardiac death (15,16). Further analysis has suggested that prolonged ischemia is a critical factor for predicting events (17). If mismatches of supply and demand in patients with critical coronary stenoses are the underlying substrate for these events, then either coronary revascularization or tight hemodynamic management should reduce morbidity (Fig. 1). The use of β-adrenergic blockade has been associated with a reduction in perioperative myocardial ischemia and a significantly improved long-term survival (18,19). Statins and their lipid-modifying and antiinflammatory properties were associated with a reduction in operative mortality in patients undergoing major noncardiac vascular surgery (20). Maintenance of normothermia significantly decreased the rate of cardiac complications in a randomized clinical trial of intraoperative forced-air warming (21). Anemia (hematocrit <28%) was associated with an increased incidence of cardiac morbidity in a small cohort study (22). All of these factors could contribute to ischemia, which, if prolonged, may lead to infarction. Yet symptomatic cardiac events and cardiac death may result from acute coronary thrombosis of a noncritical stenosis. Plaque rupture and acute coronary thrombosis and occlusion occur in preexisting critical and noncritical coronary lesions. Downstream myocardium in the latter case may be at greater risk than myocardium supplied by a significantly obstructed coronary artery, because there is unlikely to be an established collateral circulation (4). Preoperative evaluation of significant preoperative coronary disease fails in this instance in identifying a high-risk event. Value may be gained by affecting the coagulation profile of surgery (23). It is unclear which surgical procedures and which anesthetics are associated with an increased propensity for arterial thrombosis.

CARDIAC RISK INDICES

Does treating the risk factor change the risk? Many studies have adopted the approach of defining a cohort of patients, identifying risk factors, and using multivariate modeling to determine those

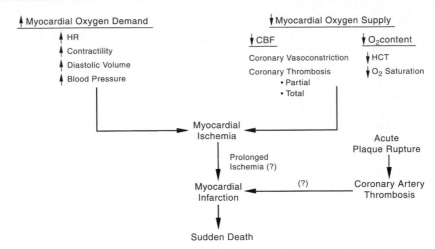

Fig. 1. Pathophysiology of acute coronary syndromes during the perioperative period. In the setting of a coronary stenosis, the normal ability of vasculature to adjust flow and meet an increase in myocardial oxygen demand is limited. Even if demand is steady, acute decreases in oxygen supply can occur. Both conditions may lead to myocardial ischemia. Prolonged ischemia, in turn, may lead to infarction, although an alternative hypothesis implicates plaque rupture and thrombus formation at a noncritical stenosis. HR, heart rate; CBF, coronary blood flow; HCT, hematocrit.

factors associated with increased risk. A major limitation was the assumption that the intraoperative period is a "black box," and that care is not modified by knowledge of the risk factor. Once a risk factor is identified, anesthesiologists will often attempt risk modification in an attempt to reduce risk, such as the use of β-blockers in the setting of known coronary artery disease. Risk modification is not without controversy. In only a few instances has risk modification been associated with improved outcome. Caution is heeded when risk modification poses a significant risk of its own. In the aggressive management of blood glucose levels after surgery in the intensive care unit, for example, despite hourly checks, the incidence of hypoglycemia increased 10-fold *(11)*.

There are numerous specific disease states that increase perioperative risk. Cardiovascular disease is the most extensively studied, with the goal of identifying patients at greatest risk for fatal and nonfatal myocardial infarctions. In 1977, Goldman and colleagues at Massachusetts General Hospital *(24)* used multivariate logistic regression to demonstrate that nine clinical factors were associated with increased morbidity and mortality in a population of 1001 patients over the age of 45 yr (Table 1). Each of these risk factors was associated with a given weight in the logistic regression equation, which was converted into a point system to calculate the Goldman Cardiac Risk Index. A higher point total resulted in a higher risk index and greater likelihood of a cardiac event. The validity of this classic study has not survived the test of time, as perioperative care has improved outcome and decreased complications. Hence, the current relevance of the Goldman Index is that risk stratification is a dynamic process. We have made substantial strides toward improvements in cardiovascular outcomes since 1977 and anticipate further advances in the years to come.

Other investigators have attempted to develop risk indices. Detsky studied a cohort of individuals who were referred to an internal medicine service for preoperative evaluation (Table 2) *(25)*. Many of the factors identified by Goldman were confirmed or slightly modified in the Detsky index, although angina was added to the risk factors. Detsky realized that the nature of the planned operation affected the risk of a complication. Detsky advocated the calculation of a pretest probability of complication based upon the type of surgery, after which the Modified Risk Index is applied using a nomogram. The Detsky index, defined in 1987, has been advocated as the starting point for risk stratification for the American College of Physicians Guidelines on preoperative evaluation published a decade later *(26)*. Hence, the overall probability of complications can be estimated as a function of both the surgical procedure and patient disease.

Table 1
Computation of the Cardiac Risk Index

Criteria	Multivariate discriminant function coefficient	"Points"
I. History:		
a. Age >70 yr	0.191	5
b. MI in previous 6 mo	0.384	10
II. Physical examination:		
a. S_3 gallop or JVD	0.451	11
b. Important VAS	0.119	3
III. Electrocardiogram:		
a. Rhythm other than sinus or PACs on last preoperative ECG	0.283	7
b. >5 PVCs/min documented at any time before operation	0.278	7
IV. General status:		
PO_2 < 60 or PCO_2 > 50 mmHg, K < 3.0 or HCO_3 < 20 mEq/L,	0.132	3
BUN > 50 or Cr > 3.0 mg/dL, abnormal SGOT, signs of		
chronic liver disease, or patient bedridden from noncardiac causes		3
V. Operation:		
a. Intraperitoneal, intrathoracic, or aortic operation	0.123	3
b. Emergency operation	0.167	4
Total possible		53 points

MI, myocardial infarction; JVD, jugular vein distention; VAS, valvular aortic stenosis; PACs, premature atrial contractions; ECG, electrocardiogram; PVCs, premature ventricular contractions; PO_2, partial pressure of oxygen; PCO_2, partial pressure of carbon dioxide; K, potassium; HCO_3, bicarbonate; BUN, blood urea nitrogen; Cr, creatinine; SGOT, serum glutamic oxalacetic transaminases. (From ref. *24* with permission.)

Table 2
Modified Cardiac Risk Index by Detsky et al.

Variables	Points
Angina	
Class IV	20
Class III	10
Unstable angina <3 mo	10
Suspected critical aortic stenosis	20
Myocardial infarction	
<6 mo	10
>6 mo	5
Alveolar pulmonary edema	
<1 wk	10
Ever	5
Emergency surgery	10
Sinus plus atrial premature beats or rhythm other than sinus on preop ECG	5
>5 PVCs at any time before surgery	5
Poor general medical status	5
Age >70 yr	5

Reproduced with permission from ref. *25*.

In an attempt to update the original Cardiac Risk Index, investigators at Brigham and Women's Hospital studied 4315 patients aged 50 yr undergoing elective major noncardiac procedures in a tertiary-care teaching hospital *(27)*. Six independent predictors of complications were identified and included in a Revised Cardiac Risk Index: high-risk type of surgery, history of ischemic heart

Table 3
Clinical Predictors of Increased Perioperative Cardiovascular Risk
(Myocardial Infarction, Congestive Heart Failure, Death)

Major
  Unstable coronary syndromes
    Recent myocardial infarction[a] with evidence of important ischemic risk by clinical symptoms or
      noninvasive study
    Unstable or sever[b] angina (Canadian Class III or IV)[c]
  Decompensated congestive heart failure
  Significant arrhythmias
    High-grade atrioventricular block
    Symptomatic ventricular arrhythmias in the presence of underlying heart disease
    Supraventricular arrhythmias with uncontrolled ventricular rate
    Severe valvular disease
Intermediate
  Mild angina pectoris (Canadian Class I or II)
  Prior myocardial infarction by history or pathological Q waves
  Compensated or prior congestive heart failure
  Diabetes mellitus
  Chronic renal insufficiency
Minor
  Advanced age
  Abnormal ECG (left ventricular hypertrophy, left bundle branch block, ST-T abnormalities)
  Rhythm other than sinus (e.g., atrial fibrillation)
  Low functional capacity (e.g., inability to climb one flight of stairs with a bag of groceries)
  History of stroke
  Uncontrolled systemic hypertension

ECG indicates electrocardiogram.
[a]The American College of Cardiology National Database Library defines recent MI as greater than 7 d but less than
or equal to 1 mo (30 d).
[b]May include "stable" angina in patients who are unusually sedentary.
[c]Campeau L. Grading of angina pectoris. *Circulation* 1976;54:522–523.
ECG, electrocardiogram. (Reproduced with permission from ref. *6*.)

disease, history of congestive heart failure, history of cerebrovascular disease, preoperative treatment with insulin, and preoperative serum creatinine >2.0 mg/dL. Rates of major cardiac complication increased with an increasing number of risk factors.

CLINICAL RISK FACTORS (TABLE 3)

In virtually all studies, the presence of active congestive heart failure (CHF) is associated with the highest perioperative risk. The American College of Cardiology/American Heart Association Guidelines differentiate active CHF, which is considered a major risk factor, from compensated CHF, which is considered an intermediate risk factor.

Time from a prior MI has traditionally been an important predictor of perioperative risk. The more recent the myocardial infarction, particularly within 3 to 6 mo, the greater the perioperative risk *(28–30)*. However, like the Goldman Index, medicine has changed and outcomes are improved. The classic Rao paper published in 1983 cited a reinfarction rate of nearly 30% if noncoronary surgery occurred within 3 mo of a prior infarction. These catastrophic events had a very high mortality rate. With the advent of dedicated postoperative intensive care units, more vigilant monitoring, and early intervention, the postoperative reinfarction rate has decreased to almost an order of magnitude less *(31)*. The ACC/AHA Guidelines advocate the use of 30 d as the acute period, with high risk continuing up to 6 to 8 wk *(6)*. After that time, a prior MI places the patient in the intermediate clinical risk category and further evaluation depends on clinical symptoms.

The presence of angina has not consistently been established as a risk factor. However, the presence of unstable angina was associated with a 28% incidence of perioperative MI *(3)*. Such patients would benefit from the delay of surgery and stability of the coronary symptoms. For patients with chronic stable angina, exercise tolerance appears to be a good method of assessing risk. The ACC/AHA Guidelines advocate the use of the Canadian Cardiovascular Society Classification as a means of stratifying risk, with those in class III or IV at high risk, and class I and II considered intermediate risk.

Risk Factors for Coronary Artery Disease

Hypertension has not been found to be an independent risk factor for perioperative myocardial infarction, heart failure, or arrhythmia in the vast majority of studies, but was shown to be predictive of perioperative myocardial ischemia. The history of hypertension should be a cue to the practitioner to target the cardiovascular system in preoperative questioning and evaluation. The patient with a sustained diastolic blood pressure greater than 110 mmHg often triggers a delay in surgery, although the data do not support such an assertion *(32,33)*. In fact, none of the patients with "uncontrolled systemic hypertension" sustained a major cardiac event, and the authors *(33)* simply state that surgery is safe with hypertension up to a diastolic of 110 mmHg. Patients with a diastolic blood pressure greater than 110 mmHg may be at risk for hemodynamic lability, but there appears to be no increased risk of postoperative complications *(32)*. They are more likely to develop hypotension and hypertension during anesthesia and surgery, but no evidence suggests they are at increased risk of MI. Isolated systolic hypertension was shown in one study of coronary artery bypass grafting (CABG) to be associated with a 30% increase in cardiovascular complications *(34)*. Chronic hypertension may increase cardiac risk simply because coronary artery disease is more prevalent in this patient cohort. Left ventricular hypertrophy, particularly with a strain pattern, has been associated with an increased risk of perioperative myocardial ischemia *(35)*.

Diabetes has been associated with a high incidence of perioperative cardiac morbidity in several studies, particularly those involving vascular surgery patients *(36)*. Diabetics have a high incidence of both silent ischemia and silent myocardial infarction *(37)*. Based on the preponderance of evidence regarding the high incidence of cardiac morbidity in diabetic patients, particularly those with concomitant peripheral vascular disease, the ACC/AHA Guidelines consider diabetes a moderate risk. As mentioned above, aggressive glucose control during surgery and postoperatively appears to affect outcome in patients who remain in the intensive care unit for several days.

IMPORTANCE OF SURGICAL PROCEDURE

It is well recognized that the surgical procedure itself significantly influences perioperative risk. In virtually every study performed, emergency surgery is associated with additional risk. The mechanism of this phenomenon has eluded explanation. Plausible mechanisms include that the underlying emergent or volatile condition is more vulnerable to the perturbations and stresses of surgery. Perhaps the care team is less prepared for emergency surgery compared with the elective case with an unhurried review and plan. The risk related to the surgical procedure is often a function of both the underlying disease processes and the stress related to the specific procedure. Vascular surgical procedures are represents among the highest risk group of the noncardiac procedures. Although aortic reconstructive surgery has traditionally been considered the highest-risk vascular procedure, infrainguinal vascular procedures have a similar rate of cardiac morbidity, likely due to an increased severity of coronary disease in the infrainguinal patients *(38)*.

In contrast to the high-risk vascular operations, the perioperative complication rate is very low for superficial procedures. Backer et al. evaluated the rate of perioperative myocardial reinfarction in patients undergoing ophthalmologic surgery and demonstrated that the rate of perioperative cardiac morbidity was extremely low, even in patients with a recent myocardial infarction *(39)*. Virtually all studies have confirmed that ophthalmologic surgery is very safe under anesthesia, further supporting the premise that risk is not independent of the operation. Warner et al. studied patients undergoing ambulatory surgery, and reported no anesthetic deaths in more than 45,000 cases *(40)*.

Table 4
Cardiac Risk[a] Stratification for Noncardiac Surgical Procedures

High	(Reported cardiac risk often >5%
	Emergent major operations, particularly in the elderly
	Aortic and other major vascular
	Peripheral vascular
	Anticipated prolonged surgical procedures associated with large fluid shifts and/or blood loss
Intermediate	(Reported cardiac risk generally <5%)
	Carotid endarterectomy
	Head and neck
	Intraperitoneal and intrathoracic
	Orthopedic
	Prostate
Low[b]	(Reported cardiac risk generally <1%)
	Endoscopic procedures
	Superficial procedure
	Cataract
	Breast

[a]Combined incidence of cardiac death and nonfatal myocardial infarction.
[b]Do not generally require further preoperative cardiac testing. (Reproduced with permission from ref. 6.)

The association of invasive surgery and increased complications is a major impetus for increasing minimally invasive operations.

Eagle and colleagues evaluated the contribution of coronary artery disease and its treatment on perioperative cardiac morbidity and mortality by surgical procedure (41). They evaluated patients enrolled in the Coronary Artery Surgery Study who had documented coronary artery disease and received either medical therapy or coronary revascularization and then underwent noncardiac surgery during the subsequent 10-yr period. The rates of perioperative myocardial infarction and death were determined, and the surgical procedures were divided into three broad categories. Major vascular surgery was again demonstrated to be associated with the highest risk, with a combined morbidity and mortality greater than 10%. Procedures associated with a combined complication rate greater than or equal to 4% included intraabdominal, thoracic, and head and neck surgeries. In all of these cases, patients who had prior CABG had a significantly lower combined morbidity and mortality than the medically treated group. Low risk procedures included breast, skin, urologic, and orthopedic surgery. These broad groups of surgical procedures were the basis for defining surgical risk in the AHA/ACC Guidelines on Perioperative Cardiovascular Evaluation for Noncardiac Surgery (Table 4) (6).

IMPORTANCE OF EXERCISE TOLERANCE

There is disagreement on the value of using exercise tolerance as a means of determining perioperative risk. Specifically, the AHA/ACC Guidelines advocate its use, while the American College of Physicians Guidelines suggest there is insufficient evidence for its use. A lack of evidence does not translate into evidence of a lack of effect, and most clinicians have advocated its use. Several studies demonstrate that the ability to raise heart rate on a stress test is the strongest predictor of perioperative outcome (42). Excellent exercise tolerance, even in patients with stable angina, suggests that the myocardium can undergo the stress of surgery without becoming dysfunctional. Exercise tolerance can be assessed with formal treadmill testing or with a questionnaire that assesses activities of daily living (Table 5) (6). The inability to walk four blocks and climb two flights of stairs increased the incidence of cardiovascular complications during surgery twofold compared to patients with improved functional status (43). Hence, exercise capacity can determine the need for further diagnostic testing.

Table 5
Estimated Energy Requirement for Various Activities[a]

| 1 MET | Can you take care of yourself?
Eat, dress, or use the toilet?
Walk indoors around the house?
Walk a block or two on level ground
    at 2–3 mph or 3.2–4.8 km/h?
Do light work around the house like
    dusting or washing dishes? | 4 METs | Climb a flight of stairs or walk up a hill?
Walk on level ground at 4 mph or 6.4 km/h?
Run a short distance?
Do heavy work around the house like
    scrubbing floors or lifting or moving heavy
    furniture?
Participate in moderate recreational activities
    like golf, bowling, dancing, doubles tennis,
    or throwing a baseball or football? |
| | | >10 METs | Participate in strenuous sports like swimming,
    singles tennis, football, basketball, or
    skiing? |

[a]Adapted from the Duke Activity Status Index and AHA Exercise Standards.
MET, metabolic equivalent. (Reproduced with permission from ref. 6.)

Approach to the Patient

The American College of Cardiology/American Heart Association Task Force has published Guidelines on Perioperative Evaluation of the Cardiac Patient Undergoing Noncardiac Surgery based on the available evidence and expert opinion. The approach advocated integrates clinical history (Table 3), surgery specific risk, and exercise tolerance (Fig. 2) (6). First, the clinician must evaluate the urgency of the surgery and the appropriateness of a formal preoperative assessment. Next, determine whether the patient has undergone a previous revascularization procedure or coronary evaluation. Patients with unstable coronary syndromes should be identified, and appropriate treatment instituted. Finally, the decision to undergo further testing depends on the interaction of the clinical risk factors, surgery-specific risk, and functional capacity. For patients at intermediate clinical risk, both the exercise tolerance and the extent of the surgery are taken into account with regard to the need for further testing.

The authors of the guidelines suggest that all patients undergoing aortic or infrainguinal bypass surgery should be considered at high surgical risk, and therefore further evaluation should be considered. In an editorial in *Annals of Internal Medicine*, two of the authors of the guidelines (Fleisher and Eagle) suggest that routine preoperative testing of all major vascular patients would lead to a high incidence of false positive test, and advocate a more Bayesian approach (44).

The American College of Physicians Guidelines apply an evidence-based approach (26). The initial decision point is the assessment of risk using the Detsky modification of the Cardiac Risk Index. If the patient is class II or III, he or she considered high-risk. If they are class I, the presence of other clinical factors, according to work by Eagle and colleagues (36) or Vanzetto and colleagues (45), are used to further stratify risk. Those with multiple markers for cardiovascular disease according to these risk indices and those undergoing major vascular surgery are considered appropriate for further diagnostic testing by either dipyridamole imaging or dobutamine stress echocardiography.

Coronary Revascularization

Patients who survive CABG are at decreased risk for subsequent noncardiac surgery (46). While there are few data to support the notion of coronary revascularization solely for the purpose of improving perioperative outcome, it is true that for specific patient subsets long-term survival may be enhanced by revascularization. Rihal et al. utilized the Coronary Artery Surgery Study database and found that CABG significantly improved survival in those patients with both peripheral vascular disease and triple-vessel coronary disease, especially the group with decreased ventricular function (47). In contrast, McFalls and colleagues demonstrated no difference in 30-d and 2.7-yr outcomes in patients with mild to moderate coronary artery disease undergoing vascular surgery who were randomized to medical therapy versus coronary revascularization (48).

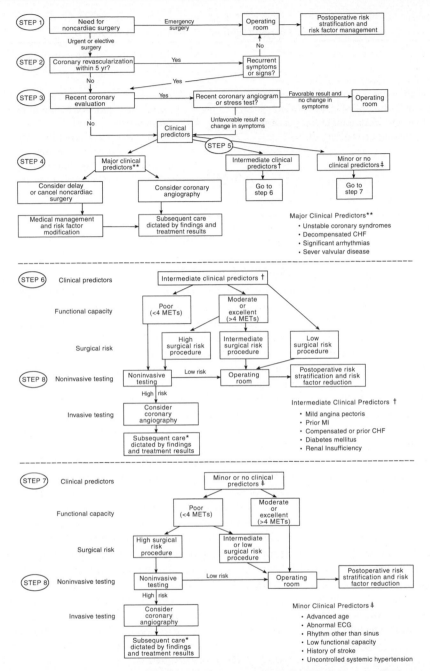

Fig. 2. The American Heart Association/American College of Cardiology Task Force on Perioperative Evaluation of Cardiac Patients Undergoing Noncardiac Surgery has proposed an algorithm for decisions regarding the need for further evaluation. This represents one of multiple algorithms proposed in the literature. It is based on expert opinion, and incorporates six steps. First, the clinician must evaluate the urgency of the surgery and the appropriateness of a formal preoperative assessment. Next, he or she must determine whether the patient has had a previous revascularization procedure or coronary evaluation. Patients with unstable coronary syndromes should be identified, and appropriate treatment should be instituted. The decision to have further testing depends on the interaction of the clinical risk factors, surgery-specific risk, and functional capacity. (Adapted with permission from the ACC/AHA Guidelines for Perioperative Cardiovascular Evaluation for Noncardiac Surgery [ref. 6].)

The value of percutaneous transluminal coronary angioplasty (PTCA), drug-eluting stents, atherectomy, and aggressive risk modification are well established in the nonsurgical population. In several series, a low incidence of cardiovascular complications was observed in patients undergoing "prophylactic" PTCA before vascular surgery, but it is difficult to determine the expected complication rate in a comparison group with single- or double-vessel disease (49,50). For perioperative MIs that result from plaque rupture and coronary thrombosis in noncritical lesions, as seen in the ambulatory setting, single-vessel PTCA of more critical stenoses will theoretically have minimal benefit. Ellis et al. studied 21 patients who had coronary angiography before major vascular surgery and sustained a perioperative cardiac event (4). None of the myocardial infarctions occurred in areas distal to a critical stenosis, while approximately one third occurred distal to noncritical stenoses (4). An administrative dataset from Washington State was analyzed to assess the value of preoperative PTCA using a case-controlled approach (51). Patients who had undergone a PTCA more than 6 wk prior to noncardiac surgery had an improved outcome compared to matched controls with coronary artery disease, while no difference in outcome was observed if the period between PTCA and noncardiac surgery was less than 6 wk. Although analysis of administrative datasets has some inherent limitations related to an inability to determine the potential selection bias for those being treated, these data suggest that "prophylactic" PTCA simply to get the patient through surgery may be of minimal or no benefit. Coronary stent placement may be a unique issue. In a case series of 39 patients who had undergone coronary stent placement within 1 mo of noncardiac surgery there was a significant incidence of perioperative death and major bleed for patients who had surgery within 14 d of stent placement (53). Wilson and colleagues identified 207 patients who underwent surgery in the 2 mo following successful coronary stent placement (54). Eight patients died or suffered a myocardial infarction or stent thrombosis among the 168 patients undergoing surgery 6 wk after stent placement. No events occurred in the 39 patients undergoing surgery 7 to 9 wk after stent placement. These data suggest that, whenever possible, noncardiac surgery should be delayed 6 wk after stent placement, by which time stents are generally endothelialized, and a course of antiplatelet therapy to prevent stent thrombosis has been completed.

Boersma and colleagues reevaluated the value of dobutamine stress echocardiography with respect to the extent of wall motion abnormalities and use of β-blockers during surgery for the entire cohort of patients screened for the Dutch Echocardiographic Cardiac Risk Evaluation Applying Stress Echocardiography (DECREASE) trial (55). They assigned one point for each of the following characteristics: age ≥70 years, current angina, myocardial infarction, congestive heart failure, prior cerebrovascular accident, diabetes mellitus, and renal failure. As the total of number of clinical risk factors increases, perioperative cardiac event rates also increase. When the risk of death or myocardial infarction was stratified by perioperative β-blocker usage, there was no significant improvement in those without any of the prior risk factors. In those with a risk factor score between 0 and 3, which represented over half of all patients, the rate of cardiac events was reduced from 3% to 0.9%. Most importantly, in those without at least three risk factors, comprising 70% of the population, β-blocker therapy was very effective in reducing cardiac events in those with new wall motion abnormalities in 1 to 4 segments (33% vs 2.8%), having smaller effect in those without new wall motion abnormalities (5.8% vs 2%), but had no effect in those patients with new wall motion abnormalities in ≥5 segments. The group with extensive wall motion abnormalities may be the group to consider for coronary revascularization.

Risks vs Benefits of Coronary Revascularization

An alternative approach to determining the optimal strategy for medical care in the absence of clinical trials is construction of a decision analysis. Three decision analyses have been published on the issue of cardiovascular testing before major vascular surgery (52,56,57). All assumed that patients with significant coronary artery disease would undergo coronary artery bypass grafting prior to noncardiac surgery. Using decision analysis modeling, preoperative testing for the purpose of coronary revascularization is not the optimal strategy if perioperative morbidity and mortality is low *(52,56,57)*. The primary cost (both in dollars and morbidity) of preoperative testing and revascularization is the revascularization procedure itself. Therefore, the indications for revascularization, and thus the frequency of its use, have a significant impact on the model. However, potential long-term benefits of coronary revascularization in this population were included in only one analysis. If long-term survival is enhanced by revascularization, then it may lead to improved overall outcome and be a cost-effective intervention *(57)*. Hence, a patient's age should be included in the equation. An 80-yr-old diabetic patient with significant comorbid diseases may gain few additional life-years and may actually have a decrease in the quality of the final years by undergoing CABG. In contrast, a 55-yr-old man with an abdominal aortic aneurysm and left main disease would have a substantial increase in both the length and quality of his life from preoperative cardiovascular testing and coronary revascularization. Therefore, identification of appropriate patients with significant disease or left main stenosis amenable to surgery with an acceptable risk should undergo revascularization before high-risk noncardiac surgery.

CHOICE OF DIAGNOSTIC TEST

Exercise electrocardiography is a useful test to diagnose CAD, but is rarely indicated preoperatively since it requires the patient to have a good exercise capacity (therefore not requiring testing). There have been a number of studies that suggest that preoperative ambulatory electrocardiography for silent myocardial ischemia is a sensitive and specific test for perioperative cardiac events; however, there are two major problems. The majority of patients at highest risk have electrocardiograms that prohibit the accurate diagnosis of silent ischemia, and attempts to relate the amount of preoperative ischemia and degree of risk have not been conclusive. In a study comparing preoperative ambulatory electrocardiography to dipyridamole thallium imaging, those patients with a greater number of minutes of preoperative ischemia did not have an increased perioperative and long-term risk compared with those with a shorter duration of preoperative ischemia *(56)*.

For patients who are unable to exercise, particularly those undergoing major vascular surgery with claudication, pharmacologic stress testing has been advocated. A redistribution defect on dipyridamole thallium imaging in vascular patients predicts postoperative cardiac event, with the larger the defect the more serious the risk. The negative predictive value of dipyridamole thallium imaging has consistently been high (above 90%), although the positive predictive value has decreased over time, related to the overall decrease in perioperative cardiac morbidity. The test is best utilized, and has its best predictive value, in those at moderate clinical risk: patients with multiple risk factors undergoing major vascular surgery *(45)*. Patients at greatest risk have larger areas of reversible defect or increased lung uptake on thallium imaging, and were associated with both an increased incidence of perioperative cardiac morbidity and decreased survival at 2 yr after surgery *(57)*.

Dobutamine stress echocardiography has very good positive and negative predicative values and may most closely mimic the hyperdynamic state seen during the perioperative period. Those patients at greatest risk develop new regional wall motion abnormalities at lower heart rates *(58)*. Similar to the findings of Eagle et al. for dipyridamole thallium imaging, dobutamine stress echocardiography has its best predictive value in those at moderate clinical risk. In two meta-analyses, dobutamine stress echocardiography had the best predictive value, but there was much overlap with dipyridamole imaging *(59,61)*. Other modalities to noninvasively assess coronary burden, such as MRI and CT imaging to quantify coronary calcium, have not been validated as markers for perioperative risk stratification.

SUMMARY

Increasing emphasis is placed on the patient's symptoms and exercise tolerance. If a patient has reduced exercise tolerance, angina pectoris, heart failure, or anginal equivalents, then further cardiovascular evaluation is warranted whether or not the patient is preparing for surgery. If the patient with risk factors for coronary artery disease has excellent exercise tolerance and is asymptomatic, then a further diagnostic workup is not indicated. The perioperative physicians may elect to add β-blockers in an attempt to decrease the incidence of tachycardia and associated perioperative ischemia. Atenolol and bisoprolol have been shown to decrease cardiovascular morbidity when started preoperatively in patients undergoing noncardiac surgery *(6,61)*, although achievement of therapeutic levels (as assessed by heart rate control) may be critical to achieving the effect. If there is no indication for stress testing or cardiac catheterization in the absence of surgery, then why should a planned operation trigger the testing? Exercise stress testing is a helpful adjunct in the triage of the high risk patient. High risk is defined by symptoms and activity–exercise tolerance in the context of the planned operation. Preoperative evaluation should focus on obtaining information regarding the extent and stability of the cardiovascular system in order to modify perioperative management. The decision to perform further evaluation and diagnostic testing depends on the interactions of patients and surgery-specific factors, as well as exercise capacity.

REFERENCES

1. Bugar JM, Ghali WA, Lemaire JB, Quan H, Canadian Perioperative Research Network. Utilization of a preoperative assessment clinic in a tertiary center. Clin Invest Med 2002;25:11–18.
2. Gowda RM, Misra D, Tranbaugh RF, et al. Endovascular stent grafting of descending thoracic aortic aneurysms. Chest 2003;124:714–719.
3. Shah KB, Kleinman BS, Rao T, et al. Angina and other risk factors in patients with cardiac diseases undergoing noncardiac operations. Anesth Analg 1990;70:240–247.
4. Ellis SG, Hertzer NR, Young JR, et al. Angiographic correlates of cardiac death and myocardial infarction complicating major nonthoracic vascular surgery. Am J Cardiol 1996;77:1126–1128.
5. Sandham JD, Hull RD, Brant RF, et al. A randomized, controlled trial of the use of pulmonary-artery catheters in high-risk surgical patients. N Engl J Med 2003;348:5–14.
6. Eagle K, Brundage B, Chaitman B, et al. Guidelines for perioperative cardiovascular evaluation of noncardiac surgery. A report of the American Heart Association/American College of Cardiology Task Force on Assessment of Diagnostic and Therapeutic Cardiovascular Procedures. Circulation 1996;93:1278–1317.
7. Cohn SL, Goldman L. Preoperative risk evaluation and perioperative management of patients with coronary artery disease. Med Clin North Am 2003;87:111–136.
8. Phillip B, Pastor D, Bellows W, Leung J. The prevalence of preoperative diastolic filling abnormalities in geriatric surgical patients. Anesth Analg 2003;97:1214–1221.
9. Redfield M, Jacobsen S, Burnett JC Jr, et al. Burden of systolic and diastolic ventricular dysfunction in the community: appreciating the scope of the heart failure epidemic. JAMA 2003;289:194–202.
10. Baum VC, Perloff JK. Anesthetic implications of adults with congenital heart disease. Anesth Analg 1992;76:1342–1358.
11. Van den Gerghe G, Wouters P, Weekers F, et al. Intensive insulin therapy in critically ill patients. N Engl J Med 2001;345:1359–1367.
12. Toller WG, Kersten JR, Pagel PS, et al. Sevoflurane reduces myocardial infarct size and decreases the time threshold for ischemic preconditioning in dogs. Anesthesiology 1999;91:1437–1446.
13. Chen Q, Camara AK, An J, et al. Sevoflurane preconditioning before moderate hypothermic ischemia protects against cytosolic [Ca(2+)] loading and myocardial damage in part via mitochondrial K(ATP) channels. Anesthesiology 2002;97:912–920.
14. Agnew NM, Pennefather SH, Russell GN. Isoflurane and coronary heart disease. Anaesthesia 2002;57:338–347.
15. Mangano DT, Browner WS, Hollenberg M, et al. Association of perioperative myocardial ischemia with cardiac morbidity and mortality in men undergoing noncardiac surgery. N Engl J Med 1990;323:1781–1788.
16. Raby KE, Barry J, Creager MA, Cook EF, Weisberg MC, Goldman L. Detection and significance of intraoperative and postoperative myocardial ischemia in peripheral vascular surgery. JAMA 1992;268:222–227.
17. Fleisher LA, Nelson AH, Rosenbaum SH. Postoperative myocardial ischemia: etiology of cardiac morbidity or manifestation of underlying disease. J Clin Anesth 1995;7:97–102.
18. Mangano DT, Layug EL, Wallace A, Tateo I. Effect of atenolol on mortality and cardiovascular morbidity after noncardiac surgery. Multicenter Study of Perioperative Ischemia Research Group. N Engl J Med 1996;335:1713–1720.
19. Wallace A, Layug B, Tateo I, et al. Prophylactic atenolol reduces postoperative myocardial ischemia. McSPI Research Group. Anesthesiology 1998;88:7–17.
20. Poldermans D, Bax JJ, Kertai MD, et al. Statins are associated with a reduced incidence of perioperative mortality in patients undergoing major noncardiac vascular surgery. Circulation 2003;107:1848–1851.
21. Frank SM, Fleisher LA, Breslow MJ, et al. Perioperative maintenance of normothermia reduces the incidence of morbid cardiac events. A randomized clinical trial. JAMA 1997;277:1127–1134.
22. Nelson AH, Fleisher LA, Rosenbaum SH. Relationship between postoperative anemia and cardiac morbidity in high-risk vascular patients in the intensive care unit. Crit Care Med 1993;21:860–866.

23. Rosenfeld BA, Beattie C, Christopherson R, et al. The effects of different anesthetic regimens on fibrinolysis and the development of postoperative arterial thrombosis. Perioperative Ischemia Randomized Anesthesia Trial Study Group. Anesthesiology 1993;79:435–443.

24. Goldman L, Caldera DL, Nussbaum SR, et al. Multifactorial index of cardiac risk in noncardiac surgical procedures. N Engl J Med 1977;297:845–850.

25. Detsky A, Abrams H, McLaughlin J, et al. Predicting cardiac complications in patients undergoing noncardiac surgery. J Gen Intern Med 1986;1:211–219.

26. Palda VA, Detsky AS. Perioperative assessment and management of risk from coronary artery disease. Ann Intern Med 1997;127:313–328.

27. Lee TH, Marcantonio ER, Mangione CM, et al. Derivation and prospective validation of a simple index for prediction of cardiac risk of major noncardiac surgery. Circulation 1999;100:1043–1049.

28. Tarhan S, Moffitt EA, Taylor WF, Giuliani ER. Myocardial infarction after general anesthesia. JAMA 1972;220:1451–1454.

29. Rao TK, Jacobs KH, El-Etr AA. Reinfarction following anesthesia in patients with myocardial infarction. Anesthesiology 1983;59:499–505.

30. Shah KB, Kleinman BS, Sami H, et al. Reevaluation of perioperative myocardial infarction in patients with prior myocardial infarction undergoing noncardiac operations. Anesth Analg 1990;71:231–235.

31. Ryan TJ, Anderson JL, Antman EM, et al. ACC/AHA guidelines for the management of patients with acute myocardial infarction: executive summary. A report of the American College of Cardiology/American Heart Association Task Force on Practice Guidelines (Committee on Management of Acute Myocardial Infarction). Circulation 1996;94:2341–2350.

32. Weksler N, Klein M, Szendro G, et al. The dilemma of immediate preoperative hypertension: to treat and operate, or to postpone surgery? J Clin Anesth 2003;15:179–183.

33. Goldman L, Caldera DL. Risks of general anesthesia and elective operation in the hypertensive patient. Anesthesiology 1979;50:285–292.

34. Aronson S, Boisvert D, Lapp W. Isolated systolic hypertension is associated with adverse outcomes from coronary artery bypass grafting surgery. Anesth Analg 2002;94:1079–1084.

35. Hollenberg M, Mangano DT, Browner WS, et al. Predictors of postoperative myocardial ischemia in patients undergoing noncardiac surgery. The Study of Perioperative Ischemia Research Group. JAMA 1992;268:205–209.

36. Eagle KA, Coley CM, Newell JB, et al. Combining clinical and thallium data optimizes preoperative assessment of cardiac risk before major vascular surgery. Ann Int Med 1989;110:859–866.

37. Kannel W, Abbott R. Incidence and prognosis of unrecognized myocardial infarction: an update on the Framingham Study. N Engl J Med 1984;311:1144–1147.

38. L'Italien GL, Cambria RP, Cutler BS, et al. Comparative early and late cardiac morbidity among patients requiring different vascular surgery procedures. J Vasc Surg 1995;21:935–944.

39. Backer CL, Tinker JH, Robertson DM, Vlietstra RE. Myocardial reinfarction following local anesthesia for ophthalmic surgery. Anesth Analg 1980;59:257–262.

40. Warner MA, Shields SE, Chute CG. Major morbidity and mortality within 1 month of ambulatory surgery and anesthesia. JAMA 1993;270:1437–1441.

41. Eagle KA, Rihal CS, Mickel MC, et al. Cardiac risk of noncardiac surgery: influence of coronary disease and type of surgery in 3368 operations. CASS Investigators and University of Michigan Heart Care Program. Coronary Artery Surgery Study. Circulation 1997;96:1882–1887.

42. McPhail N, Calvin JE, Shariatmadar A, et al. The use of preoperative exercise testing to predict cardiac complications after arterial reconstruction. J Vasc Surg 1988;7:60–68.

43. Reilly DF, McNeely MJ, Doerner D, et al. Self-reported exercise tolerance and the risk of serious perioperative complications. Arch Intern Med 1999;159:2185–2192.

44. Fleisher LA, Eagle KA. Screening for cardiac disease in patients having noncardiac surgery. Ann Intern Med 1996;124:767–772.

45. Vanzetto G, Machecourt J, Blendea D, et al. Additive value of thallium single-photon emission computed tomography myocardial imaging for prediction of perioperative events in clinically selected high cardiac risk patients having abdominal aortic surgery. Am J Cardiol 1996;77:143–148.

46. Huber KC, Evans MA, Bresnahan JF, et al. Outcome of noncardiac operations in patients with severe coronary artery disease successfully treated preoperatively with coronary angioplasty. Mayo Clin Proc 1992;67:15–21.

47. Rihal CS, Eagle KA, Mickel MC, et al. Surgical therapy for coronary artery disease among patients with combined coronary artery and peripheral vascular disease. Circulation 1995;91:46–53.

48. McFalls EO, Ward HB, Moritz TE, et al. Coronary artery revascularization before major elective vascular surgery. N Engl J Med 2004;351:2795–2804.

49. Elmore J, Hallett J, Gibbons R, et al. Myocardial revascularization before abdominal aortic aneurysmorrhaphy: effect of coronary angioplasty. Mayo Clin Proc 1993;68:637–641.

50. Gottlieb A, Banous M, Sprung J, et al. Perioperative cardiovascular morbidity in patients with coronary artery disease undergoing vascular surgery after percutaneous transluminal coronary angioplasty. J Cardiothor Vas Anes 1998;12:501–506.

51. van Norman GA, Posner KL, Wright IH, Spiess BD. Adverse cardiac outcomes after noncardiac surgery in patients with prior PTCA compared to patients with nonrevascularized CAD and no CAD. Circulation 1997;96:I–734.

52. Fleisher LA, Skolnick ED, Holroyd KJ, Lehmann HP. Coronary artery revascularization before abdominal aortic aneurysm surgery: a decision analytic approach. Anesth Analg 1994;79:661–669.
53. Kaluza GL, Joseph J, Lee JR, et al. Catastrophic outcomes of noncardiac surgery soon after coronary stenting. J Am Coll Cardiol 2000;35:1288–1294.
54. Wilson SH, Fasseas P, Orford JL, et al. Clinical outcome of patients undergoing noncardiac surgery in the two months following coronary stenting. J Am Coll Cardiol 2003;42:234–240.
55. Boersma E, Poldermans D, Bax JJ, et al. Predictors of cardiac events after major vascular surgery: role of clinical characteristics, dobutamine echocardiography, and beta-blocker therapy. JAMA 2001;285:1865 1873.
56. Mason JJ, Owens DK, Harris RA, et al. The role of coronary angiography and coronary revascularization before noncardiac surgery. JAMA 1995;273:1919–1925.
57. Glance LG. Selective preoperative cardiac screening improves five-year survival in patients undergoing major vascular surgery: a cost-effectiveness analysis. J Cardiothorac Vasc Anesth 1999;13:265–271.
58. Fleisher LA, Rosenbaum SH, Nelson AH, et al. Preoperative dipyridamole thallium imaging and Holter monitoring as a predictor of perioperative cardiac events and long tem outcome. Anesthesiology 1995;83:906–917.
59. Poldermans D, Arnese M, Fioretti PM, et al. Improved cardiac risk stratification in major vascular surgery with dobutamine-atropine stress echocardiography. J Am Coll Cardiol 1995;26:648–653.
60. Mantha S, Roizen MF, Barnard J, et al. Relative effectiveness of four preoperative tests for predicting adverse cardiac outcomes after vascular surgery: a meta-analysis. Anesth Analg 1994;79:422–433.
61. Shaw LJ, Eagle KA, Gersh BJ, Miller DD. Meta-analysis of intravenous dipyridamole-thallium-201 imaging (1985 to 1994) and dobutamine echocardiography (1991 to 1994) for risk stratification before vascular surgery. J Am Coll Cardiol 1996;27:787–798.

RECOMMENDED READING

Mangano DT. Assessment of the patient with cardiac disease: an anesthesiologist's paradigm. Anesthesiology 1999;91: 1521–1526.
Eagle KA, Berger PB, Calkins H, et al. ACC/AHA guideline update for perioperative cardiovascular evaluation for noncardiac surgery—executive summary: a report of the American College of Cardiology/American Heart Association Task Force on Practice Guidelines (Committee to Update the 1996 Guidelines on Perioperative Cardiovascular Evaluation for Noncardiac Surgery). J Am Coll Cardiol 2002;39:542–553.
Fleisher LA, Eagle KA. Clinical practice: lowering cardiac risk in noncardiac surgery. N Engl J Med 2001;345:1677–1682.
Boersma E, Poldermans D, Bax JJ, et al. Predictors of cardiac events after major vascular surgery: role of clinical characteristics, dobutamine echocardiography, and beta-blocker therapy. JAMA 2001;285:1865–1873.

42   Cardiovascular Gene
and Cell Therapy

Eddy Kizana, MB BS, *Federica del Monte,* MD, PhD,
Sian E. Harding, PhD, *and Roger J. Hajjar,* MD

INTRODUCTION

Cardiovascular disease is a major cause of morbidity and mortality in contemporary societies. Although progress in conventional treatment modalities is making steady and incremental gains to reduce this disease burden, there remains a need to explore new and potentially therapeutic approaches. Gene therapy, for example, was initially envisioned as a treatment strategy for inherited monogenic disorders. It is now apparent that gene therapy has broader potential that also includes acquired polygenic diseases, such as atherosclerosis and heart failure. Advances in the understanding of the molecular basis of conditions such as these, together with the evolution of increasingly efficient gene transfer technology, has placed some cardiovascular pathophysiologies within reach of gene-based therapy.

As shown in Fig. 1, myocardial dysfunction induced by genetic or specific disease states such as coronary artery disease, hypertension, diabetes, infection, or inflammation results in a myocardium that has a mixture of permanently lost myocytes, diseased and dysfunctional myocytes, and nondiseased myocytes. The presence of nondiseased myocytes is especially relevant in myocardial infarction and coronary artery disease where myocardial dysfunction is patchy. However, these nondiseased myocytes are under bombardment from hormonal and physical stresses that can induce apoptosis and cell death or render them dysfunctional. The targets for stem-cell therapy are the permanently lost myocytes, while the targets for gene therapy are the dysfunctional myocytes and the prevention of the nondiseased myocytes from becoming lost or diseased.

In this review, we highlight the following new strategies for the treatment of myocardial diseases: (1) gene transfer to modulate cardiac function and (2) cell transplantation to repair damaged myocardium.

This chapter focuses on gene and cell therapy strategies that have targeted diseases of the cardiovascular system. Gene and vector delivery systems are presented from the perspective of designing a successful cardiovascular gene therapy protocol. The molecular targets for therapeutic intervention are then systematically reviewed according to individual pathophysiologies. These strategies are discussed mindful of the constraints of contemporary gene transfer technology and the demands imposed by the pathophysiology of interest. This is done with the aim of instilling in the mind of the reader the likelihood of successful therapeutic intervention with any given strategy.

GENERAL CONSIDERATIONS

When targeting a pathophysiology for gene and cell transfer intervention a number of factors need to be considered. These include target cell and transgene biology, and the demands imposed

From: *Essential Cardiology: Principles and Practice, 2nd Ed.*
Edited by: C. Rosendorff © Humana Press Inc., Totowa, NJ

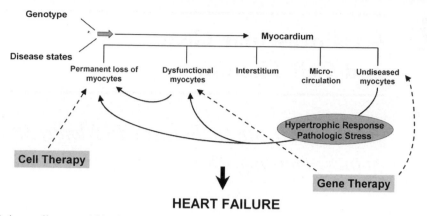

Fig. 1. Various cell types within the myocardium of failing hearts and the targets for gene and cell therapy.

by the pathophysiology of interest. In addition, the choice of gene and vector delivery systems and the approach to gene transfer, ex vivo or in vivo, also have a bearing on the outcome. It is helpful from the outset to address a number of generic questions that encompass these considerations.

How many target cells need to be gene-modified for phenotypic correction?

This question is of overriding importance because its answer will rapidly determine the likelihood of a positive outcome. It addresses the proportion of target cells within the tissue of interest that need to be successfully gene-modified in order to favorably affect the pathophysiology in question. The creation of a biological pacemaker requires the focal genetic-modification of only a modest number of cells within the heart. In contrast, restoring myocardial contractility in the context of heart failure has a higher threshold for correction and requires the successful gene transfer to a majority of target cells.

What is the required temporal pattern of transgene expression?

The natural history of the target disease will have the greatest bearing on the temporal requirement of transgene expression. The required pattern of transgene expression will determine the choice of gene transfer system that can be employed for a desired outcome. The strategy of transient expression of angiogenic factors by plasmid-mediated gene transfer has proven successful in relieving myocardial ischemia. Likewise, the requirement for persistent transgene expression for conditions such as heart failure is inherent in the irreversible nature of the underlying pathophysiology.

Is it possible to employ an ex vivo approach?

An ex vivo approach can be used only when the target cell can be harvested and maintained in culture. Hence postmitotic cardiomyocytes would not be suitable for this approach. Vascular endothelial cells and autologous stem cells, on the other hand, can be grown and genetically modified ex vivo prior to implantation. The benefit of an ex vivo approach is the avoidance of genetic modification of nontarget cells and any adverse consequences as a result. In addition, target cell number can be significantly expanded prior to administration.

GENE DELIVERY SYSTEMS

Gene delivery systems can be classified into two main groups, nonviral physicochemical systems and recombinant viral systems (1,2). The strengths of nonviral systems include the ease of vector production, reduced limitation on expression cassette size, and relatively minimal biosafety risks. The limitations include low transfection efficiency and transient effect due to intracellular degradation.

Nonviral Vectors

Nonviral vectors can be loosely grouped as plasmid DNA, liposome-DNA complexes (lipoplexes), and polymer-DNA complexes (polyplexes) *(3)*. Oligonucleotides and their analogs, either alone or in complexes, are also an example of nonviral vector-mediated gene transfer. Almost half of the human cardiovascular gene therapy protocols in North America are based on plasmid-mediated gene transfer *(4)*. Although myocardial plasmid-mediated gene transfer is relatively inefficient, it has been the vector system on which several therapeutic angiogenesis trials have been based. In this setting, transient secretion of angiogenic factors by a modest number of gene-modified cells is sufficient for the desired phenotypic effect. The use of synthetic oligonucleotides to modulate gene expression in biological systems has immense research and therapeutic potential. Therapeutic oligonucleotides take multiple forms that include antisense molecules, transcription factor decoys, catalytic oligonucleotides, and chimeroplasts. The therapeutic potential of each of these has been explored in cardiovascular disease models and examples of these are given in the subsequent text.

Viral Vectors

The predominant use of viral vector systems in preclinical models of gene therapy is a reflection of the increased gene-transfer efficiencies achievable with these systems. This efficiency is conferred as a result of including elements of parental virus biology that secure a favorable fate for the transferred gene. The four most developed and commonly used viral vector systems will be covered in the following discussion. Other virus-based systems are based on herpes simplex virus (HSV-1), semliki forest virus (SFV), and baculovirus *(5)*.

ADENOVIRAL VECTORS

Recombinant human adenoviral vectors are the most commonly vectors in preclinical gene therapy models and in clinical cardiovascular gene therapy protocols *(4)*. The strengths of this vector system that underlie its widespread use include the relative ease of production, high functional vector titers achievable, and broad target cell tropism, particularly within the cardiovascular system. All major cardiac cell types can be efficiently transduced by adenoviral vectors, both in vitro and in vivo. With regard to cardiomyocytes, efficient in vivo transduction has been demonstrated in gene therapy models from several mammalian species. In these models, the pattern of myocardial transduction reflects the method of vector delivery. For example, direct myocardial injection results in intense transduction at the site of injection *(6)*, whereas intracoronary delivery results in more widespread transduction in the distribution of the vessel *(7)*.

The adenovirus uses the Coxsackie adenovirus receptor to enter the target as shown in Fig. 2. β-Integrins are also involved in this process of cell entry. In a recent study, it was shown that a decrease in the β-integrins is responsible for the decreased efficiency in adenoviral gene transfer in aging cardiac myocytes *(8)*.

A number of maneuvers have been shown to enhance gene transfer efficiency of adenoviral vectors to the myocardium following intracoronary delivery. Physical approaches include methods that rely on catheter-based or surgically induced transcoronary pressure gradients to increase gene delivery to the myocardium *(9)* or the application of ultrasound energy to disperse circulating vector as it traverses the myocardium *(10,11)*. Chemical approaches include the use of vasodilatory and permeabilizing agents that facilitate transfer of vector form the vascular lumen to the myocardium *(12)*. Target cells within the cardiovascular system also include vascular endothelial and smooth muscle cells. In the presence of an intact endothelium, intravascular delivery of adenoviral vectors will result in preferential gene delivery to the endothelial cells. Smooth muscle cells, in contrast, can be transduced with moderate efficiency only after vessel injury *(6,13)*. Adenoviral vectors have a widely appreciated capacity for evoking intense immune and inflammatory reactions. In animal models, adenoviral vectors have been reported to cause myocardial and vascular inflammation, endothelial cell dysfunction, vasoproliferation, and intravascular thrombus formation. Additional

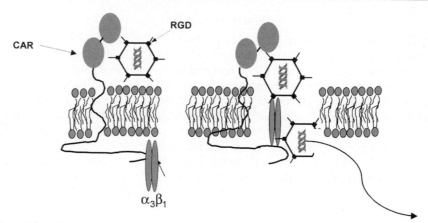

Fig. 2. Coxsackie and adenovirus receptor (CAR) is the entry point for the adenovirus into a mammalian cell followed by a pull-down facilitated by the β-integrins that play a critical role in the internalization of the adenovirus.

constraints on the clinical use of these vectors include the preexistence of neutralizing antibodies to commonly used vectors; the *de novo* development of these antibodies precludes readministration of the same vector serotype.

ADENO-ASSOCIATED VIRUS VECTORS

Recombinant adeno-associated virus (rAAV) vectors are derived from the dependent parvovirus AAV type 2. This vector system has a number of clinically favorable attributes such as lack of parental agent pathogenicity and vector-related cytotoxicity, minimal immunogenecity, and the capacity for stable long-term transgene expression through genomic integration and/or stable episome maintenance *(14)*. These vectors are tropic for striated muscle and can confer stable long-term transgene expression in skeletal and cardiac muscle in immunocompetent hosts *(15)*. Major limitations of rAAV vector systems include the production of high-titer vector stocks of consistent purity and bioactivity, a limited packaging capacity of 4.8 kb, and the potential for preexistent neutralizing antibodies in human populations. Recently a number of additional AAV serotypes have been described. Pseudotyping the AAV type-2 genome with capsids from these may avoid the problem of neutralizing antibodies. In addition, pseudotyping rAAV-2 genomes modifies vector tropism and has been found to enhance skeletal muscle transduction when capsid serotypes 1 and 5 are used *(16–18)*. The tropism of cardiovascular tissues for pseudotyped AAV vectors is under investigation, with early in vitro data suggesting superiority of AAV-2 with regard to vascular endothelial and smooth muscle transduction. This pattern of widespread and stable transgene expression is able to rescue the cardiomyopathy phenotype in genetically predisposed animals *(19)*. Intravascular delivery of AAV-2 results in poor transduction of endothelial cells. Smooth muscle cells, however, can be transduced following intraluminal vector delivery, even in the presence of an intact endothelium *(20)*.

RETROVIRUS VECTORS

Retroviral vectors based on Moloney murine leukemia virus (MoMLV) were developed two decades ago. These vectors have been used widely in preclinical models and first entered human clinical trials in 1989. More recently this vector has been used in the successful French trial of gene therapy for X-linked severe combined immunodeficiency (X-SCID) *(21)*. The main limitations of retroviral vectors are an inability to transduce nondividing cells and low-titer vector stocks. In keeping with the requirement for cell division, postmitotic cardiomyocytes and quiescent cell populations, such as intact vascular endothelial and smooth muscle cells, cannot be efficiently transduced by these vectors. As a result, many investigators have sought the overcome this block by inducing the in vivo proliferation in target cells or by employing an ex vivo strategy *(22)*. Due to these limitations, the use of this vector system in cardiovascular models has fallen dramatically. This has occurred in conjunction with the increased use of adenoviral vectors and other integrating vectors that are capable of transducing nondividing cells such as rAAV and lentiviral vectors.

Recently, 2 out of 10 children from the French X-SCID trial developed premalignant clonal T-cell proliferation that was directly attributable to dysregulation of a gene at the proviral integration site *(23)*. The risk of insertional mutagenesis with integrating vector use had previously been considered minimal, a view now under revision. As a result of this development there has been renewed interest in integrating vector design to improve biosafety. Modifications such as the use self-inactivating vectors, the introduction of insulator sequences, and targeting of genome integration sites are potential ways of reducing the risk of insertional mutagenesis.

LENTIVIRUS VECTORS

Lentiviral vectors, similar to MoMLV-based retroviral vectors, transduce target cells by genomic integration. In contrast to retroviral vectors, these vectors are capable of transducing mitotically quiescent cells, a property that broadens the range of target cells, particularly within the cardiovascular system. The first developed, and most commonly used, lentiviral vector system is based on the human immunodeficiency virus type 1 (HIV-1) *(24)*. Concerns regarding the pathogenecity of the parental virus underlie the drive to explore nonhuman-based lentiviral vector systems. Vector modifications addressing biosafety concerns associated with contemporary HIV-1-derived lentiviral vectors include the deletion of all accessory protein genes from the packaging system, separation of packaging elements into multiple plasmids, and the use of a chimeric 5' long terminal repeat (LTR) and a self-inactivating 3' LTR in the vector plasmid *(25)*.

Design of the Expression Cassette

The basic components of an expression cassette include promoter/enhancer elements, the gene(s) of interest and an appropriate mRNA stabilizing polyadenylation signal. Other frequently employed *cis*-acting elements include internal ribosome entry site (IRES) sequences to allow expression of two or more genes without the need for an additional promoter, and introns and posttranscriptional regulatory elements to improve transgene expression. Of these, promoter selection has received greatest attention in the literature.

Models of gene therapy generally employ expression cassettes containing strong viral promoters that are constitutively active in a wide spectrum of cells. Spatial and temporal regulation of transgene expression can be achieved by the choice of promoter. Tissue-specific promoters can be used to restrict transgene expression to the desired target cell population and avoid unintended cells such as antigen-presenting cells. For example, cardiomyocyte-specific promoters such as α-myosin heavy chain have been employed to restrict gene expression to the myocardium. Similarly, the smooth muscle-specific promoter SM22α has been demonstrated to restrict gene expression to cells of this type. Promoters subject to pharmacological or physiological regulation can be used to achieve the desired temporal pattern of transgene expression. Ligand-dependent regulatory systems are the subject of intense study, but have not been widely used in cardiovascular gene therapy models *(26–28)*. Systems exploiting physiological regulation can be designed to incorporate promoters with transcriptional activity that is contigent upon signals provided by the pathophysiology of interest. Hypoxia, intravascular shear stress, and left ventricular strain have all been used in models of this type of regulation.

VECTOR DELIVERY

Once a molecular target and gene delivery system have been chosen, the next step is to deliver the vector to the site of interest within the cardiovascular system. There are several approaches to vector delivery in rodents, as shown in Fig. 3. Many of these are of relevance only to animal

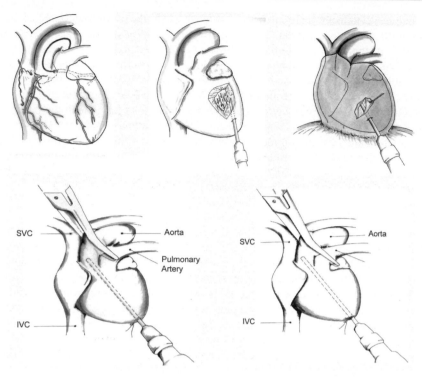

Fig. 3. Different methods of gene transfer in rodents: (1) coronary injection; (2) myocardial injection; (3) pericardial injection; (4) aortic clamping, pulmonary and aortic clamping while injecting in the aortic root.

models, while others rely on percutaneous and surgical techniques that are readily transferable into clinical practice. The method of vector delivery employed is determined mainly by the target pathophysiology.

Catheter-Based Vessel Wall Delivery

The development of catheter-based gene transfer to the vessel wall was based on existing angioplasty techniques employed in peripheral and coronary artery interventions. Gene transfer in this context has largely targeted post-intervention restenosis in animal models of vascular injury. Injury often occurred in normal peripheral arterial segments. The significance of this system as a model for gene transfer to atherosclerotic or restenotic human arteries is unknown. The diseased human artery is likely to impose several barriers to successful gene transfer to the vessel wall, and these are not recreated in animal models. The experience with gene transfer to human arteries is, however, limited; hence the continued requirement for animal models in refining vector delivery techniques. As a result several catheters have been tried over the years. Successive catheters have been designed to enhance focal gene delivery to the artery wall, to limit catheter-induced injury, and to minimize downstream effects such as myocardial ischemia and systemic dissemination of vector *(29,30)*. Examples of these catheters include the double-balloon, the Dispatch™, the hydrogel-coated balloon, and various porous balloon catheters.

Catheter-Based Myocardial Delivery

Percutaneous catheter-based gene delivery to the myocardium in vivo can be achieved by the intracoronary route, by endocardial delivery, or by retroinfusion of the coronary veins. Variable transduction efficiencies have been reported after intracoronary vector delivery. This variability in transduction is due to a number of factors, which include differences between animal species, biocompatibility of catheter and vector, pharmacological agents used to permeabilize vasculature, and vector-related variables such as titer. These factors need to be optimized when the target pathophysiology demands high transduction efficiencies. Viral vectors based on adenovirus, rAAV, and lentivirus have all been reported to result in gene-transfer efficiencies approximating 50%. The latter two are capable of conferring long-term transgene expression. However, only the former two vectors have been shown to rescue the heart failure phenotype in genetically predisposed animals when the appropriate anti-heart failure transgene is expressed. In contrast, other pathophysiologies require only focal gene transfer for phenotypic effect. For example, gene delivery to AV node via the intracoronary route resulted in gene transfer to 50% of AV nodal cells and physiological slowing of electrical conduction *(31)*. In contrast, percutaneous endocardial delivery is limited to focal gene transfer to the myocardium. This method of vector delivery and pattern of gene transfer lends itself most readily to applications such as therapeutic angiogenesis *(32)* and, to a lesser extent, focal arrhythmia therapy *(33)*. Gene delivery can be achieved using steerable needle-tip catheters through which vector may be injected to predetermined regions of endocardium. The catheter tip can be guided by fluoroscopy or by intracardiac echocardiography, both of which have been used safely in large animal models. The nonfluoroscopic electromechanical mapping system is even more suited to endocardial gene transfer approach. This system is capable of identifying ischemic myocardium and also guiding delivery catheters for gene-transfer interventions such as therapeutic angiogenesis. Importantly, the feasibility, safety, and potential efficacy of this approach have been established in phase I clinical trials of patients with medically refractory severe angina secondary to multivessel coronary artery disease unsuitable for revascularisation by conventional means *(34, 35)*. A novel catheter-based technique for myocardial gene delivery has recently been reported. This approach consists of the retrograde infusion of vector via the coronary veins and can result in gene transfer efficiencies comparable with intracoronary injection *(36)*. This approach has been validated in a porcine model of acute myocardial injury. In this study, transfer of decoy NF-κB oligonucelotides to acutely ischemic myocardium resulted in limitation of infarct size and retention of regional myocardial contractility *(37)*. The ability to deliver genes to myocardium through disease-free veins while bypassing diseased arteries that are likely to impede vector delivery is a clinically attractive attribute of this vector delivery strategy.

Direct Myocardial Delivery

Direct injection of vector into the myocardium of an intact animal can be achieved via the transthoracic or subxiphisternal approaches. Use of this method in the literature has been restricted to small animal models *(38)*. The usual target in this context is the myocardium or the left ventricular cavity. Injection of the latter results not only in myocardium delivery via coronary perfusion, but also in systemic vector spread. In certain conditions, such as hypertension, systemic delivery might be desirable. Direct myocardial vector delivery in small animals can result in moderate transduction efficiencies. In larger animals, however, the amount of accessible myocardium is restricted and hence significantly limits gene transfer efficiency.

Pericardial Delivery

Myocardial gene delivery has been attempted via the pericardial space. The rationale underlying this approach is the anatomical proximity between the pericardium and the myocardium, and the accessibility of the pericardial sac for percutaneous vector delivery. Myocardial transduction by this approach has been reported to be low, with vector mostly transducing pericardial cells *(39)*. Gene-transfer efficiency, however, can be significantly improved by the coadministration of proteolytic enzymes that disrupt the pericardial cellular and extracellular barriers to the myocardium *(39)*. An alternate strategy involves vector delivery to the pericardial space before the cell-lined pericardial sac has developed. This strategy has been tried in 5-d-old neonatal mice and has been reported to result in high transduction rates after subxiphisternal vector delivery, with acceptably low procedural mortality *(40)*. Other investigators have taken advantage of the ability of vectors to transduce pericardial cells following intrapericardial delivery. Transgene expression from these cells can be utilized as a platform for therapeutic protein production and delivery. An example of this is the secretion and paracrine effect of angiogenic factors from gene-modified pericardial cells.

Surgical Delivery

Surgical gene delivery is considered to be the most invasive approach because of the significant morbidity associated with achieving access to the myocardium. In the context of human gene therapy, surgical vector delivery can potentially be performed at open cardiac surgery, thorascopically or during the ex vivo phase of cardiac allografting. The choice of surgical approach will largely depend on the clinical setting and the availability of noninvasive or percutaneous alternatives. All these approaches have been successfully used in preclinical animal models of myocardial gene transfer. Of note, early-phase therapeutic angiogenesis trials involving surgical protocols have been initiated in human subjects with chronic refractory angina. Gene delivery to the myocardium by multiple direct injections in open-chested small animals is a well-established technique *(38)*. This results in a pattern of moderate but multifocal transgene expression. Improved and more widespread myocardial transduction can be achieved using a recently described method of vector delivery *(9)*. This method entails delivery into the aortic root via a catheter introduced into the LV cavity and advanced cranially into the aortic root, while the ascending aorta and pulmonary artery are transiently occluded. This method relies on the production of a transcoronary myocardial perfusion gradient for vector delivery. Variations on this method include avoidance of pulmonary artery occlusion, occluding the distal rather than the ascending aorta, the use of hypothermia to prolong cross-clamp times, and pharmacological induction of asystole. More recent developments avoid surgery and rely on balloon catheters for aortic and right-heart occlusion while maintaining the ability to deliver vector into the proximal aorta *(11,41–43)*. The successful application of this method in small animal models has the potential to be extrapolated into the clinic within the context of cardiac surgery that requires aortic cross-clamping and cardiopulmonary bypass.

Catheter-Based Antegrade Intracoronary
Viral Gene Delivery With Coronary Venous Blockade

An efficient and homogenous method for gene delivery during percutaneous coronary intervention would be very beneficial, without the need for an invasive procedure. There have been a number of gene delivery methods used in large animals by percutaneous delivery techniques. The first is the antegrade coronary gene delivery with coronary artery occlusion and coronary sinus occlusion in rabbits. The second is selective pressure-regulated retroinfusion of coronary veins during coronary artery occlusion in swine. The brief interruption of coronary flow and a high-pressure condition during viral delivery seems to be very important to increase diffuse and homogenous gene distribution. More recently, a percutaneous and clinically applicable catheter-based gene delivery method was developed that allows selective antegrade myocardial gene transfer with concomitant specific coronary vein blockade and a high gene expression in targeted myocardium, as shown in Fig. 4.

TARGETS FOR INTERVENTION

The number of molecular targets for each pathophysiology is likely to increase with advances in the knowledge of the molecular basis of cardiovascular disease. With this in mind, the reader should be aware that the remaining part of this chapter is not meant to be exhaustive, but rather representative of the molecular targets that have been pursued in the literature *(42)*. These targets are grouped according to the tissue of interest and include the myocardium, the vasculature, and the cardiac conducting system.

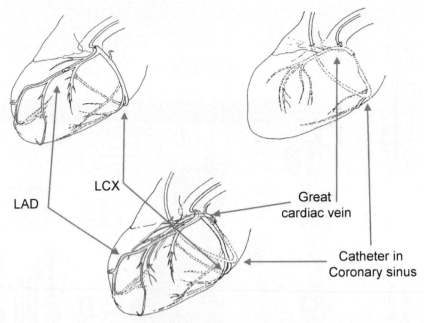

Fig. 4. A 7-Fr sheath is placed in the right femoral artery and an 8-Fr sheath is placed in the right femoral vein using a standard Seldinger technique. A 5-Fr wedge-balloon is advanced to the great cardiac vein or anterior interventricular vein. For both the LAD and LCX territories, the myocardium was preconditioned with a 1-min arterial balloon occlusion. The anterior interventricular vein was occluded during LAD delivery and similarly, the GCV at the entrance of the middle cardiac vein is occluded during LCX delivery. With both the arterial and venous balloons inflated (total 3 min), and following an intracoronary adenosine (25 μg) injection to increase cellular permeability, antegrade injection through the center lumen of the angioplasty balloon with either an adenoviral solution (1 mL of viral solution).

MYOCARDIUM

Heart failure is a major health problem in the modern world. Despite significant gains in medical and surgical treatment of this condition, the disease burden continues to increase, particularly as the population ages. Late-stage heart failure has a poor prognosis and effective treatment is limited to transplantation and the use of mechanical assist devices. These treatment options are severely constrained due to the perennial shortage of donor hearts and the restricted availability of costly mechanical devices. Faced with these challenges, researchers have vigorously explored novel therapeutic options, including gene-based treatments. Consequently many animal models of gene therapy for heart failure have begun to emerge *(41)*. In the following section a systematic overview of the more promising molecular targets is provided. In Fig. 5, we summarize the different transporters and protein within the myocardial cell that have been targeted by gene transfer.

β-Adrenergic Signaling Cascade

The main role of the β-adrenergic receptor (βAR) signaling cascade is to regulate heart rate and contractility in response to agonist catecholamines. Binding of an agonist activates the heterotrimeric G protein second messenger system, which, in the context of the cardiomyocyte, results in stimulatory G protein α-subunit ($G_{\alpha S}$) dissociation. This stimulates adenylyl cyclase (AC) to increase cyclic adenosine monophosphate (cAMP) production, which then activates protein kinase A (PKA). The PKA-dependent phosphorylation of several downstream targets, such as troponin-I, phospholamban (PLB), and L-type calcium channels, mediates the physiological effects of βAR stimulation. Chronic heart failure is associated with increased sympathetic outflow. While initially this is com-

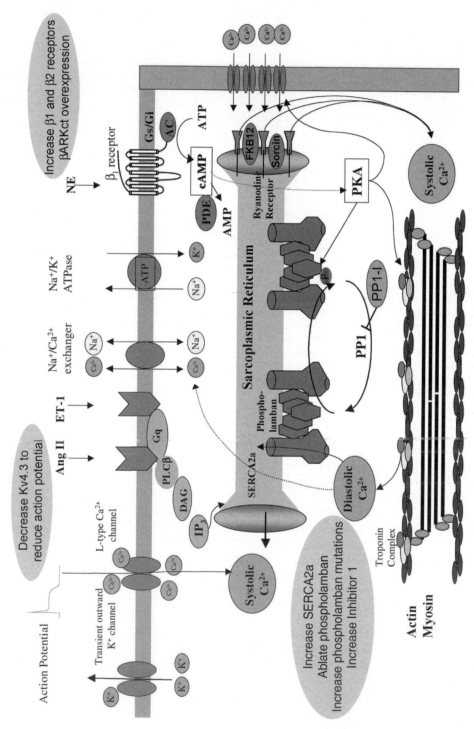

Fig. 5. Excitation–contraction coupling in failing cardiomyocytes.

pensatory, in the long term chronic βAR stimulation contributes to worsening of the pathophysiology. A number of alterations in the βAR signaling cascade have been described in this context; these include βAR downregulation, upregulation of βAR kinase (βARK), and increased inhibitory G protein α-subunit ($G_{\alpha i}$) function *(44)*. Together, these alterations desensitize βARs and diminish signaling through this pathway. Several gene-based approaches have been reported to successfully restore this signaling defect and, as a result, rescue the heart failure phenotype. These observations were initially made in transgenic mice and then reproduced by somatic gene transfer in animal models of inherited and acquired heart failure. Transgenic mice with augmented βAR signaling, through either βAR or βARK inhibitor (βARKct) overexpression, display increased baseline and stimulated contractility. When these mice were crossbred with genetic mouse models of heart failure, the resultant mice were rescued from the heart failure phenotype. Of note, in these crossbreeding experiments the βARKct-overexpressing mouse outperformed the βAR mouse. This suggests that reversing desensitization of βARs is mechanistically more important than just overexpressing them. Additional information gleaned from these experiments is that threshold overexpression levels exist for βARs above which cardiomyopathy ensues. Moreover, different thresholds exist for different βARs, with β_1ARs having a much lower toxicity threshold than β_2ARs. Several in vivo gene transfer strategies have evolved from the transgenic mouse experiments. For example, both β_2AR and βARKct have been reported to result in augmented or rescued βAR signaling following adenovirus-mediated transfer of each gene to normal or dysfunctional rabbit cardiomyocytes, respectively. Similarly, in vivo adenovirus-mediated β_2AR or βARKct gene transfer to the normal rabbit heart resulted in increased contractility following transcoronary vector delivery. More importantly, gene transfer of the adenoviral vector encoding βARKct was reported to have beneficial effects in a rabbit myocardial infarct (MI) model. This benefit varied according to the timing of vector delivery. If vector was delivered at the time of MI, heart failure was prevented; if delivered 3 wk after MI, at a time when heart failure is established, then βARKct gene transfer was capable of reversing this pathophysiology *(45)*. More recently, gene transfer of βARKct in cardiac myocytes isolated from patients with congestive heart failure has shown restoration of contractile function.

In contrast with the small animal gene transfer data, the clinical experience with pharmacological agents suggests that genetically augmenting βAR signaling may be prove to be detrimental in the setting of chronic heart failure. For example, ionotropic βAR agonists increased, whereas βAR antagonists decreased, mortality in patients with heart failure, suggesting that βAR desensitization occurs as a protective mechanism against the toxic effects of chronic sympathetic discharge *(46)*. As a result, controversy abounds in the scientific literature as to the perceived benefits and potential dangers of the gene-based approaches to augmenting βAR. The key to reconciling these discrepancies is probably in the basic science that underpins the diverse signaling and consequent physiological effects of the βAR subtypes. Until these important differences are understood this approach to gene therapy of heart failure is best viewed with cautious optimism.

CALCIUM-HANDLING PROTEINS

The intracellular handling of calcium is central to the process of excitation-contraction coupling in muscle cells. In cardiomyocytes, membrane excitation results in the entry of calcium via the L-type calcium channel. This triggers release of intracellular stores of calcium from the sarcoplasmic reticulum (SR) via the ryanodine receptor, a calcium release channel. The resulting rise in intracellular calcium causes sarcomeric shortening and muscle contraction. Conversely, muscle relaxation is initiated by a fall in intracellular calcium, a process that is largely driven by sarcoplasmic endoreticulum Ca-ATPase (SERCA)-mediated reuptake of calcium into the SR. The activity of SERCA is modulated by phospholamban (PLN), an SR transmembrane protein. Unphosphorylated PLN inhibits SERCA function, whereas PKA-dependent phosphorylation, relieves this inhibitory effect. Increased SERCA activity, as a result of PLN phosphorylation, results in increased SR calcium reuptake and subsequent release. This is the mechanism by which βAR signaling, with PKA activation and PLN phosphorylation, results in increased cardiac contractility. Several calcium-handling protein defects have been described in the context of chronic heart failure. Of these, increasing

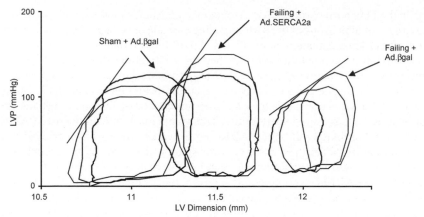

Fig. 6. In a rat model of pressure overload hypertrophy in transition to failure (after 20–24 wk of banding), gene transfer of SERCA2a restores end-systolic pressure-volume relationship, increases stroke volume and decreases end-diastolic volume.

SERCA function or decreasing the inhibitory effect of PLN have been the subject of most gene transfer approaches targeting altered calcium physiology *(41)*. The net effect of either overexpressing SERCA2a or downregulating PLN function is to restore a favourable PLN to SERCA2a ratio, a measure that seems to be of greater physiological relevance than either change alone. Support for these approaches, like the βAR signaling strategies, comes from transgenic mice where overexpression of SERCA or PLN ablation has been reported to result in favorable changes in cardiac hemodynamics and to prevent dilated cardiomyopathy in crossbred genetically predisposed mice, respectively.

In experiments targeting SERCA function, restoration of the calcium transient morphology in cardiomyocytes isolated from failing human hearts has been reported after adenovirus-mediated gene transfer of SERCA *(43,47)*. In vivo transcoronary gene transfer of the same adenoviral vector to pressure-loaded myopathic rat hearts was also found to result in restoration of SERCA2a levels, improved cardiac hemodynamics, and increased animal survival *(43,47)*. In fact as shown in Fig. 6, gene transfer of SERCA2a in an animal model of heart failure resulted in a restoration of the end-systolic pressure-volume relationship, a decrease in end-diastolic volume, and an increase in stroke volume. Furthermore, survival in this animal model was improved from 9% to 64%, as depicted in Fig. 7. Ablation of PLN function has been achieved by either antisense or dominant-negative approaches. Both approaches have been validated in vitro. Of note, normalization of the calcium transient morphology and restoration of cell contractility has been reported in cardiomyocytes isolated from failing human hearts after adenovirus-mediated PLN antisense gene transfer *(48)*. These in vitro findings have been extended in a cardiomyopathic hamster model. Improved calcium handling, cardiac hemodynamics, and retardation of the progression to heart failure were reported following transcoronary delivery of rAAV encoding a dominant-negative form of PLN *(19)*. The excitement generated by this study, which utilized clinically meaningful gene and vector delivery methods, has recently been tempered by the discovery of a dominant-negative mutation in PLN as a cause of human dilated cardiomyopathy. Additionally, inconsistencies have recently been described in the ability of PLN knockout mice to rescue heart failure in crossbred genetic heart failure models. These latter developments have raise doubts about using PLN ablation as a universal approach to treat all forms of heart failure.

MYOCARDIAL PROTECTION STRATEGIES

Myocardial protection by gene transfer encompasses a diverse range of strategies aimed at preventing cardiac cell injury and death. Offending pathophysiologies cause cell death by inflammatory, immunological, or oxidant stress-dependent pathways. Cardiac cells respond by activating

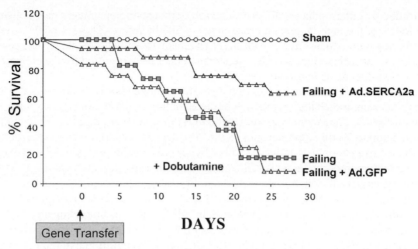

Fig. 7. In a rat model of pressure overload hypertrophy in transition to failure (after 20–24 wk of banding), gene transfer of SERCA2a improves survival from 8–9% to 64%.

endogenous protective mechanisms or by undergoing apoptotic and nonapoptotic cell death. Gene-transfer approaches have demonstrated a capacity for protecting the myocardium and promoting survival in cardiac cells confronted with the aforementioned insults. Generically, these include anti-inflammatory, immunoinhibitory, antioxidant, and antiapoptotic or prosurvival approaches.

The transcription factor NF-κB has been the most common molecular target of antiinflammatory approaches in ischemia-reperfusion myocardial injury models. The attractiveness of this target lies in the ability of NF-κB to modulate the activity of several downstream genes involved in inflammation. Its role in mediating inflammation in the context of ischemia-reperfusion injury has been demonstrated by blocking its activity using decoy oligonucleotides. In a rat MI model, for example, reduced infarct size was reported after transcoronary delivery of oligonucleotides packaged in HVJ-liposomes (49). This benefit was conferred irrespective of whether delivery occured before coronary occlusion or after reperfusion. These positive findings were reproduced in a preclinical porcine model of ischemia-reperfusion injury, following retrograde coronary venous delivery of the abovementioned oligonucleotides packaged in liposomes (37). In addition to these, the anti-inflammatory benefits of NF-κB decoy therapy have also been demonstrated in animal models of myocarditis and cardiac allografting.

Gene based immunoinhibitory strategies for myocardial protection includes the use of immunomodulatory cytokines, inhibition of inflammatory cytokines, and blockade of T-cell costimulation. These approaches have been tested mainly in the context of experimental myocarditis and cardiac allografting. In small animal models of myocarditis, improved histological and functional outcomes have been reported after peripheral skeletal muscle delivery of plasmid-encoding genes for interleukin (IL)-10, IL-1 receptor antagonist, and murine interferon A6. Similarly, in cardiac allograft animal models, gene transfer of immunomodulatory cytokines IL-4, IL-10, IL-14 and tumor growth factor (TGF)-β, have been reported to prolong graft survival. Finally, inhibition of T-cell costimulatory activation by gene transfer of blocking antibodies has also been demonstrated to reverse the pathological features of autoimmune myocarditis and markedly prolong allograft survival in small animal models.

There is a growing literature on the role of oxidative stress in cardiovascular disease. "Stress" occurs when excess amounts of reactive oxygen species (ROS) are generated and overwhelm the endogenous antioxidant systems, resulting in cell death or dysfunction. Gene-based approaches to antioxidant therapy were initially guided by enzyme-based interventions and more recently by the promising findings from experiments involving transgenic mice. In general, an antioxidant effect can be afforded by either reducing ROS production or increasing enzymatic metabolism of these species. Models of the latter approach predominate in the literature. These models usually entail gene transfer of an antioxidant enyme to the myocardium of an animal subjected to ischaemia-reperfusion injury. Myocardial protection after gene transfer has been reported for the enzymes manganese superoxide dismutase and hemoxygenase-1.

Apoptotic myocardial cell death contributes to the pathogenesis of heart failure, irrespective of etiology. As such, molecular targets within the signaling and effector pathways for apoptosis have been pursued in gene therapy models of heart failure, in an attempt to attenuate the burden of cell death. Support for this approach includes in vitro data demonstrating that rat cardiomyocytes can be protected from apoptosis-inducing p53 or hypoxia after adenovirus-mediated over-expression of Bcl-2 (antiapoptotic effector) or PI-3 kinase and Akt (prosurvival signaling), respectively. In small animal models of ischemia-reperfusion injury, adenovirus-mediated gene transfer of Akt has been reported to significantly reduce the number of apoptotic cells in the region of injury, limit infarct size, and preserve cardiac hemodynamics. In a different model targeting an apoptotic effector molecule, pacing-induced heart failure was prevented by the intracoronary delivery of adenoviral vector encoding p35, a caspase-3 inhibitor. Undoubtedly, additional antiapoptotic and cell-survival pathways will be targeted. A notable recent development is the discovery of an endogenous glycoprotein (gp) 130 receptor-mediated antiapoptotic pathway *(50,51)*. The IL-6 family of cytokines ordinarily signals via this receptor to improve cell survival. Cardiac-restricted ablation of this molecule has been shown to markedly increase the rate of apoptosis after pressure-loading the heart. This observation not only highlights the protective role of this signaling pathway against the development of heart failure, but also provides a novel molecular target for therapy of heart failure.

MOLECULAR AND CELLULAR CARDIOMYOPLASTY

The term *cardiomyoplasty* has been used in the literature to describe the process of converting scarred noncontractile myocardium into functional muscle. The molecular approach involves the use of MyoD, a skeletal myogenic transcription factor, capable of forcing myogenesis in non-muscle cells such as fibroblasts. In vivo MyoD gene transfer into infarcted myocardium resulted in poor rates of myogenic conversion. These rates were increased by ex vivo gene transfer to fibroblasts, prior to implantation of these cells into damaged myocardium. However, the functional outcomes of this approach have not been assessed. The use of MyoD for molecular cardiomyoplasty is unlikely to be successful due to the biological differences between skeletal and cardiac muscle. Cellular cardiomyoplasty, on the other hand, involves the transplantation of cells capable of restoring contractile function in damaged myocardium and appears promising. This approach has been the subject of intense investigation with positive preclinical data culminating in phase I clinical trials in Europe and North America. As several excellent reviews of this topic have appeared in the literature, the following discussion is limited to gene transfer in the context of cell transplantation for cardiac repair.

Cells for cardiomyoplasty can be genetically manipulated to confer diverse biological effects. For example, high rates of death have been observed in certain cell types after transplantation into damaged myocardium. Targeting this problem, improved survival of engrafted mesenchymal stem cells has been reported after retroviral-mediated ex vivo gene transfer of Akt, a pro-survival kinase *(52)*. Conversely, other cell types result in large grafts due to uncontrolled proliferation. Preliminary in vitro work has been reported to result in exogenous control of proliferation in gene-modified skeletal myoblasts by expressing a chimeric receptor that emulates mitogenic signaling following the administration of a synthetic ligand. Moreover, some cells types have been gene-modified in attempt to confer a capacity for functional integration with host tissue. An example of this is the expression of connexin-43, a gap junction protein in skeletal myoblasts. Skeletal, in contrast with cardiac, muscle lacks the capacity for gap junctional intercellular communication. This physiological property is essential for efficient electrical conduction. Finally, transferring a strategy employed for allograft protection, cells can be be rendered resistant to host immune responses by overexpressing CTLA4-Ig, an antibody capable of blocking T-cell costimulatory activation and prolonging graft survival. In addition to altering the biology of transplanted cells, grafts can be gene-modified to function as a platform for therapeutic recombinant protein delivery. The most prevalent example of this is the expression of angiogenic cytokines from different cell types *(53)*. In general, a benefit of the combined gene and cell approach, beyond that of either alone, has been reported in small animal models. Of some concern, however, is a report of local angioma formation, cachexia, and premature animal death following implantation of skeletal myoblasts, expressing retroviral-mediated VEGF, into normal murine hearts *(54)*.

Coronary Vasculature

Atherosclerosis is the most prevalent pathological process affecting human adult coronary and peripheral arteries. This underlies the predominance of vascular disease as a cause of mortality in modern societies. Management of this disease includes risk factor modification, the use of pharmacological agents, and revascularization procedures. Subsets of patients, ineligible for revascularization, continue to experience clinical manifestations of myocardial and peripheral limb ischemia despite maximal medical therapy. This pathophysiology of refractory and nonrevascularizable tissue ischemia has been targeted by a gene therapy strategy known generically as therapeutic angiogenesis. Further groups of patients develop recurrent symptoms after revascularization due to remodeling of the vessel postintervention. This remodeling results in restenosis of the target artery or bypass conduit. The high rates of restenosis after intervention and unsatisfactory treatment options have lead to several gene-based approaches targeting this pathophysiology. An additional gene transfer target has been the process of thrombosis that not only contributes to the pathogenesis of atheroscelerosis, but also causes many of the complicating acute clinical syndromes. In the following section therapeutic angiogenesis, antirestenosis, and antithrombosis gene therapy models will be discussed.

THERAPEUTIC ANGIOGENESIS

Therapeutic angiogenesis has become the favored intervention among a number of emerging nonconventional revascularization strategies. The reasons for this prominence include the efficiency with which angiogenic cytokines induce new-vessel formation, the reliance on simple gene transfer technology to achieve this, the low threshold for phenotypic effect, and the availability of techniques that facilitate vector delivery in the clinical setting.

Angiogenesis and consequent relief from muscle ischemia have been demonstrated using plasmid and adenoviral vector-mediated gene transfer. The transient pattern of gene expression conferred is sufficient to correct this pathophysiology. Similar outcomes have been reported when integrating vectors, such as rAAV, are used. Stable and long-term transgene expression in this context, however, has the potential to result in adverse effects (discussed below). One potential solution to this problem, which retains the benefits of an integrating vector, is to engineer a hypoxia-responsive promoter element in the expression cassette *(55–57)*. The application of therapeutic angiogenesis to peripheral vascular disease (PVD) has evolved ahead of the use of this technology in ischemic heart disease (IHD). While gene therapy is an important advance in the treatment of critical limb ischemia (CLI) due to PVD, this disease also represents a model system of end-stage vascular insufficiency that lends itself to gene-based interventions and the objective assessment of therapeutic endpoints. Successful peripheral interventions can potentially be extrapolated to the treatment of refractory myocardial ischemia. Preclinical and early-phase clinical studies have consistently yielded positive results after intraarterial or intramuscular plasmid-mediated delivery of recombinant angiogenic cytokines in the context of PVD *(58,59)*. Recent phase II studies, however, soberly report clinical improvements in patients with PVD treated with either adenoviral vector encoding vascular endothelial growth factor $(VEGF)_{121}$ or $VEGF_{165}$ in an adenoviral or liposomal vector that did not exceed that of placebo control *(60,61)*. There was, however, improvement in vascularity, as measured angiographically. Data from these studies emphasize the importance of appropriate controls in assessing the efficacy of new therapeutic interventions. A number of study parameters can be varied in redesigning trials of this type. Variables such as patient selection and number, measured endpoints, choice of angiogenic factor or combination of factors, dose and type of vector, and method of delivery all have a bearing on the outcome of the study. Undoubtedly, the design of future studies will incorporate these variations. The late Dr. Jeffrey Isner initiated the first clinical trial of therapeutic angiogenesis for myocardial ischemia. These patients with refractory symptoms were treated with plasmid-encoded $VEGF_{165}$ by direct injection via a mini-thoracotomy. This group of patients had improved symptoms and myocardial perfusion as documented by nuclear perfusion scans and electromechanical maps *(34)*. This group has since reported successful therapeutic angiogenesis in early-phase trials using a catheter-based transendocardial approach. Ischemic myocardium was identified and the anatomical position of the catheter tip guided by the electromechanical mapping system. Patients receiving $VEGF_{165}$ by this approach have been reported to achieve both subjective and objective improvements when compared to patients receiving placebo injections.

ANTIRESTENOSIS STRATEGIES

The treatment of postintervention restenosis is poised to be revolutionized with the development of cytostatic drug-eluting intracoronary stents. These stents have been reported to totally abolish clinical restenosis rates following coronary angioplasty, a problem that has plagued vascular intervention since its inception. The role of gene-based treatments, as a result of this remarkable advance, is likely to be limited. Conceivably, gene therapy may have a role in situations in which drug-eluting stents cannot be used or in the treatment of long-term stent-related complications, potentially borne out with extended follow-up of patients receiving drug-eluting stents. Gene-based interventions have been vigorously explored in animal models targeting the pathology of vascular smooth muscle hyperplasia and extracellular matrix deposition. These processes underlie neointima formation and vessel restenosis. The results of antirestenotic interventions in these models have consistently provided positive outcomes, lending support for a genetic strategy. Also supporting gene therapy as a treatment modality is the focal nature of the pathophysiology together with amenability to noninvasive vector delivery techniques. Sadly, despite promising preclinical results, gene-based treatments have not translated into benefit in the small number of patients treated in clinical trials to date. One possible reason for this discrepancy is the inability of animal models to recapitulate the pathology seen in restenosis that occurs in the context of atherosclerotic human arteries.

The clinical experience with gene-based interventions for restenosis is limited. The first clinical trial demonstrated a positive 12-mo clinical outcome for composite endpoints in patients undergoing bypass vein grafting for obstructive PVD. Randomly assigned patients received decoy E2F oligonucleotides, delivered by an ex vivo approach during graft harvest. Similarly, the ITALICS trial for the prevention of restenosis in patients undergoing coronary intervention also used an oligonucleotide-based strategy. In contrast, the rate of restenosis in patients receiving intracoronary antisense oligonucleotide to the protooncogene *c-myc* was not reduced in comparison with control patients. Also reporting a lack of effect is the KAT trial, in which intracoronary VEGF gene transfer failed to reduce restenosis rates in patients undergoing coronary intervention. These mixed results have been generated from a limited number of trial patients. Ongoing larger trials will hopefully allow more definitive conclusions to be drawn regarding the efficacy of gene-based antirestenosis therapy.

ANTITHROMBOTIC STRATEGIES

Focal genetic manipulation of the biochemical factors that modulate thrombosis has a number of possible applications in cardiovascular disease. Manipulations of this type have the potential to create a local environment of reduced thrombogenecity without affecting systemic coagulation parameters. Conventional pharmacological agents, on the other hand, have attendant bleeding risks due to their systemic action. It is the avoidance of bleeding complications that has provided some of the motivation for gene transfer research in this area. Additional impetus is derived from the knowledge that thrombosis contributes to the pathogenesis of atherosclerosis and its complications. The coagulation cascade has been targeted in a number of gene-transfer studies. Reduced local thrombus production and unchanged systemic coagulation parameters have been reported following adenovirus-mediated transfer of the genes for hirudin, thrombomodulin, and tissue-factor pathway inhibitor. In these models thrombosis is induced by either injury or stasis. In vivo testing of this system is pending. Reduced thrombus formation has also been reported following gene transfer of cyclooxygenase-1 and nitric oxide synthase in carotid and coronary artery injury models. An antiplatelet effect was thought to underlie the antithrombotic effect of gene transfer in these latter studies. Moreover, molecules with fibrinolytic activity such as tissue-type plasminogen activator or surface-anchored urokinase have also been demonstrated to confer local antithrombotic effects in gene transfer models, again without altering systemic coagulation. Among other biological effects, molecules such as NO and angiogenic factors have the potential to reduce the prothrombotic tendency associated with vessel injury by improve endothelial cell function and reendothelialization.

Cardiac Conducting System and Arrhythmias

The genetic manipulation of the physiological processes that underlie cardiac excitability and electrical impulse generation and conduction is a small but exciting component within the broader context of gene therapy for cardiovascular disease. Manipulations of this type are achieved by either focal or global myocardial delivery. Examples of physiological effects amenable to focal gene transfer include the creation of biological pacemakers and the modulation of conduction throughout the AV node or reentrant arrhythmia circuits. The threshold for achieving these physiological effects is potentially low due to the requirement for focal genetic modification. In contrast, pathophysiologies affecting the entire heart, such as genetic forms of long-QT syndrome, impose demands similar to those of myocardial-based pathophysiologies and are currently limited by inefficient gene transfer.

Impulse Generation and Biological Pacemakers

Electronic pacemakers are highly effective treatment for bradyarrhythmias. These devices, however, are prone to lead failure and battery depletion that necessitate repeat procedures. The burden of repeat procedures is greatest in those who receive pacemakers at a relatively young age. For this reason the creation of biological pacemakers is conceptually meritorious and deserving of further investigation. The first approach involved the overexpression of $\beta_2 AR$ in cardiomyocytes and right atrium in vivo. The effect of this was to enhance chronotropy. This approach, however, did not confer a capacity for spontaneous diastolic depolarization in gene-modified cells, the hallmark of pacemaker cells. The next approach and the first study to report the generation of a biological pacemaker employed a dominant-negative molecular approach to reduce the current Ik_1. This current normally suppresses diastolic depolarization by anchoring the cell membrane at a negative resting potential. Adenovirus-mediated transfer of the mutant gene resulted in the generation of dominant escape ventricular rhythms, following transcoronary vector delivery to guinea pig hearts.

Modulating Impulse Conduction

Cardiac impulse conduction can be modulated by altering either cardiomyocyte excitability or intercellular coupling. To date genetic manipulations have targeted the former electrophysiological property in order to affect electrical conduction. The only published in vivo model reported slowing of AV nodal conduction following focal gene transfer and overexpression of the inhibitory G protein ($G_{\alpha i2}$) (31). In this porcine model, adenoviral vector was delivered to the AV node by selective catheterization of the AV nodal artery. The biological effect of $G_{\alpha i2}$ overexpression is to emulate βAR blockade. As a result, gene transfer induced prolongation of PR and AH intervals and also reduced the ventricular response rate to adrenergic stimulation and induced atrial fibrillation. Additional approaches to slowing conduction are preliminary and include the in vitro data from cocultures of cardiomyocytes and fibroblasts that have been genetically engineered to express a repolarizing current. This study reported slowing of electrical propagation in cardiomyocytes cultured with these gene-modified fibroblasts.

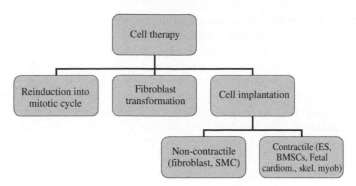

Fig. 8. Different strategies for cell therapy.

TARGETING REPOLARIZATION

Abnormalities of repolarization resulting from inherited or acquired ion-channel defects can give rise to potentially fatal ventricular arrhythmias *(62–66)*. Advances in the understanding of the molecular basis of these arrhythmic syndromes have increased the prospect of gene-based treatments. In vitro studies have confirmed the capacity for this technology to correct the cellular electrophysiological abnormality of prolonged APD that is common to many of these syndromes. Extending these findings, in vivo gene transfer has also been reported to result in potentially important physiological effects such as shortening of the QT interval in genetically normal guinea pig hearts. More recently, phenotypic correction has been reported in a transgenic mouse model of long-QT syndrome, after gene transfer restored the dysfunctional ion channel *(62–66)*.

CELL THERAPY

Cell Therapy in Myocardial Diseases

Although the target of cell therapy (also known as cellular cardiomyoplasty) has now spread to nonischemic cardiomyopathy, the basic concept of cell therapy is to replace postinfarction scar tissue with contractile cells and to restore the contractile function in the area. There seems to be three distinct approaches, as shown in Fig. 8, including (1) reinduction of residual cardiomyocytes to a mitotic cycle and expansion of the number of contractile elements, (2) transformation of in-scar fibroblasts into contractile cells, and (3) injection of exogenous contractile cells into the scar.

REINDUCTION OF RESIDUAL CARDIOMYOCYTES
TO MITOTIC CYCLE AND EXPANSION OF NUMBER OF CONTRACTILE ELEMENTS

Recently it has been shown that while most adult myocytes are terminally differentiated and irreversibly withdraw from the cell cycle, there are some myocytes able to reenter the cell cycle with a probability that increased significantly in certain pathological conditions *(67)*. Now it is likely that even the adult heart contains cardiomyocytes having proliferative capacity. Nevertheless, the expression of Ki-67, which is a maker of cell cycle entry, was detected in only a small population of myocytes in the adjacent region to the infarct. The proliferation is extremely limited at only 0.08% mitotic index in the adjacent region to the infarct *(67)*. Consequently, the proliferative capacity is obviously not enough to compensate for massive cell loss by a large infarct. However, this evidence also raises the possibility that increasing the number of the remaining cardiomyocytes may be a therapeutic alternative to replace damaged myocardium. To date, some attempts to stimulate cardiomyocyte DNA replication have been reported. It is known that progression of the mammalian cell cycle is regulated by a family of cyclins and cyclin-dependent kinases (CDKs). In particular, the cyclin D1 plays an important role for promoting cell cycle of G1-to-S phase progression by inactivating the action of the retinoblastoma protein (Rb) through phosphorylation.

TRANSFORMATION OF IN-SCAR FIBROBLASTS INTO CONTRACTILE CELLS BY OVEREXPRESSION OF MyoD

So far, no specific transcription factor for cardiac myogenesis exists. Meanwhile, in skeletal muscle, the MyoD family of basic helix-loop-helix proteins is well known to function as master genes for induction of the skeletal muscle differentiation program. Therefore, studies about the transformation of scar tissue have focused on the conversion into skeletal muscle. Tam et al. first indicated the feasibility that overexpression of MyoD gene in vitro may convert cardiac fibroblasts into skeletal muscle cells showing myotubes, myosin heavy chain (MHC) and myocyte-specific enhancer factor 2 (MEF2). Although the in vivo conversion of fibroblasts to skeletal muscles required high doses of adenoviral vectors, MyoD gene transfer induced skeletal muscle differentiation in the scar formation of infarcted heart (68). However, in canine myocardial infarction models, the transfection of MyoD was limited and the converted cells showed the expression of skeletal MHC, but no morphological myotubes. Accordingly, this concept is still controversial. In addition, it should be mentioned that further investigation of specific cardiac myogenic factors must be required for successful transformation strategy.

INJECTION OF EXOGENOUS CONTRACTILE CELLS INTO THE SCAR

Form a clinical standpoint, transplantation of cells has looked more realistic than other approaches. Although most studies have focused on ischemic, segmental cardiomyopathies, some reports suggested that this technique can apply to congestive heart failure due to idiopathic or doxorubicin-induced globally dilated cardiomyopathies. The candidate for implanted cells can be broadly divided into noncontractile cells, such as fibroblast and smooth muscle cell (SMC), and contractile cells. Noncontracting cells are implanted for the purpose of preventing the deterioration of post-infarct diastolic function, while contracting cells are expected to improve both systolic and diastolic function. Furthermore, contractile cells are divided into two cell types, namely naturally contractile cells and potentially contractile cells. The former includes fetal and neonatal cardiomyocytes, and skeletal myoblasts. On the other hand, the latter is represented by embryonic stem (ES) cells and bone marrow cells (also known as adult stem cells).

NONCONTRACTING CELL TRANSPLANTATION

Fibroblast Cell as Source for Cell Transplantation. Fibroblast cells are an attractive cell source for cell transplantation as well as the target for transformation strategy. This is because fibroblasts are autologous, abundant, and easily expandable. It is also easy to harvest from several organs, including skin and pericardium. These properties are particularly important for elderly patients because of their limited availability of adult stem cells and myoblasts. As already mentioned in the transformation to skeletal muscles, several attempts with in vivo gene transfer of MyoD using direct injection required a high dose of viral vectors and yielded a low efficiency of the conversion into skeletal muscle.

Smooth Muscle Cell Transplantation. A number of studies have shown that smooth muscle cell (SMC) transplantation improved both systolic and diastolic function in rat MI model and in hamster dilated cardiomyopathy models because implanted cells increased wall tension and elasticity. These studies indicated that injected SMC may prevent the deterioration of systolic dysfunction by attenuating systolic overstretch of native viable cardiomyocytes and diastolic dysfunction, or rather ventricular enlargement by limiting ventricular expansion. In addition, SMCs have the following technical and biological advantages: the possibility of autotransplantation, the ability to proliferate more easily than skeletal myoblasts, the elastic property, long-term steadiness of the contractile property (termed tonus contraction), and the hyperplasic response of SMC to the increased stretch.

NATURALLY CONTRACTILE CELLS

Fetal and Neonatal Cardiomyocytes. In cellular cardiomyoplasty, the primary candidate was fetal and neonatal myocytes because these cells have the ability to differentiate into an adult matured cardiomyocyte phenotype, but at the same time, they still retain a certain ability to proliferate. Soonpaa et al. first demonstrated that grafted fetal cardiomyocytes were detected over 2 mo in normal mouse hearts (69). Interestingly, in this fundamental study, grafted fetal cardiomyocytes in normal mice hearts showed nascent intercalated disks connected with the host myocardium. Similarly, Murry's group indicated that both grafted fetal and neonatal cardiomyocytes formed matured myocardium in rat hearts 2 mo after the injection (70). In some cases in this study, graft cells formed gap and adhesion junctions with host cardiomyocytes, suggesting electromechanical coupling. Theoretically, successful cell transplantation, which contributes to the improvement of cardiac function, depends crucially on integration into the host and differentiation toward the adult phenotype. In this regard, fetal and neonatal cardiomyocytes seem to be quite promising candidates. It must be mentioned, however, that as far as clinical perspective is concerned, ethical issues could severely hinder the application with other hurdles to be overcome, including availability and immunogenicity.

Skeletal Myoblasts

Skeletal myoblasts, which are also known as satellite cells, are myogenic precursors and normally exist in a quiescent state under the basal membrane of skeletal muscle fibres. These cells are rapidly mobilized into the injured area and proliferate and fuse to regenerate the damaged fibers. Skeletal myoblasts have some advantages as a source for cell transplantation, such as (1) autologous origin, (2) relatively easy to multiply to large numbers from a small biopsy, (3) low tumoregenicity because of well-differentiated myogenic lineage, and (4) high resistance to ischemia. In experimental studies, it has been detected that grafted myoblasts differentiated into typical multinucleated myotubes and substituted the postinfarct fibrosis. However, so far no studies have shown reliable evidence of transdifferentiation of injected myoblasts into cardiomyocytes, despite some forms of phenotype (change myosin pattern), which can be an adaptation to the myocardial environment. In addition, most studies of skeletal myoblast transplantation failed to show the existence of gap junction of injected cells with host myocytes in vivo. Furthermore, in vitro study by Murry's group reported that although cultured skeletal myoblasts express N-cadherin and connexin-43, which is known as the major protein for gap junctions, the expression decreased after intramyocardial implantation in vivo (71). Recently, Menasché's group has shown some conclusive results that skeletal myoblasts retained the typical electrical membrane properties and functional and electrophysiological independence after transplantation (72). In contrast to these negative results of the graft-host coupling, the improvement of cardiac function after skeletal myoblast transplantation has been continuously demonstrated in many animal models and even clinical cases in both the short and long term. Menasché et al. has repeatedly indicated that functional improvement could be mechanistically linked to engrafted skeletal myoblasts and has proposed three possible mechanisms. First, the elastic properties of implanted cells may provide a scaffold strengthening the ventricular wall and subsequently limiting postinfarct scar expansion in a similar way to the SMC implants. In this regard, it is consistent that the grafted skeletal myoblasts have a protective effect against excessive remodeling. Second, intrinsic contractile function of skeletal myoblasts may be directly involved in the improvement of the systolic function. In a 1-yr follow-up study, functional parameters of sheep hearts remained significantly improved in both systole and diastole that were detected 4 mo after the transplantation. Similarly, Menasché reported that postoperative echocardiography showed 63% of the myoblast-transplanted infarcted segments demonstrated new-onset systolic thickening. Therefore, despite many negative results of skeletal myoblast-to-host cardiomyocyte coupling, this possibility still remains. Lastly, the engrafted myoblast may act as a source of growth and/or angiogenic factors. It has been reported that hepatocyte growth factor/scatter factor (HGF) was detected in skeletal myoblasts. In addition, since the expression of HGF in myocardial ischemia and reperfusion has antiapoptotic and antifibrotic effects, this factor has been targeted as a new therapeutic alternative for ischemic heart disease. The precise role of HGF is not completely clear, but it is quite possible that grafted skeletal myoblasts secret HGF and have a positive effect on the host cardiomyocytes including recruiting resident cardiac stem cells and stimulating regeneration of cardiomyocytes. This hypothesis is also supported by the result of long-term follow-up after skeletal transplantation, which shows that, despite the decrease in the number of grafted cells in the heart, the functional improvement still remains 1 yr after the transplantation. The first clinical report of the cell-based therapy was in 2001 by Menasché et al. *(73)*. The result of this first phase I trial was much awaited. This trial served a major dual purpose—the feasibility and safety of autologous skeletal myoblast transplantation in patients with severe ischemic cardiomyopathy. The result and the protocol have been kept brief, so the reader is referred to the excellent clinical report and editorial comment recently published. The cell-based therapy was performed for 10 patients. The criteria of patient selection are (1) impairment of left ventricular function: ejection fraction ≤0.35, (2) previous history of myocardial infarction with a residual discrete, akinetic, and nonviable scar in the left ventricle, and (3) indication for concomitant coronary artery bypass grafting (CABG) in another segment of the ventricle, which is dependent, viable, but ischemic, not in cell-implanted area. Skeletal muscle was harvested from the patient's thigh under local anaesthesia. The sample was upscaled to at least 5×10^8 cells containing ≥50% myoblasts and ≥70% viable cells. All patients had cell transplantation of 8.7×10^8 cells on average, which was concomitant with two or three bypass grafts. The whole process from the muscle biopsy to the operation was done within 2 to 3 wk. Among 10 patients, there was one early death and one noncardiac death during the follow-up, but no perioperative complication related to the cell preparation and the transplantation, except for ventricular arrhythmia. It could be fair to say, therefore, that the result is quite encouraging in terms of feasibility and safety of the procedure. The authors carefully concluded that the scale-up of cell number was more than enough to improve the cardiac function, and the transplantation was relatively safe. It would be impossible to completely rule out the effect of the concomitant revascularization. Nevertheless, it is noteworthy that at about 11-mo follow-up, 63% of cases showed a new-onset systolic wall thickening in implanted scar area. In addition, patients also showed a significant improvement of New York Heart Association functional class (from 2.7 to 1.6) and left ventricular ejection fraction (from 24% to 32%). Concerning ventricular tachycardia (VT) after the transplantation, whether the arrhythmia directly connects with the transplantation or not is not clear. It should be mentioned, however, that all four cases out of nine showed sustained VT and had the implantation of an automatic internal cardiodefibrillator (AICD). All in all, this phase I trial has shown the real possibility of cell-based therapy to treat human heart failure, at the same time it has opened our eyes to the drawbacks, such as the possibility of arrhythmia after the transplantation. Now the clinical trial has moved to phase II, aiming at assessing the safety and efficacy with placebo-control group in multiple centers.

POTENTIALLY CONTRACTILE CELLS: EMBRYONIC STEM CELLS AND BONE MARROW CELLS

Myogenic stem cells that have potential for differentiation into cardiomyocytes could be divided into two categories, namely, embryonic stem (ES) cells and adult stem cells, which are contained in bone marrow. ES cells derived from the inner cell mass of blastocyst-stage embryos are characterized by the ability to proliferate unlimitedly and undifferentiatedly and to be pluripotent, which means having the capability to differentiate into every somatic cell type of the adult organism. Therefore, these cells are expected to be an ideal source of cells for the repair of damaged myocardium. Mouse ES cells in vitro form an aggregate termed *embryonic bodies*. In general, within 10 d 80 to 100% of them have spontaneously contracting areas, but the fraction of the contracting areas is small. The methods to generate essentially pure cardiomyocyte cultures have been reported by several groups. Klug et al. reported that more than 99% purified cultured and genetically selected mouse cardiomyocytes formed stable intracardiac grafts with a normal myocardial structure, showing the formation of intercalated disks and gap junctions when transplanted into the healthy mouse heart *(74)*. Like mouse ES cells, human ES cells are also characterized by immortality, expression of specific transcription factors and cell surface molecules, and the ability to differentiate into all cell types. The pluripotent stem cells express a variety of receptors for growth factors. In particular, transforming growth factor β-1 (TGF-β1) and activin-A are known to promote differentiation into mesodermal derivatives such as muscle cells. Differentiation of cardiomyocytes from human ES cell and electrical coupling and synchronous contraction of the human stem cell-derived cardiomyocytes with rat cardiomyocytes in coculture can also be achieved. In addition, in rat heart infarction models, implanted ES cells survived and differentiated into mature cardiomyocytes 6 wk after the transplantation and as a result of that, cardiac function was improved. Moreover, a recent study reported the improvement remained in the long term (32 wk). Undoubtedly, these studies have indicated that ES cells could provide enormous potential for cell therapy in heart failure because ES cells theoretically have the unlimited availability as a source of cardiomyocytes even for humans. Grafted ES cells are also expected to form electrical coupling with the host cardiomyocytes and improve global cardiac function. It could be fair to say, however, that there still remain a number of major issues to be overcome for clinical application of human ES cells. Firstly, the allogeneic origin of these cells raises immunological problems, and antirejection strategies including immuno-suppressive drugs could be required. Secondly, the efficacy and culture conditions for cardiomyo-cyte differentiation should be more optimized. Thirdly, the immorality of undifferentiated stem cells, which can form cell types other than cardiomyocytes, is a huge benefit, but also may cause tumoregenicity. Last but not least, like fetal and neonatal cardiomyocytes, moral and ethical issues could be the greatest obstacle to clinical application.

Bone Marrow Stem Cells (Adult Stem Cells). Recently, bone marrow cells, i.e., stem cells derived from the bone marrow, have been focused on as a source of cell transplantation into the heart. Like ES cells, the so-called adult stem cell is also expected to have the capacity of unlimited, undifferentiated proliferation and to be able to develop into different types of cells including cardiomyocytes. To date, since there is no universally acceptable characterization and definition of the stem cells and progenitor cells, these cells have a variety of names, for instance, "marrow progenitor cells," "stromal stem cells," "marrow stromal cells," "marrow mononuclear cells," and "mesenchymal stem cells." In this review, we will use "bone marrow stem cells" (BMSCs) as the term for these cells, which seem pluripotent and have the ability to differentiate into various phe-notypes. In contrast to ES cell, BMSCs appear to be an ideal cell source for cardiac repair because these cells, having great plasticity, can be collected from patients without evoking ethical and moral questions and creating problems of immunological reaction. Although the precise angiogenic and myogenic effects after the transplantation of BMSCs are still unclear, most experimental studies showed the differentiation into cardiomyocytes with the improvement of global cardiac function in acute or chronic infarcted heart models and even in the nonischemic heart. There are several studies showing the induction of differentiation of BMSCs into cardiomyocytes by treating with 5-azacytid-ine and the investigation of additional inducing factors for the differentiation has been explored.

It is noteworthy that in contrast to clinical studies of skeletal myoblast transplantation, these studies reported no patients with ventricular arrhythmia, including sustained VT. Still, it should also be mentioned that the condition and cell types of these clinical studies are varied and long-term follow-up must be done. In addition, the following questions must be answered for clinical appli-cation to treating heart failure: first, which component of bone marrow cells, such as stromal cells and/or hematopoietic progenitors, is suitable for a cell source of cardiomyocytes; second, how to scale the population of bone marrow cells up without affecting cell plasticity. According to the study by Jackson et al., the percentage of the donor stem cell-derived cardiomyocytes is 0.02% and obviously not enough to improve the damaged heart function *(75)*. It is consistent with recent reports suggesting that the main effect of bone marrow cell transplantation on the improvement of regional heart function is angiogenesis by the paracrine effect of bone marrow cells, not direct effects on contraction. It is certain that the paracrine effects are likely to trigger the differentiation of adult stem cells into cardiomyocytes, stimulate host myocytes to reentry of a cell cycle, and induce a cardiomyogenic lineage of bone marrow cells or circulating progenitor cells to injured sites. Even so, scale-up of BMSCs will be vital to improve cardiac function directly.

DELIVERY SYSTEMS FOR CELL THERAPY IN HEART FAILURE

Theoretically, the fundamental basis of delivery systems to target cardiovascular tissues is not different between gene therapy and cell therapy. So far, in experimental and clinical studies of gene and cell therapy for heart disease, a variety of delivery methods have been reported, but the methods are physiologically categorized into two major methods, such as injection using the coronary circulation including intracoronary injection (ICI) and retrograde injection via coronary sinus (RCI), or direct injection (DI) including epicardial and endocardial approaches. In addition, each delivery method can be applicable to interventional and less invasive or ordinary surgical approaches. Whether the delivered material is genes or cells, the functional efficacy to treat heart disease depends on how efficiently they can settle in the targeted tissue and how settled materials can function as expected. In this regard, both gene and cell therapy in heart disease still have no sufficient delivery systems. Furthermore, all systems have the same potential risk, namely, untoward effects on non-target organs. Therefore, it is of paramount importance to obtain biodistribution data from clinical studies and defining biodistribution and excretion of injected material is essential for the safe progression to clinical studies.

SURVIVAL AND FUNCTIONAL EFFECT IN CELL DELIVERY

In cell therapy, there is no significant difference between delivery methods in experimental studies. Today, the delivery of skeletal myoblasts in clinical trials has been done by multiple DI via epicardial approach under direct vision, whereas in BMSC transplantation various methods including multiple DI via epicardial approach, ordinary coronary transluminal angioplasty catheter, and endoventricular injection using the NOGA myostar injection catheter have been used. Not surprisingly, clinical delivery procedures have a tendency to become less invasive. It should be mentioned, however, that whatever the method for cell delivery is, the obstacle is still the lack of sufficient functional efficacy. The settlement of injected cells seems to be easier than that of vectors in cardiac gene delivery because injected cells, which are biologically bigger than viruses, may have the ability to permeate through endothelial barriers. Therefore, the survival rate could be mainly involved with the low functional efficacy. Theoretically, the survival of grafted cells can be influenced by physical factors and biological ones. The former may include cell loss during injection due to technical errors and cell death due to high-pressure injection. In addition, washing out by coronary flow and contractile force within the injected area may affect the survival of grafted cells. On the other hand, biological factors may be composed of inflammatory reaction, environmental hypoxia, and apoptosis. Among studies that have investigated the survival of grafted cells, some discrepancies have existed regarding the major factors for cell survival. Several quantitative studies after cell therapy, of which most used neonatal cardiomyocytes, have been reported. Zhang et al. reported that the survival rate was reduced by 53% in granulation tissue and by 86% in normal myocardium at day 1, and eventually 90% of cells lost over the first week with half the cell death occurring over the first 24 h *(76)*. This is similar to another study by Murry et al. reporting that 32% of the survival rate 1 d after the transplantation rapidly decreased to 1 to 10% at 7 d *(77)*. In addition, this study showed that dead graft cells electron-microscopically had several findings of irreversible ischemic injury and apoptosis and that there was an increase in the fraction of dying cells with increasing cell number. These results indicate that ischemia may play a major role in cell death despite the fact that acute host inflammation remains as another possibility. In contrast to these studies, some studies demonstrated that viability of engrafted cells in infarcted myocardium has been demonstrated for up to 6 to 7 mo after transplantation of fetal and neonatal cardiomyocytes with the survival rate of 60% in infarcted rat heart models. These studies appear to support the hypothesis that physical factors mainly affect the fate of grafted cells and can explain why grafted cells in the infarct model showed better survival rate (60% 6 mo after transplantation) than that in the noninfarcted model. Moreover, in skeletal myoblast implantation, the increase in the number of injected cells was correlated with the improvement of cardiac function.

CONCLUSION AND FUTURE PROSPECTS

The clinical cardiovascular cell and gene therapy experience is very limited. The available data, however, emphasize the importance of randomized placebo-controlled trials in assessing the efficacy of novel treatments. Larger trials of this type are in progress and the results of these are eagerly awaited. Meanwhile, the large volume of preclinical data is likely to continue to expand with increases in knowledge of the molecular basis of cardiovascular disease. Importantly, the accumulation of this data provides the scientific basis for which to pursue the human evaluation of novel gene-based therapies. With regard to gene transfer technology, recent serious adverse reactions in young human subjects have been attributed to the vector employed. As a result, efforts to improve vector biosafety have been appropriately revitalized. With these efforts, vectors will hopefully undergo modifications to further improve biosafety, in addition to gene transfer efficiency. Conventional treatment modalities have made significant advances over the last decade in the areas of pharmacotherapy, vascular intervention, surgery, and implantable devices. The modest success of gene therapy in cardiovascular disease, thus far has been in filling a therapeutic need lacking effective therapy. Future success will depend on either exceeding conventional therapies or finding effective gene-based therapies for additional niches.

ACKNOWLEDGMENTS

This work was supported in part by grants from the NIH (HL069842 to Dr. del Monte, HL-057623 and HL 071763 to Dr. Hajjar). Dr. Hajjar is a Paul Beeson Scholar of the American Federation of Aging Research.

REFERENCES

1. Nishikawa M, Huang L. Nonviral vectors in the new millennium: delivery barriers in gene transfer. Hum Gene Ther 2001;12:861–870.
2. Kay MA, Glorioso JC, Naldini L. Viral vectors for gene therapy: the art of turning infectious agents into vehicles of therapeutics. Nat Med 2001;7:33–40.
3. Felgner PL. Nonviral strategies for gene therapy. Sci Am 1997;276:102–106.
4. Isner JM. Myocardial gene therapy. Nature 2002;415:234–239.
5. Wahlfors J, Morgan RA. Semliki Forest virus vectors for gene transfer. Methods Mol Med 2003;76:493–502.
6. Guzman RJ, Hirschowitz EA, Brody SL, et al. In vivo suppression of injury-induced vascular smooth muscle cell accumulation using adenovirus-mediated transfer of the herpes simplex virus thymidine kinase gene. Proc Natl Acad Sci USA 1994;91:10,732–10,736.
7. Barr E, Carroll J, Kalynych AM, et al. Efficient catheter-mediated gene transfer into the heart using replication-defective adenovirus. Gene Ther 1994;1:51–58.
8. Communal C, Huq F, Lebeche D, et al. Decreased efficiency of adenovirus-mediated gene transfer in aging cardiomyocytes. Circulation 2003;107:1170–1175.
9. Hajjar RJ, Schmidt U, Matsui T, et al. Modulation of ventricular function through gene transfer in vivo. Proc Natl Acad Sci USA 1998;95:5251–5256.
10. Shohet RV, Chen S, Zhou YT, et al. Echocardiographic destruction of albumin microbubbles directs gene delivery to the myocardium. Circulation 2000;101:2554–2556.
11. Beeri R, Guerrero JL, Supple G, et al. New efficient catheter-based system for myocardial gene delivery. Circulation 2002;106:1756–1759.
12. Donahue JK, Kikkawa K, Johns DC, et al. Ultrarapid, highly efficient viral gene transfer to the heart. Proc Natl Acad Sci USA 1997;94:4664–4668.
13. Lemarchand P, Jones M, Yamada I, Crystal RG. In vivo gene transfer and expression in normal uninjured blood vessels using replication-deficient recombinant adenovirus vectors. Circ Res 1993;72:1132–1138.
14. Monahan PE, Samulski RJ. AAV vectors: is clinical success on the horizon? Gene Ther 2000;7:24–30.
15. Xiao X, Li J, Samulski RJ. Production of high-titer recombinant adeno-associated virus vectors in the absence of helper adenovirus. J Virol 1998;72:2224–2232.
16. Hildinger M, Auricchio A, Gao G, et al. Hybrid vectors based on adeno-associated virus serotypes 2 and 5 for muscle-directed gene transfer. J Virol 2001;75:6199–6203.
17. Chao H, Mao L, Bruce AT, Walsh CE. Sustained expression of human factor VIII in mice using a parvovirus-based vector. Blood 2000;95:1594–1599.
18. Rutledge EA, Halbert CL, Russell DW. Infectious clones and vectors derived from adeno-associated virus (AAV) serotypes other than AAV type 2. J Virol 1998;72:309–319.
19. Hoshijima M, Ikeda Y, Iwanaga Y, et al. Chronic suppression of heart-failure progression by a pseudophosphorylated mutant of phospholamban via in vivo cardiac rAAV gene delivery. Nat Med 2002;8:864–871.
20. Richter M, Iwata A, Nyhuis J, et al. Adeno-associated virus vector transduction of vascular smooth muscle cells in vivo. Physiol Genomics 2000;2:117–127.
21. Cavazzana-Calvo M, Hacein-Bey S, de Saint Basile G, et al. Gene therapy of human severe combined immuno-deficiency (SCID)-X1 disease [see comment]. Science 2000;288:669–672.

22. Nabel EG, Barry J, Rocco MB, et al. Effects of dosing intervals on the development of tolerance to high dose transdermal nitroglycerin [see comment]. Am J Cardiol 1989;63:663–669.

23. Hacein-Bey-Abina S, de Saint Basile G, Cavazzana-Calvo M. Gene therapy of X-linked severe combined immunodeficiency. Methods Mol Biol 2003;215:247–259.

24. Trono D. Lentiviral vectors: turning a deadly foe into a therapeutic agent. Gene Ther 2000;7:20–23.

25. Galimi F, Verma IM. Opportunities for the use of lentiviral vectors in human gene therapy. Curr Top Microbiol Immunol 2002;261:245–254.

26. Agha-Mohammadi S, Lotze MT. Regulatable systems: applications in gene therapy and replicating viruses. J Clin Invest 2000;105:1177–1183.

27. Agha-Mohammadi S, Lotze MT. Immunomodulation of cancer: potential use of selectively replicating agents. J Clin Invest 2000;105:1173–1176.

28. Rosenberg SA, Blaese RM, Brenner MK, et al. Human gene marker/therapy clinical protocols. Hum Gene Ther 2000; 11:919–979.

29. Feldman LJ, Pastore CJ, Aubailly N, et al. Improved efficiency of arterial gene transfer by use of poloxamer 407 as a vehicle for adenoviral vectors. Gene Ther 1997;4:189–198.

30. Feldman LJ, Steg G. Optimal techniques for arterial gene transfer. Cardiovasc Res 1997;35:391–404.

31. Donahue JK, Heldman AW, Fraser H, et al. Focal modification of electrical conduction in the heart by viral gene transfer. Nat Med 2000;6:1395–1398.

32. Koransky ML, Robbins RC, Blau HM. VEGF gene delivery for treatment of ischemic cardiovascular disease. Trends Cardiovasc Med 2002;12:108–114.

33. Edelberg JM, Huang DT, Josephson ME, Rosenberg RD. Molecular enhancement of porcine cardiac chronotropy. Heart (Brit Cardiac Soc) 2001;86:559–562.

34. Losordo DW, Kawamoto A. Biological revascularization and the interventional molecular cardiologist: bypass for the next generation [comment]. Circulation 2002;106:3002–3005.

35. Isner JM, Vale PR, Symes JF, Losordo DW. Assessment of risks associated with cardiovascular gene therapy in human subjects. Circ Res 2001;89:389–400.

36. Boekstegers P, von Degenfeld G, Giehrl W, et al. Myocardial gene transfer by selective pressure-regulated retroinfusion of coronary veins. Gene Ther 2000;7:232–240.

37. Kupatt C, Wichels R, Deiss M, et al. Retroinfusion of NFkappaB decoy oligonucleotide extends cardioprotection achieved by CD18 inhibition in a preclinical study of myocardial ischemia and retroinfusion in pigs. Gene Ther 2002; 9:518–526.

38. Guzman RJ, Lemarchand P, Crystal RG, et al. Efficient gene transfer into myocardium by direct injection of adenovirus vectors. Circ Res 1993;73:1202–1207.

39. Fromes Y, Salmon A, Wang X, et al. Gene delivery to the myocardium by intrapericardial injection. Gene Ther 1999; 6:683–688.

40. Christensen G, Minamisawa S, Gruber PJ, et al. High-efficiency, long-term cardiac expression of foreign genes in living mouse embryos and neonates. Circulation 2000;101:178–184.

41. Hajjar RJ, del Monte F, Matsui T, Rosenzweig A. Prospects for gene therapy for heart failure. Circ Res 2000;86: 616–621.

42. Hajjar RJ. The promise of gene therapy as a therapeutic modality in heart failure. Journal Medical Libanais—Lebanese Med J 2000;48:86–88.

43. del Monte F, Williams E, Lebeche D, et al. Improvement in survival and cardiac metabolism after gene transfer of sarcoplasmic reticulum Ca(2+)-ATPase in a rat model of heart failure. Circulation 2001;104:1424–1429.

44. Bristow MR. Why does the myocardium fail? Insights from basic science. Lancet 1998;352 Suppl 1:SI8–S14.

45. Shah AS, White DC, Emani S, et al. In vivo ventricular gene delivery of a beta-adrenergic receptor kinase inhibitor to the failing heart reverses cardiac dysfunction. Circulation 2001;103:1311–1316.

46. Port JD, Bristow MR. Altered beta-adrenergic receptor gene regulation and signaling in chronic heart failure. J Mol Cell Cardiol 2001;33:887–905.

47. del Monte F, Harding SE, Schmidt U, et al. Restoration of contractile function in isolated cardiomyocytes from failing human hearts by gene transfer of SERCA2a. Circulation 1999;100:2308–2311.

48. del Monte F, Harding SE, Dec GW, et al. Targeting phospholamban by gene transfer in human heart failure. Circulation 2002;105:904–907.

49. Morishita R, Aoki M, Nakamura S, et al. Potential role of a novel vascular modulator, hepatocyte growth factor (HGF), in cardiovascular disease: characterization and regulation of local HGF system. J Atheroscl Thromb 1997; 4:12–19.

50. Hirota H, Chen J, Betz UA, et al. Loss of a gp130 cardiac muscle cell survival pathway is a critical event in the onset of heart failure during biomechanical stress. Cell 1999;97:189–198.

51. Hirota J, Furuichi T, Mikoshiba K. Inositol 1,4,5-trisphosphate receptor type 1 is a substrate for caspase-3 and is cleaved during apoptosis in a caspase-3-dependent manner. J Biol Chem 1999;274:34,433–34,437.

52. Mangi AA, Noiseux N, Kong D, et al. Mesenchymal stem cells modified with Akt prevent remodeling and restore performance of infarcted hearts [see comment]. Nat Med 2003;9:1195–1201.

53. Nabel EG. Stem cells combined with gene transfer for therapeutic vasculogenesis: magic bullets? [comment]. Circulation 2002;105:672–674.

54. Lee LY, Patel SR, Hackett NR, et al. Focal angiogen therapy using intramyocardial delivery of an adenovirus vector coding for vascular endothelial growth factor 121. Ann Thorac Surg 2000;69:14–23; discussion 23–24.

55. Harvey BG, Maroni J, O'Donoghue KA, et al. Safety of local delivery of low- and intermediate-dose adenovirus gene transfer vectors to individuals with a spectrum of morbid conditions. Hum Gene Ther 2002;13:15–63.
56. Ailawadi M, Lee JM, Lee S, et al. Adenovirus vector-mediated transfer of the vascular endothelial growth factor cDNA to healing abdominal fascia enhances vascularity and bursting strength in mice with normal and impaired wound healing. Surgery 2002;131:219–227.
57. Leotta E, Patejunas G, Murphy G, et al. Gene therapy with adenovirus-mediated myocardial transfer of vascular endothelial growth factor 121 improves cardiac performance in a pacing model of congestive heart failure. J Thorac Cardiovasc Surg 2002;123:1101–1113.
58. Isner JM. Vascular endothelial growth factor: gene therapy and therapeutic angiogenesis. Am J Cardiol 1998;82: 63S–64S.
59. Baumgartner I, Isner JM. Stimulation of peripheral angiogenesis by vascular endothelial growth factor (VEGF). Vasa 1998;27:201–206.
60. Makinen K, Manninen H, Hedman M, et al. Increased vascularity detected by digital subtraction angiography after VEGF gene transfer to human lower limb artery: a randomized, placebo-controlled, double-blinded phase II study. Mol Ther: J Am Soc Gene Ther 2002;6:127–133.
61. Manninen HI, Makinen K. Gene therapy techniques for peripheral arterial disease. Cardiovasc Intervent Radiol 2002; 25:98–108.
62. Marban E. Cardiac channelopathies. Nature 2002;415:213–218.
63. Ennis IL, Li RA, Murphy AM, et al. Dual gene therapy with SERCA1 and Kir2.1 abbreviates excitation without suppressing contractility. J Clin Invest 2002;109:393–400.
64. Mazhari R, Nuss HB, Armoundas AA, et al. Ectopic expression of KCNE3 accelerates cardiac repolarization and abbreviates the QT interval. J Clin Invest 2002;109:1083–1090.
65. Marban E, Nuss HB, Donahue JK. Gene therapy for cardiac arrhythmias. Cold Spring Harbor Sympos Quant Biol 2002;67:527–531.
66. Miake J, Marban E, Nuss HB. Biological pacemaker created by gene transfer. Nature 2002;419:132–133.
67. Beltrami AP, Urbanck K, Kajstura J, et al. Evidence that human cardiac myocytes divide after myocardial infarction. N Engl J Med 2001;344:1750–1757.
68. Murry CE, Kay MA, Bartosek T, et al. Muscle differentiation during repair of myocardial necrosis in rats via gene transfer with MyoD. J Clin Invest 1996;98:2209–2217.
69. Koh GY, Soonpaa MH, Klug MG, et al. Stable fetal cardiomyocyte grafts in the hearts of dystrophic mice and dogs. J Clin Invest 1995;96:2034–2042.
70. Reinecke H, Zhang M, Bartosek T, et al. Survival, integration, and differentiation of cardiomyocyte grafts: a study in normal and injured rat hearts. Circulation 1999;100:193–202.
71. Reinecke H., MacDonald GH, Hauschka SD, et al. Electromechanical coupling between skeletal and cardiac muscle. Implications for infarct repair. J Cell Biol 2000;149:731–740.
72. Leobon B, Garcin I, Menasche P, et al. Myoblasts transplanted into rat infarcted myocardium are functionally isolated from their host. Proc Natl Acad Sci USA 2003;100:7808–7811.
73. Menasche P, Hagege AA, Scorsin M, et al. Myoblast transplantation for heart failure. Lancet 2001;357:279-280.
74. Klug MG, Soonpaa MH, Koh GY, et al. Genetically selected cardiomyocytes from differentiating embronic stem cells form stable intracardiac grafts. J Clin Invest 1996;98:216–224.
75. Jackson KA, Majka SM, Wang H, et al. Regeneration of ischemic cardiac muscle and vascular endothelium by adult stem cells. J Clin Invest 2001;107:1395–1402.
76. Zhang M, Methot D, Poppa V, et al. Cardiomyocyte grafting for cardiac repair: graft cell death and anti-death strategies. J Mol Cell Cardiol 2001;33:907–921.
77. Murry CE, Whitney ML, Reinecke H, Muscle cell grafting for the treatment and prevention of heart failure. J Card Fail 2002;8(6 Suppl):S532–S541.

RECOMMENDED READING

Hacein-Bey-Abina S, de Saint Basile G, Cavazzana-Calvo M. Gene therapy of X-linked severe combined immunodeficiency. Methods Mol Biol 2003;215:247–259.
Hajjar RJ, del Monte F, Matsui T, Rosenzweig A. Prospects for gene therapy for heart failure. Circ Res 2000;86:616–621.
Isner JM. Myocardial gene therapy. Nature 2002;415:234–239.
Kay MA, Glorioso JC, Naldini L. Viral vectors for gene therapy: the art of turning infectious agents into vehicles of therapeutics. Nat Med 2001;7:33–40.
Marban E. Cardiac channelopathies. Nature 2002;415:213–218.

43 Preventive Cardiology

Michael Miller, MD

INTRODUCTION

Since the inaugural edition of this book, an increased awareness in preventing and treating heart disease has been spawned by revisions of cholesterol, hypertension and diabetes guidelines. As national guidelines have recently dictated, there is a trend in the direction of "the lower the better" for each of these risk factors. However, the past several years have also witnessed the emergence of diagnostic biomarkers of atherothrombosis that include C-reactive protein and noninvasive surrogates of atherosclerosis, such as carotid intima-media thickness and coronary calcification. In contrast, therapies that were previously deemed to have an important role in offsetting coronary heart disease (CHD) risk (e.g., antioxidant vitamins and hormone replacement therapy) have been shown to exert no beneficial impact. As our understanding of cardiovascular preventive measures continues to evolve, the goal of this chapter is to focus on the most important advances in this relatively new field with an emphasizes on clinical endpoint data influencing both initial and secondary cardiovascular events.

IDENTIFICATION OF HIGH CHD RISK

In 2001, the National Cholesterol Education Program (NCEP) published a strategy for identifying high-risk subjects defined as coronary risk equivalence based on preexisting vascular disease, diabetes mellitus or a high Framingham risk score *(1)*. While the Framingham risk score is useful in this regard, there are at least two groups at high risk who are not currently classified as a risk equivalent. These include impaired renal function (e.g., glomerular flow rate (GFR) <60 mL/min) and metabolic syndrome. To this end, the National Kidney Foundation has endorsed a target low-density lipoprotein (LDL) goal of less than 100 mg/dL in renal insufficient patients, irrespective of other CHD risk factors (http://www.kidney.org/professionals/doqi/kdoqi/toc.htm). Moreover, recent data evaluating metabolic syndrome (Table 1) have also identified significant increased all-cause mortality attributable to the presence of this syndrome (Fig. 1) *(2)*. A second shortcoming relates to the omission of other factors not considered in calculating Framingham risk (e.g., family history of premature CHD). Despite these concerns, nearly 75% of CHD can still be explained by traditional risk factors included in the Framingham risk score *(3)*. As such, the focus of intensive therapies should continue to be aimed at reducing LDL cholesterol (LDL-C), blood pressure, and elevated glucose.

LDL-C: HOW LOW SHOULD WE GO?

Barring monogenic abnormalities that result in inborn errors of lipoprotein metabolism, total cholesterol (TC) and LDL-C approx 70 and 30 mg/dL, respectively, at birth. These levels nearly double between 6 and 12 mo of age *(4)*, providing the foundation for "physiologic" TC and LDL-C anticipated in humans throughout life. In fact, it has been well established that CHD risk begins to accentuate as TC levels exceed 150 mg/dL and that societies at the lowest risk of CHD also maintain

From: *Essential Cardiology: Principles and Practice, 2nd Ed.*
Edited by: C. Rosendorff © Humana Press Inc., Totowa, NJ

Table 1
Criteria Defining Metabolic Syndrome
(Presence of Three or More)

1. Increased waist circumference (Men >40 in., women >35 in.
2. Elevated triglycerides (≥150 mg/dL)
3. Low HDL-C (<40 in men, <50 mg/dL in women)
4. Elevated blood pressure (≥130/85 mmHg)
5. Elevated blood glucose (≥110 mg/dL)

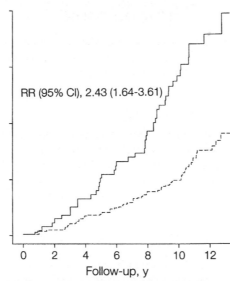

RR (95% CI), 2.43 (1.64-3.61)

Follow-up, y

Fig. 1. Unadjusted Kaplan-Meier hazard curves. Bottom of legend: RR, relative risk; CI, confidence interval. Curves for men with vs without the metabolic syndrome based on factor analysis (men in the highest quarter of the distribution of the metabolic syndrome factor were considered to have the metabolic syndrome). Median follow-up (range) for survivors was 11.6 (9.1–13.7) yr. Relative risks were determined by age-adjusted Cox proportional hazards regression analysis. (From ref. 2. Copyright 2002 American Medical Association.)

physiologic lipid levels (non-HDL <100 mg/dL). Early clinical trials focused on proving the cholesterol hypothesis, that is, whether lowering TC and LDL-C reduces CHD event rates. During the past several years, however, the aim has been to refine how low LDL-C can safely and effectively be reduced. To that end, recent data suggest that even the present designated acceptable target goal for LDL-C in CHD or CHD risk equivalents (e.g., 100 mg/dL or less) may still be too high. Two trials that have tested this hypothesis are the REVERSAL (Reversal of Atherosclerosis with Aggressive Lipid Lowering) and PROVE-IT (Pravastatin or Atorvastatin Evaluation and Infection Therapy Thrombolysis) trials *(5,6)*. In both studies, LDL-C was reduced to either the NCEP target (~100 mg/dL) or lower (60–80 mg/dL). REVERSAL demonstrated halting of atheromatous progression in the intensively treated (80 mg/d atorvastatin) compared to the conventionally treated group (40 mg/d pravastatin) as assessed by intravascular ultrasound (IVUS). The PROVE-IT study found a 16% reduction in CHD death or major endpoint ($p = 0.005$) between the groups ($n = 4162$) (Fig. 2). Two larger clinical endpoint trials whose anticipated release is 2005, TNT (Treat to New Targets) and SEARCH (Study of the Effectiveness of Additional Reductions in Cholesterol and Homocysteine) are expected to seal the fate as to whether further LDL-C cutpoints are warranted. These data coupled with the demonstration that hypertensive subjects (without necessarily CHD risk equivalence) benefit from LDL lowering below 100 mg/dL as suggested in ASCOT (Anglo-Scandinavian Cardiac Outcomes Trial), suggest that cutpoints may be lowered at various designated risks *(7)*. For example, Table 2 shows present target LDL-C and non-HDL cutpoints of the present NCEP guidelines and potential anticipated changes for the next revision pending results of ongoing trials.

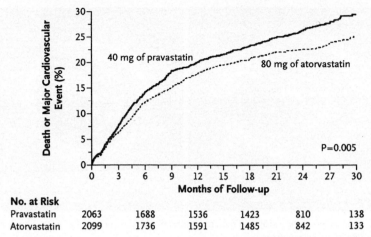

Fig. 2. Kaplan–Meier estimates of the incidence of the primary endpoint of death from any cause or a major cardiovascular event. (From ref. *6*. Copyright 2004 Massachusetts Medical Society.)

Table 2
Present NCEP Guidelines and Proposed Revisions

	Present guidelines		Proposed revisions	
Risk category	*LDL goal (mg/dL)*	*non-HDL*	*LDL goal (mg/dL)*	*non-HDL*
CHD and CHD risk equivalents[a]	<100	<130	<70[b]	<100
Multiple CHD risk factors (2+)	<130	<160	<100[c]	<130
0–1 risk factor	<160	<190	<130	<160

[a]May include renal insufficiency (50% or greater reduction in GFR) and metabolic syndrome in future revisions.
[b]Based on REVERSAL and PROVE-IT data. Pending results of TNT and SEARCH.
[c]Based on ASCOT.

HDL-C: AN EMERGING THERAPEUTIC TARGET

Although it is well recognized that HDL-C is inversely correlated with CHD and that risk is augmented even in the setting of a "normal" LDL-C, NCEP has assigned HDL-C as a tertiary therapeutic target owing to the relative paucity of data demonstrating an independent effect of HDL raising on reducing CHD event rates. That may change however, in view of recent data and development of newer HDL-raising drugs. In HATS (HDL Atherosclerosis Intervention Trial) ($n = 160$), the combination of niacin (2–4 g/d) and simvastatin (10–20 mg/d), which increased HDL by 30% and decreased LDL by 35%, blunted progression of arteriographic disease and reduced CHD events by more than 70% (*8*). More recently, five weekly intravenous injections of an ApoA-I mimetic, resulted in 4% reduction in atheroma volume as assessed by IVUS (Fig. 3), supporting proof of concept that HDL is a primary mediator of reverse cholesterol transport and that reversal of coronary atherosclerosis may reflect efficiency of this process (*9*). Thus, if ongoing clinical trials demonstrate that the rise in HDL-C (that results, for example, from cholesterol ester transport protein [CETP] inhibition), translates into reduced CHD event rates, it is likely that NCEP will reassess HDL raising as an additional primary or secondary therapeutic target.

NONLIPID CHD BIOMARKERS

Though nonlipid biomarkers represent potentially important contributors to enhanced CHD event rates, there are currently limited data demonstrating that reduction of these parameters confers additional benefits beyond that achieved through hygienic and pharmacotherapies aimed at

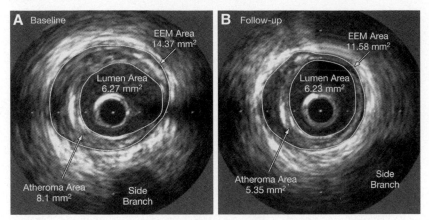

Fig. 3. Example of atheroma regression in a patient who received high-dose ETC-216. (From ref. *9.* Copyright 2003 American Medical Association.)

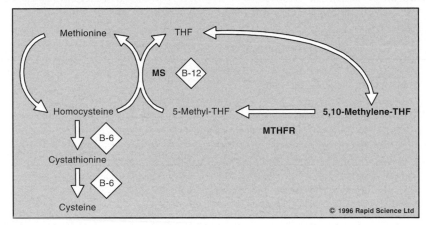

Fig. 4. Simplified scheme of homocysteine metabolism, focusing on remethylation. MS, methionine synthase; MTHFR, methylenetetrahydrofolate reductase; THF, tetrahydrofolate. (From ref. *63.* Copyright 1998 Lippincott Williams & Wilkins.)

improving lipids, blood pressure, and glycemic control. The most extensively studied of these atherogenic markers are homocysteine and C-reactive protein. Personality factors such as mental stress and depression have also been evaluated in CHD risk assessment and deserve mention.

Homocysteine

The metabolism of homocysteine begins with its precursor, the essential amino acid methionine. Methionine is converted to homocysteine following intermediary metabolism to S-adenosylmethionine and S-adenosylhomocysteine. Cystathione β-synthase initiates a series of reactions that converts homocysteine to cysteine; Vitamin B_6 serves as cofactor for these reactions. Alternatively, homocysteine may be remethylated via transfer of a methyl group from 5-methyltetrahydrofolate, a reaction catalyzed by methionine synthase (MS) with vitamin B_{12} as cofactor or by transfer of a methyl group by betaine (Fig. 4). An excess of homocysteine may result from abnormalities in the genes encoding cystathione β-synthase or 5,10 methyltetrahydrofolate reductase (MTHFR). Cystathione β-synthase deficiency is an autosomal recessive disorder characterized by connective tissue abnormalities, including skeletal and ocular deformaties that may be the consequence of homocysteine induced alterations in matrix protein (e.g. collagen, fibrillin) crosslinking; it bears clinical resemblance to Marfan's syndrome. However, in contrast to Marfan's, there is neither joint laxity, aortic root enlargement, nor mitral valve prolapse. Pulmonary emboli represents a common

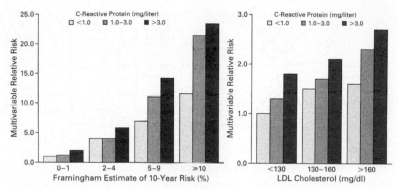

Fig. 5. Multivariable-adjusted relative risks of cardiovascular disease according to levels of C-reactive protein and the estimated 10-yr risk based on the Framingham risk score as currently defined by the National Cholesterol Education Program and according to levels of C-reactive protein and categories of LDL cholesterol. To convert values for LDL cholesterol to mmol/L, multiply by 0.02586. (From ref. *14*. Copyright 2002 Massachusetts Medical Society.)

cause of death and may occur in up to 50% of untreated cases by age 30. Despite genotypic heterogeneity between North American and European populations, a common polymorphism in the MTHFR gene (677C → T) has been associated with a 16% increased likelihood of CHD *(10)*.

Acquired causes of elevated homocysteine include systemic diseases such as renal failure (reduced catabolism of homocysteine), psoriasis, acute lymphoblastic leukemia (increased cell turnover), and hypothyroidism. Transplant recipients also have elevated levels owing to cyclosporine inhibition of folate-induced remethylation. Pharmaceuticals that have an impact on homocysteine include those that interfere with folate-induced remethylation (e.g., methotrexate, anticonvulsants) or folate absorption (bile-acid sequestrants) as well as substances that block methionine synthase (nitric oxide) or increase SAM (niacin). As homocysteine levels exceed 10 μmol/L, the risk of CHD events increases. Homocysteine is believed to be directly injurious to the endothelium by facilitating LDL modification *(11)*. However, while observational studies have suggested that intake of folate and vitamins B_6 and B_{12} reduce stroke incidence *(12)*, at least one recent randomized study failed to show clinical benefit in stroke survivors *(13)*.

C-Reactive Protein

C-reactive protein (CRP) predicts CHD independent of LDL-C and has gained increased recognition in CHD risk assessment. Using high-sensitivity assays, three categories of risk have been defined: low (<1 mg/L), intermediate (1–3 mg/dL), and high (>3 mg/L) the latter of which raises the 10-yr Framingham Risk to the CHD equivalent range *(14)* (Fig. 5).

However, a recent AHA position statement did not endorse widespread screening, in part because of the lack of evidence demonstrating the independent benefit of CRP lowering on CHD event rate reduction *(15)*. CRP is hepatically synthesized in response to the upregulation of peripheral cytokines, including interleukin-6 (IL-6) elaborated by adipocytes. As such, elevated CRP is tightly correlated with body mass index, obesity *(16)*, and other measures of metabolic syndrome. Therapies that reduce CRP levels include weight-reducing measures (e.g., diet and exercise), and medications including lipid-lowering drugs (statins, niacin), aspirin (325 mg/d), and thiazolidene diones (TZDs). The extent to which reducing elevated CRP in otherwise normolipidemic impacts on initial CHD events is the subject of a clinical trial (e.g., JUPITER); positive outcome may elevate the utility of CRP screening for intermediate risk patients in the future.

Mental Stress

A paradigm of how acute mental stress may lead to CAD events is shown in Fig. 6. A paradoxical vasoconstrictor response following intracoronary acetylcholine was observed in patients asked to

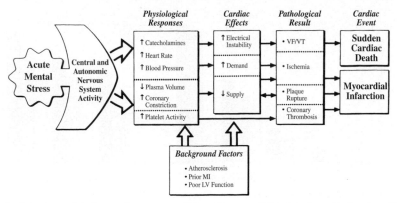

Fig. 6. Pathophysiologic model of mental stress as a trigger of myocardial ischemia and infarction. (From ref. *64.*)

perform mental arithmetic *(17)*. Other studies have extended these findings by demonstrating wall motion abnormalities, transient reduction in ventricular function, and silent ischemia in response to mental stress *(18)*. Most recently, these findings have been extended to include a reduced likelihood of silent ischemia during high positive emotional periods (e.g., happiness) compared with negative emotions such as tension, frustration, and sadness.

Depression

As many as 20% of myocardial infarction (MI) survivors experience major depression and the risk of mortality quadruples within the first year following a CHD event *(19)*. A recent meta-analysis suggests that depression may be a predictor of initial CHD events, even after adjusting for other covariates *(20)*. An overactive hypothalamic-pituitary-adrenocortical axis in depressed subjects leads to enhanced cortisol production and mediation of proatherothrombotic activity (e.g., platelet activation and systemic inflammation) *(21,22)* coupled with reduced heart rate variability, which are believed to contribute to accelerated CHD event rates *(23)*. Tricyclic antidepressants are often contraindicated in CHD patients owing to potential deleterious CV effects including tachyarrhythmias, prolongation of the QT interval and orthostatic hypotension. In contrast, selective serotonin reuptake inhibitors (SSRIs) have few if any untoward cardiovascular side effects and are the drugs of choice *(24)*.

DIAGNOSTIC STRATEGIES

Of the numerous emerging noninvasive diagnostic tools under evaluation, carotid intima-media thickening and coronary calcification have been the most investigated to date.

Carotid Intima-Media Thickness

Measurement of common carotid artery (CCA) intima-media thickness (IMT) remains the most validated noninvasive surrogate for detection of early atherosclerosis because of its high reproducibility and low variability. CCA IMT is highly correlated with existing CHD and predictive of future CHD events in subjects without symptomatic disease *(25)*. The mean CCA IMT in 55-yr-old men and women are 0.70 and 0.64 mm, respectively, with an average annual cross-sectional change approximating 0.008 mm/yr *(26)*. However, high-risk groups such as FH may have up to a fivefold greater rate of CCA IMT progression compared to the lower-risk subjects. Statin therapy may reduce or reverse CCA IMT progression and it appears that the lower LDL (or non-HDL) achieved, the greater the effect, mirroring similar observations using IVUS *(27)*.

Coronary Artery Calcification

Another noninvasive method employed for detection of subclinical CHD is scanning for coronary artery calcification (Fig. 7). While the majority of published studies to date have evaluated

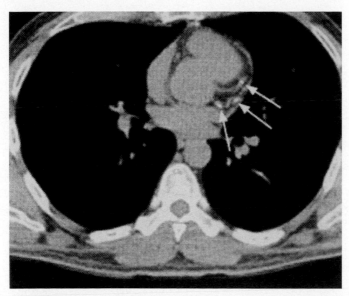

Fig. 7. Electron-beam computed tomographic image obtained in a 49-yr-old man. The patient's total calcium score is 70. Three areas of calcification (arrows) are visible in the regions of the coronary arteries—one in the left anterior descending artery and two in the left circumflex artery. (From ref. *65.*)

electron-beam CT, helical or multislice CT scanners are more readily available in hospitals and are being more widely used. Although the degree of calcification correlates with anatomic abnormalities as assessed by coronary arteriography, highly calcified vessels are often stable and are not predictive as the culprit lesion in acute coronary syndromes (ACS) or MI. Nevertheless, high calcium scores (age and gender adjusted calcium exceeding the 75th percentile) are associated with a greater presence of noncalcified, highly thrombogenic lipid-rich lesions at high risk of rupture/ erosion, which result in a fourfold or greater increased likelihood of MI. Because of significant retest variability in calcium scores, a standardized measuring system was recently developed by the International Consortium for Standardization in Coronary Artery Calcium. This new standard uses 100 mg/cc as the threshold for a positive scan and is applicable across the spectrum of devices used to measure coronary calcium. While calcium scanning is presently not recommended as a screening tool for diagnosing CHD based on the 2000 ACC/AHA Consensus Statement, recent data suggest that this test may be most useful in modifying CHD risk prediction with Framingham risk scores in the intermediate range (10–20%) but not at lower risk ranges. Nonetheless, the highest scores (>300) were associated with the greatest likelihood of CHD events across all strata of Framingham risk (Fig. 8) *(28).* The ongoing Multi-Ethnic Study of Atherosclerosis (MESA) will evaluate the utility of coronary calcium scanning in 6000 men and women to determine the association of baseline risk factors with the progression of coronary calcium, and association of progression of coronary calcium with clinical CVD events. It will be equally important to assess the impact of intensive secondary preventive therapies on calcium progression rates and confirm whether intensive lipid lowering regresses calcified lesions in hyperlipidemic subjects as previously suggested *(29).*

HYGIENIC THERAPIES: THE OBESITY EPIDEMIC

Poor diet and inactivity are now responsible for 400,000 deaths in the US, accounting for 1 in 6 deaths and second only to tobacco as the leading preventable cause of mortality (Table 3) *(30).* In fact, since 1990, death rates resulting from obesity have climbed 33% compared to the approx 9% increase related to smoking. Based on current trends, poor hygienic measures will overtake tobacco as the top cause of preventable death by 2010. Likely explanations include fast-food life-

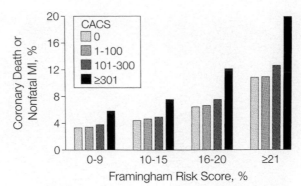

Fig. 8. Predicted 7-year event rates from COX regression model for CHD death or nonfatal MI for categories of Framingham risk score or coronary artery calcium score (CACS). (From ref. *28*. Copyright 2004 American Medical Association.)

Table 3
Trends in Percentage of Total Preventable Deaths
in the US Between 1990 and 2000

	1990	*2000*
Tobacco use	19%	18.1%
Poor diet/physical inactivity	14%	16.6%
Alcohol consumption	5%	3.5%
Microbial agents	4%	3.1%
Toxic agents	3%	2.3%
Car accidents	1%	1.8%
Gun-related deaths	2%	1.2%
AIDS	1%	0.8%
Drug use	<1%	0.7%

Data from ref. *30*.

styles, increases in food portion sizes, decline in school physical education programs, and sedentary activities including more weekly hours spent on computers and television. Obesity, defined as body mass index (BMI) >30 kg/m^2, is epidemic in the US with nearly half of the states reporting an obesity prevalence of at least 20% (Fig. 9) *(31)*. Moreover, with aging, intrinsic basal metabolic rate (BMR) defined as energy expenditure at rest falls at an approximate rate of 5 Kcal/d per year. Not surprisingly, weight gain in adults has averaged approx 10 lb during the past decade. Thus, even before discussing specific dietary measures, reduction in total caloric intake and or increased energy expenditure should be a top priority in CHD risk reduction strategies.

NUTRITIONAL ASPECTS OF PREVENTIVE CARDIOLOGY

Important Lessons From Our Paleolithic Ancestors

Barring monogenic abnormalities (e.g., FH), a diet low in saturated and *trans* fats translates into a low risk of CHD, as exemplified by today's industrialized societies. A comparison of the dietary composition of the foods consumed by the descendants of modern preliterate societies (e.g., our paleolithic ancestors) with present Westernized countries is outlined in Table 4.

The reduced percentage of fat consumed in Stone Age societies reflects a predominantly low intake of saturated fat and, of course, no *trans* fats. Wild game, the primary source of fat in Stone Age societies, has been found to contain considerably less carcass fat (4%) compared with domesticated livestock (30%). Equally important was the absence of dairy products from the diet of our paleolithic ancestors; the processing of milk products was developed during the agricultural revo-

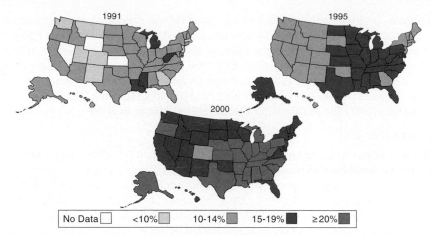

Fig. 9. Prevalence of obesity between 1991 and 2000 among adults in the United States. (From ref. *66*. Copyright 2000 American Medical Association.)

Table 4
Comparison Between Late Paleolithic and Contemporary American Diets

Energy (%)	Late paleolithic diet	Contemporary american diet
Carbohydrate	46	46
Fat	21	42
Protein	33	12
P:S ratio	1.4:1	0.44
Cholesterol (mg)	520	300–500
Fiber (g)	100–150	<20
Sodium (mg)	<700	2300–6900

Modified from ref. *60, 61.*

lution within the past 5000 yr. Harvesting of tobacco also occurred during this period. Thus, not only was the relative intake of fat reduced in these preagrarian societies, but the percentage of saturated fat consumption was also low, as reflected in the polyunsaturated to saturated fat (P:S) ratio. It is noteworthy that fiber intake was considerably higher and sodium intake lower compared with modern-day societies. Taken together, the earlier dietary habits support the notion that atherothrombosis was an uncommon occurrence.

Impact of Dietary Fat in Cardiovascular Disease Prevention

SATURATED FAT

It has been well established that diets high in saturated fat (>40% of caloric intake) are associated with an increased tendency to atherothrombosis. Nearly 35 yr ago, Connor demonstrated the impact of saturated fatty acids on coagulation and thrombosis *(32)*. Saturated fatty acids may also inhibit LDL-C receptor activity, thereby raising LDL-C *(33)*. In general, for each 1% rise in saturated fat there is a 2.7 mg/dL increase in total cholesterol. Of the major saturated fats, only stearate is believed to have a neutral effect on cholesterol levels.

TRANS FATTY ACIDS

Trans fatty acids are present in animal and dairy fats and in polyunsaturated vegetable oils that are (partially) hydrogenated to increase product stability and shelf-life. Substitution of *trans* fatty acids for *cis* fatty acids (e.g., oleic acid) raises LDL, TG, and Lp(a) and reduces HDL *(34)*. *Trans* fats represent ~20% of total dietary fat; common sources include shortening used in baked products (e.g., doughnuts, cookies), packaged foods (e.g., potato chips, crackers), and margarines. Recent data have now demonstrated that the link between *trans* fatty acids and abnormal lipids and lipoproteins extends to enhanced CHD event rates, as shown in the Framingham Heart Study *(35)*, Alpha-Tocopherol Beta-Carotene study (ATBC) *(36)*, and the Nurses Health Study (NHS) *(37)*. NHS was the most comprehensive of the *trans* fat studies; it observed that each 2% increase in *trans* fatty acid intake was associated with a near-doubling of CHD rates. The FDA has mandated that food manufacturers list the amount of *trans* fats beginning in 2006.

Monounsaturated Fat

The Mediterranean diet gained prominence following publication of the Seven Countries Study, which disclosed a significantly lower incidence of CAD in southern European countries (e.g., Italy, Spain) compared with North America. The primary fatty acid, oleate, reduces VLDL-C and LDL-C and may reduce macrophage uptake of LDL-C by inhibiting oxidation. In addition to olive oil, the Mediterranean diet also includes a high concentration of fruits and vegetables (an excellent source of antioxidant vitamins and flavonoids), supplemented with fish, poultry, and occasionally red meat. Alcoholic beverages (particularly red wine) and nuts are consumed in the Mediterranean diet. Milk products, when consumed, are often in the form of grated cheese added to pasta. Eggs (up to 4) are also consumed weekly. In addition to its palatability, the Mediterranean diet has been the only diet to demonstrate CHD reduction. In the Lyon Diet Heart Study, subjects randomized to this diet experienced a 73% reduction in CAD deaths and nonfatal MI and a 70% reduction in overall mortality during the initial 27-mo period *(38)* with benefits extending to 4 yr (Fig. 10). It has also been suggested that diabetic patients benefit from a Mediterranean rather than a high-carbohydrate, low-fat diet. As carbohydrate intake exceeds 65% of total caloric intake, VLDL-C production is increased, thereby raising plasma TG level. Even 55% carbohydrate diets have been associated with elevated TG, reduced HDL levels, and potential deterioration of glycemic control *(39)*. In addition to olive oil, other important sources of monounsaturated fats are avocados and nuts *(40)*. Avocados are rich in vitamins E and C, while nuts provide a rich source of antioxidants, including the phytonutrient ellagic acid (walnuts, pecans), Vitamin E (almonds, peanuts), and omega-3 fatty acids (walnuts).

Diets Rich in Omega-3 Fatty Acids

Omega-3 fatty acids are long-chain polyunsaturated fats that contain the first double bond at the third position adjacent to the methyl terminal of the molecule. As a precursor of arachidonic acid, they may be incorporated through the cyclooxygenase or leukotriene pathway (Fig. 11), providing both antiplatelet and antiinflammatory effects. The clinical impact of these fatty acids was demonstrated in Greenland Eskimos whose diet of predominantly fatty fish was enriched with omega-3s (e.g., whale, salmon, herring, and mackerel). Dyerberg and Bang *(40a)* found that these individuals had a increased bleeding time and a low incidence of CAD and astutely attributed these effects to a high content of omega-3 fatty acids such as eicosapentanoic acid (EPA) (C20:5-3) and dicosahexanoic acid (C22:4-3). In addition, significant TG lowering (20–50%) was also observed owing to reduced hepatic VLDL-C secretion. Both observational (e.g., Diet and Reinfarction Trial) *(41)* and randomized clinical trials (e.g., GISSI) *(42)* of patients with CHD, omega-3 fatty acid supplements significantly reduced CV events (death, nonfatal heart attacks, nonfatal strokes). Omega-3 fatty acids are believed to reduce sudden cardiac death by inhibiting L-type calcium channels and voltage-dependent sodium currents *(43)*. In view of the cardioprotective effects of fish, the AHA/ACC has endorsed consumption of 1 g of omega-3-containing fish daily either in the form of fish-oil capsules or consumption of oily fish *(44)*. Table 5 lists the content of omega-3 among fish consumed in the US. Generally, for each 1 g of EPA/DHA, there is also a 10% reduction in TG; often 2 to 4 g are needed in hyperTG patients. High doses should be used particularly cautiously in CHD patients receiving aspirin (>162 mg/d) and/or clopidogrel. Fish-oil capsules should be refrigerated or frozen after opening to minimize oxidation and fishy odor eructation. Capsules recently tested by *Consumer Reports* are free of mercury and other contaminants.

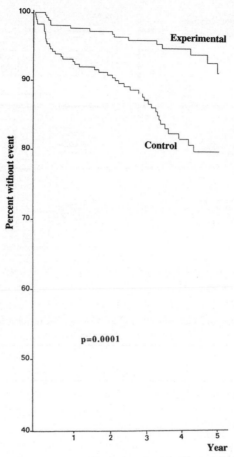

Fig. 10. Survival curves between the experimental and control groups in the Lyon Diet Heart Study. (From ref. *67*.)

WEIGHT-LOSS DIETS: LOW-CARB VS LOW-FAT

Weight loss is most sustainable if performed on a gradual basis. Small changes in diet and exercise patterns will enhance the likelihood of achieving the recommended reductions approximating 1 lb/wk. Table 6 provides examples of modest hygienic measures that enable a net negative balance of 500 kcal/d in an average 70-kg adult. A primary concern with various weight-loss programs is the induction phase, where water loss accounts for the precipitous weight drop. For example, in low-carbohydrate, high-protein diets, weight loss is rapid because for each gram of glycogen depleted, 2 to 4 g of intracellular water are mobilized, resulting in rapid weight (e.g., water) loss. If carbohydrate restriction is severe (less than 60 g), ketosis ensues, leading to nausea, reduced appetite, and hyperuricemia as ketones compete with uric acid for renal tubular excretion *(45)*. Diets low in total and saturated fat were popularized by Pritikin; he reduced his dietary fat intake following an MI and reportedly had minimal evidence of coronary disease on postmortem examination. The Lifestyle Heart Trial also evaluated the efficacy of a very-low-fat diet (10% of caloric intake) in concert with lifestyle changes (aerobic exercise, stress management training, smoking cessation, and group support) on arteriographic progression in patients with preexisting CAD. The dietary component of the treated (experimental) group consisted primarily of fruits, vegetables, grains, legumes, and soybean products. Red meat, poultry, and fish consumption was not permitted. After 1 yr, the experimental group evidenced reduced progression and slight regression of lesions *(46)*. At the 5-yr follow-up, total fat intake represented 8.5% of calories, LDL-C was reduced 20%,

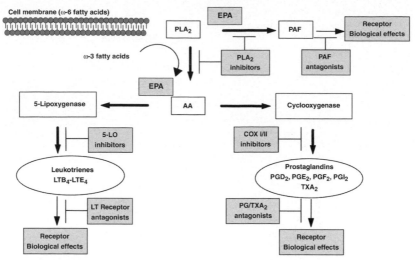

Fig. 11. Eicosanoid and platelet-activating factor. (From ref. *68*.)

Table 5
Total Fat and Content of Highest Omega-3-Containing Fish
(Grams per 3.6-oz Serving)

Fish	Total fat	Omega-3 content per 100 g
Sardines, in sardine oil	15.5	3.3
Atlantic mackerel	13.9	2.5
Pacific herring	13.9	1.7
Atlantic herring	9.0	1.6
Lake trout	9.7	1.6
Anchovy	4.8	1.4
Chinook salmon	10.4	1.4
Sablefish	15.3	1.4
Bluefish	6.5	1.2
Sockeye salmon	8.6	1.2
Atlantic salmon	5.4	1.2
Pink salmon	8.6	1.2

Modified from ref. *62*.

and reduced coronary arteriographic progression compared to the control group became more apparent. Nevertheless, there were still 25 cardiac events among the 28 experimental patients during the 5-yr follow-up period *(47)*. As the TG level in the experimental group was elevated (mean TG = 258 mg/dL), these results suggest that intensive lifestyle measures may not be sufficient in optimizing CAD event reduction. Other low-fat nonpharmacologic trials, including the St. Thomas Arteriographic Regression Study (STARS) (27% fat), and the Heidelberg Exercise/Diet Study (<20% fat), also resulted in reduced arteriographic progression of CAD in patients assigned to the intervention group. While evidence supports reduction of total fat intake to less than 40% of total caloric burden, it remains unclear whether very-low-fat diets (<10% fat) as consumed in the Lifestyle Heart Diet offer any advantages to more palatable diets offered by the Mediterraneans (25–35% fat), the paleolithic diet (21% fat; *see* above), or an American Heart Association diet supplemented with lipid-lowering therapy. The combination of intensive diet, exercise, and lipid-lowering agents may yield the most favorable responses on TC, LDL, and TG (Fig. 12) but the relative impact on CAD event rates has been established only for a Mediterranean approach.

Table 6
5 Ways to Offset 500 Kcal Daily in a 70-kg Adult

Eliminate	+	Add
1 4 oz bagel (250 cal)		45 min walk at 4 mph (250 cal)
2 1 candy bar (250 cal)		55 min yoga (250 cal)
3 16 oz soda (200 cal)		50 min low-impact aerobics (300 cal)
4 2 oz whole wheat pretzels (200 cal)		35 min jogging (300 cal)
5 2 slices of bread (150 cal)		40 min stationary bicycling (moderate) (350 cal)

Sources: USDA National Nutrient Database (http://www.nal.usda.gov/fnic/foodcomp/index.html) and DiscoverFitness. Com (http://www.discoverfitness.com/MET_value_table_.html).

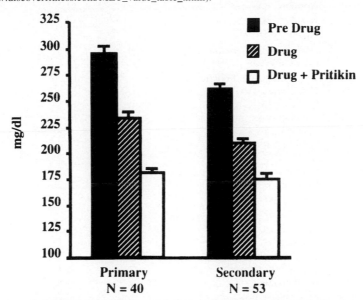

Fig. 12. Total serum cholesterol values before and after cholesterol-lowering drug therapy and then with the addition of the Pritikin diet and exercise program for both primary and secondary prevention groups. All three values were significantly different ($p < 0.01$) for both groups. (From ref. *69.* Copyright 1997 Excerpta Medica, Inc.)

CARDIOPROTECTIVE NUTRIENTS

In recent years, polyphenols found in a variety of foods have been linked to cardioprotective health. This broad group of antioxidant compounds includes flavonoids, which are plant-derived pigments responsible for bright colored chemical components present in fruits and vegetables. Epidemiologic studies have evaluated the clinical significance of two flavonoid subclasses, flav-an-3-ols (e.g., catechins) and flavanols (e.g., quercetin, myricetin), the former of which represent powerful antioxidants with greater potency than vitamins A, C, and E. In the Zutphen elderly prospective study of 800 seniors (65–84 yr old), the highest intake of catechins was inversely associated with CHD death after adjustment for other covariates (RR = 0.48; 95% CI: 0.28, 0.82), so that for each 50-mg intake there was a corresponding 25% reduction in CHD events *(48).* Rich sources of catechins are listed in Table 7; quercetin and myricetin are also potent antioxidants. In a prospective study of 10,000 Finnish men and women, a 20% reduced incidence of type 2 diabetes mellitus coincided with higher quercetin and myricetin intake; quercetin was also found to be inversely related to CHD mortality *(49).* Most recently, a major fraction of the total flavonoid content was analyzed in more than 40 different foods *(50).* In the US, the mean daily intake of these antioxidants approximated 60 mg/d with the majority obtained from three primary sources, apples (32%), chocolate (18%), and grapes (18%). Examples of the flavonoid content in selected nuts is shown in Fig. 13.

Table 7
Selected Foods With High Flavonoid Content
From the 2003 USDA Database (mg/100 g or /100 mL)

High catechin-containing foods	
Tea, green, brewed	133
Tea, black, brewed	114
Chocolate bar, dark	53
Blackberries	19
Chocolate bar, milk	13
Red table wine	12
Cherries, raw	12
Apricots, raw	11
Raspberries	9
Apples, with skin	9
High quercetin-containing foods	
Cocoa powder	20
Onions, cooked, boiled	19
Cranberries, raw	14
Onions, raw	13
Lingonberries, raw	12
Spinach, raw	4.9
Apples, with skin	4.4
Barley	3.8
Celery	3.5
Broccoli, raw	3.2
Blueberries	3.1
High myricetin-containing foods	
Cranberries, raw	4.3
Rutabagas	2.13
Black currant juice	1.9
Tea, green, brewed	1.1
Blueberries	0.82
Red table wine	0.7
Grape juice	0.6
Grapes, black, green, or white	0.45
Tea, black, brewed	0.45

In the Nurses Study of 86,000 women aged 34 to 59, frequent intake of nuts (1 oz or greater at least 5 times weekly) was associated with a 35% reduction in fatal CAD events and nonfatal MI compared with women who did not (or rarely) consume nuts *(51)*. Overall, the most concentrated source of antioxidant units were found in cinnamon, and two recent studies suggest that polyphenolic polymers potentiate insulin action, which in turn may improve glycemic control in diabetic patients *(52, 53)*. Taken together, identification of potential cardioprotective nutrients provides an excellent opportunity to further explore the critical yet underemphasized role of diet in the prevention of CHD.

Impact of Exercise in Cardiovascular Disease Prevention

Individuals with a high aerobic capacity have a lower incidence of CAD compared with sedentary subjects. While it has been widely touted that the most well-conditioned athletes present with the lowest case-fatality rates of MI *(54)*, moderate levels of physical activity have also been associated with favorably reduced rates. These activities must persist throughout life; a high school athlete who foregoes exercise in later life is not protected from the subsequent development of CAD *(55)*. Exercise is beneficial throughout all age groups. In fact, regular exercise in the elderly (walking or cycling for 20 min three times weekly) resulted in a 30% reduction in CHD and total mortality. In addition, moderate physical activity may also reduce stroke rates. In the Harvard Alumni Health Study, an approx 50% reduction in stroke was observed in men (mean age = 58 yr)

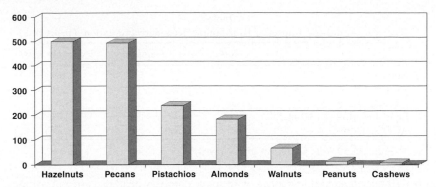

Fig. 13. Flavonoid content in selected nuts (mg/100 mg proanthocyanidins). (Adapted from ref. *50.*)

who expended 2000 to 3000 kcal of energy weekly. This can easily be achieved with one hour of brisk walking (3–4 mph) daily. We also recommend wearing a pedometer with a minimum of 10,000 steps taken daily. Finally, light weight lifting exerts an additional 20 to 25% reduction in CHD event rates and is independent of other cardioprotective measures *(56).*

ABCs of CHD Prevention

In addition to quitting smoking, physical activity, and weight management, other important considerations in maximizing secondary preventive efforts are antiplatelet agents, angiotensin-converting enzyme (ACE) inhibitors, β-blockers, and cholesterol-lowering therapies (covered in more depth in previous chapters).

ANTIPLATELET AGENTS

Aspirin reduces the risk of CHD by 20 to 25% in high-risk patients and remains the first-line antiplatelet drug because of its relative safety, low cost, and cost-effectiveness. However, the FDA recently denied Bayer's petition for routine aspirin use in primary prevention because of the lack of data demonstrating reduction in CHD mortality or ischemic stroke. Previous studies have indicated that the platelet ADP inhibitor clopidogrel reduces CHD events by 10% compared with aspirin in acute coronary syndromes or non-ST segment elevation MI *(57).* Moreover, in patients undergoing percutaneous coronary intervention (PCI), the combination of clopidogrel and aspirin was shown to be more effective in reducing MI or CHD death than aspirin alone (OR 0.23, 95% CI 0.11–0.49, $p = 0.0001$). In the Clopidogrel in Unstable Angina to Prevent Recurrent Ischemic Events (CURE) trial ($n = 12,000$), the combination of aspirin and clopidogrel treated for 9 mo (in subjects not having PCI) resulted in a 20% reduction in the primary endpoint (MI, CVA, CHD death). While risk of bleeding was generally higher, the most favorable combination included use of low-dose (75 mg/d) aspirin. In the smaller subgroup of PCI subjects ($n = 2100$), pretreatment with clopidogrel resulted in a 30% reduction in the primary endpoint. Continuation of clopidogrel for up to 1 yr following PCI continued to show benefit, as indicated by a 27% reduction in MI and stroke. Ongoing studies will determine whether longer-term combination treatment (e.g., 1–3 yr) remains cardioprotective. In addition to use for ACS and as pre- and post-PCI therapy, 75 mg/d clopidogrel is a suitable replacement for aspirin in allergic or sensitive patients and in those who have experienced atherothrombotic events on aspirin.

ACE INHIBITORS

Randomized controlled trials in MI survivors have revealed significant reductions in recurrent cardiovascular events and mortality (20–25%) with ACE inhibitor use. The HOPE study extended the benefit of ACE inhibition using ramipril in high-risk subjects (CHD and diabetics) even without markedly compromised EF (>40%). Most recently, the EUROPA (Reduction Cardiac Events with Perindopril in Stable Coronary Artery) study showed that ACE inhibition resulted in 20%

Table 8
Potential Cumulative Impact of Four Simple Secondary Prevention Treatments

	Relative-risk reduction	*2-yr event rate*
None	...	8%
Aspirin	25%	6%
β-blockers	25%	4.5%
Lipid lowering (50-60 mg/dL)	30%	3%
ACE inhibitors	25%	2.3%

From ref. *59*. With permission from Elsevier.

reduction in CHD death and MI in patients with stable coronary heart disease and without CHF. In this population, ACE inhibition is cost-effective, as 4 yr of therapy is expected to prevent one event for every 50 treated patients *(58)*.

β-Blockers

β-Blockers are very effective agents for reducing recurrent MI events (15–25%), sudden cardiac death (30–35%), and overall mortality (20%). Hemodynamically stable post-MI patients with compromised ventricular function (<40%) also benefit from β-blocker use.

Potential Cumulative Effect of Secondary Preventive Measures

The impact of established strategies on offsetting CHD events is shown in Table 8.

Among high-risk patients, defined as an annual CHD event rate of 4%, employing all these strategies along with smoking cessation would reduce the risk by an estimated 80% and thereby reduce event rates to a level observed in low-risk subjects. Overall and with few exceptions, CHD remains largely avertable in the US and even among genetically susceptible individuals, effective strategies are now available to prevent initial and recurrent CHD events *(59)*.

REFERENCES

1. Expert Panel on Detection, Evaluation, and Treatment of High Blood Cholesterol in Adults. Executive summary of the Third Report of The National Cholesterol Education Program (NCEP) Expert Panel on Detection, Evaluation, and Treatment of High Blood Cholesterol in Adults (Adult Treatment Panel III). JAMA 2001;285:2486–2497.
2. Lakka HM, Laaksonen DE, Lakka TA, et al. The metabolic syndrome and total and cardiovascular disease mortality in middle-aged men. JAMA 2002;288:2709–2716.
3. Greenland P, Knoll MD, Stamler J, et al. Major risk factors as antecedents of fatal and nonfatal coronary heart disease events. JAMA 2003;290:891–897.
4. Kwiterovich PO Jr. Biochemical, clinical, epidemiologic, genetic, and pathologic data in the pediatric age group relevant to the cholesterol hypothesis. Pediatrics 1986;78:349–362.
5. Nissen SE, Tuzcu EM, Schoenhagen P, et al. Effect of intensive compared with moderate lipid-lowering therapy on progression of coronary atherosclerosis: a randomized controlled trial. JAMA 2004;291:1071–1080.
6. Cannon CP, Braunwald E, McCabe CH, et al. Comparison of intensive and moderate lipid lowering with statins after acute coronary syndromes. N Engl J Med 2004;350;1495–1504.
7. Sever PS, Dahlof B, Poulter NR, et al. Prevention of coronary and stroke events with atorvastatin in hypertensive patients who have average or lower-than-average cholesterol concentrations, in the Anglo-Scandinavian Cardiac Outcomes Trial—Lipid Lowering Arm (ASCOT-LLA): a multicentre randomized controlled trial. Lancet 2003;361: 1149–1158.
8. Brown BG, Zhao XQ, Chait A, et al. Simvastatin and niacin, antioxidant vitamins, or the combination for the prevention of coronary disease. N Engl J Med 2001;345:1583–1592.
9. Nissen SE, Tsunoda T, Tuzcu EM, et al. Effect of recombinant ApoA-I Milano on coronary atherosclerosis in patients with acute coronary syndromes: a randomized controlled trial. JAMA 2003;290:2292–2300.
10. Klerk M, Verhoef P, Clarke R, et al. MTHFR Studies Collaboration Group. MTHFR 677C→T polymorphism and risk of coronary heart disease: a meta-analysis. JAMA 2002;288:2023–2031.
11. Wang H, Jiang X, Yang F, et al. Hyperhomocysteinemia accelerates atherosclerosis in cystathionine beta-synthase and apolipoprotein E double knock-out mice with and without dietary perturbation. Blood 2003;101:3901–3907.
12. He K, Merchant A, Rimm EB, et al. Folate, vitamin B6, and B12 intakes in relation to risk of stroke among men. Stroke 2004;35:169–174.
13. Toole JF, Malinow MR, Chambless LE, et al. Lowering homocysteine in patients with ischemic stroke to prevent recurrent stroke, myocardial infarction, and death: the Vitamin Intervention for Stroke Prevention (VISP) randomized controlled trial. JAMA 2004;291:565–575.

14. Ridker PM, Rifai N, Rose L, et al. Comparison of C-reactive protein and low-density lipoprotein cholesterol levels in the prediction of first cardiovascular events. N Engl J Med 2002;347:1557–1565.
15. Pearson TA, Mensah GA, Alexander RW, et al. Centers for Disease Control and Prevention; American Heart Association. Markers of inflammation and cardiovascular disease: application to clinical and public health practice: a statement for healthcare professionals from the Centers for Disease Control and Prevention and the American Heart Association. Circulation 2003;107:499–511.
16. Ford ES. Body mass index, diabetes, and C-reactive protein among US adults. Diabetes Care 1999;22:1971–1977.
17. Yeung AC, Vekshtein VI, Krantz DS, et al. The effect of atherosclerosis on the vasomotor responses of coronary arteries to mental stress. N Engl J Med 1991:325;1551–1556.
18. Jain D, Shaker SM, Burg M, et al. Effects of mental stress on left ventricular and peripheral vascular performance in patients with coronary artery disease. J Am Coll Cardiol 1998;31:1314–1322.
19. Carney RM, Freedland KE, Miller GE, Jaffe AS. Depression as a risk factor for cardiac mortality and morbidity: a review of potential mechanisms. J Psychosom Res 2002;53:897–902.
20. Rugulies R. Depression as a predictor for coronary heart disease. a review and meta-analysis. Am J Prev Med 2002; 23:51–61.
21. Musselman DL, Tomer A, Manatunga AK, et al. Exaggerated platelet reactivity in major depression. Am J Psychiatry 1996;153:1313–1317.
22. Dentino AN, Pieper CF, Rao MK, et al. Association of interleukin-6 and other biologic variables with depression in older people living in the community. J Am Geriatr Soc 1999;47:6–11.
23. Pratt LA, Ford DE, Crum RM, et al. Depression, psychotropic medication, and risk of myocardial infarction. Prospective data from the Baltimore ECA follow-up. Circulation 1996;94:3123–3129.
24. Zellweger MJ, Osterwalder RH, Langewitz W, Pfisterer ME. Coronary artery disease and depression. Eur Heart J 2004;25:3–9.
25. O'Leary DH, Polak JF, Kronmal RA, et al. Carotid-artery intima and media thickness as a risk factor for myocardial infarction and stroke in older adults. Cardiovascular Health Study Collaborative Research Group. N Engl J Med 1999;340:14–22.
26. Howard G, Sharrett AR, Heiss G, et al. Carotid artery intimal-medial thickness distribution in general populations as evaluated by B-mode ultrasound. ARIC Investigators. Stroke 1993;24:1297–1304.
27. Kastelein JJ, Wiegman A, de Groot E. Surrogate markers of atherosclerosis: impact of statins. Atheroscler Suppl 2003; 4:31–36.
28. Greenland P, LaBree L, Azen SP, et al. Coronary artery calcium score combined with Framingham score for risk prediction in asymptomatic individuals. JAMA 2004;291:210–215.
29. Callister TQ, Raggi P, Cooil B, et al. Effect of HMG-CoA reductase inhibitors on coronary artery disease as assessed by electron-beam computed tomography. N Engl J Med 1998;339:1972–1978.
30. Mokdad AH, Marks JS, Stroup DF, Gerberding JL. Actual causes of death in the United States, 2000. JAMA 2004; 291:1238–1245.
31. Mokdad AH, Serdula MK, Dietz WH, et al. The spread of the obesity epidemic in the United States, 1991–1998. JAMA 1999;282:1519–1522.
32. Connor WE, Hoak JC, Warner ED. The effects of fatty acids on blood coagulation and thrombosis. Thromb Diath Haemorrh Suppl 1965;17:89–102.
33. Dietschy JM. Dietary fatty acids and the regulation of plasma low density lipoprotein cholesterol concentrations. J Nutr 1998;128:444S–448S.
34. Mensink RP, Katan MB. Effect of dietary *trans* fatty acids on high-density and low density lipoprotein cholesterol levels in healthy subjects. N Engl J Med 1990;323:439–445.
35. Gillman MW, Cupples LA, Gagnon D, et al. Margarine intake and subsequent coronary heart disease in men. Epidemiology 1997;8:144–149.
36. Pietinen P, Ascherio A, Korhonen P, et al. Intake of fatty acids and risk of coronary heart disease in a cohort of Finnish men. The Alpha-Tocopherol, Beta-Carotene Cancer Prevention Study. Am J Epidemiol 1997;145:876–887.
37. Willett WC, Stampfer MJ, Colditz GA. Intake of trans fatty acids and risk of coronary heart disease among women. Lancet 1993;341:581–585.
38. de Lorgeril M, Renaud S, Marmelle N, et al. Mediterranean alpha-linolenic acid-rich diet in secondary prevention of coronary heart disease. Lancet 1994;343:1454–1459.
39. Garg A, Bantle JP, Henry RR, et al. Effects of varying carbohydrate content of diet in patients with non-insulin-dependent diabetes mellitus. JAMA 1994;271:1421–1428.
40. Kris-Etherton PM, Yu-Poth S, Sabate J, et al. Nuts and their bioactive constituents: effects on serum lipids and other factors that affect disease risk. Am J Clin Nutr 1999;70(Suppl):504–511.
40a. Dyerberg J, Bang HO. Haemostatic function and platelet polyunsaturated fatty acids in Eskimos. 1979. Nutrition 1995;11:475.
41. Burr ML, Fehily AM, Gilbert JF, et al. Effects of changes in fat, fish and fibre intakes on death and myocardial reinfarction: diet and reinfarction trial (DART). Lancet 1989;334:757–761.
42. Anonymous. Dietary supplementation with n-3 polyunsaturated fatty acids and vitamin E after myocardial infarction: results of the GISSI-Prevenzione trial. Gruppo Italiano per lo Studio della Sopravvivenza nell'Infarto miocardico. Lancet 1999;354:447–455.
43. Leaf A. Diet and sudden cardiac death. J Nutr Health Aging 2001;5:173–178.

44. Kris-Etherton PM, Harris WS, Appel LJ. AHA Nutrition Committee. American Heart Association. Omega-3 fatty acids and cardiovascular disease: new recommendations from the American Heart Association. Arterioscler Thromb Vasc Biol 2003;23:151–152.

45. Denke M. Metabolic effects of high-protein, low-carbohydrate diets. Am J Cardiol 2001;88:59–61.

46. Ornish D, Brown SE, Scherwitz LW, et al. Can lifestyle changes reverse coronary heart disease ? The Lifestyle Heart Trial. Lancet 1990;336:129–133.

47. Ornish D, Scherwitz LW, Billings JH, et al. Intensive lifestyle changes for reversal of coronary heart disease. JAMA 1998;280:2001–2007.

48. Arts I, Hollman P, Feskens E, et al. The Zutphen Elderly Study. Am J Clin Nutr 2001;74:227–232.

49. Knekt P, Kumpulainen J, Järvinen R, et al. Flavonoid intake and risk of chronic diseases. Am J Clin Nut 2002;76: 560–568.

50. Gu L, Kelm MA, Hammerstone JF. Concentrations of proanthocyanidins in common foods and estimations of normal consumption. J Nutr 2004;134:613–617.

51. Hu FB, Willett WC. Optimal diets for prevention of coronary heart disease. JAMA 2002;288:2569–2578.

52. Khan A, Safdar M, Ali Khan MM, et al. Cinnamon improves glucose and lipids of people with type 2 diabetes. Diabetes Care 2003;26:3215–3218.

53. Anderson RA, Broadhurst CL, Polansky MM, et al. Isolation and characterization of polyphenol type-A polymers from cinnamon with insulin-like biological activity. J Agric Food Chem 2004;52:65–70.

54. Paffenbargar RS Jr, Hyde RT, Wing AL, et al. The association of changes in physical activity level and other lifestyle characteristics with mortality among men. N Engl J Med 1993;328:538–545.

55. Byers T. Body weight and mortality. N Engl J Med 1995;333:723–724.

56. Tanasescu M, Leitzmann MF, Rimm EB, et al. Exercise type and intensity in relation to coronary heart disease in men. JAMA 2002;288:1994–2000.

57. Wodlinger AM, Pieper JA. The role of clopidogrel in the management of acute coronary syndromes. Clin Ther 2003; 25:2155–2181.

58. Fuller JA. Combine EUROPA and HOPE. Lancet 2003;362:1937.

59. Yusuf S. Two decades of progress in preventing vascular disease. Lancet 2002;360:2–3.

60. Eaton SB, Konner M, Shostak M. Stone agers in the fast lane: chronic degenerative diseases in evolutionary perspective. Am J Med 1988;84:739–749. Review.

61. Eaton SB, Eaton SB 3rd, Konner MJ, Shostak M. An evolutionary perspective enhances understanding of human nutritional requirements. J Nutr 1996;126:1732–1740. Review. No abstract available.

62. Connor SL, Connor WE. Are fish oils beneficial in the prevention and treatment of coronary artery disease? Am J Clin Nutr 1997;66(Suppl):1020S–1031S.

63. Verhoef P, Stampfer MJ, Rimm EB. Folate and coronary heart disease. Curr Opin Lipidol 1998;9:17–22.

64. Krantz DS, Kop WJ, Santiago HT, Gottdiener JS. Mental stress as a trigger of myocardial ischemia and infarction. Cardiol Clin 1996;14:271–287.

65. Greenland P, Gaziano JM. Clinical practice. Selecting asymptomatic patients for coronary computed tomography or electrocardiographic exercise testing. N Engl J Med 2003;349:465–473.

66. Mokdad AH, Serdula MK, Dietz WH, Bowman BA, Marks JS, Koplan JP. The continuing epidemic of obesity in the United States. JAMA 2000;284:1650–1651.

67. de Lorgeril M, Salen P, Martin JL, Monjaud I, Delave J, Mamelle N. Mediterranean diet, traditional risk factors, and the rate of cardiovascular complications after myocardial infarction: final report of the Lyon Diet Heart Study. Circulation 1999;99:779–785.

68. Heller A, Koch T, Schmeck J, van Ackern K. Lipid mediators in inflammatory disorders. Drugs 1998;55:487–496.

69. Barnard RJ, DiLauro SC, Inkeles SB. Effects of intensive diet and exercise intervention in patients taking cholesterol-lowering drugs. Am J Cardiol 1997;79:1112–1114.

RECOMMENDED READING

Ascherio A, Hennekens CH, Buring JE, et al. *Trans* fatty acid intake and risk of myocardial infarction. Circulation 1994; 89:94–101.

Bijnen FCH, Caspersen CJ, Feskens EJM, et al. Physical activity and 10-year mortality from cardiovascular diseases and all causes. Arch Intern Med 1998;158:1499–1505.

Harris WS. Fish oils and plasma lipid and lipoprotein metabolism in humans: a critical review. J Lipid Res 1989;30: 785–807.

Katan MB, Grundy SM, Willett WC. Beyond low fat diets. N Engl J Med 1999;337:563–566.

Kris-Etherton PM, Krummel D, Russell ME, et al. National Cholesterol Education Program. The effect of diet on plasma lipids, lipoproteins, and coronary heart disease. J Am Diet Assoc 1988;88:1373–1400.

Mayer EM, Jacobsen DW, Robinson K. Homocysteine and coronary atherosclerosis. J Am Coll Cardiol 1996;27:517–527.

O'Rourke RA, Brundage BH, Froelicher VF, et al. American College of Cardiology/American Heart Association Expert Consensus Document on electron-beam computed tomography for the diagnosis and prognosis of coronary artery disease. J Am Coll Cardiol 2001;36:326–340.

Redberg RF, Vogel RA, Criqui MH, et al. 34th Bethesda Conference: Task force #3—What is the spectrum of current and emerging techniques for the noninvasive measurement of atherosclerosis? J Am Coll Cardiol 2003;41:1886–1898.

44

Peripheral Arterial Disease

James J. Jang, MD
and Jonathan L. Halperin, MD

INTRODUCTION

The most widely recognized peripheral vascular disease in adults *is obstructive atherosclerosis of the extremities or peripheral arterial disease (PAD)*. The traditional term "arteriosclerosis obliterans" distinguishes the development of obstructive lesions from normal aging by which the arteries increase in diameter, rigidity, and calcium content *(1)*. The disease was defined in 1958 by the World Health Organization as a "variable combination of changes of the intima or arteries (as distinguished from arterioles) consisting of the focal accumulation of lipids, complex carbohydrates, blood and blood products, fibrous tissue and calcium deposits, and associated with medial changes" *(2)*.

EPIDEMIOLOGY

By the time symptoms of obstructive arterial disease develop there is usually at least 50% narrowing of the vascular lumen. Based on a 26-yr longitudinal surveillance of the Framingham Heart Study cohort of 5209 subjects, the annual incidence of symptomatic ischemic arterial obstructive disease was 0.26% for men and 0.12% in women *(3)*. The incidence increased with age until age 75 yr, with about a twofold male predominance at all ages (Fig. 1). The peak incidence of symptomatic limb arterial obstructive disease occurred in males in the sixth and seventh decades of life. Fewer than 10% of nondiabetic cases younger than 60 yr were females. The incidence in women beyond menopause rose quickly toward that in men. Lower extremity vascular disease causes considerable morbidity among women, particularly in those following menopause. In a cross-sectional study involving 1601 healthy elderly women (mean age 71 yr, range 65–93 yr), the prevalence of lower extremity arterial disease assessed by ankle-brachial index (ABI) ranged from 2.9% in those aged 65 to 69 yr to 15.5% in those aged 80 yr or older *(4)*. Approximately 20% of those with disease had symptoms of claudication.

The prevalence of arterial obstructive disease exceeds that of symptomatic ischemia *(5)*. Since patients often present with atypical limb symptoms or without claudication, the frequency of PAD diagnosis is generally considerably lower than the prevalence of the disease. Based on the ABI, the prevalence of PAD in unselected populations 25 to 65 yr old was 0.7% for females and 1.3% for males. The prevalence of disease depends, however, on the threshold ABI selected *(6)*. The national cross-sectional survey of the PAD Awareness, Risk, and Treatment; New Resources for Survival (PARTNERS) program, in which PAD diagnosis was defined by ABI $\leq$0.9, found the disease was detected in 29% of patients who were either 50 to 69 yr old with risk factors of tobacco smoking or diabetes mellitus or $\geq$70 yr old regardless of risk factors *(7)*. More than 70% of the primary care physicians who participated were unaware that their patients had PAD before screening in the PARTNERS study *(7)*.

From: *Essential Cardiology: Principles and Practice, 2nd Ed.*
Edited by: C. Rosendorff © Humana Press Inc., Totowa, NJ

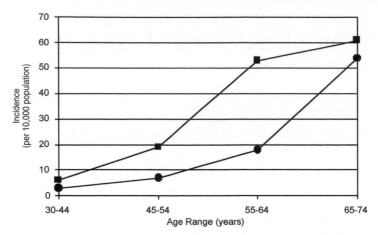

Fig. 1. Age-specific annual incidence: intermittent claudication. (Adapted from ref. *83*.)

The prevalence of asymptomatic atherosclerosis is highest in elderly patients, in whom gangrene is frequently the initial symptom because coexisting conditions limit ambulation *(8)*. In the Rotterdam Study of 7715 subjects aged ≥55 yr, the prevalence of PAD was 19.1% based on ABI <0.9 *(9)*. Symptoms of intermittent claudication were reported by only 6.3% *(9)*. In an elderly nursing home population, the prevalence of severe obstructive arterial disease (ABI <0.7) was approx 50%, and this predicted increased mortality compared to patients without signs of disease *(10)*. Among patients older than 90 yr, the second most common surgical operation is lower extremity amputation for limb arterial disease or gangrene.

RISK FACTORS

Like other manifestations of atherosclerosis, the prevalence of peripheral arterial disease is related to hyperlipidemia, diabetes mellitus, hypertension, and tobacco smoking, which modify the effects of age, gender, and heredity. It is difficult to separate data pertaining to atherosclerotic disease in the peripheral circulation from observations of coronary artery disease, but there is little reason to suspect substantial difference based on the anatomic site of involvement *(3)*. Specific risk factors appear additive and better predict relative risk than absolute risk. Overall, a risk profile made up of the major cardiovascular risk factors correlates better with intermittent claudication than with clinical manifestations of coronary heart disease.

Hyperlipidemia

The prevalence of hyperlipoproteinemia in patients with PAD ranges in various studies from 31 to 57%, while intermittent claudication is more than twice as common in patients with serum cholesterol levels higher than 260 mg/dL than in those without hyperlipidemia*(11)*. The Edinburgh Artery Study demonstrated that PAD was directly associated with elevated serum cholesterol levels and inversely related to high-density lipoprotein (HDL) levels *(12)*. In addition, the development of PAD is independently associated with elevations in lipid peroxides, such as oxidized low-density lipoproteins (LDL) and very-low-density lipoproteins (VLDL) *(13,14)*.

Diabetes Mellitus

Peripheral atherosclerosis develops more commonly in diabetic patients, with a predilection for the tibial and peroneal arteries between the knees and ankles, for which revascularization procedures are more difficult. While the incidence of femoropopliteal arterial obstructive disease is similar to that in the nondiabetic population, aortoiliac occlusive disease may actually occur less frequently in diabetics. The risk of developing PAD appears related to the duration of non-insulin-dependent diabetes mellitus *(15)*. Diabetes raises the risk of ischemic gangrene 20-fold and that of surgical amputation fourfold *(16)*. Coexisting sensory and autonomic neuropathy, lack of reflex hyperemia, loss of pain sensation, and arteriovenous shunting contribute to ischemic complications in diabetics.

Hypertension

The frequency and severity of atherosclerotic disease and its coronary and cerebral complications are increased in hypertensive patients. In the Framingham study cohort, hypertension increased the risk of PAD 2.5- to 4-fold in men and women, respectively *(3)*. Autopsy studies have demonstrated more extensive atherosclerosis of the aortoiliac arteries in hypertensive men than in age-matched normotensive controls. In women, this difference is more generalized along the course of the arterial tree. Limb arterial obstructive disease occurs twice as frequently as coronary artery disease among hypertensive individuals.

Tobacco Smoking

The Framingham Heart Study found a relationship between the number of cigarettes smoked and the incidence of intermittent claudication *(17)*. Multivariate analysis found that tobacco smoking was the strongest single risk factor for development of symptomatic obstructive arterial disease *(17)*. From the Framingham Offspring Study, for each 10-pack-yr increment of smoking, there was a 1.3-fold increased incidence of PAD *(18)*. The occurrence of intermittent claudication is twice as frequent in smokers as in nonsmokers. In males with symptomatic atherosclerotic disease of the limb vessels, the majority of patients report smoking cigarettes at the onset of the clinical phase of the disease. Smoking is clearly associated with an increase in amputations and bypass graft occlusions *(19,20)*. Seventy-three to 90% of patients with limb arterial disease are smokers, such that it is distinctly rare to encounter a young female with the disease who does not smoke cigarettes. Pathophysiologic mechanisms from tobacco smoking involve vasoconstriction, lipid metabolism, and thrombogenicity *(21)*.

Additional Risk Factors

Hereditary disorders associated with ischemic complications in the limbs include homocysteinuria, oxalosis, inhibitors of von Willebrand factor, and inherited states associated with increased thrombogenicity. The latter is more closely associated with venous than with arterial diseases.

HISTOPATHOLOGY

Histopathologically, peripheral arteriosclerosis obliterans is identical to atherosclerosis that affects the aorta and its branches, including the coronary, visceral, cervical, and cerebral arteries. The basic lesion is the atherosclerotic plaque that produces *localized stenosis* of the lumen with or without areas of complete *arterial occlusion*. Deposition of thrombus and subsequently progressive fibrosis occur in eccentric layers. Fragmentation of the internal elastic lamina typically occurs and areas of intraplaque hemorrhage and calcification characterize the advanced lesion.

Segmental lesions usually produce stenosis or occlusion of large and medium-sized arteries. After the thoracoabdominal aorta, the coronary arteries are most commonly affected by atherosclerosis, followed by the iliofemoral, carotid, renal, mesenteric, vertebrobasilar, tibial-peroneal, subclavian, brachial, radial, and ulnar arteries. Even in advanced cases, smaller arteries of the digits are generally spared, though these may become obstructed by thrombus when there is proximal atherosclerotic disease. Patients with intermittent claudication may have disease at multiple arterial levels. In symptomatic patients, approx 80% have *femoropopliteal* disease, approx 30% have lesions at the *aortoiliac* level, and up to 40% have *tibial-peroneal* obstruction. Involvement of the distal vessels is most frequent in diabetics and in the elderly.

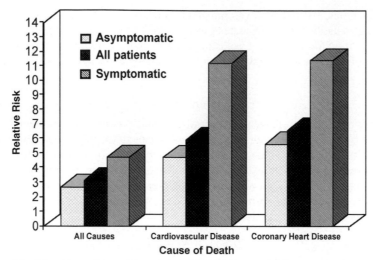

Fig. 2. Relative risk of death in patients with peripheral arterial disease (PAD) compared with patients without PAD: all-cause mortality, cardiovascular and coronary mortality are shown for asymptomatic, symptomatic, and all patients. (Adapted from ref. *24*.)

NATURAL HISTORY AND PROGNOSIS

The clinical courses of patients with PAD vary markedly, with abrupt vascular occlusion in some cases and chronic progression in others. In patients with aortoiliac disease, a copious collateral circulation tends to develop with a generally favorable prognosis in terms of limb outcome. Patients with distal tibial-peroneal disease have a distinctly poorer outcome, encountering amputation at annual rate of 1.4% *(22)*.

Followed without surgical intervention, yearly mortality averages over 5%, with death usually due to coronary or cerebral vascular disease. In the Framingham Heart Study, the relative mortality risk imposed by symptomatic PAD without cardiovascular comorbidity was 1.3 for men and 2.1 for women; total mortality ratios were 2.2 and 4.1, respectively. In patients with severely symptomatic PAD the rate of coronary heart disease (defined angiographically as >70% stenosis of at least one coronary vessel) was nearly 90%. About 50% of these patients had decreased left ventricular function *(23)*. Symptomatic PAD raises the risk of myocardial infarction, coronary, and cardiovascular death five- to sixfold (Fig. 2) *(24)*. In a 15-yr study of 2777 patients with claudication, over 66% of mortality was attributable to cardiovascular disease *(25)*. Angina and history of myocardial infarction were not predictive of increased mortality. Instead, reduced ABI at rest and following exercise, diabetes mellitus, and age were significant predictors *(25)*.

Remission of intermittent claudication is common. Among patients followed 4 or more yr from onset of symptoms in the Framingham study, 45% became asymptomatic *(26)*. In a Mayo Clinic study, 24% of nondiabetic patients with PAD affecting the superficial femoral artery had symptomatic improvement, while 69% experienced no progression of symptoms and clinical deterioration developed in only 7% *(27,28)*. According to the TransAtlantic Inter-Society Consensus (TASC) working group, only 5% of patients with intermittent claudication require surgical or endovascular intervention and approx 2% need major amputation over a 5-yr period *(29)*.

CLINICAL PRESENTATION

Intermittent Claudication

The cardinal symptom of obstructive arterial disease in the lower extremities is *intermittent claudication*. Typically, patients describe calf pain, since the gastrocnemius musculature has the greatest

Table 1
Differential Diagnosis of Exertional Calf Pain

Obstructive arterial disease
Neurogenic pseudoclaudication
Venous claudication
Muscular disorders

oxygen consumption of any muscle group in the leg during ambulation. Some patients report aching, heaviness, fatigue, or numbness when walking, but distress is usually relieved within a few minutes of rest. Ischemic claudication must be distinguished from other conditions producing exertional calf pain (Table 1). Among 460 patients with PAD evaluated in the Walking and Leg Circulation study, only 32.6% had intermittent claudication; the remainder had either no exertional leg symptoms, atypical leg pain, or rest pain *(30)*. Diabetic patients with distal tibial or peroneal arterial obstruction may describe ankle or foot pain while walking; this may be difficult to distinguish from ischemic neuropathy. With proximal aortoiliac disease, thigh, hip, or buttock claudication or low back pain may develop while walking, usually preceded by calf pain. Bilateral "high claudication" accompanying impotency and global atrophy of the lower extremities characterizes the *Leriche syndrome*, associated with aortoiliac disease.

Multiple factors contribute to leg discomfort during exercise in patients with PAD. Hemodynamically significant arterial stenosis may reduce pressure and flow minimally at rest while the pressure gradient across the stenosis increases during exercise. Extravascular compression by exercising muscle and lack of flow-mediated vasodilation in atherosclerotic vessels may further blunt limb blood flow. Discomfort may be related to activation of local chemoreceptors due to accumulation of lactate or other metabolites as a result of ischemia.

Initial and absolute claudication thresholds are best expressed in terms of pace and incline. Ambient environmental conditions such as temperature and wind, training, and recruitment of muscle groups in less ischemic zones all influence walking capacity and have therapeutic implications in maintaining overall cardiovascular conditioning.

Critical Limb Ischemia

When the minimal nutritional requirements of resting skin, muscle, nerves and bone are not met, *ischemic rest pain, ulceration*, and *gangrene* ensue, any of which translates to a poor prognosis. Clinically, limb ischemia at rest is manifested first in the cutaneous tissues of the foot, where factors regulating perfusion differ from those governing calf muscle circulation. Reflexive sympathetically mediated vasoconstrictor activity may reduce foot blood flow even under conditions of ischemia. With tissue necrosis there is typically severe pain that is worse at night with limb elevation and improves upon standing. With advanced neuropathy, ulceration and gangrene may occur painlessly. Other symptoms of ischemia at rest include hypesthesia, cold sensitivity, muscular weakness, joint stiffness, and contracture.

Severe ischemia of this kind usually demands angiographic examination and therapeutic intervention by percutaneous angioplasty or surgical revascularization. When these procedures are not feasible, gangrene commonly ensues and leads to amputation, though remission has been described even at this advanced stage of disease. Critical limb ischemia results in some 150,000 amputations annually in the United States, with perioperative mortality rates of 5 to 10% for below-knee and up to 50% for above-knee amputations.

Acute Arterial Occlusion

The major causes of acute arterial occlusion are trauma, arterial thrombosis, and arterial embolism. Traumatic occlusion is usually associated with external compression, transection, or laceration. Increasingly, the clinical spectrum of traumatic arterial occlusive disease includes iatrogenic

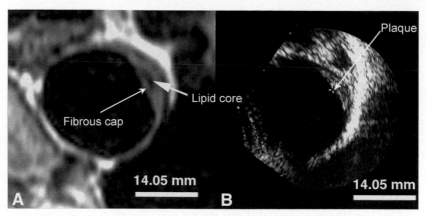

Fig. 3. Magnetic resonance, T2-weighted (**A**) and transesophageal echocardiographic (**B**) images of a 4.5-mm fibroatheromatous aortic plaque showing the eccentric lesion with fibrous cap and lipid-laden core. (From ref. *84.*)

cases, most commonly associated with indwelling intravascular diagnostic or therapeutic cannulation. Atraumatic acute arterial occlusion includes systemic embolism, usually cardiogenic, but occasionally derived from mural thrombi within aneurysms of the aorta, and thrombosis superimposed on chronic atherosclerosis or other intrinsic arterial disease. Systemic disorders of coagulation associated with arterial thrombosis include those associated with anticardiolipin antibodies, circulating lupus anticoagulants, and heparin-associated thrombocytopenia.

Arterial Embolism

Nearly 85% of systemic arterial emboli arise from thrombi in the chambers of the left side of the heart. Atrial fibrillation accounts for about half the cases and ventricular thrombi for most of the remainder. Infective (particularly fungal) endocarditis, cardiac tumors, invasive lesions of the pulmonary venous system, mural thrombi within aortic aneurysms, ulcerated proximal atherosclerotic lesions, vascular grafts, arteritis, and traumatic arterial lesions represent additional sources of embolism.

Microembolism of atherosclerotic debris consisting of lipid and thrombotic material may originate in the aorta or more distal arteries and lead to occlusion of small distal limb arteries. The source may involve either aneurysmal disease or irregular ulceration of diffusely atherosclerotic vessels that are not dilated. Transesophageal echocardiography and magnetic resonance imaging have identified such atherosclerotic lesions (Fig. 3) *(31).* The syndrome, designated *atheroembolism,* is often labeled "blue toe syndrome" when the feet are affected, and is characterized by unilateral or bilateral, painful, cyanotic toes in the presence of palpable pedal pulses (Fig. 4). The lateral and plantar aspects of the feet are frequently involved and manifest as livedo reticularis and petechiae on feet and legs. The violaceous parts generally blanch with pressure, and the surrounding skin may appear normally perfused. Calf pain and gastrocnemius muscle tenderness is often present as a result of embolic occlusion of small intramuscular vessels. Fever, eosinophilia, and acceleration of the erythrocyte sedimentation rate may signal an inflammatory reaction to atheroembolism, which may be difficult to distinguish from acute vasculitis.

Atheroembolism implies a physically unstable proximal atherosclerotic lesion that may be at risk for acute thrombotic arterial occlusion depending on the diameter of the arterial segment involved and other factors governing flow. Antithrombotic therapy should be given in the form of platelet inhibitor or anticoagulant medication. Although angioplasty and stent grafting are sometimes effective, intravascular catheterization may provoke embolism. The most definitive approach is removal or exclusion of the source from the circulation. When the lower limbs are ischemic, aortobifemoral bypass is often required; but an alternative approach is axillobifemoral extraanatomic

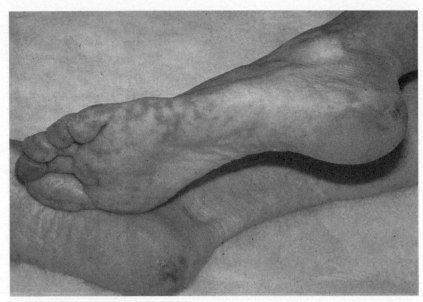

Fig. 4. Typical appearance of atheromatous embolism involving the feet. There is livedo reticularis along the lateral aspect of the foot and cyanosis of several toes. (From ref. *85.*)

bypass with ligation of the external iliac arteries proximal to the point of anastomosis. When renal embolism occurs, more proximal aortic reconstruction may be necessary. The risks of proximal aortic procedures are considerable, particularly when severe atherosclerosis involves the entire length of the aorta accompanied by a malignant syndrome of cerebral, mesenteric, and limb ischemia.

DIFFERENTIAL DIAGNOSIS

Exertional calf pain may be produced by both nonatherosclerotic arterial obstructive diseases and conditions unrelated to the arterial circulation (Table 1). Among the latter are *neurogenic pseudo-claudication* (a form of lumbosacral radiculopathy), in which ambulation provokes nerve root irritation with pain referred to the posterior aspect of the lower extremity. Characteristic symptoms include pain upon walking just a few steps without progression to ischemia at rest, relief on bending forward at the waist, and reproduction of symptoms by straight leg-raising.

Venous claudication illustrates the role of venous pressure as a factor in regional circulatory resistance. Exertional leg pain (especially near the medial aspect of the leg above the ankle) results from insufficiency of the musculovenous pumping mechanism that normally reduces distal venous pressure during ambulation. Venous hypertension contributes to increased local vascular resistance and this causes exertional ischemia. Venous claudication is uncommon and usually occurs in patients with concomitant arterial insufficiency.

In patients with *McArdle's syndrome,* skeletal muscle metabolites accumulate due to phosphorylase deficiency, evoking exercise intolerance in the absence of an ischemia-inducing substrate. Similar metabolites, including but not limited to lactic acid, may be responsible for the pain of intermittent claudication due to obstructive arterial disease.

Obstructive arterial diseases other than atherosclerosis that may produce intermittent claudication include *fibromuscular dysplasia* (FMD), *thromboangiitis obliterans* (Buerger's disease) and other arteritides, arterial entrapment syndromes (most commonly caused by the gastrocnemius muscles) and extravascular compressive lesions, adventitial cysts and tumors, and thromboembolic lesions (Table 2). The most prevalent of these diseases is *fibromuscular dysplasia*, a hyperplastic disorder that usually affects medium-sized and small arteries in Caucasian females *(32).* The renal

Table 2
Differential Diagnosis of Obstructive Arterial Disease

Arteriosclerosis obliterans
Fibromuscular dysplasia
Vasculitis
Vascular entrapment or compression
Adventitial cysts and tumors
Thrombosis and embolism

Table 3
**Trophic Signs of Ischemia in Patients
With Peripheral Arterial Disease of the Extremities**

Chronic arterial obstructive disease
Hair loss
Subcutaneous atrophy
Thickened nails
Dependent rubor
Acute ischemia
Ulceration
Petechiae
Calf tenderness
Dependent edema

and carotid arteries are most frequently involved, but the disorder has also been described in the mesenteric, coronary, subclavian, and iliac arteries. Three histologic varieties have been delineated, based on which layer of the arterial wall displays the predominant features of the process. Medial fibroplasias, the most common FMD, are characterized angiographically by a "string of beads" appearance, representing multiple thickened fibromuscular ridges alternating with thin areas of the arterial wall. The etiology is unknown, but pathogenic concepts include influence of female sex hormones, vascular microtrauma, and genetic factors. The natural history in limb arteries is less well defined than in the renal and carotid arteries, where progression of stenosis occurs over 5 yr in a third of cases. Clinical manifestations such as intermittent claudication, rest pain, coldness, and cyanosis of the limb and even microembolism are similar to atherosclerosis. In addition to surgical reconstruction, percutaneous angioplasty has been employed for management of FMD. Balloon dilation with or without intravascular stenting has been successfully accomplished with relatively low inflation pressures.

Buerger's disease (thromboangiitis obliterans) is a nonatherosclerotic segmental inflammatory obliterative disease most commonly affecting small- and medium-sized arteries and veins in both the upper and lower extremities *(33)*. Though the disease was once considered confined to young males, in recent clinical series up to a third of the cases occurred in women. Most patients are heavy users of tobacco, usually cigarette smokers, and antigenic cross-reactivity between type III vascular collagen and a component of tobacco smoke has been considered etiologically important *(34)*. Distinctive pathological findings distinguish this disorder from other arterial occlusive diseases. Successful therapy requires abstinence from tobacco.

PHYSICAL FINDINGS

Trophic signs of chronic limb ischemia include subcutaneous atrophy, brittle toenails, hair loss, pallor, coolness, or dependent rubor (Table 3). Other visible changes reflect sympathetic denervation and sensorimotor neuropathy. Severe ischemia produces petechiae, regional edema, tenderness, ulceration, or gangrene. The level of arterial obstruction may be judged by palpation of the femoral,

Table 4
Elevation and Dependency Tests
in the Evaluation of Acral Ischemia

	Color return (s)	Venous filling (s)
Normal	10	10–15
Adequate collaterals	15–25	15–30
Severe ischemia	>35	>40

Table 5
Noninvasive Laboratory Evaluation
of Peripheral Arterial Disease

Doppler sphygmomanometry
Segmental pressure measurement
Pulse volume recording
Venous-occlusion plethysmography
Radionuclide mapping
Duplex ultrasound imaging
Magnetic resonance angiography
Computed tomographic angiography

popliteal, posterior tibial, and dorsalis pedis pulses. Vascular bruits denote turbulent flow but do not indicate the severity of stenosis.

Cutaneous perfusion may be estimated by the color and temperature of the feet during elevation above heart level at rest and following exercise. The rate of hyperemic color return and venous filling in the foot upon dependency reflect collateral perfusion (Table 4). When this does not meet minimal tissue perfusion requirements, cutaneous ulceration is frequent. *Arterial ulcers* caused by arterial disease are often as small as 3 to 5 mm in diameter, have irregular borders and pale bases, usually involve the tips of the toes or the heel of the foot, are typically painful on elevation, and are most bothersome at night. The clinical course of these ulcers is often one of rapid progression to extensive gangrene. *Vasospasm* may produce cutaneous ischemia leading to ulceration of the digits in patients with *Raynaud's phenomenon* or chronic *pernio*. Diabetics, who are prone to combined peripheral sensory neuropathy and ischemic disease, often develop deep *neurotrophic ulcers* from trauma or pressure on the plantar surface. In patients with severe hypertension, painful *Hines ulcers* related to arteriolar obliteration tend to occur near the lateral malleoli. *Vasculitic ulcers* are characterized by arteriolar thickening, with or without superimposed thrombosis. Hematologic disorders such as the hemoglobinopathies, hereditary spherocytosis, dysproteinemias, and myeloproliferative diseases may be associated with cutaneous infarction, venous thrombosis, and microvascular occlusion. *Chronic venous stasis* usually produces indolent or recurrent ulceration near the medial malleoli that are more painful during dependency, which helps distinguish them from ulcers due to arterial disease. A host of systemic diseases may also be associated with cutaneous ulceration in the lower extremities, such as tumors (i.e., Kaposi's sarcoma), syphilitic chancre and gumma, tuberculous lupus vulgaris, and pyoderma gangrenosum. Factitious and traumatic ulcers may also mimic those induced by obstructive arterial disease *(35)*.

NONINVASIVE EVALUATION (TABLE 5)

Doppler Sphygmomanometry

Doppler sphygmomanometry has become part of the initial bedside vascular examination for determination of the ABI. Normally, systolic arterial pressure at the ankle exceeds that at the brachial artery. An ABI ≤0.9 at rest indicates hemodynamically significant arterial obstruction proximal

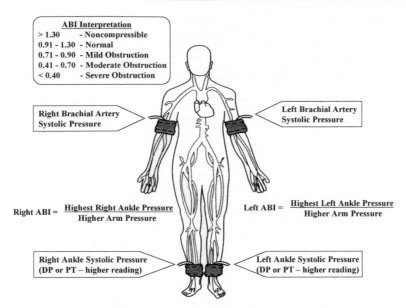

Fig. 5. Measurement of ankle-brachial index (ABI).

to the pneumatic leg cuff. In general, ABI may exceed 0.9 in individuals with obstructive disease in the absence of symptoms; values between 0.5 and 0.9 at rest are typical in patients with intermittent claudication, and values below 0.5 are frequently associated with ischemic rest pain, ulceration, and gangrene threatening the viability of the limb (Fig. 5).

Advanced calcific atherosclerosis of vessels beneath the cuff resists compression producing overestimation of regional perfusion pressure. This constitutes the major limitation of sphygmomanometry, and may falsely elevate the ABI in patients with diabetes mellitus or end-stage renal disease. Ankle-brachial indices may be normal at rest despite hemodynamically significant arterial stenosis, yet decline following calf muscle exercise. Postexercise systolic ankle pressure readings below 90 mmHg are typical of patients with intermittent claudication, and values below 60 mmHg are typical of ulcerative ischemia at rest *(36)*.

Segmental Pressure Measurements

To localize segmental arterial lesions, pneumatic cuffs are applied to determine systolic pressure at several levels, based on the principle that pressure drops distal to the level of obstruction. *Segmental pressure measurements* are subject to the same limitations as Doppler sphygmomanometry. Segmental compression cuffs combined with the Doppler ultrasound device, *photoplethysmograph*, or other flow detectors are subject to error related to arterial rigidity.

Pulse volume recordings overcome some of these limitations. The amplitude of the pulse volume wave reflects local arterial pressure, vascular wall compliance, the number of arterial vessels beneath the cuff, and the severity of atherosclerotic disease. The normal pulse is characterized by a sharp systolic upstroke that rises rapidly to a peak, and then drops off slowly toward the baseline. The downslope curves toward the baseline and usually contains a dicrotic notch and secondary wave that is midway between the peak and the baseline. The pulse recording distal to an arterial obstruction is more rounded, the anacrotic slope is reduced, the crest is delayed, the catacrotic limb descends more gradually, and the dicrotic wave is lost.

The pulse volume recorder has the advantage of revealing distortions in pulse wave contour even in patients with vascular calcification. The pulse waveforms appear depressed and altered even when arteries are noncompressible. The *pulsatility index*, representing the ratio of pulse amplitude to mean volume obtained by integration of the deflection, is abnormally low even when systolic pressure readings are falsely elevated. The value of these observations is enhanced by exercise testing, which also provides a quantitative estimate of functional capacity. In addition, exercise testing enables the physician to distinguish PAD from disorders producing similar symptoms, since the ABI declines following exercise in those with arterial obstructive disease.

Ultrasound Velocity Spectroscopy and Imaging

Doppler velocity analysis of normal arteries reveals a triphasic signal. Rapid acceleration to peak systolic velocity occurs along a narrow frequency spectrum, end-systolic deceleration culminates in protodiastolic flow reversal, and antegrade flow resumes in mid-diastole. Peak systolic velocities diminish with advancing age. Arterial obstruction proximal to the probe transforms the waveform by loss of the reversed flow component and attenuation of all parts of the spectrum, with delayed upstroke and decreased amplitude.

Duplex ultrasound scanning combines B-mode and pulsed-Doppler ultrasound analysis to examine arterial configuration and localize velocity information at sites of stenosis. Flow through a stenosis is accelerated, and turbulence is detected as spectral broadening of the velocities, instead of the narrow band seen with normal flow. Microprocessor-based systems for calculation of blood cell velocities allow accurate estimation of instantaneous pressure gradients and degrees of stenosis *(37)*. Duplex scanning is more sensitive and specific than segmental blood pressure measurements for detection of restenosis following vascular interventional procedures.

The clinical vascular noninvasive laboratory is subject to misconceptions that predispose to misuse. Among these are that findings can establish indications for specific therapeutic procedures, since clinical decisions are best based on symptoms and the physical appearance of the limb. Noninvasive vascular measurements reflect the severity of ischemia, the contribution of obstructive arterial factors to symptoms, and the hemodynamic significance of lesions at various points. It is important that in formulating management decisions, noninvasive testing aid rather than replace the medical history, physical examination, and clinical judgment.

Magnetic Resonance Angiography

Magnetic resonance angiography obviates arterial catheterization and exposure to iodinated contrast material and may identify runoff vessels not visualized by conventional angiography *(38)*. Magnetic resonance (MR) imaging methods are currently emerging to characterize the arterial wall and atherosclerotic lesions. In the magnetic field, water molecules are excited by a radiofrequency (RF) pulse generating a secondary signal that is detected and measured digitally and displayed as images that distinguish fine details of tissue architecture and composition. Plaque dimensions and composition are assessed using T1-weighted, proton density, and T2-weighted images and techniques of real-time, cine MR angiography are under development. Currently, MR imaging is limited in assessing restenosis in arteries following angioplasty and stenting.

Contrast Angiography

The diagnosis of arterial obstructive disease does not generally require invasive techniques, and most patients with intermittent claudication should not undergo angiographic examination. *Contrast angiography* is indicated for mapping the extent and location of arterial pathology prior to a revascularization procedure. Such testing should be reserved for patients in whom the diagnosis is in doubt or as a prelude to vascular intervention when conservative approaches are not satisfactory. Aortic injection of contrast material in patients with aortoiliac occlusive disease can be accomplished either by the *retrograde transfemoral, translumbar,* or *transaxillary* approach. Aortic injection of contrast material provides visualization of the aorta and proximal limb vessels, but definition of the circulation distal to the popliteal trifurcations may be compromised by dilution of proximally injected contrast. In patients with femoropopliteal obstructive disease, antegrade or retrograde transfemoral angiography can be confined to the involved extremity with fine definition of the distal vasculature.

Computer-enhanced *digital subtraction angiography* may be useful in patients with localized stenosis either to minimize the volume of contrast material injected or to improve image resolution. The technique may be employed with either intravenous or intraarterial contrast injection, especially for postoperative examination of anastomotic segments, but is not an effective means of visualizing large regions of the arterial tree.

MEDICAL THERAPY

The principles of patient management for PAD involve measures directed at protection of affected tissues, preservation of functional capacity, avoidance of disease progression or acute arterial thrombosis, restoration of blood flow, and prevention of mortality. These principles can be categorized as local measures, treatment of associated risk factors, drug therapy for claudication, and antithrombotic agents.

Local Measures

Local measures to reduce skin breakdown and infection are particularly important in diabetics and in patients with severely impaired perfusion. The feet should be kept clean. Moisturizing cream applied to prevent fissuring must be selected to avoid irritant effects. Well-fitted shoes reduce the risk of pressure-induced necrosis. Stockings made of absorbent fibers are recommended. The skin of the feet should be inspected frequently so minor abrasions may be promptly tended. Elastic support stockings may restrict cutaneous blood flow and should be avoided. In patients with ischemia at rest, conservative measures such as positioning the affected limb below heart level increases oxygen tension in ischemic tissues. When edema is present, the limb should be kept horizontal to enhance healing. The heels should be protected from pressure against the bedsheets with sheepskin padding. Blankets should be cradled over a foot-board to reduce friction. Separation of the toes with cotton helps protect against intertriginous friction. Unless purulence is present, dryness is preferred to soaks except for intermittent cleansing. Gentle warmth is recommended to minimize vasoconstriction. Antimicrobial treatment of fungal onycholysis reduces skin breakdown and superinfection. Topical medications should be used cautiously to avoid inflammatory reactions. Open sores should be cultured and roentgenograms performed on affected limbs to detect possible osteomyelitis. Antibiotic medication is less effective when delivery to ischemic tissue is impaired. Passive physical therapy may proceed to progressive weight-bearing and ambulation, with attention to foot care and properly fitted footwear, using soft, cotton stockings and nonconstrictive shoes.

Risk Factor Modification

Modification of associated risk factors may reduce the likelihood of progression of atherosclerotic disease, as discussed earlier in this chapter. Accordingly, attention should be directed toward correction of dyslipidemia, treatment of diabetes mellitus, control of hypertension, cessation of cigarette smoking, and exercise training.

TREATMENT OF DYSLIPIDEMIA

Lipid-lowering therapy with HMG-CoA-reductase inhibitors ("statins") have favorable effects in patients with intermittent claudication *(39)*. In addition to improving lipid profiles, statin treatment improves walking distance in patients with PAD and decrease the risk of developing new or worsening intermittent claudication *(40–42)*.

TREATMENT OF DIABETES MELLITUS

Aggressive control of blood glucose reduces the incidence of microvascular complications, but data are insufficient regarding the efficacy of this strategy on the progression and complications of peripheral atherosclerosis *(43)*. In the UK Prospective Diabetes Study, aggressive blood-glucose control was not associated with statistically significant reduction in myocardial infarction, amputation, and death associated with PAD *(44)*.

HYPERTENSION TREATMENT

Meta-analysis has shown approx 40% reduction in the risk of stroke and 10 to 15% reduction in the risk of myocardial infarction with antihypertensive treatment, but specific effects of therapy on peripheral manifestations of atherosclerosis have not been quantified *(45)*. Treatment with the angiotensin-converting enzyme inhibitor ramipril was associated with a 27% relative risk reduction in stroke, myocardial infarction, and death in the subgroup of PAD patients enrolled in the Heart Outcomes Prevention Evaluation (HOPE) trial *(46)*.

SMOKING CESSATION

Clinical prognosis for those with arterial obstructive disease of the extremities seems related to tobacco use. Among smokers with intermittent claudication, 11% of those who continued to smoke required amputation, while this fate befell none who quit *(47)*. Patients with intermittent claudication who stopped smoking had twice the survival benefit of those who continued to smoke at 5 and 10 yr *(48,49)*.

EXERCISE TRAINING

Exercise training improves walking capacity and functional capacity among patients with obstructive arterial disease over a period of several months, but most studies have not identified consistent improvement in measured indices of perfusion and data from well-controlled prospective trials are scant *(50)*. Studies involving animals in which arterial obstructions have been created support the view that regular muscular exercise increases collateral development, but in the clinical setting functional improvement may depend on other factors in muscle metabolism or ergonomics.

TREATMENT OF HYPERHOMOCYSTEINEMIA

Hyperhomocysteinemia is strongly associated with peripheral atherosclerosis. Treatment with B-complex vitamins including folic acid, pyridoxine, and cyanocobalamin reduces homocysteine levels, but there are no conclusive data about the efficacy of treatment on the clinical consequences of atherosclerosis.

Drug Therapy to Reduce Ischemia and Claudication

VASODILATOR DRUGS

In contrast to their usefulness for treatment of patients with angina pectoris, vasodilator drugs have been disappointing for relief of intermittent claudication. In patients with limb ischemia, the goal is to increase the work capacity of exercising muscle. An obstructive arterial lesion producing critical stenosis limits blood supply and reduces distal perfusion pressure. Intramuscular arterioles normally dilate in response to the metabolic demands of exercise. In patients with proximal stenotic arterial disease, flow augmentation is blunted and distal pressure falls during exercise. This process leads to accumulation of the ischemic metabolites that mediate claudication. The distal vasculature virtually collapses under the compressive force of exercising skeletal muscle, and this mechanism cannot be mitigated by arteriolar vasodilator therapy.

The history of limb arterial disease is replete with therapeutic agents that achieve popularity for awhile before falling into disrepute and disuse when adequate studies confirm their ineffectiveness. β-*Adrenergic agonists, α-adrenergic antagonists, nitrates*, and other vasodilator drugs have been evaluated in such clinical trials. No vasodilator agent increases blood flow in exercising skeletal muscle subtended by significant arterial obstructive lesions, or improves symptoms of intermittent claudication and objective measures of exercise capacity *(51)*.

PHARMACOLOGICAL ENHANCEMENT OF COLLATERAL FLOW

An alternative tactic for patients with obstructive arterial disease involving major limb arteries is augmentation of collateral perfusion. This is the rationale behind the use of the selective serotonin antagonist, *ketanserin*, which in one study increased collateral blood flow in patients with obstructive lesions. In a multicenter trial involving patients with intermittent claudication, however, treadmill exercise performance was no better 1 yr after treatment with ketanserin than with placebo *(52)*.

Hemorheologic Agents

Abnormal rheology is present in many patients with atherosclerotic disease. Oral *pentoxifylline* is in clinical use to improve the walking capacity of patients with intermittent claudication related to obstructive arterial disease, based upon salutary results in several clinical trials *(53)*. In vitro, abnormally reduced erythrocyte flexibility of blood obtained from patients with claudication is partially corrected, and skeletal muscle oxygen tension has been reported to rise at rest following treatment with pentoxifylline. Improved blood fluidity in vivo has not been conclusively demonstrated, however, in patients with intermittent claudication treated with pentoxifylline. Vascular resistance during reactive hyperemia showed no improvement after administration of pentoxifylline compared with placebo in a study of patients with stable intermittent claudication. This result suggests that the hemorheologic effects of the drug were not sufficient to reduce the impedance to blood flow. In fact, pentoxifylline has not been shown to have conclusive clinical benefits *(54)*.

Metabolic Agents

Cilostazol, an inhibitor of phosphodiesterase-III with vasodilator, antiplatelet, and vascular smooth muscle cell inhibitory actions, was approved by the US Food and Drug Administration in 1999 for treatment of patients with intermittent claudication. The mechanism of its effect is not well understood. Cilostazol has been compared to placebo in eight controlled trials involving more than 2000 patients and in two studies to pentoxifylline (the only other drug approved in the US for treatment of patients with intermittent claudication). Primary endpoints were the distances patients could walk on a treadmill before the onset of claudication pain (initial claudication distance, ICD) and before pain became intolerable (absolute claudication distance, ACD). In six of the eight studies, ICD and ACD were significantly improved with cilostazol compared with placebo. In one study, cilostazol was superior to pentoxifylline; in the other comparison with pentoxifylline, neither drug was superior to placebo *(55)*. In general, 100 mg cilostazol twice daily was superior to a lower dose of 50 mg twice daily. There are no data bearing on longer-term aspects of treatment, such as limb preservation, rate of disease progression, and so on. Several other phosphodiesterase inhibitors (such as milrinone and vesnarinone) have been associated with increased mortality when used as inotropic agents in patients with severe (NYHA class III–IV) congestive heart failure, and cilostazol is presently contraindicated in patients with a history of cardiac failure *(56)*.

Propionyl L-carnitine reportedly facilitates transfer of acetylated compounds and fatty acids across mitochondrial membranes, leading to enhanced energy storage. Accumulation of acylcarnitines in ischemic skeletal muscle correlates with impairment of exercise performance and may reflect abnormal oxidative metabolism *(57)*. Increased substrate availability has been suggested as the mechanism by which proprionyl-L-carnitine supplementation may improve walking capacity in patients with intermittent claudication, as suggested by results from a European multicenter trial, but results have been inconsistent in different populations and larger studies are needed *(58)*.

The mechanism by which *prostaglandin E₁* (PGE_1) and *prostacyclin* (PGI_2), which are potent vasodilators and inhibitors of platelet aggregation, relieve ischemic rest pain and promote healing of ulcers remains controversial. Intravenous or intraarterial infusions of PGE_1 and PGI_2 have effects on blood flow and exercise capacity that persist for weeks to months, but intravenous administration has yielded inconsistent results *(59)*. The major drawback to this type of prostaglandin therapy is the short half-lives of these drugs, but oral analogs are under development. Overall, prostacyclins may provide temporary relief of ischemic rest pain in patients with severe arterial insufficiency, best when given intraarterially, but it is unknown whether this therapy will prevent amputation in patients not amenable to revascularization.

Recently, a few novel agents have been studied to improve walking capacity for PAD patients. L-arginine, a substrate for nitric oxide, increased pain-free and total walking distances in patients with intermittent claudication after 2 wk of administration *(60)*. Avasimibe, an inhibitor of acyl coenzyme A-cholesterol acyltransferase (ACAT), given in a dose of 50 mg daily for 52 wk demonstrated a trend toward improved walking distances that did not reach statistical significance *(61)*.

ANGIOGENESIS

Therapeutic angiogenesis involves administration of vascular growth factors, usually as recombinant protein or DNA to augment the collateral blood supply to ischemic tissues. Recent clinical trials of angiogenic growth factors have given inconclusive results. The Therapeutic Angiogenesis with Recombinant Fibroblast Growth Factor-2 for Intermittent Claudication (TRAFFIC) study demonstrated that intraarterial administration of recombinant fibroblast growth factor-2 (rFGF-2) improved walking distance in patients with intermittent claudication *(62)*. The Regional Angiogenesis with Vascular Endothelial growth factor (RAVE) trial, however, did not show improvement in peak walking time in patients with PAD treated with intramuscular vascular endothelial growth factor (VEGF) *(63)*. In a recent study, injection of bone marrow-mononuclear cells into the legs of patients with PAD improved ABI, measurements of tissue oxygenation made by transcutaneous oximetry, and peak walking times 24 wk following implantation *(64)*.

IMMUNE MODULATION THERAPY

A novel and investigational therapeutic technique known as *immune modulation therapy* (IMT) has recently been shown in a clinical trial to increase claudication distance in 70 patients with severe walking impairment (less than 100 m) *(65)*. IMT involves the administration of ex vivo processed autologous blood to induce a cascade of events with the intent of reducing in vascular inflammation and progression of atherosclerosis. A larger multicenter trial of this technique, the Study of Immune Modulation Therapy in Peripheral Arterial Disease and Intermittent Claudication Outcomes (SIM-PADICO), is presently in progress.

Antithrombotic Therapy

Antithrombotic therapy should be considered part of the management of patients with PAD. In those with chronic disease, the goal is to prevent progression of the obliterative process leading to thrombotic occlusion of arteries and to reduce coronary and cerebrovascular events and mortality. Following limb revascularization, the objective is to prevent thrombotic complications and preserve the patency of reconstruction. In those with acute arterial occlusion resulting from embolism or thrombosis, therapy is directed toward preventing propagation of thrombus and recurrent embolism. Available approaches include *anticoagulant medications, platelet inhibitor* agents, *thrombolytic* substances, and *direct inhibitors of thrombin*. A combination of approaches is warranted for high-risk patients.

There is no conclusive evidence that antithrombotic therapy alters the clinical course of vascular insufficiency related to arteriosclerosis obliterans, although some reports have suggested a benefit of anticoagulant or platelet inhibitor agents. Only recently have data emerged indicating that antithrombotic therapy delays the progression of atherosclerotic lesions. In double-blind studies involving several hundred patients, serial angiography revealed less pronounced progression of arterial disease in those randomly assigned to platelet inhibitor medication (*aspirin* or the combination of *aspirin plus dipyridamole*) than in those given placebo *(66)*. The role of platelet-inhibitor medication in retarding progression of the atherosclerotic plaque has been demonstrated over a longer period in patients with coronary artery disease.

Intermittent claudication carries important prognostic weight in terms of other atherothrombotic cardiovascular events. Aspirin therapy has been convincingly demonstrated to reduce the risks of myocardial infarction, ischemic stroke, and vascular death in patients with atherosclerosis. The Antiplatelet Trialists Collaboration (ATC), a meta-analysis of more than 100 randomized clinical trials involving about 70,000 participants, concluded that aspirin reduces these vascular events by about 25%, regardless of dose *(68)*. Nonfatal myocardial infarctions and strokes were reduced by about one third, while vascular deaths by about one sixth *(67)*. From the ATC, 9214 PAD patients were reassessed and found to have a 23% reduction in vascular events with antiplatelet therapy *(68)*.

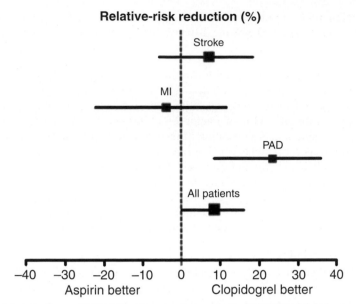

Fig. 6. Relative-risk reduction and 95% CI by disease subgroup in the CAPRIE trial. MI, myocardial infarction; PAD, peripheral arterial disease. (From ref. *69.*)

The thienopyridine derivatives *ticlopidine* and *clopidogrel* antagonize the platelet adenosine diphosphate receptor. In Clopidogrel versus Aspirin in Patients of Ischaemic Events (CAPRIE) a large, multicenter trial, 75 mg/d clopidogrel was compared with 325 mg/d aspirin over a mean follow-up of 1.5 yr in 19,185 patients with clinical atherosclerosis *(69).* Participants included survivors of myocardial infarction or nondisabling stroke as well as those with symptomatic peripheral arterial disease; the primary endpoint was a composite of ischemic stroke, myocardial infarction, or vascular death. Patients treated with clopidogrel had a 5.32% annual risk of primary events compared with 5.83% for those treated with aspirin (a statistically significant relative risk reduction of 8.7%). Most benefit was confined to the 6452 patients entered on the basis of peripheral arterial disease, in whom the relative risk reduction for occurrence of primary vascular events was 24% ($p = 0.0028$) (Fig. 6). The benefit of combination clopidogrel and aspirin versus aspirin alone is currently under investigation in patients at high cardiovascular risk, including PAD, in the Clopidogrel for High Atherothrombotic Risk and Ischemic Stabilization, Management, and Avoidance (CHARISMA) trial.

Insufficient data have been forthcoming to validate an advantage to long-term anticoagulation for patients with PAD. The incidence of ischemic events was lower, and survival was greater, among selected anticoagulated patients following femoropopliteal bypass surgery than in a control group *(70).* The ABI declined more gradually in anticoagulated patients, and graft patency was prolonged out to 12 yr, but this falls short of confirming delayed progression of atherosclerotic vascular disease. In fact, oral anticoagulation given to 2690 patients with PAD undergoing infrainguinal grafting did not reduce graft occlusion as compared with aspirin *(71).*

INTERVENTIONAL ANGIOGRAPHY

Considerable success has attended transluminal dilation for correction of iliac arterial stenoses, but patency rates are lower in the femoral and popliteal arteries. Initial and long-term success is related to the acuity of ischemic symptoms, morphologic features of the atherosclerotic segment (i.e., the length of obstruction, relation to anatomic branch points, and condition of the distal artery), and comorbid conditions (e.g., diabetes, active smoking). Experience with obstructions distal to the popliteal trifurcation has been disappointing, but "steerable" devices drawn from coronary catheterization enhance outcome in selected cases. In view of the limitation of dilation techniques, various alternative recanalization tools have been developed. Currently, endovascular techniques used to treat atherosclerosis obliterans include percutaneous atherectomy, angioplasty, stents, and thrombolysis.

Antithrombotic therapy prior to catheter intervention is advocated in conjunction with balloon angioplasty procedures to reduce thrombus formation and the associated risk of occlusion at the dilated site. Current practice tends toward pre- and postprocedural administration of aspirin plus ticlopidine or clopidigrel, and intraprocedural administration of heparin, followed by maintenance therapy with aspirin or clopidogrel. Despite this widespread practice, the benefits of antiplatelet or anticoagulant therapy in conjunction with percutaneous interventions of peripheral arterial lesions have not been proven. Some reviewers reported no difference in reocclusion rates with antiplatelet or anticoagulant therapy following peripheral angioplasty (72), but a meta-analysis found increased patency and lower amputation rates with antiplatelet therapy (73).

Transcatheter Atherectomy and Endovascular Stents

Extraction of atherothrombotic material using the Simpson rotating blade device or abrasion and pulverization methods intends to remove atheromatous material and leave the remaining surface smooth. Unlike other methods of angioplasty, atherectomy appears well suited to eccentric atherosclerotic lesions associated with calcification (74). For stenoses at the femoropopliteal level, angiographic success has been reported in 87 to 93% of the lesions removed; recurrent symptoms occurred in 31% of patients during 6 mo of clinical follow-up (75). Additionally, atherectomy for infrapopliteal occlusive disease has demonstrated an overwhelming high restenosis rate (91%) at 6 mo postintervention (76). Therefore, atherectomy is not recommended for routine peripheral atherosclerotic lesions except for possible limb salvage.

Patency rates following angioplasty and endovascular stent deployment in iliac arterial stenosis were 92% at 9 mo and clinical benefit has been reported to extend for 2 yr (77). Results with infrainguinal endovascular stents have not been as favorable, however, with restenosis or reocclusion rates of approx 50% in the femoropopliteal segment. Infrainguinal endovascular angioplasty with or without stents has been an accepted practice for salvage of critically ischemic limbs. The TASC working group recommends that endovascular interventions for iliac and femoropopliteal arterial occlusions that are <3 cm in length (type A) (Fig. 7) (30). Percutaneous angioplasty with stenting of long segment superficial femoral arterial disease has had poor restenosis and reocclusion rates (78).

Endovascular brachytherapy and drug-eluting stents have recently been reported to possibly decrease restenosis rates in intervened femoropopliteal and infrapopliteal arterial occlusions (79, 80). However, long-term prospective clinical trials are necessary to determine the utility of these techniques compared to conventional therapy.

Intraarterial Thrombolysis

Catheter-directed, intraarterial thrombolytic therapy has been used as an adjunct to revascularization for management of both acute and chronic critical limb ischemia. Several studies have compared thrombolytic therapy with surgical revascularization in patients with acute peripheral arterial insufficiency and have shown comparable rates of mortality and limb salvage (81,82). In the Thrombolysis or Peripheral Arterial Surgery (TOPAS) trial, administration of urokinase versus surgery had similar amputation-free survival at 12 mo (81). However the Surgery versus Thrombolysis for Ischemia of the Lower Extremity (STILE) trial showed higher reoccurrence for limb ischemia with lysis compared to surgery (82). In both studies, lysis was equal to or possibly superior to surgery for arterial occlusions <14 d in duration (81,82). Although the rate of successful reperfusion (50–80%) is higher with local intraarterial than with systemic (intravenous) thrombolytic therapy, local infusions allow concurrent angiographic definition of effectiveness and define regional vascular disease so that angioplasty may be incorporated to prevent reocclusion. Bleeding or thromboembolism up to 20% of cases may complicate protracted periods of indwelling arterial catheterization. Thrombolytic therapy may be particularly useful in cases of thrombotic distal arterial occlusion in the forearm, hand, ankle, and foot, where surgical access is difficult.

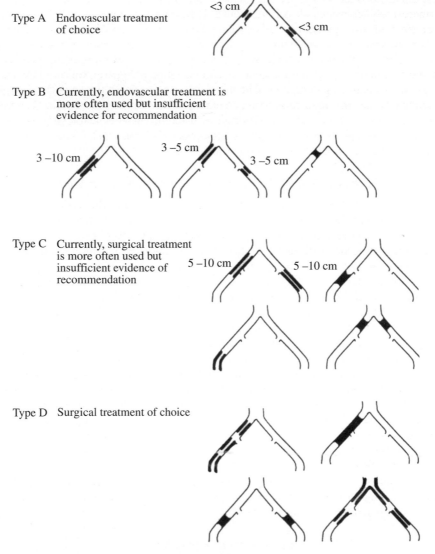

Fig. 7. The TransAtlantic Inter-Society Consensus (TASC) recommendations in the interventional management of iliac lesions. (Adapted from ref. *29*.)

SURGICAL THERAPY

Surgical intervention is not indicated for the majority of patients with stable intermittent claudication who have sufficient collateral blood supply to meet the nutritional requirement of resting limb tissue. It is an indicated procedure if patients fail maximum aggressive medical management and have severe functional impairment. The most pressing indication for surgical revascularization is ischemic rest pain, ulceration, or gangrene amenable to arterial reconstruction when more limited measures, including angioplasty, are insufficient, unsafe, or not feasible. Since most patients with intermittent claudication remain stable or improve with time, surgical intervention becomes appropriate when the disease process becomes severely debilitating or progressive.

Beyond the severity of ischemia and associated symptoms, the anatomic pathology is important in deciding whether surgery should be undertaken. In general, the syndromic approach to disease classification reflects the success of surgical bypass procedures. The TASC working group recommends that diffuse, multiple iliac lesions, and complete common femoral, superficial femoral, popliteal, or proximal trifurcation arterial occlusions be treated with surgery (type D) (Fig. 7) *(30)*. Revascularization for aortoiliac obstructive disease is associated with approx 85% patency rates at 5 to 10 yr; for femoropopliteal reconstruction, around a 70% patency rate at 5 yr; and for distal anastomosis located beyond the popliteal trifurcation, a patency rate in the range of 40 to 60% after 2 yr. This aspect should be interpreted in the context of a patient's overall functional status and medical condition, with particular reference to risk imposed by associated coronary or cerebrovascular disease.

REFERENCES

1. Wilens SL. The nature of diffuse intimal thickening of arteries. Am J Pathol 1951;27:825–839.
2. World Health Organization Study Group. Classification of atherosclerotic lesions: report of a study group. WHO Tech Rep Ser 1958;143:1–20.
3. Kannel WB, McGee DL. Update on some epidemiologic features of intermittent claudication: The Framingham Study. J Am Geriatr Soc 1985;33:13.
4. Vogt MT, Cauley JA, Kuller LH, Hulley SB. Prevalence and correlates of lower extremity arterial disease in elderly women. Am J Epidemiol 1993;137:559–568.
5. Criqui MH, Froner A, Barrett-Connor E, et al. The prevalence of peripheral arterial disease in a defined population. Circulation 1985;71:510–515.
6. Hiatt WR, Hoag S, Hamman RF. Effect of diagnostic criteria on the prevalence of peripheral arterial disease: the San Luis Valley Diabetes Study. Circulation 1995;91:1472–1479.
7. Hirsch AT, Criqui MH, Treat-Jacobson D, et al. Peripheral arterial disease detection, awareness, and treatment in primary care. JAMA 2001;286:1317–1324.
8. Mathiesen FR, Mune O. Arterial insufficiency in the lower extremities of elderly patients. Acta Chir Scand P Suppl 1966;357:78.
9. Meijer WT, Hoes AW, Rutgers D, et al. Peripheral arterial disease in the elderly: the Rotterdam Study. Arterioscler Thromb Vasc Biol 1998;18:185–192.
10. Paris BEC, Libow LS, Halperin JL, Mulvihill MN. The prevalence and one-year outcome of limb arterial obstructive disease in a nursing home population. J Am Geriatr Soc 1988;36:607–612.
11. Greenhalgh RM, Rosengarten DS, Mervart I, et al. Serum lipids and lipoproteins in peripheral vascular disease. Lancet 1971;3:947.
12. Fowkes FG, Housley E, Riemersma RA, et al. Smoking, lipids, glucose intolerance, and blood pressure as risk factors for peripheral atherosclerosis compared with ischemic heart disease in the Edinburgh Artery Study. Am J Epidemiol 1992;135:331–340.
13. Sanderson KJ, van Rij AM, Wade CR, et al. Lipid peroxidation of circulating low density lipoproteins with age, smoking and in peripheral vascular disease. Atherosclerosis 1995;118:45–51.
14. Harris LM, Armstrong D, Browne R, et al. Premature peripheral vascular disease: clinical profile and abnormal lipid peroxidation. Cardiovasc Surg 1998;6:188–193.
15. Katsilambros NL, Tsapogas PC, Arvanitis MP, et al. Risk factors for lower extremity arterial disease in non-insulin-dependent diabetic persons. Diabet Med 1996;13:243–246.
16. Strandness DE Jr, Priest RE, Gibbon GE. Combined clinical and pathologic study of diabetic and nondiabetic peripheral arterial disease. Diabetes 1964;13:366–372.
17. Kannel WB, McGee D, Gordon T. A general cardiovascular risk profile: The Framingham Study. Am J Cardiol 1976; 38:46.
18. Murabito JM, Evans JC, Nieto K, et al. Prevalence and clinical correlates of peripheral arterial disease in the Framingham Offspring Study. Am Heart J 2002;143:961–965.
19. Stewart CP. The influence of smoking on the level of lower limb amputation. Prosthet Orthot Int 1987;11:113–116.
20. Ameli FM, Stein M, Prosser RJ, et al. Effects of cigarette smoking on outcome of femoral popliteal bypass for limb salvage. J Cardiovasc Surg (Torino) 1989;30:591–596.
21. Coffman JD, Javett SL. Blood flow in the human calf during tobacco smoking. Circulation 1963;28:932.
22. Imparato AM, Kim G, Davidson T, et al. Intermittent claudication: its natural course. Surgery 1975;78:795.
23. Hertzer NR, Young JR, Kramer JR, et al. Routine coronary angiography prior to elective aortic reconstruction. Arch Surg 1979;114:1336.
24. Criqui M, Langer RD, Fronek A, et al. Mortality over a period of 10 years in patients ith peripheral arterial disease. N Engl J Med 1992;328:381–386.
25. Muluk SC, Muluk VS, Kelley ME, et al. Outcome events in patients with claudication: a 15-year study in 2777 patients. J Vasc Surg 2001;33:251–257.
26. The Framingham Study: an Epidemiologic Investigation of Cardiovascular Disease. US Government Printing Office, Section 25, 1970.
27. Schadt DC, Hines EA Jr, Juergens JL, et al. Chronic atherosclerotic occlusion of the femoral artery. JAMA 1961; 175:937.

28. Coffman JD. Intermittent claudication: be conservative. N Engl J Med 1991;325:577–578.
29. Dormandy JA, Rutherford RB. Management of peripheral arterial disease (PAD). TASC Working Group. Trans-Atlantic Inter-Society Concensus (TASC). J Vasc Surg 2000;31:S1–S296.
30. McDermott MM, Greenland P, Liu K, et al. The ankle brachial index is associated with leg function and physical activity: the Walking and Leg Circulation Study. Ann Intern Med 2002;136:873–883.
31. Montgomery DH, Ververis JJ, McGorisk G, et al. Natural history of severe atheromatous disease of the thoracic aorta: a transesophageal echocardiographic study. J Am Coll Cardiol 1996;27:95–101.
32. Slovut DP, Olin JW. Fibromuscular dysplasia. N Engl J Med 2004;350:1862–1871.
33. Olin JW. Thromboangiitis obliterans (Buerger's disease). N Engl J Med 2000;343:864–869.
34. Adar R, Papa MZ, Halpern Z, et al. Cellular sensitivity to collagen in thromboangiitis obliterans. N Engl J Med 1983;308:1113–1116.
35. Thiele B. Evaluation of ulceration of the lower extremities. Vasc Diag Ther 1980;1:33.
36. Karmody A, Wittmore AD, Baker JD, Ernst CB. Suggested standards for reports dealing with lower extremity ischemia. J Vasc Surg 1986;4:80–94.
37. Halperin JL. Noninvasive vascular laboratory evaluation: applications for laser angioplasty. In: Sanborn TA, ed. Laser Angioplasty. AR Liss, New York, 1989, pp. 7–14.
38. Owen RS, Carpenter JP, Baum RA, et al. Magnetic resonance imaging of angiographically occult runoff vessels in peripheral arterial occlusive disease. N Engl J Med 1992;326:1577–1581.
39. Pedersen TR, Kjekshus J, Pyorala K, et al. Effect of simvastatin on ischemic signs and symptoms in the Scandinavian Simvastatin Survival Study (4S). Am J Cardiol 1998;81:333–338.
40. Regensteiner JG, Hiatt WR. Current medical therapies for patients with peripheral arterial disease: a critical review. Am J Med 2002;112:49–57.
41. Mondillo S, Ballo P, Barbati R, et al. Effects of simvastatin on walking performance and symptoms of intermittent claudication in hypercholesterolemic patients with peripheral vascular disease. Am J Med 2003;114:359–364.
42. Pedersen TR, Kjekshus J, Pyorala K, et al. Effect of simvastatin on ischemic signs and symptoms in the Scandinavian simvastatin survival study (4S). Am J Cardiol 1998;81:333–335.
43. Diabetes Control and Complications Trial Research Group. The effect of intensive treatment of diabetes on the development and progression of long-term complications in insulin-dependent diabetes mellitus. N Engl J Med 1993;329:977–986.
44. Intensive blood-glucose control with sulphonylureas or insulin compared with conventional treatment and risk of complications in patients with type 2 diabetes (UKPDS 33). UK Prospective Diabetes Study (UKPDS) Group. Lancet 1998;352:837–853.
45. Hansson L, Zanchetti A, Carruthers SG, et al. Effects of intensive blood-pressure lowering and low-dose aspirin in patients with hypertension: principal results of the Hypertension Optimal Treatment (HOT) randomised trial. HOT Study Group. Lancet 1998;351:1755–1762.
46. Yusuf S, Sleight P, Pogue J, et al. Effects of an angiotensin-converting-enzyme inhibitor, ramipril, on cardiovascular events in high-risk patients. The Heart Outcomes Prevention Evaluation Study Investigators. N Engl J Med 2000;342:145–153.
47. Lassila R, Lepantalo M. Cigarette smoking and the outcome after lower limb arterial surgery. Acta Chir Scand 1988;154:635–640.
48. Faulkner KW, House AK, Castleden WM. The effect of cessation of smoking on the accumulative survival rates of patients with symptomatic peripheral vascular disease. Med J Aust 1983;1:217–219.
49. Jonason T, Bergstrom R. Cessation of smoking in patients with intermittent claudication. Effects on the risk of peripheral vascular complications, myocardial infarction and mortality. Acta Med Scand 1987;221:253–260.
50. Skinner JS, Strandness DE Jr. Exercise and intermittent claudication: II. Effect of physical training. Circulation 1967;36:23.
51. Coffman JD, Mannick JA. Failure of vasodilator drugs in arteriosclerosis obliterans. Ann Intern Med 1972;76:35–59.
52. PACK Claudication Substudy Investigators. Randomized placebo-controlled, double-blind trial of ketanserin in claudicants: changes in claudication distance and ankle systolic pressure. Circulation 1989;80:1544–1548.
53. Porter JM, Cutler BS, Lee BY, et al. Pentoxifylline efficacy in the treatment of intermittent claudication: multicenter controlled double-blind trial with objective assessment of chronic occlusive arterial disease patients. Am Heart J 1982;104:66–72.
54. Girolami B, Bernardi E, Prins MH, et al. Treatment of intermittent claudication with physical training, smoking cessation, pentoxifylline, or nafronyl: a meta-analysis. Arch Intern Med 1999;159:337–345.
55. Dawson DL, Cutler BS, Hiatt WR, et al. A comparison of cilostazol and pentoxifylline for treating intermittent claudication. Am J Med 2000;109:523–530.
56. Dawson DL, Cutler BS, Meissner MH, et al. Cilostazol has beneficial effects in treatment of intermittent claudication. Circulation 1998;98:678–686.
57. Hiatt WR, Nawaz D, Brass EP. Carnitine metabolism during exercise in patients with peripheral arterial disease. J Appl Physiol 1987;74:236–240.
58. Brevetti G, Chiariello M, Ferulano G, et al. Increases in walking distance in patients with peripheral vascular disease treated with L-carnitine: a double-blind, cross-over study. Circulation 1988;77:767–773.
59. The ICAI (Ischemia Cronica degli Arti Inferiore) Study Group. Prostanoids for chronic critical limb ischemia: a randomized, controlled, open-label trial with prostaglandin E$_1$. Ann Intern Med 1999;130:412–421.

60. Maxwell AJ, Anderson BE, Cooke JP. Nutritional therapy for peripheral arterial disease: a double-blind, placebo-controlled, randomized trial of HeartBar. Vasc Med 2000;5:11–19.
61. Hiatt WR, Klepack E, Nehler M, et al. Effects of avasimide in claudicants with peripheral arterial disease. J Am Coll Cardiol 2003;41(Suppl A), p. 304A.
62. Lederman RJ, Mendelsohn FO, Anderson RD, et al. Therapeutic angiogenesis with recombinant fibroblast growth factor-2 for intermittent claudication (the TRAFFIC study): a randomised trial. Lancet 2002;359:2053–2058.
63. Rajagopalan S, Mohler ER III, Lederman RJ, et al. Regional angiogenesis with vascular endothelial growth factor in peripheral arterial disease: a phase II randomized, double-blind, controlled study of adenoviral delivery of vascular endothelial growth factor 121 in patients with disabling intermittent claudication. Circulation 2003;108: 1933–1938.
64. Tateishi-Yuyama E, Matsubara H, Murohara T, et al. Therapeutic angiogenesis for patients with limb ischaemia by autologous transplantation of bone-marrow cells: a pilot study and a randomised controlled trial. Lancet 2002; 360:427–435.
65. McGrath C, Robb R, Lucas AJ, et al. A randomised, double blind, placebo-controlled study to determine the efficacy of immune modulation therapy in the treatment of patients suffering from peripheral arterial occlusive disease with intermittent claudication. Eur J Vasc Endovasc Surg 2002;23:381–387.
66. Goldhaber SZ, Manson JE, Stampfer MJ, et al. Low-dose aspirin and subsequent arterial surgery in the Physicians' Health Study. Lancet 1992;340:143–145.
67. Antiplatelet Trialists Collaboration. Collaborative overview of randomised trials of antiplatelet therapy. Prevention of death, myocardial infarction, and stroke by prolonged antiplatelet therapy in various categories of patients. Br Med J 1994;308:81–101.
68. Collaborative meta-analysis of randomised trials of antiplatelet therapy for prevention of death, myocardial infarction, and stroke in high risk patients. BMJ 2002;324:71–86.
69. CAPRIE steering committee. A randomised, blinded trial of clopidogrel versus aspirin in patients at risk of ischemic events (CAPRIE). Lancet 1996;348:1329–1339.
70. Kretschmer G, Herbst F, Prager M, et al. A decade of oral anticoagulant treatment to maintain autologous vein grafts for femoropopliteal atherosclerosis. Arch Surg 1992;127:1112–1115.
71. Efficacy of oral anticoagulants compared with aspirin after infrainguinal bypass surgery (The Dutch Bypass Oral Anticoagulants or Aspirin Study): a randomised trial. Lancet 2000;355:346–351.
72. Watson HR, Bergqvist D. Antithrombotic agents for peripheral transluminal angioplasty; a review of the studies, methods, and evidence for use. Eur J Vasc Endovasc Surg 2000;19:445–450.
73. Girolami B, Bernardi E, Prins MH, et al. Antiplatelet therapy and other interventions after revascularization procedures in patients with peripheral arterial disease: a meta-analysis. Eur J Vasc Endovasc Surg 2000;19:370–380.
74. Zacca NM, Raizner AE, Noon GP, et al. Treatment of symptomatic peripheral atherosclerotic disease with a rotational atherectomy device. Am J Cardiol 1989;63:77–80.
75. vonPolnitz A, Nerlich A, Berger H, et al. Percutaneous peripheral atherectomy: angiographic and clinical followup of 60 patients. J Am Coll Cardiol 1990;15:682–688.
76. Jahnke T, Link J, Muller-Hulsbeck S, et al. Treatment of infrapopliteal occlusive disease by high-speed rotational atherectomy: initial and mid-term results. J Vasc Interv Radiol 2001;12:221–226.
77. Palmaz JC, Laborde JC, Rivera FJ, et al. Stenting of the iliac arteries with the Palmaz stent: experience from a multicenter trial of cardiovascular intervention. Radiology 1992;15:291–297.
78. Gray BH, Sullivan TM, Childs MB, et al. High incidence of restenosis/reocclusion of stents in the percutaneous treatment of long-segment superficial femoral artery disease after suboptimal angioplasty. J Vasc Surg 1997;25: 74–83.
79. Krueger K, Landwehr P, Bendel M, et al. Endovascular gamma irradiation of femoropopliteal de novo stenoses immediately after PTA: interim results of prospective randomized controlled trial. Radiology 2002;224:519–528.
80. Duda SH, Pusich B, Richter G, et al. Sirolimus-eluting stents for the treatment of obstructive superficial femoral artery disease. Six-month results. Circulation 2002;106:1505–1509.
81. Ouriel K, Veith FJ, Sasahara AA. Comparison of recombinant urokinase with vascular surgery as initial treatment for acute arterial occlusion of the legs. N Engl J Med 1998;338:1105–1111.
82. Weaver FA, Comerota AJ, Youngblood M, et al. Surgical revascularization versus thrombolysis for nonembolic lower extremity native artery occlusions: results of a prospective randomized trial. The STILE Investigators. Survey versus Thrombolysis for Ischemia of the Lower Extremity. J Vasc Surg 1996;24:513–521.
83. Kannel WB, Skinner JJ Jr, Schwartz MJ, Shurtleff D. Intermittent claudication. Incidence in the Framingham Study. Circulation 1970;41:875–883.
84. Fayad ZA, Nahar T, Fallon JT, et al. In vivo magnetic resonance evaluation of atherosclerotic plaques in the human thoracic aorta: a comparison with transesophageal echocardiography. Circulation 2000;101:2503–2509.
85. Bartholomew JR, Olin JW. Atheromatous embolization. In: Young JR, Olin JW, Bartholomew JR, eds. Peripheral Vascular Diseases, 2nd ed. C.V. Mosby, St. Louis, MO, 1996.

RECOMMENDED READING

Spittell JA. Peripheral Vascular Disease for Cardiologists. A Clinical Approach. Blackwell Publishing/Futura Division, New York, 2004.

Dormandy JA, Rutherford RB. Management of peripheral arterial disease (PAD). TASC Working Group. TransAtlantic Inter-Society Concensus (TASC). J Vasc Surg 2000;31:S1–S296.

Hirsch AT, Criqui MH, Treat-Jacobson D, et al. Peripheral arterial disease detection, awareness, and treatment in primary care. JAMA 2001;286:1317–1324.

Halperin JL, Creager MA. Arterial obstructive diseases of the extremities. In: Loscalzo J, Creager MA, Dzau VJ, eds. Vascular Medicine: A Textbook of Vascular Biology and Diseases, 2nd ed. Little, Brown, Boston, 1996, pp. 825–854.

Hirsch AT, ed. An office-based approach to the diagnosis and treatment of peripheral arterial disease, Parts I-III. Am J Med Continuing Education Series. Excerpta Medica, Belle Mead, MD, 1998–1999.

Jackson MR, Clagett GP. Antithrombotic therapy in peripheral arterial occlusive disease. Chest 1998;114:666S–682S.

CAPRIE Steering Committee (on behalf of the CAPRIE Study Group). A randomised, blinded, trial of clopidogrel versus aspirin in patients at risk of ischaemic events (CAPRIE). Lancet 1996;348:1329–1339.

Spittell JA, ed. Clinical Vascular Disease. F.A. Davis, Philadelphia, 1983.

INDEX

Entries in boldface type signify complete chapters. Pages followed by *f* indicate figures; pages followed by *t* indicate tables.

single ventricle, 402
tetralogy of Fallot, 400–401
total anomalous pulmonary venous
connection, 402
transposition of great arteries, 400
treatment principles, 398, 400
tricuspid atresia, 401
truncus arteriosus, 402
Cyclic AMP (cAMP)
β–adrenergic receptor signaling defects, 53
arrhythmia modulation, 289, 292–293
synthesis, 58
vasodilation mechanism, 58
Cyclic GMP (cGMP), signaling, 68, 68f
Cytokines
atherosclerosis role, 413
heart failure role, 365–366, 366t

D

DAD. *See* Delayed afterdepolarization
DCM. *See* Dilated cardiomyopathy
D–dimer test, 670–671, 673
DECREASE trial, 757
Deep venous thrombosis (DVT)
diagnosis, 670–671, 672f
filter management, 669–670, 671f
management
embolectomy, 678
fondaparinux, 677
heparin, 676
supportive therapy, 674, 676
thrombolytic therapy, 678
warfarin, 676–677
ximeltagatran, 677–678
prevention, 669–670
risk factors, 669, 670t
Delayed afterdepolarization (DAD), 290f, 292–
293
DeMusset's sign, 102t
Depression
preventive cardiology, 792, 794
reduction by exercise, 535–536
Diabetes
cardiovascular disease risk, 6–7, 7t
dyslipidemia management, 434–435
hypertension management, 633–634
peripheral arterial disease
management, 818
risks, 808–809
Diastasis, 37, 51
Diastole
atrial function, 51–52
chronic renal disease dysfunction, 740–741
definition, 37–38

distensibility and compliance, 53
heart failure dysfunction, 52–53
hypertrophic dysfunction, 52
imaging of dysfunction, 277–278
phases, 51, 52f
pressure–volume curves, 38, 39f
relaxation, 50–51
Diastolic murmur, 110–111, 111f
Diet. *See* Nutrition
Digital subtraction angiography, peripheral
arterial disease, 818
Digoxin
delayed afterdepolarization induction, 292,
292t
electrocardiography of toxicity, 135
exercise testing effects, 178
heart failure management, 380, 382
elderly patients, 719
pulmonary hypertension management, 668
Dihydropyridine receptor, 30
Dilated cardiomyopathy (DCM)
causes, 641, 643t, 644t
echocardiography, 159–160, 642, 642t
evaluation, 642
heart failure, 350–351, 352t
natural history, 642
peripartum cardiomyopathy, 697–698
survival, 645f
treatment, 642
Diltiazem
angina pectoris management, 460
supraventricular tachycardia management,
308t
Vaughan–Williams classification, 307t
Diphenhydramine, contrast allergy prophylaxis,
202t
Dipyridamole
nuclear perfusion stress imaging, 226, 228t
peripheral arterial disease management, 821
Diuretics. *See also specific drugs*
adverse effects, 376
combination therapy, 375
heart failure management, 373, 374t, 375–
376
elderly patients, 719
hypertension management
indications and contraindications, 624t
initial choice for therapy, 622–623
preeclampsia management, 702
pulmonary hypertension management, 668
refractory patients, 375
renal parenchymal hypertension management
loop diuretics, 735–736
thiazide diuretics, 735